Student Resource CD-ROM for *Klossner:* Introductory Maternity Nursing

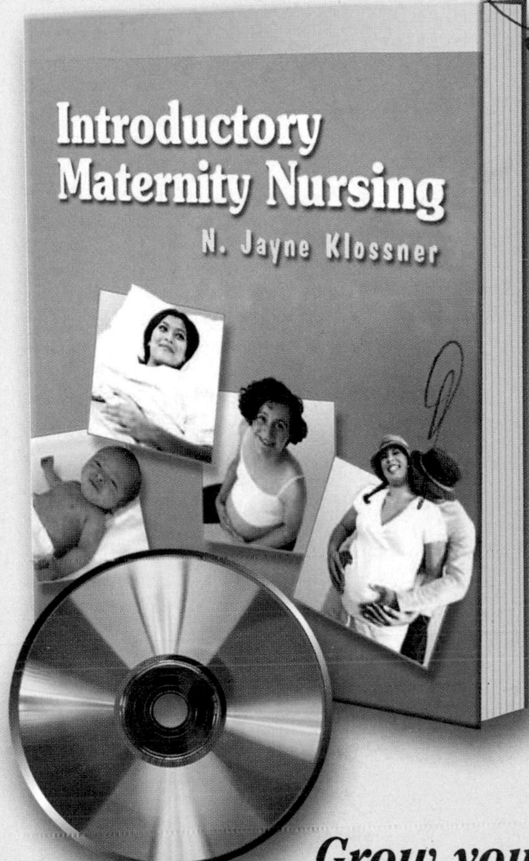

This reliable resource accompanies the text and provides additional tools to help you succeed!

A FREE CDROM in the front of the book includes:

- **Video Clips** help you apply content to practice!
  - **Administering nursing comfort** measures during labor
  - **A delivery** in progress

AND

- **A Connection Website**: provides additional learning tools and resources!

Grow your knowledge and develop clinical skills!

If you like the videos on thc front of book CDROM, check out:

NEW! Coming in July 2005

Lippincott's Maternity Nursing Video Series

From prenatal care, through labor and delivery, to postpartum care…these informative and dynamic videos address each phase of effective maternal-neonatal nursing in a documentary presentation that makes complex concepts easy to grasp and retain. Each 45-minute program focuses on a critical phase of maternity nursing care.

AND

Lippincott's Pediatric Nursing Video Series

This documentary style video series focuses on nursing care, including growth and development, communicating with children and families, and caring for ill children. Each video focuses on the five age groups—Infants, Toddlers, Pre-Schoolers, School Agers, and Adolescents— highlighted by nurse, patient, and family interviews.

Put these skill-builders to work for you…
ORDER TODAY!

Call TOLL FREE 1-800-638-3030
Visit us on the Web at LWW.com/nursing or nursingcenter.com
Or visit your local health science bookstore

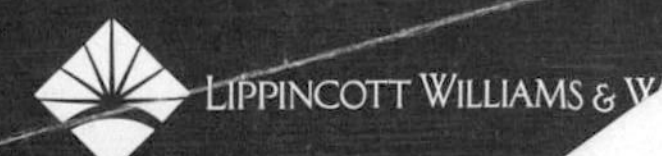

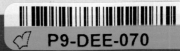

Introductory
Maternity
Nursing

Suzette Williams
240-462-2092

Introductory Maternity Nursing

N. Jayne Klossner, MSN, RNC
Director of Women's Services
North Central Baptist Hospital
Part of Baptist Health System
San Antonio, Texas

LIPPINCOTT WILLIAMS & WILKINS
A **Wolters Kluwer** Company
Philadelphia • Baltimore • New York • London
Buenos Aires • Hong Kong • Sydney • Tokyo

Acquisitions Editor: Elizabeth Nieginski
Developmental Editor: Danielle DiPalma
Editorial Assistant: Josh Levandoski
Senior Production Editor: Sandra Cherrey Scheinin
Director of Nursing Production: Helen Ewan
Managing Editor/Production: Erika Kors
Art Director: Carolyn O'Brien
Senior Manufacturing Manager: William Alberti
Indexer: Coughlin Indexing Services, Inc.
Compositor: TechBooks
Printer: R.R. Donnelley

9 8 7 6 5 4 3

Library of Congress Cataloging-in-Publication Data

Klossner, N. Jayne.
Introductory maternity nursing / N. Jayne Klossner.
p. ; cm.
Includes bibliographical references and index.
ISBN 0-7817-6237-5 (alk. paper)
1. Maternity nursing. I. Title.
[DNLM: 1. Maternal-Child Nursing—methods. WY 157.3 K66i 2006]
I. Title.
RG951.K566 2006
618.2'0231—dc22 2004027096

Care has been taken to confirm the accuracy of the information presented and to describe generally accepted practices. However, the authors, editors, and publisher are not responsible for errors or omissions or for any consequences from application of the information in this book and make no warranty, express or implied, with respect to the content of the publication.

The authors, editors, and publisher have exerted every effort to ensure that drug selection and dosage set forth in this text are in accordance with the current recommendations and practice at the time of publication. However, in view of ongoing research, changes in government regulations, and the constant flow of information relating to drug therapy and drug reactions, the reader is urged to check the package insert for each drug for any change in indications and dosage and for added warnings and precautions. This is particularly important when the recommended agent is a new or infrequently employed drug.

Some drugs and medical devices presented in this publication have Food and Drug Administration (FDA) clearance for limited use in restricted research settings. It is the responsibility of the health care provider to ascertain the FDA status of each drug or device planned for use in his or her clinical practice.

LWW.com

RRS0910

Dedication

To Kevin

My husband, my partner, my friend—I love you with all my heart

To Katelyn

My "Baby Girl" for understanding all those nights I was at the computer during your high school years. We made it!

To Joshua and Jonathan

My sons for the support and love you have given me from wherever you may be!

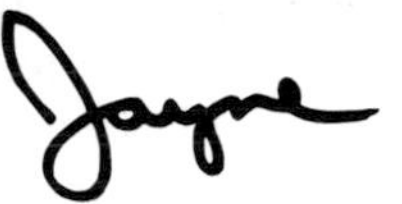

Contributors

Martha Dianne DeBarros, BS. in Ed., LCCE, IBCLC
Coordinator
Family Education Services and Lactation Center
St. Luke's Baptist Women's Center
San Antonio, Texas

Karen Edmondson, RN
Instructor
University of South Carolina, Spartanburg
Mary Black School of Nursing
Spartanburg, South Carolina

Maryann Foley, RN, BSN
Independent Clinical Consultant
Flourtown, Pennsylvania

Margaret Dextraze Humm, RN, MSN, CNS
Clinical Nurse Specialist for Maternal-Child Health
St. Luke's Baptist Women's Center
San Antonio, Texas

Barbara Gonzalez Pino, PhD
Associate Professor
University of Texas at San Antonio
San Antonio, Texas

Cynthia Kincheloe RN, BSN, MSN
NICU Staff Nurse
Presbyterian Hospital
Albuquerque, New Mexico
Former Instructor
Albuquerque T-VI
Albuquerque, New Mexico

Frank Pino, PhD
Professor
University of Texas at San Antonio
San Antonio, Texas

Reviewers

Margaret D. Cole, RN, DSN
Associate Professor of Nursing
Spring Hill College
Mobile, Alabama

Karen R. Ferguson, RNC, BSN, MSN
Nursing Instructor
Calhoun Community College
Decatur, Alabama

Donna J. Gatlin, RN, BSN, MA
Nursing Instructor
Paris Junior College
Paris, Texas

Joy Green-Hadden, MSN, RN, FNP-C
Family Nurse Practitioner
Case Western University
Knoxville, Tennessee

Margaret J. Henry, RN, BSN
Assistant Professor of Nursing
Belmont Technical College
St. Clairsville, Ohio

Debra Lea Jenks, RN, MSN, PhD
Assistant Professor
Milwaukee School of Engineering
Milwaukee, Wisconsin

John A. McCarter, RN, BSN, MSN
Adjunct Pediatric Clinical Instructor
University of South Alabama College of Nursing
Mobile, Alabama

Audrey N. McLarty RN
Staff Nurse, Childbirth Educator
Huntsville Hospital for Women & Children
Huntsville, Alabama

Nancy Mizzoni, RN, MSN, CPNP
Associate Professor
Middlesex Community College
Lowell, Massachusetts

Vicki Nees, RNC, MSN, APRN-BC
Associate Professor
Ivy Tech State College
Lafayette, Indiana

Jan Peek, RN, MSN
Chairperson, Nursing Department
Calhoun Community College
Decatur, Alabama

Lisa Richwine, RN, BSN
LPN Instructor
Ivy Tech State College
Lafayette, Indiana

Gayle Sewell, RN, MN
Nursing Instructor
North Central Kansas Technical College
Beloit, Kansas

Russlyn A. St. John, RN, MSN
Associate Professor
St. Charles Community College
St. Peters, Missouri

Margaret C. Stone, RN (LPN), BSN, MSN
Associate Professor
North Shore Community College
Danvers, Massachusetts

Roselena Thorpe, RN, PhD
Professor and Department Chairperson Nursing
Community College of Allegheny County
Pittsburgh, Pennsylvania

Preface

This first edition of *Introductory Maternity Nursing* reflects the underlying philosophy of love, caring, and support for the childbearing woman, the newborn, and the families of these individuals. The content has been developed according to the most current information available. In this text we recognize that cultural sensitivity and awareness are important aspects of caring for the childbearing families. We also recognize that many pregnant women and newborns live in families other than traditional two-parent family homes and therefore refer to teaching and supporting the childbearing clients and family caregivers of newborns in all situations and family structures.

Maternal–newborn health care has seen a shift from the hospital setting into community and home settings. More responsibility has fallen on the family and family caregivers to care for the pregnant woman or ill newborn. We stress teaching the patient and family, with an emphasis on prevention. The nursing process has been used as the foundation for presenting nursing care. Implementation information is presented in a narrative format to enable the discussion from which planning, goal setting, and evaluation can be put into action. The newest and most current NANDA terminology has been used for the possible nursing diagnoses for health care concerns.

Our goal in this text is to keep the readability of the text at a level with which the student can be comfortable. In recognition of the limited time that the student has and the frustrations that can result from having to turn to a dictionary or glossary for words that are unfamiliar, we have attempted to identify all possible unfamiliar terms and define them within the text. This increases the reading ease for the student, decreasing the time necessary to complete the assigned reading and enhancing the understanding of the information. A four-color format, current photos, drawings, tables, and diagrams will further aid the student in using this edition.

This text offers the instructor and student of maternity nursing a user-friendly, comprehensive quick reference to features in the text, including the Family Teaching Tips, Nursing Care Plans, Nursing Procedures, and Personal Glimpses.

RECURRING FEATURES

In an effort to provide the instructor and student with a text that is informative, exciting, and easy to use, we have incorporated a number of special features throughout the text, many of which are included in each chapter.

Chapter Outlines

A basic outline of what will be covered in the chapter is presented at the beginning of each chapter. This roadmap helps students in recognizing the focus of the chapter.

Student Objectives

Measurable student-oriented objectives are included at the beginning of each chapter. These help to guide the student in recognizing what is important and why, and they provide the instructor with guidance for evaluating the student's understanding of the information presented in the chapter.

Key Terms

A list of terms that may be unfamiliar to students and that are considered essential to the chapter's understanding is at the beginning of each chapter. The first appearance in the chapter of each of these terms is in boldface type, with the definition included in the text. All key terms can be found in a glossary at the end of the text.

Nursing Process

The nursing process serves as an organizing structure for the discussion of nursing care covered in the text. This feature provides the student with a foundation from which individualized nursing care plans can be developed. Each Nursing Process section includes the nurse's role in caring for the patient and family and also includes nursing assessment, relevant nursing diagnoses, outcome identification and planning, implementation, and evaluation of the goals and expected outcomes. Emphasis is placed on the importance of involving the pregnant woman and family caregivers in the assessment process. In the Nursing Process sections we have used current NANDA-approved nursing diagnoses. These are used to represent appropriate concerns for a particular condition, but we do not attempt to include all diagnoses that could be identified. The student will find the goals specific, measurable, and realistic and will be able to relate the goals to patient situations and care plan development. The expected outcomes and evaluation provide a goal for each nursing diagnosis and criteria to measure the successful accomplishment of that goal.

Nursing Care Plans

Throughout the text Nursing Care Plans are presented to provide the student with a model to follow in using the information from the nursing process to develop specific nursing care plans. To make the care plans more meaningful, a scenario has been constructed for each one.

Nursing Procedures

Needed equipment and step-by-step procedures are found to help the students understand the procedures. These can be easily used in a clinical setting to perform nursing procedures.

Family Teaching Tips

Information that the student can use in teaching the maternity patient and family caregivers is presented in highlighted boxes ready for use.

Clinical Secrets

These present a recurring cartoon nurse who provides brief clinical pearls. The student will find these valuable in caring for patients in clinical settings. Safety concerns and important issues to consider are highlighted.

Personal Glimpse With Learning Opportunity

Personal Glimpses are presented in every chapter. These are actual first-person narratives, unedited, just as the individual wrote them. Personal Glimpses help the student have a view of an experience an individual has had in a given situation and of that person's feelings about or during the incident. These are presented to enhance the student's understanding and appreciation of the feelings of others. A Learning Opportunity at the end of each Personal Glimpse encourages students to think of how they might react or respond in the situation presented. These further enhance the student's critical thinking.

Cultural Snapshot

These boxes highlight issues and topics that may have cultural considerations. The student is encouraged to think about cultural differences and the importance of accepting the attitudes and beliefs of individuals from cultures other than his or her own.

Tables, Drawings, and Photographs

These important aspects of the text have been developed in an effort to help the student visualize the content covered. Many color photographs in a variety of settings are included.

Key Points

We have selected key points to help the student focus on the important aspects of the chapter. These provide a quick review of essential elements of the chapter. The Key Points are structured to recap each student objective stated at the beginning of the chapter.

References, Selected Readings and Websites

This section offers the student additional information on topics and conditions discussed in the chapter. The websites also provide resource information that the student can share with patients and families. Throughout the text, websites are included as resources for the student to access available sites discussing certain conditions, diseases and disorders, as well as offering support and information for families.

LEARNING OPPORTUNITIES

In order to offer students opportunities to check their understanding of material they have read and studied, many learning opportunities are provided throughout the text.

Test Yourself

These questions are found in each chapter and are designed to test understanding and recall of the material presented. The student will quickly determine if a review of what he or she just read is needed.

Workbook

At the end of each chapter the student will find a workbook section that includes

- **NCLEX–Style Review Questions** are written to test the student's ability to apply the material from the chapter. These questions use the client–nurse format to encourage the student to critically think about patient situations as well as the nurse's response or action. Innovative style questions have been included.
- **Study Activities** include interactive activities requiring the student to participate in the learning process. Important material from the chapter has been incorporated into this section to help the student review and synthesize the chapter content. The instructor will find many of the activities appropriate for individual or class assignments.
- **Internet Activities.** Many chapters include an Internet activity within the Study Activities that helps the student explore the Internet. Each activity takes the student step by step into a site where he or she can access new and updated information as well as resources to share with patients and families. Some include fun activities to use with pediatric patients. These activities may require the use of Acrobat Reader. This can be downloaded free of charge for the student to readily view the site.
- **Critical Thinking: What Would You Do?** Critical thinking real-life situations encourage the student to think about the chapter content in practical terms. These situations require the student to incorporate knowledge gained from the chapter and apply it to real-life problems. Questions provide the student with opportunities to problem solve, think critically, and discover his or her own ideas and feelings. The instructor also can use them as a tool to stimulate class discussion. Dosage Calculations are found in the Workbook section of each pediatric chapter where diseases and disorders are covered. This section offers the student practice in dosage calculations that can be directly applied in a clinical setting.

ORGANIZATION

The text is divided into six units to provide an orderly approach to the content. The first unit helps build a foundation for the student beginning the study of maternity and newborn nursing. This unit introduces the student to caring for the childbearing woman and for newborns in various settings.

Foundational topics are presented in the first chapters of each unit followed by chapters that feature the application of knowledge within the nursing process. Maternity topics that address the low-risk woman are covered first in Units 2 to 5. Unit 6 addresses issues related to at-risk pregnancy, childbirth, and newborn care. The instructor may choose to teach the normal content of pregnancy followed by the at-risk pregnancy chapters, if desired. However, the author designed the content so that normal considerations would be covered first followed by discussion of the at-risk woman, fetus, and neonate. This grouping ensures that all normal content is covered before any at-risk topics are addressed, which cuts down on the need for parenthetical content in the at-risk chapters. It also encourages the student to review the normal chapters when studying the at-risk content. This repetition of content is designed to help cement the student's understanding of the material. In Unit 6 the at-risk disorders are organized so that an explanation of the disorder is covered first followed by a discussion of medical treatment and nursing care.

Unit 1, Overview of Maternal and Newborn Nursing Care

Unit 1 introduces the student in Chapter 1 to a brief history of maternal and newborn nursing, and discusses current trends in maternal–newborn health care and maternal–newborn health status issues and concerns. A brief discussion of the nursing process is included. Chapter 2 follows with a discussion of the family, its structure, and family factors that influence childbearing and child rearing. The chapter introduces community-based health care and discusses the various settings in the community through which health care is provided for the maternity client and the newborn.

Unit 2, Foundations of Maternity Nursing

Unit 2 introduces the student in Chapter 3 to male and female reproductive anatomy, which is essential to the understanding of maternity nursing. The menstrual cycle and the sexual response cycle are also addressed. (Note: Pelvic anatomy is addressed in Chapter 8 and breast anatomy in Chapter 14.) Chapter 4 continues with a discussion of special reproductive issues to include family planning, elective termination of pregnancy, and issues of fertility.

Unit 3, Pregnancy

Unit 3 begins in Chapter 5 with a discussion of fetal development from fertilization through the fetal period. Chapter 6 introduces the student to diagnosis of pregnancy, physiologic and psychological adaptation of the woman during pregnancy. The chapter ends by outlining nutritional requirements of pregnancy. Chapter 7 covers the nurse's role in prenatal care and assessment of fetal well-being during pregnancy.

Unit 4, Labor and Birth

Unit 4 begins with a discussion of the labor process in Chapter 8. The four components of birth, the process of labor, and maternal and fetal adaptation to labor are covered. Female pelvic anatomy is discussed here. Chapter 9 introduces the student to concepts of pain management during labor and birth. The chapter begins with an overview of the characteristics and nature of labor pain as well as general principles of labor pain management. Nonpharmacologic and pharmacologic methods of pain management are reviewed. Chapter 10 covers the nurse's role during labor and birth to include assessment of the fetus through fetal monitoring and other methods. The nurse's role in each stage of labor is covered within the framework of the nursing process. The nurse-controlled delivery is also covered in this chapter. Chapter 11 discusses cesarean birth, version, cervical ripening procedures, induction and augmentation of labor, amnioinfusion, assisted delivery (including episiotomy, vacuum, and forceps delivery), and vaginal birth after cesarean.

Unit 5, Postpartum and Newborn

Unit 5 begins with a discussion of normal postpartum adaptation, nursing assessment, and nursing care in Chapter 12. Chapter 13 covers topics related to normal transition of the neonate to extrauterine life, general characteristics of the neonate, and the initial nursing assessment of the newborn. Chapter 14 delves into issues of infant nutrition. Breast-feeding and formula feeding are presented along with tips on choosing a feeding method, as well as advantages and disadvantages of each method. Physiology of breast-feeding, including breast anatomy, is covered here. The nurse's role in assisting the woman who is breast-feeding and the woman who is formula feeding is also discussed. Chapter 15 presents the nurse's role in caring for the normal newborn and includes nursing care considerations in the stabilization and transition of the newborn, normal newborn care, assessment and facilitation of family interaction and adjustment, and discharge considerations. An emphasis is placed on teaching the new parents to care for their newborn.

Unit 6, Childbearing At Risk

Unit 6 begins with a focus on pregnancy at risk. Chapter 16 focuses on the pregnancy that is placed at risk by pre-existing and chronic medical conditions of the woman. This chapter covers the major medical conditions, such as diabetes and heart disease, as well as exposure to substances harmful to the fetus, threats from intimate partner violence, and age-related concerns on either end of the age spectrum. Chapter 17 introduces the student to the pregnancy that becomes at risk because of pregnancy-related complications and disorders. Threats from hyperemesis, bleeding disorders of pregnancy, hypertensive disorders, and blood incompatibilities are presented. Chapter 18 covers topics associated with the at-risk labor, such as dysfunctional labor, preterm labor, post-term labor, placental abnormalities, and emergencies associated with labor and birth. Chapter 19 looks at the postpartum woman at risk. Postpartum hemorrhage, subinvolution, infection, thrombophlebitis, malattachment, grief reaction, and postpartum depression and psychosis are addressed. In Chapter 20 gestational concerns and acquired disorders of the newborn are discussed. Chapter 21 addresses congenital disorders of the newborn, including congenital malformations, inborn errors of metabolism, and chromosomal abnormalities.

Glossaries, Workbook Answers, and Appendices

The text concludes with a **Glossary** of key terms and an **English-Spanish Glossary** of maternity and pediatric phrases. Additionally, **Answers to Workbook Questions** are provided. Ten appendices are included at the back of the text and contain important information for the nursing student in maternity and pediatrics courses. Appendices include:

Appendix A: Standard and Transmission-Based Precautions
Appendix B: NANDA-Approved Nursing Diagnoses
Appendix C: JCAHO List of "Do Not Use" Abbreviations
Appendix D: Good Sources of Essential Nutrients
Appendix E: Breast-feeding and Medication Use
Appendix F: Cervical Dilation Chart
Appendix G: Temperature and Weight Conversion Charts

TEACHING/LEARNING PACKAGE

Instructor's Resource CD-ROM

This essential resource for instructors offers a number of tools to assist you with teaching your course:

- The Instructor's Manual features Lecture Outlines, Teaching Strategies for both the classroom and clinical setting, and unique Critical Thinking Assignments with sample answers.

- PowerPoint presentations for every chapter provide an easy way for you to integrate the textbook with your students' classroom experience, either via slide shows or handouts.
- The Image Bank lets you use the photographs and illustrations from this textbook in your PowerPoint slides or as you see fit in your course.
- The Test Generator lets you put together exclusive new tests from a bank containing over 200 questions, to help you in assessing your students' understanding of the material.

Front-of-Book CD-ROM

This free Front-of-Book CD-ROM features video clips of labor and delivery.

Contact your sales representative or visit LWW.com/Nursing for details and ordering information.

Acknowledgments

Many people were involved in the creation of this first edition of **Introductory Maternity Nursing.** I worked with some of these individuals on a frequent and ongoing basis, while others, I do not even know their names. With gratitude and appreciation I would like to thank every person on our team from Lippincott, Williams & Wilkins, whether they had a small or a large part in the process of publishing this textbook.

I especially want to express my appreciation to:

Danielle DiPalma, Developmental Editor, for being the solid foundation and support for this book. I thank her for her never-wavering belief that this text would be written and her dedication and commitment to ensure that would happen. Danielle, you are fantastic!

Sarah Kyle, Developmental Editor, for her attention to detail and excellent suggestions. I thank her for contributing material and for pitching in when the going got tough to help us meet our deadlines. Sarah, you are amazing!

Maryann Foley, Development Editor, for stepping in with her expertise and knowledge to help fine tune and complete the newborn chapters.

Elizabeth Nieginski, Senior Acquisitions Editor, for her support behind the scenes managing the business aspects of the project.

Katherine Rothwell and Josh Levandoski, Editorial Assistants, for their enthusiasm and help obtaining reviews and assisting with the many necessary administrative tasks.

Sandy Cherrey Scheinin, Senior Production Editor, for her help in the final editing process.

Michelle Clark, Ancillary Editor, for her work on the instructor's resource materials.

Cynthia Kincheloe for her excellent work writing two of the maternity chapters.

Doctors Frank and Barbara Pino for their wonderful work on the translation of the English-Spanish glossary, despite being asked at the last minute.

Joe Mitchell for his patience and beautiful photography.

Peggy Humm for facilitating and organizing the photo shoot at St. Luke's Baptist Hospital.

Megan Klim, Development Editor, for her help with the photo shoot.

Doug Dobbs, if it weren't for him, I would never have known that Lippincott Williams & Wilkins wanted to do this project.

All of the women, children, families, and nurses who were models for the photos.

Kevin, thank you from the bottom of the heart for all the support you have given me throughout this project. You have shown your love in so very many ways. Thank you for picking up the slack at home with the bills, chores, moving, and in the countless other ways that you have shown your support. Thank you for directly contributing to this project by taking photos and doing an initial edit of some chapters before I submitted them to Sarah. Thank you for making me laugh and helping me keep my sense of humor when it seemed the book would never be finished. Your encouragement and love have been my anchor. Thank you, Frannie Rettig, for your faith in me that I could do this project when I first took it on. And a special thanks to Donna Guenther for keeping everything together at work, and to Janeen Koti for taking the pager and other responsibilities, which enabled me to concentrate on the book when I needed to. Thanks to Kathy Eichner, Susan Monahan, Mark Clayton, and all my employees for your encouraging words and for understanding when I needed to rearrange my schedule to meet deadlines. I couldn't have done it without you!

N. Jayne Klossner

Contents

UNIT 1

Overview of Maternal and Newborn Nursing Care 1

UNIT 2

Foundations of Maternity Nursing 39

Quick Reference to Features

FAMILY TEACHING TIPS

NURSING PROCEDURES

NURSING CARE PLANS

UNIT 1

Overview of Maternal and Newborn Nursing Care

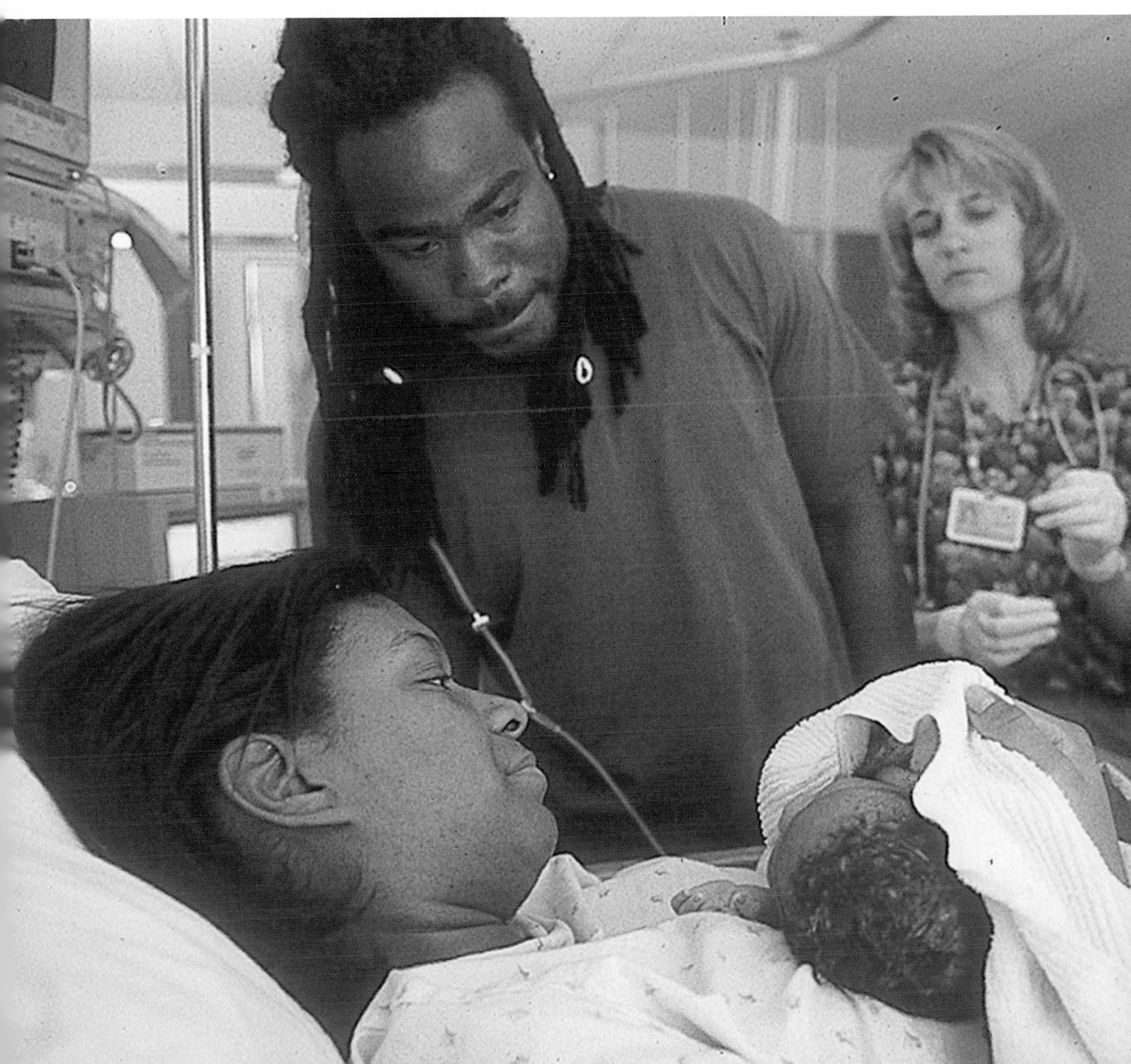

The Nurse's Role in a Changing Maternal–Newborn Health Care Environment

STUDENT OBJECTIVES

On completion of this chapter, the student should be able to

1. Discuss factors influencing the development of maternity and newborn care in the United States.
2. Describe how current trends in maternal–newborn care have affected the delivery of care to mothers and infants in the United States.
3. Name three ways that nurses contribute to cost containment in the United States.
4. Examine the maternal–infant health status in the United States.
5. Discuss two possible reasons the United States ranks low compared with other developed countries in terms of infant mortality rate.
6. Discuss major objectives of Healthy People 2010 as they relate to maternal and newborn nursing.
7. List new roles the nurse is expected to assume when providing maternal and newborn nursing care.
8. Discuss how the nurse uses critical thinking skills in maternal and newborn nursing.
9. List the five steps of the nursing process.
10. Explain the importance of complete and accurate documentation.

KEY TERMS

actual nursing diagnoses
capitation
case management
couplet care
dependent nursing actions
fetal mortality rate
independent nursing actions
infant mortality rate
interdependent nursing actions
maternal mortality rate
mortality rates
morbidity
neonatal
neonatal mortality rate
neonate
nursing process
objective data
outcomes
perinatal
perinatal mortality rate
prospective payment system
puerperal fever
risk nursing diagnoses
subjective data
utilization review
viable
wellness nursing diagnoses

The nurse preparing to care for today's and tomorrow's childbearing families faces vastly different responsibilities and challenges than did the maternal and newborn nurse of even a decade ago. Nurses and other health professionals are becoming increasingly concerned with much more than the care of at-risk pregnancies and sick newborns. Health teaching; preventing illness; and promoting optimal (most desirable or satisfactory) physical, developmental, and emotional health have become a significant part of contemporary nursing.

Scientific and technological advances have reduced the incidence of communicable disease and helped to control metabolic disorders such as diabetes. As a result, more health care is provided outside the hospital. Patients now receive health care in the home, at clinics, and from their primary care provider. Prenatal diagnosis of birth defects, transfusions, other treatments for the unborn fetus, and improved life-support systems for premature infants are but a few examples of the rapid progress in newborn care.

Controversy continues to rage about choices in family planning. In January 1973, a Supreme Court decision declared abortion legal anywhere in the United States. In 1981, efforts were made to convince Congress that legislation should be passed to make all abortions illegal on the alleged grounds that the fetus is a person and, therefore, has the right to life. In the 1990s, bitter debate between "pro-life" and "pro-choice" groups raged and seems likely to continue for many years.

Tremendous sociologic changes have affected attitudes toward, and concepts in, maternal–newborn health. American society is largely suburban, with a population of highly mobile persons and families. The women's movement has focused new attention on the needs of families in which the mother works outside the home. Escalating divorce rates, changes in attitudes toward sexual roles, and general acceptance of unmarried mothers have increased the number of single-parent families. Many people have come to regard health care as a right, not a privilege, and expect to receive fair value for their investment. In addition, the demand for financial responsibility in health care has contributed to shortened hospital stays and alternative methods of health care delivery.

The reduction in the incidence of communicable and infectious diseases has made it possible to devote more attention to such critical problems as preterm birth, congenital anomalies, child abuse, and illnesses during pregnancy. Research in these areas continues; as these findings become available, nurses will be among the practitioners who will help translate this research into improved health care for pregnant women, newborns, and families.

However, nurses' ability to translate the relevant medical research into practice is based on their understanding of the predictable but variable phases of pregnancy and of a newborn's growth and development, and on their understanding of and sensitivity to the importance of family interactions.

CHANGING CONCEPTS IN MATERNAL–NEWBORN HEALTH CARE

Maternity care has changed dramatically throughout the years as attitudes and opinions have altered. Historically, maternity care was a function of lay midwives, and most births occurred in the home setting. As knowledge increased about birth interventions and physicians developed methods of infection prevention, the family physician became the provider of choice for prenatal care, and hospitals, instead of homes, became the accepted place to give birth.

In today's society, as the health care consumer has become more knowledgeable, two different trends can be noted. On one hand, as lawsuits have become more common with large judgments being leveled against practitioners, maternity care has become increasingly specialized. Obstetricians often provide routine prenatal and delivery care. The at-risk client is frequently followed by a perinatologist, a physician who specializes in the care of women with high-risk pregnancies. Neonatologists provide expert specialized care to at-risk newborns. On the other hand, the consumer movement has pushed for birth to be viewed as a natural process in which little intervention is required. Therefore, the midwife has once again come to be accepted as a provider of maternity care, and some women elect to deliver at home or in birthing centers, which provide a home-like atmosphere. The development of, and current trends in, maternal and newborn health care are discussed briefly in the following sections.

Development of Maternity Care

In colonial times, most births occurred at home. The lay midwife, who had no formal education, attended the woman throughout labor and birth. Experience and knowledge about childbirth was shared among the women of the community. Childbirth was truly a woman's affair.

As physicians became educated in the practice of midwifery and began to use instruments such as forceps, to which the midwives had no access, physicians began to replace lay midwives as the attendant at deliveries. Few women became physicians because of the cultural pressures for a woman to fulfill the roles of housewife and mother.

Another change that occurred was that physicians began to increasingly rely on interventions to assist the natural process of labor and hasten delivery. Lay midwives mainly provided support and encouragement to a woman during her labor and relied on nature to take its course. Therefore, as more physicians began to attend deliveries, labor came to be viewed as an illness, or at the very least, a dangerous condition that required the skillful intervention of a physician. Two major developments greatly influenced the way maternity care was practiced in the United States—acceptance of the germ theory and development of anesthesia to decrease the pain of childbirth.

Acceptance of the Germ Theory

Before it was known how infection was transmitted, it was common for a woman to develop **puerperal fever**, an illness marked by high fever caused by infection of the reproductive tract after the birth of a child. Puerperal fever was often fatal. Although rates of infection and mortality were much higher in hospitals, women who delivered at home also were susceptible to puerperal fever.

In the late 1700s, Alexander Gordon, a Scottish physician, was the first to recognize that puerperal fever was an infection transmitted to patients by physicians and nurses as they moved between treating patients with puerperal fever and attending births or caring for women who had already delivered. The work of two other men, Oliver Wendell Holmes and Ignaz Philip Semmelweis, confirmed Gordon's infection theory and began the development of interventions to stop the transmission of puerperal fever.

In 1842, Oliver Wendell Holmes, the famous American poet, physician, and professor of anatomy and physiology at Harvard University, wrote an essay on puerperal fever based on conclusions he made after observing physicians in clinical practice. He strongly advocated that a physician who performed autopsies on individuals who died of infection[1] should not attend women during childbirth. Ignaz Philip Semmelweis (1818–1865), a German-Hungarian physician, made similar observations in his practice. He noticed a dramatic difference in rates of puerperal fever between two maternity wards, one in which medical students practiced, the other run by midwives. The death rate in the ward attended by medical students was two to three times higher than that of the ward in which the midwives delivered. Semmelweis noticed that the only difference between the two wards was that the medical students would dissect cadavers, then go immediately to the maternity ward to examine patients. The midwives, of course, did not dissect cadavers. Then a physician friend of Semmelweis died from a cut he sustained while examining a woman who died of puerperal fever. These observations convinced Semmelweis that the infection was carried on the hands of the physicians. He began requiring medical students to wash their hands in a chlorinated lime solution between examinations. Immediately the mortality rate fell from approximately 18% to 1%, equivalent to the death rate in the midwives' ward.

The medical community largely ignored Holmes' advice and Semmelweis' work. Efforts to prevent the spread of infection did not begin in earnest until Louis Pasteur, a French chemist and microbiologist, proved that microorganisms cause infection. Joseph Lister, a British surgeon, embraced Pasteur's theory. Lister used carbolic acid as an antiseptic during surgery and greatly improved the survival rates of his surgical patients. His research and persistence led to general acceptance of the germ theory by physicians in Europe and the United States. As antiseptic techniques were applied to the childbirth process, maternal mortality rates fell.

Easing the Pain of Childbirth

The development and use of anesthesia during childbirth was the change that most influenced wealthy and middle-class women to begin delivering their children in hospitals, rather than at home. In the 1920s and 1930s, a method called "twilight sleep" greatly increased the number of women who chose to deliver in hospitals. Morphine and scopolamine were administered at the beginning of labor to induce twilight sleep. Morphine eased the pain of labor and scopolamine, an amnesiac, induced a hypnotic-like state and caused the woman to be unable to recall the pain of labor. This development allowed women to enjoy painless childbirth and gave the physician more control over the birth process. Therefore, the hospital came to be viewed as the safest and most humane place in which to deliver a baby.

Development of Newborn (Neonatal) Care

The term "neonatology" (study of newborns from birth through 28 days of life), was first coined by Alexander Schaffer in 1960; however, interest in the

[1] He specified puerperal fever, erysipelas, and peritonitis as types of infection that could be transmitted and cause puerperal fever in a woman who had just delivered.

unique needs of the newborn, in particular the premature newborn, can be traced back to the 17th century. It was not until the mid 1800s, however, that serious inquiry by the medical community into the special needs of newborns began in earnest. Neonatology, considered a subspecialty of pediatrics, is an outgrowth of pediatrics and obstetrics.

Pediatric Roots

In colonial times, epidemics were common, and many children died in infancy. In some cases, disease wiped out entire families. Sick children often were cared for by the adults in the family or by a neighbor with a reputation of being able to care for the sick. The first children's hospital opened in Philadelphia in 1855. Until that point in Western civilization, hospitalized children and infants were cared for in hospitals as adults were, often in the same bed. Unfortunately early institutions for children were notorious for their unsanitary conditions, neglect, and lack of proper infant nutrition. Well into the 19th century, mortality rates were commonly 50% to 100% among institutionalized infants and children in asylums or hospitals.

Pioneers who began to apply principles of sanitation to decrease the infant and child mortality rates include Arthur Jacobi, a Prussian-born physician who is generally recognized as the father of pediatrics. Dr. Jacobi and others are credited with decreasing the death rate of children in the early 1900s by initiating the practices of boiling milk and isolating children with infectious conditions.

Unfortunately, general acceptance of the germ theory by the medical community led to a heavy emphasis on asepsis to the detriment of sensory stimulation and nurturing. In fact, after World War I, a period of strict asepsis began in children's hospitals. Infants were placed in individual cubicles, and nurses were strictly forbidden to pick them up, except when absolutely necessary. Crib sides were draped with clean sheets, leaving infants with nothing to do but stare at the ceiling. The importance of sensory stimulation appears not to have been recognized. Parents were allowed to visit for a brief time (half an hour to 1 hour) each week, and they were forbidden to pick up their babies under penalty of having their visiting privileges revoked.

Despite these precautions, high infant mortality rates continued. One of the first people to suspect the cause was Joseph Brennaman, a physician at Children's Memorial Hospital in Chicago. In 1932, he suggested that the infants suffered from a lack of stimulation; other concerned child specialists became interested. In the 1940s, Ren Spitz published the results of studies that supported his contention that deprivation of maternal care caused a state of dazed stupor in an infant. He believed this condition could become irreversible if the child were not returned to the mother promptly. He termed this state "anaclitic depression." He also coined the term *hospitalism*, which he defined as "a vitiated condition of the body due to long confinement in the hospital" (*vitiated* means feeble or weak). Later the term came to be used almost entirely to denote the harmful effects of institutional care on infants. Another physician, Bakwin, found that infants hospitalized for a long time actually developed physical symptoms that he attributed to a lack of emotional stimulation and a lack of feeding satisfaction.

Working under the auspices of the World Health Organization (WHO), John Bowlby of London thoroughly explored the subject of maternal deprivation. His 1951 study, which received worldwide attention, revealed the negative results of the separation of child and mother due to hospitalization. Bowlby's work, together with that of associate John Robertson, led to a re-evaluation and liberalization of hospital visiting policies for infants and children.

In the 1970s and 1980s, Marshall Klaus and John Kennell, physicians at Rainbow Babies and Children's Hospital in Cleveland, carried out important studies on the effect of the separation of newborns and parents. They established that this early separation may have long-term effects on family relationships and that offering the new family an opportunity to be together at birth and for a significant period after birth may provide benefits that last well into early childhood (Fig. 1-1). These findings also have helped to modify hospital policies. Hospital regulations changed slowly, but gradually they began to reflect the needs of children and their families. Isolation practices have been relaxed for children who do not have infectious diseases, and parents are encouraged to visit as often as possible and to touch, hold, and care for their infants.

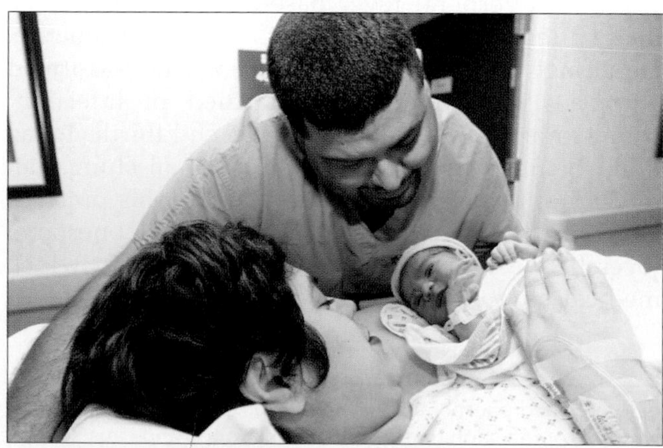

● ***Figure 1.1*** The mother, father, and infant son soon after birth. Photo by Joe Mitchell.

Development of the Modern Neonatal Intensive Care Unit (NICU)

At the same time an interest in pediatrics and the newborn was developing, obstetricians were becoming more interested in care of the newborn, or **neonate** (newborn from birth through 28 days, or one month, of life), in particular, the premature newborn. Until that time it was generally expected that premature neonates, referred to as "weaklings," and neonates with congenital malformations would die. No particular care was taken to salvage these tiny, sick newborns. In the late 1800s obstetrician, Pierre Budin and his pupil Couney pioneered incubator care of premature neonates, demonstrating that special care of these newborns could increase their survival rates (Avery, 1999).

In 1925, Dr. Alfred P. Hart published the first report on the use of exchange transfusions to treat severe neonatal jaundice, a practice that was soon adopted worldwide (University of Toronto, undated). By the 1950s premature care in neonatal intensive care units (NICUs) focused on resuscitation, thermoregulation, careful feeding techniques, simple transfusions, and exchange transfusions. Care of respiratory distress was supportive (Avery, 1999).

During the 1960s cardiac and respiratory monitors were developed. Feeding of neonates too sick to suck was accomplished by nasogastric tubes. Increased laboratory monitoring and measurement of blood gases became possible. Antibiotics were used to treat neonatal sepsis. By the 1970s the use of umbilical catheters and arterial pressure transducers was routine. In addition to nasogastric tubes, transpyloric and intravenous feedings were begun. Fetal surgery for congenital malformations became possible. In the 1980s transcutaneous (through the skin) monitoring of oxygen saturation levels and carbon dioxide levels began. Treatment of respiratory disease in the tiniest neonates became much more sophisticated and successful. By the 1990s, NICUs were highly sophisticated technological marvels and neonates who once had been considered unsalvageable began to survive (Avery, 1999). Attention started turning toward improving the quality of life, a trend that continues today.

CURRENT TRENDS IN MATERNAL–NEWBORN HEALTH CARE

Family-Centered Care

Childbirth came to be viewed as a safe and natural process as maternal and infant mortality rates began to fall. Women questioned the need for intense intervention in every birth. Also in question were the effects that medications and anesthesia had on the fetus. Many women began to insist on natural childbirth methods that allowed nature to take its course with minimal medical involvement. Some women voiced the desire for increased control over decisions about the timing and extent of interventions during labor and birth.

These efforts throughout the 1970s, 1980s, and 1990s led to family-centered maternity care, which eventually became the norm for American hospitals. Physicians and other health care providers began to respect the rights of women to participate in planning the type of care to be given during labor and birth. Husbands were at first allowed, and then encouraged, to participate in the birth process. Siblings were allowed greater access to their mother and the new baby. Birthing rooms and later labor, delivery, and recovery rooms (LDR) replaced the old assembly-line system of moving from a labor room, to a delivery room, to a recovery room. **Couplet care,** in which the mother and newborn remain together and receive care from one nurse, became the norm for postpartum care.

Regionalized Care

During the past several decades there has been a definite trend toward centralization and regionalization of maternity and neonatal services. Providing high-quality medical care for the at-risk patient necessitated transporting the pregnant woman or the newborn to medical teaching centers with the best resources for diagnosis and treatment. To contribute to economic responsibility by avoiding duplication of services and equipment, the most intricate and expensive services and the most highly specialized personnel were made available in the centralized location: perinatologists, neonatologists, pediatric neurologists, neonatal nurse practitioners, and clinical nurse specialists. In these large regional centers are found geneticists, at-risk antenatal units, neonatal intensive care units, computed tomography scanners, and other highly specialized equipment and units.

Regionalized care often takes the maternity and neonatal patient far from home. Family caregivers must travel a longer distance to visit than if the patient were at a local suburban hospital. Family-centered care becomes even more important under these circumstances. Measures are taken to keep the hospitalization as brief as possible and the family close and directly involved in the patient's care. For the newborn in particular, separation from the family is traumatic and may actually retard recovery. Many of these regionalized centers (tertiary care hospitals) have accommodations where families may stay during the hospitalization of the pregnant woman and the neonate.

Advances in Research

Huge technological and scientific advances were made at the same time the movement for family-centered care was gaining momentum. It became possible to save premature and low–birth-weight infants who previously would not have survived. Diagnostic techniques were perfected. Surgical techniques to intervene on the fetus while in utero were developed. New research and techniques have made it possible to detect and treat children born with congenital problems and disorders almost immediately after birth. These are only a few examples of the research that has been done.

Questions that influence maternity care are guiding many biomedical research projects today. Two areas of intense scientific inquiry are the prediction and prevention of preterm labor and the causes, prevention, and treatment of pregnancy-induced hypertension, a condition exclusively found in pregnancy marked by high blood pressure, edema, and loss of protein in the urine. Progress in the prevention and/or treatment of these disorders would decrease maternal and infant mortality rates significantly.

Gene therapy is used to treat certain immune disorders. Scientists are studying ways to prevent and treat genetic disorders with gene therapy, which likely will be possible in the near future. Many animal, human, and stem cell studies are being done to better understand and treat a variety of obstetric disorders. Much progress has been made in understanding and treating infertility. Other examples of current studies include the identification of genes that are responsible for the unique characteristics of Down's syndrome and therapies to treat intrauterine growth retardation (IUGR), a condition in which the fetus fails to gain sufficient weight.

Bioethical Issues

An ethical issue is one in which there is no one "right" solution that applies to all instances of the issue. Ethical decision making is a complex process that should involve many groups of individuals with varying experiences and perspectives. Recent scientific and medical advances have raised bioethical issues that did not exist in times past. Examples of bioethical issues that are present in our world today include the Human Genome Project, prenatal genetic testing, surrogate motherhood, and rationing of health care.

The Human Genome Project (HGP) was started in 1990 with the purpose of studying all of the human genes and how they function. New concepts and ideas regarding many aspects of health and disease emerge as the project continues. Identification of gene mutations in people who may be carriers of genetic disorders or who may be at risk for developing inherited disorders later in life has been a big part of the research findings in the project. Genetic testing and counseling is one area that has been greatly affected by the HGP. A predisposition to certain diseases that become evident in adulthood is also being studied through the HGP. The ability to study the human gene and factors related to the inheritance of disease and disorders has an impact on the future health of all individuals.

Today it is possible to know many things about a child before the child is born. Ultrasound can reveal the gender of the fetus and certain abnormalities early in pregnancy. Amniocentesis and chorionic villus sampling show the entire genetic code of the fetus. In this way, many chromosomal abnormalities can be diagnosed during the first trimester. Decisions can be made about continuing with the pregnancy or preparing to cope with a child who has a genetic disorder. Some parents want to know everything possible before the child is born, whereas others do not wish to interfere with the natural order of things and decline any type of prenatal testing.

Many ethical questions can be raised regarding prenatal testing. Is it right to end a pregnancy because a child has a mild genetic abnormality? Will we become a society in which a child can be chosen or rejected for life based on his or her genetic code? Is it right to bring a child into the world with a severe defect, which may cause him and his caregivers untold pain and suffering? Is it OK to make life and death decisions based on quality of life? Or is any form of life sacred regardless of the quality? These and other questions have been raised in light of technology that makes prenatal diagnosis possible.

Did you know? Many professional organizations have developed position statements that list guiding principles to be used when making certain ethical decisions. The American Academy of Pediatrics (AAP) has developed guidelines to be used when surrogacy options are being explored. For example, the AAP recommends that the rules surrounding adoption be used to guide decision making in surrogacy cases. This principle helps to safeguard the rights of the child in this unusual situation.

Surrogacy is an arrangement whereby a woman or a couple who is infertile contract with a fertile woman to carry a child. The fetus may result from in vitro fertilization techniques; embryos created from such techniques are subsequently implanted in the surrogate woman's womb to be carried to term.

At other times the surrogate mother is impregnated by artificial insemination with the sperm of the man or with the sperm of an unknown donor.

Surrogate motherhood is a situation fraught with ethical dilemmas. Some of the questions that surround this issue include: Who has the right to make decisions about the pregnancy? Who is legally obligated for the unborn child? What if one or the other of the parties changes their minds before the end of the pregnancy? What if the infant is born with a genetic disorder that leaves him physically or mentally disabled?

A phenomenon that some have referred to as "rationing of health care" is on the rise. On the one hand, there have been enormous advances in knowledge, technology, and the ability to intervene to change outcomes. Some conditions that were untreatable in the past can now be treated and even cured. On the other hand, individuals who live in poverty are less likely than persons of higher socioeconomic status to have access to these treatments and cures. Examples of ethical questions that arise in this situation include: To which services should all citizens have access regardless of ability to pay? What services are appropriate to exclude if the consumer cannot afford payment?

Demographic Trends

Several demographic trends are influencing the delivery of maternal–newborn health care in the United States. The aging of society and the tendency of American families to have fewer children have caused a shift in focus from the needs of women and newborns to those of the elderly. This trend has shifted fund allocation away from health care programs and research that enhance the health care of women and children.

The growing percentage of minority populations in relation to white, non-Hispanic populations in the United States will continue to affect health care. Nurses and other health care providers are expected to provide culturally appropriate care. The use of nontraditional methods of healing and over-the-counter herbal remedies must be assessed and integrated into the plan of care. More and more nurses are expected to accommodate the unique needs of these populations.

Poverty

One social issue that greatly influences maternity and newborn care is the problem of poverty. A woman who lives in poverty is less likely to have access to adequate prenatal care. Poverty also has a negative impact on the ability of a woman and her children to be adequately nourished and sheltered. A woman who lives in poverty is at risk for substance abuse and exposure to diseases such as tuberculosis, human immunodeficiency virus /acquired immunodeficiency syndrome (HIV/AIDS), and other sexually transmitted infections. Each of these factors has been linked to adverse outcomes for childbearing women and their children.

Cost Containment

Cost containment refers to strategies developed to reduce inefficiencies in the health care system. Inefficiencies can occur in the way health care is used by consumers. For example, taking a pregnant woman to the emergency department (ED) for treatment of constipation is inappropriate use. It would be more efficient for the woman's constipation to be treated at a clinic.

Inefficiencies also can relate to the setting in which health care is given. For example, in the past all surgical patients were admitted to the hospital the night, or sometimes even several days, before the scheduled procedure. This practice was found to be an inefficient use of the hospital setting. It was discovered that the patient could be prepared for surgery more efficiently on an outpatient basis without reducing quality.

Inefficiencies also can exist in the way health services are produced. For example, a neonatal intensive care unit (NICU) is a highly specialized, costly unit to operate. If every hospital in a large city were to operate a NICU, this would be an inefficient production of health services. It is more cost effective to have one large NICU for the entire region.

Cost Containment Strategies

There is no dispute that health care costs continue to increase at a rate out of proportion to the cost of living. This situation has challenged local, state, and federal governments; insurance payers; and providers and consumers of health care to cope with skyrocketing costs while maintaining quality of care. Some major strategies that have been implemented to help control costs include prospective payment systems, managed care, capitation, cost sharing, cost shifting, and alternative delivery systems.

Prospective Payment Systems. A **prospective payment system** predetermines rates to be paid to the health care provider to care for patients with certain classifications of diseases. These rates are paid regardless of the costs that the health care provider actually incurs. This system tends to encourage efficient production and use of resources. Prospective payment systems were developed by the government in an attempt to control Medicare costs. These systems include diagnosis-related groups (DRGs) for inpatient billing; ambulatory payment classifications (APCs); home health, inpatient rehabilitation facility, and skilled nursing facility prospective payment systems.

Managed Care. Managed care is a system that integrates management and coordination of care with financing in an attempt to improve cost effectiveness, use, quality, and outcomes. Managed care evolved from the old "fee-for-service" type of health insurance, in which providers of care were paid the amount they billed to provide a service. Under managed care plans, both the provider of service and the consumer have responsibilities to help control costs. The main types of managed care plans—health maintenance organizations (HMOs), preferred provider organizations (PPOs), and point-of-service (POS) plans—are discussed in the section "Payment for Health Services."

Capitation. Capitation is one method managed care plans have used to reduce costs. The health care plan pays a fixed amount per person to the health care provider to provide services for enrollees. This amount is negotiated up front, and the health care provider is obligated to provide care for the negotiated amount, regardless of the actual number or nature of the services provided.

Cost Sharing and Cost Shifting. Cost sharing refers to the costs that the patient incurs when using his health insurance plan. Examples of cost sharing are co-payments and deductibles. When costs go up, health insurance plans often increase the amount of deductibles and co-payments before they raise the price of the insurance premium. Cost shifting is a strategy in which the cost of providing uncompensated care for uninsured individuals is passed onto people who are insured. Often cost shifting results in higher premiums, co-pays, and deductibles.

Alternative Delivery Systems. Another way to control costs is to provide alternative delivery systems. In this situation, alternatives to expensive inpatient services are provided. Many hospitals found that it was more cost efficient to send a patient home earlier and provide follow-up care using a home health agency. Skilled and intermediate nursing and rehabilitation facilities and hospice programs are other examples of alternative delivery systems.

Nursing Contribution to Cost Containment

Specific cost containment strategies that nurses have been instrumental in implementing include health promotion and case management. Nurses are the primary providers of **utilization review**, which is a systematic evaluation of services delivered by a health care provider to determine appropriateness and quality of care, as well as medical necessity of the services provided.

Nurses have long advocated health promotion activities as a valuable way to maintain quality of life and control health care costs. Health promotion involves helping people to make lifestyle changes to move them to a higher level of wellness. Health promotion includes all aspects of health: physical, mental, emotional, social, and spiritual. Many nurses and nursing organizations lobby for increased spending on health promotion and illness prevention activities. For example, nurses may testify at a public hearing that it is more cost effective to provide comprehensive prenatal care for low income women than to pay high "back end" costs of highly specialized care in a NICU for a preterm baby.

Although nurses are not the only licensed professionals qualified to provide case management, many case managers are nurses. **Case management** involves monitoring and coordinating care for individuals who need high-cost or extensive health care services. An at-risk pregnant woman with diabetes is a good candidate for case management because she requires frequent monitoring of blood sugars and coordination of several health care providers.

PAYMENT FOR HEALTH SERVICES

Access to and use of health care services often is facilitated by health care insurance. Typically, families with health care insurance are more likely to have a primary care provider and to participate in appropriate preventive care (Healthy People 2010, 2001). Statistics provided by Healthy People 2010 show that more than 44 million people in the United States do not have health insurance. Of this number, 11 million are children.

Most employment facilities provide some form of medical insurance for employees and their families; or families may elect to purchase their own insurance apart from an employer. This type of insurance is known as private insurance, whether it is provided by an employer or purchased directly by the health care consumer. For those who are uninsured, the federal and state governments have provided means to access health care services. In addition, specialized services are available, which may be funded by local, state, or federal governments or may be administered by private organizations.

Private Insurance

Private insurance can be acquired through work benefits or through individual means. The policyholder pays a monthly fee for the insurance coverage. The policyholder is responsible for paying the preset co-payment for any health services needed. Before the onset of managed care, medical services traditionally were paid for on a fee-for-service basis. Physicians billed for their services, and insurance providers paid whatever was charged. However, as technological advances were made and costs skyrocketed, managed care was created in an effort to contain costs and make health care affordable. Managed care insurance plans include HMOs and PPOs (Box 1-1).

Federally Funded Sources

Medicaid

Medicaid was founded in 1965 under Title XIX of the Social Security Act. This federal program supplies block grants to states to provide health care for certain individuals who have low incomes. On average, the federal government contributes approximately 57% of the monies needed to finance the program. The states must fund the remaining 43% (National Association of State Budget Officers, undated). Under broad federal guidelines, each state develops and administers its own Medicaid program; therefore, eligibility requirements and application processes vary from state to state. Pregnant women and children who meet the income guidelines qualify for this program (Health Care Financing Administration, undated).

Although Medicaid has helped address the problem of access to health care for some childbearing women and some children, the process for applying is often complex and confusing. Many women and children who qualify do not benefit from the program. Concerned citizen groups in many states are working to modify the application process and find ways to assist eligible individuals to apply for and receive Medicaid.

State Child Health Insurance Program

Many families make too much money to qualify for Medicaid; however, health insurance is not available or affordable to them. Because of this problem, many pregnant women and children do not get adequate health care, particularly preventive care, such as prenatal care, well-child visits, and immunizations. In response to this need, the federal government instituted another block grant program to states under Title XXI of the Social Security Act. The State Child Health Insurance Program, also known by its acronym "SCHIP"

BOX 1.1 Managed Care Plans

Health Maintenance Organizations (HMOs)
With an HMO, contracts are made with selected health care providers and health care facilities to provide services to its policyholders for a fixed amount of money paid in advance for a specified set of time. The policyholder and insured family members choose health care providers and facilities from the list of those specifically associated with their HMO. The providers and facilities are closely evaluated for any unnecessary health care services.

Preferred Provider Organizations (PPOs)
PPOs consist of selected health care professionals and facilities who are under contract with insurance companies, employers, or third party payers to provide medical and surgical services to policyholders and insured family members. The policyholder has more choices for service providers when they choose a PPO versus a HMO. In addition, the services under a PPO are not fixed or prepaid. Should the policyholder choose to access services from a provider outside the PPO list of professionals and facilities, this may increase the policyholder's out-of-pocket expense for services rendered.

Some insurance companies provide physicians fixed amounts to provide health care to individuals, regardless of the actual costs involved. This system discourages physicians from ordering costly laboratory and diagnostic tests or from giving treatments of questionable therapeutic benefit. It has also encouraged physicians to see more patients, which decreases the amount of time available to individual patients.

Managed care has had multiple effects on individual consumers of health care. Consumers pay higher premiums with higher deductibles and co-payment amounts. At the same time, they have fewer choices. The consumer may choose from a limited number of providers that belong to a HMO or who are "in network" if the insurance plan is set up as a PPO. Review panels chosen by the HMO or PPO have the right to review and decline services deemed unnecessary. Usually the consumer cannot appeal these decisions. This situation has led to a consumer movement for the right to sue these companies when decisions negatively affect the individual's health.

This is not to say that all of the effects have been negative. Managed care has provoked the health care industry to be more cost conscious and fiscally temperate. Health care providers are less likely to order expensive tests and procedures unless there is an unmistakable benefit. However, health care costs, particularly pharmaceutical costs, have continued to increase out of proportion to other costs of living.

or simply "CHIP," was enacted in 1997 as part of the Balanced Budget Act.

SCHIP provides health insurance to newborns and children in low-income families who do not otherwise qualify for Medicaid and are uninsured. Premiums and co-payment amounts are kept to a minimum and are based on a sliding scale according to total family income. Emphasis is placed on preventive care and health promotion in addition to treatment for illness and disease. One of the requirements for states to participate in SCHIP is that each state must develop an outreach program to inform and enroll eligible families and children.

Special Supplemental Nutrition Program for Women, Infants, and Children

One federally funded program that continues to successfully meet its goal to enhance nutritional status for women and children is the Special Supplemental Nutrition Program for Women, Infants, and Children (WIC). WIC began serving low-income, nutritionally at-risk pregnant, breast-feeding, and postpartum women and their children (as old as 5 years) in 1974. The Food and Nutrition Service administers this grant program, which distributes monies to state agencies to provide benefits to eligible citizens.

WIC services are provided in local health departments, hospitals, and clinics in all 50 states. Women and their children must first meet income eligibility requirements, and then they are screened by a trained health professional (such as a nurse, social worker, or physician) for nutritional risk factors based on federal guidelines (Fig. 1-2). Nutritional risk factors are categorized as medically based risk and diet-based risk. Examples of medical risk factors include conditions such as young maternal age, anemia, poor pregnancy outcomes, and being underweight. Diet-based risk includes diets with deficiencies in any of the major food groups, vitamins, or minerals. Because there are not unlimited funds available, at-risk women are screened according to predetermined categories of priority.

Here's how you can help!

Provide the patient and family with a list of available community health care resources before the patient leaves the hospital or the clinic. This information can be of great help, especially if the family needs financial assistance to afford adequate medical treatment.

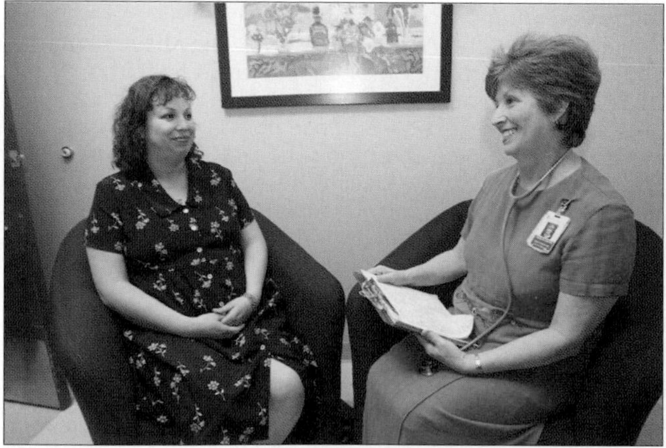

● ***Figure 1.2*** A trained registered nurse screens a pregnant woman at a WIC clinic. If the woman meets income and nutritional eligibility requirements, she may receive vouchers to purchase nutritious foods.

The program is one of the federal government's success stories. It is currently estimated to be serving all eligible infants and 90% of all other eligible participants. Eligible women and their children receive food vouchers to redeem at participating grocery stores. The vouchers can be used to purchase foods that are high in at least one of the following nutrients: protein, iron, calcium, and vitamins A and C. Fortified cereals, milk, eggs, cheese, peanut butter, and legumes are examples of eligible foods. Although women are encouraged to breast-feed, if they choose to bottle-feed, their infants can receive formula assistance to 6 months of age.

Test Yourself

- Name two major developments that contributed to the modernization of maternity care in the United States.
- The work of which pediatric reformer led to the liberalization of hospital visiting policies for pediatric patients in the 1950s?
- Define "prospective payment system."

MATERNAL–INFANT HEALTH TODAY

One way to measure the health status of a nation is to determine **mortality rates** of childbearing women, infants, and children. Mortality rates are statistics recorded as the ratio of deaths in a given category to the number of individuals in that category of the population. The statistics that are of interest to the maternity and neonatal nurse are maternal, fetal, neonatal, **perinatal** (the period surrounding birth, from conception throughout pregnancy and birth), and infant mortality rates. **Morbidity** refers to the number of persons afflicted with the same disease condition per a certain number of populations.

Maternal–Infant Health Status

Several definitions are required to better understand perinatal mortality rates. A **viable** fetus is one that is able to live outside of the uterus. In most states the law prescribes 20 weeks of gestation the arbitrary divider between viability and nonviability. The **fetal mortality rate** is calculated by dividing the number of deaths that occur in utero (during pregnancy) at 20 or more weeks of gestation (i.e., when the fetus is considered viable) by the number of live births plus fetal deaths.[2] **Neonatal** is the adjective used to describe the time period from birth through the first 28 days or 1 month of life. Therefore, the **neonatal mortality rate** is expressed as the number of infant deaths during the first 28 days of life for every 1,000 live births. **Perinatal mortality** encompasses the number of fetal/neonatal deaths that occur from 28 weeks of gestation through the first 7 days of life. The perinatal mortality rate is expressed as the number of deaths (as previously described) per 1,000 live births, plus fetal deaths that occur from 28 weeks of gestation and beyond. The **infant mortality rate** is the number of deaths during the first 12 months of life, which includes neonatal mortality. The **maternal mortality rate** refers to the number of maternal deaths per 100,000 live births caused by a pregnancy-related complication that occurs during pregnancy or during the 42 days after pregnancy. The leading causes of infant and maternal deaths are listed in Box 1-2. All death statistics relating to the fetus, neonate, and infant are reported as the number of deaths for every 1,000 live births. Maternal deaths are reported per 100,000 live births because they are uncommon.

Both infant and maternal mortality rates have fallen dramatically since the early 1900s (Figs. 1-3 and 1-4). At that time, for every 1,000 live births, approximately 100 infants died before they reached their first birthday. In 1999 that number had dropped to 7.1 deaths per 1,000 live births—a decline greater than 90%! Maternal mortality rates at the turn of the century were from 600 to 900 deaths per 100,000 live births and decreased to 7.7 deaths per 100,000 live births by 1997. This represents a greater than 99% decline in the maternal mortality rate (Centers for Disease Control, 1999).

Notwithstanding these remarkable advances, much work remains to be done. The United States lags behind 21 other industrialized nations in maternal mortality statistics. Since 1982, the maternal mortality rate has hovered between 7 and 8 deaths per 100,000 live births. The Healthy People 2000 goal[3] of 3.3 maternal

[2] Fetal deaths are often referred to as "stillbirths" in lay terminology.

BOX 1.2 Leading Causes of Infant and Maternal Mortality in the United States

Infant Mortality

The three leading causes of infant death for the year 2000 (the latest year for which data are available) are listed in descending order.

1. Congenital malformations, deformations, and chromosomal abnormalities (21%)
2. Disorders related to short gestation and low birth weight (16%)
3. Sudden infant death syndrome (SIDS) (9%)*

Maternal Mortality

The three leading causes of pregnancy-related death for the years 1991 to 1999 (the latest year for which data are available) are listed in descending order.

1. Embolism (20%)
2. Hemorrhage (17%)
3. Pregnancy-related hypertension (16%)†

*Source: Centers for Disease Control. (2002). *National vital statistics report, 50*(12). Retrieved July 13, 2003, from http://www.cdc.gov/nchs/data/nvsr/nvsr50/nvsr50_12.pdf

†Source: Centers for Disease Control. (2003). *Fact sheet. Pregnancy-related mortality surveillance—United States, 1991–1999.* Retrieved July 13, 2003, from http://www.cdc.gov/od/oc/media/pressrel/fs030220.htm

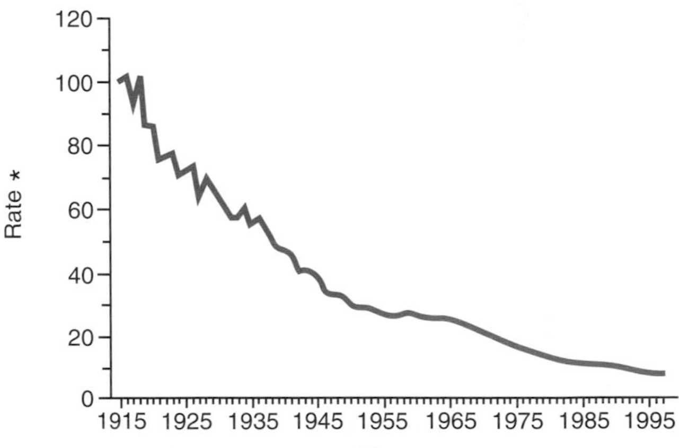

● ***Figure 1.3*** United States infant mortality rate by year (1915–1997). Centres for Disease Control. (1999). Healthier mothers and babies. *MMWR: Morbidity and Mortality Weekly Report, 48*(38), 849–856. Retrieved March 3, 2002, from http://www.cdc.gov/mmwr/PDF/wk/mm4838.pdf

[3] Healthy People 2000 were national health goals set in 1987. For further information on the Healthy People initiative see the website: http://www.health.gov/healthypeople/

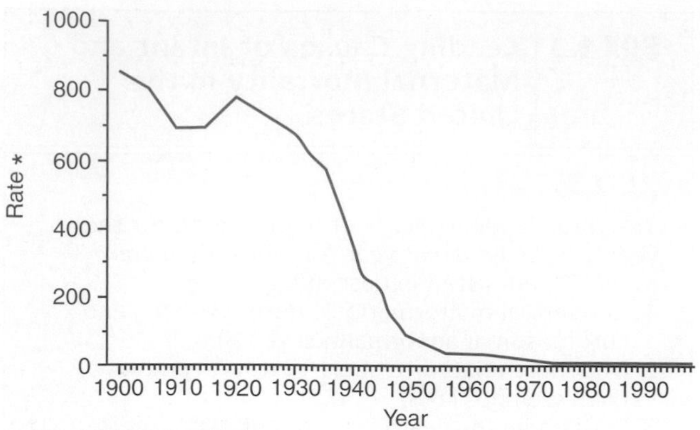

● ***Figure 1.4*** United States maternal mortality rate by year (1900–1997).
Centres for Disease Control. (1999). Healthier mothers and babies. *MMWR: Morbidity and Mortality Weekly Report, 48*(38), 849–856. Retrieved March 3, 2002, from http://www.cdc.gov/mmwr/PDF/wk/mm4838.pdf

deaths per 100,000 live births set in 1987 has not been reached (Centers for Disease Control, 1998).

In addition, there is a racial disparity in maternal mortality rates. The maternal mortality rate of black women for the years 1982 to 1996 hovers between 18 and 22 deaths per 100,000 live births, whereas white women have a mortality rate of 5 to 6 during the same period. A black woman is almost twice as likely as a white woman to experience a complication of pregnancy and is four times more likely to die of a complication of pregnancy. If the disparity were to be eliminated, the overall rate would fall from 7.5 to less than 6 per 100,000 live births (Centers for Disease Control, 1998).

The U.S. infant mortality rate lags behind that of many other industrialized nations. Preliminary statistics from 2002 indicate that the U.S. infant mortality rate is 6.69; nearly twice that of Iceland, the country with the lowest reported rate, which is 3.53 (*The World Factbook*, 2002). Many factors may be associated with high infant mortality rates and poor health. Low birth weight and late or nonexistent prenatal care are main factors in the poor rankings in infant mortality. Other major factors that compromise infants' health include congenital anomalies, sudden infant death syndrome, respiratory distress syndrome, and increasing rates of HIV. Low birth weight and other causes of infant death and chronic illness are often linked to maternal factors, such as lack of prenatal care, smoking, use of alcohol and illicit drugs, pregnancy before age 18 or after age 40, poor nutrition, lower socioeconomic status, lower educational levels, and environmental hazards.

Both infant and maternal mortality rates are much higher among nonwhite populations; studies repeatedly attribute high mortality rates to lack of adequate prenatal care and an increased birth rate among the high-risk group of adolescent girls and young women 15 to 19 years of age. The lack of adequate financial resources, insurance, and education regarding birth control and health care in general contributes to this situation.

Addressing Maternal–Infant Health Status

Box 1-3 shows the Centers for Disease Control (CDC) recommendations of ways to continue to decrease maternal and infant mortality. Other major steps toward addressing the issue of maternal–infant health status are discussed in this chapter.

National Commission to Prevent Infant Mortality

In 1986, Congress established the National Commission to Prevent Infant Mortality and charged it with the responsibility of creating a national strategic plan to reduce infant mortality and morbidity rates in the United States. In 1988, the Commission's first report, *Death Before Life: The Tragedy of Infant Mortality,* listed two primary objectives: to make the health of mothers and babies a national priority and to provide universal access to care for all pregnant women and children. The Commission concluded that educating the nation about the health needs of mothers and babies would cause a national response to the problem and that women would have to be given information and motivation to reduce infant mortality and morbidity rates. The Commission also stated that barriers of finances, geography, education, social position, behavior, and program administration problems must be eliminated to provide universal access to health care. In February 1990, the Commission published *Troubling Trends: The Health of the Next Generation,* which concluded that early prenatal care, along with smoking cessation, pregnancy planning, and nutrition counseling and food supplementation, would result in heavier and healthier infants. The Commission has been successful in its objective of decreasing infant mortality.

Healthy People 2010

In 1990, a national consortium of more than 300 organizations developed a set of objectives for the year 2000, *Healthy People 2000.* Prevention of illness, or health promotion, was the underlying goal of these objectives. States were encouraged to set their own objectives. Priority areas specifically affecting children were identified. These objectives were reviewed mid-decade; although there had been progress in some goals, much remained to be accomplished. The initiative has continued, and *Healthy People 2010* outlines

BOX 1.3 Opportunities to Reduce Maternal and Infant Mortality

Prevention measures to reduce maternal and infant mortality and to promote the health of all childbearing-aged women and their newborns should start before conception and continue through the postpartum period. Some of these prevention measures include the following:

Before Conception

- Screen women for health risks and pre-existing chronic conditions, such as diabetes, hypertension, and sexually transmitted diseases.
- Counsel women about contraception and provide access to effective family planning services (to prevent unintended pregnancies and unnecessary abortions).
- Counsel women about the benefits of good nutrition; encourage women especially to consume adequate amounts of folic acid supplements (to prevent neural tube defects) and iron.
- Advise women to avoid alcohol, tobacco, and illicit drugs.
- Advise women about the value of regular physical exercise.

During Pregnancy

- Provide women with early access to high-quality care throughout pregnancy, labor, and delivery. Such care includes risk-appropriate care, treatment for complications, and the use of antenatal corticosteroids when appropriate.
- Monitor and, when appropriate, treat pre-existing chronic conditions.
- Screen for and, when appropriate, treat reproductive tract infections including bacterial vaginosis, group B streptococcus infections, and human immunodeficiency virus.
- Vaccinate women against influenza, if appropriate.
- Continue counseling against use of tobacco, alcohol, and illicit drugs.
- Continue counseling about nutrition and physical exercise.
- Educate women about the early signs of pregnancy-related problems.

During Postpartum Period

- Vaccinate newborns at age-appropriate times.
- Provide information about well-baby care and benefits of breast-feeding.
- Warn parents about exposing infants to secondhand smoke.
- Counsel parents about placing infants to sleep on their backs.
- Educate parents about how to protect their infants from exposure to infectious diseases and harmful substances.

From Centers for Disease Control. (1999). Healthier mothers and babies. *MMWR: Morbidity and Mortality Weekly Report, 48*(38), 849–856. Retrieved March 3, 2002, from http://www.cdc.gov/mmwr/PDF/wk/mm4838.pdf

two basic goals for health promotion and disease prevention. Goal one is to increase quality and years of healthy life; goal two is to eliminate health disparities (Healthy People 2010, 2001). These goals are divided further into focus areas and attainment objectives. Many of the focus areas and objectives directly relate to pregnant women and children and their health care (Box 1-4). Nurses caring for pregnant women and children use these objectives as underlying guidelines in planning care.

Test Yourself

- What deaths are covered under the term "perinatal mortality?"
- Name the number one cause of maternal mortality in the United States.
- Name the two basic goals for health promotion and disease prevention outlined by Healthy People 2010.

THE NURSE'S CHANGING ROLE IN MATERNAL–NEWBORN HEALTH CARE

The image of nursing has changed, and the horizons and responsibilities have broadened tremendously in recent years. The primary thrust of health care is toward prevention. In addition to the treatment of disease and physical problems, modern maternal–newborn care addresses prenatal care, growth and development, and anticipatory guidance on maturational and common health problems. Teaching also is an important aspect of caring for the childbearing family. Clients are educated on a variety of topics, from follow-up of immunizations to other, more traditional aspects of health.

Nurses at all levels are legally accountable for their actions and assume new responsibilities and accountability with every advance in education. Nurses practicing in maternity and newborn settings at all levels must keep up to date with education and information on how to help their patients and where to direct families for help when other resources are needed. When the nurse functions as a teacher, adviser, and resource person, it is

BOX 1.4 Healthy People 2010: Focus Areas Related to Childbearing Women and Children

Focus Area: Access to Quality Health Services
Goal: Improve access to comprehensive, high-quality health care services.
Persons with health insurance
Single toll-free number for poison control centers
Special needs for children
Early (starting in the first trimester) and consistent prenatal care

Focus Area: Educational and Community-Based Programs
Goal: Increase the quality, availability, and effectiveness of education and community-based programs designed to prevent disease and improve health and quality of life.
School health education
School nurse-to-student ratio
Community health promotion programs
Patient and family education
Culturally appropriate and linguistically competent community health promotion programs

Focus Area: Environmental Health
Goal: Promote health for all through a healthy environment.
Safe drinking water
Elevated blood lead levels in children
School policies to protect against environmental hazards
Toxic pollutants

Focus Area: Family Planning
Goal: Improve pregnancy planning and spacing and prevent unintended pregnancy.
Adolescent pregnancy
Abstinence before age 15 and among adolescents age 15 to 17 years
Birth spacing
Contraceptive use
Male involvement in pregnancy prevention
Pregnancy prevention and sexually transmitted disease (STD) protection
Insurance coverage for contraceptive supplies and services
Problems in becoming pregnant and maintaining a pregnancy

Focus Area: HIV
Goal: Prevent HIV infection and its related illness and death.
Condom use
Screening for STDs and immunization for hepatitis B
Perinatally acquired HIV infection

Focus Area: Immunization and Infectious Diseases
Goal: Prevent disease, disability, and death from infectious disease, including vaccine-preventable diseases.
Hepatitis B and bacterial meningitis in infants and young children
Antibiotics prescribed for ear infections
Vaccination coverage and strategies

Focus Area: Injury and Violence Prevention
Goal: Reduce injuries, disabilities, and deaths due to unintentional injuries and violence.
Child fatality review
Deaths from firearms, poisoning, suffocation, motor vehicle crashes
Child restraints
Drownings
Maltreatment and maltreatment fatalities of children

Focus Area: Maternal, Infant, and Child Health
Goal: Improve the health and well-being of women, infants, children, and families.
Fetal, infant, child, adolescent deaths
Maternal deaths and illnesses
Prenatal and obstetric care
Low birth-weight and very low–birth-weight, preterm births
Developmental disabilities and neural tube defects
Prenatal substance exposure
Fetal alcohol syndrome
Breast-feeding
Newborn screening

Focus Area: Nutrition and Overweight
Goal: Promote health and reduce chronic disease associated with diet and weight.
Overweight or obesity in children and adolescents
Iron deficiency in young children and in females of childbearing age
Anemia in low-income pregnant females
Iron deficiency in pregnant females

Focus Area: Physical Fitness and Activity
Goal: Improve health, fitness, and quality of life through daily physical activity.
Physical activity in children and adolescents

Focus Area: Sexually Transmitted Diseases
Goal: Promote responsible sexual behaviors, increase access to quality services to prevent STDs and their complications.
Responsible adolescent sexual behavior
STD complications affecting females
STD complications affecting the fetus and newborn
Screening of pregnant women

Focus Area: Substance Abuse
Goal: Reduce substance abuse to protect the health, safety, and quality of life for all, especially children.
Adverse consequences of substance use and abuse
Substance use and abuse

Focus Area: Tobacco Use
Goal: Reduce illness, disability, and death related to tobacco use and exposure to secondhand smoke.
Adolescent tobacco use, age, and initiation of tobacco use
Smoking cessation by adolescents
Exposure to tobacco smoke at home among children

Focus Area: Vision and Hearing
Goal: Improve the visual and hearing health of the nation.
Vision screening for children
Impairment in children and adolescents
Newborn hearing screening, evaluation, and intervention
Otitis media
Noise-induced hearing loss in children

Adapted from National Center for Health Statistics. (2001). *Healthy people 2010.* Hyattsville, MD, Author.

important that the information and advice provided be correct, pertinent, and useful to the person in need.

Advanced practice nurses, in particular the certified nurse midwife (CNM) and nurse practitioners—family, neonatal, and women's health—have taken a significant place in caring for childbearing families. The family nurse practitioner (FNP) provides primary care for women and their families. When pregnancy occurs, the FNP usually refers the woman to a CNM or obstetrician for prenatal care. The neonatal nurse practitioner (NNP) specializes in the care of the neonate. NNPs are employed by hospital NICUs and by neonatologists to provide care for premature and other sick newborns. The women's health nurse practitioner (WHNP) specializes in primary care of the woman. In addition, clinical nurse specialists (CNS) are nurses with advanced education prepared to provide care at any stage of illness or wellness.

Health teaching is one of the most important aspects of promoting wellness. Nurses are often in a position to do incidental teaching, as well as more organized formal teaching. Nurses also must be aware that they serve as role models to others in practicing good health habits. Some examples of possible teaching opportunities include those in a work environment, such as helping the family of an ill neonate understand a diagnosis or proposed treatment, understanding medications, and providing teaching materials to families. In the community, the nurse can be an advocate for healthy living practices and policies or can serve as a volunteer in community organizations to promote healthy growth and development and anticipatory guidance. Nurses can become involved in the community to offer knowledge and expertise in wellness practices. They should use every opportunity to contribute to and encourage healthy living practices.

Throughout this text, teaching opportunities are identified and teaching suggestions supplied. Nurses are encouraged to use these suggestions as a foundation for further teaching. However, during any teaching the nurse must be alert to the abilities of the family to understand the material being presented. By using methods of feedback, questions and answers, and demonstrations when appropriate, the nurse can confirm that the information is understood. This also gives the nurse the opportunity to reinforce any areas of weak information. With experience, nurses can become very competent teachers.

CRITICAL THINKING

Along with teaching, it is important for the nurse to use clinical judgment and purposeful thought and reasoning to make decisions that lead to positive outcomes for the maternal and pediatric patient. This process is called critical thinking. The nurse takes data collected and uses skills and knowledge to make a conscious plan to care for the patient and family. As the plan is carried out, the nurse continues to evaluate and revise the care of the patient, keeping the desired outcomes always in mind. By using critical thinking, the nurse can be more proficient and effective at meeting the needs of the patient. Critical thinking is based on a systematic process and is used as the nurse follows and uses the nursing process.

THE NURSING PROCESS

The **nursing process** is a proven form of problem solving based on the scientific method. The nursing process consists of five components:

- Assessment
- Nursing diagnosis
- Outcome identification and planning
- Implementation
- Evaluation

Based on the data collected during the assessment, nursing diagnoses are determined, nursing care is planned and implemented, and the results are evaluated. The process does not end here but continues through reassessment, establishment of new diagnoses, additional plans, implementation, and evaluation until all the patient's nursing problems are identified and dealt with (Fig. 1-5).

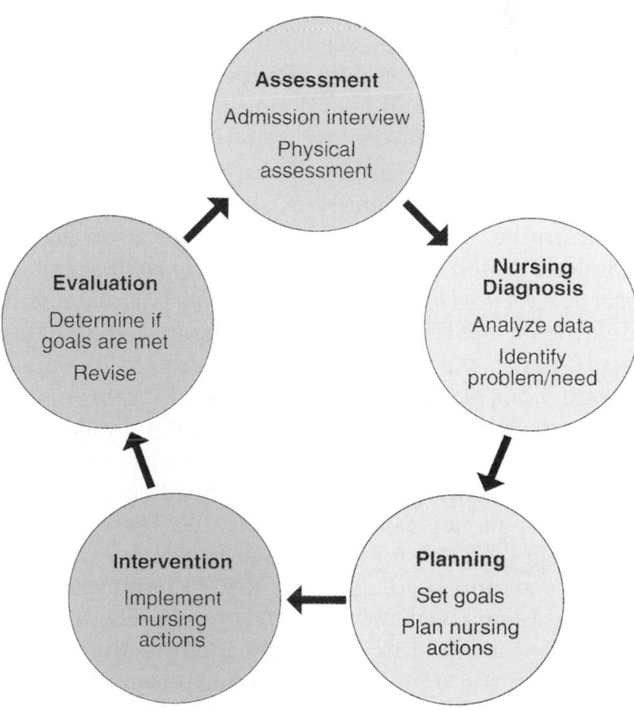

● ***Figure 1.5*** Diagram of the Nursing Process.

Assessment

Nursing assessment is a skill that must be practiced and perfected through study and experience. The practical nurse collects data and contributes to the child's assessment. The nurse must be skilled in understanding the concepts of verbal and nonverbal communication; concepts of growth and development; anatomy, physiology, and pathophysiology; and the influence of cultural heritage and family social structure. Data collected during the assessment of the pregnant woman and family form the basis of all nursing care.

Assessment and data collection begin with the admission interview and physical examination. During this phase, a relationship of trust begins to build between the nurse and the family. This relationship forms more quickly when the nurse is sensitive to the family's cultural background. Careful listening and recording of **subjective data** (data spoken by the woman or family) and careful observation and recording of **objective data** (observable by the nurse) are essential to obtaining a complete picture.

Nursing Diagnosis

The process of determining a nursing diagnosis begins with the analysis of information (data) gathered during the assessment. Along with the registered nurse or other health care professional, the practical nurse participates in the development of a nursing diagnosis based on actual or potential health problems that fall within the range of nursing practice. These diagnoses are not medical diagnoses but are based on the individual response to a disease process, condition, or situation. Nursing diagnoses change as the patient's responses change; therefore, diagnoses are in a continual state of re-evaluation and modification.

Nursing diagnoses are subdivided into three types: actual, risk, and wellness diagnoses. **Actual nursing diagnoses** identify existing health problems. For example, a woman in labor may have an actual diagnosis stated as *Acute Pain related to contractions of labor as evidenced by verbal reports of pain.* This statement identifies a health problem the woman actually has (acute pain), the factor that contributes to its cause (contractions of labor), and the signs and symptoms, in this case, verbal reports. This is an actual nursing diagnosis because of the presence of signs and symptoms.

Risk nursing diagnoses identify health problems to which the patient is especially vulnerable. These identify patients at high risk for a particular problem. An example of a risk nursing diagnosis is *Risk for Injury related to uncontrolled muscular activity secondary to seizure.*

Wellness nursing diagnoses identify the potential of a person, family, or community to move from one level of wellness to a higher level. For example, a wellness diagnosis for a family adapting well to the birth of a second child might be *Readiness for Enhanced Family Coping.*

The North American Nursing Diagnosis Association (NANDA) first published an approved list of nursing diagnoses in 1973; since then the list has been revised and expanded periodically. Nursing diagnoses continue to be developed and revised to keep them current and useful in describing what nurses contribute to health care.

Outcome Identification and Planning

To plan nursing care for the patient, data must be collected (assessment) and analyzed (nursing diagnosis) and outcomes identified in cooperation with the patient and family. These **outcomes** (goals) should be specific, stated in measurable terms, and include a time frame. The goal must be realistic, patient focused, and attainable. After mutual goal setting has been accomplished, nursing actions are proposed. Although a number of possible diagnoses may be identified, the nurse must review them, rank them by urgency, and select those that require the most immediate attention.

After selecting the first goals to accomplish, the nurse must propose nursing interventions to achieve them. This is the planning aspect of the nursing process. These nursing interventions may be based on clinical experience, knowledge of the health problem, standards of care, standard care plans, or other resources. The interventions should be discussed with the patient and family to determine if they are practical and workable. Proposed interventions are modified to fit the individual patient. If standardized care plans are used, they must be individualized to reflect the patient's age and developmental level, cognitive level, and family, economic, and cultural influences. Expected outcomes are set with specific measurable criteria and time lines.

Implementation

Implementation is the process of putting the nursing care plan into action. These actions may be independent, dependent, or interdependent. **Independent nursing actions** are actions that may be performed based on the nurse's own clinical judgment, for example, initiating protective skin care for an area that might break down. **Dependent nursing actions,** such as administering analgesics for pain, are actions that the nurse performs as a result of a physician's order. **Interdependent nursing actions** are actions that the nurse must accomplish in conjunction with other health team members, such as meal planning with the dietary therapist.

Evaluation

Evaluation is a vital part of the nursing process. The practical nurse participates with other members of the health care team in the patient's evaluation. Evaluation measures the success or failure of the nursing plan of care. Like assessment, evaluation is an ongoing process. Evaluation is achieved by determining if the identified outcomes have been met. The criteria of the nursing outcomes determine if the interventions were effective. If the goals have not been met in the specified time, or if implementation is unsuccessful, a particular intervention may need to be reassessed and revised. Possibly the outcome criterion is unrealistic and needs to be discarded or adjusted. The patient and the family must be assessed to determine progress adequately. Both objective data (measurable) and subjective data (based on responses from the patient and family) are used in the evaluation.

DOCUMENTATION

One of the most important parts of nursing care is recording information about the patient on the permanent record. This record, the patient's chart, is a legal document and must be accurate and complete. Nursing care provided and responses to care are included. In maternity and newborn settings, documentation is extremely important because those records can be used in legal situations many years after they are written. These records include the nurse's observations and findings, and they help explain and justify the actions taken.

Documentation may be done in various forms, including admission assessments, nurse's or progress notes, graphic sheets, checklists, medication records, and discharge teaching or summaries. Many health care settings use computerized or bedside documentation records. Whatever the system or form used, concise, factual information is charted. Everything written must be legible and clear and include the date and time. Nursing actions such as medication administration must be documented as soon as possible after the intervention to ensure the action is communicated, especially in the care of childbearing women and newborns.

Test Yourself

- During the nursing process, analysis of information (data) gathered during the assessment is done in order to determine the ________________________ ____________________ (two words).
- In which part of the nursing process is it determined whether or not identified outcomes have been met?
- Name at least one important criterion that must be met when health information is documented.

KEY POINTS

- Two major developments that forever changed the way maternity care was given in the United States were acceptance of the germ theory that led to decreased deaths from infection and the development of obstetric anesthesia to ease the pain of childbirth.
- The concept of family-centered care developed in conjunction with the consumer movement that led childbirth to be viewed as a safe and natural process.
- Regionalization of care contributes to economic responsibility by avoiding duplication of services and expensive equipment.
- Recent advances in research have led to new ethical dilemmas that must be addressed by health care providers. Examples include the Human Genome Project, prenatal genetic testing, surrogate motherhood, and rationing of health care.
- The increase in the number of older Americans, the tendency for American families to limit the number of children, and budget deficiencies have influenced a shift in focus away from programs for childbearing women and their infants.
- Poverty and the "rationing of health care" are social issues that have a negative impact on the health of childbearing women *and newborns* and increase the chance that complications will occur.
- Ethical dilemmas are by definition difficult to decide and involve complex choices and conflicts. Ethical decisions should always be made after careful consideration and with input from a variety of sources.
- Rising health care costs and shrinking budgets have led to attempts to reform health care. Managed care has become the norm of American health care. Attempts to contain health care costs have led to the development of prospective payment systems (such as HMOs and PPOs) and capitation. Nurses have been especially helpful with the cost-containment strategies of utilization review, critical pathways, and case management.
- Health care reform has led to changes in the Medicaid program and the development of SCHIP, low cost insurance for low-income children whose parents make too much money to qualify for Medicaid.

- One way in which the health status of a nation is measured is through morbidity (illness) and mortality (death) rates. Measures particularly useful to maternity and neonatal health include perinatal, maternal, and neonatal mortality rates.
- The three leading causes of infant mortality are congenital disorders, prematurity and low birth weight, and sudden infant death syndrome. The three leading causes of maternal mortality are embolism, hemorrhage, and pregnancy-induced hypertension.
- Although its infant mortality rate is improving, the United States still remains behind most other industrialized countries. Lack of or inadequate prenatal care is believed to be one major cause of this problem.
- *Healthy People 2010* sets goals for health care with a focus on health promotion and prevention of illness as the nation approaches the year 2010.
- The role of the nurse has changed to include the responsibilities of teacher, adviser, resource person, and researcher, as well as caregiver.
- The nurse uses critical thinking skills to take data collected and use it to develop a plan to meet the desired outcomes for the maternity and neonatal patient.
- The nursing process is essential in the problem-solving process necessary to plan nursing care. The five steps of the nursing process include assessment, nursing diagnosis, outcome identification and planning, implementation, and evaluation.
- Accurate and timely documentation is essential for providing a legal record of care given. This is particularly important to the maternity and neonatal nurse because legal action can occur many years after an event.

REFERENCES AND SELECTED READINGS

Books and Journals

Avery, G. B. (1999). Neonatology: Perspective at the end of the twentieth century. In G. B Avery, M. A. Fletcher, & M. G. MacDonald (Eds.), *Neonatology: Pathophysiology & management of the newborn* (5th ed., pp. 3–7). Philadelphia: Lippincott Williams & Wilkins.

Butz, A. M., Pulsifer, M., Marano, N., Belcher H., Lears, M. K., & Royall, R. (2001). Effectiveness of a home intervention for perceived child behavioral problems and parenting stress in children with in utero drug exposure. *Archives of Pediatrics & Adolescent Medicine, 155*(9), 1029–1037.

Carr, I. (Undated). Dying to have a baby: The history of childbirth. Retrieved February 24, 2002, from http://www.umanitoba.ca/outreach/manitoba_womens_health/hist1.htm

Centers for Disease Control. (1999). Healthier mothers and babies. *MMWR: Morbidity and Mortality Weekly Report, 48*(38), 849-856. Retrieved March 3, 2002, from http://www.cdc.gov/mmwr/PDF/wk/mm4838.pdf

Centers for Disease Control. (1998). Maternal mortality—United States, 1982–1996. *MMWR: Morbidity and Mortality Weekly Report, 47*(34), 705–707. Retrieved March 3, 2002, from http://www.cdc.gov/mmwr/PDF/wk/mm4734.pdf

Corrarino, J. E., Williams, C., Campbell, W. S., Amrhein, E., LoPiano, L., & Kalachik, D. (2000). Linking substance-abusing pregnant women to drug treatment services: A pilot program. *Journal of Obstetric, Gynecologic, and Neonatal Nursing (JOGNN), 29*(4), 369–376.

Cunningham, F. G., Gant, N. F., Leveno, K. J., Gilstrap III, L. C., Hauth, J. C., & Wenstrom, K. D. (2001). *Williams obstetrics* (21st ed.). New York: McGraw-Hill Medical Publishing Division.

Eckenrode, J., Ganzel, B., Henderson, C. R., Smith, E., Olds, D. L., Powers, J., et al. (2000). Preventing child abuse and neglect with a program of nurse home visitation: The limiting effects of domestic violence [Abstract]. *The Journal of the American Medical Association (JAMA), 284*(11), 1385–1391.

Encyclopedia Britannica Article. (Undated). Pasteur, Louis. Retrieved February 24, 2002, from http://www.britannica.com/eb/article?idxref=55613

Encyclopedia Britannica Article. (Undated). Semmelweis, Ignaz Philipp. Retrieved February 24, 2002 from http://www.britannica.com/eb/article?eu=68445&tocid=0&query=%22puerperal%20fever%22

Health Care Financing Administration. (Undated). Overview of the Medicaid Program. Retrieved March 13, 2002, from http://www.hcfa.gov/medicaid/mover.htm

Healthy People Consortium. (2000). *Healthy people 2000 fact sheet*. Retrieved June 30, 2002, from http://odphp.osophs.dhhs.gov/pubs/hp2000/hp2kfact.htm

Kitzman, H., Olds, D. L., Sidora, K., Henderson, C. R., Hanks, C., Cole, R., et al. (2000). Enduring effects of nurse home visitation on maternal life course: A 3-year follow-up of a randomized trial. *The Journal of the American Medical Association (JAMA), 283*(15), 1983–1989.

Koniak-Griffin, D., Mathenge, C., Anderson, N. L., & Verzemnieks, I. (1999). An early intervention program for adolescent mothers: A nursing demonstration project. *Journal of Obstetric, Gynecologic, and Neonatal Nursing (JOGNN / NAACOG), 28*(1), 51–59. (Abstract).

Lieu, T. A., Braveman, P. A., Escobar, G. J., Fischer, A. F., Jensvold, N. G., & Capra, A. M. (2000). A randomized comparison of home and clinic follow-up visits after early postpartum hospital discharge. *Pediatrics 105*(5), 1058–65.

Morrell, C. J., Spiby, H., Stewart, P., Walters, S., & Morgan, A. (2000). Costs and benefits of community postnatal support workers: A randomized controlled trial. *Health Technology Assessment 4*(6), 1–100.

National Association of State Budget Officers. (Undated). *Medicaid*. Retrieved March 13, 2002, from http://www.nasbo.org/Policy_Resources/Medicaid/medicaid.htm

Olds, D. L., Eckenrode, J., Henderson, C. R., Kitzman, H., Powers, J., Cole, R., et al. (1997). Long-term effects of home visitation on maternal life course and child abuse and neglect: Fifteen-year follow-up of a randomized trial.

The Journal of the American Medical Association (JAMA), 278(8), 637-643.

University of Pennsylvania Health System. (Undated). *A century of obstetrics*. Retrieved January 20, 2002, from http://www.obgyn.upenn.edu/History/clinobhis.html

University of Toronto. (Undated). Neonatology—history. Retrieved September 11, 2004, from http://www.utoronto.ca/paedadm/division/neon/history.html

The World Factbook. (2002). Infant mortality rate. Retrieved July 13, 2003, from http://www.bartleby.com/151/a28.html

Wertz, R. W., & Wertz, D. C. (1989). *Lying-in: A history of childbirth in America, expanded edition*. Yale University Press: New Haven & London.

Websites

www.health.gov/healthypeople

www.dhhs.gov

http://www.fns.usda.gov/wic/AboutWIC.htm

WORKBOOK

NCLEX-STYLE REVIEW QUESTIONS

1. Preventing and treating infections during childbirth have reduced maternal and perinatal mortality rates. Of the following, which scientific advancement has done the *most* to improve neonatal mortality statistics?
   a. Control of puerperal fever
   b. Use of anesthesia during labor
   c. Enforcement of strict rules in hospitals
   d. Treatment advances for preterm infants
2. The nursing process is a scientific method and proven form of which process?
   a. Cost containment
   b. Problem solving
   c. Oral communication
   d. Health teaching
3. The nurse collects data and begins to develop a trust relationship with the patient in which step of the nursing process?
   a. Assessment
   b. Planning
   c. Implementation
   d. Evaluation
4. The nurse carries out the nursing care for the patient in which step of the nursing process?
   a. Assessment
   b. Planning
   c. Implementation
   d. Evaluation

STUDY ACTIVITIES

1. Choose the three social issues you think have the highest impact on health care concerns of women and infants. Using these issues, complete the following table.

	How Does This Issue Affect Women's and Infants' Health Care?	What Is the Nurse's Role in Dealing With This Issue?
Social issue		
Social issue		
Social issue		

2. Go to the following Internet site: http://web.health.gov/healthypeople/. At "Healthy People—Leading Health Indicators," click on "What are the Leading Health Indicators?"
   a. Make a list of the leading health indicators.
   b. Hit the back arrow and return to "Leading Health Indicators." Click on "Resources for Individual Action." What is a resource site you could share with a family caregiver regarding health care access?
   c. What is a resource site you could share with someone needing information on injury or violence?

CRITICAL THINKING: What Would You Do?

1. A new mother tells you that her husband makes a few dollars an hour over the minimum wage, so her new baby is not eligible for Medicaid. She sighs and wonders aloud how she is going to pay for the medical bills. What would you say to the new mother? Does she have any options? If so, what are they?
2. While working, you overhear an older nurse complaining about family caregivers "being underfoot so much and interfering with care of the newborn." Describe how you would defend open visiting for family caregivers to this person.

Family-Centered and Community-Based Maternal and Newborn Nursing

2

STUDENT OBJECTIVES

On completion of this chapter, the student should be able to

1. Identify the primary purpose of the family in society.
2. Discuss the functions of the family.
3. Discuss the types of family structure.
4. List four factors that have contributed to the growing number of single-parent families.
5. Describe how children are affected by family size and sibling order.
6. Explain the trend for families to spend less time together.
7. Identify the focus of community-based health care.
8. Describe advantages of community-based health care for the pregnant woman, child, and family.
9. Differentiate between primary, secondary, and tertiary prevention and give one example of each.
10. List the skills needed by a community health nurse.
11. Explain the information a nurse needs to successfully teach a group of individuals.

KEY TERMS

blended family
case management
client advocacy
cohabitation family
communal family
community-based nursing
cultural competency
extended family
nuclear family
primary prevention
secondary prevention
single-parent family
socialization
stepfamily
tertiary prevention

Each person is a member of a family and a member of many social groups, such as church, school, and work. Families and social groups together make up the fabric of the larger society. It is within the context of the family and the community that an individual presents herself to receive health care. It is critical for maternity and newborn nurses to recognize the context of the patient's needs within the patient's family and community.

THE FAMILY AS A SOCIAL UNIT

The arrival of a baby alters forever the primary social unit—a family—in which all members influence and are influenced by each other. Each subsequent child joining that family continues the process of reshaping the individual members and the family unit. In addition, the community affects family members as individuals and as a family unit.

Nursing care of women and newborns demands a solid understanding of normal patterns of growth and development—physical, psychological, social, and intellectual (cognitive)—and an awareness of the many factors that influence those patterns. It also demands an appreciation for the uniqueness of each individual and each family. For nursing care to be complete and as effective as possible, the identified patient must be considered as a member of a family and a larger community.

Throughout history, family structure has evolved in response to ongoing social and economic changes. Today's families may only faintly resemble the nuclear families of 30 or 40 years ago, in which the father worked outside the home and the mother cared for the children at home. It is estimated that in 60% to 70% of today's families with school-age children, only one parent lives at home. More than 50% of American women with a child younger than age 1 year work outside the home. Changes such as these create bigger demands on parents and have contributed to the growing demands on public institutions to fill the gaps. "Blended" families or stepfamilies have created other major changes in family structure and interactions within the family. Divorce, abandonment, and delayed childbearing are all contributing factors.

Family Function

The family is civilization's oldest and most basic social unit. The family's primary purpose is to ensure survival of the unit and its individual members and to continue the society and its knowledge, customs, values, and beliefs. It establishes a primary connection with a group responsible for a person until that person becomes independent.

Although family structure varies among different cultures, its functions are similar. The family's functions in relation to society are twofold: to reproduce and socialize offspring. For each family member the family functions to provide sustenance and support in the five areas of wholeness: physical, emotional, intellectual, social, and spiritual.

Physical Sustenance

The family is responsible for meeting each member's basic needs for food, clothing, shelter, and protection from harm, including illness. The family determines which needs have priority and what resources will be used to meet those needs. Sometimes families need help obtaining the proper resources. For instance, a pregnant woman's nutritional needs might be partially fulfilled through a community program. Some families need help learning to set priorities. For example, very young parents may benefit from parenting classes to help them set priorities for infant and child care.

The work necessary to meet the family's needs was once clearly divided between mother and father, with the mother providing total care for the children and the father providing the resources to make care possible. These attitudes have changed so that in a two-parent family, each parent has an opportunity to share in the joys and trials of child care and other aspects of family living. In the **single-parent family,** one person must assume all these responsibilities.

Don't be quick to judge! Sometimes it is difficult to remember how many responsibilities a single parent has. You may be able to help the parent find a Big Brother or Big Sister program in your community. In these programs an older teen or young adult "adopts" a child and provides special social opportunities for him. For instance, the Big Brother may take the child to a ball game.

Emotional Support

The process of parental attachment to a child begins before birth and continues throughout life. This process is enhanced when early interaction is encouraged between the new parents and the newborn.

Research studies continue to support the importance of early parent–child relationships to emotional adjustment in later life. As little as a few hours may constitute a critical period in the emotional bond between parent and child. Although specific results of these studies are controversial, it is generally agreed that young children are highly sensitive to psychological influences, and those influences may have long-range positive or negative effects.

Within the family, children learn who they are and how their behavior affects other family members.

Children observe and imitate the behavior of family members, learning quickly which behaviors are rewarded and which are punished. Participation in a family is a child's primary rehearsal for parenthood. How parents treat the child has a powerful influence on how the child will treat future children. Studies show that many abusive parents were abused by their parents as children.

Intellectual Stimulation

Many experts suggest that parents read to their unborn children and play music to provide early stimulation. It is unknown when the fetus can actually hear, but it is clear that the newborn recognizes and is comforted by his parents' voices.

The need for intellectual development continues throughout life. The small infant needs to have input through his five senses to develop optimally. Many parents buy brightly colored toys and play frequently with their infants to facilitate this stimulation. Talking and reading to the infant and small child is another way parents fulfill this function.

Socialization

Within the family, a child learns the rules of the society and the culture in which the family lives: its language, values, ethics, and acceptable behaviors. This process, called **socialization,** is accomplished by training, education, and role modeling. The family teaches children acceptable ways of meeting physical needs, such as eating and elimination, and certain skills, such as dressing oneself. The family educates children about relationships with other people inside and outside the family. Children learn what is permitted and approved within their society and what is forbidden.

Each family determines how goals are to be accomplished based on its principles and values. Family patterns of communication, methods of conflict resolution, coping strategies, and disciplinary methods develop over time and contribute to a family's sense of order.

Spirituality

Spirituality addresses meaning in life. The values and principles of each family are based in large part upon its spiritual foundation. Although spirituality may be expressed through religion, this is not the only way it is defined. Cultivating in children an appreciation for the arts (literature, music, theater, dance, and visual art) gives them the basis from which to begin their own spiritual journey.

Family Structure

Various traditional and nontraditional family structures exist. The traditional structures that occur in many cultures are the nuclear family and the extended family. Nontraditional variations include the single-parent family, the communal family, the stepfamily, and the gay or lesbian family.The adoptive family can be either a traditional or a nontraditional structure.

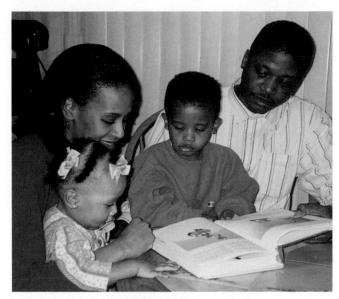

● ***Figure 2.1*** The nuclear family is an important and prominent type of family structure in American society. This nuclear family enjoys reading together.

Nuclear Family

The **nuclear family** is composed of a man, a woman, and their children (either biological or adopted) who share a common household (Fig. 2-1). This was once the typical American family structure; now fewer than one-third of families in the United States fit this pattern. The nuclear family is a more mobile and independent unit than an extended family but is often part of a network of related nuclear families within close geographic proximity.

Extended Family

Typical of agricultural societies, the **extended family** consists of one or more nuclear families plus other relatives, often crossing generations to include grandparents, aunts, uncles, and cousins. The needs of indiviual members are subordinate to the needs of the group, and children are considered an economic asset. Grandparents aid in child rearing, and children learn respect for their elders by observing their parents' behavior toward the older generation.

Here's an important tip. In some cultures the extended family continues to play an important role in everyday life. It may be challenging, but when the extended family comes to visit the new mother and newborn, it is important to work with them to accommodate their needs.

A PERSONAL GLIMPSE

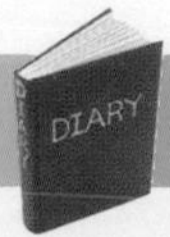

Living with both my mother and grandmother definitely has its advantages. Even though I had a male figure around me while I was growing up, it wasn't really the same as having a father who would always be there. I lived with my aunt and her family along with my mother and my grandmother. I had my uncle or cousin to turn to if I needed advice that my mother or my grandmother couldn't give me. However, my uncle wasn't always around, neither was my cousin, so a lot of my questions were left unanswered. Questions that I didn't think anybody else other than a man could answer. I learned a lot of things on my own, whether it was by experience or by asking somebody else.

Things are different now. It's only my mother, my grandmother, and myself. As I grow older, I'm finding that I can open up to the both of them a lot more. There is no reason to keep secrets. I can tell them anything and they understand. Actually they are a lot more understanding than I thought they would be about certain things. Every day I'm realizing that I can tell them anything.

People often ask me what it is like not knowing about my father. They ask me if I'm curious about my father. And I say, "Of course I'm curious. Who wouldn't be?" I also tell them that love is a lot stronger than curiosity. I love and care about my mother and grandmother more than anything in this world. No one father could ever give me as much love and devotion as the two of them give me. And I wouldn't give that up for anything.

Juan, age 15 years

LEARNING OPPORTUNITY: Where would you direct this mother in your community to go to find opportunities for her son to interact with male adults who could be positive role models for him? What are the reasons it would be important for this child to have appropriate adult male role models? If someone other than the biological parent has raised a child, What are some of the reasons these individuals seek their biological parents?

Single-Parent Family

Rising divorce rates, the women's movement, increasing acceptance of children born out of wedlock, and changes in adoption laws reflecting a more liberal attitude toward adoption have combined to produce a growing number of single-parent families. About 23% of households in the United States are included in this category, and most are headed by women (United States Bureau of Census, 2000). Although this family situation places a heavy burden on the parent, no conclusive evidence is available to show its effects on children. At some time in their lives, more than 50% of children in the United States may be part of a single-parent family.

Communal Family

During the early 1960s, increasing numbers of young adults began to challenge the values and traditions of the American social system. One result of that challenge was the establishing of communal groups and collectives, or **communal families.** This alternative structure occurs in many settings and may favor either a primitive or a modern lifestyle. Members of a communal family share responsibility for homemaking and child rearing; all children are the collective responsibility of adult members. Not actually a new family structure, the communal family is a variation of the extended family. The number of communal family units has decreased in recent years.

Gay or Lesbian Family

In the gay or lesbian family, two people of the same sex live together, bound by formal or informal commitment, with or without children. Children may be the result of a prior heterosexual mating or a product of the foster-child system, adoption, artifcial insemination, or surrogacy. Although these families often face complex issues, including discrimination, studies of children in such families show that they are not harmed by membership in this type of family (Gottman, 1990).

Did you know? The children of a gay or lesbian family are no more likely to become homosexual than are children of heterosexual families.

Stepfamily or Blended Family

The **stepfamily** is made up of the custodial parent and children and a new spouse. As the divorce rate has climbed, the number of stepfamilies has increased. If both partners in the marriage bring children from a previous marriage into the household, the family is usually termed a **blended family.** The stress that remarriage of the custodial parent places on a child seems to depend in part on the child's age. Initially there is an increase in the number of problems in children of all ages. However, younger children apparently can form an attachment to the new parent and accept that person in the parenting role better than can adolescents. Adolescents, already engaged in searching for identity and exploring their own sexuality, may view the presence of a nonbiological parent as an intrusion. When children from each partner's former marriage are brought into the family, the incidence of problems increases. Second marriages often produce children of that union, which contributes to the adjustment problems of the family members. However, remarriage may provide the stability of a two-parent family, which may offer additional resources for the child. Each family is unique and has its own set of challenges and advantages.

Cohabitation Family

In the nuclear family, the parents are married; in the **cohabitation family,** couples live together but are not married. The children in this family may be children of earlier unions, or they may be a result of this union. These families may be long lasting, and the cohabitating couple may eventually marry, but sometimes such families are less stable because the relationships may be temporary. In any family situation with frequent changes in the adult relationships, children may feel a sense of insecurity.

Adoptive Family

The adoptive family, whether a traditional or nontraditional family structure, falls into a category of its own. The parents, child, and siblings in the adoptive family all have challenges that differ from other family structures. A variety of methods of adoption are available, including the use of agencies, international sources, and private adoptions. Paperwork, interviews, home visits, long periods of waiting, and often large sums of money all contribute to the potential stress and anxiety a family who decides to adopt a child goes through. Sometimes adopted children have health, developmental, or emotional concerns. Many have been in a series of foster homes or have come from abusive situations. The family who adopts a child of another culture may have to deal with the prejudices of friends and family. These factors add to the challenges the adoptive family faces.

Some research shows that "open adoption," in which the identity of the birth and adoptive parents is not kept a secret, is less traumatic for the birth mother, child, and adoptive family. Legal issues must be worked out in advance to decrease the painful situations that can occur if a birth mother changes her mind about giving up her child for adoption.

The newly adopted child should be given a complete physical examination soon after the adoption. Basic information regarding the child's health, growth, and development is obtained so any problems or concerns can be discussed with the adoptive family. The feelings of the parents as well as the siblings need to be explored and support given. Throughout childhood and into adulthood adopted children often continue to have questions and need emotional support from health care personnel.

Test Yourself

- Name the two main purposes of the family in relation to society.
- What are the five areas of wholeness?
- What are the two traditional family structures?

Family Factors That Influence Childbearing and Child Rearing

Family Size

The number of children in the family has a significant impact on family interactions. The smaller the family, the more time there is for individual attention to each child. Children in small families, particularly only children, often spend more time with adults and, therefore, relate better with adults than with peers. Only children tend to be more advanced in language development and intellectual achievement.

Understandably a large family emphasizes the group more than the child. Less time is available for parental attention to each child. There is greater interdependence among these children and less dependence on the parents (Fig. 2-2).

Sibling Order and Gender

Whether a child is the firstborn, a middle child, or the youngest also makes a difference in the child's relationships and behavior. Firstborn children command a great deal of attention from parents and grandparents

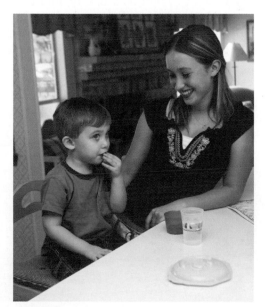

● ***Figure 2.2*** Children from large families learn to care for one another. Many older children are expected to help with homework and prepare after-school snacks. Photo by Joe Mitchell.

and also are affected by their parents' inexperience, anxieties, and uncertainties. Often the parents' expectations for the oldest child are greater than for subsequent children. Generally firstborn children are greater achievers than their siblings.

With second and subsequent children, parents tend to be more relaxed and permissive. These children are likely to be more relaxed and are slower to develop language skills. They often identify more with peers than with parents.

Sexual identity in relation to siblings also affects a child's development. Girls raised with older brothers tend to have more male-associated interests than do girls raised with older sisters. Boys raised with older brothers tend to be more aggressive than are boys with older sisters (Craig, 1992).

Parental Behavior

Many factors have contributed to the change in the traditional mother-at-home, father-at-work image of the American family (Fig. 2-3). Sixty-five percent of American mothers of children younger than age 18 years work outside the home. Some mothers work because they are the family's only source of income, others because the family's economic status demands a second income, and still others because the woman's career is highly valued. More than half of all children between ages 3 and 5 years spend part of their day being cared for by someone other than their parents.

Many factors contribute to the trend for families to spend less time together. Both parents may work; the children participate in many school activities; family members watch television, rather than talking together at mealtime, or eat fast food or individual meals without sitting down together as a family; and there is an emphasis on the acquisition of material goods, rather than the development of relationships. All these factors contribute to a breakdown in family communication, and they are typical of many families. Their impact on today's children, the parents of tomorrow, is unknown.

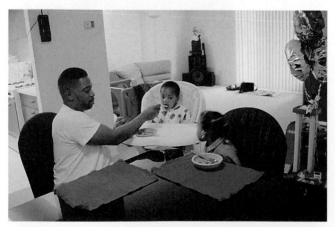

● ***Figure 2.3*** In some American families, traditional roles are being reversed. The father cares for the children while the mother is at work.

Divorce

From 1970 to 1990, the number of divorces increased every year. Although there has been a slight decrease in this number in recent years, more than 1 million children younger than age 18 years have been involved in a divorce each year. Although obviously these children are affected, it is difficult to determine the exact extent of the damage. Children whose lives were seriously disrupted before a divorce may feel relieved, at least initially, when the situation is resolved. Others who were unaware of parental conflict and felt that their lives were happy may feel frightened and abandoned. All these emotions depend on the children involved, their ages, and the kind of care and relationships they experience with their parents after the divorce.

Children may go through many emotions when a divorce occurs. Feelings of grief, anger, rejection, and self-worthlessness are common. These emotions may follow the children for years, even into adulthood, even though children may understand the reason for the divorce. In addition, the parents, either custodial or noncustodial, may try to influence the child's thinking about the other parent, placing the child in an emotional trap. If the noncustodial parent does not keep in regular contact with the child, feelings of rejection may be overwhelming. The child often desperately wants a sign of that parent's continuing love.

Culture

Each person is the product of a family, a culture, and a community. In some cultures, family life is gentle, permissive, and loving; in others, unquestioning obedience is demanded of children, and pain and hardship are to be endured stoically. The child may be from a cultural group that places a high value on children, giving them lots of attention from many relatives and friends, or the child may be from a group that has taught the child from early childhood to fend for oneself (Fig. 2-4).

The timing and number of children desired by the childbearing family are culturally influenced. Values and beliefs about birth control, abortion, and sexual practices influence the choices individuals and couples make about childbearing.

Culture also determines the family's health beliefs and practices. Respect for a person's cultural heritage and individuality is an essential part of nursing care. To plan culturally appropriate and acceptable care, nurses need to understand the health practices and lifestyle of families from various cultures. Rather than memorizing a list of generalized facts regarding different cultures, it is more useful for the nurse to develop

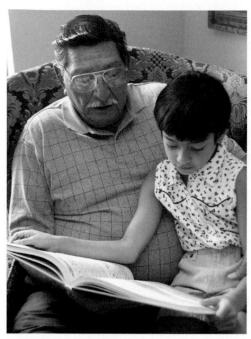

● *Figure 2.4* Many cultural preferences are seen in families. In some cultures, extended family members such as grandparents participate in raising children. Photo by Joe Mitchell.

cultural competency, the capacity to work effectively with people by integrating the elements of their culture into nursing care (Snow, 1996). To develop cultural competency, the nurse must first understand cultural influences on his or her life. The nurse must recognize surface cultural influences (e.g., language, food, clothing), as well as hidden cultural influences (e.g., communication styles, beliefs, attitudes, values, perceptions). Then the nurse may recognize and accept the different attitudes, behaviors, and values of another person's culture.

Integrating cultural attitudes toward food, cleanliness, respect, and freedom are of utmost importance. The nurse must be especially sensitive to the fears of the woman who is separated from her own culture during child birth and finds the food, language, people, and surroundings of the health care facility totally alien. Cultural competency promotes cooperation from the woman and family and minimizes frustration.

Test Yourself

- Name one way that family size affects a child's development.
- What are two factors that contribute to American families spending less time together?
- Define cultural competency.

HEALTH CARE SHIFT: FROM HOSPITAL TO COMMUNITY

In the last century, health care has gone through a number of changes. The sophisticated health care currently available is extremely expensive and has strained health care funding to a point where other health care approaches have become necessary. This need for change has led to the emergence of community-based health care and an emphasis on wellness and preventive health care.

The shift to community-based health care has impacted normal and at-risk maternity care. Many women with limited resources choose to obtain prenatal care from local health department clinics. A pregnant woman who develops complications can sometimes receive care at home with the assistance of a nurse case manager who helps to coordinate her care. This allows the woman to receive high quality care at a lower cost than if she were to require hospitalization. Community-based programs such as Women, Infants, and Children (WIC) provide nutritional screening and assistance for the low-income pregnant woman and her small children.

Community-Based Nursing

Community-based nursing focuses on prevention and is directed toward persons and families within a community. The goals are to help persons meet their health care needs and to maintain continuity of care as they move through the various health care settings available to them.

The role of the nurse who works in the community is different from that of the hospital nurse. Generally the nurse in the community focuses on **primary prevention**, health promoting activities that help prevent the development of illness or injury. This level of prevention includes teaching regarding safety, diet, rest, exercise, and disease prevention through immunizations and emphasizes the nursing role of teacher and client advocate. An example of primary prevention is a nurse in a maternity clinic giving teaching tips on proper nutrition during pregnancy.

In some community settings, the nurse's role focuses on **secondary prevention**, health screening activities that aid in early diagnosis and encourage prompt treatment before long-term negative effects are realized. Such settings are clinics, home care nursing, and schools. The nurse participates in screening measures such as height, weight, hearing, and vision. During client assessments and follow-up, the nurse compiles a health history and collects data, including vital signs, blood work, and other diagnostic tests as ordered by the health care practitioner. One example of secondary prevention is a community clinic nurse's identification of a pregnant adolescent who is gaining insufficient weight and is possibly anemic. The nurse works with the family caregiver to review the family's dietary habits and nutritional state. This would help determine if the problem is limited to the pregnant adolescent or if other family members are also malnourished and if there is lack of knowledge or inadequate means. After finding these answers, the nurse can help the family caregiver provide better nutrition for the family and focus on nutritional issues unique to the pregnant adolescent.

Tertiary prevention, health-promoting activities that focus on rehabilitation and teaching to prevent further injury or illness, occurs in special settings. For example, the at-risk infant might be helped through special intervention programs, group homes, or selected outpatient settings focusing on rehabilitation, such as an orthopedic clinic.

Such a broad selection of settings and roles places the nurse in a remarkable situation. Pregnant women and infants are seen in settings familiar to them—homes, schools, or community centers. Although involved in direct care, the nurse in the community spends a great part of his or her time as a communicator, teacher, administrator, and manager.

Community Care Settings for the Maternity Client

Prenatal and Postpartum Home Health Care

Nurses often made home visits in the early days of public health nursing. Through the years, it gradually became expected that patients would come to clinics and offices for care. Recently, in an effort to meet the challenges of cost-containment and poor access to care, some organizations and researchers have reinstituted home visits by nurses.

Current evidence shows that low-risk mothers and infants do not have better health outcomes when nurses or specially trained workers go to the home for follow-up social support and care, but the mothers report being happier with the care that they receive (Lieu et al., 2000; Morrell, Spiby, Stewart, Walters, & Morgan, 2000). The most positive results occur when nurses make in-home visits to at-risk populations, such as adolescent and poverty-stricken mothers.

When at-risk women are assessed and receive intervention from nurses in their homes during pregnancy and the postpartum period, some researchers have found both short- and long-term positive effects. In general these positive effects include a lower incidence of child abuse and neglect, longer periods of time between pregnancies, fewer overall pregnancies, less dependence on welfare, and fewer reports of criminal behavior and drug and alcohol abuse (Corrarino et al., 2000; Eckenrode et al., 2000; Kitzman et al., 2000; Olds et al., 1997). Some researchers have also found decreased incidence of preterm births and fewer infant hospitalization days when at-risk mothers receive planned nursing intervention, which includes home visits during pregnancy (Koniak-Griffin, Mathenge, Anderson, & Verzemnieks, 1999).

Settings for Birth

Choosing the setting in which to give birth has been guided by cultural beliefs, political beliefs, and personal preferences throughout the years. For example, on the United States western frontier during the mid- and late-1800s, women gave birth in their homes, attended by female family members or female neighbors. These women cared for the older children, helped with chores, and stayed with the new mother during the early postpartum period, when possible. Today, in most parts of the world, the choices of birth settings are primarily home, birthing centers, and hospitals (Fig. 2-5).

Home. In the early 20th century, home births were the norm before the availability of anesthesia and pain medication in the hospital setting. Today home births occur rarely. A woman may choose to deliver at home for a variety of reasons. She may desire a more comfortable setting, more control over birthing conditions and positions, or to prevent nonmedically indicated interventions. In addition, a woman may prefer to give birth at home so that she can take care of her healthy newborn, rather than experiencing periods of separation while her baby is cared for in a hospital nursery.

Midwives usually attend births at home; physicians rarely do. Some are lay midwives, often trained through apprenticeships with experienced lay midwives. Others are formally trained certified nurse midwives (CNMs) who practice independently in home settings and clinics with physician backup for consultation and referral. Laws in individual states regulate the practice of midwifery.

The safety of giving birth at home is debated. According to Ackerman-Liebrich, et al. (1996), "healthy low-risk women who wish to deliver at home have no increased risk either to themselves or to their babies." In a study of outcomes of 11,788 planned home births attended by CNMs (Anderson & Murphy, 1995), the researchers concluded that home birth can be an acceptable delivery option for low-risk women, if it is planned and attended by "qualified care providers." A newer study (Janssen et al., 2002) evaluating the safety of home births attended by trained midwives concludes that there are no increased risks with home births; however, the results of this

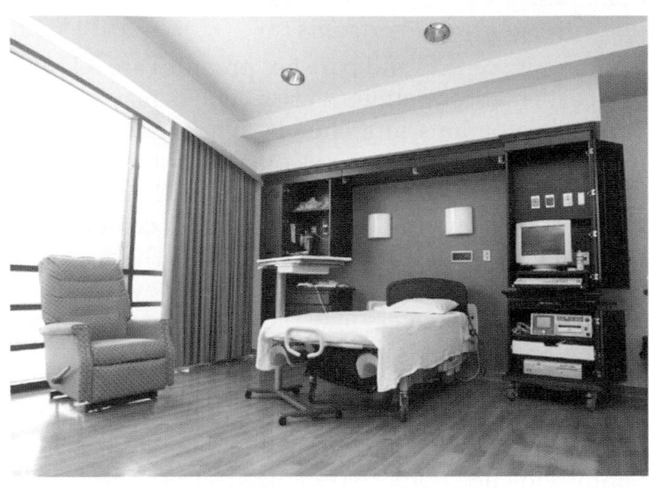

A

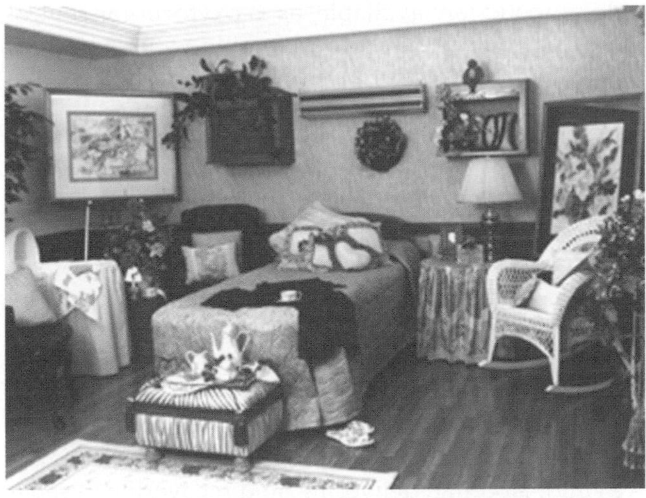

B

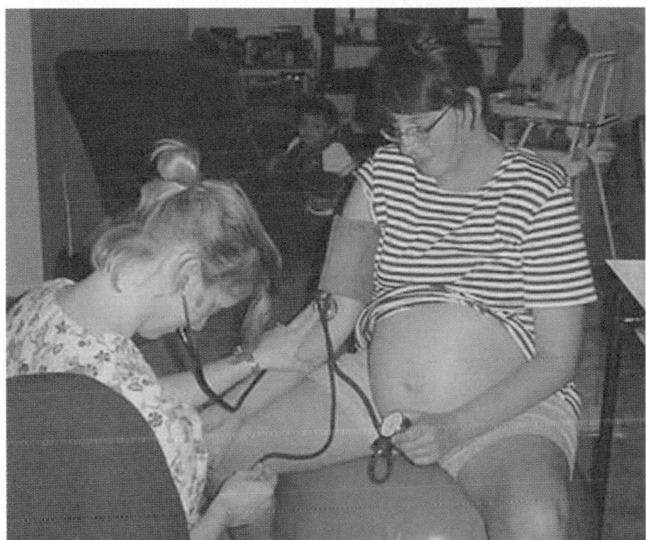

C

● ***Figure 2.5*** (Birth setting collage). There are many different settings in which a woman can choose to give birth. These decisions are influenced by preferences regarding methods of pain control and general beliefs about how a birth should be managed. (**A**) Hospital LDRP (**B**) Birthing center (**C**) Home setting. Photos by Joe Mitchell.

study have been widely criticized for researcher bias. The American College of Obstetricians and Gynecologists (2002) reports that newborns born at home tend to be at higher risk for very low Apgar scores; there is a strong association between newborn death and nulliparous women attempting to deliver at home; and that planned home births are associated with prolonged labor and postpartum hemorrhage. The latest Cochrane Review pertaining to home versus hospital birth (Olsen & Jewell, 2000) concluded that at present there is insufficient evidence indicating that one setting is superior to the other for low-risk women.

Birthing Centers. Since the early 1980s, birthing centers have increased in popularity and availability in some areas of the United States. The environment is usually comfortable with furnishings and lighting designed to make the laboring woman and her family feel welcome. There often are family areas (e.g., kitchens and sitting rooms) and bathrooms with showers and/or whirlpool tubs. A variety of health care professionals may be employed by a birthing center, including registered nurses (RNs), CNMs, licensed practical nurses (LPNs), and doulas (specialized birth attendants). Medical interventions are rarely done, so physicians are seldom present. However, birthing centers often are affiliated with a variety of obstetricians and pediatricians as consultants.

Only low-risk women are accepted as patients after being screened by the birthing center. Most birthing centers have medical equipment such as intravenous lines, fluids, oxygen, newborn resuscitation equipment, infant warmers, and local anesthesia for repair of tears or infrequently performed episiotomies.

Mild narcotics are available, as is oxytocin for control of postpartum bleeding. If a laboring woman decides she wants an epidural anesthesia, or if she presents with complications determining her to be at risk, she is transported to a hospital.

Hospitals. Childbirth in a hospital setting began to be accepted as the norm by the 1920s. By 1950, the vast majority of births in the United States took place in hospitals. Today, 99% of births in the United States are in hospitals, with 92% attended by medical doctors (MDs). Doctors of osteopathic medicine (DOs) and midwives attend most of the other 8% of births in U.S. hospitals.

Until the 1970s giving birth in a hospital required enduring uncomfortable procedures (e.g., enemas, shaving); laboring, delivering, and recovering in separate rooms; and separation from the newborn until several hours after birth. Patients began to be more consumer oriented in the mid-1970s. They began to "shop around" for more family-centered maternity care, which included more time with their babies and less time moving from room to room. Hospital administrators and physicians began to listen to consumer needs, and hospital policies began to change. As a result, in many hospitals the trend is to promote family-centered maternity care in more home-like settings. Most hospitals today offer combination labor-delivery-recovery rooms (LDRs). The rooms are larger to accommodate family support and to allow health care professionals enough room to attend the birth. In addition, LDRs are aesthetically appealing, with home-like furnishings, wallpaper, softer lighting, and showers in the bathrooms.

Some hospitals have initiated combination labor-delivery-recovery-postpartum rooms (LDRPs), thus further reducing the number of locations to which a woman is moved during her hospital stay. Couplet care, another concept that some hospitals have embraced, places the healthy mother in the same room with her newborn as long as there is no medical indication for them to be separated. One nurse is responsible for the care of both. This practice encourages early bonding and provides time for new parents to learn to care for their newborns before discharge. Parents learn to recognize their newborns' cues and therefore are better prepared to care for their newborns at home.

Test Yourself

- Define primary prevention.
- Give one example of tertiary prevention.
- List three childbirth settings.

Community Centers, Parishes, and Intervention Programs

Community centers and parishes provide care relevant to a particular community. Parish centers may sponsor outreach programs in a church, synagogue, or other religious setting. The services offered by these centers are designed to meet community needs. For example, in areas with many homeless persons, centers may provide basic health care and nutrition. These centers may also provide food, clothing, money, or other resources. Other centers may provide childcare classes for new mothers or young families.

Some communities offer walk-in or residential clinics for special purposes such as teen pregnancy, alcohol and drug abuse, nutritional guidance, and family violence. Other specialized clinics offer programs on HIV/AIDS, cancer, and mental health; provide maternal and well-baby care; and offer day care services for children or the elderly.

Many communities also have services provided by volunteer service organizations such as the Lions, Rotary Club, Shriners, or Kiwanis. Some of these organizations have specific goals. For example, the Shriners sponsor clinics for children with orthopedic problems.

In any community center, there are people who can benefit from the services of health care professionals. Often the health services focus on education and other primary prevention practices. Nurses help design safety, exercise, and nutrition programs; provide basic immunization services; conduct parenting classes; organize crisis intervention programs for youth and teens; and help organize health fairs. The health care staff may be paid or may work on a volunteer basis, or there may be a combination of paid and volunteer staff.

Skills of the Community-Based Nurse

The nursing process serves as the foundation of nursing care in the community, just as it does in a health care facility. Communication with the patient and family is essential. Teaching is a fundamental part of community-based care because of the emphasis on health promotion and preventive health care. Case management is necessary to coordinate care and monitor case progress through the health care system.

The Nursing Process

The focus of the community-based nurse is the patient within the context of the family. In the initial family assessment interview, the nurse determines how various family members affect the pregnant woman or the newborn. The nurse may obtain additional information by picking up on cues in the environment. Upon completion of data collection and assessment, the RN and health care team focus on identifying the nursing diagnoses based on the family's strengths, weaknesses, and needs. Family interaction and cooperation leads to collaborative goal setting and proposed interventions. The ongoing nursing process requires that these interventions be evaluated as the cycle continues.

Communication

Positive, effective communication is fundamental to the nursing process and the care of childbearing families in the community. Establishing rapport with the woman and the family, understanding and appropriately responding to cultural practices, and being sensitive to needs all require good communication skills.

Teaching

Here's an idea. When teaching a group with which you are unfamiliar, ask the group leader for demographic information to help develop an appropriate teaching plan.

Teaching and health education are key components of community-based nursing care. Health care often involves teaching families, small groups of children, family caregivers, members of extended families, and large groups of children, on various topics that focus on primary prevention (Fig. 2-6).

To teach a group successfully, the nurse must know the needs of the target population and have the appropriate teaching skills, strategies, and resources. When the nurse is familiar with the group, he already has important information, such as age, educational level, ethnic and gender mix, language barriers, and any previous teaching the group has had on the subject. The nurse should review growth and developmental principles to identify the appropriate level of information, learning activities, and average attention span. Additional information includes any available teaching resources, group size, seating arrangements, and other advantages or restrictions of the environment. For instance, the nurse may want to find out

- Are the chairs movable for small-group discussions?
- Is there a videocassette recorder to show a video?
- Will a lot of noise disturb others in the building?

A successful group teaching experience relies on a prepared nurse educator.

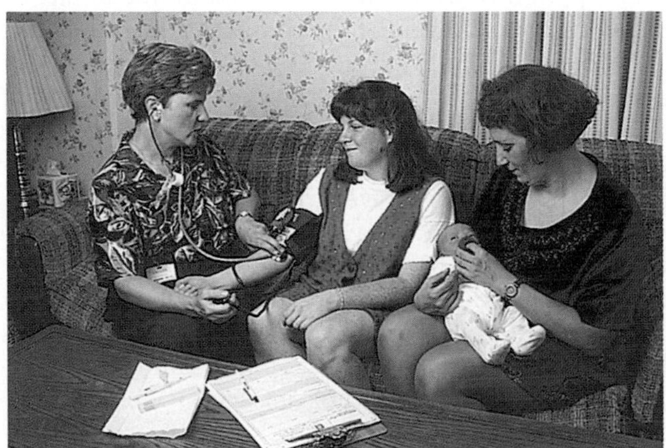

● ***Figure 2.6*** The nurse providing postpartum and newborn care in the home takes the opportunity to provide patient education.

Case Management

Case management, a systematic process that ensures that a client's multiple health and service needs are met, may be a formal or an informal process. In formalized case management, the agency or insurer who pays for the health care services predetermines the contact with the client. In other settings, the nurse may determine the needed follow-up and either provide the services or assist with referrals to obtain services.

If case management is formalized, the insurer pays for nursing services. The case manager's role is clearly outlined with care plans, protocols, and limits to service determined by the insurer. In community agencies where nursing services are part of the overall service (for instance, schools or group homes), the intensity of follow-up is determined by the agency's philosophy, available resources, and the nurse's perception of the role and her individual skills.

Client Advocacy

Client advocacy is speaking or acting on behalf of others to help them gain greater independence and to make the health care delivery system more responsive and relevant to their needs. The nurse working in a community setting may often develop a long-standing relationship with childbearing and child rearing families because of the continuous nature of client contact in an outpatient, school, or other setting. This type of relationship may allow the nurse to discover broader health and welfare issues. Examples of interventions include

- Teaching a family about the services for which the pregnant woman or newborn is eligible.
- Assisting the family to apply for Medicaid or other forms of health care reimbursement.
- Identifying inexpensive or free transportation services to medical appointments.
- Making telephone calls to establish eligibility for and to acquire special equipment for a special needs newborn.

Examples of client advocacy are limitless and include health and social welfare services that intertwine in ways that families cannot manage alone. One example is assistance with referrals and acquisition of needed resources. As a member of a team of health care professionals, the nurse assists with the referral process. This process focuses on the childbearing or child rearing family obtaining the appropriate services and resources. Actions taken are geared toward improving the family's health or quality of life. The nurse must be knowledgeable about community resources, contact persons, details of appropriate applications, and other required documentation.

The Challenge of Community-Based Nursing

There are differences between caring for families in a hospital or clinic and caring for them in community settings. Community-based work requires a different set of skills.

The Unique Aspects of Community-Based Nursing

Community-based nursing practice is autonomous. The nurse must be self-reliant to be successful. There may not be many other health care practitioners with whom to consult; those available may be physically distant. To provide families with high-quality care, the nurse must have well-developed assessment and decision-making skills.

Community practice tends to be more holistic. The individual is viewed as an integrated whole mind, body, and spirit interacting with the environment. The community nurse must consider the effects of the mother's or newborn's health on family functioning, the newborn's developmental progress, and the multiple services the family needs to improve the quality of life.

A final difference is the focus on wellness. Some community settings have a population of at-risk pregnant women and newborns with an illness or diagnosis in common, such as diabetes or prematurity. Working with these groups involves managing the disease or limitations with a wellness focus. For instance, the focus might be on teaching a group of pregnant women with diabetes about diabetic diets.

In most areas where the community nurse works, the focus is on wellness. Women and newborns are basically well but may be going through a growth and developmental crises. The nurse intervenes to ease the transition from one developmental stage to another. The nurse provides anticipatory guidance to family caregivers and emphasizes preventive health practices. Teaching health-promotion practices to pregnant women and their families is another activity of primary importance.

Issues Facing Pregnant Women, Newborns, and Families

Nurses who work in the community encounter the complex issues facing childbearing and child rearing families. Nursing care given to pregnant women, newborns, and families within their own environments allows the nurse to better understand their unique needs.

Poverty is a major issue that affects all aspects of recovery and responses to care. For many families, a lack of resources hinders compliance and takes its toll on the health of all family members. Services and resources may be inaccessible because of cost, location, or lack of transportation. Sometimes family caregivers see such services as unnecessary. Poverty, lack of information, questionable decisions about priorities, and ineffective coping skills affect the health of pregnant women, newborns, and families in significant ways. The results are often seen in emergency departments, neonatal intensive care units (NICUs), and in acute care beds of women's units.

The community nurse must explore these issues with the family caregivers. When a pregnant woman delays prenatal care, what issues surround this behavior? When a family does not follow up with a newborn's appointment for a bilirubin checkup, what factors influenced their decision?

Test Yourself

- Name two settings, other than the hospital, in which a woman can give birth.
- Define client advocacy.
- Name three unique aspects of community-based nursing.

Rewards of Community-Based Nursing

The nurse in community-based settings sees the client over a period of time. This allows the nurse to have a broader understanding of the context within which the individual and family lives. The clinic nurse may see the same family for different problems over a period of many years. A nurse in a home for pregnant teens works with a young mother throughout her pregnancy and takes pleasure in the birth of a healthy baby.

Community nurses work in many ways to prevent unnecessary hospitalization. Examples of health problems that the community nurse seeks to prevent include an infant who fails to thrive because the parents do not know that infants need specific amounts of formula, or a pregnant teen who contracts HIV because she does not practice safe sex.

The community nurse helps families develop the skills and knowledge they need to make decisions that affect their lives and those of other family members. In this way, families can learn and practice preventive health care. With a focus on wellness, the community nurse provides a service that eventually improves the health of the entire community.

KEY POINTS

- The family is the basic social unit. It provides for survival and teaches the knowledge, customs, values, and beliefs of the family's culture.
- The basic functions of the family are to reproduce and socialize children to function within the larger society. To meet the needs of individual members, the family also functions to provide support in the five areas of wholeness: physical, emotional, intellectual, social, and spiritual.
- The nuclear family and the extended family are the two types of traditional family structures that exist in most cultures. The single-parent family, communal family, gay or lesbian family, and cohabitation family are four examples of nontraditional family structures.
- Mobility, changing attitudes about children born out of wedlock and divorce, women working outside the home, and changes in adoption laws all have contributed to an increase in single-parent families.
- Family size affects the child's development. Children from small families receive more individual attention and tend to relate better to adults. Children from large families develop interdependency skills.
- Birth order also influences development. First-born children tend to be high achievers. Subsequent children are often more relaxed and are slower to develop language skills.
- Families tend to spend less time together than in the past for many reasons—both parents may work, the children participate in many school activities, families often do not eat together, and there is an emphasis on acquisition of material goods, rather than the development of relationships.
- Community-based health care focuses on wellness and prevention and is directed toward helping persons and families meet their health care needs.
- Community-based health care is advantageous for the pregnant woman, newborn, and family because it allows the individual to receive care within the context of the community and culture. It also identifies and meets needs within the community, which may allow for less costly care than that provided in a hospital setting.
- Primary prevention focuses on preventing illness and injury. An example is a nurse in a maternity clinic giving teaching tips on proper nutrition during pregnancy.
- Secondary prevention involves health screening activities that aid in early diagnosis and encourage prompt treatment before long-term negative effects are realized.
- Tertiary prevention involves health-promoting activities that focus on rehabilitation and teaching to prevent additional injury or illness. The nurse assists the family to find resources so that proper care and medical monitoring can continue to prevent the development of additional problems.
- The community-based nurse uses the nursing process to plan and provide care to families and groups, communicate effectively and teach individuals and groups, perform case management, and practice client advocacy.
- An effective community nurse educator must identify and assess the target population by determining the age, educational level, ethnic and gender mix, language barriers, and any previous teaching the group may have had. The nurse must assess each audience and gear the teaching appropriately.
- The community nurse functions as an advocate by taking actions geared toward improving the woman's or newborn's health or quality of life.

REFERENCES AND SELECTED READINGS

Books and Journals

Acherman-Liebrich, U., Voegli, T. Gunter-Witt, K., Kunz, I., Zullig, M., et al. (1996). Home versus hospital deliveries: Follow up study of matched pairs for procedures and outcome. Zurich study team. *BMJ: British Medical Journal, 313*(7068), 1313–1318.

Ahmann, E., & Johnson, B. H. (2001). Family matters: New guidance materials promote family-centered change in health care institutions. *Pediatric Nursing, 27*(2), 173–175.

Allender, J. A., & Spradley, B. W. (2000). *Community health nursing* (5th ed.). Philadelphia: Lippincott Williams & Wilkins.

American College of Obstetricians and Gynecologists. (2002, July 31). Home births double risk of newborn death. *ACOG News Release*. Retrieved June 7, 2003, from http://www.acog.org/from_home/publications/press_releases/nr07-31-02-3.cfm

Anderson, R. E., & Murphy, P. A. (1995). Outcomes of 11,788 planned home births attended by certified nurse-midwives: A retrospective descriptive study. *Journal of Nurse Midwifery, 40*(6), 468–473, 483–492.

Clayton, M. (2000). Health and social policy: Influences on family-centered care. *Pediatric Nursing, 12*(8), 31–33.

Corrarino, J. E., Williams, C., Campbell, W. S., Amrhein, E., LoPiano, L., Kalachick, D. (2000). Linking substance-abusing pregnant women to drug treatment services: A pilot program. *JOGNN: Journal of Obstetric, Gynecologic, and Neonatal Nursing, 29*(4), 369–376.

Craig, G. (1992). *Human development* (6th ed.). Englewood Cliffs, NJ: Prentice-Hall.

Eckenrode, J., Ganzel, B., Henderson, C. R., Smith, E., Olds, D. L., Powers, J., et al. (2000). Preventing child abuse and neglect with a program of nurse home visitation: The limiting effects of domestic violence. *The Journal of the American Medical Association (JAMA), 284*(11), 1385–1391.

Fuller, Q. (2000). Cultural competence in pediatric nursing. *Nursing Spectrum*. Available at: http://community.nursingspectrum.com/MagazineArticles.

Gottman, J. (1990). Children of gay and lesbian parents. In F. W. Bozett, M. Sussman (Eds.), *Homosexuality and family relations*. New York: Harrington Park.

Hunt, R. (2001). *Introduction to community-based nursing* (2nd ed.). Philadelphia: Lippincott Williams & Wilkins.

Janssen, P. A., Lee, S. K., Ryan, E. M., Etches, D. J., Farquharson, D. F., Peacock, D., Klein, M. C. (2002). *CMAJ: Canadian Medical Association Journal, 166*(3), 315.

Kitzman, H., Olds, D. L., Sidora, K., Henderson, C. R., Hanks, C., Cole, R., et al. (2000). Enduring effects of nurse home visitation on maternal life course: A 3-year follow-up of a randomized trial. *The Journal of the American Medical Association (JAMA), 283*(15), 1983–1989.

Koniak-Griffin, D., Mathenge, C., Anderson, N. L., & Verzemnieks, I. (1999). An early intervention program for adolescent mothers: A nursing demonstration project [Abstract]. *Journal of Obstetric, Gynecologic, and Neonatal Nursing (JOGNN), 28*(1), 51–59.

Lieu, T. A., Braveman, P. A., Escobar, G. J., Fischer, A. F., Jensvold, N. G., Capra, A. M. (2000). A randomized comparison of home and clinic follow-up visits after early postpartum hospital discharge. *Pediatrics, 105*(5), 1058.

Monsen, R. B. (2001). Raising kids, grandparents bear a burden. *Journal of Pediatric Nursing, 16*(2), 130–131.

Morrell, C. J., Spiby, H., Stewart, P., Walters, S., & Morgan, A. (2000). Costs and benefits of community postnatal support workers: Randomised controlled trial. *BMJ: British Medical Journal, 321*(7261), 593.

Olds, D. L., Eckenrode, J., Henderson, C. R., Kitzman, H., Powers, J., Cole, R., et al. (1997). Long-term effects of home visitation on maternal life course and child abuse and neglect: Fifteen-year follow-up of a randomized trial [Abstract]. *The Journal of the American Medical Association (JAMA), 278*(8): 637.

Olsen, O., & Jewell, M. D. (2000). Home versus hospital birth. *Cochrane Database of Systematic Reviews*. Retrieved June 1, 2003, from http://www.medscape.com/viewarticle/453976

Patterson, G. J. (1996). Lesbian and gay parenthood. *Handbook of parenting*. Hillsdale, NJ: Lawrence Erlbaum Associates.

Snow, C. (1996). Cultural sensitivity workshop. Philadelphia: Nationality Service Council, United Way.

United States Bureau of Census. (2000). *Statistical abstract of the United States: 2000*. Washington DC: Superintendent of Documents.

Woodring, B. C. (2000). Family matters: If you have taught, have the child and family learned? *Pediatric Nursing, 26*(5), 505–509.

Websites

Cultural Competence—available at www.air.org/cecp/cultural.

Minority Health—available at www.omhrc.gov/omh-home.htm.

Ethnic and Racial Health Disparities—available at http://raceandhealth.hhs.gov

www.health.discovery.com

www.kidshealth.org/kid

www.kinderstart.com

WORKBOOK

NCLEX-STYLE REVIEW QUESTIONS

1. In working with families, the nurse recognizes that different family structures exist. Which of the following examples best describes a blended family? A family in which
   a. the adult members share in homemaking as well as in child rearing.
   b. the partners in the marriage bring children from a previous marriage into the household.
   c. grandparents live in the same house with the grandchildren and their parents.
   d. partners of the same sex share a household and raise children together.
2. The nurse is caring for a Korean woman who is in labor with her first child. Which of the following is the best example of cultural competency? The nurse
   a. asks an Asian colleague to take care of the woman.
   b. bases her nursing care on knowledge she obtained when previously caring for a Korean family.
   c. performs a search on Korean culture on the Internet to determine the type of food to order.
   d. seeks information from a variety of sources and includes the woman and family in planning care.
3. Which of the following is the best example of primary prevention? The nurse
   a. advises a woman who wants to become pregnant to stop smoking.
   b. answers a pregnant woman's questions about birth settings.
   c. assists the family of a premature baby to learn to work with an apnea monitor.
   d. screens a pregnant woman for high blood pressure.
4. A woman expresses an interest in giving birth at home. Which reply by the nurse is best?
   a. "If you deliver at home, you can't have an epidural."
   b. "Studies have shown that it isn't safe to have your baby at home."
   c. "What is it that most interests you about a home birth?"
   d. "Your doctor doesn't deliver in the home setting. Maybe you should reconsider."
5. When a nurse is doing teaching in a community-based setting, it is *most* important for the nurse to
   a. ask questions about the histories of those present.
   b. use posters that everyone in the group can read.
   c. tell the participants about the nurse's background.
   d. know the needs of the audience.

STUDY ACTIVITIES

1. Survey your community to discover the community-based health care providers available. Use the information you found to complete the following table.

Community-Based Health Care Providers	How Are They Funded?	What Types of Health Care for Families Do They Provide?

2. Using the information you obtained above, evaluate your community's health care services by answering the following:
   a. Does your community have adequate health care services for childbearing and child rearing families?
   b. Are funding concerns an issue for your community? In what ways?
   c. What other services do you think are needed to care for the childbearing and child rearing families in your community?
3. Select a community-based setting and outline the services that a nurse in that setting should

ideally provide. Include the resources needed to provide the services.

4. Go to the following Internet site: http://www.culturediversity.org. At "Transcultural Nursing," click on "Cultural Competency."
   a. What is the definition of cultural competence?
   b. What are the five essential elements necessary for an organization to become culturally competent?
   c. What are the four major challenges to attaining cultural competency?

CRITICAL THINKING: What Would You Do?

Apply your knowledge of the family and the nurse's role in the community to the following situations.

1. You are making a home visit to the Andrews family because their newborn needs home phototherapy treatment for 3 to 5 days. You find 6-year-old Samantha ill with bronchitis. Both parents smoke. Outline a teaching plan for these caregivers regarding the health of their family.
2. Mrs. Perez, a high school teacher, asks you to teach a unit on responsible sex.
   a. Identify the information you will need from Mrs. Perez.
   b. Describe how you will present the lesson to these adolescents.

UNIT 2

Foundations of Maternity Nursing

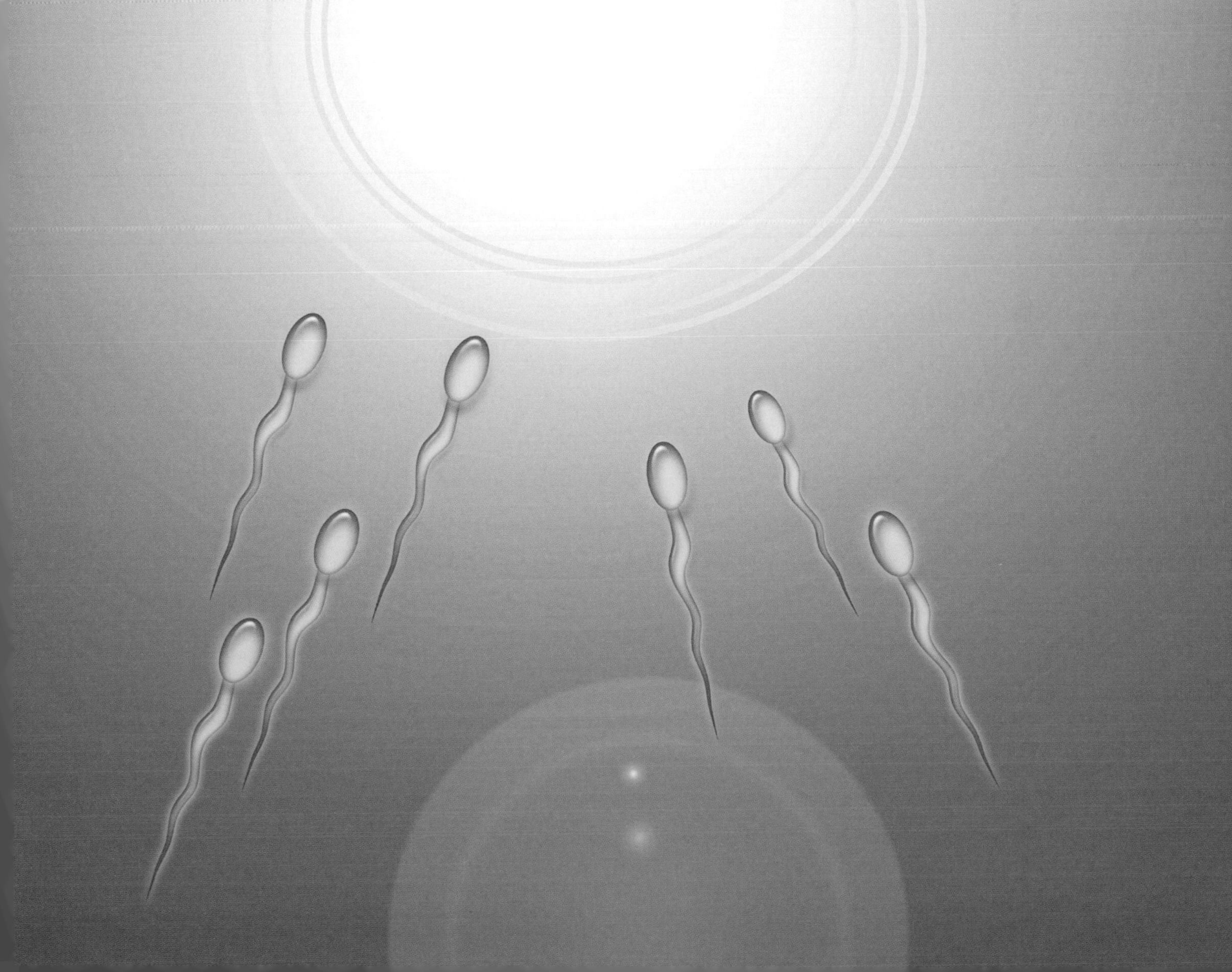

Structure and Function of the Reproductive System

3

STUDENT OBJECTIVES

On completion of this chapter, the student should be able to

1. Explain two major functions of the reproductive system.
2. Label an anatomic drawing of the female and male reproductive systems, including external genitalia and internal anatomy.
3. Discuss major functions of each reproductive structure, gland, and organ.
4. Trace the path of sperm through the male reproductive system, from the site of formation to ejaculation from the body.
5. Describe the process of semen production.
6. Compare hormonal regulation of male reproductive function with that of the female.
7. Illustrate the inter-relationships of the ovarian and uterine cycles and the overall menstrual cycle.
8. Compare the sexual response cycle of the male to that of the female.

KEY TERMS

climacteric
corpus luteum
endometrium
epididymis
gametes
menarche
mons pubis
myometrium
ovulation
prepuce
seminiferous tubules
spermatogenesis
vas deferens
vestibule
vulva

The obstetric nurse is called upon to counsel prospective parents before and throughout pregnancy and childbirth. To accomplish this task, the nurse must have a working knowledge of reproductive anatomy and physiology and the menstrual cycle. This knowledge guides the nurse in choosing appropriate interventions for the childbearing woman and her family.

The main purpose of the male and female reproductive systems is to produce offspring. Male testes produce and female ovaries contain **gametes** or sex cells, spermatozoa (sperm) in the male and ova (eggs) in the female. Each gamete contains one half of the genetic material needed to produce a human baby. However, as you will see some of the structures in the reproductive tract serve dual purposes. Most often these alternate functions have to do with urinary elimination because the urinary system is connected closely with the reproductive system.

You will notice that most structures in the reproductive tract are paired (e.g., testes, ovaries, labia majora, labia minora) and that male and female reproductive systems are complementary; for example, male testes and female ovaries; male scrotum and female labia majora; and male glans penis and female clitoris. It is important to know that the pituitary gland governs reproductive hormone production and function (Fig. 3-1).

MALE REPRODUCTIVE SYSTEM

Sometimes the man's contribution to childbirth is not fully appreciated because of the focus on the pregnant woman and her growing fetus. However, the father's role is crucial to this process. His genetic material not only determines the sex of the unborn child, but also influences numerous other inherited traits. The male reproductive anatomy consists of external reproductive organs and internal reproductive organs. The purpose of the male reproductive tract is to allow for sexual intimacy and reproduction of offspring, and to provide a conduit for urinary elimination.

External Genitalia

The man's external reproductive organs, the external genitalia, consist of the penis and scrotum (Fig. 3-2).

Penis

The penis serves a dual role as the male organ of reproduction and as the external organ of urinary elimination. The penis is composed of a bulbous head, the glans penis or glans, and a shaft. The glans is the most sensitive area on the penis because this is where the greatest concentration of nerve endings is found. This part of the penis is analogous to the clitoris in the female. At birth a layer of tissue, the **prepuce** or foreskin, covers the glans.

Make a note of this. It is the prepuce that is removed in the surgical procedure called circumcision. Some parents choose to have this procedure done within the first few days of their son's life. Others choose to leave their male babies uncircumcised. Circumcision can be performed on adult males, usually for medical reasons; however, this procedure is not often done in adulthood.

The shaft of the penis (Fig. 3-2) is made up of three columns of erectile tissue: the paired cavernous bodies (corpus cavernosa) and the spongy body (corpus spongiosum). The cavernous bodies are parallel, and the spongy body lies atop them in the midline. The spongy body is cradled in the channel created where the cavernous bodies meet. Each column is encased in a thick sheath called the tunica albuginea. Two layers of fascia encircle all three columns along the length of the shaft. The fascia gives the penis support, allowing it to become a firm structure during sexual stimulation.

The erectile tissue is well supplied with blood vessels and nerves. When the penis is stimulated sexually, parasympathetic nerves cause the veins in the shaft to dilate. The sinuses within the erectile tissue fill up with blood causing an erection. The erect penis is capable of penetrating the female vagina for the purposes of sexual fulfillment and intimacy. If the erect penis is stimulated to ejaculation within the vagina, the reproductive function of depositing sperm in the female reproductive tract occurs.

The urethra passes through the shaft of the penis within the spongy body. It functions to eliminate urine from the bladder and to transport semen to the woman's vagina during ejaculation.

Scrotum

The scrotum is an external sac that houses the testes in two internal compartments. The main functions of the scrotum are to protect the testes from trauma and to regulate the temperature within the testes, a process that is extremely important to the production of healthy male gametes. The ideal temperature within the scrotum is approximately 96°F, just slightly lower than normal body temperature. The skin of the scrotum is greatly pigmented and folded into furrows called rugae. When either the environmental or body temperature is hot, the cremaster muscle within the scrotal sac remains relaxed so that the testes dangle down, away

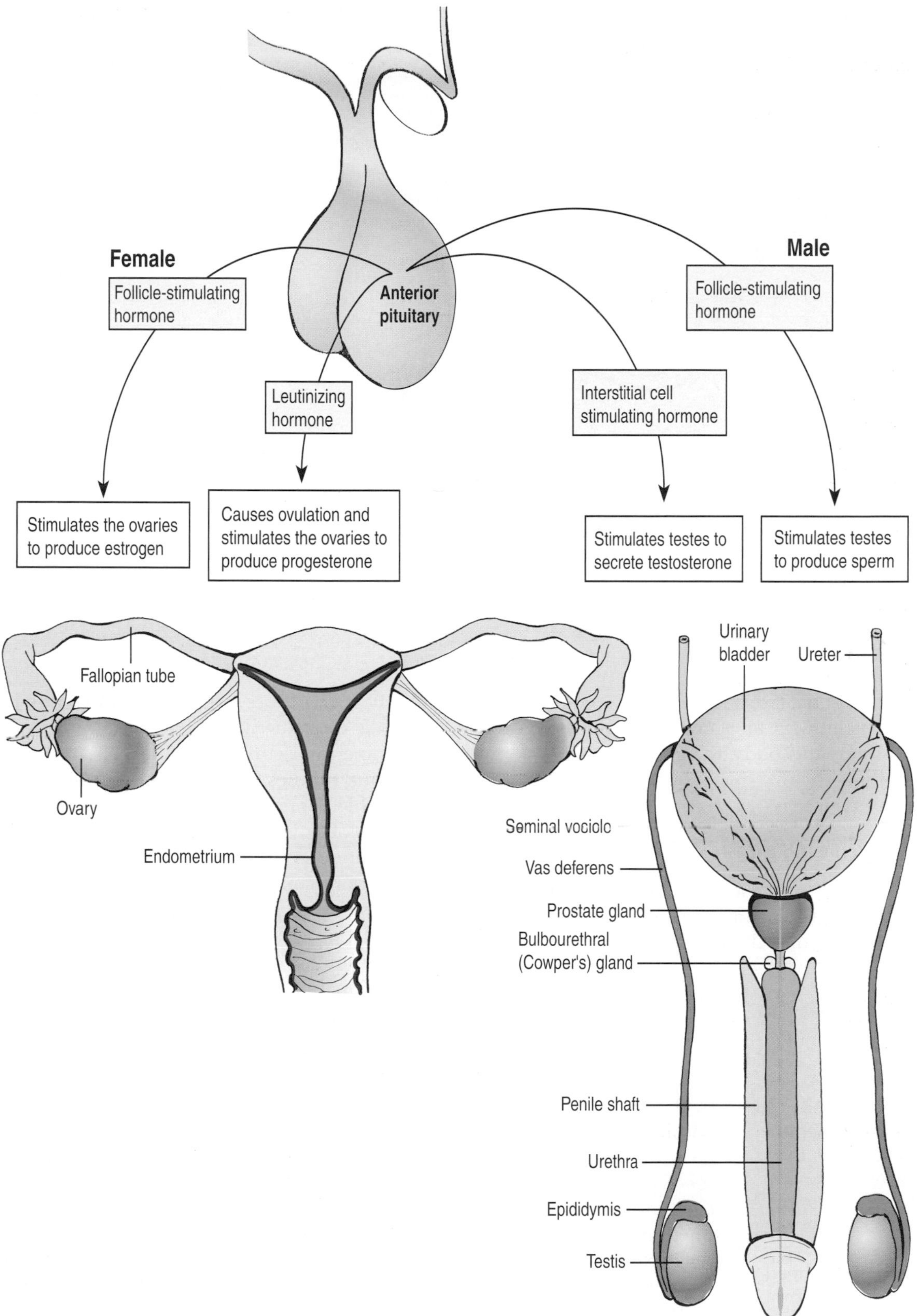

● ***Figure 3.1*** Hormones of the anterior pituitary stimulate the reproductive system in the male and the female.

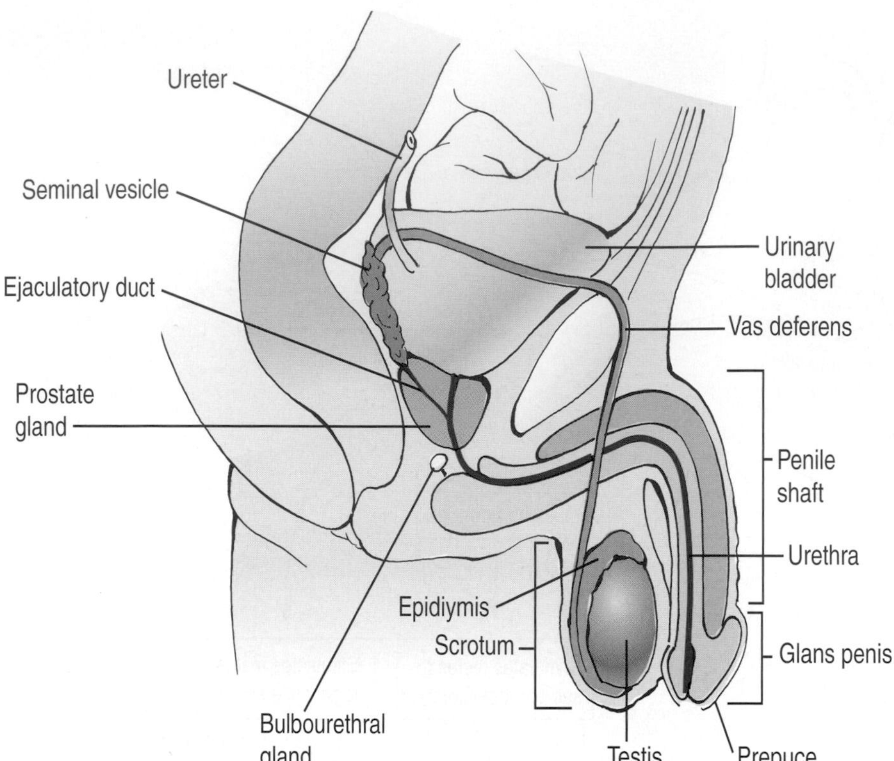

● ***Figure 3.2*** Male reproductive anatomy.

from the warmth of the body. If the temperature is cold, the cremaster muscle contracts, an action that pulls the scrotum in toward the man's body, thereby increasing the temperature in the testicles.

Internal Reproductive Organs

Male internal reproductive organs include the testes and a system of glands and ducts that are involved in the formation of nutrient plasma and the transport of semen out of the man's body (Fig. 3-3).

This is an important teaching tip. The temperature within the testes should be slightly lower than core body temperature. When the temperature is too hot, sperm are not produced efficiently. A simple act such as wearing constrictive clothing (e.g., tight jeans) for prolonged periods can lead to low sperm counts and male infertility because the scrotal contents are held too close to the body and the temperature within the testes becomes too hot for optimal sperm production.

Testes

The testes, two oval organs, one within each scrotal sac (Fig. 3-4), serve two important functions: production of male sex hormones, androgens, and formation and maturation of spermatozoa. Each testis is about 4 centimeters long by 2.5 centimeters wide and is divided into lobes. The lobes contain **seminiferous tubules,** tiny coils of tissue in which **spermatogenesis**, production of sperm, occurs. Interstitial cells surround the seminiferous tubules and produce the androgen testosterone, which is necessary for the maturation of sperm. A system of tiny tubes called the rete testis lead from the seminiferous tubules to the **epididymis**, an intricate network of coiled ducts on the posterior portion of each testis that is approximately 6 meters (20 feet) in length. It is here that sperm mature. Refer to Table 3-1 for a summary of the hormones that influence male reproduction. Box 3-1 depicts how to perform testicular self-examination (TSE). This procedure is recommended monthly for all men age 15 years and older to detect early changes associated with testicular cancer.

Ductal System

The **vas deferens** is the muscular tube in which sperm begin their journey out of the man's body. It connects the epididymis with the ejaculatory duct. The vas deferens is sheathed in the spermatic cord, which also contains the blood vessels, nerves, and lymphatics that serve the testes. The left spermatic cord is usually longer than the right so that the left testis hangs lower than the right.

The spermatic cord (and vas deferens contained within it) leads into the abdominal cavity through the inguinal canal, arches over the urinary bladder, and then curves downward on the posterior side of the

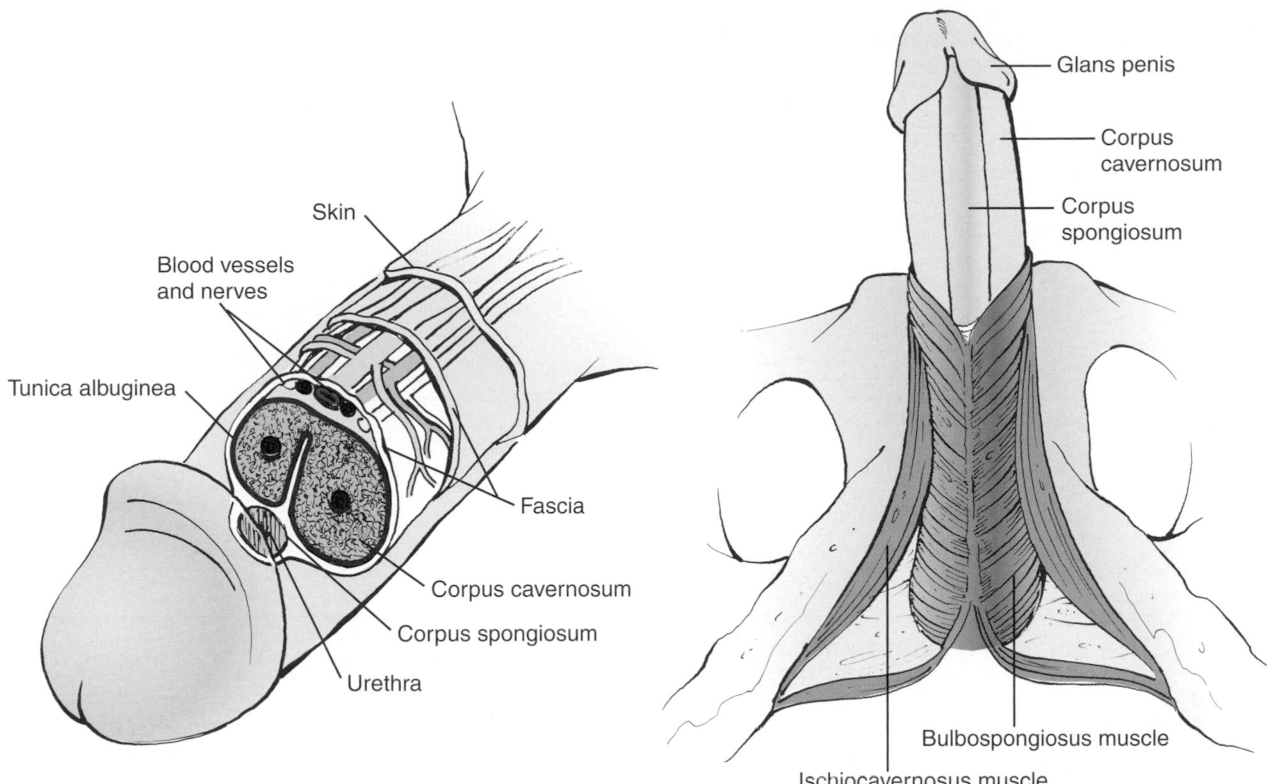

Notice the three columns of erectile tissue. These are well supplied with blood and nerve tissue. The cavernous bodies (corpus cavernosa) contain sinuses that fill with blood during an erection. The urethra traverses the shaft encased within the spongy body (corpus spongiosum).

This view of the ventral aspect shows how the spongy body lies in relation to the cavernous bodies. Notice how the root of the penis is anchored to the pelvis by the tough connective tissue and muscle.

● ***Figure 3.3*** Internal structure of the penis.

bladder. It is at this point that the vas deferens joins with the ejaculatory duct. The paired ejaculatory ducts then connect with the single urethra, which transports the sperm out of the man's penis during ejaculation.

Accessory Glands and Semen

The seminal vesicles are paired glands that empty an alkaline, fructose-rich fluid into the ejaculatory ducts during ejaculation. The prostate is a muscular gland that surrounds the first part of the urethra as it exits the urinary bladder. It is approximately the size of a chestnut. Prostatic fluid is alkaline and is secreted when the prostate contracts during ejaculation. The bulbourethral (Cowper's) glands secrete an alkaline fluid that coats the last part of the urethra during ejaculation.

The alkaline fluids secreted by these glands are nutrient plasmas with several key functions, including

- Enhancement of sperm motility (i.e., ability to move)
- Nourishment of sperm (i.e., provides a ready source of energy with the simple sugar fructose)

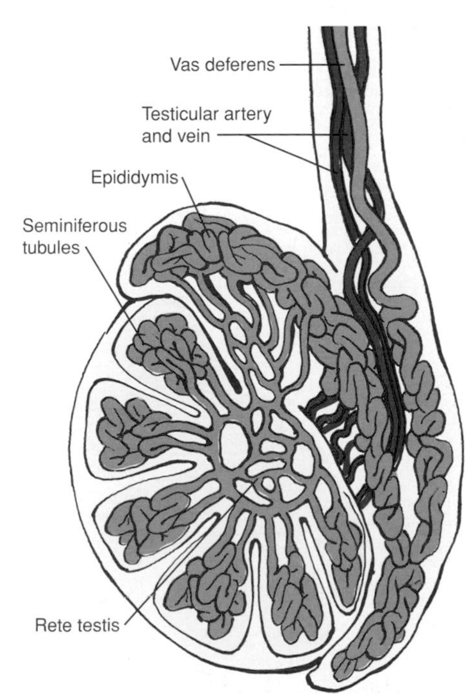

● ***Figure 3.4*** Internal structure of a testis.

TABLE 3.1 Hormonal Control of Male Reproductive Functions

Hormone	Source	Reproductive Functions
Follicle-stimulating hormone (FSH)	Anterior pituitary	• Stimulates production of sperm in the seminiferous tubules
Interstitial cell-stimulating hormone (ICSH)[1]	Anterior pituitary	• Stimulates the interstitial cells to secrete testosterone
Testosterone	Interstitial cells	• Assists sperm to mature • Influences the development of secondary sex characteristics (facial and pubic hair growth, deepening of the voice, growth of the penis)

[1]Homologous to luteinizing hormone (LH) in the female.

BOX 3.1 Testicular Self-examination (TSE)

The National Institutes for Health recommend that men (starting at age 15) perform TSE once monthly for early detection of testicular tumors or abnormalities. The examination should be performed after a warm bath or shower. The warmth relaxes the scrotal skin, which makes it easier to detect abnormalities. There are four steps to a complete examination.

1. Inspection of scrotal sac. The man stands in front of a mirror and checks for swelling on the scrotal skin. It is normal for one testicle to hang lower than the other.
2. Palpation of testicles. The man examines each testicle with both hands. The index and middle finger are placed under the testicle, and the thumb is placed on top. The testicle is then rolled between the fingers and thumbs. The procedure is repeated on the other testicle. Pain should not be felt during the exam. Cancerous lumps are usually found on the sides of the testicle, but can also appear in the front.
3. Palpation of the epididymis. The man then palpates the epididymis, a cordlike structure found on the top and back of each testicle. Lumps on the epididymis are not cancerous.
4. Examination by a physician. If a suspicious lump or swelling is noted, the man is instructed to see a physician, preferably a urologist, as soon as possible. TSE should be done in association with annual health examinations.

Signs of testicular cancer include

- Small, painless lump in a testicle.
- Enlargement of a testicle. It is normal for one testicle to be slightly larger than the other.
- Significant loss in size of a testicle.
- A feeling of scrotal heaviness.
- A dull ache in the lower abdomen or groin.
- Testicular or scrotal pain or discomfort.
- Sudden accumulation of blood or fluid in the scrotum.
- Enlargement or tenderness of the breasts.

TABLE 3.2 A Sperm's Journey Through the Male Reproductive Tract

Event	Site
Formation of sperm	Seminiferous tubules (paired)
Maturation of sperm	Epididymis (paired)
Path into the abdominal cavity	Vas deferens (paired)
Connecting duct between vas deferens and urethra	Ejaculatory duct (paired)
Path out of the man's body	Urethra (single)

- Protection of sperm (i.e., sperm are maintained in an alkaline environment to protect them from the acidic environment of the vagina)

The alkaline fluids and sperm combination is a thick, whitish secretion termed semen or seminal fluid. An average human ejaculate has a volume of 1 to 5 mL and contains several hundred million sperm. Table 3-2 describes (in order) the journey of sperm from formation in the seminiferous tubules to the path out of the body via the urethra.

Test Yourself

- What is the general term that refers to male and female sex cells?
- Name two important functions of the testes.
- Trace a sperm through the male reproductive tract to outside of the body beginning at the seminiferous tubules. Name all the ducts and glands along the way.

FEMALE REPRODUCTIVE SYSTEM

The external genitalia, or **vulva,** and internal reproductive organs compose the female reproductive tract. The purpose of the female reproductive tract is to allow for sexual intimacy and fulfillment and to produce children through the processes of conception, pregnancy, and childbirth. Each part of the female reproductive tract contributes in some way to these purposes.

The mammary glands and bony pelvis are also part of female reproductive anatomy. Breast anatomy is discussed with infant nutrition and lactation in Chapter 14, and the bony pelvis is described in Chapter 8. Box 3-2 explains how to do a self-breast examination, an important procedure to detect breast cancer in the early stages.

External Genitalia (Vulva)

The external genitalia consist of the mons pubis, labia majora and minora, clitoris, vestibule, and perineum. Figure 3-5 illustrates these structures.

Mons Pubis

The **mons pubis**, or mons, is a rounded fatty pad located atop the symphysis pubis. Coarse pubic hair and skin cover the mons. The function of the mons is to protect the pelvic bones during sexual intercourse.

Labia Major and Minora

The labia majora (singular: labium major) are paired fatty tissue folds that extend anteriorly from the mons pubis and then join posteriorly to the true perineum. Labia majora are covered with pubic hair, are vascular, and contain oil and sweat glands. Inside the labia majora are the labia minora (singular: labium minor), paired erectile tissue folds that extend anteriorly from the clitoris and then join posteriorly to the fourchette, a tissue fold that is formed where the labia minora meet posteriorly. The labia minora are thinner than the labia majora, are hairless, contain oil glands, and are sensitive to stimulation.

Clitoris

At the apex of the labia minora is a hooded body composed of erectile tissue called the clitoris. The clitoris, similar to the glans penis, is highly sensitive and allows the woman to experience sexual pleasure and orgasm during sexual stimulation. The hooded structure over the clitoris is called the prepuce.

Vestibule

The area between the labia minora is called the **vestibule**. The urethral meatus (opening to the urethra),

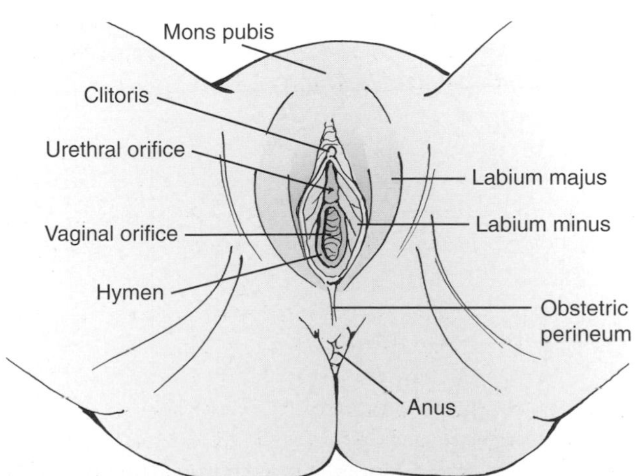

● ***Figure 3.5*** Female external genitalia.

BOX 3.2 Breast Self-examination (BSE)

BSE is recommended once monthly for early detection of breast tumors or abnormalities. The examination should be performed approximately 1 week after the menstrual period ends, or if the woman is no longer having menstrual periods, then on a particular day each month that is easy for her to remember, such as the first day of the month. BSE is part of a comprehensive breast-screening program, which includes yearly clinical breast exams and mammography for women who are 40 years of age and older.

There are five steps to a complete examination.

1. Inspection of breast tissue with arms on hips. The woman stands in front of a mirror with the shoulders straight and the arms on her hips. She checks for any change in size, shape, or color, and for visible swelling or dimpling of breast tissue. It is normal for one breast to be slightly larger than the other.

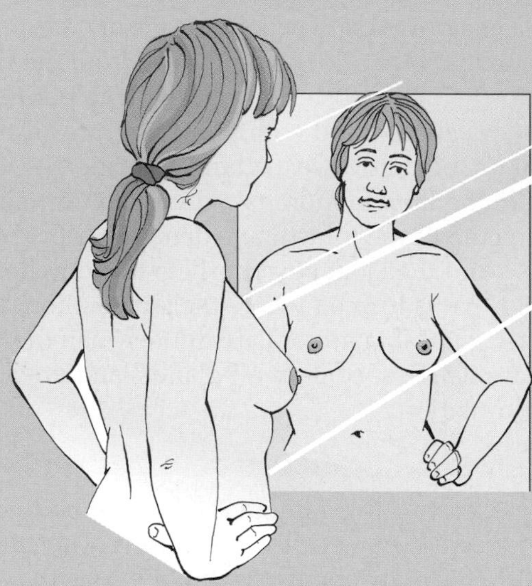

2. Inspection of breast tissue with arms raised. The woman continues in front of the mirror and raises both arms. She looks for the same changes as described in Step 1.

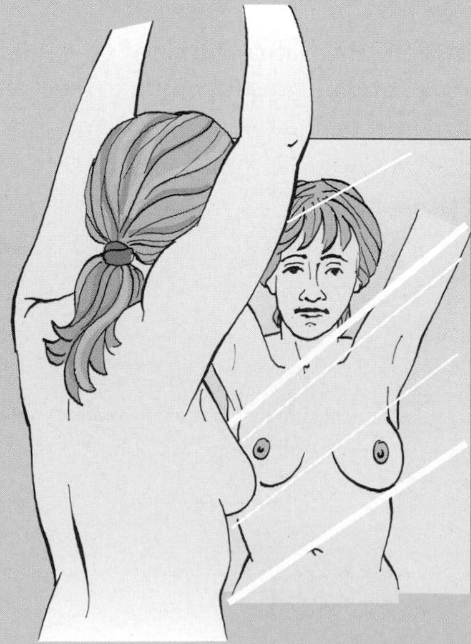

3. Palpation of the nipple for discharge. The woman continues in front of the mirror, and then squeezes the nipple tissue, attempting to elicit a discharge. Any fluid (in a nonpregnant, nonlactating woman) is abnormal.
4. Palpation of breast tissue lying down. The woman lies down on a firm surface. She uses her right hand to exam her left breast and her left hand to examine her right breast. She should use a firm, smooth touch with the first few fingers of the hand. The fingers should be kept flat and held together.
   a. The entire breast should be covered, from the collarbone to the top of the abdomen, and from the armpit to the breast cleavage. (The armpit is an area that is frequently missed.)
   b. The woman should use a pattern to ensure that all breast tissue is covered. Some women use a circular pattern, beginning at the nipple and working outward in ever-larger circles until all breast tissue is palpated. Another method is to move the fingers up and down in vertical rows.
   c. The woman should use light palpation, then deep palpation in each area, so that superficial and deep abnormalities can be detected.

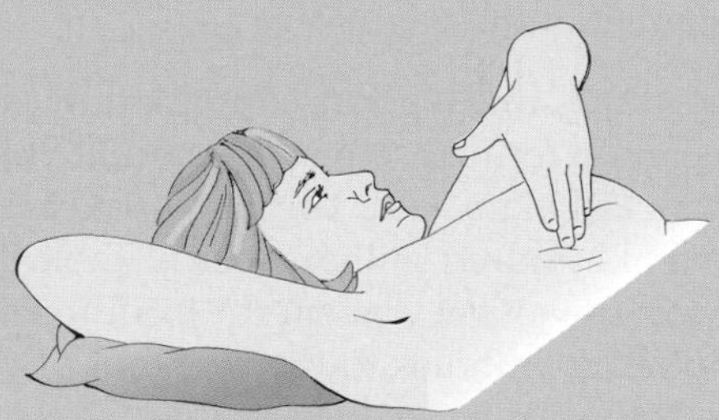

5. Palpation of breast tissue standing up. The entire process used in Step 4 is repeated in Step 5, only this time the woman is in the standing position. Many women find it helpful to perform this part of the exam in the shower.

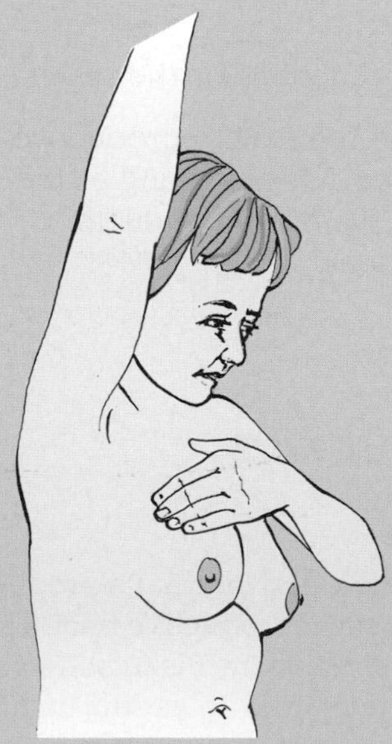

Signs of breast cancer include

- Dimpling, puckering, or swelling of breast tissue.
- Breast pain.
- Nipple discharge.
- Change in position of a nipple.
- Breast lump or mass.

A PERSONAL GLIMPSE

For the first 12 years of my marriage I never experienced an orgasm. My husband and I married very young, just out of high school. In the early years of marriage sex was okay but never great for me. Then after three kids and no sleep, I really did not enjoy sex. I began to think there was something wrong with me. Why couldn't I enjoy sex when everyone else seemed to enjoy it? I began to speak confidentially with my nurse practitioner at my obstetrician's office. She had delivered two of my kids and I trusted her completely. I explained my concerns to her. She said that this is a very normal concern and that I was right to come see her. She said she would perform a physical examination to rule out any physical reasons for my lack of interest in, and enjoyment of, sex. A few days after the examination we sat in her office and talked. She told me that I was in great physical shape, my lab work looked fine, and my reproductive tract was healthy. She asked what kind of stimulation my husband provided before intercourse. I said none. She explained that this could be the reason I did not enjoy sex. She explained in detail how the female clitoris was designed and how it functions to bring sexual pleasure and orgasm during sexual stimulation. She showed me drawings of where it is located on my body and described how it changes during sexual stimulation. She encouraged me to locate it on my own body and ask my husband to stimulate that area during sexual intercourse. I took her advice and now I really enjoy sex with my husband. I wish someone had explained female reproductive anatomy to me earlier in my marriage.

Donna

LEARNING OPPORTUNITY: How does knowledge of the reproductive tract help nurses take care of women who desire greater sexual satisfaction?

paraurethral (Skene's) glands, vaginal opening or introitus, and Bartholin glands are located within the vestibule. The paraurethral and Bartholin glands are each paired glands whose secretions moisten the delicate vaginal mucosa and raise the pH of vaginal fluid during sexual intercourse to enhance sperm motility.

The hymen is an avascular fold of tissue located around or partially around the introitus. It varies in shape from woman to woman and throughout an individual woman's reproductive life span. In times past an intact hymen was believed to be evidence of female virginity. However, the hymen can be torn in ways other than sexual intercourse, such as during heavy physical exertion or with the use of tampons, so the appearance of this tissue is not a reliable method of ascertaining virginity.

Be careful! It is easy to confuse the clitoris with the urethral meatus. When you are preparing to catheterize a woman, use your finger and thumb to carefully part the labia minora, and then locate the urethral meatus below the clitoris and above the vaginal opening. If you touch the sensitive tissue of the clitoris with the catheter, you may cause the woman pain.

Perineum

The true perineum is a band of fibrous, muscular tissue that extends from the posterior portion of the labia majora to the anus. Several sets of superficial and deep muscle groups meet at the perineum to provide support for pelvic structures. The perineum and muscles of the pelvic floor are capable of great expansion during childbirth to allow for delivery of the fetus. These structures are also subject to the stresses and trauma of childbirth. The perineum is the site in which an episiotomy is sometimes done. Uncontrolled tearing and lacerations can also occur. If these are not properly repaired, or if they do not heal appropriately, the woman may experience stress incontinence or prolapse of pelvic organs later in life.

Internal Reproductive Organs

The internal reproductive organs include the vagina, uterus, fallopian tubes, and ovaries. Figure 3-6 illustrates the internal reproductive structures.

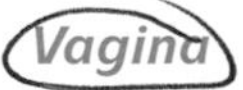

Vagina

The vagina, or birth canal, is a muscular tube that leads from the vulva to the uterus. The opening lies within the vestibule from which it slopes up and backward to the cervix. Because the walls of the vagina extend beyond the uterine cervix, the cervix dips into the

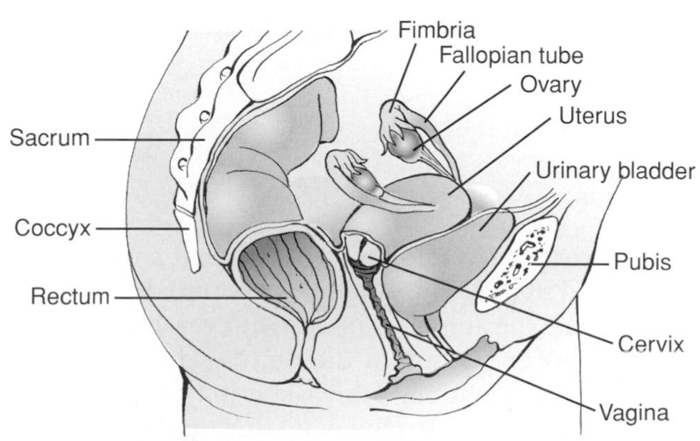

● ***Figure 3.6*** Internal female anatomy.

vagina and forms fornices, which are arch-like structures or pockets. The posterior fornix is largest because the posterior vaginal wall is longer than the anterior wall (approximately 9 and 7 centimeters long, respectively). Because of its location and size, the posterior fornix provides the physician ready access to the peritoneal cavity when invasive procedures are needed.

The vagina serves several important functions. The inner folds, or rugae, allow the vagina to stretch during birth to accommodate a full-term infant. In addition, normally, the vagina maintains an acidic pH of 4 to 5, which protects the vagina from infection. The vagina receives the penis during sexual intercourse and serves as the exit point for menstrual flow.

This is a good client teaching point. The acidic environment of the vagina is protective. Any change that alters the pH, particularly if the pH increases (becomes more alkaline), multiplies the risk for irritation and infection. Douching, tampons, or sanitary pads that contain deodorant, and antibiotic therapy (through the bloodstream) are examples of substances that can affect the pH of the vagina.

Uterus

The uterus, or womb, is a hollow, pear-shaped, muscular structure located within the pelvic cavity between the bladder and the rectum. The anterior surface is over the superior portion of the bladder, separated by the vesicouterine pouch, a fold of peritoneum. In the nonpregnant woman, the uterus is approximately 7.5 centimeters long by 5.0 centimeters wide (at the widest portion) and weighs approximately 40 grams. It is normally tipped forward and rests just above the urinary bladder (see Fig. 3-6). The main structures that provide support and hold the uterus in position are the broad ligaments laterally and the round ligament anteriorly. The functions of the uterus are to prepare for pregnancy each month, protect and nourish the growing child when pregnancy occurs, and to aid in childbirth. The uterus (Fig. 3-7) is divided into four sections:

- cervix
- uterine isthmus
- corpus
- fundus

The cervix is a tubular structure that connects the vagina and uterus. The outer os (opening) dips into the vagina, and the inner os opens into the uterine isthmus, the lower portion of the uterus. The cervix normally has a tiny slit that allows sperm to enter and the menstrual flow to exit. However, during childbirth the cervix must thin and open fully so that the baby can be born. The ciliated epithelium that lines the inner walls of the cervix produces mucus that lubricates the vaginal canal and serves to protect the uterus from ascending infectious agents.

The uterine isthmus is a narrow neck portion or corridor that connects the cervix to the main body of the uterus. During pregnancy and childbirth the uterine isthmus is referred to as the lower uterine segment. This is the thinnest portion of the uterus and does not participate in the muscular contractions of labor. Because it is the thinnest portion, this is the area of the uterus that is most likely to rupture during the stress of labor.

The corpus is the main body of the uterus, and the fundus is the topmost section. The walls of the corpus and fundus are made up of three layers. The perimetrium is the tough outer layer of connective tissue that supports the uterus. The middle layer is the **myometrium**, a muscular layer that is responsible for the contractions of labor. The muscle fibers of the myometrium wrap around the uterus in three directions: obliquely, laterally, and longitudinally. This muscle configuration allows for tremendous expulsive force during labor and birth. The vascular mucosal inner layer is called the **endometrium**. This is the tissue that changes under hormonal influence every month in preparation for possible conception and pregnancy.

The principal support for the uterus is provided by four paired ligaments (see Fig. 3-7), which anchor the uterus at the base (cervical region), leaving the upper portion (corpus) free in the pelvic cavity. The broad ligament is a sheet of peritoneum that attaches the lower sides of the uterus to the sidewalls of the pelvis. The right and left cardinal ligaments anchor the walls of the cervix and vagina to the lateral pelvic walls. The round ligaments are paired fibromuscular bands that tip the uterus forward and hold it in an anteflexed position. They extend from the anterior/lateral portions of the uterus to the labia majora. The round ligaments are homologous to the spermatic cord in the male. The uterosacral ligaments anchor the lower posterior portion of the uterus to the sacrum.

Fallopian Tubes

The paired fallopian tubes (also known as oviducts) are tiny, muscular corridors that arise from a lateral position on the superior surface of the uterus near the fundus and extend out on either side toward the ovaries. They are 8 to 14 centimeters in length. Each fallopian tube is divided into three sections. The isthmus, which means a neck or narrow section, is the medial one third of the tube that connects to the uterus. The ampulla, middle portion of the tube, connects the isthmus with the infundibulum, the outer portion that opens into the lower abdominal cavity. At the outer edges of the infundibulum are fimbriae,

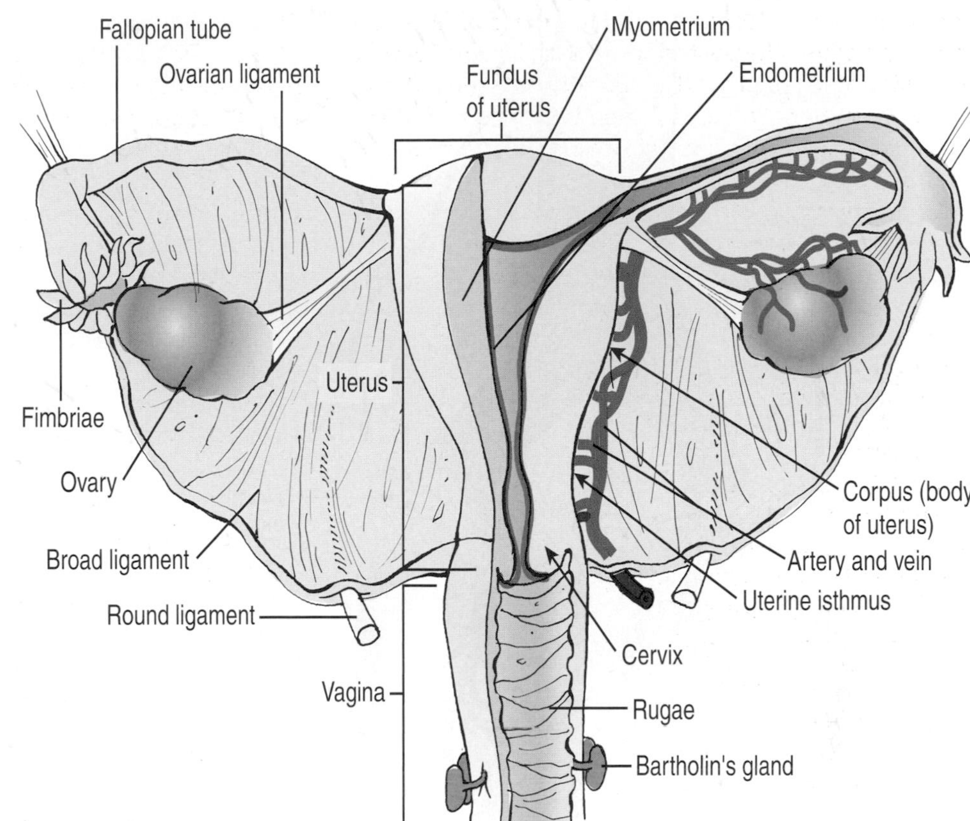

● ***Figure 3.7*** Anterior view of the female reproductive tract. The right fallopian tube and ovary, uterus, and vagina are shown in a cross-sectional view to demonstrate the internal structure of these organs.

fingerlike projections that undulate gently over the ovaries.

The tubes have a critical role in the process of conception. When an egg is released from the ovary, the undulating movements of the fimbriae attract the egg toward the fallopian tube. Once within the tube, muscular contractions and beating of tiny cilia propel the egg toward the uterus. If sperm are present, fertilization of the egg is possible. Fertilization most frequently occurs in the ampulla of the tube. The tubes secrete lipids and glycogen to provide nourishment to the fertilized egg as it makes its way to the uterus. The functions of the fallopian tubes are to provide a site for fertilization, a passageway, and a nourishing, warm environment for the fertilized egg to travel to the uterus.

You do the math. If one ovum matures every month during the childbearing years (from age 12 through 50), a woman would only use 456 ova. Even if that number were doubled to accommodate two eggs per cycle (a situation that sometimes results in twins), she would still use only 912 ova. Because on average a baby girl is born with 2 million immature ova, there are significantly more available than will ever be used.

Ovaries

The ovaries, two sex glands homologous to the male testes, are located on either side of the uterus. They are similar to almonds in size and shape. The ovaries are supported by the broad and ovarian ligaments. The female is born with all the ova (eggs) that she will ever have. Typically, females are born with approximately 2 million eggs, many of which will deteriorate during childhood. The remaining ova are usually released one per month during ovulation until the woman's reproductive years are over. The function of the ovaries is to produce the female hormones estrogen and progesterone, which are responsible for female secondary sex characteristics and for regulating the menstrual cycle in response to anterior pituitary hormones (see discussion in the Menstrual Cycle section).

Blood Supply for the Pelvic Organs

The pelvic organs have a rich blood supply (Fig. 3-8). The internal iliac artery arises from the common iliac artery and supplies the pelvic organs, gluteal region, hip, and medial thigh. The vagina and uterus are supplied by the vaginal and uterine arteries, respectively, both of which arise from the anterior division of the internal iliac artery. The ovarian artery, which supplies the ovaries and oviducts, branches directly from the abdominal aorta. The internal pudendal artery is the primary blood

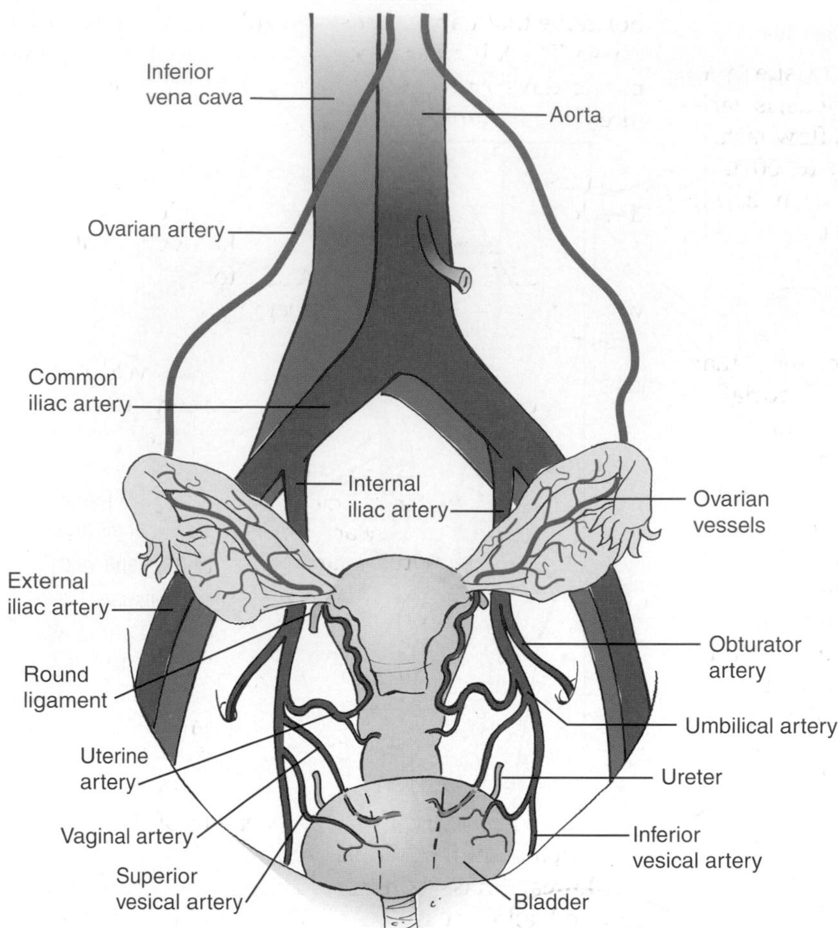

● ***Figure 3.8*** Pelvic blood supply.

supply to the perineum. This artery branches from the anterior division of the internal iliac artery and supplies the anus, superficial and deep perineal muscles, clitoris, and posterior aspect of the labia majora.

Several major veins drain the tissues of the pelvic organs. The ovarian vein, which drains the ovary, the distal part of the fallopian tube, and ureter, intersects directly with the inferior vena cava on the right and on the left connects with the left renal vein. The uterus, fallopian tubes, and vagina are drained by the uterine and vaginal venous plexus, respectively. A plexus is a network of veins that forms multiple tributaries. These plexuses connect with the uterine and vaginal veins to drain into the internal iliac vein. The external and internal pudendal veins allow deoxygenated blood from the perineal region to flow into the femoral, great saphenous, and internal iliac veins.

Test Yourself

- What structures are found in the vestibule?
- Name and describe the four divisions of the uterus.
- What important function do the ovaries fulfill?

REPRODUCTIVE FUNCTION

Puberty

Puberty is the time of life in which the individual becomes capable of sexual reproduction. Puberty occurs on average between the ages of 10 and 14 years. This phase is marked by maturation of the reproductive organs and development of secondary sex characteristics, external physical evidence of sexual maturity. Secondary sex characteristics include female breast development, growth of pubic and axillary hair, growth of external genitals (labia and penis), appearance of facial hair, and deepening of the voice in the male.

The changes associated with puberty happen in response to hypothalamic and pituitary hormones. Secondary sex characteristics develop in an orderly sequence, although the timing may be varied between individuals. Breast budding in the female is usually the first physical sign noted and occurs between the ages of 10 and 12 years on average. Appearance of pubic hair usually occurs just before **menarche**, the first menstrual period. Menarche is most frequently experienced between the ages of 12 and 14 years.

Menstruation

Menstruation, the casting away of blood, tissue, and debris from the uterus as the inner lining sheds, is variable in amount and duration. On average, flow lasts 4 to 6 days, with a total blood loss of 25 to 60 mL. Although this loss is seemingly negligible, with time it can contribute to low iron stores and anemia.

Menstrual Cycle

The menstrual cycle refers to the recurring changes that take place in a woman's reproductive tract associated with menstruation and intermenstruation. The menstrual cycle encompasses the events that transpire in the woman's reproductive organs between the beginnings of two menstrual periods. Hormones from the ovaries and the pituitary gland regulate these cyclical changes. The average cycle lasts 28 days, approximately one month; however, there are great variations between women, and an individual woman's cycle may vary in duration from cycle to cycle. For ease of understanding, the following discussion of the menstrual cycle is based on the average 28-day cycle.

Don't get lost in the details! The menstrual cycle is also referred to as the female reproductive cycle because the overarching goal is to produce human offspring. At any given time, a woman in her reproductive years is in some phase of the menstrual cycle unless pregnancy occurs, in which case the goal of the menstrual cycle has been met. When you understand the menstrual cycle, you will then be able to understand the process of conception, and you will be better prepared to counsel families on how to prevent pregnancy or how to increase the probability that pregnancy will occur.

There are two main components of the menstrual cycle, the changes that happen in the ovaries in response to pituitary hormones, the ovarian cycle, and the variations that take place in the uterus, the uterine cycle. We will discuss each cycle separately, but it is important to remember that both cycles work together simultaneously to produce the menstrual cycle (Fig. 3-9). Changes in cervical mucus also take place during the course of the menstrual cycle; these changes are discussed below.

Ovarian Cycle

Cyclical changes in the ovaries occur in response to two anterior pituitary hormones: follicle-stimulating hormone (FSH) and luteinizing hormone (LH). Each of the two phases of the ovarian cycle is named for the hormone that has the most control over that particular phase. The follicular phase, controlled by FSH, encompasses days 1 to 14 of a 28-day cycle. LH controls the luteal phase, which includes days 15 to 28.

Follicular Phase. At the beginning of each menstrual cycle, a follicle on one of the ovaries begins to develop in response to rising levels of FSH. The follicle produces estrogen, which causes the ovum contained within the follicle to mature. As the follicle grows, it fills with estrogen-rich fluid and begins to resemble a tiny blister on the surface of the ovary.

When the pituitary gland detects high levels of estrogen from the mature follicle, it releases a surge of LH. This sudden increase in LH causes the follicle to burst open, releasing the mature ovum into the abdominal cavity, a process called **ovulation**. Ovulation occurs on day 14 of a 28-day cycle. As the ovum floats along the surface of the ovary, the gentle beating of the fimbriae draws it toward the fallopian tube.

Remember, all of the ova already exist within the ovaries; however, they are in an immature state. In order to ripen, or mature, an ovum needs a stimulus. FSH is the messenger from the pituitary that provides the required stimulus.

Luteal Phase. After ovulation, LH levels remain elevated and cause the remnants of the follicle to develop into a yellow body called the **corpus luteum**. In addition to producing estrogen, the corpus luteum secretes a hormone called progesterone. If fertilization does not take place, the corpus luteum begins to degenerate, and estrogen and progesterone levels fall. This process leads back to day 1 of the cycle, and the follicular phase begins anew.

Test Yourself

- Which hormone is responsible for ovulation?
- What is the main purpose of FSH?
- What structure produces progesterone?

Uterine Cycle

The uterine cycle refers to the changes that are found in the uterine lining of the uterus. These changes come about in response to the ovarian hormones estrogen and progesterone. There are four phases to this cycle: menstrual, proliferative, secretory, and ischemic.

Menstrual Phase. Day 1 of the menstrual cycle is marked by the onset of menstruation. During the menstrual phase of the uterine cycle, the uterine lining is

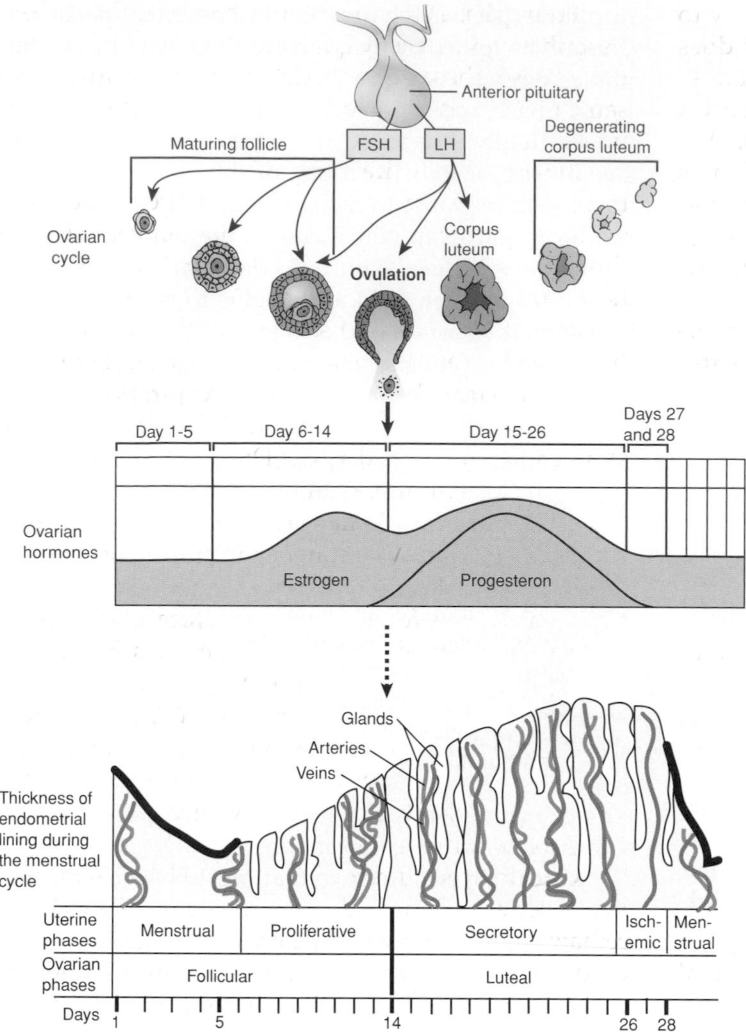

● ***Figure 3.9*** A 28-day (average) menstrual cycle. The anterior pituitary hormones control the ovarian cycle. The ovaries produce hormones that control the uterine cycle.

shed because of low levels of progesterone and estrogen. At the same time, a follicle is beginning to develop and starts producing estrogen. The menstrual phase ends when the menstrual period stops on approximately day 5.

Proliferative Phase. When estrogen levels are high enough, the endometrium begins to regenerate. Estrogen stimulates blood vessels to develop. The blood vessels in turn bring nutrients and oxygen to the uterine lining, and it begins to grow and become thicker. The proliferative phase ends with ovulation on day 14.

Secretory Phase. After ovulation, the corpus luteum begins to produce progesterone. This hormone causes the uterine lining to become rich in nutrients in preparation for pregnancy. Estrogen levels also remain high so that the lining is maintained. If pregnancy does not transpire, the corpus luteum gradually degenerates, and the woman enters the ischemic phase of the menstrual cycle.

Ischemic Phase. On days 27 and 28, estrogen and progesterone levels fall because the corpus luteum is no longer producing them. Without these hormones to maintain the blood vessel network, the uterine lining becomes ischemic. When the lining starts to slough, the woman has come full cycle and is once again at day 1 of the menstrual cycle.

Test Yourself

- What is the main function of estrogen during the menstrual cycle?
- Which hormone is active only during the secretory phase of the uterine cycle?
- What happens to the uterine lining during the ischemic phase?
- What causes the ischemic phase to occur?

Cervical Mucus Changes

Changes in cervical mucus take place over the course of the menstrual cycle. Some women use these characteristics to help determine when ovulation is likely to happen. During the menstrual phase the cervix does not produce mucus. Gradually, as hormonal changes transpire and the proliferative phase begins, the cervix begins to produce a tacky, crumbly type of mucus that is yellow or white. As the time of ovulation draws near, the mucus becomes progressively clear, thin, and lubricative, with the properties of raw egg white. At the peak of fertility (i.e., during ovulation), the mucus has a distensible, stretchable quality called spinnbarkheit (see Chapter 4 for further discussion of cervical mucus changes that indicate ovulation). After ovulation the mucus again becomes scanty, thick, and opaque.

Menopause

Menopause refers to the time in a woman's life when reproductive capability ends. Gradually the ovaries cease to function, and hormone levels fall. The woman begins to experience irregular menstrual cycles until finally they come to an end. The interlude surrounding menopause in which these changes take place is called the **climacteric**. The average age at which menopause occurs is between 47 and 55 years.

SEXUAL RESPONSE CYCLE

Sexuality is part of our human nature. We are sexual beings with sexual needs. Nature has provided us with the capacity to give and receive pleasure through the process of sexual stimulation. Therefore, a discussion of reproduction would be incomplete without mention of the physiology of sexual response.

There are two underlying physiologic responses to sexual stimulation in both men and women: vasocongestion and myotonia (muscular tension). These two processes are fundamental to almost all physiologic responses that take place during sexual arousal.

Vasocongestion occurs in the pelvic organs during sexual excitement because the arteries dilate, allowing inflow of blood that is greater than venous capacity to drain the area. The result is widespread congestion of the pelvic tissues. Vasocongestion leads to erection of the penis and clitoris, vaginal lubrication, and engorgement of the labia and testicles. Other tissue, such as the nipples and earlobes, may also be affected.

Myotonia is present throughout the body during sexual arousal and orgasm. It is evident in voluntary and involuntary contractions. Facial grimacing, spasmodic contractions of the hands and feet, and the involuntary muscular contractions during orgasm are the most notable examples of myotonia.

Four phases of the sexual response have been described: excitement, plateau, orgasm, and resolution. These phases occur in both sexes and follow the same general patterns regardless of the method of sexual stimulation.

During the excitement phase, the woman's clitoris becomes engorged and enlarged, the labia majora separate, and the labia minora increase in size. The uterus increases in size and begins to elevate. For the man, excitement leads to erection of the penis, thickening of the scrotal sac, and testicular elevation. In both sexes excitement is marked by an increase in heart rate, blood pressure, and respirations. Some individuals experience a "sex flush," reddening of the skin on the chest and neck. Duration of the excitement phase is from several minutes to several hours.

There is no set event that marks the beginning of the plateau phase. Vasocongestion and myotonia continue, and the heart rate and blood pressure remain elevated. For the female, the outer third of the vagina becomes engorged, the clitoris retracts behind its hood, and the labia minora deepen in color. The uterus is fully elevated in the pelvic cavity. The head of the penis in the male becomes further engorged, and the testes remain engorged and elevated. The plateau phase is typically a few seconds to several minutes in duration.

Orgasm, the climax of sexual response, is marked by a series of muscular contractions. The clitoris remains retracted behind the hood, and the outer third of the vagina, rectal sphincter, and uterus undergo rhythmic contractions. The male experiences contractions of the urethra, base of the penis, and rectal muscles, as well as emission and expulsion of semen.

During resolution, the muscles gradually relax and there is a reversal of vasocongestion. The heart rate, blood pressure, and breathing return to normal rates. The clitoris descends, and the labia and internal organs return to their prearoused positions and color. The male loses his erection, the testes descend, and the scrotum thins.

KEY POINTS

- Two major functions of the reproductive system are to produce offspring and to provide the experience of pleasure through physical intimacy.
- The testes and ovaries are responsible for the production of sex cells, or gametes.
- Male external genitalia include the penis and scrotum. The penis serves to eliminate urine from the bladder and functions to deposit sperm in the female reproductive tract for the purposes of reproduction. The scrotum regulates the temperature and protects the testes from trauma.

- The testes and ductal system compose the man's internal reproductive tract. Spermatogenesis occurs in the testes, and the ductal system serves as the exit route for sperm from the man's body.
- Sperm are formed in the seminiferous tubules and mature in the epididymis. During ejaculation, sperm travel from the epididymis through the paired vas deferens and ejaculatory ducts to the urethra and out of the body.
- Sperm need an alkaline environment and an energy source to be motile. The seminal vesicles (paired), prostate gland, and the bulbourethral glands (paired) contribute alkaline secretions to semen. The seminal vesicles also contribute fructose, an energy source for sperm.
- Testosterone, FSH, and interstitial cell-stimulating hormone (ICSH) are the male hormones responsible for production of sperm and the development of secondary sex characteristics.
- Female external genitalia, or vulva, includes the mons pubis, labia majora, labia minora, clitoris, urethral meatus, vaginal opening, and Bartholin glands. The vestibule is the area within the boundaries of the labia minora and includes the urethral meatus, vaginal opening, and Bartholin glands.
- The vagina is an internal reproductive organ that functions as the female organ for sexual intercourse, exit point for the menstrual flow, and as the birth canal. Rugae, or folds, allow for stretching during the birth process.
- The main divisions of the uterus are the cervix, isthmus, corpus, and fundus. The walls of the uterus have three layers: perimetrium (protective cover), myometrium (muscle), and endometrium (lining).
- The fallopian tubes lead from the uterus toward the ovaries. The isthmus is the narrow portion near the uterus. The ampulla is the middle portion, and the infundibulum is the outer portion close to the ovaries. Fimbriae on the infundibulum make wave-like motions over the ovary, a process that guides the ovum toward the fallopian tube.
- The ovaries are homologous to the male testes. The ovarian hormones, estrogen and progesterone, play a major role in the menstrual cycle and in the development of secondary sex characteristics in the female.
- The menstrual cycle begins with day 1, the start of menstrual flow. It encompasses the ovarian cycle and the uterine cycle. FSH and LH from the pituitary govern the ovarian cycle, and estrogen and progesterone from the ovaries guide the uterine cycle.
- The sexual response cycle is divided into four phases: excitement, plateau, orgasm, and resolution. Vasocongestion and myotonia are the primary physiologic processes that contribute to sexual response in both the male and female.

REFERENCES AND SELECTED READINGS

Books and Journals

Cunningham, F. G., Gant, N. F., Leveno, K. J., Gilstrap, L. C. III, Hauth, J. C., & Wenstrom, K. D. (2001). Anatomy of the reproductive tract. In *Williams obstetrics* (21st ed., pp. 31–61). New York: McGraw-Hill Medical Publishing Division.

Mattson, S., & Smith, J. E. (Eds.). (2000). *Core curriculum for maternal–newborn nursing*. AWHONN publication (2nd ed.). Philadelphia: WB Saunders.

Pillitteri, A. (1999). Reproductive and sexual health. In *Maternal & child health nursing: Care of the childbearing & childrearing family* (3rd ed., pp. 61–94). Philadelphia: Lippincott Williams & Wilkins.

Scanlon, V. C., & Sanders, T. (1999). *Essentials of anatomy and physiology* (3rd ed.). Philadelphia: F.A. Davis.

Websites

Male

http://www.healthac.org/male.html

http://www.nlm.nih.gov/medlineplus/ency/imagepages/1113.htm

Female

http://www.nlm.nih.gov/medlineplus/ency/imagepages/1112.htm

Menstrual Cycle

http://www.people.virginia.edu/~rjh9u/menscyc3.html

http://anatomy.med.unsw.edu.au/cbl/embryo/wwwhuman/MCycle/MCycle.htm

http://www.abington-repromed.com/cycle.html

WORKBOOK

NCLEX-STYLE REVIEW QUESTIONS

1. You are teaching a male client about the male reproductive system. You ask him which gland provides the sugar that gives the sperm energy to move. Which answer indicates that he correctly understands your teaching?
   a. Bartholin gland
   b. Bulbourethral gland
   c. Epididymis
   d Seminal vesicles
2. The vagina is a hostile environment for sperm. What characteristic of semen protects sperm from the vaginal environment?
   a. Acidic fluid
   b. Alkaline fluid
   c. Presence of testosterone
   d. Secretions from seminiferous tubules
3. You are preparing to perform a urinary catheterization on a female client. In which location will you expect to find the urinary meatus?
   a. Above the clitoris
   b. Below the vaginal opening
   c. On the true perineum
   d Within the vestibule
4. You are caring for a woman in labor. The doctor is concerned that the uterus might rupture. Which part of the uterus requires the closest assessment because it is the thinnest part of the uterus?
   a. Corpus
   b. Fundus
   c. Inner cervical os
   d. Lower uterine segment
5. Which ovarian hormone predominates during the proliferative phase of the uterine cycle?
   a. FSH
   b. LH
   c. Estrogen
   d. Progesterone

STUDY ACTIVITIES

1. In each row of the table you will find either a male or a female reproductive organ listed. In the column that is missing information, fill in the name of the homologous reproductive organ.

Male Reproductive Organ	Female Reproductive Organ
Glans penis	
	Round ligaments
	Ovaries
Foreskin or prepuce	

2. Go to the following Internet site: http://www-medlib.med.utah.edu/WebPath/webpath.html
   a. Click on "Systemic Pathology"
   b. Click on "Female Genital Tract Pathology"
   c. Look for pictures of a normal uterus, fallopian tubes, ovaries, and cervix.
3. Explain the step-by-step procedure for testicular self-examination. List important points to be covered when teaching TSE and why each step is important.
4. In your clinical group, have a discussion as to why it is important for a nurse to understand the menstrual cycle.

CRITICAL THINKING: What Would You Do?

Apply your knowledge of reproductive anatomy and physiology to the following situation.

1. Doug and Nancy, a young married couple, ages 26 and 22 years, respectively, have not been using any contraception for the past year, but Nancy has not become pregnant. Doug is a rancher and dresses in cowboy gear, including tight jeans. He works in a hot, humid environment for 10 to 12 hours almost every day.
   a. Using your knowledge about male reproductive anatomy, what is one possible reason pregnancy has not occurred?
   b. What advice might be helpful for Doug to increase the likelihood that pregnancy will occur?
2. Nancy complains of frequent vaginal infections. During an office interview, Nancy tells you that she douches at least once per week.
   a. What other questions should you ask regarding Nancy's hygiene habits?
   b. What advice might be helpful for Nancy to decrease her risk for vaginal infections?

Special Issues of Reproduction and Women's Health Care

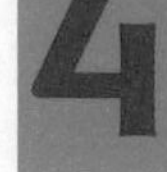

STUDENT OBJECTIVES

On completion of this chapter, the student should be able to

1. Describe recommendations for health screening for women.
2. Differentiate between dysmenorrhea and premenstrual syndrome (PMS).
3. Explain the clinical manifestations, treatment, and nursing care for endometriosis.
4. Discuss risk factors for pelvic inflammatory disease (PID).
5. Explain causes and risk factors for pelvic support disorders.
6. Discuss the significance of family planning.
7. Compare and contrast methods of contraception.
8. Explain advantages and disadvantages for each method of contraception.
9. List possible causes for fertility problems.
10. Identify diagnostic testing used related to fertility problems.
11. Discuss treatment options available for fertility problems.
12. Discuss the psychosocial sequelae related to fertility problems.
13. Identify major considerations for the perimenopausal and postmenopausal woman.

KEY TERMS

abstinence
amenorrhea
coitus interruptus
dysmenorrhea
dyspareunia
elective abortion
endometriosis
gestational surrogate
induced abortion
infertility
menorrhagia
metrorrhagia
perimenopause
postcoital test
spinnbarkeit
therapeutic abortion

The focus of this chapter is to examine issues related to women's health and reproduction. Women's health issues include preventive health care, menstrual disorders, pelvic infections, disorders of the uterus and ovaries, and pelvic support disorders. Issues related to the reproductive life cycle include family planning and contraception, elective termination of pregnancy, infertility, and menopause. Friends and family members often turn to the nurse as a resource for questions about women's health issues, becoming pregnant, contraception, or infertility. Therefore, the nurse's role in women's health and reproductive life cycle issues also is discussed.

Several Healthy People 2010 goals relate to the topics in this chapter. Selected goals include

- Reducing breast and cervical cancer deaths by increasing the number of females who comply with screening recommendations.
- Increasing the proportion of pregnancies that are intended from 51% to 70%.
- Promoting responsible sexual behaviors, strengthening community capacity, and increasing access to quality services to prevent sexually transmitted infections (STIs) and their complications.
- Reducing the proportion of adults aged 50 years and older with osteoporosis from 10% to 8%.

WOMEN'S HEALTH ISSUES

Women's health issues encompass a broad variety of topics. Current research is highlighting the unique needs of women in relation to medical–surgical conditions, such as diabetes, heart disease, and stroke. Although these topics are critical to the overall health of women, this chapter focuses on conditions that occur universally, or near universally, in women.

HEALTH SCREENING FOR WOMEN

Health promotion is a broad concept that involves educating and assisting individuals to make behavior and lifestyle modifications for the prevention or early detection and treatment of disease. Because nurses are trusted health care professionals, individuals and families often turn to them for information and advice on health-related matters. As a result, health promotion for women is an area in which the nurse can have great influence.

Health screening is a component of a comprehensive health promotion plan. Screening tests do not diagnose disease. Instead, a positive result indicates the need for more thorough testing. The following discussion encompasses screening procedures that promote the early detection of disorders that are unique to, or occur commonly in, women.

Breast Cancer Screening

Breast cancer is the second most commonly diagnosed malignancy in women in the Western world.[1] Each year in the United States there are more than 200,000 new cases diagnosed and more than 40,000 deaths caused by breast cancer (American Cancer Society, 2004). A palpable mass is the most common "first" sign or symptom associated with breast disease. Recommended screening for early identification of breast cancer consists of a three-pronged approach: breast self-awareness, clinical breast examination, and mammography. Detection of breast cancer before axillary node involvement increases the chance for survival. It is the role of the nurse to educate women regarding the importance of each screening test and recommended techniques for breast self-examination.

The American Cancer Society (ACS) recommends that women get regular screening to detect signs of breast cancer in the very early stages, if possible. The recommendations vary according to age. The woman in her 20s and 30s should have a clinical breast examination at least every 3 years. When the woman reaches 40 years of age, she should schedule a yearly clinical breast examination, and she should have a yearly mammogram. Breast self-examination (BSE) is a self-scheduled, step-by-step approach the woman uses to check her breasts. In the past it was recommended that BSE be performed on a monthly basis. The ACS now presents BSE as optional because current research indicates that performing BSE does not decrease mortality associated with breast cancer. However, the ACS recommends that each woman know how her breasts normally look and feel, and if changes are found, to immediately report them to a physician. (Refer to Chapter 3, Box 3-2 for instructions on how BSE is done.)

Mammography is a screening tool that uses very–low-dose x-ray for examination of breast tissue. Mammography is useful in the early detection of cancer because it can detect a breast tumor 2 years before the woman or the primary care provider can palpate it. The ACS recommends yearly mammograms for women older than 40 years.

For this procedure the breast is placed on a platform and then compressed firmly between the platform and a plastic paddle (Fig. 4-1). Routine views include a top-to-bottom and a side view. The compression can be uncomfortable for some women. It is usually recommended to schedule the examination for the week after the menstrual period, when the breasts are less tender, to minimize discomfort.

---

[1] Nonmelanoma skin cancers are the most common type of cancer found in women.

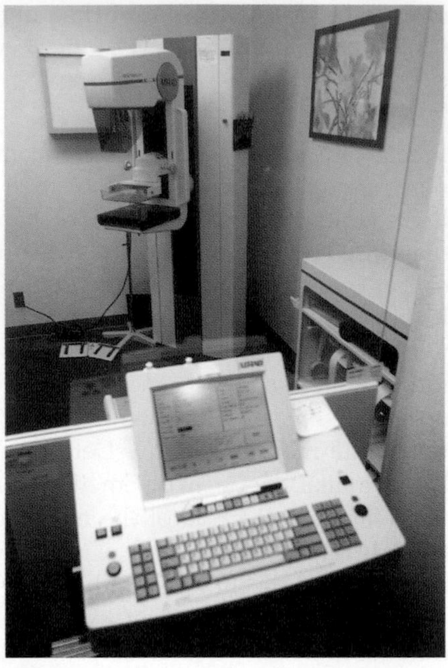

A

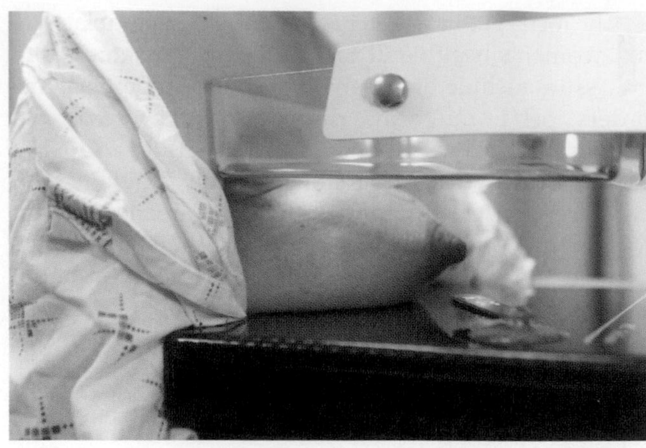

B

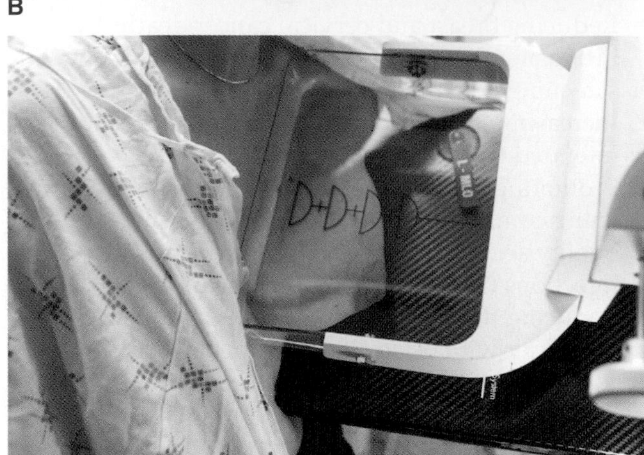

C

● ***Figure 4.1*** Mammography. (**A**) Mammography equipment. (**B**) A top-to-bottom view of the breast. (**C**) A side view of the breast.

Pelvic Examination and Pap Smear

Every woman should have a yearly physical examination. A pelvic examination should be part of the total physical examination. A pelvic examination is done to detect changes associated with certain gynecologic conditions, such as infection, inflammation, pelvic pain, cancer, and other disorders. The Papanicolaou test (Pap smear) may be done in conjunction with the pelvic examination.

The pelvic examination begins with the woman in lithotomy position. The structures of the vulva are visualized and palpated. Then a speculum is inserted to visualize the walls of the vagina and the cervix. When the cervix is clearly visible, the primary care provider swabs the cervix. Secretions can be cultured to diagnose pelvic infection. Cell samples are obtained for the Pap smear. A bimanual examination follows the speculum examination. The practitioner inserts two lubricated fingers into the vagina with one hand and uses the other hand to palpate uterine and ovarian structures through the abdominal wall. A rectal examination to test for fecal occult blood and/or to palpate the rectovaginal wall is usually done at the end of the examination.

The Pap smear is an important screening tool for cervical cancer. In fact, the incidence of cervical cancer has decreased by 50% since practitioners began to routinely perform Pap smears in the 1970s (Katz, 2003) because precancerous changes are caught early and promptly treated. The American College of Obstetricians and Gynecologists' (ACOG's) newly revised guidelines recommend that the initial Pap smear be done approximately 3 years after the woman first has sexual intercourse or by 21 years of age, whichever comes first. Subsequent Pap smears should occur annually in women younger than 30 years of age. Healthy women age 30 and older may require a Pap smear only every 2 to 3 years. The woman who has the human immunodeficiency virus (HIV) or is otherwise immunocompromised, and the woman who was exposed to diethylstilbestrol (DES) in utero should continue to have annual Pap smears. ACOG continues to recommend annual pelvic examinations for all women, even when a Pap smear is not required.

Vulvar Self-Examination

Some primary care practitioners recommend that women older than 18 years (and those younger who are sexually active) should perform a monthly self-examination of the external genitalia. As with BSE, the major value of the monthly vulvar self-examination is that the woman will become familiar with her own normal anatomy. Using a hand mirror and an adequate light source, the woman should inspect her vulva for any lesions, growths, reddened areas, unusual discharge, or changes in skin color. Any changes in sensation, such as itching or pain, should also be noted. The woman should be cautioned that, although most changes are not cancerous, all changes should be reported to her primary care practitioner for evaluation.

COMMON DISORDERS OF THE FEMALE REPRODUCTIVE TRACT

There are several female reproductive tract disorders that occur commonly. Many involve disorders of menstruation. Others are related to or caused by infections or decreased support of the pelvic floor.

Menstrual Disturbances

Disturbances of the menstrual cycle may be related to increased or decreased frequency, and absent, excessive, or irregular bleeding. Pain may also be part of the symptomatology. Nursing intervention will depend on the cause and treatment of the disorder but may include providing information about recommended treatments or prescribed medications, caring for the woman before and after a procedure, and providing emotional support and reassurance.

Amenorrhea

Amenorrhea refers to the absence of menstruation. A 16-year-old girl, who is developing normally and yet does not experience menarche (the first menstrual period), is said to have *primary amenorrhea*. *Secondary amenorrhea* is defined as cessation of menstrual periods after they have occurred previously.

The presence of regular menstrual periods is a sign of health. Regular menses signal that the pituitary and ovarian connection are working together properly and that appropriate amounts of sex hormones are present.

Because pregnancy is the most common cause of amenorrhea in women of reproductive age, a pregnancy test is often the first test performed when a woman presents with this symptom. Once pregnancy is ruled out as a cause, a thorough review of systems is indicated.

Endocrine symptoms, such as hot flashes, night sweats, and vaginal dryness, associated with amenorrhea often indicate ovarian dysfunction. There are many factors that can cause the ovaries to stop working prematurely. These include history of radiation therapy or chemotherapy to treat cancer and unknown causes. Systemic symptoms may indicate disorders of the hypothalamus and pituitary. Factors that can interfere with normal hypothalamic function include excessive exercise; endocrine disorders, such as hyper- or hypothyroidism; human immunodeficiency virus/acquired immunodeficiency syndrome (HIV/AIDS); malnutrition; and major psychiatric disorders.

If there are no associated endocrine symptoms, the problem may be in the outflow tract. The ovaries may be functioning normally, but the endometrium may be scarred by adhesions (Asherman syndrome), so it does not respond to ovarian stimulation. Imperforate hymen or underdevelopment of the lower reproductive tract does not allow the menstrual flow to escape.

Medical intervention is based on a thorough assessment by physical examination, history taking, and laboratory testing to identify the underlying cause. Specific treatment is related to the underlying cause.

Atypical Uterine Bleeding

There are several types of atypical (abnormal) uterine bleeding. Heavy or prolonged bleeding, **menorrhagia**, is the most common menstrual complaint and can lead to anemia, if left untreated. **Metrorrhagia** refers to menstrual bleeding that is normal in amount but occurs at irregular intervals between menstrual periods. Metrorrhagia that occurs with hormonal contraceptives is called break-through bleeding. This type of bleeding frequently decreases over time.

Many of the factors that contribute to amenorrhea can also cause menorrhagia, including ovarian dysfunction. A thorough history and physical are indicated to rule out systemic causes. Other uterine conditions, such as polyps and fibroids, can cause menorrhagia. When causative factors cannot be found, a trial of oral progestin therapy may be initiated. If this therapy does not work, the primary care practitioner might insert an intrauterine device that releases progestin into the uterine cavity. The advantage of this therapy is that the hormones are released directly into the uterine cavity, so systemic levels remain low. Another therapy that may be used if traditional measures do not work is endometrial ablation, removal of the uterine lining. Hysterectomy, surgical removal of the uterus, remains a treatment option when other measures have failed.

This is worth noting. Pregnancy is the most common cause of abnormal bleeding during the reproductive years. Bear in mind that any woman of childbearing age who presents with atypical or irregular bleeding may be pregnant.

Dysmenorrhea

Dysmenorrhea is defined as painful or difficult menses. Primary dysmenorrhea refers to painful menstrual periods that cannot be attributed to a disease process. Secondary dysmenorrhea is painful menses secondary to pelvic pathology. This discussion focuses on primary dysmenorrhea, which is the more common of the two conditions. Secondary dysmenorrhea is discussed in conjunction with other disease states with which it occurs.

Don't get confused. Primary dysmenorrhea is not the same thing as premenstrual syndrome (PMS). A woman can have both conditions, but they are separate entities.

Primary dysmenorrhea is attributed to the action of prostaglandins on the uterus during ovulatory cycles. Prostaglandins contribute to dysmenorrhea in two ways. They cause the uterus to contract, which leads to painful cramping; and they decrease blood flow to the myometrium, which contributes to lactic acid buildup and additional pain.

Primary dysmenorrhea affects as many as 50% of women during their childbearing years (Alzubaidi, Calis, & Nelson, 2003). It occurs at a higher rate in younger women who have not borne children. As age and parity increase, the incidence of primary dysmenorrhea decreases. Risk factors that increase the severity of symptoms include earlier age at menarche, long and/or heavy menstrual flow, smoking, and a family history of the condition.

Clinical Manifestations

Primary dysmenorrhea typically begins within 6 months to 2 years after menarche. Severe intermittent cramping in association with constant pain in the lower abdomen, which may radiate to the lower back or upper thighs, is descriptive of the major symptoms. General malaise, fatigue, dizziness, nausea and vomiting, diarrhea, and headache frequently accompany the spasmodic cramping. Symptoms usually begin shortly before or with the onset of menstrual flow.

The primary care provider must rule out secondary dysmenorrhea before treatment can be initiated. A thorough history and physical and a pelvic examination are done, along with a variety of diagnostic procedures, to identify any underlying causes. If a causative factor is found, treatment is initiated to cure the underlying condition or control its symptoms. When no secondary cause is found, primary dysmenorrhea is diagnosed.

Treatment

The most effective treatments to date have been nonsteroidal anti-inflammatory drugs (NSAIDs) and oral contraceptives (birth control pills), given alone or in combination. NSAIDs, such as ibuprofen, naproxen, and meclofenamate, reduce symptoms by lowering prostaglandin levels and intrauterine pressure. NSAIDs are most effective when taken around the clock as soon as menstrual flow begins. They are less effective when taken on an as-needed basis. Gastrointestinal distress is the most common side effect.

Oral contraceptives relieve symptoms by inhibiting ovulation, which thins the endometrial lining and decreases prostaglandin production. Sometimes NSAIDs must be taken together with oral contraceptives to obtain adequate symptom control.

Alternative therapies that sometimes decrease dysmenorrhea include relaxation and massage, yoga, acupuncture, and herbal or homeopathic remedies.

Nursing Care

Nursing care of the woman with primary dysmenorrhea is directed toward education regarding the condition and its treatment and toward the effective relief of pain. Explain medication actions, common side effects, measures to reduce side effects, and timing of administration. Reassure the woman that sometimes medications have to be switched several times before the best therapy for her symptoms is determined. Reinforce that she should take her NSAIDs on a schedule, rather than waiting until the pain begins or becomes severe.

Several nonmedication interventions can help relieve the pain associated with dysmenorrhea. Heat can be soothing. Suggest the use of hot baths or heating pads. Sometimes changing positions can be helpful. Some women report relief when they assume a knee-chest position. Pain is usually less severe when the woman is in good general health. Encourage adequate exercise, diet, rest, and hygiene.

Test Yourself

- Define amenorrhea.
- What is the medical term for irregular menstrual flow?
- What is the difference between primary and secondary dysmenorrhea?

Premenstrual Syndrome

It is estimated that about 60% of all women experience premenstrual syndrome (PMS). PMS is characterized by physical and behavioral symptoms that occur cyclically during the last half of the menstrual cycle. Most likely to affect women in their 30s, it can occur as early as adolescence or as late as in the perimenopausal years.

Premenstrual dysphoric disorder (PMDD) is a more severe form of PMS. PMDD includes all of the physical symptoms of PMS with additional and more debilitating emotional symptoms. Approximately 5% of menstruating women are thought to experience PMDD.

Clinical Manifestations

PMS presents with a wide variety of symptoms, which may be physical, behavioral, or both (see Box 4-1). The symptoms can be highly distressing for the woman and her family. In making a diagnosis of PMS, the crucial component is the cyclical nature of the symptoms, as indicated in the following diagnostic criteria:

- Signs/symptoms must occur during the last half of the menstrual cycle.
- The woman should be asymptomatic before ovulation, and there must be at least 7 symptom-free days in each cycle.
- Symptoms reported must be severe enough to affect relationships, work, and daily lifestyle.
- Diagnosis must be made based on symptoms charted as they occur, rather than depending on recall of past experiences. PMS diaries are used for this purpose.

Typically, the severity of symptoms progresses over time. In the early stages of PMS, women describe symptoms beginning a few days before their period that stop when bleeding begins. With time, symptoms begin to appear 1 to 2 weeks before the onset of menses. Some women describe a cluster of symptoms occurring at the time of ovulation, followed by a symptom-free week, then a recurrence of symptoms a week before menses. PMS should not be equated with dysmenorrhea. Many women with symptoms of PMS have pain-free periods.

BOX 4.1 Signs and Symptoms of Premenstrual Syndrome (PMS)

Physical Symptoms
- Edema
- Weight gain
- Abdominal bloating
- Abdominal cramping
- Constipation
- Hot flashes
- Breast swelling and pain
- Headache, migraine
- Acne
- Rhinitis
- Exacerbation of pre-existing conditions (e.g., arthritis, lupus, ulcers)
- Heart palpitations
- Hives
- Joint swelling and pain
- Sore throat
- Urinary difficulties
- Seizures
- Asthma
- Bruising
- Coordination difficulties
- Back pain
- Fainting
- Nausea
- Alcohol intolerance

Behavioral Symptoms
- Aggressive behavior
- Emotional lability
- Confusion
- Depression
- Increased appetite
- Food cravings (salt, sweet) and binges
- Fatigue, lethargy
- Poor concentration
- Sex drive changes
- Suicidal thoughts
- Withdrawal from others
- Anxiety
- Rage
- Sleeplessness

Treatment

The cause of PMS remains unknown and is considered to be multifactorial, rather than arising from a single "cause." Pregnancy and menopause are the only true cures for PMS. Treatment is focused on alleviating the specific signs and symptoms. Vitamin B_6, calcium, and magnesium supplementation have been shown to be beneficial in some studies. Hormonal suppression of ovulation can be helpful, but side effects limit their long-term usefulness. Mild diuretics may reduce bloating. NSAIDs have been shown to relieve PMS symptoms. Naproxen sodium 500 mg/day is particularly beneficial. Antianxiety medications and stress-reduction techniques may also be prescribed.

PMDD responds to treatments similar to those used for PMS. In addition, low-dose antidepressant therapy during the last half of the cycle has been effective in treating the severe mood swings and other emotional problems that interfere with work productivity and social relationships.

Nursing Care

Assist the woman to find ways to decrease stress. Encourage regular exercise, even when she is experiencing symptoms. Exercise has been shown to decrease symptom severity. Encourage the reduction or elimination of caffeine and alcohol. Explain that limiting salt intake can decrease the symptoms of bloating. Family Teaching Tips: Relief Measures for PMS describes additional relief measures the nurse may recommend for the woman with PMS.

Endometriosis

Endometriosis is a painful reproductive and immunologic disorder in which tissue implants resembling endometrium grow outside of the uterus. The tissue implants respond to cyclic hormonal changes in a manner similar to that of endometrial tissue, causing menstrual-like internal bleeding that leads to inflammation,

FAMILY TEACHING TIPS

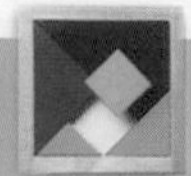

Relief Measures for PMS

DIET

- Reduce (or eliminate) caffeine intake (including coffee, tea, colas, and chocolate).
- Avoid simple sugars (as in candy, cakes, cookies).
- Reduce salt intake (pickles, fast foods, chips).
- Avoid alcohol.
- Drink 2 quarts of noncaffeinated fluid, preferably water, each day.
- Eat six small meals (to stabilize blood glucose levels).

EXERCISE

- Do aerobic exercise, such as walking or jogging, several times each week.

STRESS MANAGEMENT

- Note your pattern of PMS symptoms and alter your schedule to minimize stressors when symptoms are most severe.
- Utilize interventions such as relaxation techniques, massage, and warm baths.

SLEEP AND REST

- Maintain a regular sleep schedule.
- Drink a glass of milk before bedtime.
- Schedule exercise for early morning or early afternoon.
- Give yourself a quiet time to relax just before going to bed.

scarring, and adhesions in the pelvic and abdominal cavities. The condition occurs in 7% to 10% of women and is a leading cause of infertility and chronic pelvic pain. As many as 50% of the hysterectomies performed in the United States are done in an attempt to treat this debilitating disease.

Clinical Manifestations

Some women with advanced endometriosis are essentially asymptomatic and are unaware of the disease until the condition is observed during abdominal or pelvic surgery. Other women may experience debilitating, almost continuous pelvic pain, with only minimal abnormal tissue growth. Symptoms are typically most pronounced right before the onset of the period.

Cyclic pelvic pain that occurs in conjunction with menses is a classic symptom, as is menorrhagia. The pain and bleeding can involve the bladder, leading to hematuria, or can affect the bowel, leading to blood in the stools and painful defecation. Chronic pelvic pain, dysmenorrhea, and **dyspareunia**, painful intercourse, are other common symptoms. Although endometriosis appears to play a role in infertility for some women, others experience no apparent difficulty with conception.

Physical examination reveals pelvic tenderness, particularly during menses. Laparoscopy is the primary diagnostic tool for endometriosis. Advantages are that the characteristic endometrial lesions can be directly visualized and biopsies taken. Disadvantages include that laparoscopy is an invasive surgical technique.

Treatment

Medical therapy is aimed at suppressing ovulation and inducing an artificial menopause, with resulting suppression of abnormal tissue and relief of pain and other associated symptoms. This objective can be accomplished through the use of oral contraceptives; gonadotropin-releasing hormone (GnRH) agonists, such as goserelin and leuprolide; or danazol, a synthetic steroid analog (androgen) that inhibits luteinizing hormone (LH) and follicle-stimulating hormone (FSH). Side effects include symptoms associated with menopause, such as labile emotions, hot flashes, and vaginal dryness.

Surgical intervention can be conservative (reproductive function is maintained), semiconservative (destroys reproductive function, but maintains ovarian function), or radical, which involves removal of the uterus and ovaries. The goal of conservative surgery is to destroy the abnormal tissue while preserving reproductive ability. Laser or electrodiathermy techniques are used to ablate (destroy) the lesions.

Nursing Care

Pain is a common nursing diagnosis for the woman with endometriosis. Evaluate the character and severity of pain. Assist the woman to find ways to cope with and decrease pain. Encourage the use of analgesics, as ordered.

Provide emotional support. Allow the woman to ventilate. She may particularly have this need if the endometriosis is causing infertility problems. Encourage the woman to ask questions. Assist the woman and her family to make treatment decisions by providing information regarding treatment options to include advantages, disadvantages, possible risks, and likely outcomes of each option.

Infectious Disorders

Infections of the reproductive tract can cause permanent damage, such as infertility and chronic pelvic pain. Organisms that are transmitted sexually cause many of these infections. Sexually transmitted infections (STIs) are discussed in the pediatric portion of the text and in Chapters 16 and 40. Toxic shock syndrome (TSS) and pelvic inflammatory disease (PID) are covered in this section.

Toxic Shock Syndrome

Toxic shock syndrome (TSS) is a rare illness caused by an exotoxin produced by the bacteria *Staphylococcus aureus*. TSS was first recognized in 1978; the majority of cases occurred in women who were using certain types of high-absorbency tampons. Shortly thereafter, changes were made to the composition and absorbency of tampons, and TSS cases declined dramatically. However, women who use tampons, diaphragms, or contraceptive sponges are still at risk for the illness.

TSS starts suddenly with a high fever (greater than 102°F), nausea, vomiting, abdominal pain, a rapid drop in blood pressure, watery diarrhea, headache, sore throat, and muscle aches. Within 24 hours, a sunburn-like rash develops. The mucous membranes may turn a deep red. Treatment requires hospitalization, often in an intensive care setting, intravenous (IV) fluids, and antibiotics.

Nurses can be helpful in the prevention of TSS. Teach the woman who uses tampons to wash her hands thoroughly before and after inserting or removing tampons. She should use the lowest absorbency that will handle her menstrual flow, change tampons frequently (at least every 2 to 3 hours), or alternate tampons with sanitary napkins. Between periods, tampons should be stored away from heat and moisture, to help prevent bacterial growth. Any vaginal device, such as a diaphragm or vaginal sponge, should be removed frequently and cleaned.

Pelvic Inflammatory Disease

Pelvic inflammatory disease (PID) is a broad term used to refer to inflammation of any portion of a woman's reproductive tract, such as uterus, fallopian tubes, or ovaries. PID occurs most commonly in association with untreated STIs, in particular gonorrhea and chlamydia. Untreated PID can lead to scarring, ectopic (tubal) pregnancy, and chronic pelvic pain. Peritonitis and sepsis are other life-threatening complications. Each year in the United States more than 1 million women will have an acute episode of PID. Rates are highest for adolescent girls who have multiple sexual partners and do not use condoms.

Clinical Manifestations

Major symptoms include lower abdominal pain and abnormal vaginal discharge. Other symptoms include chills, fever, vomiting, dyspareunia, menorrhagia, dysmenorrhea, fatigue, loss of appetite, backache, and painful or frequent urination. Some women are asymptomatic but can still experience permanent damage.

Diagnosis is made by history and physical to include a pelvic examination. Generally specimens are collected and cultured for STIs. Other tests that may be ordered include ultrasound, endometrial biopsy, or laparoscopy.

Treatment

Often the exact organism cannot be cultured, so primary care practitioners prescribe at least two wide-spectrum antibiotics. Sometimes two courses of antibiotics are necessary. Approximately 75% of cases of PID can be treated on an outpatient basis. Occasionally, the woman must be hospitalized for the administration of IV antibiotics. Sex partners of the woman with PID must also be treated with antibiotics, even if they have no symptoms.

Nursing Care

Patient teaching is an important nursing function for the woman with PID. Discuss the transmission, treatment, and prevention of infection. Encourage the woman to take all of her antibiotics, even after she starts to feel better. Explain the use of any pain medications that are prescribed. Explain how important it is for her partner to be treated, as well. Instruct the woman to avoid sexual intercourse until the full course of antibiotics has been taken and her partner has been treated.

Instruct her on ways to prevent STIs and PID in the future because the more frequently she experiences these infections, the more likely the infection will lead to scarring and infertility. The best way to prevent PID is to avoid sexual intercourse or to remain in a monogamous relationship—in which both partners are sexually faithful to the other. The next best way is for the woman's partner to use latex condoms for every act of sexual intercourse. Diaphragms and other barrier methods afford some protection but are not as reliable as condoms. Douching should be avoided because it can force bacteria into the reproductive tract.

Disorders of the Uterus and Ovaries

Cervical Polyps

Cervical polyps are benign tumors that hang on a stem-like pedicle and protrude through the cervical os. Cervical polyps are associated with infection and chronic inflammation. Postcoital (after intercourse) bleeding, metrorrhagia, menorrhagia, and leukorrhea (white or yellow vaginal discharge) are associated symptoms. Cervical polyps can be visualized during a speculum examination of the cervix and may be removed during the procedure. Tissue is sent to pathology for microscopic examination. Antibiotics are usually prescribed prophylactically after the polyps are removed.

Uterine Fibroids

Uterine leiomyomata, or fibroids, as they are commonly called, are benign estrogen-responsive tumors of the uterine wall that regress with menopause. Many are asymptomatic; however, the tumors can enlarge and cause pelvic pressure, pain, and menstrual irregularities. Diagnosis is made via transvaginal or abdominal ultrasound, hysterosalpingogram (injection of dye into the uterine cavity through a cannula in the cervix, followed by x-ray), or hysteroscopy (insertion of a scope through the cervical canal into the uterine cavity).

Therapy depends on the symptoms and whether or not the woman wishes to retain fertility. Because estrogen and progesterone stimulate fibroid growth, hormonal contraceptives are not recommended for treatment. The presence of uterine fibroids is the most common reason cited for hysterectomy and may be the treatment of choice if future pregnancy is not desired. A less radical procedure, myomectomy, can be done via a hysteroscopic procedure. Laparoscopy can also be used to remove multiple fibroids. Myomectomy and laparoscopy can preserve fertility in some patients. A newer procedure, uterine fibroid embolization, also known as uterine artery embolization, uses a technique similar to heart catheterization to introduce a catheter into the uterine artery and then inject a substance that flows to the arteries supplying the fibroids and blocks them. The fibroids shrink after the procedure because of decreased blood supply.

Ovarian Cysts

Two types of functional ovarian cysts can develop: follicular and luteal. The type is dependent upon when in the menstrual cycle the cyst develops. Most ovarian cysts develop during the childbearing years; however, cysts are possible at any time in the female life cycle.

Ovarian cysts are usually benign but can lead to complications, such as hemorrhage (which can be life threatening), ovarian torsion (twisting), inflammation, necrosis, and bacterial infection leading to septic shock. Pelvic adhesions, infertility, and chronic pelvic pain syndrome are chronic complications that can occur. Transvaginal and abdominal ultrasound done simultaneously is the most effective method for diagnosing an ovarian cyst. Laparoscopy allows for diagnosis and removal of cysts. Medical therapy is accomplished with oral contraceptives, which regulate the menstrual cycle and may cause regression of a cyst or prevention of additional cyst formation.

Pelvic Support Disorders

The pelvic organs are held in place by three types of support: endopelvic fascia, ligaments, and paired muscle groups of the pelvic floor. These support structures function like a hammock to support the urethra, bladder, small intestine, rectum, uterus, and vagina. Problems occur when these support structures relax or weaken, causing the organs to drop down or protrude through the vaginal wall.

Pelvic support disorders are named according to the affected organ:

- Cystocele occurs when the bladder bulges into the front wall of the vagina.
- Rectocele occurs when the rectum protrudes into the back wall of the vagina.
- Enterocele occurs when the small intestine and peritoneum jut downward between the uterus and rectum.
- Uterine prolapse occurs when the uterus drops down into the vagina.

Figure 4-2 illustrates pelvic support disorders.

The most common causes of pelvic support disorders are pregnancy, vaginal birth, and aging. Some medical experts think cesarean birth may be protective against pelvic support disorders, although this theory is controversial. Other causes include obesity, chronic coughing, frequent straining during bowel movements, heavy lifting, hysterectomy, nerve disorders, injuries, and tumors.

Clinical Manifestations

Pelvic support disorders are basically hernias in which organs prolapse (abnormally protrude) through the weakened tissues of the support structure. Common symptoms are a feeling of heaviness or pressure in the vaginal area, or a feeling that something is dropping out of the vagina. Symptoms tend to occur when the woman is upright and may be relieved when she is in the recumbent position. Dyspareunia is sometimes present. In mild cases, the woman may be asymptomatic. Some symptoms are specific to a certain type of prolapse. A cystocele may lead to urinary incontinence, whereas a rectocele may cause constipation.

Diagnosis of pelvic floor disorders is usually made during a pelvic examination. The primary care practitioner may ask the woman to cough or bear down during the examination. The woman may also be examined while standing. Other tests may be done to test bladder or bowel functioning.

Treatment

Treatment is based on the type of pelvic floor dysfunction, the severity of the dysfunction, and symptoms the woman is experiencing. For mild cases that are asymptomatic, no treatment may be necessary. Often, when treatment is recommended, it is helpful to start with less invasive techniques and then progress to more invasive techniques, as needed.

Kegel exercises can be done to strengthen pelvic floor muscles and improve tone. A pessary is a device that comes in various sizes and shapes that can be inserted into the vagina to hold pelvic organs in place. It must be fitted by the primary care practitioner and taken out periodically by the woman to be cleaned with soap and water and then reinserted.

Surgical techniques are often necessary to treat pelvic support disorders. Hysterectomy may be done

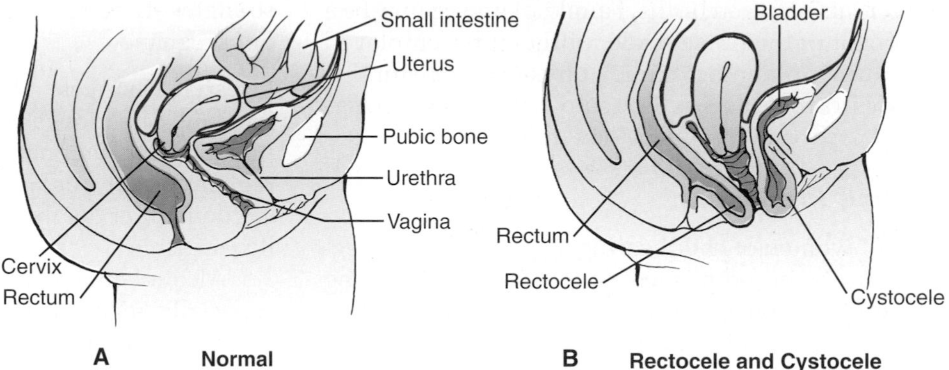

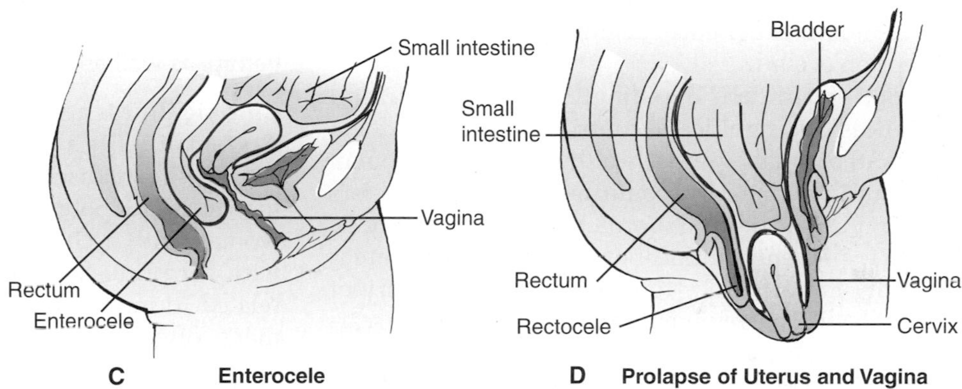

● ***Figure 4.2*** Pelvic support disorders. (**A**) Normal pelvic anatomy. (**B**) A cystocele occurs when the bladder bulges into the anterior vaginal wall. A rectocele develops when the muscles of the posterior vaginal wall weaken and the rectum and posterior vaginal wall protrude into the vagina. (**C**) An enterocele occurs when the small intestine and peritoneum protrude between the uterus and rectum into the posterior vaginal wall. (**D**) Prolapse of the uterus occurs when the uterus drops down into the vagina.

for uterine prolapse. During hysterectomy, other pelvic support disorders may also be repaired.

Nursing Care

Teach the woman to do Kegel exercises regularly. The muscles used to stop the stream of urine are tightly squeezed and held tightly while the woman counts to 10. The exercise is repeated 10 to 20 times in a row several times per day. A woman can perform Kegel exercises discreetly wherever she happens to be. They can be performed while sitting, standing, or lying down.

Teach the woman to recognize signs of urinary tract infection (UTI): pain or burning upon urination, urinary frequency and urgency, and cloudy urine. The woman with a cystocele is at higher risk for UTI. Other measures to prevent infection are to drink plenty of fluids, including fruit juices, to wipe from front to back after using the bathroom, and to get enough rest.

Test Yourself

- Name five symptoms of PMS.
- What is endometriosis?
- List three ways to prevent PID.

REPRODUCTIVE LIFE CYCLE ISSUES

Life cycle issues related to reproduction are present throughout the life span. Major milestones include prenatal differentiation of reproductive organs, growth and development of reproductive organs during childhood, maturation of the reproductive system in adolescence, reproductive capability during early and middle adulthood, declining reproductive capability during middle adulthood, and the end of reproductive capability in late middle to older adulthood. This section addresses issues directly related to reproductive functioning.

FAMILY PLANNING

Family planning consists of two complementary components: planning pregnancy and preventing pregnancy. Family planning gives the woman control over the number of children she wishes to have and allows her to determine when births will occur in relation to each other and in relation to her age and/or the age of the father. Women and couples can avoid unwanted pregnancies, bring about wanted births, and control the intervals between births. Family planning may be a component of the nurse's role for the nurse employed in a family planning clinic, physician or nurse—midwife practice, and in the acute care setting, such as in the postpartum or gynecology units.

Planning Pregnancy

For most women of childbearing age, planning a pregnancy can be accomplished simply by discontinuing the use of contraception. However, pregnancy planning should include "prepregnancy" planning. The condition of the woman before pregnancy affects pregnancy outcome. Therefore, a healthy pregnancy begins well in advance of conception. Pregnancy can be seen as a 12-month experience, beginning 3 months before conception occurs.

Good health and avoiding exposure to harmful substances are significant contributing factors for a successful pregnancy and a healthy baby. If the woman waits until pregnancy is confirmed to remedy factors that can put her or an unborn child at risk, it may be too late to prevent complications. Preconception care is especially important for the woman with a history of problems with a previous pregnancy, such as miscarriage or preterm labor or birth. In many cases causative factors can be identified and treated, reducing the risk for problems in subsequent pregnancies. Preconception care is equally important for the woman with a chronic medical condition, family history of genetic disorders, or any other factor that might increase the risk associated with pregnancy and childbirth.

Areas of Focus for Pregnancy Planning

Because a woman may not realize she is pregnant during the early and vulnerable weeks of fetal development, any woman of childbearing age should be aware of health problems or medication regimens that may adversely affect pregnancy and the birth of a healthy baby. There are several key areas upon which the woman and her partner should focus while planning for a pregnancy. These areas include nutrition and exercise, lifestyle changes, chronic illness and genetic disorders, and medications.

Nutrition and Exercise

It is recommended for women to optimize their intake of folic acid several months before becoming pregnant. Folate occurs naturally in foods such as dark green leafy vegetables and legumes. Ideally, daily dietary intake should supply a minimum of 400 micrograms. If needed, folic acid supplements can be taken to meet daily requirements.

Regular aerobic exercise conditions the heart, lungs, muscles, and other organs in preparation for the increased demands of pregnancy. Exercise can also be helpful in building up low-back and abdominal strength—two areas that can cause discomfort throughout pregnancy.

Lifestyle Changes

Smoking cessation is an important consideration when planning for pregnancy. Women who smoke are at higher risk for miscarriage, lower infant birth weight, sudden infant death syndrome, and infant respiratory illnesses.

Alcohol intake can affect the developing child, especially in the earliest weeks of pregnancy. Fetal alcohol syndrome is now recognized as a cause of serious and irreversible birth defects, particularly mental underdevelopment. The level of alcohol intake that causes birth defects to occur is unknown, so women of childbearing age are advised to abstain from alcohol before, as well as during, pregnancy.

Chronic Illness and Genetic Disorders

A woman with a chronic illness, such as diabetes, asthma, heart disease, or high blood pressure, is at higher risk for poor pregnancy outcome. Therefore, the woman with a chronic disorder will need to consult with her primary care physician about possible risks related to medications or therapies. Medication regimens often can be adjusted before pregnancy to decrease the risk to the woman and her fetus.

Referral for genetic counseling may be indicated for the following reasons: The woman or her partner has a genetic disorder. Either partner is known to be a carrier for a genetic condition. A previous child was born with a genetic syndrome or when there is a strong family history of a genetically transmitted disorder.

Medications

Be very careful! In no case should a woman discontinue or change her prescribed medication regimen without discussing it first with her primary care provider, even if she suspects she is pregnant. In some conditions, the risk to the baby or mother of an uncontrolled medical condition outweighs the possible risk of medication side effects.

Many medications cross the placenta easily and can cause birth defects. Prepregnancy planning includes assessment of medications the woman is taking. This assessment allows for timely adjustments in dosage or alterations in choice of medication.

Nursing Care

Nurses, especially those working in settings such as clinics or doctors' offices or in public health, play an important role in pregnancy planning and preconception care. A major nursing focus of preconception care is education and counseling, which may be offered

BOX 4.2 Nursing Assessment for Preconception Care

Nursing assessment for preconception care includes a complete health history for the woman and her partner, addressing specific concerns such as

- **Lifestyle:** tobacco, alcohol, caffeine, and drug use; prescription or over-the-counter medication use; exposure to toxins such as chemicals or radiation; exercise and rest patterns
- **Nutrition:** a 1- to 3-day meal diary; behaviors such as eating nonfood substances or binging or purging; special diets; dietary supplements; food intolerances; current weight and recent weight loss or gain
- **Medical history:** chronic diseases such as diabetes, hypertension, kidney disease, cardiac disease, asthma, and thyroid disease
- **Infectious disease history:** sexually transmitted infections (STIs); immune status related to rubella; risk for exposure to cytomegalovirus (CMV) or toxoplasmosis; risk for HIV/AIDS or hepatitis B
- **Reproductive history:** sexual history; menstrual, uterine, or cervical abnormalities; previous miscarriage or fetal deaths; previous preterm births; infants with birth weight less than 5½ pounds; infants requiring care in a neonatal intensive care unit (NICU); infants with birth defects or congenital anomalies
- **Family history:** genetic disease or birth defects such as cystic fibrosis, sickle-cell anemia, and phenylketonuria (PKU); consanguinity with partner; ethnic or racial background
- **Sociocultural history:** cultural/religious concerns; support systems; financial needs; the couples' relationship and readiness for parenting; availability of family or other support system; maternal age; socioeconomic status; readiness for pregnancy

through individual counseling or in traditional classroom settings. The nurse also may be responsible for gathering the woman's and her partner's health histories, including current health status and lifestyle practices (Box 4-2).

Nursing interventions include anticipatory guidance or teaching, discussing issues such as risk behaviors or risk factors and corrective or preventative measures. Nutrition and exercise are important concerns for the woman planning to become pregnant. Advise the woman to consume a nutritious diet that provides all essential nutrients, with emphasis on calcium, iron, folic acid, protein, B-complex vitamins, vitamin C, and magnesium. Exercise that includes aerobic conditioning and muscle toning will improve circulation and general health. The woman should continue her current exercise plan or establish a routine beginning at least 3 months before she plans to become pregnant. Encourage the woman who is trying to become

FAMILY TEACHING TIPS

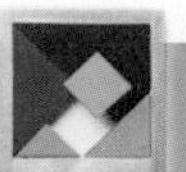

Pregnancy Planning

At least 3 months before attempting to conceive:

- Stop or considerably reduce smoking.
- Stop or considerably reduce alcohol consumption.
- Stop use of recreational drugs.
- Eat a healthy diet that is rich in protein, calcium, iron, and zinc.
- Avoid raw meats. Be sure to thoroughly wash your hands before and after handling raw meat.
- Take folic acid tablets (400 micrograms per day) to supplement the folate in a diet that includes leafy green vegetables, beans, and whole-wheat breads. Vitamin B complex is also beneficial.
- Begin a regular exercise program that includes aerobic conditioning.
- Share with your primary care provider any family history of genetic disorders or history of recurrent pregnancy loss.
- Know your rubella and varicella (chickenpox) immunity status and get vaccinated several months in advance of conception, if susceptible to either disease.
- Avoid exposure to X-rays.
- Consult your primary care provider about existing medical conditions or medications.

pregnant to follow the recommendations in Family Teaching Tips: Pregnancy Planning.

Preventing Pregnancy

Planning pregnancy means that steps must be taken to prevent pregnancy when it is not desired. Serious negative health consequences may result from unplanned pregnancy. Also, it has been estimated that up to one-half of all unplanned pregnancies are terminated by induced abortion (Mishell, Burkman, Shulman, Westhoff, & Wysocki, 2002). Even so, approximately 50% of pregnancies in the United States are unplanned. Of those that are unplanned, more than half of the couples were using some form of contraception when conception occurred (Hutti, 2003).

When pregnancy happens despite contraceptive use, either the method is imperfect (method failure) or the individual does not use the method perfectly (user error). Contraceptive methods are graded based on their perfect use and typical use failure rates. Perfect use describes a contraceptive method that is used exactly as directed 100% of the time. Typical use accommodates humans' tendency to forget or make errors. Generally speaking, perfect use has a lower associated failure rate than does typical use. Table 4-1 compares the failure rates of major contraceptive methods.

TABLE 4.1 Comparison of Selected Contraceptive Methods: Failure Rates and STI Protection

The failure rate is reported as a percentage. The number listed represents the number of women who become pregnant for every 100 women who use the method.

Contraceptive Method	Failure Rates With Typical Use*	Failure Rates With Perfect Use†	Protection From STIs When Used Correctly
Natural Methods			
Unprotected intercourse (leaving it to chance)	15%	15%	None
Abstinence	Unknown	0%	Completely protective
Coitus interruptus (withdrawal)	27%	4%	May offer some protection
Fertility awareness methods (FAM)	12%–22%	1%–5%	None
Barrier Methods			
Spermicides (nonoxynol-9)	2%–59%	6%	May actually increase risk by causing genital irritation
Male condom	15%	2%	Highly protective
Female condom	21%	5%	Offers fair protection
Diaphragm	16%	6%	Offers some protection
Cervical cap (nulliparous woman)	16%	9%	Offers some protection
Cervical cap (multiparous woman)	32%	26%	Offers some protection
Hormonal Methods			
Combination (estrogen/progestin) oral contraceptives (COCs)	5%	0.1%	None
Progestin-only pills (POPs or the "mini-pill")	5%	0.5%	None
Every-3-months hormonal injections (Depo-Provera)	3%	0.3%	None
Combined monthly hormonal injections (Lunelle)	3%	0.05%	None
Single rod hormonal implant (Implanon)	0%‡	0%	None
Hormonal implant (Norplant)	0.05%	0.05%	None
Transdermal patch (Ortho Evra)	0.8%	0.6%	None
Vaginal ring (NuvaRing)	0.65%	0.65%	
Intrauterine Devices			
IUD (copper)	0.8%	0.6%	None
IUD (levonorgestrel-releasing system)	0.1%	0.1%	None
Sterilization			
Female sterilization (tubal ligation)	0.5%	0.5%	None
Male sterilization (vasectomy)	0.15%	0.10%	None

* Typical use refers to percentage of women who have an accidental pregnancy during the first year of using the method in a typical manner.

† Perfect use refers to the percentage of women who experience an accidental pregnancy during the first year while using the method as directed 100% of the time.

‡ No pregnancies have been reported to date with Implanon, although women are cautioned that no method of birth control is 100% effective (Hutti, 2003).

Table adapted from the following sources: Managing Contraception (produced by The Bridging the Gap Foundation) http://www.sexualetiquette101.com/§; Planned Parenthood website (www.plannedparenthood.org)§; Cwiak, C., & Zieman, M. (2003). New methods in contraception: A review of their advantages and disadvantages. *Women's Health in Primary Care, 6*(10), 473–478; Fehring, R. J. (2004). The future of professional education in natural family planning. *JOGNN, 33*(2), 34–43; Hutti, M. H. (2003). New and emerging contraceptive methods: Nurses can help women make wise choices. *AWHONN Lifelines,* 7(1), 32–39; Nissl, J. (2003). Healthwise knowledgebase topic: Hormone injections for birth control. Palo Alto Medical Foundation: A Sutter Health Affiliate. Melnikow, J., Hatcher, R.A., & Jones, K. (Medical reviewers). Retrieved April 10, 2004, from http://www.pamf.org/teen/healthinfo/index.cfm?section=healthinfo& page=article&sgml_id=hw239088.

§All website references were retrieved April 2004.

The woman who wishes to defer or avoid pregnancy has a wide variety of contraceptive methods from which to choose. An ideal method of contraception is one that is effective, easy to understand and use, and acceptable to both partners. There should be minimal side effects and low risk of sequelae. Ideally, the contraceptive should not be related directly with lovemaking and should not interfere with sexual pleasure. It should be inexpensive and easy to maintain. Protection from sexually transmitted infections (STIs) is an additional consideration. Reversible methods should allow the couple to conceive readily after discontinuing use of the method.

Natural Methods

A natural contraceptive method refers to any method that does not use hormones, pharmaceutical compounds, or physical barriers that block sperm from entering the uterus. Natural methods of birth control include abstinence, coitus interruptus, and natural family planning.

Abstinence

Abstinence, as related to birth control, means refraining from vaginal sexual intercourse. Abstinence can include other means of sexual stimulation, such as oral sex. Complete, or strict, abstinence refers to the avoidance of all sexual contact. Abstinence is a normal and acceptable alternative to sexual intercourse, especially for teens and singles in noncommittal relationships. The use of complete abstinence as a method of birth control has no cost, is readily available, and is the only 100% effective method for preventing pregnancy and STIs. A major drawback is that it can be difficult to maintain abstinence. A couple may make a rash decision during the heat of passion, which may leave the woman without a means of preventing pregnancy.

Coitus Interruptus

Coitus interruptus, also called withdrawal, requires the man to pull the penis out of the vagina before ejaculation to avoid depositing sperm in or near the vagina. However, the pre-ejaculate fluid may contain sperm, so pregnancy can occur. Effectiveness is dependent on the male partner's ability to withdraw his penis before ejaculation.

One advantage of coitus interruptus is that it provides some level of protection when no other method is available. However, the disadvantages are many. This is an unreliable method of birth control (see Table 4-1), and it offers no protection from STIs. This method requires a great deal of self-control on the part of the male partner and cannot be used if the man ejaculates prematurely. It is not recommended for sexually inexperienced men or adolescents (Planned Parenthood, Undated).

Fertility Awareness Methods

Fertility awareness methods (FAM) refer to all methods that use the identification of fertile and infertile phases of a woman's cycle to plan or prevent pregnancy. Such methods involve observing and charting the signs and symptoms of the menstrual cycle (e.g., menstrual bleeding, cervical mucus changes, and variations in basal body temperature) through the use of one or a combination of several methods to determine the woman's fertile period. Then abstinence or a barrier contraceptive method is used during days identified as fertile to reduce the risk of pregnancy. FAM is also used to plan pregnancy.

FAM is the only method of birth control that requires the cooperation of both partners. Many couples who prefer a natural, mutual method of preventing pregnancy find cooperation to be an empowering component of the method, giving them control of their fertility and encouraging shared responsibility. Advantages of these methods are that they are inexpensive, do not require the use of artificial devices or drugs, and have no harmful side effects. Disadvantages include that the method requires discipline to use and can seem cumbersome for a woman or couple with a busy lifestyle. It also has a high failure rate during the first year with typical use.

A foundational component for practicing FAM is knowledge about the menstrual cycle. Guidelines derive from the assumption that ovulation occurs exactly 14 days before the onset of the next menstrual cycle, and that the fertile window extends 3 to 4 days before and after ovulation, or in other words, between days 10 and 17 of the menstrual cycle. Four methods used to anticipate the fertile window are:

1. Calendar method
2. Basal body temperature method
3. Cervical mucus method
4. Symptothermal method

In addition to these four methods, some couples use an ovulation predictor test to determine ovulation and thus the fertile period.

Calendar Method. With the calendar method, fertile days are determined by an accurate charting of the length of the menstrual cycle over a period of 6 months. The number of days per cycle is counted, beginning on the first day of menses. The beginning of the fertile period is determined by subtracting 18 days from the length of the shortest cycle. The end of the fertile days is determined by subtracting 11 days from the length of the longest cycle. An example of how the fertile period is calculated using this method is found in Box 4-3. To avoid pregnancy, the couple abstains from sexual intercourse or uses a barrier method during the identified fertile period.

The major drawbacks of this method are that the couple is using data about past cycles to predict what

BOX 4.3 Calculation of Fertile Window Using the Calendar Method

A woman keeps track of the length of her menstrual cycles for at least 6 months. Then she calculates her fertile window by subtracting 18 days from her shortest cycle and 11 days from her longest cycle. For a woman whose shortest cycle is 24 days and longest cycle is 28 days, the calculation would be as follows:

Shortest cycle	Longest cycle
24	28
−18	−11
6	17

Therefore, the woman's fertile window would be days 6 to 17 of her menstrual cycle. She and her partner would then use abstinence or a barrier method to prevent pregnancy during the fertile window.

will happen in the future, and they are counting on the regularity of what can be an unpredictable event. In reality, the timing of the fertile period can be highly variable, even for women who consider their cycles to be regular. Wilcox, Dunson, and Baird (2000) found that more than 70% of women are in their fertile period before day 10 and/or after day 17 of their menstrual cycle. Thus, there are very few days during the menstrual cycle during which some women are not potentially fertile.

The method is contraindicated for women who do not have regular cycles, such as women who are anovulatory (absence of ovulation), adolescents, women approaching menopause, and women who have recently given birth.

Basal Body Temperature Method. The basal body temperature (BBT) is the lowest normal temperature of a healthy person, taken immediately after waking and before getting out of bed. The BBT method is based on the principle of identifying the shift in body temperature that occurs normally around the time of ovulation.

The BBT ranges from 36.2°C to 36.3°C during menses, and for about 5 to 7 days after. At about the time of ovulation, a slight drop in temperature may be observed, followed by a slight rise (approximately 0.2°C to 0.4°C) after ovulation in response to increasing progesterone levels. This temperature elevation persists until 2 to 4 days before menstruation. The BBT then drops to the lower levels recorded during the previous cycle, unless pregnancy occurs. The drop and subsequent rise in BBT is called the thermal shift.

To prevent conception, the couple avoids unprotected intercourse from the day the BBT drops through the fourth day of temperature elevation. The BBT must be charted daily on a graph for an entire month to accurately perceive a pattern in BBT. Confounding factors such as fatigue, infection, anxiety, awakening late, getting fewer than 3 hours sleep, jet lag, alcohol consumption, and sleeping in a heated waterbed or using an electric heating blanket, may all cause temperature fluctuation, altering the expected pattern. Because so many factors can interfere, BBT alone is not a reliable method for predicting ovulation but should be used along with the calendar or cervical mucus methods.

Cervical Mucus Method. The cervical mucus method, also called the Billings method or the Creighton ovulation method, requires recognition and interpretation of characteristic changes in the amount and consistency of cervical mucus through the menstrual cycle. Accurate assessment of cervical mucus requires that the mucus be free of contraceptive gel or foam, semen, blood, or abnormal vaginal discharge for at least one full cycle.

Before ovulation cervical mucus is thick and does not stretch easily. This quality inhibits sperm from entering the cervix. Just before ovulation, changes occur that facilitate the viability and motility of sperm, allowing the sperm to survive in the female reproductive tract until ovulation. Cervical mucus becomes more abundant and thinner with an elastic quality. It feels somewhat slippery and can be stretched 5 centimeters or more between the thumb and forefinger, a quality referred to as **spinnbarkeit** (Fig. 4-3). These cervical mucus changes indicate the period of maximum fertility.

Observation begins on the last day of menses and is done several times a day for several cycles. Because

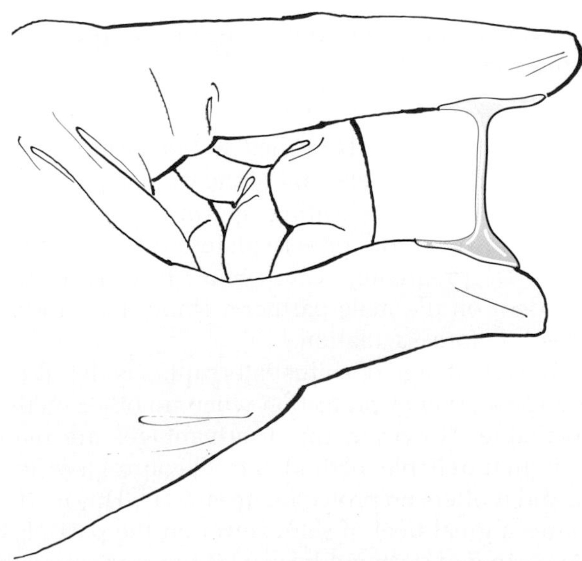

● ***Figure 4.3*** Spinnbarkeit refers to the stretchable, distensible quality of cervical mucus around the time of ovulation. Some fertility awareness methods (FAM) rely on this quality to help determine when ovulation has occurred.

mucus can be obtained at the vaginal introitus, there is no need to attempt to reach into the vagina to the cervix. Confounding factors include the presence of sperm, contraceptive gels or foam, vaginal discharge, use of douches or vaginal deodorants, sexual arousal, and medications such as antihistamines. Although self-evaluation of cervical mucus can help the woman to predict ovulation, the effectiveness of this method is enhanced when it is used in combination with the calendar and/or BBT methods. This method may be unacceptable for the woman who is uncomfortable touching her genitals.

Symptothermal Method. The symptothermal method is a combination of the calendar, BBT, and cervical mucus methods, along with an awareness of other signs of fertility. The woman acquires fertility awareness as she understands the secondary physiologic and psychological symptoms marking the phases of her cycle. These secondary symptoms include increased libido, midcycle spotting, mittelschmerz (unilateral lower abdominal pain in the ovary region associated with ovulation), pelvic fullness or tenderness, and vulvar fullness. The woman may palpate the cervix to assess for changes that normally occur with ovulation. The cervical os dilates slightly, the cervix softens and rises in the vagina, and cervical mucus becomes abundant with a slippery consistency. Calendar calculations and cervical mucus changes are used to approximate the beginning of the fertile period. Changes in cervical mucus and BBT are used to predict the end of the fertile period. Some studies have demonstrated a lower failure rate when multiple indicators are used to predict the fertile window (Fehring, 2004).

Ovulation Predictor Test. The Ovulation Predictor Test is a handheld device that detects metabolites of luteinizing hormone (LH) and estrogen in the urine. LH levels surge during the 12 to 24 hours before ovulation, and the test is designed to detect the increase. The home kit supplies testing materials for testing the urine over several days during a cycle. A positive reaction for LH is indicated by an easily read color change. Currently in the United States, the device is used to determine ovulation so that the woman can increase her changes of becoming pregnant. However, research is ongoing to determine the usefulness of the device as a contraceptive method.

Other Natural Methods

Other natural methods used to try to prevent pregnancy include douching after intercourse and breast-feeding. Douching is not reliable for preventing pregnancy; on the contrary, it may actually increase the chance of pregnancy by propelling sperm farther into the birth canal. Breast-feeding suppresses ovulation only if the woman is nursing at least 10 feedings per 24-hour period. Ovulation is suppressed by the release of prolactin, which stimulates milk production. Should the woman supplement with bottle feedings or solid foods, milk production and prolactin secretion will decrease, which may allow ovulation to occur.

Barrier Methods

Barrier methods of contraception provide a physical barrier, chemical barrier, or both to prevent sperm from entering the cervical os. Types of barrier methods of contraception include spermicidal gels or foams, condoms, diaphragms, and cervical caps. Spermicidal gels or foams are used frequently in conjunction with condoms, diaphragms, and cervical caps to increase effectiveness (see Table 4-1). Many barrier method contraceptives have the added benefit of providing at least some protection against STIs.

Spermicides

Spermicides provide a physical barrier that prevents sperm penetration and a chemical barrier that kills the sperm. The most commonly used chemical spermicide in the United States is nonoxynol-9 (N-9). Spermicides are available as aerosol foams, foaming tablets, suppositories, films, creams, and gels. Most of these products are designed to be inserted vaginally immediately before or within a few hours before engaging in vaginal sexual intercourse.

Although early research seemed to indicate that N-9 provided some protection against STIs, the World Health Organization (WHO) and Centers for Disease Control (CDC) recommend against relying on N-9 products for this protection. In fact, the WHO and CDC warn that spermicide use might actually increase the risk of STIs by creating irritation and breakdown of the protective vaginal or anal mucosa. N-9 is appropriate for contraceptive use in the woman who is at low risk for contracting HIV and who does not engage in multiple daily acts of vaginal or anal intercourse (Planned Parenthood, 2002). The effectiveness of spermicides can be greatly increased by combining them with other physical barrier methods, such as the condom, diaphragm, or cervical cap.

Advantages include that this method is readily available without a prescription. Spermicides can be inserted several hours before vaginal sexual intercourse and so can be used discreetly by the woman. Some disadvantages are that effectiveness rates are highly variable (see Table 4-1) and the method does not protect against (and may actually enhance) the transmission of STIs.

Male Condom

The male condom is a thin, stretchable sheath that covers the erect penis during sexual intercourse. A condom functions as a contraceptive by collecting semen before, during, and after ejaculation to prevent sperm from entering the vagina and causing pregnancy. The majority of condoms are made of latex rubber, although a small percentage is composed of other substances, such as natural membrane or polyurethane. Additional features in condoms manufactured in the United States include shape, and the addition of lubricants and spermicides. One feature related to shape is the presence or absence of a sperm reservoir tip. Some condoms are contoured, rippled, or have a roughened surface to enhance vaginal stimulation. A thinner sheath increases heat transmission and penile sensitivity. Some condoms are prelubricated with a wet jelly or a dry powder, and some have spermicide added to the interior or exterior surface. Effectiveness is dependent upon correct and consistent application and usage (see Table 4-1).

One significant advantage is the protection condoms afford against STIs. Condoms can be used as an additional protective measure against the transmission of HIV and other STIs, even when another method of contraception is used for birth control (such as oral contraceptives or barrier methods). Other advantages include low cost, easy availability, no prescription or physician visit needed, and condoms can be put on as part of sexual play. Some men find condom use helpful in preventing premature ejaculation or maintaining an erection for a longer period of time.

There are also disadvantages. The condom can break, which decreases its effectiveness. Some couples find that condoms decrease sexual sensation. Condom use can also be perceived as inhibiting spontaneity, or the man may feel self-conscious. Another potential disadvantage is latex allergy; however, polyurethane condoms can be used if this is an issue (see Family Teaching Tips: Safe Condom Use in Chapter 27).

Female Condom

The female condom, or vaginal sheath, is a thin tube made of polyurethane, with flexible rings at both ends. The closed end is inserted into the vagina and anchored around the cervix. The open end covers the labia. Like the male condom, the female condom collects sperm before, during, and after ejaculation to protect against pregnancy and STIs. The condom can be applied before intercourse, a feature that may increase spontaneity. Before intercourse, a spermicide can be added, if not already present. The female condom comes in one size and, like the male condom, is available without a prescription.

Advantages of the female condom are that it can be inserted before intercourse, an erection is not necessary to keep the condom in place, individuals who are allergic to latex can use it, and the external ring may supply clitoral stimulation. Reported disadvantages are that the condom may be difficult to apply, makes noise, causes vaginal or penile irritation, or it may slip into the vagina during vigorous intercourse, a condition that decreases its effectiveness.

Diaphragm and Cervical Cap

The diaphragm is a shallow dome-shaped latex rubber device with a flexible, circular wire rim that fits over the cervix. The wire rim may be flat, coiled, arcing, or wide seal. A diaphragm works by mechanically blocking sperm from entering the cervix. Spermicide, which must be used with the diaphragm to provide optimal protection, interferes with sperm motility.

Diaphragms are available by prescription in a wide range of diameters between 50 and 90 millimeters. They require special fitting by a trained practitioner. The woman must apply spermicidal jelly or cream to the rim and center of the diaphragm before inserting and positioning the diaphragm over the cervix (Fig. 4-4). A diaphragm may be inserted several hours before intercourse, and must be left in place over the cervix for at least 6 hours afterward to allow the spermicide time to destroy the sperm. If the device is inserted and more than 6 hours passes before sexual intercourse, or if intercourse is repeated, the woman should leave the diaphragm in place and insert another application of spermicidal cream, jelly, or foam into the vagina. A diaphragm should not be left in place for longer than 24 hours.

The cervical cap is much smaller than the diaphragm and is available in four sizes between 21 and 31 millimeters. Its rubber dome has a firm, pliable rim that fits snugly around the base of the cervix, close to the junction of the cervix and the vaginal fornices. The device should remain in place 6 to 8 hours after the last act of intercourse, but not longer than 48 hours. The seal of the cap provides a mechanical barrier. Spermicide applied in the center of the cap provides an additional chemical barrier.

The typical failure rates for both devices are similar for nulliparous women. However, the failure rate of the cervical cap in the multiparous woman is quite high (see Table 4-1). A primary health care provider must specifically fit the diaphragm or cervical cap to each woman. Both devices must be refitted after pregnancy (whether it ends in miscarriage, abortion, or delivery), abdominal or pelvic surgery, and weight gain or loss of 10 or more pounds. The woman must learn how to insert and remove the cap or diaphragm correctly and to verify proper placement. Before insertion, the woman should check either device for pinholes or weakened areas by holding it up to the light.

Here's a teaching tip for diaphragm use. Additional spermicidal jelly or cream must be inserted into the vagina if the woman has intercourse again within 6 hours. With the cervical cap, using additional spermicide for repeated episodes of intercourse is optional.

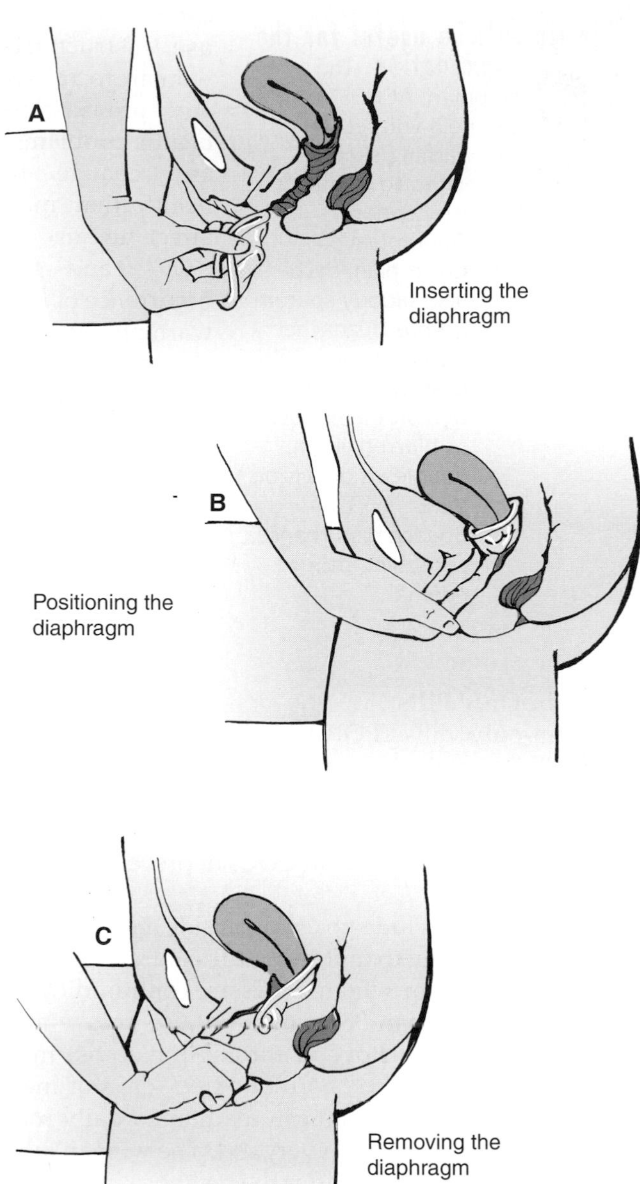

● ***Figure 4.4*** Application of a diaphragm. (**A**) To insert, fold the diaphragm in half, separate the labia with one hand, then insert upwards and back into the vagina. (**B**) To position, make certain the diaphragm securely covers the cervix. (**C**) To remove, hook a finger over the top of the rim and bring the diaphragm down and out.

Typical advantages for the use of diaphragms and cervical caps are that both devices offer some protection against STIs and pelvic inflammatory disease (PID). Both may be inserted ahead of time and are not easily felt by either partner, and therefore do not readily interfere with the spontaneity of love-making. Both methods can be used during breast-feeding and are immediately reversible.

Disadvantages unique to the diaphragm are that some sexual positions, penis sizes, and vigorous thrusting techniques can dislodge the device during intercourse, thus decreasing its effectiveness. Also, some women develop frequent bladder infections or cannot use the diaphragm because of poor vaginal tone. Disadvantages of both methods are that they can be difficult to insert and the woman must feel comfortable touching her genitals. Also, in rare instances women have developed toxic shock syndrome (TSS) with the use of these devices.

Hormonal Methods

Hormonal methods of contraception include oral contraceptives, implants, injections, vaginal ring, and transdermal patches. Depending on their hormonal composition, all hormonal methods prevent or suppress ovulation; thicken cervical mucus, making it resistant to sperm penetration; and create an inhospitable uterine environment, preventing implantation of any fertilized ovum, although this third mechanism of action is reported to occur rarely.

Advantages of hormonal contraceptives are that they are highly effective in preventing pregnancy (see Table 4-1) when used consistently and correctly. Several hormonal methods provide noncontraceptive health benefits, such as menstrual cycle improvements, management of perimenopause, and protection against certain cancers, ovarian cysts, ectopic pregnancy, pelvic inflammatory disease (PID), and acne (Davidson, 2003).

Although efficacious in preventing pregnancy, there are disadvantages to the use of hormonal methods of contraception. Sixty percent of new users discontinue hormonal methods during the first year of use because of experienced or perceived side effects (Hutti, 2003). In addition, hormonal contraceptives do not offer protection from STIs, including HIV, for either partner. Therefore, condoms should be used if STI protection is desired.

Combination Oral Contraceptives

Combination oral contraceptives (COCs), also known as "the pill," are the most commonly used reversible method of contraception (Mishell et al., 2002). COCs can be monophasic or phasic. Monophasic pills provide fixed doses of estrogen and progestin, whereas phasic pills (biphasic, triphasic, and multiphasic) are formulated to alter the amount of progestin, and in some cases, estrogen, within each cycle. Phasic preparations reduce the total dosage of hormones in a cycle, without sacrificing effectiveness. COCs are available in 21- or 28-day packs. If the woman uses a 21-day pack, she takes a pill each day for 21 days, then stops for 7 days. With the 28-day pack, a pill is taken daily throughout the cycle. The last 7 pills of the 28-pill pack are inert but help maintain the habit of taking the daily pill. Menstruation occurs during the time of pill withdrawal or when the inert pills are taken. Some practitioners are prescribing longer regimens of COCs to suppress menstruation while also providing birth control. COCs should be taken at the same time each day.

If taken daily as prescribed, COCs provide a high contraception effectiveness rate (see Table 4-1). In addition, COCs therapy offers many noncontraceptive benefits, in particular menstrual cycle improvements, including a decrease in menstrual blood loss, reduction in the occurrence of iron-deficiency anemia, regulation of irregular cycles, lessening of the symptoms of dysmenorrhea (painful menstrual periods), and lower incidence of premenstrual syndrome. COCs offer protection against endometrial adenocarcinoma and, perhaps, ovarian cancer. They are associated with a reduced incidence of benign breast disease, protection against the development of functional ovarian cysts and some types of pelvic inflammatory disease, and a decreased risk for ectopic pregnancy.

Disadvantages of COCs include no protection from HIV and other STIs. In addition, the woman must remember to take the pill every day. A large percentage of women stop using COCs because of side effects. Common side effects include nausea, headache, breast tenderness, weight gain, breakthrough spotting or bleeding, and amenorrhea. These side effects usually decrease over time and are less common with lower-dose preparations. COCs may promote growth of breast cancer, although they probably do not cause breast cancer. Another disadvantage is the expense. COCs require a visit to the primary care provider or clinic and are available by prescription only.

Some women should not use COCs, or use them only with great caution. Box 4-4 outlines contraindications for their use. Instruct the woman to report any pre-existing health problems, any change in health that may affect her use of COCs, and the occurrence of any warning signs, including severe abdominal or chest pain, dyspnea, headache, weakness, numbness, blurred or double vision, speech disturbances, or severe leg pain and edema.

This tip will be useful for the examination. The acronym "ACHES" can help you recall warning signs related to using oral contraception:

- **A**bdominal pain
- **C**hest pain, dyspnea, bloody sputum
- Severe **H**eadache, weakness or numbness in extremities
- **E**ye problems such as blurred vision, double vision, vision loss
- **S**peech disturbance, severe leg pain or edema

BOX 4.4 Contraindications for Using Combination Oral Contraceptives (COCs)

Women who should not use COCs include those who have any of the following conditions or lifestyle patterns:

- Thromboembolic disorders
- History of heart disease or cerebral vascular accident
- Estrogen-dependent cancer or breast cancer
- Impaired liver function
- Undiagnosed vaginal bleeding
- A confirmed pregnancy or a strong suspicion of pregnancy
- A smoking pattern of more than 15 cigarettes per day in women older than 35 years

Progestin-Only Pills

Progestin-only pills (POPs), also referred to as the "mini-pill," contain only one hormone: progestin. Its major effect is to thicken the cervical mucus and make the endometrium inhospitable to implantation. POPs are slightly less effective than COCs in preventing ovulation.

Advantages include no estrogen side effects, so the woman is less likely to quit using the contraceptive. In addition, women for whom COCs are contraindicated (e.g., those older than 35 years who also smoke and those who have a history of thrombophlebitis) may take POPs. There are no "hormone-free" days or inert pills to take, so the woman can maintain a daily routine of taking the same pill every day. The woman who is lactating can take POPs after the newborn is 6 weeks old. POPs decrease dysmenorrhea and the pain sometimes associated with ovulation.

Menstrual irregularities are one disadvantage of POPs, although periods are usually very short and scanty, which some women find desirable. POPs must be taken every day at the same time of day without fail because their main action (thickening cervical mucus) lasts only 22 to 24 hours. As with COCs, POPs do not provide STI protection and require a primary care provider visit and a prescription.

Hormonal Injections

There are two types of hormonal injection therapies available: a progestin-only agent, depot medroxyprogesterone acetate (DMPA or Depo-Provera); and a combination estrogen/progestin product, medroxyprogesterone acetate with estradiol cypionate (MPA/E2C or Lunelle). Both products provide a level of contraceptive protection similar to that of COCs (see Table 4-1).

As with other hormonal contraceptive methods, hormonal injections do not provide protection against STIs.

Depot Medroxyprogesterone Acetate: Depo-Provera. Depo-Provera consists of a slow-release form of progestin that prevents ovulation. Intramuscular injections are administered four times a year (i.e., each injection provides 3 months of protection). The first shot is given in the first 5 days of the menstrual period. After that the woman must schedule appointments every 11 to 13 weeks for an injection.

Advantages are that the woman does not have to remember to take a pill on a daily basis, and she does not have to use a product at the time of sexual intercourse. Depo-Provera provides the woman with a high level of privacy. No one has to know she is using this method of birth control, unless she chooses to share this information. Lactating mothers can use Depo-Provera. Other advantages include prevention of ectopic pregnancy, and improvement of premenstrual syndrome, depression, and the pain associated with endometriosis.

Take it easy! When administering an injection of Depo-Provera, do not massage the site. This could hasten absorption of the hormone and cause a shorter period of effective contraception.

Disadvantages include prolonged amenorrhea. Many women stop menstruating after the third Depo-Provera injection. This effect is not harmful, and some women may even consider it an advantage. In addition to menstrual irregularities, the most common side effects are weight gain, headache, and nervousness. Sometimes depression and premenstrual symptoms worsen. Another potential disadvantage is the length of time it takes (an average of 10 months) before fertility returns after discontinuing the method. Some women have allergic reactions, although this is rare. Depo-Provera may lower the woman's estrogen levels, leading to loss of bone mineral density and increased risk of fractures. Some research has shown an increase in LDL ("bad") cholesterol and a decrease in HDL ("good") cholesterol levels. Contraindications for using Depo-Provera include pregnancy, history of breast cancer, stroke, or liver disease.

Combined Monthly Injection (Lunelle). Lunelle is a combination progestin/estrogen product that is given via monthly intramuscular injection. Lunelle works by preventing ovulation and by causing cervical mucus to thicken and the endometrial lining to thin. Advantages to Lunelle as compared with Depo-Provera are that a regular menstrual pattern is maintained, estrogen levels remain within normal limits, and fertility returns within 2 to 3 months after stopping the method. As with Depo-Provera, Lunelle provides privacy for the woman's contraceptive choice.

Disadvantages include repeated injections and returning for an office visit every month. Lunelle may cause breast tenderness and is not recommended for breast-feeding women. Some menstrual irregularities are normal at first but usually resolve after the first month or two of use. Weight gain has been reported but less than with Depo-Provera.

Hormonal Implants

The hormonal implant currently available in the United States is Implanon, a single etonogestrel (progestin-only) rod implant. The implant is a small, flexible, plastic rod about the size of a matchstick. It is inserted under local anesthesia just under the skin on the inside of the upper arm. Insertion takes approximately 1 minute. Removal requires a small incision and takes about 3 minutes (Hutti, 2003). Contraceptive protection is provided for 3 years.

Implanon is an extremely effective method of birth control (see Table 4-1). Although no contraceptive method can claim to prevent pregnancy 100% of the time, in more than 70,000 cycles of use to date there have been no pregnancies reported with this method (Hutti, 2003). Other advantages include there are no daily pills to remember and no interference with sexual activity to use the method. Fertility returns quickly (within 3 months) after the implant is removed. Implanon frequently improves symptoms of dysmenorrhea and appears to be safe for lactating women.

Disadvantages include weight gain, which is the most common reason women stop using this method of birth control. Irregular bleeding patterns, acne, breast pain, vaginitis, pharyngitis, and headaches are other side effects sometimes experienced with Implanon. No protection from STIs is provided.

Norplant, a six-rod levonorgestrel implant system, was removed from the United States market in 2002. It was designed to last 5 years; therefore, some women continue to use this method of birth control until it must be removed after 5 years. Removal is a minor surgical procedure and may be difficult or painful. The rods have a tendency to break during removal. Common side effects include irregular menses, headaches, nervousness, mood changes, nausea, skin changes, and vertigo.

Transdermal Patch

The transdermal patch (Ortho Evra) supplies continuous levels of estrogen and progestin. It is available as a prescription and can be placed on the lower abdomen, upper outer arm, buttock, or upper torso, excluding the breasts. The patch is placed on the skin continuously for 3 weeks, and then removed for 1 week to allow menses to occur. Each new patch should be applied on the same day of the week. No more than one patch should be worn at a time.

Individuals who use the patch are more likely to be compliant with the method than with COCs or POPs because there is no daily requirement. It is a highly effective form of birth control (see Table 4-1). Disadvantages include decreased effectiveness in women who weigh more than 198 pounds. The most common side effects include breast symptoms, headache, application site reactions, nausea, upper respiratory tract infections, and dysmenorrhea (Hutti, 2003).

Vaginal Ring

The vaginal ring contraceptive (NuvaRing) is a soft, flexible ring, approximately 2 inches in diameter that contains estrogen and progestin. It is placed into the vagina once a month, during which time it releases low levels of hormones. Lower dosing is possible because it works in the vagina. The ring must be removed after 21 days to allow menstruation.

Advantages include low estrogen exposure with high effectiveness. There is a low incidence of hormone-related side effects, such as headaches, nausea, and breast tenderness. It is easy to insert and generally discreet to use. Disadvantages include that a woman must feel comfortable touching her genitals, some women or their partners may be able to sense the ring during intercourse, and the device may cause increased vaginal discharge.

Intrauterine Device

The intrauterine device (IUD) is a small T-shaped device that is inserted into the uterine cavity. Two types of IUDs are currently approved for use in the United States, each containing a chemically active substance (either copper or progestin). The copper-bearing device is effective for 4 to 10 years, and the progestin-releasing device for 5 to 7 years. As a safety measure, IUDs are also saturated with barium sulfate for radiopacity. Each month the woman must check for presence of the string in the vagina to confirm continued placement of the device.

The copper-bearing IUD acts by damaging sperm in transit through the uterus. Few viable sperm are able to reach the ovum, thus preventing fertilization. The progestin-bearing device affects the cervical mucus and endometrial development. The effect is local and causes no disruption of ovulation. The absence of estrogen makes the IUD a more appropriate contraceptive for women older than 35 years, heavy smokers, and for women with hypertension, vascular disease, or familial diabetes.

The IUD offers continuous protection from unwanted pregnancy without the need to remember a daily pill or engage in other manipulations between coital acts. The IUD can be placed at any time during the menstrual cycle after obtaining a negative pregnancy test. It can be placed immediately after childbirth or after an abortion. When pregnancy is desired, the care provider removes the device. The progestin-bearing device offers the added benefits of decreasing dysmenorrhea and is useful for decreasing bleeding in women with menorrhagia (abnormally long or heavy menstrual periods).

Side effects include cramping and bleeding upon insertion of the device. Common reasons for removal of the copper device include dysmenorrhea and increased menstrual flow. Headache, breast tenderness, and acne are common side effects of the progestin-releasing device. Risks include uterine perforation, pelvic inflammatory disease, bacterial vaginosis, and infection (the IUD offers no protection against STIs). Complications, which may transpire should pregnancy occur, include spontaneous abortion, ectopic pregnancy, or a preterm birth.

Here's another memory trick!

The acronym "PAINS" can help you remember the signs of potential complications related to IUDs.

- **P**eriod late, abnormal spotting or bleeding
- **A**bdominal pain, pain with intercourse
- **I**nfection exposure, abnormal vaginal discharge
- **N**ot feeling well, fever, chills
- **S**tring missing, shorter or longer

Sterilization

Sterilization is a permanent method of birth control obtained via a surgical procedure. Although in some instances reversal may be accomplished, the procedure to do so is expensive and often not successful. The incidence of successful pregnancy after reanastomosis of a tubal ligation is just 15%, and the fertility rate after vasectomy reversal is as low as 16%. Therefore, surgical sterilization procedures should be considered permanent.

Female Sterilization

Female sterilization, by tubal ligation or tubal occlusion, involves blocking or ligating (tying) the fallopian tubes. The procedure may be done immediately after giving birth (within 24 to 48 hours), at the time of an abortion, or during any phase of the menstrual cycle. It can be done using electrocautery or by application of bands or clips via a laparoscopic or minilaparotomy technique. In 2002, the Food and Drug Administration (FDA) approved injection of an occlusive material into the tubes using a transcervical approach (nonsurgical sterilization).

During a minilaparotomy, a small vertical incision is made in the abdominal wall near the umbilicus. The surgeon brings each tube through the incision and cauterizes the tube, which destroys the tissue. An alternative is to ligate and then cut each tube. The procedure may be done under regional anesthetic, or general anesthesia may be used. Oral analgesics are usually sufficient to relieve postoperative discomfort. Although female sterilization is considered a minor surgical procedure, the postoperative recovery period is about 1 to 2 days. The woman is instructed to report bleeding or signs of infection.

Nonsurgical sterilization (Essure Permanent Birth Control System) is accomplished by using hysteroscopy to guide a tiny metallic implant through the vagina, uterus, and into each fallopian tube. Flexible coils hold the implant in place, and mesh material embedded in the coils of the device causes irritation in the tubes, which respond by causing scar tissue to grow and eventually completely occlude the tubes. Alternative methods of birth control must be used for 3 months after the procedure to allow time for scar tissue to form and the method to be completely effective at preventing pregnancy.

Advantages of the Essure system include a less invasive procedure than a surgical approach and avoidance of general anesthesia. The procedure can be performed in a physician's office or clinic. The most common side effects are cramping and nausea and vomiting. Serious, but infrequently occurring, side effects include expulsion of the implant and uterine perforation.

Male Sterilization

Male sterilization, or vasectomy, can be done with a local anesthetic on an outpatient basis. The procedure takes about 20 minutes to perform. A small incision is made on each side of the scrotum over the spermatic cord. Each vas deferens is then ligated and cut. The surgeon may cauterize the cut ends of the vas deferens and then bury them in the scrotal fascia to reduce the chance of spontaneous reanastomosis. The skin incisions are closed, often with a single suture, and a dressing is applied.

Some pain, bruising, and swelling are to be expected after the surgery. Rest, the application of an ice pack, scrotal support, and a mild oral analgesic are effective comfort measures. Moderate inactivity may be recommended for 1 to 2 days because of scrotal tenderness. The skin sutures are removed about 4 to 7 days after surgery. The man should report any signs of bleeding or infection.

Sexual intercourse may be resumed as desired; however, with vasectomy, sterilization is not immediate because sperm remain in the system distal to the ligation. It takes approximately 1 month for the sperm to be purged from the man's system. Therefore, it is necessary for the couple to use another method of birth control until a negative sperm count verifies sterility. Vasectomy has no effect on the man's ability to achieve or maintain erection or on the volume of ejaculate. In addition, there is no interference with the production of testosterone, so secondary sexual characteristics are not affected.

Emergency Contraception

Emergency contraception refers to methods used to prevent pregnancy after unprotected intercourse. Emergency contraception was first used to protect rape victims from pregnancy. It can also be used if a condom breaks or unplanned unprotected sexual intercourse occurs. It is not recommended that emergency contraception be used as the only way of preventing pregnancy in sexually active individuals. It is much more effective to use a consistent form of birth control. It is also important to recognize that emergency contraception is not an "abortion pill." Emergency contraception works to prevent pregnancy from occurring.

Oral contraceptives or mifepristone (RU 486) may be prescribed as a "morning-after pill" to reduce the risk of pregnancy in the event of unprotected intercourse. A larger than usual dose is prescribed, with the exact dosage dependent upon the type of pill. The first dose is given within the first 72 hours after intercourse, followed by a second dose 12 hours after the first.

The copper IUD can be inserted as long as 5 days after unprotected intercourse. One advantage of this method is that it is very effective at preventing pregnancy. However, it should not be used in women who are at high risk for STIs because it can lead to infection, PID, and infertility in these women.

● Nursing Process for Assisting the Couple to Choose a Contraceptive Method

Providing care related to contraception is a collaborative process, involving a variety of health care personnel. The nurse often is working with a physician, certified nurse–midwife, nurse practitioner, family planning counselor, and social worker. Roles for each team member may vary across settings and may overlap within a specific setting. The nurse may be involved in history taking, teaching, and counseling, as well as assisting during physical assessment. Communication among team members and clear protocols for physical assessment, counseling, and teaching are essential to provide quality care. The quality of all family planning care is dependent on the ability of health care team members to work together as professional colleagues.

Steps toward developing excellence in practice include clarifying one's own feelings about family planning, maintaining a current knowledge base through independent study and continuing education activities, awareness of current standards of practice, evaluating current societal norms, and striving to avoid allowing personal prejudices to influence nursing care. Application of the nursing process provides a framework for the nurse working with women and their partners desiring a method of contraception.

ASSESSMENT

Assessment is an essential initial step for identifying the needs and desires of the woman and her partner regarding contraception. The assessment should be conducted in an unhurried and accepting atmosphere with adequate privacy to make the woman and her partner feel comfortable. It is important to treat the couple with respect, accepting their feelings and beliefs, even when these feelings and beliefs differ from the nurse's personal perspective. The assessment includes gathering physiologic, psychoemotional, sociocultural, and cognitive data related to the issue of preventing pregnancy.

The physician or nurse practitioner takes the patient's medical, reproductive, and contraceptive history. Examples of contraception-related questions include:

- What types of contraception were used in the past?
- What problems occurred?
- What did the couple like or dislike about the method?
- What were factors contributing to discontinuing use of the previous method?

The physician or nurse practitioner also performs a physical examination, which includes a general medical examination, a complete gynecologic examination, and routine diagnostic laboratory testing. This information assists in identifying any contraindications to a specific birth control method.

The nurse or family planning counselor often performs the psychoemotional, sociocultural, and cognitive assessments. Psychoemotional data should include information about the couple's feelings regarding their sexuality, family planning in general, and specific methods of contraception. To develop a long-range plan of care, it is important to discuss the couple's goals for their family, regarding the number of children they want and the preferred spacing of those children. Are both partners equally motivated? Studies have indicated that the woman's perception of her partner's support is a major predictor of her use or nonuse of any particular method. Other important issues helpful in identifying the optimal contraceptive method include the woman's self-image, level of comfort with her body, and willingness to touch her genitals.

Sociocultural issues such as family background, religious beliefs, or cultural taboos may influence the couple's compliance with a particular method for contraception. It is important to identify myths or sexual practices related to culture. Social data that should be identified include information about the nature of the woman's sexual activity, such as the number of partners, and her desire for partner involvement in birth control. It is important to assess the relationship between the woman and her partner(s) and the level/quality of communication they share because this influences the choice and subsequent use of contraception. Financial issues may also have an influence on the choice of contraceptive method.

It is important to assess the couple's level of understanding about the reproductive cycle and their knowledge of varied types of birth control available. Many couples have a knowledge base regarding contraception gleaned from other sources, such as popular magazines, television, or the Internet. It is not unusual for new information to be disseminated by the lay media even before publication in professional journals. Identifying the couple's educational needs can be done as part of an interview or by using assessment questionnaires. Such assessment tools will help the nurse to quickly evaluate the couple's knowledge about birth control methods and identify educational needs, as well as personal preferences.

SELECTED NURSING DIAGNOSES

- Deficient Knowledge, lack of information related to reproductive cycle and birth control methods
- Decisional Conflict related to:
  - contraceptive alternatives
  - unwillingness of sexual partner to agree on birth control method
  - possibility of contraceptive method side effects
- Ineffective Sexuality Patterns related to interference with normal sexuality patterns or discomfort caused by the contraceptive method

OUTCOME IDENTIFICATION AND PLANNING

Appropriate goals may include that the woman and her partner will express adequate knowledge of the reproductive cycle and contraceptive methods; that a method of contraception suitable to their needs and lifestyle will be chosen; and that the woman and her partner will express satisfaction with their pattern of sexual expression. Other goals and interventions are planned according to the individual needs of the woman and her partner.

IMPLEMENTATION

Nursing interventions are chosen based on the assessment data, goals, and plan of care. The physician, or nurse practitioner will perform physical interventions, such as the fitting of diaphragms or cervical caps, or insertion of an IUD. Nursing interventions will be concerned primarily with psychoemotional, sociocultural, or cognitive needs of the woman and her partner.

Providing Teaching

Teaching must be presented in an unbiased manner, dispelling myths and misinformation, and providing needed information. Information may be presented through either group teaching sessions or individual discussion, depending on the needs and preferences of the couple. For example, if a couple has already decided on a specific method of contraception, a group session discussing all methods may not be appropriate. In any case, it is imperative to provide complete and accurate information, regardless of the teaching format. Any discussion of contraceptive methods should include the following information:

- A description of the method, including an example or illustration
- The mode of action, showing how the method acts to prevent pregnancy
- The effectiveness or failure rate of the method and causes for method failure
- Requirements for use, such as how to obtain the method, implementation, and necessary compliance
- How the method will affect love-making, such as when the method should be implemented in relation to coitus, and possible effects on coitus
- Medical and emotional advantages and disadvantages
- Risks, contraindications, side effects, drug interactions, warning signs, and any factors related to safe use
- Effectiveness of the method to protect against STIs and HIV
- Costs of the method, both initially and for the long term
- Reversibility or irreversibility of the method, including how to discontinue the method and the length of time until the return of fertility

Addressing Emotional or Sociocultural Needs

Discussion of emotional or sociocultural needs may be better addressed in private, individualized teaching sessions. This allows the couple to freely express feelings, opinions, and concerns, and ask questions about intimate, personal aspects of their lives. Religious, cultural, social, and financial concerns can be explored. In addition, the nurse will be better able to assess the couple's understanding and acceptance of the chosen method. The nurse should establish a trusting relationship with the couple, provide a warm and accepting atmosphere, and remain sensitive to their needs and concerns.

Assisting With Follow-up

After the woman and her partner have chosen a method, follow-up is important to determine satisfaction with the method and ability to use the method correctly. Often a follow-up telephone call is appropriate. Ask the woman how things are going using the chosen method. Inquire regarding adverse effects or any problems she is having that might cause her to quit using the method. Each office visit is another opportunity to explore with the woman regarding how she is doing and her satisfaction level. Periodically ask the woman to explain the steps of the chosen method and correct any misperceptions.

EVALUATION: GOALS AND EXPECTED OUTCOMES

- **Goal:** The woman and her partner will express adequate knowledge of the reproductive cycle and contraceptive methods.
  Expected Outcomes:
  - Describes the physical signs indicating fertile and infertile periods of the woman's menstrual cycle.
  - Verbalizes understanding about contraceptive methods.
- **Goal:** The woman and her partner will choose a method of contraception suitable to their needs and lifestyle.
  Expected Outcomes:
  - Discusses attitudes and feelings about contraception in general and about specific birth control methods.
  - Asks questions and expresses concerns related to using different birth control methods.
- **Goal:** The woman and her partner will express satisfaction with their pattern of sexual expression using the chosen birth control method.
  Expected Outcomes:
  - Voices satisfaction with the chosen method.

- Encounters no adverse reactions or complications related to the chosen birth control method.
- Demonstrates successful use of the selected birth control method through prevention of unplanned pregnancy.

INDUCED ABORTION

An **induced abortion** is the purposeful interruption of pregnancy before 20 weeks' gestation. A **therapeutic abortion** is a pregnancy termination performed for reasons related to maternal or fetal health or disease. The term **elective abortion** refers to an abortion performed at the woman's request that does not involve preservation of health. Most women who have abortions are Caucasian, younger than 24 years of age, and unmarried. Sixty percent of women who have abortions report using a contraceptive method that failed.

The type of abortion procedure used depends on the gestational age of the fetus. Table 4-2 briefly describes several of the more common abortion procedure techniques and special considerations associated with each procedure.

Nursing care roles and responsibilities vary, depending upon the setting, method of termination used, and the client's needs. In some settings, the nurse and physician may be the only health care providers involved. In others, care providers may include social workers or counselors. In either situation, the nurse's role is central to achieving optimal client care outcomes. It is important to examine personal beliefs and values related to abortion before assuming responsibility for the care of women choosing to have an abortion. The nurse must be able to provide compassionate and nonjudgmental care.

Document the amount and character of bleeding after the abortion procedure. Save anything that appears to be tissue or clots. A pad count with an estimation of pad saturation provides a more accurate record of blood loss. Assess the woman's vital signs frequently, as for other postoperative care, and observe for signs and symptoms of hypovolemic shock. Hematocrit testing is usually done before discharge. Rh immune globulin should be administered to the woman who is Rh negative.

Postabortion teaching should include information about signs and symptoms of possible complications, including elevated temperature, continued/excessive vaginal bleeding, malodorous vaginal discharge, and abdominal pain. Any adverse effects should be reported immediately. Advise the woman to delay sexual intercourse for 1 to 2 weeks. Contraception counseling and instructions about follow-up care and appointments are important.

Test Yourself

- Name the two complementary components to family planning.
- List one advantage and one disadvantage to the use of coitus interruptus as a birth control method.
- List one fertility awareness method and one barrier method of birth control.

INFERTILITY

Infertility is commonly defined as the inability to conceive after a year or more of regular and unprotected intercourse, or the inability to carry a pregnancy to term. Infertility affects approximately 10% to 15% of couples in the United States, a rate that has remained stable for the past 50 years (Garcia, Nelson, & Wallach, 2003). There are two main types of infertility: primary and secondary. A couple who has never been able to conceive is diagnosed with primary infertility; whereas, a couple who has been able to conceive in the past but is currently unable to do so is diagnosed with secondary infertility.

For the majority of couples who engage in frequent, unprotected intercourse, the chance for conception is about 60% at 6 months, 90% at 12 months, and 95% at 24 months. Because the chances of conception are affected by the frequency of intercourse, if a couple has intercourse only one time per week for 6 months, there is only a 15% chance of pregnancy. If the couple increases intercourse frequency to four times a week around the time of ovulation, the chance of conception increases to 83%. Research has shown that the optimal timing for sexual intercourse when conception is desired is every 48 hours at midcycle. Counseling about the timing and frequency of intercourse and the expected time of ovulation often can resolve problems of infertility.

Causes of Infertility

For conception to occur many factors have to work together perfectly. Viable sperm have to be deposited in the female reproductive tract. The passageway through the woman's cervix, uterus, and fallopian tubes has to be clear for sperm to negotiate the journey toward the egg. Ovulation has to occur. The egg must be swept into a fallopian tube. The egg must be fertilized within 12 to 24 hours after ovulation, before it begins to disintegrate. After fertilization, the egg must travel down the fallopian tube to the uterus and implant. Any factor that prevents the sperm and egg from meeting or interferes with the fertilized egg traveling to and implanting in the uterine lining can result in infertility.

TABLE 4.2 Selected Induced Abortion Techniques

Method	Procedure	Special Considerations
Surgical techniques		
Menstrual aspiration	The endometrial cavity is aspirated with a flexible cannula and syringe within 1 to 3 weeks after a missed menstrual period.	• A positive pregnancy test must confirm pregnancy before the procedure is done. • Possible complications include implanted zygote missed during procedure, ectopic pregnancy not recognized, and uterine perforation (rare).
Dilatation and curettage (D&C)	1. Cervix is dilated with a blunt instrument or laminaria. 2. A sharp instrument, called a curette, is used to scrape the endometrium and remove uterine contents. 3. Suction may be used during the procedure to aspirate uterine contents.	• Primary procedure used in United States. • Used for 1st trimester terminations (up to 14 weeks). • Possible complications include uterine perforation, cervical laceration, hemorrhage, incomplete removal of products of conception, and infection.
Dilatation and evacuation (D&E)	Procedure is similar to D&C; however, wider dilation of the cervix is done to facilitate removal of the fetus and placenta.	• D&E is the surgical technique of choice for 2nd trimester abortions. • Complications are the same as for D&C.
Medical Techniques		
Mifepristone (RU 486)	One dose (600 mg) of this oral antiprogesterone is given alone or in conjunction with prostaglandins.	• Effective for 1st trimester (7 weeks and less) abortions. • Common side effects are nausea, vomiting, and gastrointestinal cramping. • Complications include hemorrhage secondary to incomplete expulsion of pregnancy or intra-abdominal hemorrhage secondary to rupture of an unrecognized tubal pregnancy.
Oxytocin	High-dose intravenous oxytocin is titrated until an effective uterine contraction pattern is established.	• Used for 2nd trimester abortions. • Oxytocin has an effectiveness rate similar to that of prostaglandins with fewer side effects. • The nurse must carefully monitor the uterine contraction pattern to avoid excessive stimulation.
Intra-amniotic hyperosmotic fluid infusion	Hyperosmotic saline or urea solutions are injected into the amniotic sac.	• Used infrequently to induce 2nd trimester abortions. • There is a high incidence of adverse side effects and complications associated with this procedure, including death.
Prostaglandins	Prostaglandins can be administered by • Vaginal suppository • Gel inserted by catheter into the cervical canal and lower uterus • Intramuscular injection • Injected into the amniotic sac • Oral route	• Frequently used to induce 2nd trimester abortions. • Side effects include fever, vomiting, diarrhea, and uterine hyperstimulation.

There are multiple factors that can contribute to the inability of a couple to conceive. Female factors alone account for approximately 48% of cases of infertility; whereas, male factors alone are causal in approximately 19% of cases. The interaction of both female and male factors is responsible for 17%, unknown factors for 10%, and other causes for 6% of the cases of infertility (Garcia et al., 2003).

If a couple is having trouble conceiving, it is helpful for them to review their health histories to identify risk factors for infertility (Box 4-5). Female-specific risk factors include any condition or situation that interferes

BOX 4.5 Risk Factors for Infertility

Risk Factors That Affect Both the Male and Female

Behavioral Factors
- Cigarette or marijuana smoking
- Alcohol use (even in moderation)
- Excessive exercise
- Being 10% to 15% over or under ideal body weight
- Multiple sexual partners (increases risk for STIs)

Occupational and Environmental Factors
Exposure to
- High environmental temperatures
- Certain chemicals
- Radiation
- Heavy electromagnetic or microwave emissions

Emotional Factors
- High stress levels
- Depression

Female-Specific Risk Factors

Factors That May Interfere With Ovulation
- Advancing age*
- Chronic medical conditions and/or associated treatments; examples include
  - Diabetes mellitus
  - Thyroid dysfunction
  - Systemic lupus erythematosus (SLE)
  - Rheumatoid arthritis
  - Hypertension
  - Asthma
- Hormonal imbalance, may be signaled by any of the following
  - Menstrual irregularities
  - Menorrhagia (prolonged or excessive bleeding)
  - Hirsutism
  - Acne
- Ovarian cysts

Factors That May Interfere With Travel of Sperm or Egg Through Female Genital Tract
- Surgical or invasive procedures involving the cervix or uterus, such as
  - Cone biopsy
  - Cryosurgery
  - Dilatation and curettage
  - Myomectomy
- In utero diethylstilbestrol (DES) exposure
- Any surgical procedure directly involving the fallopian tubes (may cause scarring and narrowing of the lumen of the tube)
- Any pelvic surgery (could lead to adhesions and scarring)
- Endometriosis
- Ectopic pregnancy
- History of STIs or pelvic inflammatory disease (PID)

Factors That May Interfere With Implantation
- More than one induced abortion
- Using an IUD for contraception (can lead to scarring)
- Hormonal imbalance

Male-Specific Risk Factors

Factors That May Interfere With Sperm Viability
- Prescription medications for ulcers or psoriasis
- DES exposure in utero
- Exposure of the genitals to hot temperatures
  - Hot tubs
  - Steam rooms
  - Tight clothing
- Cryptorchidism
- Prostatitis
- Varicocele
- Genital tract infection
- Mumps after puberty

Factors That May Interfere With Sperm Deposit in Female Genital Tract
- Erectile dysfunction
- Retrograde ejaculation (semen is released into male bladder, rather than ejected from the penis during ejaculation)
- History of hernia repair
- Hypospadias
- Vasectomy

* Female fertility declines with advancing age. A woman in her 30s is 30% less fertile than one in her 20s.

with ovulation, patency of the cervix or fallopian tubes, or ability of the fertilized ovum to implant in the uterine lining. Male-specific risk factors include anything that can cause decreased or abnormal sperm production or any factor that prevents sperm from being deposited in the female reproductive tract.

Initial Evaluation of Infertility

Frequently the woman presents to her primary care provider with her concerns when she has been unable to conceive. The primary care provider or gynecologist performs the initial evaluation. If complex problems are found, or the problem is not readily identifiable, the woman and her partner are then referred to a reproductive endocrinologist for additional evaluation and treatment.

Because of the high incidence of multiple contributing factors, evaluation of infertility should include both partners, even when the problem seems to be "obvious." Evaluation begins with a thorough history and physical examination for both partners to identify evidence of conditions that may be affecting fertility. Important health history information includes:

- The woman's menstrual pattern
- Number of pregnancies with the current partner or any other partner, and the pregnancy outcomes
- Identification of any sexual dysfunction for both partners

- History of STIs or genital tract surgery or trauma for both partners
- Lifestyle issues, such as alcohol consumption, tobacco use, recreational drug use, occupation, and patterns of physical activity for both partners
- Chronic medical conditions and treatment for both partners
- The couple's pattern of intercourse as related to the woman's ovulatory cycle
- Length of time the couple has had unprotected intercourse
- Natural techniques or home tests the couple has already used

In addition to the above-mentioned health history, the primary care practitioner will do a complete review of systems to help identify any endocrinologic or immunologic issues that might contribute to infertility. A thorough physical examination is done. A gynecologist may evaluate the female partner, whereas the male partner is frequently referred to an urologist for initial evaluation.

The woman's physical examination includes a pelvic examination, Pap smear, cultures for gonorrhea and chlamydia, and a bimanual examination (see Chapter 6). A pelvic ultrasound is part of the initial examination. The male examination includes determining if any genital tract abnormalities are present. Results of the initial evaluation are discussed with the couple. Plans for a more comprehensive evaluation, if needed, are explained.

A PERSONAL GLIMPSE

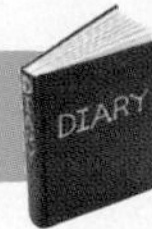

My husband and I had been married 5 years when we decided to start a family. I tried to get pregnant for 8 months without success. My aunt advised me to get a physical examination. Reluctantly I called to make an appointment. The physician couldn't see me for several months, so I booked the appointment with the Women's Health Nurse Practitioner. She performed a thorough physical exam. She told me that nothing appeared to be wrong with my reproductive tract. She said that many couples don't get pregnant right away. She instructed me that healthy living habits were good not only for a healthy heart, but also for a healthy reproductive tract. She advised me to start a regular program of exercise and to eat a well-balanced diet. She told me that stress can interfere with getting pregnant, and she referred me for yoga lessons after I indicated to her that I had always wanted to learn yoga. I followed her advice, and 6 months later I was pregnant.

Sylvia

LEARNING OPPORTUNITY: What advice can nurses give to couples who want to start a family? How does knowledge of the reproductive tract help nurses take care of women who want to get pregnant?

Comprehensive Evaluation and Diagnostic Testing

Diagnostic testing for infertility usually begins with the simplest testing methods and moves toward the more complex and invasive methods. The couple should be told that diagnostic testing is done in relation to the woman's menstrual cycle. It may take up to two menstrual cycles to complete the testing (Garcia et al., 2003).

Frequently, male infertility factors are evaluated first because the testing is often simpler than that for female testing. The first diagnostic test is almost always a semen analysis. For this procedure, semen is collected via masturbation or in a special condom during intercourse if masturbation is unacceptable to the couple. Optimal results are obtained when the man has abstained from sexual release for 3 to 5 days before the test. The entire ejaculate is collected in a sterile container and must be delivered to the laboratory no later than 30 minutes after collection. The sample is examined for semen volume and quality, and for numbers, shape, motility, and viability of the sperm. Frequently two to three samples, collected at least 2 to 3 days apart, are analyzed. If the semen analysis results are normal, the diagnostic testing then focuses on the female partner.

If the semen analysis results are abnormal, the analysis may be repeated 1 month later to rule out short-term causes or inadequate specimen collection. Additional tests of male fertility that may be performed include endocrine hormonal analysis. Serum levels of four hormones—follicle-stimulating hormone (FSH), luteinizing hormone (LH), testosterone, and prolactin—are evaluated. Transrectal (through the rectum) or scrotal ultrasonography may be done to identify structural abnormalities that could interfere with fertility. Sperm function tests are sometimes done to determine the ability of the sperm to penetrate and fertilize the egg. Testicular biopsy may be performed to obtain a sample of testicular tissue for analysis. The results of this analysis can often pinpoint the cause of male infertility.

Comprehensive fertility evaluation of the woman often begins with the least invasive techniques. The **postcoital test,** which evaluates the interaction of the man's sperm with the woman's cervical mucus, is frequently done. The timing of the test is critical for accurate results. The methods used to predict ovulation for FAM (i.e., BBT, cervical mucus changes, and/or a urinary LH kit) are used. When it has been determined that ovulation is about to occur, the couple is asked to have vaginal intercourse without lubricants. A sample of cervical mucus is collected 8 to 12 hours afterward and evaluated for mucus characteristics, a sperm count, and evaluation of sperm motility. Endocrine testing is useful. Serum hormone levels of estrogen, progesterone, thyroid-stimulating hormone, prolactin, and androgen are drawn to determine if endocrine abnormalities are present.

More invasive techniques include hysterosalpingogram, hysteroscopy, and laparoscopy. A hysterosalpingogram allows for identification of an obstruction anywhere along the tract. A hysteroscopy facilitates direct visualization of the endometrial cavity. This method can be used to diagnose and treat some endometrial conditions. Laparoscopy is usually the last test performed because it involves surgical and anesthetic risk and cost. This procedure provides for direct visualization of the pelvic cavity, which frequently allows for accurate diagnosis of the cause of infertility.

Management of Infertility

The appropriate therapy for infertility is chosen based on the underlying causes identified during diagnostic testing, duration of infertility, and the woman's age. As with testing, therapies begin with the simplest and least invasive and progress toward the more complex, as needed. Possible interventions include medication administration, surgical procedures, insemination techniques, advanced reproductive techniques, and other parenting/childbirth options.

Treatment of Cervical Factors

The easiest, most successful therapy for cervical abnormalities is intrauterine insemination. In this procedure, the physician inserts sperm directly into the uterus near the time of ovulation. More than one insemination may be performed to ensure that insemination coincides with ovulation. Sperm can be from the woman's partner, homologous insemination, or from a donor, heterologous insemination. The woman is placed in the dorsal lithotomy position and a speculum is inserted into the vagina. After the cervix is cleansed, the specimen is placed in a 1-mL syringe attached to a thin, flexible catheter, which is advanced through the cervix until it reaches the upper uterus. Care is taken not to injure the endometrium or induce bleeding. The semen specimen is injected slowly into the uterus, and the catheter is withdrawn. The woman is typically instructed to remain supine for at least 10 minutes after the insemination.

Treatment of Endometrial Factors

Most endometrial causes of infertility are treated by various surgical techniques. Hysteroscopy, laparoscopy, or laparotomy may be done, followed by a hysterosalpingogram to evaluate effectiveness of treatment. If the woman has endometriosis, it is treated as described previously in the chapter.

Treatment of Ovarian Factors

Medications to stimulate ovulation, also known as fertility drugs, are the treatment of choice when lack of ovulation is the cause of infertility. All have side effects and potential complications, which can be severe. Multifetal pregnancy is also common with these medications. Clomiphene citrate (Clomid, Serophene), human menopause gonadotropins (Pergonal, Humegon, Repronex), synthetic gonadotropin-releasing hormone (GnRH), and pure FSH are examples of fertility drugs used to treat ovarian dysfunction.

Treatment of Male Factors

If a varicocele is the cause of low sperm production, it is repaired surgically. If the cause of a low sperm count is unknown and FSH, LH, and testosterone levels are normal, then the man is treated with Clomid to increase sperm production. Alternatively, intrauterine insemination of the woman is done.

Assisted/Advanced Reproductive Therapies

The first advanced reproductive therapy (ART) to be successful in humans, in vitro fertilization, resulted in the 1978 delivery of Louise Brown. Since that time additional therapies have been developed, and indications for ARTs have been expanded to include conditions that heretofore would have been considered impossible to treat.

The four leading ARTs are in vitro fertilization (IVF), gamete intrafallopian transfer (GIFT), tubal embryo transfer (TET), and intracytoplasmic sperm injection (ICSI). The nurse's role in this area is to provide the couple with balanced and accurate information regarding the risks and benefits of the technologies available to facilitate their decision-making process (Box 4-6).

BOX 4.6 Ethical and Legal Issues Related to Advanced Reproductive Therapies (ARTs)

Research in the area of ARTs has resulted in additional technologies that, while giving new hope to couples who once considered their infertility irreversible, are also creating ethical and legal dilemmas for all concerned. Common ethical and legal questions include:

- Who should have the right to reproduce?
- Should ARTs be limited to married couples?
- Who owns the embryos produced?
- Should embryos be frozen for later use?
- Who are the parents?
- Do the biologic donors or surrogates have custodial rights?
- Should donors only be anonymous?
- Should fetal reduction techniques be done when ARTs results in multifetal gestation?

In Vitro Fertilization

IVF is a relatively common procedure that is used when the woman has absent or blocked fallopian tubes; when the man has a low sperm count; or when the etiology of infertility is unknown. IVF involves several steps. The procedure begins with administration of fertility drugs to the woman to stimulate ovulation. After one or more ova (eggs) are harvested from the ovary, the ova are fertilized by sperm in the laboratory and placed in a growth medium, where they develop for 48 to 72 hours. The embryos are then transferred to the uterus. In general, only three to four embryos are placed in the woman's uterus to reduce the risk of multifetal gestation.

Gamete Intrafallopian Transfer

In GIFT, the harvested ova are aspirated into a catheter containing prepared sperm. The ova are then transferred into the fallopian tube, where fertilization can take place. One prerequisite for the procedure is that the woman must have at least one patent fallopian tube. A success rate of 20% to 30% has been reported for this procedure.

Tubal Embryo Transfer

The TET procedure, also called zygote intrafallopian transfer (ZIFT), is a combination of IVF and GIFT. The ova are fertilized as in IVF; however, the embryos are returned to the fallopian tube versus the uterus. Success rates for TET are similar to the success rates for GIFT.

Intracytoplasmic Sperm Injection

ICSI is the latest development to give hope to the male with very low sperm counts. Fertilization is possible with only one sperm. The sperm is obtained by masturbation, testicular biopsy, or aspiration. Stroking the distal portion of the tail then paralyzes it. After the ovum is harvested, the sperm is placed into a microneedle (tail first), and then injected into the ovum. The fertilized ovum is placed into the woman's reproductive tract for implantation. Pregnancy rates are similar to those seen with IVF. An increased risk of congenital malformation and chromosomal abnormalities is associated with ICSI; however, some research studies do not demonstrate increased risk.

Surrogate Parenting

Surrogate parenting is a process by which a woman carries to term the infant of an infertile couple. A **gestational surrogate,** or surrogate mother, may donate only the use of her uterus, or she may also donate her ovum and agree to be inseminated with the male partner's sperm. Surrogate parenting has raised extensive legal and ethical issues that require counseling for both the infertile couple and the surrogate and possibly the surrogate mother's spouse and family.

Psychological Aspects of Infertility

Psychosocial sequelae related to infertility include shock, guilt, isolation, depression, and stress. The partner who has the identified problem is at most risk for feelings of guilt. It is important to avoid using words that imply blame when discussing the problem of infertility.

A couple who is having difficulty conceiving may feel isolated and "different" from others who are able to conceive. They may separate themselves from others in an attempt to avoid emotional pain. Infertility will challenge the couple's self-image, self-worth, and sense of command over events in their life. They may experience a "roller coaster" of emotions, ranging from hope to despair with each ovulatory cycle.

Infertility places stress on the couple's relationship. One or both may develop poor self-esteem and feel unworthy or unlovable. A man may find it difficult to perform sexually or provide semen specimens "on demand" at specific times. Intimacy, love, and support, essential components of a couple's sexual relationship, may be lost because intercourse takes on a "clinical" and mechanical tone.

Failure to achieve pregnancy may lead the couple to consider adoption. Adoption is a viable option for parenting, but the couple must consider some realities about pursuing this route. Many couples have preferences regarding the health status, race, and possibly other characteristics they desire in an infant. A couple may need to reflect on their willingness to adopt an older child, a child of another race, or a child with special needs. How will they feel about having minimal information about the child's background? How would they feel about knowing the child's birth mother or father? These and other questions must be asked and answered by the couple before deciding to adopt. The nurse should have information about adoption available and use positive language when discussing that option. Discussion should focus on sharing complete and balanced information and supporting the couples' feelings and decision.

Nursing Care

The major focus of nursing care related to infertility involves providing support for the couple as they undergo diagnosis and their chosen treatment option. Therapeutic communication skills are an essential component in nursing care. It is important to facilitate the couple's ability to communicate with each other and to encourage each partner to discuss his/her own feelings and be accepting of the other's. The nurse should reinforce the couple's coping strategies or assist them in exploring adaptive alternatives to poor coping, increasing their sense of control in this situation.

After the physician has told the couple about their diagnosis and potential treatment options, the nurse's major role is to provide additional information, helping them to make an informed decision. The nurse supports the couple through the decision-making process and helps them toward a resolution of infertility by either assisting with the grief process or through facilitating parenting. Providing emotional support is an essential component of care, especially when a treatment has been unsuccessful. The general goals for the couple with infertility will be aimed toward:

- Providing complete and accurate information about the diagnosis and treatment options available, including adoption, or child-free living.
- Education about human reproduction, including factors that interfere with normal conception.
- Providing support and counseling to the couple during the diagnostic and decision-making process.
- Assisting the couple during the process of treatment for infertility.
- Evaluating the need for referrals to other resources, such as psychological or pastoral counseling.

Test Yourself

- Define infertility.
- Which test of infertility is normally the first to be done?
- Describe two advanced reproductive technologies.

MENOPAUSE

Your perimenopausal patients will appreciate this tip! Encourage the woman in the perimenopausal period not to be lulled into a false sense of security. Although fertility declines, pregnancy can still occur. The woman in perimenopause should continue to use a reliable form of birth control.

Menopause, the cessation of menses, signals the end of the woman's reproductive capability. The climacteric, as defined in Chapter 3, refers to the gradual changes associated with declining ovarian function that are commonly called "the change of life." **Perimenopause** refers to the time before menopause when vasomotor symptoms (hot flashes, night sweats) and irregular menses begin. Menopause is a normal part of the life cycle and is not a disease, although associated symptoms may be distressing and require treatment.

Menopause occurs when the ovaries no longer respond to stimulation from the pituitary. During the perimenopausal period, the woman begins to experience shorter menstrual cycles and irregular bleeding. Although these changes occur normally in response to hormonal changes, all irregular bleeding should be reported to the primary care practitioner for evaluation.

Clinical Manifestations

The perimenopausal woman typically experiences a set of symptoms that are together referred to as the "climacteric syndrome." These symptoms include hot flashes, insomnia, weight gain, bloating, emotional lability, irregular menses, and headache (Bachmann, 2002).

A hot flash is a sudden feeling of warmth or intense heat that may be accompanied by reddening of the skin on the upper body. The duration is anywhere from seconds to several minutes. The average length of symptoms in the perimenopausal woman is 2 years; however, some women experience hot flashes for 5 or more years. Although the physiology is not completely understood, a hot flash is linked to low estrogen levels and periodic surges of LH.

Physical changes associated with hormone depletion include changes to the reproductive organs. The vaginal mucosa thins and becomes pale and dry. Vaginal rugae disappear, and the vaginal walls become smooth. The uterus and ovaries decrease in size. Pelvic support muscles lose tone, and pelvic support disorders may become apparent. The skin loses its elasticity, and dense breast tissue is replaced with adipose tissue.

Decreased bone mineral density is one of the changes that can have life-threatening effects on the menopausal woman. The overall effect of decreased bone mineral density is loss of bone mass, with resulting reduction of bone strength and increased risk for fracture. This systemic condition is called osteoporosis. It is important to know the risk factors for osteoporosis (Box 4-7) because this disease often has no symptoms until a serious bone fracture occurs.

Treatment

The gold standard for prevention and treatment of perimenopausal symptoms as a whole has historically been hormone replacement therapy (HRT). However, recent research is showing the HRT may not be the best option for many women. The Women's Health Initiative (WHI) study was stopped early because of the adverse effects of HRT on women's health. An

BOX 4.7 Risk Factors for Osteoporosis

- Female gender
- Caucasian or Asian ethnicity
- Slender build
- Advanced age
- Estrogen deficiency because of menopause (especially if early or surgically induced)
- Low bone mass density
- Family history of osteoporosis
- Personal history of fracture as an adult
- Smoking
- Excessive alcohol intake
- Low dietary intake of calcium
- Vitamin D deficiency
- Inactive lifestyle
- Use of glucocorticoids
- Use of anticonvulsants

increased risk for coronary heart disease, stroke, venous thromboembolism, pulmonary embolism, and breast cancer was found with HRT therapy and no decrease in cardiovascular disease (one of the focuses of the study). Many health care professionals are advising that HRT be prescribed only for the control (not prevention) of perimenopausal symptoms, and that it be used at the lowest dose possible for the shortest time possible. Benefits of HRT shown by the WHI study are a decreased risk for colorectal cancer and osteoporotic fractures.

Treatment for Hot Flashes and Sweats

Hot flashes and sweats are the most common reasons that the perimenopausal woman seeks medical treatment. To date the most effective therapy for hot flashes continues to be HRT. Hormonal alternatives to HRT include progestins alone, which have been shown to be beneficial in treating hot flashes. Nonhormonal options that show promise include the antihypertensive agent lofexidine; the anticonvulsant gabapentin; and the antidepressants paroxetine and venlafaxine.

Treatment for Osteoporosis

Bone mineral density testing is recommended for postmenopausal women as follows: women at increased risk for osteoporosis should begin screening at age 60 years, and all other women should begin screening at age 65 years. Wallace, Rogers, Keenum, Shah, and Turner (2003) recommend that the primary care practitioner schedule bone mineral density testing with annual mammograms for postmenopausal women.

HRT continues to be beneficial for reducing the risk of osteoporosis and fractures in the peri- and postmenopausal woman. However, there are other treatment options that lower the risk for fractures. These options include raloxifene, calcitonin, and bisphosphonates. Calcium and vitamin D supplementation and regular weight-bearing exercise continue to be recommended as preventive measures.

Treatment for Vaginal Atrophy and Dryness

HRT continues to be an effective treatment, although the use of local applications of estrogen-containing vaginal creams, tablets, or suppositories brings relief of symptoms with minimal systemic absorption. The woman for whom estrogen use is contraindicated may benefit from nonestrogenic vaginal lubricants.

Nursing Care

Nurses have a large role to play in health promotion for the perimenopausal and postmenopausal woman. It is important to develop rapport with the woman and to let her know that you are available to talk about her concerns. Reassure the woman of the normality of menopause.

Give the woman factual information on HRT and other therapies. It may be helpful to give her a list of resources that she can read at home. It is important that the woman be informed of the risks and benefits of any therapy so that she can make an informed decision.

There are many nursing interventions that can help the perimenopausal woman. Suggest lifestyle modifications to decrease the discomfort of hot flashes. These include dressing in lightweight clothing and dressing in layers. Regular exercise and setting the thermostat to a lower temperature may also be helpful. Suggest that she avoid spicy foods, caffeine, and alcohol.

Some common sense guidelines to prevent osteoporosis can be helpful as well. Encourage regular weight-bearing activity, such as walking and stair climbing, at least three to four times per week. The postmenopausal woman should continue to take calcium and vitamin D supplements. She should take her calcium supplements with orange juice (or another vitamin C source) and avoid caffeine, which tends to interfere with the absorption of calcium.

Safety instructions can help prevent fractures from falls inside the house. Encourage the postmenopausal woman to have her bed lowered, if possible; to eliminate throw rugs and clutter from the floors; and to use night lights throughout the house. In the bathroom it is helpful to install safety tread and safety rails. Suggest that she keep a cordless or mobile telephone close by to eliminate the temptation to run to answer the phone. All of her slippers and shoes should have tread and should provide traction and stability.

Falls outside the home can be reduced if the woman will take extra precautions after dark. Advise her to use railings whenever possible. She should clear walkways of debris and avoid walking on ice.

FAMILY TEACHING TIPS

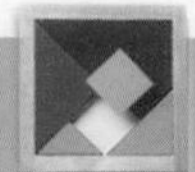

Reducing the Discomfort of Menopause

- Wear cotton clothes in layers.
- Avoid caffeine intake (e.g., colas, tea, coffee).
- Explore relaxation activities because stress exacerbates vasomotor symptoms.
- Discuss HRT with your caregiver.
- Consider nutritional supplements as recommended by your primary care practitioner to help reduce vasomotor symptoms.
- Use a water-soluble lubricant before intercourse.
- Nonprescription products, such as Replens and Lubrin, are effective for the relief of vaginal dryness.
- If using an estrogen vaginal cream, apply it at bedtime.
- Perform Kegel exercises to improve pelvic muscle tone.
- Drink at least 5 glasses of water per day. Do not count caffeine-containing drinks as part of this water intake.
- Urinate regularly; do not allow the bladder to become overdistended.
- Practice good hygiene, such as wiping from front to back, after toileting.

Review medications with the woman. She should understand how to take the medication and side effects that should be reported. She should also understand how often she should see the primary care practitioner and what routine screening examinations should be done, such as yearly mammograms and bone density measurements. Family Teaching Tips: Reducing the Discomfort of Menopause lists helpful tips to share with the woman and her family.

Test Yourself

- Define perimenopause.
- Name five symptoms that are part of the climacteric syndrome.
- Describe three things (nonpharmacologic) that the nurse can teach the older woman to do to treat or prevent hot flashes.

KEY POINTS

- Self-awareness of breast characteristics and yearly clinical breast examinations are recommended for women of all ages. Women older than 40 years should have yearly mammograms as well.
- Sexually active women younger than 30 years should have annual Pap smears. The healthy woman older than 30 years should have Pap smears every 2 to 3 years.
- Dysmenorrhea is defined as painful or difficult menses. Premenstrual syndrome (PMS) encompasses a constellation of symptoms that are cyclical in nature and progress with time.
- A classic symptom of endometriosis is cyclic pelvic pain that occurs in conjunction with menses. Therapy is aimed at suppressing ovulation and inducing an artificial menopause to suppress growth of abnormal tissue and relieve symptoms. The nurse's role is to help the woman find pain relief and provide support.
- The major risk factor for the development of pelvic inflammatory disease (PID) is untreated sexually transmitted infections (STIs). Treatment of the woman and her partner with antibiotics is recommended.
- Pelvic support disorders are caused by weakening of the structures that support the pelvic organs. Major risk factors include pregnancy, vaginal delivery, and aging.
- Family planning involves the two components of planning pregnancy and preventing pregnancy. Family planning should include prepregnancy planning, which involves focusing on nutrition and exercise, lifestyle changes, counseling and treatment for chronic illness and genetic disorders, and evaluation of medications.
- Natural methods of contraception do not use hormones or other physical barriers to prevent conception. These methods include abstinence, coitus interruptus, and fertility awareness methods (FAM). Natural methods do not require the use of artificial devices or hormones but require a great deal of education and discipline to be effective.
- Barrier methods provide a physical or chemical barrier or both to prevent pregnancy. These include spermicides, male and female condoms, the diaphragm, and cervical cap. Many barrier methods have the advantage of decreasing the risk for STIs.
- Hormonal methods of contraception include combination oral contraceptives (COCs), progestin-only pills (POPs), hormonal injections, hormonal implants, transdermal patch, and vaginal ring. Hormonal contraceptives are highly effective but do not provide reliable protection against STIs.
- Intrauterine devices (IUDs) are small objects that provide long-term pregnancy protection. They must be inserted by a primary care provider and require removal every few years. They do not provide protection against STIs.
- Female and male sterilization techniques are highly effective, permanent methods of contraception.

- Emergency contraception refers to hormonal methods used to prevent pregnancy after unprotected intercourse.
- Infertility is defined as the inability to conceive after a year of unprotected intercourse. Multiple factors contribute to infertility. Anything that interferes with the sperm and egg meeting or the fertilized egg from traveling to and implanting in the uterus can lead to infertility.
- Evaluation of infertility begins with the least invasive and complex and progresses to the more invasive and complex techniques. All infertility evaluation begins with a thorough history and physical examination of both partners. Usually the first test is a sperm analysis, and the second test is a postcoital examination.
- Treatment of infertility depends upon the identified cause. Therapeutic insemination techniques, surgical techniques to correct structural problems, medication to stimulate ovulation, and advanced reproductive therapies (ART) may all be used in the treatment of infertility.
- If infertility treatment fails, surrogate parenthood, adoption, and childless living are options.
- A couple undergoing evaluation and treatment for infertility may feel guilt, shock, isolation, depression, and stress. It is very stressful on a relationship to perform sexually "on demand," and intercourse often takes on a clinical and mechanical tone, rather than the desired traits of intimacy, love, and support.
- Menopause is a natural part of the life cycle. It is not a disease; however, the associated symptoms may need medication or other interventions.
- Hormone replacement therapy (HRT) used to be the gold standard of treatment for major menopausal-related symptoms; however, recent research has highlighted serious adverse effects that may be associated with HRT.
- Hot flashes, osteoporosis, and vaginal atrophy and dryness are the major symptoms for which women need and desire treatment and nursing care during menopause.

REFERENCES AND SELECTED READINGS

Books and Journals

Alzubaidi, N., & Calis, K. A., & Nelson, L. M. (2003). Dysmenorrhea. In A. C. Sciscione, F. Talavera, A. D. Barnes, F. B. Gaupp, & L. P. Shulman (Eds.), *eMedicine*. Retrieved April 10, 2004, from http://www.emedicine.com/med/topic606.htm

American Cancer Society. (2004). *Detailed guide: Breast cancer*. Cancer Reference Information [online]. Retrieved April 15, 2004, from http://www.cancer.org/docroot/CRI/CRI_2_3x.asp?dt=5

Bachmann, G. (2002). Menopause. In R. K. Zurawin, F. Talavera, G. F. Whitman-Elia, F. B. Gaupp, & L. P. Shulman (Eds.), *eMedicine*. Retrieved April 10, 2004, from http://www.emedicine.com/med/topic3289.htm

Chandran, L. (2004). Menstruation disorders. In E. Alderman, R. Konop, W. Wolfram, P. D. Petry, & M. Strafford (Eds.), *eMedicine*. Retrieved April 15, 2004, from http://www.emedicine.com/ped/topic2781.htm

Cwiak, C., & Zieman, M. (2003). New methods in contraception: A review of their advantages and disadvantages. *Women's Health in Primary Care, 6*(10), 473–478.

Davidson, M. R. (2003). Contraception update: The latest hormonal options. *Clinician Reviews, 13*(6), 53–59.

Fehring, R. J. (2004). The future of professional education in natural family planning. *JOGNN, 33*(2), 34–43.

Garcia, J. E., Nelson, L. M., & Wallach, E. E. (2003). Infertility. In R. K. Zurawin, F. Talavera, A. D. Barnes, F. B. Gaupp, & L. P. Shulman (Eds.), *eMedicine*. Retrieved April 10, 2004, from http://www.emedicine.com/med/topic3535.htm

Hickey, M., & Farquhar, C. M. (2003). Update on treatment of menstrual disorders. *eMJA, 178*(12), 625–629. Retrieved April 15, 2004, from http://www.mja.com.au/public/issues/178_12_160603/hic10854.fm.html

Htay, T. T., Aung, K., Carrick, J., & Papica, R. (2004). Premenstrual dysphoric disorder. R. C. Albucher, F. Talavera, D. Chlmow, H. H. Harsch, & S. Soreff (Eds.), *eMedicine*. Retrieved April 9, 2004, from http://www.emedicine.com/med/topic3357.htm

Hutti, M. H. (2003). New and emerging contraceptive methods: Nurses can help women make wise choices. *AWHONN Lifelines, 7*(1), 32–39.

Katz, A. (Ed.). (2003). Conversations with colleagues: Cervical cancer screening. *AWHONN Lifelines, 7*(6), 512–514.

Kazzi, A. A., & Roberts, R. (2001). Ovarian cysts. In D. A. Stearns, F. Talavera, M. Zwanger, J. Halamka, & W. K. Mallon (Eds.), *eMedicine*. Retrieved April 10, 2004, from http://www.emedicine.com/EMERG/topic352.htm

McCrink, A. (2003). Evaluating the female pelvic floor. *AWHONN Lifelines, 7*(6), 516–522.

Mishell, D. R., Burkman, R. T., Shulman, L. P., Westhoff, C. L., & Wysocki, S. J. (2002). Understanding contraceptive effectiveness. *Dialogues in Contraception, 7*(2), special issue.

Nissl, J. (2003). Healthwise knowledgebase topic: Hormone injections for birth control. Palo Alto Medical Foundation: A Sutter Health Affiliate. J. Melnikow, R. A. Hatcher, & K. Jones (medical reviewers). Retrieved April 10, 2004, from http://www.pamf.org/teen/healthinfo/index.cfm?section=healthinfo&page=article&sgml_id=hw239088

Planned Parenthood Federation of America. (2002). *Fact sheet: Nonoxynol-9: Benefits and risks*. Katharine Dexter McCormick Library (publisher). Retrieved April 9, 2004, from http://www.plannedparenthood.org/library/birthcontrol/020926_non9.html

Planned Parenthood Federation of America. (Undated). *Birth control*. Retrieved April 9, 2004, from http://www.plannedparenthood.org/bc/index.html

Pradhan, A., & Bachmann, G. (2003). Today's therapeutic options for hot flashes: Treatment in the post-women's health initiative era. *Women's Health in Primary Care, 6*(11), 527–533.

Shaw, J. A., & Shaw, H. A. (2002). Menorrhagia. In T. M. Price, F. Talavera, A. D. Barnes, F. B. Gaupp, & L. P. Shulman (Eds.), *eMedicine*. Retrieved April 9, 2004, from http://www.emedicine.com/med/topic1449.htm

Shulman, L. P. (2003, September). Advances in contraception: Choices to improve quality of life [special edition]. *Patient Care for the Nurse Practitioner*, 3–12.

Taylor, D., & Hwang, A. C. (2003). Mifepristone for medical abortion: Exploring a new option for nurse practitioners. *AWHONN Lifelines, 7*(6), 524–529.

Wallace, L. S., Rogers, E. S., Keenum, A. J., Shah, A. R., & Turner, L. W. (2003). Promoting osteoporosis screening in postmenopausal women. *Women's Health in Primary Care, 6*(8), 380–391.

Wilcox, A. J., Dunson, D., & Baird, D. D. (2000). The timing of the "fertile window" in the menstrual cycle: Day specific estimates from a prospective study. *British Medical Journal, 321*(7271):1259–1262.

Websites

Endometriosis

http://www.endocenter.org/

http://www.endometriosis.org/

Ovarian Cysts (Laparoscopic Images)

http://www.pta.net.au/sgeg/ovcyst.htm

Family Planning

www.plannedparenthood.org/

Infertility

http://www.resolve.org/

Osteoporosis

http://www.nof.org/

WORKBOOK

NCLEX-STYLE REVIEW QUESTIONS

1. An adolescent girl asks the nurse when she should have her first "Pap test." How should the nurse reply?
   a. "I don't know. Ask the doctor."
   b. "When you first start having sex."
   c. "As soon as possible and every year thereafter."
   d. "Three years after you first have sex, or age 21, whichever comes first."
2. A 35-year-old female reports very heavy menstrual periods. How does the nurse chart this in the medical record?
   a. "Chief complaint: dysmenorrhea."
   b. "Complains of metrorrhagia."
   c. "Reports amenorrhea."
   d. "Reports menorrhagia."
3. A woman is having severe symptoms of PMS. She asks the nurse what she can do to obtain relief from symptoms. What reply by the nurse is most likely to be helpful?
   a. "Antibiotics are necessary to treat the underlying infection."
   b. "Diuretics tend to be the most helpful medications for PMS treatment."
   c. "Don't worry. The medication the doctor has prescribed will take care of your symptoms."
   d. "In addition to taking medications, stress reduction and regular exercise are beneficial."
4. A woman with a pelvic support disorder reports all of the following. Which statement by the woman should alert the nurse to instruct the woman to come in immediately for examination by a physician.
   a. "My urine is cloudy."
   b. "I forgot to do my Kegel exercises today."
   c. "Every time I cough a little bit of urine comes out."
   d. "I took my pessary out to wash it, and forgot to put it back in."

STUDY ACTIVITIES

1. Develop a 10-minute presentation on considerations a couple should make before deciding on a method of birth control.
2. Explain how natural family planning techniques can be used to enhance the chance that a couple will get pregnant. Why can these methods be used to both prevent and enhance pregnancy?
3. Using the table below, compare natural methods of contraception.

Method	How it Works to Prevent Pregnancy	Special Nursing Considerations

CRITICAL THINKING: What Would You Do?

Apply your knowledge of infertility and its treatments to the following situation.

1. Amanda Rodriguez is a 37-year-old woman who has never before been pregnant. She put off pregnancy to pursue her career as an attorney. Now she and her husband have been trying to conceive for 2 years without success. She has come to the clinic for initial evaluation.
   a. Explain to Amanda what she can expect from today's visit.
   b. If Amanda is experiencing infertility, what type is it?
   c. Amanda confides in you that she thinks God is punishing her for waiting to start a family. She says that she should have tried to have children several years ago when all her friends were having babies. How would you reply to Amanda?
2. The physician tells Amanda that her husband will need to have a semen analysis and then a postcoital test will be done.
   a. Explain both of these procedures to Amanda.
   b. The semen analysis reveals a low sperm count. The physician recommends ICSI. Amanda asks how that procedure is done. How will you answer Amanda?

3. Apply your knowledge of menopause to the following situation: Cindy McFarland, a 52-year-old woman, comes to the clinic because she has been experiencing hot flashes. She tells you that the hot flashes are very intense and seem to last "forever." She says that her sweat drenches her clothes and she is embarrassed to go out in public.

   a. Explain the physiology of hot flashes to Cindy.

   b. What treatments will the physician likely recommend for Cindy?

   c. What other advice do you have for Cindy during this time of her life?

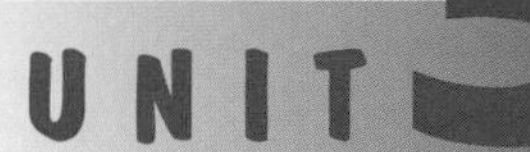

Pregnancy

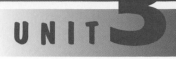

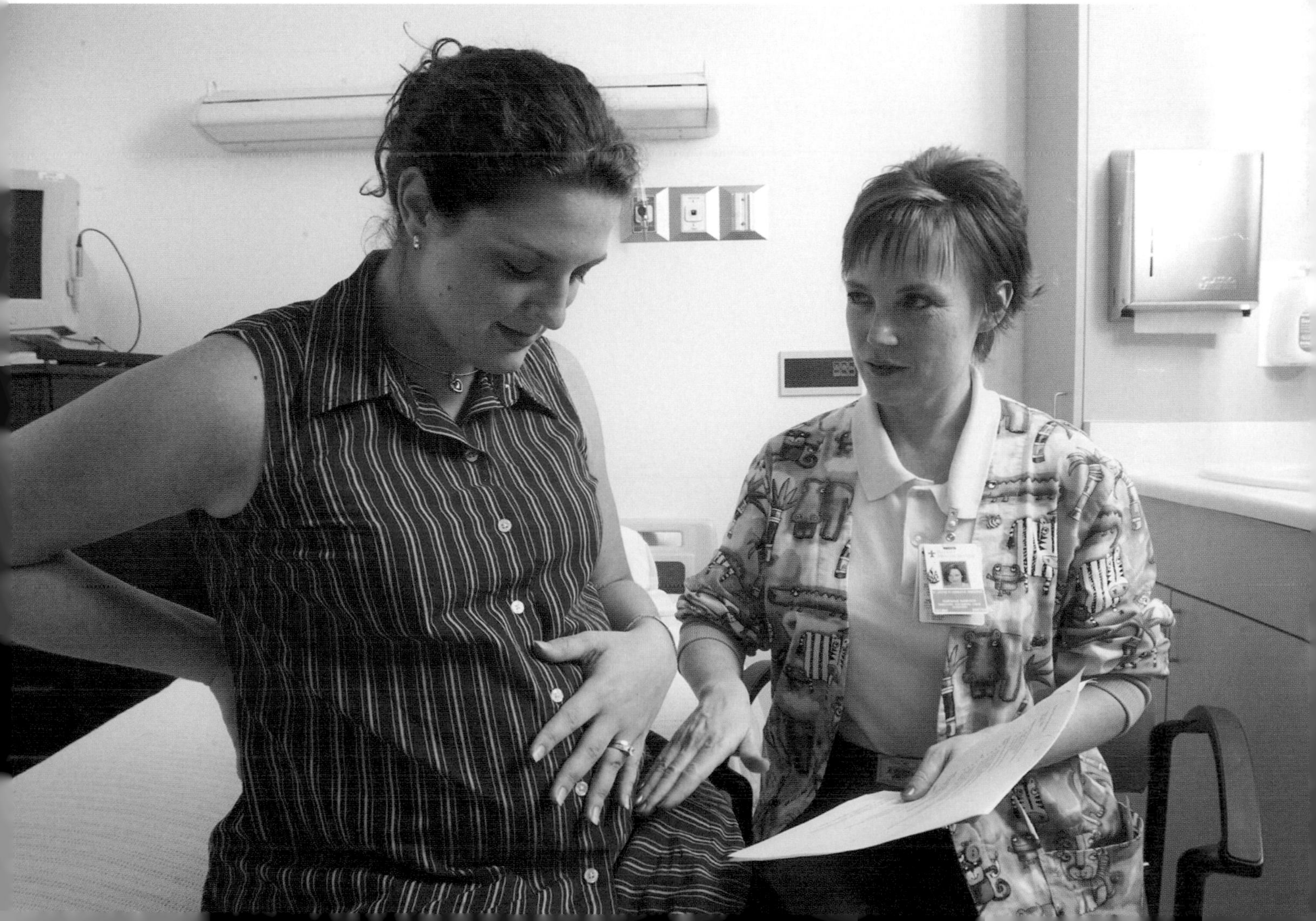

Fetal Development

STUDENT OBJECTIVES

On completion of this chapter, the student should be able to

1. Differentiate between mitosis and meiosis.
2. Describe how the process of spermatogenesis differs from oogenesis.
3. Explain how the sex of the conceptus is determined.
4. Compare the three developmental stages of pregnancy with regard to the beginning and ending time frames and major events occurring during each stage.
5. Describe the development of support structures during pregnancy.
6. Name four major functions of amniotic fluid.
7. Discuss three functions of the placenta.
8. List the steps in the process of the exchange of nutrients and wastes between the maternal and fetal bloodstreams.
9. Trace the path of fetal circulation, including the three fetal shunts.
10. Name three types of teratogens and list two examples of each kind.
11. Discuss the threat to pregnancy that occurs with ectopic pregnancy.
12. Differentiate between a monozygotic and dizygotic multifetal pregnancy.

KEY TERMS

amnion
amniotic fluid
blastocyst
chorion
chorionic villi
cleavage
decidua
dizygotic
ductus arteriosus
ductus venosus
ectopic pregnancy
embryo
fetus
foramen ovale
gametogenesis
monozygotic
morula
teratogen
Wharton's jelly
zygote

Every human being starts out as two separate germ cells, or gametes. The female gamete is the ovum, and the male gamete is the spermatozoon, or sperm for short. At conception the gametes unite to form the cell that eventually becomes the developing fetus. Human development is an ongoing process that begins at the moment of fertilization and continues even after birth. Many factors affect development. Some of these factors can cause abnormalities and birth defects. Others are part of the normal process of human development, such as gender determination. The major processes involved in human fertilization and development are discussed.

CELLULAR PROCESSES

It may seem contradictory to say that cellular division results in multiplication of cells, but that is exactly what happens in several stages of human conception and development. There are two major categories of cells and two major types of cellular division involved in the reproduction of human life.

Types of Cells

Cells are the building blocks of all organs. There are two major types of cells: soma cells, which make up the organs and tissues of the human body, and gametes, also known as germ cells or sex cells, which are found in the reproductive glands only.

The nucleus of each soma cell contains 46 chromosomes, arranged in 23 pairs. Each parent donates one chromosome of every pair. Each chromosome is composed of genes, which are defined as segments of DNA that control hereditary traits. Twenty-two of the 23 pairs of chromosomes are known as autosomes; the remaining pair determines an individual's gender.

The ovum and the sperm are, respectively, the female and male gametes. Each gamete has 23 chromosomes, exactly half of the 46 required chromosomes needed for human development.

Cellular Division

There are two types of cellular division involved in the creation of human life: mitosis and meiosis (Fig. 5-1).

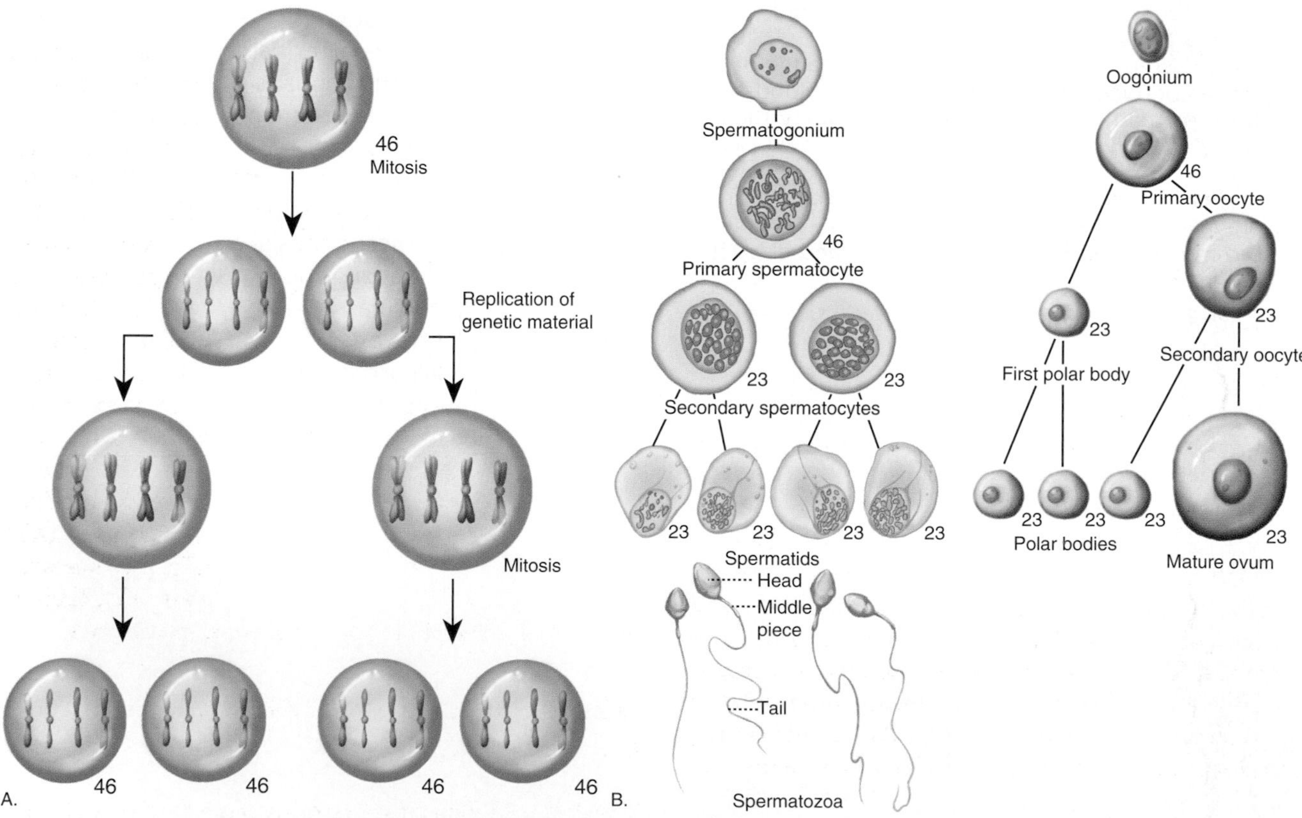

● ***Figure 5.1*** (**A**) Mitosis of the soma cell. (**B**) Gametogenesis. The various stages of spermatogenesis are indicated on the left; one spermatogonium gives rise to four spermatozoa. On the right, oogenesis is indicated; from each oogonium, one mature ovum and three abortive cells are produced. The chromosomes are reduced to one-half the number characteristic for the general body cells of the species. In humans, the number in the body cells is 46, and that in the mature spermatozoon and secondary oocyte is 23.

Mitosis

Mitosis is the process by which somatic (body) cells give birth to daughter cells. Each daughter cell contains the same number of chromosomes as the parent cell. It is the process by which the body grows and somatic cells are replaced.

Meiosis

Meiosis is the process by which gametes undergo two sequential cellular divisions of the nucleus. It is in this way that the number of chromosomes of the gametes is halved. The formation and development of gametes or germ cells by the process of meiosis is known as **gametogenesis**. Remember, each gamete has only 23 chromosomes, which is half, also known as the haploid number, of the total number of chromosomes required for human cells.

The spermatozoon and the ovum are the male and female germ cells. The ovum undergoes meiosis just before ovulation, and the male germ cell divides in the seminiferous tubules of the testes. A **zygote**, or conceptus, results when an ovum and a spermatozoon unite. The zygote has the full complement of 46 chromosomes (also called the diploid number), arranged in 23 pairs. The process of meiosis occurs in either the testes or the ovaries.

Spermatogenesis. Spermatogenesis begins at puberty in the male. In the testes, primary spermatocytes, each containing 46 chromosomes, undergo the first meiotic division, which results in two secondary spermatocytes, each with 23 chromosomes. These spermatocytes then undergo a second meiotic division, resulting in a final number of four spermatids that contain the haploid number of chromosomes (23). The spermatids undergo a change in form to become mature spermatozoa but undergo no further meiotic divisions.

Oogenesis. In the ovaries, oogenesis begins before birth but is not fully complete until the childbearing years. At birth, the female ovaries contain primary oocytes, which have completed the prophase stage of the first meiotic division. The completion of the first meiotic division occurs before ovulation. The two cells that result from this division are not identical. They are called the secondary oocyte and the first polar body. The secondary oocyte contains the haploid number of chromosomes. The first polar body soon disintegrates because it contains almost no cytoplasm. The secondary oocyte begins its second meiotic division at ovulation but does not complete the process unless it is fertilized by a sperm.

Gender Determination

Gender determination occurs at the time of fertilization. Because the spermatozoon can have either an X or a Y chromosome, it is the male that is responsible for fetal gender determination. The Y chromosome is smaller and contains mainly genes for maleness. The female ovum always contains an X chromosome, which carries several genes for other traits besides femaleness.

A female fetus (XX) will develop when the ovum unites with a spermatozoon with an X chromosome. Conversely, fertilization with a spermatozoon that contains a Y chromosome will produce a male fetus (XY) (Fig. 5-2). Research states that there is an approximately 50-50 chance of either occurrence.

This is worth noting! Many couples mistakenly believe that they can influence sex determination by using certain sexual positions, ingesting particular foods before intercourse, or timing sex to occur at specific times during the menstrual cycle. These beliefs are often rooted in folklore. Teach in a nonthreatening and respectful manner that cultural or family practices designed to control sex determination are not grounded in scientific principles.

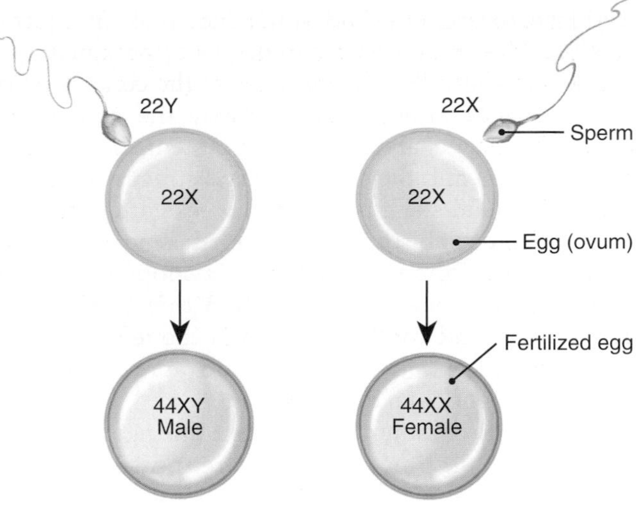

● ***Figure 5.2*** Inheritance of gender. Each ovum contains 22 autosomes and an X chromosome. Each spermatozoon (sperm) contains 22 autosomes and either an X chromosome or a Y chromosome. The gender of the zygote is determined at the time of fertilization by the combination of the sex chromosomes of the sperm (either X or Y) and the ovum (X).

DEVELOPMENTAL STAGES OF PREGNANCY

The three different stages of human development during pregnancy are:

1. Pre-embryonic
2. Embryonic
3. Fetal

The pre-embryonic stage begins at fertilization and lasts through the end of the 2nd week after fertilization. The embryonic stage begins approximately 2 weeks after fertilization and ends at the conclusion of the 8th week after fertilization. By the end of the embryonic stage, all of the organ systems have begun development and the conceptus is distinctly human in form. The fetal stage begins at 9 weeks after fertilization and ends at birth. However, birth is not the end of human development. Human development is an ongoing process of transformation that begins with fertilization and continues through the teenage years and beyond. Figure 5-3 illustrates pre-embryonic, embryonic, and fetal development.

When discussing development during pregnancy in this chapter, time references are measured in the number of weeks after fertilization, not weeks of gestation. Table 5-1 shows the corresponding time frame for postfertilization and gestational dates.

Pre-embryonic Stage

The pre-embryonic stage begins with fertilization and encompasses the first 2 weeks thereafter. Cellular division and implantation occur during this stage of development.

TABLE 5.1 Comparison of Gestational Age to Fetal Developmental Age

Stage of Development	Weeks After Fertilization	Gestational Age
Pre-embryonic	0–2 weeks	3–4 weeks' gestation
Embryonic	3–8 weeks	5–10 weeks' gestation
Fetal	9–38 weeks	11–40 weeks' gestation

Fertilization

Fertilization, also called conception, occurs when the sperm penetrates the ovum. The ovum is receptive to fertilization for approximately 24 to 48 hours after release from the ovary, and the sperm are viable for 24 to 72 hours after ejaculation into the female reproductive system. During the act of sexual intercourse, the man ejaculates approximately 300 to 600 million sperm. However, only one sperm will fertilize the mature ovum.

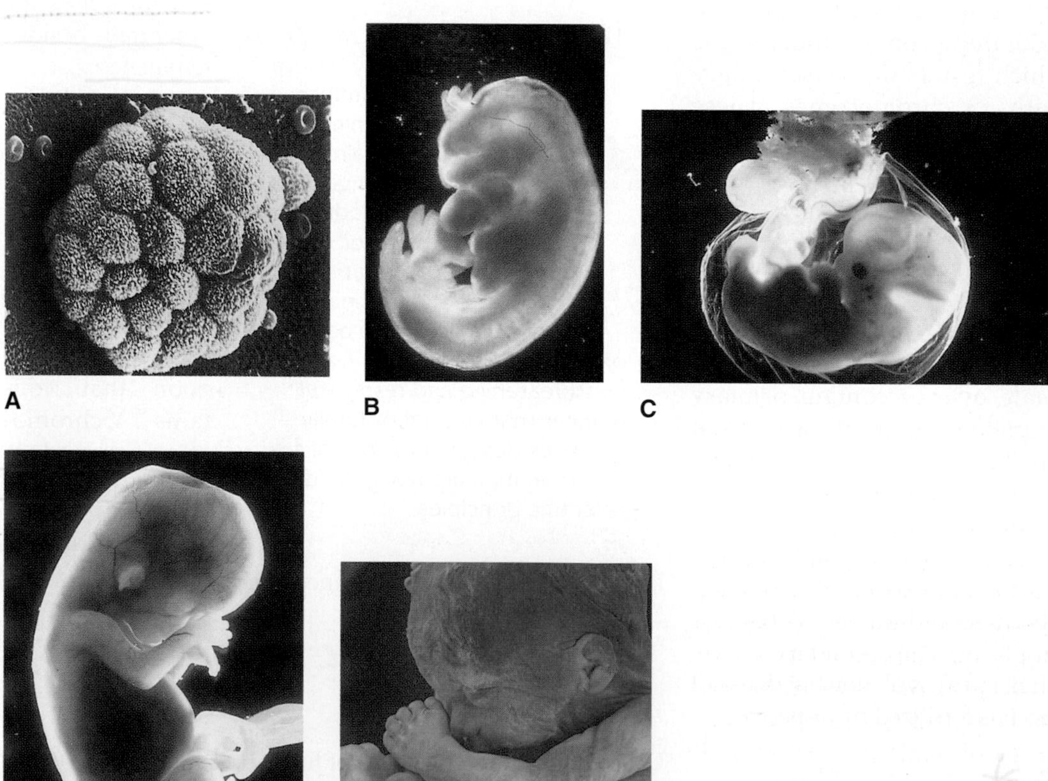

● *Figure 5.3* Pre-embyronic, embryonic, and fetal development. (**A**) Blastocyst 7 to 8 days after fertilization; (**B**) 4-week embryo; (**C**) 5-week embryo; (**D**) 6-week embryo; (**E**) 12- to 15-week fetus.

After the sperm are ejaculated into the vagina, they travel through the cervix, into the uterus, and then into the fallopian tube. Prostaglandins in the semen increase smooth muscle contractions of the uterus, thus facilitating the transport of sperm. Conception usually occurs when the ovum is in the ampulla (the outermost half) of the fallopian tube.

You do the math! If sperm are able to fertilize the ovum for as long as 72 hours after ejaculation, fertilization could potentially happen if coitus occurs 3 days before ovulation. Because the ovum can be fertilized only to a maximum of 48 hours after ovulation, fertilization can occur as long as 2 days after ovulation. Thus, the window of opportunity for conception to occur is between 3 days before until 2 days after ovulation.

Once a single sperm has penetrated the thick membrane that surrounds the ovum, called the zona pellucida, a chemical reaction occurs that causes the ovum to become impenetrable to other sperm. The chromosomes of the sperm merge with those of the ovum to complete the diploid number of 46.

Cellular Reproduction

The resulting single cell is now referred to as the zygote. The zygote begins the process of mitotic division known as **cleavage**. As the cells divide, the zygote transforms from one cell into two cells, and then each cell further divides to form a total of four cells. Each of these cells in turn divides to form a total of eight cells and so on. Each new cell contains the diploid number of chromosomes (46) beginning with the first mitotic division. All the while that cleavage is occurring, the zygote is traveling through the fallopian tube toward the uterus.

At about 3 days after fertilization, the total cell count has reached 32. The solid cell cluster is now referred to as a **morula**. The morula continues its journey toward the uterine cavity while cleavage and transformation of the cells continue. At about 5 days after fertilization, the dividing cell mass has developed a hollow, fluid-filled core and is now called a **blastocyst**. The blastocyst has an outer layer of cells, the trophoblast; a fluid-filled hollow core; and an inner cell mass. The trophoblast will go on to become the structures that nourish and protect the developing conceptus. By the end of the pre-embryonic period, the inner cell mass has become the embryonic disk, which will eventually become the fetus.

Implantation

On about the 6th day after fertilization, the trophoblast develops finger-like projections that help the blastocyst to burrow itself into the nutrient-rich endometrium. By the 10th day, the blastocyst is completely buried in the uterine lining. During the process of implantation, small cavities, called lacunae, develop around the blastocyst. Maternal blood pools in the lacunae, which allows nutrients from the woman to be exchanged for metabolic wastes from the blastocyst. The lacunae eventually become the intervillous spaces of the placenta. The tiny blastocyst begins to produce human chorionic gonadotropin (hCG), which signals the corpus luteum to continue producing progesterone to maintain the endometrial lining and the pregnancy.

Here is a teaching opportunity! Some women have a small amount of bleeding during the time of implantation, which is known as implantation bleeding. This bleeding can be mistaken for a scanty menstrual period and can lead to miscalculation of fetal age.

At this point in the woman's menstrual cycle, the endometrium is ready to support the pregnancy, and is now referred to as the **decidua**. The woman has not yet missed her menstrual period and is unaware of her pregnancy. Figure 5-4 illustrates the transport of the ovum from ovulation to fertilization and the transport of the zygote from fertilization to implantation.

Test Yourself

- Gametogenesis occurs by which type of cellular division: mitosis or meiosis?
- A male fetus carries which two sex chromosomes?
- What is the name of the single cell that results from fertilization?

Embryonic Stage

The embryonic stage lasts from the end of the 2nd week after fertilization until the end of the 8th week. This is also the time when the woman misses her first menstrual period. The developing conceptus is now called an **embryo**. By the end of the embryonic stage, all of the organ systems and major structures are present, and the embryo is fully recognizable as human in form.

During the embryonic period, the cells of the embryo multiply and tissues begin to assume specific functions, a process known as differentiation. It is

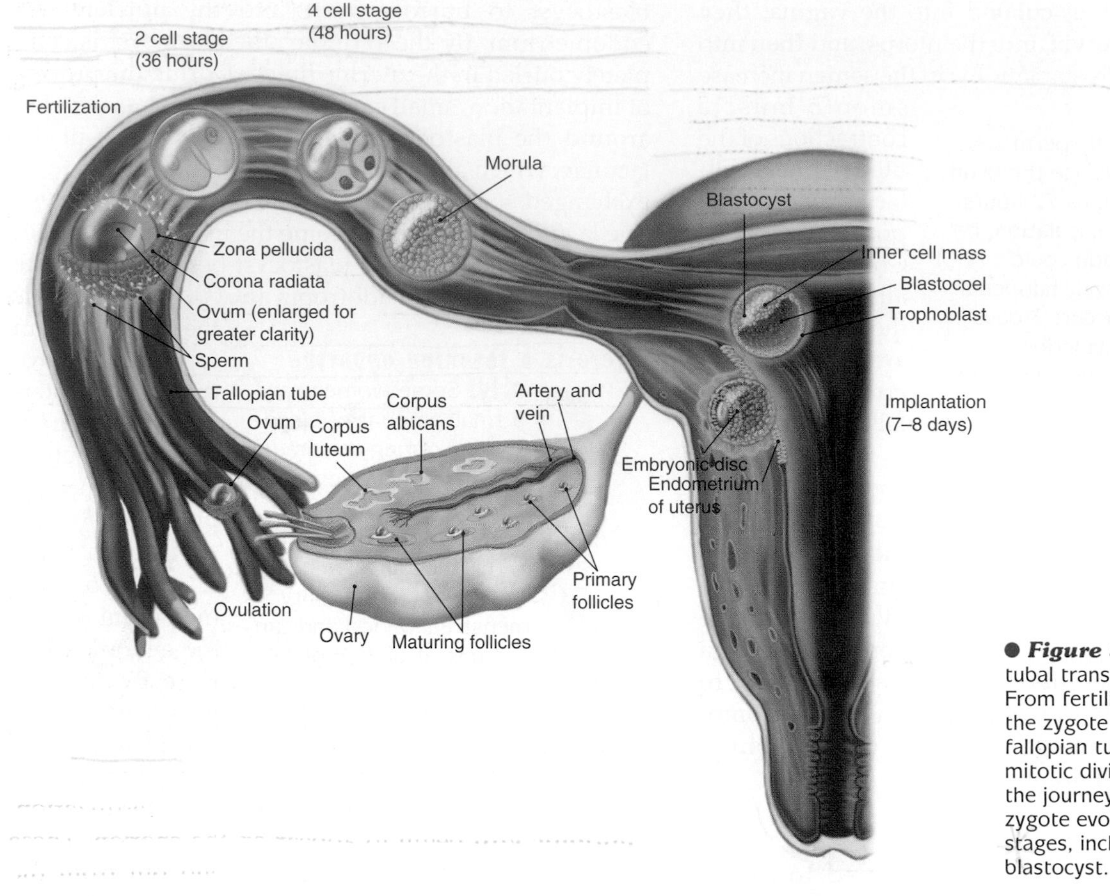

● ***Figure 5.4*** Fertilization and tubal transport of the zygote. From fertilization to implantation, the zygote travels through the fallopian tube, experiencing rapid mitotic division (cleavage). During the journey toward the uterus the zygote evolves through several stages, including morula and blastocyst.

through differentiation that tissues form rudimentary organs and organ systems.

In the 3rd week, three germ layers develop in the embryo. These layers are the ectoderm, mesoderm, and endoderm. The germ layers will become the different organs and tissues of the developing embryo. The ectoderm, which is the outer layer of cells, develops to form skin, hair, nails, and the nervous system. The mesoderm is the middle layer, which will form the skeletal, muscular, and circulatory systems. Lastly, the endoderm, which is the inner layer, will form the glands, lungs, and urinary and digestive tracts (Table 5-2).

Advise the woman who is trying to become pregnant to be very careful! Exposure to a **teratogen** (any substance or process that can interfere with normal development and lead to birth defects) during the embryonic stage produces the greatest damaging effects because it is during this time that cells are rapidly dividing and differentiating into specific body structures. (See "Teratogens and the Fetus.")

TABLE 5.2 Body Structures Developing From the Primary Germ Cells

Germ Layer	Structure Formation
Ectoderm	Skin Nervous system Nasal passages Crystalline lens of the eye Pharynx Mammary glands Salivary glands
Mesoderm	Muscles Circulatory system Bones Reproductive system Connective tissue Kidneys Ureters
Endoderm	Alimentary tract Respiratory tract Bladder Pancreas Liver

Fetal Stage

The fetal stage is from the beginning of the 9th week after fertilization and continues until birth. At this time, the developing human is referred to as the **fetus**. During the fetal stage, there is additional growth and maturation of the organs and body systems. At the beginning of this stage, the fetus is about 50 mm long and weighs about 8 grams. By the end of the fetal stage, the fetus will be about 36 cm long and weigh approximately 3,400 grams. Box 5-1 summarizes and illustrates the highlights of growth during the embryonic and fetal stages.

Test Yourself

- What is the name of the stage of development that occurs during weeks 3 to 8?
- List the three germ layers in the embryo.
- At the beginning of the fetal stage, how long is the fetus and how much does it weigh?

DEVELOPMENT OF SUPPORTIVE STRUCTURES

Fetal membranes surround the fetus in a protective sac filled with fluid that allows for protection and unrestricted growth. The fetus receives its nutrition from the woman's body, which also removes the metabolic wastes created by the fetus. This exchange is done at the placenta. The fetus and the placenta are connected by the umbilical cord. Table 5-3 summarizes characteristics of the supportive structures.

TABLE 5.3 Characteristics of Supportive Structures

Supportive Structure	Characteristics
Placenta	2–3 cm thick, thickness established by 20 weeks 15–20 cm in diameter 500–600 grams in weight Made up of 15–20 lobes called cotyledons
Amniotic fluid	About 1 liter at term Filtered and replaced every 3 hours Pale yellow to straw colored
Umbilical cord	50 cm long and 2 cm wide Blood flow through cord is about 400 mL/minute Two arteries, which carry deoxygenated blood to placenta from fetus One vein, which carries oxygen and nourishment from placenta to fetus Formed from the amnion

Fetal Membranes

A small space begins to form between the inner cell mass that will become the embryo and the tissue that has embedded into the endometrial lining. This space will become the amniotic cavity in which the fetus will grow. The amniotic cavity begins to develop around 9 days after conception. The amniotic cavity is surrounded by the **amnion**. The amnion is a thick fibrous lining, made up of several layers, that helps to protect the fetus and forms the inner part of the sac in which the fetus grows. This sac is filled with amniotic fluid. Lying against the amnion toward the exterior of the blastocyst is the **chorion**. The chorion is a second layer of thick fibrous tissue that surrounds the amnion. The amnion and chorion are not fused but lie in close contact with each other (Fig. 5-5). Together they make up the fetal membranes.

At the end of the 2nd week after fertilization, **chorionic villi** begin to appear on the chorion. These are finger-like projections that extend out from the chorion, giving it a rough appearance. Around 15 to 20 days after fertilization, cells in the chorionic villi form

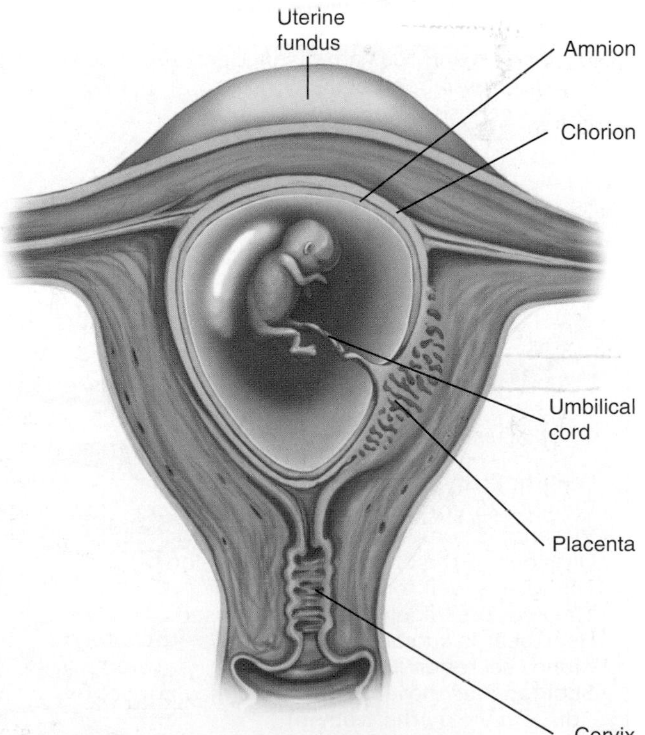

● ***Figure 5.5*** The embryo is floating in amniotic fluid surrounded by the protective fetal membranes (amnion and chorion).

BOX 5.1 Embryonic and Fetal Development

End of 4 Weeks

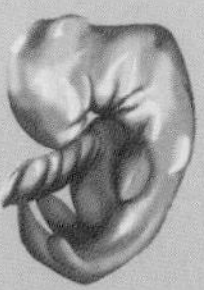

4 weeks

Chorionic villi form
The embryo is C-shaped
Length: 0.75 to 1 cm
Weight: 400 mg
Arms and legs are bud-like structures.
Rudimentary eyes, ears, and nose are discernible.
Foundations for nervous system, genitourinary system, skin, bones, and lungs are formed.

End of 8 Weeks

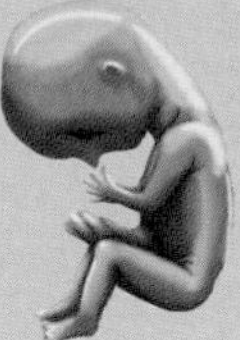

8 weeks

Length: 2.5 to 3 cm. (1 inch)
Weight: 8 grams
The head is disproportionately large as a result of brain development.
The heart, with a septum and valves, is beating rhythmically.
The fingers and toes are distinct and separated.
Sex differentiation begins.
Organogenesis is complete.

End of 12 Weeks

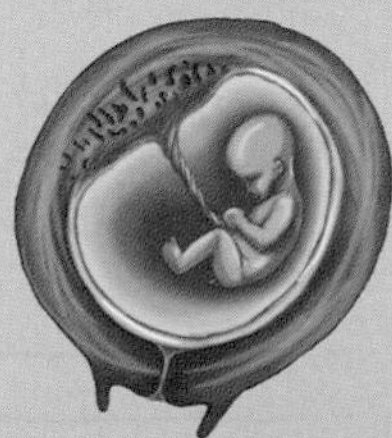

12 weeks

Length: 8 cm (3 inches)
Weight: 25 grams
Placenta is complete.
Divisions of the brain begin to develop.
The face is well formed.
The eyes are widely spaced and fused.
Heartbeat is audible by Doppler.
Kidney secretion has begun.
Spontaneous movements occur (may not yet be discernible by the woman).
Sex is discernible by outward appearance.

End of 16 Weeks

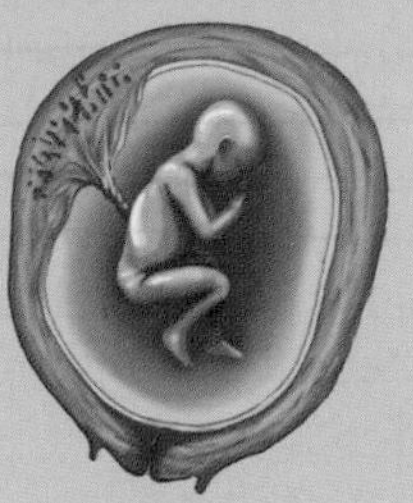

16 weeks

Length: 10 to 17 cm
Weight: 55 to 120 grams
Lungs are fully shaped.
Fetus swallows amniotic fluid.
Skeletal structure is identifiable.
Downy lanugo hair present on body.
Liver and pancreas are functioning.
Sex can be determined by ultrasound.

End of 20 Weeks

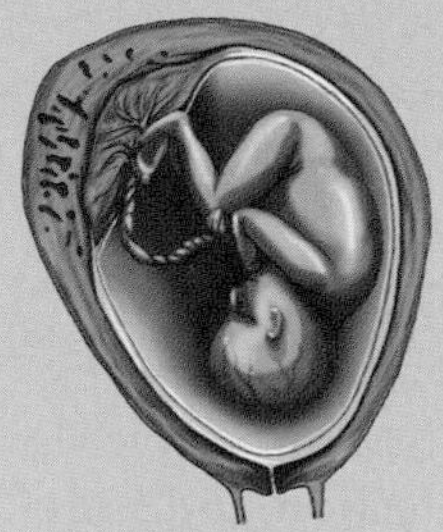

20 weeks

Length: 25 cm
Weight: 220 grams
Eyebrows and scalp hair are present.
Lanugo covers the entire body.
Vernix caseosa begins to form.
Heart sounds can be heard with a fetoscope.
Fetal movements are felt by the woman.

End of 24 Weeks

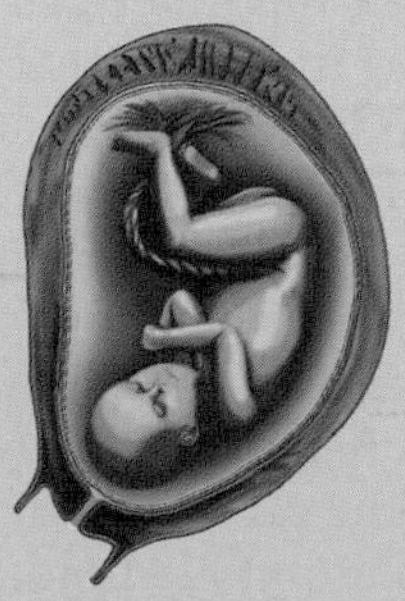

25 weeks

Length: 28 to 36 cm
Weight: 550 grams
Eyelids are now open.

BOX 5.1 (continued) **Embryonic and Fetal Development**

Pupils are capable of reacting to light.
Active production of lung surfactant begins.
Exhibits a startle reflex.
Skin is red and wrinkled, with little subcutaneous fat.
Vernix caseosa covers the skin.
May survive if born in a facility with a fully equipped neonatal intensive care unit (NICU).

End of 28 Weeks

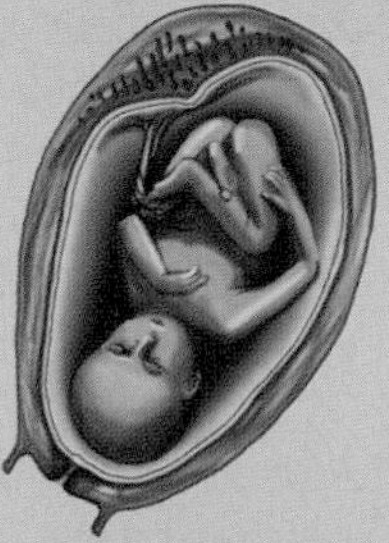

29 weeks

Length: 35 to 38 cm
Weight: 1,200 grams
Respiratory system is developed enough to provide gaseous exchange; however, the fetus needs care in a NICU in order to survive.
Adipose tissue begins to accumulate.
Male: The testes begin to descend into the scrotal sac.
Female: Clitoris is prominent and labia majora are small and do not cover the labia minora.

End of 32 Weeks

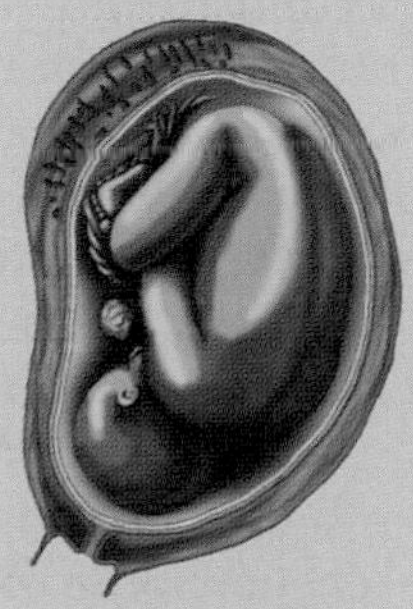

34 weeks

Length: 38 to 43 cm
Weight: 1,600 grams
The lungs are not yet fully developed, but the fetus usually does well, if born at this time.
Active Moro reflex is present.
Steady weight gain occurs.
Male: Testes descend into the scrotum. The scrotal sac has few rugae.

End of 36 Weeks

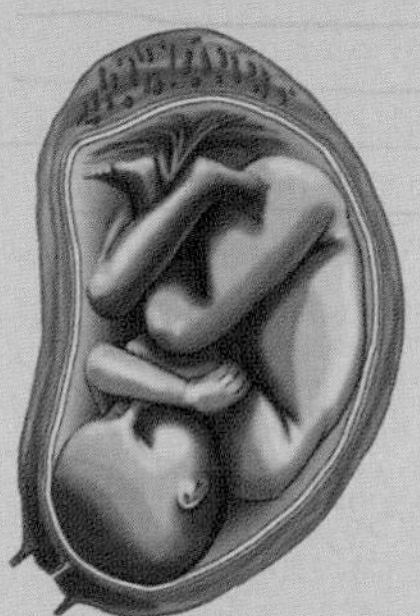

37 weeks

Length: 42 to 48 cm
Weight: 1,800 to 2,700 grams
Lanugo begins to thin.
Sole of the foot has few creases.
Birth position is usually assumed (vertex, head down).

End of 40 Weeks (Full Term)

Length: 48 to 52 cm
Weight: 3,000 grams
Vernix caseosa is evident in body folds.
Lanugo remains on the shoulders and upper back only.
Creases cover at least two thirds of the surface of the sole of the foot.
Female: The labia majora are well developed.

Adapted from: Pillitteri, A. (2003). *Maternal and child health nursing: Care of the childbearing and childrearing family* (4th ed.). Philadelphia: Lippincott Williams & Wilkins; Mattson, S., & Smith, J. E. (Eds.). (2000). *Core curriculum for maternal–newborn nursing*. AWHONN publication (2nd ed.). Philadelphia: WB Saunders; Reeder, S. J., Martin, L. L., & Koniak-Griffin, D. (1996). *Maternity nursing: Family, newborn, and women's health care* (18th ed.). Philadelphia: Lippincott-Raven; The Visible Embryo website, http://www.visembryo.com.

arterial-capillary-venous networks, which become fetal blood vessels. These capillaries pick up oxygen and nutrients from maternal blood that enters the intervillous spaces in exchange for waste products and carbon dioxide from the developing embryo.

Around the 8th week, some of the chorionic villi disintegrate, leaving a large area of the chorion that is smooth. The chorionic villi that remain increase in number and size and further branch out. The chorionic villi eventually become the fetal part of the placenta where the exchange of nutrients and wastes occurs.

Amniotic Fluid

The amniotic cavity is filled with a specialized fluid called **amniotic fluid**. Amniotic fluid serves four main functions for the fetus: physical protection, temperature regulation, provision of unrestricted movement, and symmetrical growth. Amniotic fluid is produced throughout the pregnancy by the fetal membranes. It also provides a medium that allows for fetal evaluation because it collects substances from the fetal alimentary, renal, and respiratory tracts. It is produced from maternal blood, fetal urine, and secretions from the fetal respiratory tract; 98% to 99% of amniotic fluid is water, whereas the remaining 1% to 2% is made up of electrolytes, creatinine, urea, glucose, hormones, fetal cells, lanugo (fine downy hair), and vernix caseosa (a cheesy substance that protects fetal skin).

The amniotic fluid acts as a cushion around the fetus. It protects the fetus from injury if the mother is bumped or falls. It helps to maintain a constant temperature around the fetus because the fetus is not mature enough to regulate its own temperature. Amniotic fluid allows for free movement of the fetus and aids in symmetrical growth. Lastly, it is a fluid source that the fetus drinks and then urinates. The swallowed amniotic fluid is absorbed by the fetal intestines and then urinated back into the amniotic sac.

The fetus also takes in and releases amniotic fluid when it practices fetal breathing movements. During the fetal exhalation, surfactant is released into the amniotic fluid. Surfactant is produced by the fetal lungs starting in the 28th week and helps to decrease the surface tension in the alveoli. Sampling of the amniotic fluid can help to determine if the fetal lungs are mature enough for birth.

The shed hair, epithelial cells, and sebaceous secretions from the fetus are swallowed by the fetus and help to make up the meconium that gathers in the fetal intestinal system. This is the first bowel movement the infant has after birth. If during pregnancy or labor the infant becomes stressed, the anal sphincter may relax and release meconium into the amniotic fluid. This action will cause the fluid to be stained a green color. Meconium staining of the amniotic fluid is said to have occurred if the amniotic fluid is green, instead of clear, at delivery. During the normal fetal process of swallowing and inhaling amniotic fluid in utero, the thick meconium particles can become trapped in the fetal lungs. The newborn is then at risk for meconium aspiration pneumonia.

Did you know? You can learn a lot from amniotic fluid! A procedure called amniocentesis can be performed to obtain a sample of amniotic fluid. The fluid can then be tested for surfactant, which reveals whether or not the lungs are mature enough to support respiration outside of the womb. The fluid can also be obtained for genetic testing because it contains fetal cells.

Placenta

The placenta is the organ that sustains and nourishes the growing pregnancy. The placenta has three main functions: to provide for the transfer and exchange of substances, to act as a barrier to certain substances, and to function as an endocrine gland by producing hormones. The placenta begins to develop during the 5th week after fertilization at the site of implantation. Most of the placenta is of embryonic origin, but about 20% is maternal in origin.

The placenta is made up of many lobes, or sections, called cotyledons. Each cotyledon consists of two or more main stem villi and their branches. A main stem villus consists of a branch of the umbilical vein and umbilical artery that branches out into the intervillous space. Maternal blood, from endometrial arteries, pools in the intervillous spaces.

The placenta is the exchange site for nutrients and wastes between the fetal and maternal circulatory systems. The maternal blood supply brings oxygen, water, electrolytes, vitamins, and glucose to the placenta. These nutrients are exchanged to the fetal circulation and taken to the fetus. The fetal circulation brings carbon dioxide, carbon monoxide, urea, and uric acid to be removed by the maternal circulatory system. These substances are carried across the placental membrane through simple or facilitated diffusion and active transport at the level of the chorionic villi.

The fetus receives passive immunity from the mother by transfer of maternal antibodies. Maternal antibodies to diphtheria, smallpox, and measles are transferred to the fetus. The fetus does not receive immunity to rubella, cytomegalovirus (CMV), varicella, or measles. If the woman is exposed to these infections during her pregnancy the fetus will be exposed and fetal infection may ensue. Some diseases are teratogenic (able to cause birth defects) to the fetus.

Don't pass up this teaching opportunity! Explain to the woman that she should consider that everything she takes in will pass to the fetus. Teach her to check with her primary care provider before taking any substance that is not specifically ordered for her. This warning extends to immunizations, as well.

The placenta acts as a barrier to some medications and hormones that are in the maternal blood supply. However, not all medications and substances are stopped by the placental barrier. Many of these substances cross over to the fetus.

The placenta also secretes hormones that help to sustain the pregnancy. These include progesterone, estrogen, human placental lactogen (hPL), and human chorionic gonadotropin (hCG). Progesterone is necessary to maintain the nutrient-rich endometrial lining (decidua). It also functions to keep the myometrium quiet, so that contractions do not occur prematurely, leading to loss of the pregnancy. Estrogen functions to provide a rich blood supply to the decidua and placenta. The main function of hCG is to sustain the corpus luteum at the beginning of the pregnancy. The main function of hPL is to regulate the glucose that is available for the fetus.

The well-being of the fetus is dependent upon free access of nutrients from the mother to the infant. Anomalies of the placenta or maternal–placental circulation impede fetal nourishment, which may lead to fetal growth restriction or death. Intrauterine growth restriction (IUGR) indicates fetal growth that has been slowed for some reason, resulting in a fetus that is smaller than expected for gestational age. IUGR can have many causes. Box 5-2 summarizes some of these common causes.

CULTURAL SNAPSHOT

Certain ethnic groups commonly produce offspring that are smaller than others. The fetuses of these ethnic groups are not referred to as IUGR. It is important to take into account the ethnicity and stature of both the mother and the father when evaluating an infant for IUGR.

Maternal hypertension, pregnancy-induced hypertension (PIH), or infectious agents can cause areas of infarction and subsequent calcification in the placenta. These areas lead to a decreased surface area, which decreases the amount of nutrients that can be delivered to the fetus at a given time. Vasoconstriction caused by hypertension, smoking, or illicit drug use also decreases the flow of blood to the fetus, which can lead to IUGR.

BOX 5.2 Common Causes of Intrauterine Growth Restriction (IUGR)

- Chromosomal abnormalities
- Fetal infection
- Placental infarcts
- Maternal nutritional deficiencies
- Maternal hypertension
- Pregnancy-induced hypertension (PIH)
- Maternal renal disease
- Maternal smoking
- Maternal illegal drug use
- Toxin/teratogen exposure
- Multifetal pregnancy

Umbilical Cord

The umbilical cord extends from the umbilicus of the fetus to the fetal surface of the placenta. In the cord are two arteries that bring deoxygenated blood from the fetus to the placenta and one vein that carries oxygenated and nourished blood from the placenta to the fetus. These three vessels are surrounded by a connective tissue called **Wharton's jelly,** which is a clear gelatinous substance that gives support to the cord and helps prevent compression of the cord, which could impair blood flow to the fetus.

Test Yourself

- The fetal membranes are composed of what two main structures?
- Name two functions of amniotic fluid.
- List three hormones produced by the placenta.

FETAL AND PLACENTAL CIRCULATION

Fetal Circulation

Fetal circulation differs from the pattern of human circulation that is present after birth. While in utero, the fetus is dependent upon the maternal circulation for its oxygenation, and the fetus does not use its lungs to oxygenate blood. Because the level of oxygen that is in the fetus' bloodstream is lower than maternal levels, fetal circulation aids in streaming oxygenated blood from the placenta to the major organs, especially the brain, liver, and kidneys. Fetal circulation is possible because of three major shunts that are present in the fetus but that close shortly after birth. These shunts are the ductus venosus, foramen ovale, and the ductus arteriosus.

Fetal blood flows to the placenta via the umbilical arteries. Each umbilical artery serves one half of the placenta. The arteries branch off into main stem chorionic villi that then branch down toward the decidua basalis in the intervillous spaces. The exchange of oxygen and nutrients from the woman's bloodstream for waste products from the fetus occurs at this level.

Fetal blood returns to the fetus from the placenta via the umbilical vein. In the umbilical vein, the saturation of fetal blood with oxygen is about 80%. The umbilical vein enters the fetus at the site that will be the umbilicus after birth. Approximately half of the oxygenated blood circulates from the umbilical vein to the liver, and the other half of oxygen-rich blood is shunted past the liver and flows directly into the inferior vena cava by way of the **ductus venosus**. The oxygenated blood in the inferior vena cava mixes with deoxygenated blood in the inferior vena cava that is returning to the heart from the lower limbs, abdomen, and pelvis, so that the oxygen saturation of the blood entering the right atrium is about 67%.

The majority of the blood in the right atrium is directed into the left atrium via the **foramen ovale**. The foramen ovale is a hole that connects the right and left atria so the majority of oxygenated blood can quickly pass into the left side of the fetal heart and be sent to the brain and the rest of the fetal body. Blood entering the right atrium from the superior vena cava is mostly deoxygenated. In the right atrium, this blood mixes with some of the well-oxygenated blood from the inferior vena cava, and this mixed blood enters the right ventricle, where it is then pumped to the fetal lungs via the pulmonary trunk.

In utero the fetus does not oxygenate its own blood in the lungs; therefore, blood supplied to the fetal lungs is for nourishment of the tissues only. The lungs are filled with fetal lung fluid and collapsed, which leads to high resistance. Because of this resistance, only 5% to 10% of the blood in the pulmonary artery enters the fetal lungs. The remainder of blood coming from the right ventricle enters the **ductus arteriosus**. The ductus arteriosus is a fetal shunt that links the pulmonary artery with the aorta.

In the left atrium the oxygenated blood is mixed with some deoxygenated blood that is returning to the heart from the lungs. The blood then travels to the left ventricle, where it is pumped to the aorta. The higher oxygenated blood from the ascending aorta is sent to the heart, head, and upper limbs by way of the aortic arch branch. The low oxygenated blood from the pulmonary artery enters the aorta via the ductus arteriosus below the aortic arch branch, which supplies the head and upper limbs with the highest oxygenated blood.

Blood in the abdominal aorta divides so that half of the blood supply returns to the placenta for reoxygenation while the other half goes to nourish the viscera and lower half of the body. The internal iliac arteries branch off to form the two umbilical arteries. The umbilical arteries then carry deoxygenated blood and waste products back to the placenta, which completes the fetal circulation circuit (Fig. 5-6).

At birth, when fetal blood stops being shunted to the placenta for oxygenation, rapid physiologic changes occur to allow the newborn to oxygenate his own blood by his lungs. After birth the ductus venosus, ductus arteriosus, and the umbilical vein and arteries constrict and eventually form ligaments, which remain present for the rest of the infant's life. It is possible for the ductus arteriosus to remain open, especially in premature infants or infants with hypoxia. When this shunt remains open, it is called a patent ductus arteriosus; medications or surgery may be required to close the duct. Refer to Chapter 13 for a detailed discussion of the circulatory changes that occur in the newborn.

Placental Circulation

The uterine arteries supply the uterus with maternal blood. The blood is then carried to the intervillous spaces by endometrial arteries, also known as spiral arteries. In the intervillous spaces, maternal blood flows around the chorionic villi, where nutrients and oxygen from the maternal circulation are transferred by diffusion and active transport across a thin membrane into the fetal circulation. Likewise, fetal wastes diffuse into the maternal bloodstream. Blood leaves the intervillous spaces by the endometrial veins and returns to the maternal circulatory system.

Test Yourself

- Name the three fetal shunts.
- Explain how the ductus arteriosus and foreman ovale aid the fetus in quickly getting oxygen-enriched blood to the tissues.
- By what processes do nutrients, oxygen, and wastes transfer between the pregnant woman's blood and fetal blood?

SPECIAL CONSIDERATIONS OF FETAL DEVELOPMENT

Teratogens and the Fetus

As described earlier in this chapter, teratogens are substances that cause birth defects. The severity of the defect depends upon when during development the conceptus is exposed to the teratogen (i.e., what body systems are developing at the time of exposure) and the particular teratogenic agent to which the fetus is exposed.

Effects of Teratogens on the Developing Fetus

During the pre-embryonic stage, exposure to a teratogen has an all-or-nothing effect. Either the exposure will cause death of the zygote, or there will be no effect because there is no connection between the maternal blood supply and the zygote.

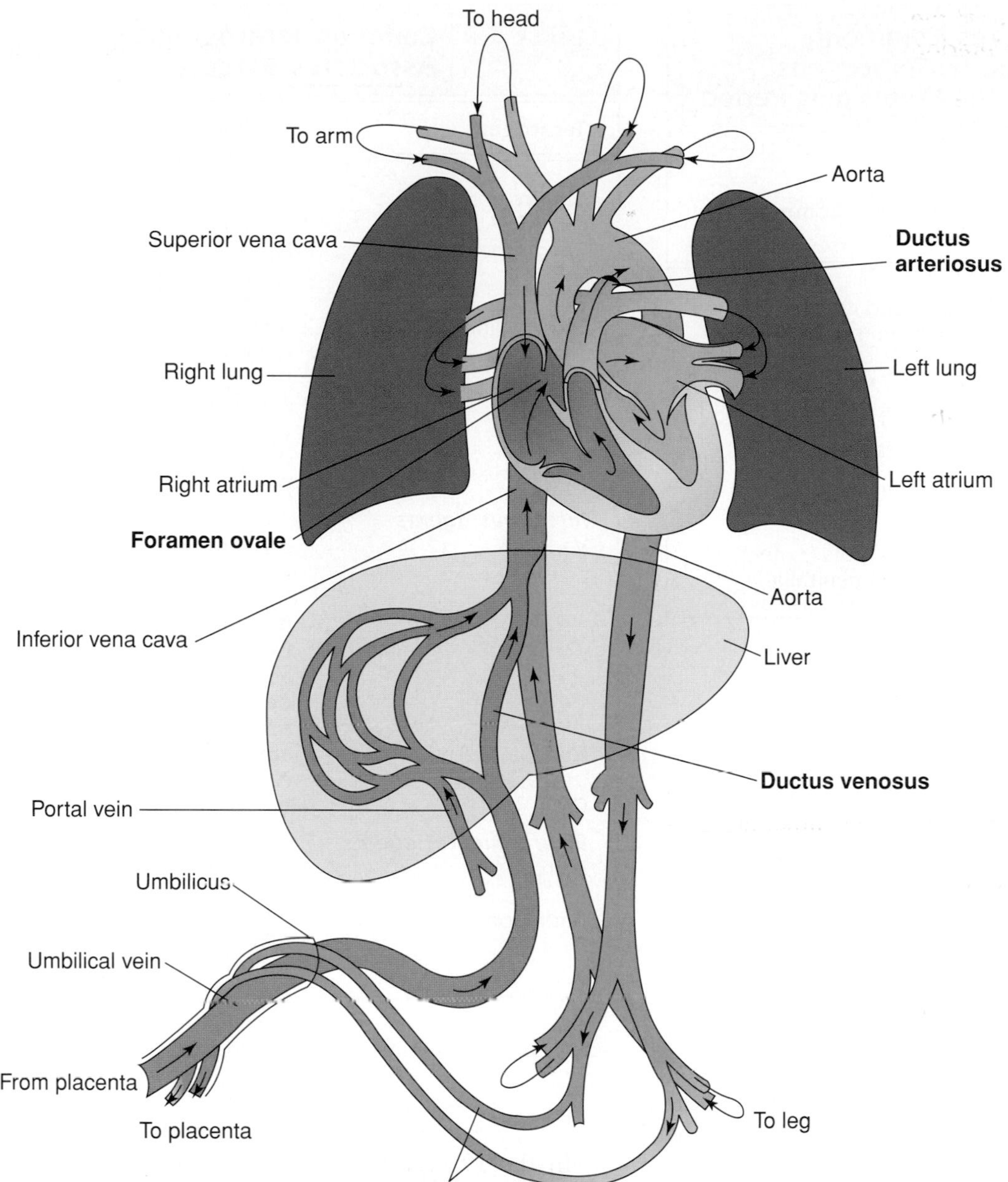

● ***Figure 5.6*** Fetal circulation. Arrows indicate the path of blood. The umbilical vein carries oxygen-rich blood from the placenta to the liver and through the ductus venosus. From there it is carried to the inferior vena cava to the right atrium of the heart. Some of the blood is shunted through the foramen ovale to the left side of the heart where it is routed to the brain and upper extremities. The rest of the blood travels down to the right ventricle and through the pulmonary artery. A small portion of the blood travels to the non-functioning lungs, while the remaining blood is shunted through the ductus arteriosus into the aorta to supply the rest of the body.

Exposure to a teratogen during the embryonic stage produces the greatest damaging effects. It is during this time that development of the primary structure and function of organs and tissues is initiated. Developing organs and body systems are highly susceptible to teratogens, and major abnormalities can result. Table 5-4 lists structures commonly affected by teratogen exposure during the embryonic period. Because the central nervous system (CNS) develops continuously throughout pregnancy, these structures are always vulnerable to teratogens.

Exposure to a teratogen during the fetal stage will have less of an effect on the fetus than exposure during the embryonic period. The effect of a teratogen during this stage may cause physiologic defects and minor structural abnormalities. The CNS and brain continue to be susceptible to damage from teratogens during the fetal period.

TABLE 5.4 Structures Commonly Affected by Teratogens During the Embryonic Period

Week of Development (# of weeks after fertilization) in Which Exposure Occurs	Structures Commonly Affected
3	Heart and central nervous system (CNS)
4	Lip, heart, arm, leg, CNS
5	Heart, eye, arm, leg, CNS
6	CNS, heart, ear, teeth
7	CNS, ear, teeth, palate, heart
8	CNS, ear, palate, heart, external genitalia

TABLE 5.5 Common Teratogens and Associated Effects

Teratogen	Possible Effect
Medications	
Dilantin	Cleft palate
Chemotherapy agents	Major congenital malformations, especially of the CNS
Tetracycline	Damage to developing dental and osseous tissue
Alcohol	Fetal alcohol syndrome (FAS) with facial defects, low birth weight, affects brain
Infectious agents	
Varicella	Fetal varicella syndrome, which ranges in severity from generalized multiorgan damage to isolated defects, such as incomplete limb development or skin scarring
Rubella (German measles)	Cataracts, deafness, and cardiac malformations
CMV	Hearing loss, microcephaly
Environmental agents	
Mercury	Neurologic damage, blindness
Radiation	Congenital malformations, mental retardation (seen in large amounts of ionizing radiation)

Types of Teratogenic Agents

Teratogens usually fall into one of three categories: an ingested, infectious, or environmental substance. Table 5-5 summarizes some of the common teratogens and their effects.

Your sensitivity can make a big difference! Guilt is a common feeling in mothers whose infants are born with a birth defect. Many defects happen before the woman knows she is pregnant. Avoid statements that imply blame. For example don't say, "You shouldn't have been around x-rays while you were pregnant."

Ingested Teratogens. Most substances ingested by the pregnant woman pass to the fetus from the maternal bloodstream through the placenta and then into the fetal circulation. Commonly ingested teratogens include prescription medications, illicit drugs, and alcohol. Some medications may be therapeutic for the mother but also have teratogenic properties. For example, phenytoin (Dilantin) is therapeutic for preventing seizures in the mother but is also known to cause cleft palate and other abnormalities in the fetus. In such a circumstance, the risk to the mother must be weighed against the risk to the developing fetus. Not all medications are teratogenic. Acetaminophen (Tylenol) is an example of a medication that, when taken as directed, is nonteratogenic. Some medications, such as heparin, are known to be unable to cross the placental barrier and thus are safe to use during pregnancy.

In the 1950s many pregnant women were prescribed thalidomide to help control morning sickness. Thalidomide was discovered to cause limb deformities in the infants who were exposed to it in utero. Thalidomide use during pregnancy was discontinued when the teratogenic effects became known.

One of the fetus' main body systems affected throughout the embryonic and fetal period is the brain and CNS. Alcohol and illicit drugs such as marijuana, cocaine, and heroin are known to affect the CNS. Infants exposed to these substances during pregnancy may be born addicted to the substance to which they were exposed. Therefore, ingestion of these substances is strongly discouraged during pregnancy.

Infectious Teratogens. If the pregnant woman develops an infection during her pregnancy, the infection can pass to the fetus and affect fetal development. Some common infections that are known to have

A PERSONAL GLIMPSE

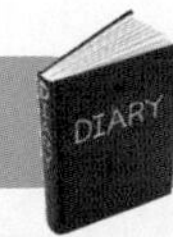

The worrying began when I found out I was pregnant with my oldest child. We hadn't been officially trying to get pregnant, and so right away I started thinking about all the things I had ingested while already pregnant. I was a 3-cup-a-day coffee drinker; I had taken several doses of Tylenol for headaches; and I remembered celebrating my birthday with a few glasses of wine. To top it all off, I hadn't been taking prenatal vitamins. I started panicking about the harm I had caused my developing baby. I immediately stopped drinking caffeine completely (which gave me very bad headaches); swore off wine for the duration; avoided taking any kind of medication for pain; never missed a day taking prenatal vitamins; and avoided eating fish, hot dogs, and lunch meat (I had heard that these foods were bad to eat during pregnancy). I was also concerned about microwave rays (and stopped using the microwave completely); cats and cat litter; gardening; being around my friends' children (they might have some lurking virus); and mold in the house. I was starting to drive my husband and myself crazy.

At my first prenatal appointment, I talked with the staff at my primary care provider's office. They gave me a brochure that listed things to avoid completely during pregnancy; things to limit during pregnancy; and things that were OK during pregnancy. It also contained practical advice for maintaining a healthy home environment during pregnancy and child rearing. I remained careful during my pregnancy, but I learned to relax a bit more and just use common sense.

Allison

LEARNING OPPORTUNITY: How can the nurse help the woman of childbearing age be aware of possible teratogens without unduly scaring her? How should the nurse advise the woman who is very worried that she may have done something to harm her unborn child before she was aware of the pregnancy?

teratogenic effects include varicella, cytomegalovirus (CMV), and rubella.

Environmental Teratogens. The pregnant woman may be exposed to substances in the environment that can have a teratogenic effect. Ionizing x-rays, radioactive substances, and certain chemicals can cause birth defects. The pregnant woman should take precautions to avoid these substances during her pregnancy. Avoiding unnecessary x-rays, or using a lead shield for unavoidable x-rays, and using gloves when handling chemicals are two ways the woman can help protect her developing fetus.

Ectopic Pregnancy

There are instances when the zygote implants in places other than the uterus. Of the implantations that occur outside of the uterine cavity, 95% occur in the fallopian tube. When the zygote implants outside the uterus, it is known as an **ectopic pregnancy**. An ectopic pregnancy that occurs in a fallopian tube is more specifically referred to as a tubal pregnancy. Usually tubal pregnancies are caused by blockage or scarring of the fallopian tubes, either from infection or trauma, such as a tubal ligation reversal. Ectopic pregnancy occurs in 19.7 of 1,000 pregnancies.

As the embryo grows in the confined space of the fallopian tube, it causes the tube to dilate. The tube will eventually rupture, unless the condition is caught in time. If the tube ruptures, it will result in maternal hemorrhage into the peritoneal cavity and can lead to maternal death. In the event of a tubal pregnancy, the affected tube and the products of conception are removed. Because there is no way to transplant the embryo into the uterine cavity and continue the pregnancy, tubal pregnancies always result in the death of the embryo. See Chapter 17 for a full discussion of ectopic pregnancy.

Multifetal Pregnancy

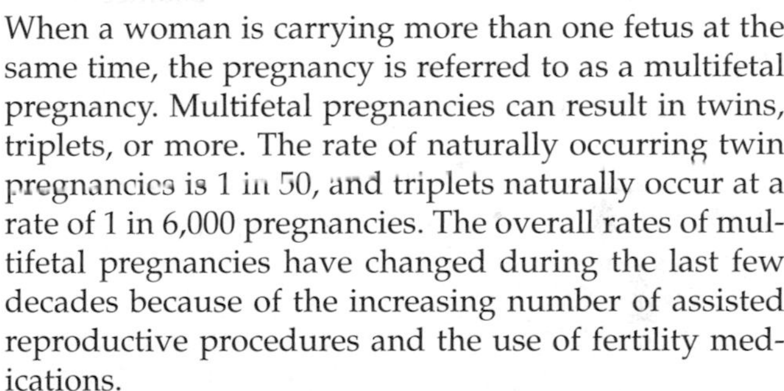

When a woman is carrying more than one fetus at the same time, the pregnancy is referred to as a multifetal pregnancy. Multifetal pregnancies can result in twins, triplets, or more. The rate of naturally occurring twin pregnancies is 1 in 50, and triplets naturally occur at a rate of 1 in 6,000 pregnancies. The overall rates of multifetal pregnancies have changed during the last few decades because of the increasing number of assisted reproductive procedures and the use of fertility medications.

Twins can be either identical or fraternal. Identical twins are derived from one zygote (one egg and one sperm divide into two zygotes shortly after fertilization), so identical twins are called **monozygotic** twins. They share the same genetic material and are always the same gender. Fraternal twins develop from separate egg and sperm fertilizations and are called **dizygotic** twins. Fraternal twins may or may not be the same gender, and their genetic material is not identical. In pregnancies that have more than two fetuses, they may have all developed from a single fertilized egg, also referred to as monozygotic, or they may have developed from separate eggs, or they may be a combination of both types (Fig. 5-7).

Twins can be classified one of three ways—diamniotic-dichorionic, diamniotic-monochorionic, and monoamniotic-monochorionic. Diamniotic-dichorionic twins each develop in their own amniotic sac. Their placentas do not share any vessels.

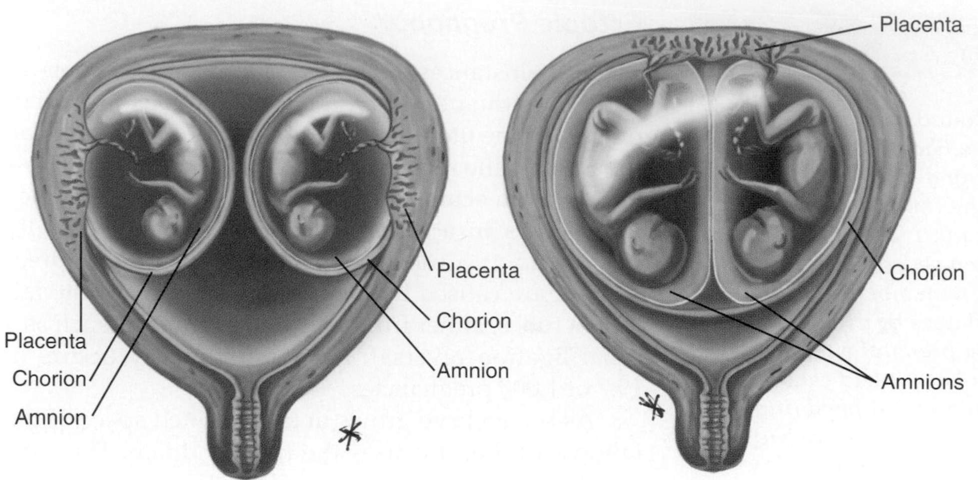

● ***Figure 5.7*** Twin pregnancy. (**A**) Fraternal (dizygotic) twins with two placentas, two amnions, and two chorions (diamniotic dichorionic). (**B**) Identical (monozygotic) twins with one placenta, two amnions, and one chorion (diamniotic monochorionic).

Diamniotic-monochorionic twins each have their own amniotic sac but share a common chorionic sac. They each have a separate placenta, but the placentas share some vessels. These types of twins are at risk for developing a condition referred to as twin-to-twin transfusion syndrome. In this syndrome, one fetus gives the other fetus part of its blood volume but does not receive any in return. Lastly, twins can be monoamniotic-monochorionic. These types of twins have one amniotic cavity that they both share. The greatest risk to these types of twins is cord entanglement. Conjoined twins occur in 1 in 50,000 to 80,000 deliveries.

Certain factors increase a woman's chance of becoming pregnant with dizygotic twins. She is more likely to have dizygotic twins if she is herself a twin or has twin siblings, if she recently stopped using oral contraceptives, if she is tall or has a large stature, or if she is of African-American heritage. The use of fertility medications, such as Clomid or Pergonal, increases a woman's chance of carrying a multifetal pregnancy. Multifetal pregnancies are at higher risk for certain conditions and need to be monitored closely (see Chapter 17).

Test Yourself

- Which organ system is susceptible throughout the pregnancy to teratogenic effects?
- Define ectopic pregnancy.
- Why are fraternal twins called dizygotic twins?

KEY POINTS

- Mitosis is the process of cell division by which two daughter cells are produced that have the diploid number of chromosomes (46). Meiosis is a special type of cell division in which cells with the haploid number of chromosomes (23) are formed.
- Spermatogenesis begins at puberty, whereas oogenesis starts during the fetal stage in the female infant and then stays in an arrested state until puberty. Spermatogenesis ends with four spermatids, each with 23 chromosomes. Oogenesis ends with one ova containing 23 chromosomes.
- Sex (or gender) determination occurs when the ovum and the sperm unite. The ovum always contributes an X chromosome, whereas the sperm contributes either an X or a Y chromosome. Two X chromosomes (XX) is female. An X and a Y chromosome (XY) is male.
- The pre-embryonic stage lasts from fertilization until the end of the 2nd week after conception. During this time the two sets of chromosomes combine, implantation occurs, and the beginning of maternal–fetal circulation occurs.
- The embryonic stage lasts from the end of the 2nd week until the end of the 8th week. During this time the organs and tissues begin to differentiate and assume specific functions. By the end of this stage all organs are developed and the embryo is distinctly human in appearance.
- The fetal stage lasts from the end of the 8th week until birth. During this time there is additional maturation and growth of already existing tissue.
- The fetal membranes are formed by the close union of the amnion and chorion. The amnion makes up the inner part of the membrane and is in contact with amniotic fluid and the fetus. The chorion is adjacent to (but not fused with) the amnion and has no contact with the fetus.
- Amniotic fluid serves as a cushion to protect the fetus from injury, a temperature control mechanism, and a medium that allows for free movement and unrestricted growth.

- The placenta transfers nutrients, such as oxygen and glucose, to the fetus while removing waste products, such as carbon dioxide and urea. The placenta acts as a barrier to some harmful substances but does not prevent most substances from passing to the fetus. The placenta has an endocrine function in that it secretes hormones that help to sustain the pregnancy. These hormones include hCG, hPL, estrogen, and progesterone.
- Maternal blood rich in oxygen and nutrients reaches the placenta at the level of the intervillous spaces that are surrounded by the chorionic villi. The chorionic villi contain the fetal blood vessels. Exchange of nutrients for wastes occurs by simple diffusion or active transport across a thin membrane that separates the fetal and maternal bloodstreams.
- Fetal blood that contains newly oxygenated blood and nutrients leaves the placenta via the umbilical vein and enters the fetal inferior vena cava via the ductus venosus. From there it travels to the right atrium, where most of the blood crosses the foramen ovale into the left atrium. The blood then travels to the aortic arch to the brain and the upper body. Some of the blood enters the right ventricle and goes to the lungs to nourish the tissues. Most of the blood that leaves the right ventricle is shunted to the aorta via the ductus arteriosus. Deoxygenated fetal blood returns to the placenta via the two umbilical arteries.
- Teratogens can be classified as ingested, infectious, or environmental. Ingested teratogens can be medications or illegal substances. Infectious teratogens include diseases such as cytomegalovirus (CMV) and rubella. Environmental teratogens include ionizing x-rays and chemicals.
- An ectopic pregnancy is one that develops outside of the uterus. Most ectopic pregnancies occur in a fallopian tube, which can rupture and lead to maternal hemorrhage and/or death. A tubal pregnancy always leads to death of the embryo, whether from tubal rupture or removal during surgery.
- Monozygotic twins are identical because they arise from one zygote and therefore share identical chromosomes. Dizygotic twins are fraternal because they arise from two separate zygotes and therefore do not share the same chromosomes.

REFERENCES AND SELECTED READINGS

Books and Journals

Blackburn, S. T., & Loper, D. L. (2002). *Maternal, fetal, and neonatal physiology: A clinical perspective* (2nd ed.). Philadelphia: WB Saunders.

Cunningham, F. G., Gant, N. F., Leveno, K. J., Gilstrap, L.C. III, Hauth, J. C., & Wenstrom, K. D. (2001). *Williams obstetrics* (21st ed.). New York: McGraw-Hill Medical Publishing Division.

Mattson, S., & Smith, J. E. (Eds.). (2000). *Core curriculum for maternal–newborn nursing*. AWHONN publication (2nd ed.). Philadelphia: WB Saunders.

Moore, K. L. (1998). *Before we are born: Essentials of embryology and birth defects*. Philadelphia: WB Saunders.

Pillitteri, A. (2003). *Maternal and child health nursing: Care of the childbearing and childrearing family* (4th ed.). Philadelphia: Lippincott Williams & Wilkins.

Potter, P. A., & Perry, A. G. (2000). *Fundamentals of nursing* (5th ed.). Oxford, UK: Elsevier Science.

Reeder, S. J., Martin, L. L., & Koniak-Griffin, D. (1996). *Maternity nursing: Family, newborn, and women's health care* (18th ed.). Philadelphia: Lippincott-Raven.

Robinson, J. N., & Abuhamad, A. Z. (2002). Determining chorionicity and amnionicity in multiple pregnancies. *Contemporary Ob/Gyn, 6*, 94–108. Retrieved November 28, 2003, from http://www.contemporaryobgyn.net

Yetter, J. F. (1998). Examination of the placenta. *American Family Physician, 57*(5), 1045. Retrieved November 28, 2003, from http://www.aafp.org/afp/980301ap/yetter.html

Websites

Visible Embryo

http://www.visembryo.com

IUGR

http://www.pediatrics.wisc.edu/childrenshosp/parents_of_preemies/IUGR.html

Teratogens

http://www.lpch.org/DiseaseHealthInfo/HealthLibrary/genetics/terathub.html

http://www.modimes.org/

Ectopic Pregnancy

http://www.aafp.org/afp/20000215/1080.html

WORKBOOK

NCLEX-STYLE REVIEW QUESTIONS

1. A mother ingests a teratogenic substance. At which stage of development will the most damage occur?
   a. Conception
   b. Pre-embryonic
   c. Embryonic
   d. Fetal
2. During which time frame does the embryonic stage last?
   a. Ovulation to conception
   b. 1 to 14 days after conception
   c. 3 through 8 weeks after conception
   d. 9 through 38 weeks after conception
3. What is the main purpose of the chorionic villi?
   a. To adhere the blastocyst to the endometrial lining
   b. To form the tissues that will become the placenta
   c. To produce amniotic fluid
   d. To provide an exchange site for the exchange of nutrients and wastes
4. Which one of the following is a fetal shunt that aids in fetal circulation?
   a. Foramen primum
   b. Foramen ovale
   c. Ductus deferens
   d. Septum secundum
5. Twins who share the same chromosomal material are classified as
   a. Monozygotic
   b. Dizygotic
   c. Fraternal
   d. Trizygotic

STUDY ACTIVITIES

1. Use the following table to compare major developmental milestones at each of the indicated gestational ages. Refer to this textbook and to the following website: http://www.visembryo.com

Gestational Age	Major Developmental Milestones
4 weeks	
8 weeks	
12 weeks	
16 weeks	
20 weeks	
28 weeks	
32 weeks	
36 weeks	

2. Talk to the following individuals in your community about teratogens. Have each person discuss several substances or processes that might be damaging to the fetus and how a pregnant woman can best protect her fetus from harm.
   a. Pharmacist
   b. Obstetrician
   c. Chemist
   d. Radiologist
3. Develop a teaching plan for an adolescent who is pregnant. Explain the processes of fertilization and development in language she will likely understand. Prepare the answers to three to four questions you anticipate she may ask you.

CRITICAL THINKING: What Would You Do?

Apply your knowledge of fetal development to the following situation.

1. Rebecca, a 25-year-old woman, has just discovered she is pregnant for the first time. She missed her first menstrual period 4 weeks ago and came to the office for a pregnancy test, which was positive.
   a. Rebecca asks you what her baby looks like right now. What will you tell her?
   b. Rebecca is worried because she has taken Tylenol several times during the past week for tension headaches. How will you advise her?

2. Rebecca comes in for her 12-week checkup. She measures larger than expected for dates, so the physician orders a sonogram.

   a. Rebecca asks you to tell her what her baby looks like at this stage. How will you answer?

   b. The sonogram shows that Rebecca is carrying twins. She wants to know whether they are identical or fraternal. How will you answer her?

Maternal Adaptation During Pregnancy

STUDENT OBJECTIVES

On completion of this chapter, the student should be able to

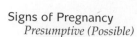

1. Differentiate between presumptive, probable, and positive signs of pregnancy.
2. Relate normal anatomy and physiology of the nonpregnant woman to that of the pregnant woman.
3. Explain expected changes in the major body systems during pregnancy.
4. Discuss maternal physiologic adaptation to pregnancy.
5. Discuss maternal psychological adaptation to pregnancy.
6. Outline components of a nutritious diet during pregnancy.

KEY TERMS

ballottement
Braxton Hicks contractions
Chadwick's sign
chloasma
colostrum
couvade syndrome
cretinism
diastasis recti abdominis
glycosuria
Goodell's sign
Hegar's sign
linea nigra
lordosis
Montgomery's tubercles
pica
pyrosis
scurvy
striae
supine hypotensive syndrome

gravida – woman pregnant
Para – # of (live) Pregnancies 20-24wks

Pregnancy is a time of adaptation and change, not only physically, but also psychologically as the woman and her partner prepare for parenthood. The body also must adapt and accommodate the needs of the growing fetus. This chapter explores the signs of pregnancy; the physiologic and psychological changes associated with pregnancy; and the changing nutritional requirements of pregnancy.

SIGNS OF PREGNANCY

The physician or certified nurse midwife (CNM) uses a combination of signs to diagnose pregnancy (Box 6-1). These signs can be categorized as presumptive, probable, and positive. The presumptive, or subjective, signs are the symptoms the woman experiences and reports to the health care provider. Each of these signs, taken alone, can have causes other than pregnancy. The same is true for probable, or objective signs, the examiner finds and reports. The only signs that are 100% diagnostic of pregnancy are the positive signs, which also are objective data noted by the examiner.

BOX 6.1 Signs of Pregnancy

After each symptom, an alternative cause (if any) other than pregnancy is suggested. All symptoms and times can vary in occurrence between individuals.

Presumptive (Possible) Signs

- 3–4 weeks+: Early breast changes (e.g., prickling and tingling sensations). Could be caused by oral contraceptives.
- 4 weeks+: Amenorrhea (missed period). May be caused by hormonal imbalance, emotional stress, or illness.
- 4–14 weeks: Morning sickness. May be related to gastrointestinal disorders, pyrexial illness, and so on.
- 6–12 weeks: Bladder irritability. Can be associated with urinary tract infection or pelvic tumor.

Probable Signs

- 4–12 weeks: Presence of hCG in blood. May be caused by hydatidiform mole.
- 6–12 weeks: Presence of hCG in urine. Choriocarcinoma is a possible cause.
- 8 weeks+: Uterine growth. May be caused by tumors.
- 16 weeks: Braxton Hicks (painless contractions). May be caused by upset stomach.
- 16–28 weeks: Ballottement of fetus. May be elicited by a tumor.

Positive Signs

- 6 weeks+: Visualization of fetus by ultrasound.
- 20–24 weeks+: Fetal heart sounds by fetal stethoscope.
- 22 weeks+: Fetal movements palpable by a trained practitioner.
- Late pregnancy: Fetal movements visible.

Adapted from material by Ian Selth, BSc Midwife. Used with permission. Retrieved November 3, 2002, from http://www.midwifery.resources.btinternet.co.uk/midwifery.htm.

Presumptive (Possible) Signs

Presumptive signs of pregnancy are subjective data that the woman reports. The most common presumptive sign of pregnancy is a missed menstrual period, or amenorrhea. There are many causes of amenorrhea. Some women have irregular periods. Emotional distress can cause a woman to skip a menstrual period. Some disorders, such as anorexia nervosa, can lead to amenorrhea. Women who perform intense exercise, such as marathon running, also can experience amenorrhea. Because so many factors, other than pregnancy, can cause a woman to miss a menstrual period, amenorrhea is classified as a presumptive or subjective sign of pregnancy.

Other presumptive signs include nausea, fatigue, swollen, tender breasts, and frequent urination. Nausea can be caused by emotional distress, a viral infection, gastritis, or a host of other problems. Anemia, lack of sleep, overexertion, or infection can lead to fatigue. Breast tissue can become swollen and tender just before a woman starts her menstrual period in response to hormonal changes. Frequent urination can result from a urinary tract infection, nervousness, or from taking in substances such as caffeine and alcohol that either act as urinary irritants or have diuretic properties.

Probable Signs

Probable signs of pregnancy are those detected by a trained examiner. These include objective data such as **Chadwick's sign**, the bluish-purplish color of the cervix, vagina, and perineum. The examiner also detects **Hegar's sign**, softening of the uterine isthmus, and **Goodell's sign**, softening of the cervix, during the speculum and digital pelvic examinations. Other objective signs include a change in the shape of the uterus, an enlarging uterus, and Braxton Hicks contractions. **Ballottement** occurs when the examiner pushes up on the uterine wall during a pelvic examination, then feels the fetus bounce back against the examiner's fingers. The reason these signs are considered probable, rather than positive, is that pelvic tumors and some types of cancers can cause similar signs.

Another probable sign is the pregnancy test. Although pregnancy tests performed in a laboratory are highly reliable (from 97% to 99%), there is still the small possibility for error. Pregnancy tests measure the presence of human chorionic gonadotropin (hCG) in the urine or the blood. hCG levels can be elevated in conditions other than pregnancy, such as hydatidiform mole and choriocarcinoma.

A woman wants confirmation of pregnancy whether she is trying to get pregnant or thinks she might be pregnant when she was not planning a pregnancy. Many women use home pregnancy tests to determine if they are pregnant. These home pregnancy tests are approximately 95% reliable when they are performed correctly and done at least 10 days after the last menstrual period. It is important for the woman to know that the home pregnancy test is more likely to be correct when it reveals a positive result than when a negative result is obtained. In other words, if the home pregnancy test is negative, she should still monitor for signs of pregnancy and repeat the test or schedule an appointment with her physician.

Several types of pregnancy tests can be done in the practitioner's office. The enzyme immunoassays (EIA) utilizing monoclonal antibodies specific for hCG can be done in approximately 10 minutes and are reliable within 7 or 8 days after ovulation. EIA can be done on urine or the woman's serum. If urine is used, it is best to have the first voided specimen of the morning because this urine is highly concentrated, making detection of hCG easier. Serum radioimmunoassay beta subunit (RIA-hCG-b) testing measures only the beta subunit of hCG. RIA testing is highly sensitive and can help diagnose pregnancy even earlier than the EIA method.

Positive Signs

Positive signs are diagnostic of pregnancy because no other condition can cause the sign. The positive sign that can be elicited earliest in the pregnancy is visualization of the gestational sac or fetus. With transvaginal ultrasound the gestational sac can be seen as early as 10 days after implantation. The fetal outline and cardiac activity are visible by abdominal ultrasound at 7 to 8 weeks.

The fetal heart beat, heard at 9 to 10 weeks with Doppler technology and by 18 to 20 weeks with a fetoscope, is a positive sign of pregnancy. Palpation of fetal movements by a trained examiner is a positive sign of pregnancy after the 20th week.

PHYSIOLOGIC ADAPTATION TO PREGNANCY

The woman's body must make tremendous changes to accommodate a pregnancy (Table 6-1). While she is pregnant her body must maintain all her vital functions and those of the growing fetus. Some changes are structural and occur because of pressure exerted by the growing fetus and expanding uterus. Other changes are hormone related. The next section discusses the physiologic changes that occur during pregnancy by body system.

Reproductive Changes

Obviously, the reproductive system changes during pregnancy. Instead of shedding endometrial tissue every month, the decidua must be maintained. The myometrium (uterine muscle) must stay relatively relaxed. If it contracts too forcefully, the pregnancy will be lost. The uterus undergoes changes immediately after conception and continues to grow and change throughout the pregnancy. The cervix, vagina, perineum, and breasts also undergo changes.

Uterus

During the first weeks after conception, the uterine muscle cells begin to hypertrophy, causing the uterus to expand. It is thought that estrogen stimulates this muscle cell hypertrophy. At first the uterine walls become thicker, but as the pregnancy progresses, the growing fetus and accessory structures began to exert pressure so that the uterus enlarges and the uterine walls become thinner. By the end of the 12th week, the uterus expands upward into the abdominal cavity. At 16 weeks, the fundus can be palpated approximately halfway between the symphysis pubis and the umbilicus. At 20 weeks, the fundus reaches the level of the umbilicus. By the end of the pregnancy, the uterus occupies much of the abdominal cavity.

Beginning in the first trimester, the uterus begins to contract sporadically. These contractions are usually painless and do not cause cervical changes. By the second trimester these contractions can be palpated. **Braxton Hicks contractions**, the painless, intermittent, "practice" contractions of pregnancy, are named after the physician who first wrote about them, Braxton Hicks. During the third trimester as the pregnancy approaches term, Braxton Hicks contractions become more frequent and can sometimes cause discomfort. As the time for labor draws near, the contractions can become somewhat regular, causing the woman to think that she is in labor. This is the cause of so-called false labor.

Blood supply to the uterus increases dramatically throughout pregnancy. Under the influence of estrogen, new blood vessels grow in the placenta and uterine walls, and vasodilation occurs in maternal vessels to allow increased blood flow to the uterus and placenta. The diameter of the uterine artery increases during pregnancy. By 20 weeks, it doubles in diameter from the nonpregnant state.

TABLE 6.1 Anatomy and Physiology Comparison: Nonpregnant to Pregnant Woman

System or Structure	Nonpregnant Characteristics	Pregnant Characteristics (At Term, Unless Otherwise Indicated)
Uterus	Weight: 70 grams	Weight: 1,100 grams
	Uterine cavity capacity: 10 mL	Uterine cavity capacity: 5 liters average, but may expand to as much as 20 liters
	Structure: Almost solid	Structure: Thin, muscular sac
	Shape: Pear shaped	Shape: Globular
	Location: Pelvis	Location: Fills the abdominal cavity
	Percentage of cardiac output supplying all abdominal organs combined: 24%	Percentage of cardiac output supplying uterus/pelvic cavity alone: 20%
Breasts	Soft, nontender tissue	Tenderness in the first few weeks of pregnancy. Nodularity of breast tissue.
	Soft, nonprominent, relatively smooth areola	Prominent areola with deepened pigmentation and prominent projections of Montgomery's tubercles.
Thyroid gland	Total gland volume: 12.1 mL	Total gland volume: 15.0 mL
Blood	Blood volume: 5 liters	Blood volume increases by 40%–50% (could be as high as 7.5 liters)
	Red blood cell volume: 2 liters	Red blood cell volume increases by as much as 30% (2.6 liters)
	Plasma volume: 3 liters	Plasma volume increases by 50% (4.5 liters)
	Hemoglobin: 12–16 g/100 mL	Hemoglobin: 11–12 g/100 mL
	Hematocrit: 36%–46%	Hematocrit: Decreases, particularly in the third trimester as plasma volume increases
	White blood cell count: 4,500–11,000/mm^3	White blood cell (WBC) count: As great as 16,000 mm^3 (in labor the WBC count can reach as high as 25,000 mm^3)
Coagulation	Fibrinogen levels: 200–400 mg/dL	Fibrinogen levels: Values may be as high as 600 mg/dL
	Factors VII, VIII, and X: Normal	Factors VII, VIII, and X: Increase by 20%–100%
		In general, pregnancy is considered to be a state of hypercoagulability.
Heart	Blood pressure in normal range: 90–140 mm Hg systolic and 60–90 mm Hg diastolic	Blood pressure decreases slightly, particularly in the second trimester
	Heart rate 60–100 beats per minute	Heart rate increases by 10–15 beats per minute
	Cardiac output: Approximately 5 liters per minute	Cardiac output increases (as much as 40%–50%) beginning by the fifth week gestation
Respiratory	Respiratory rate: 16–20 breaths per minute	Respiratory rate: Unchanged or increased by 2–3 breaths per minute
	Nasal mucosa thin and moist	Nasal mucosa edematous due to vasocongestion.
	Tidal volume (the volume of air moved during normal inspiration and expiration): 500 mL	Tidal volume: 700 mL
	Oxygen consumption normal for adult female	Oxygen consumption increases by 14%
	$PaCO_2$: 35–45 mm Hg	Average $PaCO_2$: 32 mm Hg

Cervix and Ovaries

The cervix undergoes characteristic changes under the influence of estrogen and progesterone. Vascularity is increased, and glandular tissue multiplies during pregnancy. The vascular congestion and increase in glandular tissue is responsible for Goodell's sign, Hegar's sign, and Chadwick's sign. Shortly after conception, a thick mucous plug develops in the opening of the cervix, which helps to protect the uterine cavity from infection. The mucous plug is expelled shortly before, or at the beginning of labor. Small capillaries break when the plug is expelled, causing a bloody show.

This will reassure your patient. Because the cervix increases in vascularity during pregnancy, a pelvic examination can rupture small capillaries and cause spotting afterward. After a pelvic examination, inform the woman that she can expect some spotting, particularly when she wipes after voiding. Reassure her that this spotting is normal unless the bleeding becomes heavy, like that of a menstrual period.

Follicles in the ovaries do not mature during pregnancy, and ovulation stops. The corpus luteum continues to function and produces progesterone for approximately 6 to 7 weeks. If the corpus luteum is removed or stops functioning before that time, a spontaneous abortion (miscarriage) will occur. After 7 weeks, the placenta produces enough progesterone to maintain the pregnancy.

Vagina and Perineum

The vagina and perineum are affected by hormonal changes and increased blood supply to the area. The vagina takes on a bluish-purplish hue, Chadwick's sign, because of vascular congestion. Copious secretions are produced in the vagina and cervix because of the increased blood flow to the area.

Breasts

In the first few weeks of pregnancy, the breasts become tender and the woman may feel tingling sensations. As pregnancy progresses, the breasts increase in size under the influence of estrogen. Prolactin, an anterior pituitary hormone, stimulates glandular production, causing the breast tissue to feel nodular. The areolas darken. **Montgomery's tubercles**, sebaceous glands on the areolas, produce secretions that lubricate the nipple. Montgomery's tubercles become more prominent during pregnancy. Tiny veins become visible on the surface of the breasts. **Striae**, stretch marks, sometimes appear. Striae appear reddish at first, then gradually fade to a light silvery color after childbirth.

As the mammary glands develop, the breasts begin to produce and secrete **colostrum**, a thick, yellow fluid that precedes milk production. Colostrum is sometimes referred to as the "foremilk." During the first 3 days of breast-feeding, colostrum is the nourishment the baby receives. It is rich in antibodies and protein.

Endocrine Changes

The hormonal changes that occur in pregnancy are tremendous. Rising levels of certain pregnancy hormones cause changes in almost every body system during pregnancy. The placental hormones are discussed in Chapter 5. Changes in the endocrine system itself occur during pregnancy. The pituitary gland enlarges by 135% compared with its nonpregnant size. In fact, pregnancy could not occur without the interaction of the pituitary hormones, follicle-stimulating hormone (FSH) and luteinizing hormone (LH).

Prolactin levels increase progressively during pregnancy. Although this hormone is not necessary for the successful completion of pregnancy, it is crucial for the initiation of lactation. Oxytocin, a posterior pituitary hormone, is responsible for the rhythmic uterine contractions of labor. Oxytocin stimulates the letdown reflex during breast-feeding and stimulates the uterus to continue contracting after delivery to control maternal bleeding.

Most endocrine glands are affected by the increased protein binding that occurs during pregnancy. Hyperplasia of glandular tissue and increased vascularity cause the thyroid gland to increase in size. The need for insulin is increased. Some women have borderline pancreatic activity when they are not pregnant. During pregnancy, these women develop gestational diabetes because the borderline pancreas cannot handle the increased demands placed upon it.

Test Yourself

- List three positive signs of pregnancy.
- Describe three changes that occur in breast tissue during pregnancy.
- What is the purpose of the hormone prolactin?

Hematologic Changes

Blood volume increases by approximately 40% to 45% above prepregnancy levels by the end of the third trimester. Blood plasma and red blood cells (RBCs) both increase in volume, although plasma volumes increase at a higher percentage (50%) than do RBCs (30%). This physiologic hemodilution causes a slight decrease in hemoglobin and hematocrit (H&H) levels.

The average hemoglobin level at term is 12.5 g/dL. Iron-deficiency anemia is not diagnosed until the hemoglobin levels fall below 11.0 g/dL. It is important to note that in the absence of sufficient iron, RBC volume increases by only 18%, rather than 30%.

Some blood clotting factors, such as fibrinogen and others, increase during pregnancy, making pregnancy a hypercoagulable state. However, clotting times and bleeding times remain within normal limits. As the uterus enlarges, blood return from the lower extremities is inhibited, a situation that can cause venous stasis. A combination of venous stasis and the state of hypercoagulability places the pregnant woman at risk for venous thrombosis (clot formation).

The increased blood volume and hypercoagulability of the blood serve protective functions during pregnancy. The expanded blood volume helps meet the needs of the enlarging uterus with its increased vascularity. It also helps protect the woman and the fetus from harmful effects of decreased venous return when the woman is standing or lying supine. The increased blood volume enhances the exchange of nutrients and respiratory gases between the pregnant woman and fetus. The increased blood volume and hypercoagulability serve to protect the woman from the blood loss that normally occurs during delivery.

Cardiovascular Changes

Tremendous demands are made upon the cardiovascular system during pregnancy. The heart has to handle the increased load of an expanded blood volume. It also must adjust to the demands of organ systems with increased workloads, such as the kidneys and uterus. In addition, the heart is physically pushed upward and to the left by the enlarging uterus, which may cause systolic murmurs.

Normally the blood pressure decreases slightly during pregnancy, particularly in the second trimester. The heart rate rises by 10 to 15 beats per minute on average. Cardiac output increases, beginning in the early weeks of pregnancy and continuing throughout pregnancy.

During late pregnancy the gravid uterus can compress the woman's vena cava and aorta causing the blood pressure to fall when the woman is in the supine position. This condition is called **supine hypotensive syndrome** (Fig. 6-1). The woman may feel light-headed and dizzy; her skin may exhibit pallor and clamminess. The treatment for this condition is to reposition the woman to a lateral position. The traditional position is left side-lying.

An ounce of prevention. . .
Because of the danger of supine hypotensive syndrome in late pregnancy, advise the woman to avoid the supine position. If she wishes to lie on her back, instruct her to place a pillow under her right hip to keep the uterus away from the great vessels.

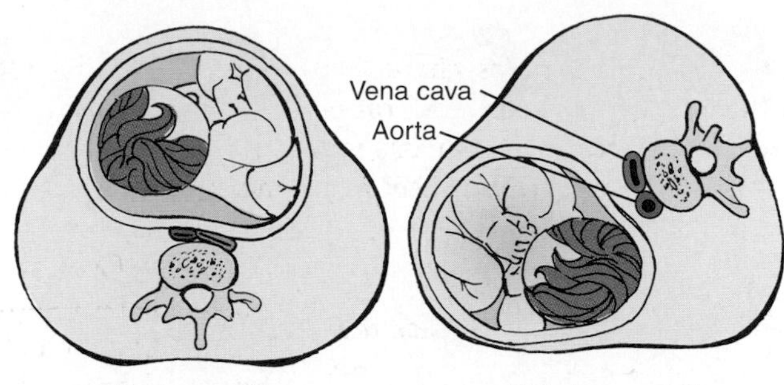

● ***Figure 6.1*** Supine hypotensive syndrome. When the woman lies flat on her back in the latter half of pregnancy, the uterus and its contents compress the aorta and vena cava against the spine. This compression decreases the amount of blood returned to the heart; therefore, the cardiac output and the blood pressure fall, leading to supine hypotensive syndrome. The cure (and prevention) is for the woman to rest on her side. As you can see in the illustration, when the pregnant woman is on her side, pressure is relieved from the great vessels and normal blood flow resumes.

Respiratory Changes

The respiratory system must accommodate to the changing needs and demands of pregnancy. Vasocongestion of the lining of the upper respiratory tract causes symptoms similar to that of the common cold. The nasal congestion and voice changes may persist throughout pregnancy. The nasal lining is more fragile, increasing the likelihood of nosebleeds. These characteristic changes to the respiratory tract lining are thought to occur under the influence of estrogen.

As the uterus enlarges, it pushes up on the diaphragm. The body compensates for this crowding by increasing the anteroposterior and transverse diameters of the chest so that total lung capacity stays approximately the same as it was before pregnancy. Ligaments that loosen under the influence of hormones (probably progesterone) allow for the increased thoracic diameters.

The woman becomes more aware of the need to breathe and may feel short of breath even when she is not. In the third trimester, pressure exerted on the diaphragm from the expanding uterus can also cause the woman to feel dyspneic.

Musculoskeletal Changes

Lordosis, an increased curvature of the spine, becomes more pronounced in the later weeks of pregnancy (Fig. 6-2) as the expanding uterus alters the center of gravity. The lordosis compensates by shifting the center of gravity back over the lower extremities.

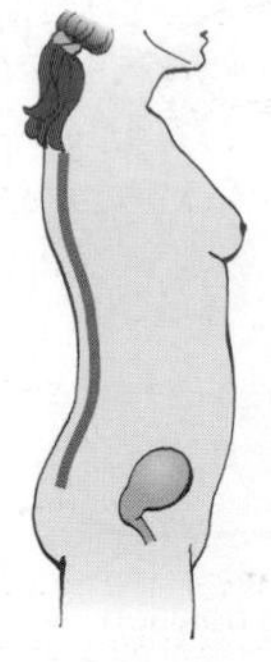

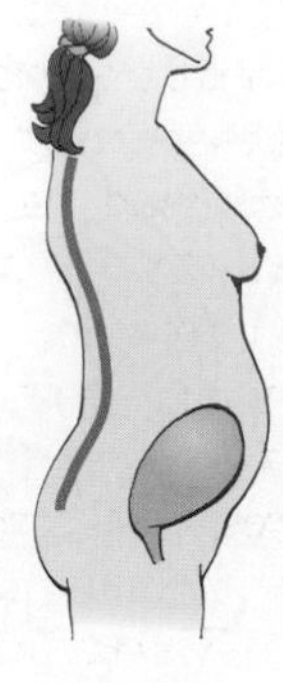

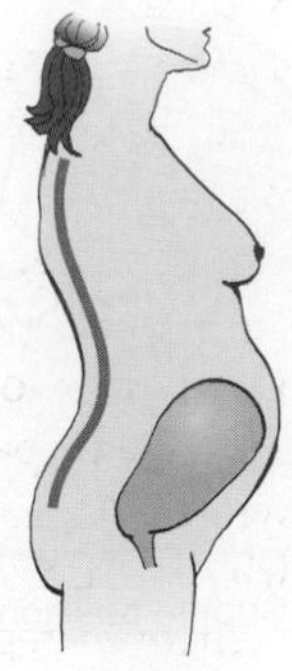

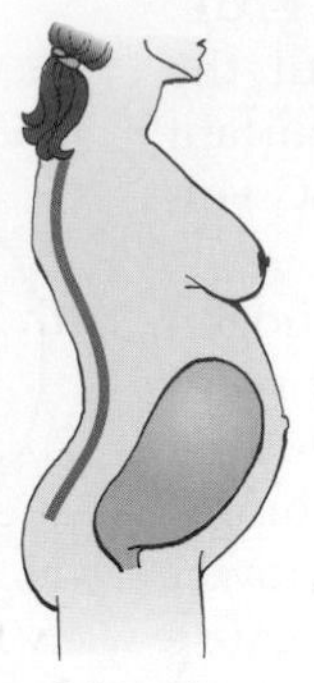

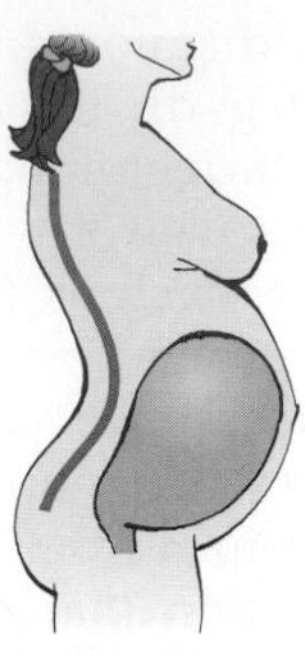

● ***Figure 6.2*** Postural changes during pregnancy. Progressive lordosis, increased curvature of the spine, is characteristic during pregnancy. Notice how the lumbar and thoracic curves become more pronounced as pregnancy progresses. This occurs to counterbalance the effect of the protruding abdomen and to keep the center of balance over the lower extremities.

The increased curvature can result in low backache. Hormonal influences on pelvic joints cause them to increase in mobility, which contributes to lower back discomfort and causes the characteristic waddling gait of pregnancy.

As the uterus enlarges, increasing pressure is put on the broad and round ligaments that support the uterus. Prolonged pressure can lead to round ligament pain. A woman who has been pregnant several times or a woman who is carrying twins is more likely to experience **diastasis recti abdominis**, separation of the rectus abdominis muscle that supports the abdomen.

Test Yourself

- By what percentage does blood volume increase during pregnancy?
- By how much is cardiac output expected to increase?
- Define diastasis recti abdominis.

Gastrointestinal Changes

Nausea and vomiting are common in the first trimester under the influence of rising human chorionic gonadotropin (hCG) levels. Occasionally a large increase in saliva production (ptyalism) occurs. The gums may become tender and bleed easily. Current scientific evidence shows no increase in the rate of tooth decay during pregnancy.

As the uterus expands upward into the abdominal cavity, the intestines are displaced to the sides and upward. The stomach is pushed upward. The lower esophageal sphincter (LES) relaxes under the influence of hormones. Pressures in the esophagus are lower than in the nonpregnant state, while pressures within the stomach are increased. These changes lead to an increased incidence of **pyrosis,** heartburn caused by acid reflux through the relaxed LES.

Displacement of the intestines and possible slowed motility of the gastrointestinal tract under the influence of progesterone may lead to delayed gastric emptying and decreased peristalsis. As a result of these changes, the pregnant woman is predisposed to constipation. Constipation and elevated pressures in the veins below the uterus contribute to an increased incidence of hemorrhoid development during pregnancy.

Progesterone interferes with normal gallbladder contraction, leading to stasis of bile. Cholestasis and increased cholesterol levels increase the risk of gallstone formation during pregnancy. Cholestasis can occur within the liver and lead to pruritus (itching).

Urinary Changes

Renal and ureteral dilation occur as a result of hormonal changes and mechanical pressure of the growing uterus on the ureters. The dilation causes an increase in kidney size, particularly on the right side. Peristalsis decreases in the urinary tract, leading to urinary stasis and a resultant increase in the risk for pyelonephritis.

The glomerular filtration rate (GFR) rises by as much as 50% because of increased cardiac output and decreased renal vascular resistance. The rise in GFR occurs as early as the 10th week and is largely responsible for the increased urinary frequency noted in the first trimester. Urinary frequency is not a common complaint in the second trimester but occurs again in the third trimester because of the pressure of the expanding uterus on the bladder.

Glycosuria, glucose in the urine, may occur normally during pregnancy because the kidney tubules are not able to reabsorb as much glucose as they were before pregnancy. However, if the woman is spilling glucose in her urine, additional tests are warranted to rule out gestational diabetes. Protein is not normally found in the urine of a pregnant woman.

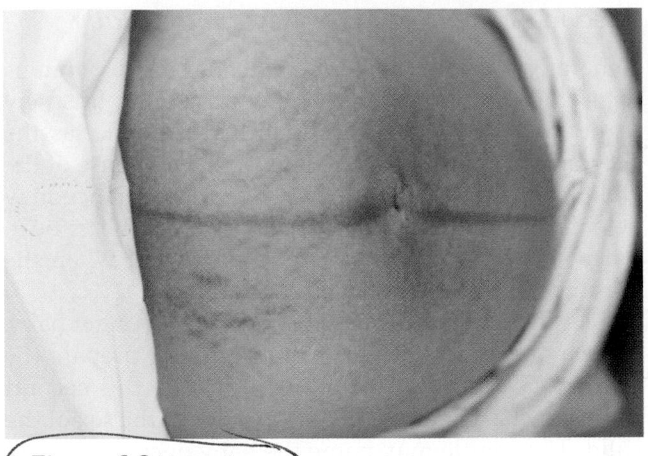

● *Figure 6.3* Linea nigra.

Integumentary Changes

Many skin changes in pregnancy result from hyperpigmentation. The so-called mask of pregnancy, known as **chloasma,** is evidenced by brown blotchy areas on the forehead, cheeks, and nose of the pregnant woman. This condition may be permanent, or it may regress between pregnancies. The condition can be stimulated with oral contraceptives. The skin in the middle of the abdomen may develop a darkened line called the **linea nigra** (Fig. 6-3). Striae (stretch marks) may develop on the abdomen in response to elevated glucocorticoid levels. As discussed in the section on breast tissue, the striae appear reddish and are more noticeable during pregnancy. After pregnancy they tend to fade and become silvery white in color.

Test Yourself

- List two reasons the pregnant woman is predisposed to pyrosis.
- Name two urinary changes normally experienced during pregnancy.
- List two conditions that result from hyperpigmentation during pregnancy.

PSYCHOLOGICAL ADAPTATION TO PREGNANCY

While adapting to rapid changes in physiology, the pregnant woman also must come to grips with her new role as parent. No matter how many children the woman has, each new pregnancy brings with it a role change. Adjusting to the role of parenting is a process that occurs throughout the pregnancy and beyond.

How a woman adjusts to her role as parent is influenced by many factors. Societal expectations and cultural values may dictate the way a woman responds to pregnancy and the idea of parenthood. Family influences are usually very strong. The way the woman was raised and the values surrounding children and parenthood in her family of origin color the way a woman adapts to pregnancy. Her own personality and ability to adapt to change will influence her response. Even her past experiences with pregnancy have an effect on the way she deals with the current pregnancy. For example, if she has a history of a stillbirth, she may not fully accept the pregnancy or begin to bond with the baby until he is born.

Social support is critical during pregnancy. If the woman is in a long-term relationship and feels supported, she will be much better prepared to handle the demands of pregnancy than if she feels alone and isolated without support. If the woman does not have a supportive partner, it is important for her to identify someone with whom she can share the experience of pregnancy. Often this will be a female friend, or perhaps the woman's own mother.

First Trimester Task: Accept the Pregnancy

Pregnancy is a development stage, and as such, psychological tasks of pregnancy have been identified. The first task of pregnancy is to accept the pregnancy. This task is usually met during the first trimester, although some women have difficulty fully accepting the pregnancy until they can feel the baby move.

Initially the woman may be shocked that she is pregnant. Or she may be ecstatic or excited. There are a myriad of emotions that a woman may experience when she first hears the news that she is pregnant. Even if the pregnancy is desired intensely, a certain amount of ambivalence is a normal initial response to pregnancy. Ambivalence refers to the feelings of uncertainty most women must deal with in the early weeks of pregnancy. The woman may have tried to get pregnant for a while before conceiving, and now that the pregnancy has occurred she may have second thoughts or doubts about her ability to be a good parent. Or the pregnancy may have been unplanned, so she must sort through her feelings about this unexpected demand that has been placed upon her.

Acceptance can be healing. Listen to your patient. Pregnancy and childbirth can stimulate many emotions. If the woman indicates that she wishes to talk, encourage her and use active listening skills. Let her know that it is normal to experience a wide array of feelings during pregnancy.

It may be helpful for her to hear that ambivalence is a healthy response because she may feel guilty about her uncertainty.

As the woman experiences the early physiologic changes of pregnancy, she gradually comes to accept that she is pregnant. She is usually introverted and focused on herself during the first trimester. The nausea associated with early pregnancy may leave her feeling sick and irritable. She may be fatigued. Often she is moody and sensitive.

It is important to be supportive of the woman's partner during this time. He (or she, if the woman is in a lesbian relationship) also must deal with feelings of ambivalence. In addition to accepting the pregnancy, the partner must learn to accept the pregnant woman as she changes with pregnancy. The mood swings, sensitivity, and irritability can make it difficult to cope. Jealousy of the unborn child can occur. It can be difficult to adjust to the introversion and self-focus of the woman. Often the partner is relieved to learn that the changes his partner is going through are normal responses to pregnancy.

A PERSONAL GLIMPSE

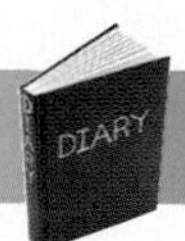

When I first found out that I was pregnant, I started shaking. I couldn't believe that I was pregnant. My husband and I didn't plan for this to happen so soon. We had wanted to wait about 8 more months before beginning our family. We weren't ready; we had only been married 5 months. We still had some financial debt to pay off and we had certain goals we wanted to meet.

We both wanted and loved children very much. In fact, we both wanted, and planned, to have three children. However, it was the timing that was wrong. I couldn't even tell my husband the news because he was away for several weeks. This added to my anxiety. Not only was I worried about my ability to be a mother, but I was worried that I may have eaten or been exposed to something harmful to my baby before knowing I was pregnant. I ended up confiding in my mother and best friends who truly helped me to calm down and get a grip.

I started to relax and accept the fact that, although my timing was off, this was pretty exciting. When I was finally able to tell my husband, he just beamed with joy. I knew in that moment that everything would be all right.

Sandra

LEARNING OPPORTUNITY: How would you advise this mother-to-be regarding her feelings when she found out that she was pregnant? How can the nurse help the woman and her family deal with the emotions that surround finding out about a pregnancy?

Second Trimester Task: Accept the Baby

Generally during the first trimester the woman is focused on the pregnancy and on accepting this new reality as being part of her identity. Gradually as the pregnancy progresses she comes to have a sense of the child as his own separate entity. This acceptance may be enhanced when she first hears the fetal heart beat, when she feels the baby move inside her, or when she sees the fetal image during a sonogram.

As she comes to accept the uniqueness of her baby, she may begin to shop for baby clothes or prepare the nursery. When ultrasound is done in the second trimester, it is generally possible to detect the sex of the child. The couple may name the baby once they know if it is a boy or a girl. But do not make the mistake of thinking that the woman has not yet accepted the baby if she does not name the baby during pregnancy. Some parents do not decide on a name until several days after the baby is born.

During the second trimester the woman may become more extroverted. She often feels much better since the nausea and fatigue of the first trimester have passed. She starts to show so that the pregnancy becomes apparent to those around her, and she may have the glow of pregnancy. Frequently the second trimester is a happy time. The woman may enjoy the extra attention and deference society gives to pregnant women.

It is important to remember that the partner is experiencing the pregnancy along with the woman. Some fathers actually experience some of the physical symptoms of pregnancy, such as nausea and vomiting, along with their partner. This phenomenon is called **couvade syndrome**. It may be easier for the man to accept his wife now that she is feeling better and is less introverted. In any event it is important to encourage the couple to communicate their needs effectively to each other. Each needs the support of the other.

Third Trimester Task: Prepare for Parenthood

Nesting instincts often begin in the third trimester. The couple may prepare the nursery and shop for baby furniture and clothes. A name may be chosen. It is during the third trimester that most childbirth classes are offered. The woman usually has a heightened interest in safe passage for herself and the baby during labor.

Toward the end of pregnancy most women begin to feel tired of being pregnant. Many discomforts of pregnancy show themselves during the third trimester. It may be difficult to get comfortable at night, and so it may be hard to get a good night's sleep. Backache and round ligament pain may be bothersome. Urinary frequency often returns as the gravid uterus presses down against the bladder. Braxton Hicks contractions may become uncomfortable and more frequent. It is important to be supportive of the woman and listen to her concerns.

It is helpful for the couple to attend childbirth preparation classes. Not only do they learn techniques to help them prepare for labor, but they are able to interact with other couples who are facing issues similar to their own. The social aspect of childbirth preparation can be a powerful source of support to the woman and her partner.

Test Yourself

- Describe two psychological characteristics normally associated with a woman in the first trimester of pregnancy.
- Which trimester of pregnancy is often the happiest for the woman?
- List two activities many women perform in the third trimester.

CHANGING NUTRITIONAL REQUIREMENTS OF PREGNANCY

Nutrition is an area that requires special attention during pregnancy, particularly during the second and third trimesters. The fetus needs nutrients and energy to build new tissue, and the woman needs nutrients to build her blood volume and maternal stores. There is an increased demand for energy and for almost every nutrient type. Most nutrient requirements can be met through careful attention to diet, although there are several nutrients that require supplementation during pregnancy.

Energy Requirements and Weight Gain

Energy requirements are increased during pregnancy because of fetal tissue development and increased maternal stores. During the first trimester, the recommended weight gain is 3 to 4 pounds total. Subsequently, for the remainder of pregnancy the recommendation is roughly 1 pound per week, for a total weight gain of 25 to 35 pounds for a woman who begins pregnancy with a normal body mass index (BMI).[1] Total weight gain recommendations vary depending upon the woman's prepregnancy BMI. A woman who is underweight when she enters pregnancy (low BMI) should gain 28 to 40 pounds, whereas a woman who has a high BMI (overweight) is recommended to gain 15 to 25 pounds during the pregnancy.

Failure to gain enough weight, and in particular gaining less than 16 pounds during pregnancy, has been associated with an increased risk of delivering a low birth-weight neonate (less than 2,500 grams or 5½ pounds). Low birth weight has consistently been associated with poor neonatal outcomes. Conversely, a woman who gains too much weight is at increased risk for delivering a macrosomic (greater than or equal to 4,000 grams or 8½ pounds) neonate. High birth-weight neonates experience complications and poor outcomes more frequently than do neonates with normal birth weights. A woman who gains too much weight also is at greater risk of requiring cesarean section.

Many women assume falsely that eating for two requires a significantly increased caloric intake. In fact, the required caloric increase during the first trimester is negligible. During the second and third trimesters, approximately 300 kilocalories per day are required above the woman's prepregnancy needs. It is important that the diet supply enough calories to meet energy needs; otherwise, protein will be broken down to supply energy, rather than to build fetal and maternal tissue.

Protein Requirements

Protein needs are increased during pregnancy because of growth and repair of fetal tissue, placenta, uterus, breasts, and maternal blood volume. It is recommended that the pregnant woman obtain adequate protein from animal sources, including milk and milk products. Milk is an excellent source of protein and calcium for the pregnant and breast-feeding woman. As stated previously, it is important for the woman to have adequate caloric intake to preserve protein stores for tissue building and repair. When protein is used to supply energy, there is less available for fetal, placental, and maternal tissue growth needs.

During the average pregnancy, approximately 1,000 grams of additional protein above the woman's basal needs are used. The fetus and placenta account for 500 grams of added protein. The other 500 grams is distributed among uterine muscle cells, mammary glandular tissue, and maternal blood in the form of hemoglobin and plasma proteins.

Mineral Requirements

Most minerals can be obtained from a varied diet without supplementation, even during pregnancy. However, it is important for a pregnant woman to get sufficient amounts of minerals to prevent deficiencies in the growing fetus and maternal stores. Table 6-2 compares the

[1] Body mass index (BMI) refers to body weight corrected for height of the person. The formula for determining BMI is: divide the person's weight (in kilograms or pounds) by her height squared (in meters or inches, respectively) then multiply by 100. Normal BMI is 19.8 to 26.

TABLE 6.2 Comparison of Recommended Daily Dietary Allowances (RDA) for Selected Vitamins and Minerals for Nonpregnant, Pregnant, and Lactating Women

Mineral/Vitamin	Function	RDA for Nonpregnant	RDA for Pregnant Women	RDA for Lactating Women	Selected Food Sources
Calcium (mg/day)	Essential role in blood clotting, muscle contraction, nerve transmission, and bone and tooth formation	1,000	1,000	1,000	Dairy products: milk, cheese, yogurt. Corn tortillas, calcium-set tofu, Chinese cabbage, kale, broccoli
Copper (μg/day)	Component of enzymes in iron metabolism	900	1,000	1,300	Organ meats, seafood, nuts, seeds, wheat bran cereals, whole grain products, cocoa products
Iodine (mg/day) Vitamin B_8	Component of thyroid hormones and prevents goiter and cretinism	150	220	290	Foods of marine origin, processed foods, iodized salt
Iron (mg/day)	Component of hemoglobin and numerous enzymes; prevents microcytic hypochromic anemia	18	27	9	Fruits, vegetables and fortified bread and grain products, such as cereal (nonheme iron sources), meat and poultry (heme iron sources)
Vitamin A (μg/day)	Required for normal vision, gene expression, reproduction, embryonic development and immune function	700	770	1,300	Liver, dairy products, fish (preformed Vitamin A sources); and carrots, sweet potatoes, mango, spinach, cantaloupe, kale, apricots (beta-carotene sources)
Vitamin B_1 (thiamin) (mg/day)	Coenzyme in the metabolism of carbohydrates and branched-chain amino acids	1.1	1.4	1.4	Enriched, fortified, or whole-brain products; bread and bread products, mixed foods whose main ingredient is grain, and ready-to-eat cereals
Vitamin B_2 (riboflavin) (mg/day)	Coenzyme in numerous redox reactions	1.1	1.4	1.6	Organ meats, milk, bread products, and fortified cereals
Vitamin B_3 (niacin) (mg/day)	Required for energy metabolism	14	18	17	Meat, fish, poultry, enriched and whole-grain breads and bread products, fortified ready-to-eat cereals

TABLE 6.2 (continued) **Comparison of Recommended Daily Dietary Allowances (RDA) for Selected Vitamins and Minerals for Nonpregnant, Pregnant, and Lactating Women**

Mineral/Vitamin	Function	RDA for Nonpregnant	RDA for Pregnant Women	RDA for Lactating Women	Selected Food Sources
Vitamin B_6 (pyroxidine) (mg/day)	Coenzyme in the metabolism of amino acids, glycogen, and sphingoid bases	1.3	1.9	2.0	Fortified cereals, organ meats, fortified soy-based meat substitutes
Vitamin B_9 (folacin, folate, folic acid) (μg/day)	Coenzyme in the metabolism of nucleic and amino acids; prevents megaloblastic anemia; in pregnancy folate deficiency is linked to an increased risk for neural tube defects	400	600	500	Enriched cereal grains, dark leafy vegetables, enriched and whole-grain breads and bread products, fortified ready-to-eat cereals
Vitamin B_{12} (Cobalamine) (μg/day)	Coenzyme in nucleic acid metabolism; prevents megaloblastic anemia	2.4	2.6	2.8	Fortified cereals, meat, fish, poultry
Vitamin C (ascorbic acid) (mg/day)	Necessary for collagen synthesis and wound healing and as a protective antioxidant	75	85	120	Citrus fruits, tomatoes, tomato juice, potatoes, Brussels sprouts, cauliflower, broccoli, strawberries, cabbage, spinach
Vitamin D (calciferol) (μg/day)	Maintain serum calcium and phosphorus concentrations	5	5	5	Fish liver oils, flesh of fatty fish, liver and fat from seals and polar bears, eggs from hens fed vitamin D fortified milk products, fortified cereals
Zinc (mg/day)	Component of multiple enzymes and proteins; involved in the regulation of gene expression	8	11	12	Fortified cereals, red meats, certain seafood

Note: The RDA is that recommended for women of childbearing age (18–50 years). Requirements for teenagers and other special groups may differ. (Source: Food and Nutrition Board, 2002.)

Recommended Daily Dietary Allowances (RDA) of selected vitamins and minerals for nonpregnant, pregnant, and lactating women of childbearing age.

Iron

Iron is necessary for the formation of hemoglobin; therefore, it is essential to the oxygen-carrying capacity of the blood. If a woman's diet is iron deficient during pregnancy, her red blood cell volume will increase by only 18%; whereas, adequate supplementation of iron results in a 30% increase in red blood cell volume. This extra "cushion" of red blood cell volume increases the amount of oxygen available at the placenta for the fetus and helps protect the woman from the effects of blood loss after delivery.

Total iron requirements of pregnancy equal 1,000 milligrams. The fetus and placenta use 300 milligrams. Two hundred milligrams are lost through various routes of excretion, even when the woman is iron deficient. Five hundred milligrams are needed to supply the additional 450 milliliters of maternal red blood cells. Almost all of these additional iron requirements are needed during the second half of pregnancy, so the need for iron is increased dramatically after 20 weeks. If the woman is iron deficient, she will develop anemia. However, the fetus will get the iron needed to manufacture its red blood cells. This is one instance in which nature robs from the woman to adequately supply the fetus.

It is almost impossible for the woman to receive an adequate amount of iron from diet alone. Therefore, it is recommended that all pregnant women receive iron supplementation in the last half of pregnancy. Sometimes the physician will elect to omit the iron supplement during the first trimester because supplemental iron often intensifies the nausea and vomiting of early pregnancy. The dose will vary depending upon the individual needs of the woman. If she enters pregnancy with normal hemoglobin and hematocrit values, she will require lower doses of iron than if she is anemic when she becomes pregnant. A woman carrying twins or an obese woman will both require higher doses of supplemental iron.

Calcium

Calcium needs are not increased above prepregnancy levels (1,000 mg/day); however, it is important for the pregnant woman to obtain sufficient amounts of calcium. Calcium is needed for a variety of bodily processes, including nerve cell transmission, muscle contraction, bone building, and blood clotting. Although no direct link has been shown between low calcium levels and the development of gestational hypertension, some studies have demonstrated a reduction in risk of gestational hypertension when pregnant women take calcium supplements (Hofmeyr, Atallah, & Duley, 2002).

Calcium continuously moves between bone and blood because a precise amount is needed in the blood to maintain normal muscle contraction (including cardiac muscle contraction). Normally the movement of calcium in and out of bones is balanced, that is there is neither a net gain nor a net loss. However, if insufficient amounts are ingested, or if calcium is not absorbed from the gastrointestinal tract, the body will take calcium from the bones to maintain blood levels. This process will also occur to meet the calcium needs of the growing fetus.

Vitamin D is necessary for adequate absorption of calcium. The amount of vitamin D obtained from 10 to 20 minutes of exposure to sunlight per day is normally sufficient. If this source is not readily available, vitamin D is also present in fortified milk products.

Phosphorus

Phosphorus is readily available in a wide variety of foods. The pregnant woman normally has no trouble obtaining sufficient amounts of this nutrient. It is worth mentioning that intake of excessive amounts of phosphorus can inhibit calcium absorption. However, calcium metabolism requires a normal amount of phosphorus to build strong bones. The key to calcium and phosphorus consumption is to keep the two nutrients in balance.

Zinc

Zinc is needed during pregnancy to provide for fetal growth and during lactation for milk production. Milk production requires higher levels of zinc than the fetus demands during pregnancy. Absorption of this mineral increases during pregnancy and lactation. However, some studies show that zinc absorption does not increase in lactating women who are taking iron supplements. These findings suggest that taking iron supplements while breast-feeding may interfere with zinc levels. Foods that contain zinc include meat, seafood, and to a lesser extent, whole grains.

Iodine

Iodine is needed for normal thyroid activity. Women with severe iodine deficiencies deliver infants with **cretinism**, a congenital condition marked by stunted growth and mental retardation. Recent studies have linked subclinical hypothyroidism with increased rates of mental retardation.

Most women in the United States get sufficient amounts of iodine, but iodine intake has been declining in the past few years. Also, during pregnancy a woman loses larger amounts of iodine in the urine than when she is not pregnant. In light of these facts, the current recommendation is for all pregnant women to use iodized salt.

Vitamin Requirements

Vitamins are known to be catalysts for many chemical reactions in the body. A varied diet that includes adequate servings from each of the food groups on the Food Guide Pyramid should supply sufficient amounts of most vitamins during pregnancy. A brief description of the function and selected food sources for each vitamin are highlighted.

Folic Acid (Vitamin B_9)

The Centers for Disease Control report that more than 4,000 pregnancies per year are affected by neural tube defects, and that more than half of these defects could be prevented with adequate folic acid intake. Because formation of the nervous system occurs during the first few weeks of pregnancy, before a woman knows she is pregnant, all women of childbearing age are well advised to include at least 400 micrograms of folic acid per day in the diet.

There are several ways to meet the dietary requirement for folic acid. The Food and Drug Administration requires that enriched grain products, such as cereals, bread, rice, and pasta, be fortified with folic acid. Natural sources of dietary folic acid include dark green leafy vegetables, legumes, citrus fruits, and most berries. Of course, folic acid supplementation is also an option, either through folic acid tablets, or a multivitamin. Prenatal vitamins contain folic acid.

Vitamin A

Vitamin A is usually found in sufficient amounts in the diets of women who live in the United States. One concern is when a pregnant woman consumes too much vitamin A. In very large amounts (levels at or above 10,000 IU or 3,000 micrograms) preformed vitamin A, found in meats (primarily liver) and some fortified foods, can cause birth defects. For this reason pregnant women are encouraged to get the majority of their vitamin A intake from beta-carotene, a substance found in fruits and vegetables with yellow, orange, and red coloration, such as carrots and sweet potatoes. Beta-carotene is converted by the body to vitamin A and is much less toxic than preformed vitamin A. The key is balanced intake of this nutrient. Too much can be toxic to the fetus but too little can stunt fetal growth and cause impaired dark adaptation and night blindness.

Vitamin C

Vitamin C is essential in the formation of collagen, a necessary ingredient to wound healing. **Scurvy**, a disease characterized by spongy gums, loosened teeth, and bleeding into the skin and mucous membranes, results from severe vitamin C deficiency. Less severe deficiencies lead to easy bruising. Vitamin C is necessary for normal fetal growth and bone formation. This vitamin also helps the body to absorb iron. Recent research is highlighting a connection between mild vitamin C deficiency and the development of gestational hypertension (University of Pittsburgh Medical Center, 2002).

Fortunately most women in the United States get adequate amounts of vitamin C in their diets. Vitamin C is found in most fresh fruits and vegetables. The best sources include citrus fruits, papaya, and strawberries. Broccoli and tomatoes are good sources of vitamin C.

Vitamin B_6

Vitamin B_6, or pyridoxine, assists in the metabolism of the macronutrients (proteins, fats, and carbohydrates), helps convert amino acids, and forms new red blood cells. This vitamin is necessary for the healthy development of the fetus' nervous system. Although increased amounts of the vitamin are needed during pregnancy, a varied diet should supply all that is needed.

Vitamin B_{12}

Vitamin B_{12}, or cobalamine, is needed to maintain healthy nerve cells and red blood cells. It is also needed to form DNA. Vitamin B_{12} occurs naturally only in animal sources, such as fish, milk, dairy products, eggs, meat, and poultry. This vitamin can also be found in fortified breakfast cereals. Most Americans get sufficient amounts of vitamin B_{12} in the diet.

The two instances in which vitamin B_{12} deficiency generally occurs are when a person lacks intrinsic factor or she is a vegan (see discussion of vegetarianism that follows). Persons who lack intrinsic factor cannot absorb vitamin B_{12}. Without intramuscular injections of the vitamin, these individuals experience pernicious anemia.

Dietary Supplementation During Pregnancy

Currently, routine multivitamin supplementation during pregnancy is not recommended by the American Academy of Pediatrics or the American College of Obstetricians and Gynecologists because it is thought that a diet that includes a variety of food types is sufficient to meet the needs of the pregnant woman. There are several exceptions. The woman who has nutritional risk factors requires a daily prenatal multivitamin supplement. Nutritional risk factors include multiple gestation, substance abuse, vegetarianism, and problems with hemoglobin formation. Some health care providers still recommend a daily vitamin supplement for all pregnant women.

Iron supplementation is recommended for all pregnant women after 28 weeks' gestation. If the woman has low hemoglobin, is obese, or is carrying twins, higher doses of iron are needed. Folic acid supplementation is also recommended during pregnancy to prevent neural tube defects. Recent studies support calcium supplementation for certain at-risk women. Women who are at risk for developing gestational hypertension and those who live in communities in which dietary calcium intake is low appear to benefit from calcium supplementation (Hofmeyr et al., 2002).

Special Nutritional Considerations

There are several situations that require unique nutritional considerations. These include vegetarianism, lactose intolerance, and pica.

Vegetarianism

There are several different categories of vegetarians. The lacto-ovo-vegetarian does not eat any flesh meats, but does include milk, eggs, and dairy products in the diet. The vegan is a strict vegetarian who does not eat milk, eggs, or any dairy product. A fruitarian only consumes fruits and nuts.

A lacto-ovo-vegetarian can easily get all of the required nutrients by careful attention to a few basic principles. Protein has always been a source of concern for vegetarian diets. Fortunately, a lacto-ovo-vegetarian can get sufficient protein by drinking milk, eating eggs, cheese, yogurt, and other dairy products, and by combining foods. Although vegetables and grains do not contain all of the essential amino acids, when they are skillfully combined, all of the essential amino acids can be obtained. The general rule is to combine a grain and a legume. For instance, a corn tortilla (grain) eaten with pinto beans (legume) provides all of the essential amino acids and qualifies as a complete protein. Other combinations include lentils and whole grain rice, peanut butter on whole wheat bread, and whole grain cereal with milk.

A vegan will need to take extra care to get enough protein because she does not use milk or dairy products. Food combining as discussed in the previous paragraph is an important nutritional strategy for the vegan. It can also help to suggest adding fortified soy milk and rice milk to the diet. Larger amounts of nuts and seeds can help offset the protein requirements. Vitamin B_{12} must be supplemented for the pregnant vegan. A fruitarian will need intensive support from her health care provider and a dietitian to meet the nutritional requirements of a healthy pregnancy. Multivitamin supplementation is necessary in this situation.

Don't get confused! A vegan can take oral forms of vitamin B_{12}. Only the woman who lacks intrinsic factor needs vitamin B_{12} injections. Without intrinsic factor, the woman cannot absorb vitamin B_{12} through the gastrointestinal system; therefore, she needs intramuscular injections.

Iron and zinc requirements are also of concern for the vegetarian. Nonmeat sources of iron are generally not absorbed as efficiently as meat sources. Therefore, the iron requirement for the vegetarian is higher. The same is true for zinc absorption and requirements.

Lactose Intolerance

Individuals of African, Hispanic, Native American, Ashkenazic Jewish, and Asian descent are more likely to have lactose intolerance than are those from a northern European heritage. Individuals with lactose intolerance lack the enzyme lactase that is necessary to break down and digest milk and milk products. Symptoms of lactase deficiency include abdominal distention, flatulence, nausea, vomiting, diarrhea, and cramps after consuming milk.

Some individuals who are lactose intolerant are able to tolerate cooked forms of milk, such as pudding or custard. Cultured or fermented dairy products, such as buttermilk, yogurt, and some cheeses may also be tolerated. Lactase may be taken with milk in the form of a chewable tablet and may allow the person to tolerate milk. Lactase-treated milk is available in most supermarkets and may be helpful.

Pica

Pica is the persistent ingestion of nonfood substances, such as clay, laundry starch, freezer frost, or dirt. It results from a craving for these substances that some women develop during pregnancy. These cravings disappear when the woman is no longer pregnant. Iron-deficiency anemia is associated with pica because many of these substances interfere with the absorption of iron. If you suspect or discover that a pregnant woman is practicing pica, tell the registered nurse (RN) or the health care provider immediately. Special counseling is indicated in this situation.

Test Yourself

- List the recommended weight gain (in pounds) for the woman with a normal body mass index.
- Describe two reasons it is important for the pregnant woman to get adequate amounts of protein.
- State the recommendations of the American Academy of Pediatrics regarding multivitamin supplementation during pregnancy.

KEY POINTS

- Presumptive signs of pregnancy, such as nausea and vomiting, can have many causes other than pregnancy. Probable signs of pregnancy are objective signs the examiner detects that point to pregnancy; however, they are not 100% indicative of pregnancy. Pregnancy tests and changes in the reproductive organs, such as Chadwick's and Hegar's signs, are probable signs of pregnancy.
- A positive sign of pregnancy is diagnostic because no other condition can cause the sign. Positive signs include visualization of the gestational sac or fetus with ultrasound, hearing the fetal heart beat with Doppler or fetoscope, and palpation of fetal movements by a trained examiner.
- Changes in anatomy and physiology that occur during pregnancy include the change of the uterus from a solid, pear-shaped, pelvic organ to a thin, globular shaped, muscular sac that fills the abdominal cavity. The thyroid gland increases in volume. Blood volume increases by 40% to 50%. Coagulation factors increase. Cardiac output increases by as much as 50%.
- The reproductive system undergoes significant changes during pregnancy. The uterus enlarges and the endometrial lining (decidua) is maintained. Blood supply to the uterus increases significantly. Increased vascularity to the reproductive tract is responsible for Goodell's, Hegar's, and Chadwick's signs.
- Endocrine system changes include enlargement of the pituitary gland, an increase in prolactin levels, and an increased need for insulin.
- Hematologic changes enhance the exchange of nutrients and gases between the woman and the fetus and protect the woman against blood loss during childbirth but predispose the woman to venous thrombosis.
- Cardiovascular changes predispose the woman to supine hypotensive syndrome if she lies on her back for prolonged periods late in pregnancy. The woman should lie on her side to prevent this syndrome.
- Respiratory system changes lead to nasal stuffiness and shortness of breath.
- Increasing lordosis, increased curvature of the spine, shifts the center of gravity and leads to a waddling gait in the last half of pregnancy.
- Gastrointestinal changes include nausea and vomiting in early pregnancy, pyrosis (heartburn) in mid and late pregnancy, constipation, and hemorrhoid formation.
- Changes in the urinary tract lead to an increased risk for pyelonephritis during pregnancy. Urinary frequency is common in the first trimester because of an increased glomerular filtration rate and again in the third trimester because of pressure of the gravid uterus on the bladder.
- Increased pigmentation, such as that seen in chloasma and the linea nigra, along with striae, are common integumentary changes.
- The psychological tasks of pregnancy include accepting the pregnancy during the first trimester, accepting the baby during the second trimester, and preparing for parenthood during the third trimester. Ambivalence is a normal feeling when pregnancy is first diagnosed. Couvade syndrome occurs when the father experiences some of the physical discomforts of pregnancy along with his partner.
- Nutritional requirements change during pregnancy. The woman needs nutrients to build extra blood volume and tissue, and the fetus needs nutrients to grow. Energy requirements are increased. A woman who enters pregnancy at normal weight should gain 25 to 35 pounds during pregnancy. A woman who is underweight should gain more, whereas a woman who is overweight should gain less. In no instance is it recommended for a woman to gain less than 15 pounds during pregnancy.
- Protein requirements increase during pregnancy. Most vitamins and minerals can be obtained without supplementation if the diet is adequate.
- After the first trimester, it is generally recommended for a woman to take an iron supplement because it is difficult to get adequate amounts of this mineral from diet alone. Although calcium needs do not increase, it is important for the pregnant woman to get sufficient amounts of this mineral.
- Folic acid supplementation is recommended to help prevent neural tube defects. Vitamin A can be toxic in large amounts. It is best to use beta-carotene (plant) sources to meet vitamin A needs during pregnancy.
- Vitamin C deficiency can lead to scurvy (severe), easy bruising, and possibly gestational hypertension.
- The woman who lacks intrinsic factor must take intramuscular injections of vitamin B_{12}, and the vegan must supplement this vitamin orally.
- Routine multivitamin supplementation is not currently recommended; however, the woman with nutritional risk factors should take prenatal vitamins. Iron and folic acid supplementation is generally recommended for all pregnant women.
- Vegetarians can receive an adequate diet with close attention to combining foods. The lacto-ovo-vegetarian can use milk and dairy products to obtain sufficient protein. The vegan can carefully combine foods (legumes and grains) to supply all of the essential amino acids and should take vitamin B_{12}

supplements. The fruitarian needs to be followed up closely by a dietitian and must take multivitamin supplements.

- When individuals lack the enzyme lactase, they are lactose intolerant. To get sufficient dairy products, these individuals can try taking lactase when they consume dairy products, or sometimes they can tolerate cooked forms of milk.
- Pica is ingestion of nonfood substances. This practice can lead to iron-deficiency anemia and other nutritional deficiencies and requires follow-up.

REFERENCES AND SELECTED READINGS

Books and Journals

Aguilera, P. A. (2001). Round ligament pain. *Emedicine*. Retrieved November 12, 2002, from http://www.emedicine.com/aaem/topic383.htm

Cunningham, F. G., Gant, N. F., Leveno, K. J., Gilstrap, L. C. III, Hauth, J. C., & Wenstrom, K. D. (2001). *Williams obstetrics* (21st ed., pp. 167—247). New York: McGraw-Hill Medical Publishing Division.

Food and Nutrition Board. (2002). *Dietary reference intakes tables*. The National Academies: Institute of Medicine. Retrieved November 11, 2002, from http://www4.nationalacademies.org/IOM/IOMHome.nsf/Pages/Food+and+Nutrition+Board

Hofmeyr, G. J., Atallah, A. N., & Duley, L. (2002). Calcium supplementation during pregnancy for preventing hypertensive disorders and related problems (Cochrane Review abstract). In The Cochrane Library, Issue 4, 2002. Oxford: Update Software. Retrieved November 11, 2002, from http://www.update-software.com/abstracts/ab001059.htm

Ladewig, P. W., London, M. L., Moberly, S., & Olds, S. B. (2002). *Contemporary maternal—newborn nursing care* (5th ed.). Upper Saddle River, NJ: Prentice Hall.

Le Hew, H. W., & Lemieux, J. (2000). Prenatal care. In A. T. Evans, & K. R. Niswander (Eds.), *Manual of obstetrics* (5th ed., pp. 19–39). Philadelphia: Lippincott Williams & Wilkins.

Mattson, S., & Smith, J. E. (Eds.). (2000). *Core curriculum for maternal–newborn nursing. AWHONN publication* (2nd ed.). Philadelphia: WB Saunders Company.

University of Pittsburgh Medical Center. (2002). Even mild vitamin C deficiency may have negative effect on vascular function. *Science Daily*. Retrieved November 11, 2002, from http://www.sciencedaily.com/releases/2002/06/020605073010.htm

Websites

Pregnancy

http://www.cfsan.fda.gov/~dms/wh-preg2.html

Pregnancy signs

http://www.thebabycorner.com/pregnancy/signs.html

http://www.fda.gov/cdrh/oivd/homeuse-pregnancy.html

Nutrition during pregnancy

http://www.4woman.gov/faq/preg-nutr.htm

http://www.vrg.org/nutrition/pregnancy.htm

WORKBOOK

NCLEX-STYLE REVIEW QUESTIONS

1. Amanda is 2 weeks late for her menstrual period. She has been feeling tired and has had bouts of nausea in the evenings. What is the classification of the pregnancy symptoms Amanda is experiencing?

   a. Positive

   b. Presumptive

   c. Probable

   d. No classification

2. Amanda makes an appointment with an obstetrician. During the exam, the obstetrician notes that the uterine isthmus is soft. What is the name of this sign, and how is it classified?

   a. Chadwick's sign; presumptive

   b. Goodell's sign; presumptive

   c. Goodell's sign; probable

   d. Hegar's sign; probable

3. Amanda is now 16 weeks pregnant. If the pregnancy is progressing as expected, where would the practitioner find the uterine fundus?

   a. Just above the pubic bone.

   b. Halfway between the pubic bone and the umbilicus.

   c. At the umbilicus.

   d. The uterine fundus would not be palpable at 16 weeks.

4. You are teaching Amanda about a proper diet during pregnancy. If Amanda understands your instructions, how will she reply when you ask her approximately how many calories per day does she need over her normal prepregnant needs?

   a. "About 300."

   b. "Approximately 500."

   c. "I need to double my calories because I'm eating for two."

   d. "I should not increase my calories while I'm pregnant."

STUDY ACTIVITIES

1. Devise a 3-day meal plan for a vegan who is pregnant. How will you meet her needs for protein, iron, calcium, and vitamin B_{12}?
2. Perform an Internet search using the key terms "pica" and "pregnancy." Share your findings with your clinical group.
3. Develop a teaching plan on the importance of folic acid for a group of women who wish to become pregnant. Be sure to address why women of childbearing age should get enough of this nutrient, how much is required, and examples of food sources.

CRITICAL THINKING: What Would You Do?

Apply your knowledge of maternal physiologic and psychological adaptation to pregnancy to the following situation.

1. Carla is 20 weeks pregnant. You are assisting the midwife during this prenatal visit.

   a. Where do you expect to find Carla's uterine fundus?

   b. You attempt to listen to the fetal heart beat with a Doppler. Do you expect to be able to hear the heart beat?

   c. Carla reports that she is excited about the pregnancy and that she and her husband have been shopping for the nursery. What do you chart regarding Carla's psychological adaptation? Is she showing evidence that she is completing the appropriate task for the trimester?

2. Carla is in the office for her 32-week checkup. She has gained a total of 20 pounds so far during her pregnancy. When you enter the room to check her vital signs you notice that she is lying on her back and she looks pale. Her blood pressure is 70/40 mm Hg.

   a. What is the likely cause of Carla's symptoms?

   b. What action do you take first, and why?

   c. How should you advise Carla regarding her weight gain?

3. Monica has just found out that she is pregnant. She is a vegan.

   a. How would you advise Monica to get enough protein in her diet?

   b. Monica complains that the iron pills her doctor prescribed are causing constipation. She asks you why she needs to take iron. How do you reply?

   c. Monica loves carrot juice, but she has heard that too much vitamin A could be unhealthy for the baby. How would you advise her?

Prenatal Care

Assessment of Maternal Well-Being During Pregnancy
- *First Prenatal Visit*
- *Subsequent Prenatal Visits*

Assessment of Fetal Well-Being During Pregnancy
- *Fetal Kick Counts*
- *Ultrasonography*
- *Doppler Flow Studies*
- *Maternal Serum Alpha-fetoprotein Screening*
- *Triple-Marker (or Multiple-Marker) Screening*
- *Amniocentesis*
- *Chorionic Villus Sampling*
- *Percutaneous Umbilical Blood Sampling*
- *Nonstress Test*
- *Vibroacoustic Stimulation*
- *Contraction Stress Test*
- *Biophysical Profile*

The Nursing Process for Prenatal Care
- *Assessment*
- *Selected Nursing Diagnoses*
- *Outcome Identification and Planning*
- *Implementation*
- *Evaluation: Goals and Expected Outcomes*

STUDENT OBJECTIVES

On completion of this chapter, the student should be able to

1. Explain the goals of early prenatal care.
2. Explain to a pregnant woman what to expect during the first prenatal visit.
3. Examine components of the obstetric history.
4. Assist the practitioner with a pelvic examination and a Papanicolaou (Pap) smear.
5. Delineate the laboratory tests that will be done during the first prenatal visit.
6. Use Nagele's rule to calculate the due date.
7. Recognize factors that put the pregnancy at risk.
8. Describe components of subsequent prenatal visits.
9. For each fetal assessment test, outline the nursing care and implications.
10. Identify common nursing diagnoses for a pregnant woman.
11. Choose appropriate nursing interventions for the pregnant woman.
12. Teach the woman how to deal with the common discomforts of pregnancy.
13. Explain to the woman normal self-care during pregnancy.
14. Assist the woman and her partner to prepare for labor, birth, and parenthood.
15. Evaluate the effectiveness of care given during pregnancy.

KEY TERMS

amniocentesis
biophysical profile
chorionic villus sampling
cordocentesis
doula
estimated date of confinement
estimated date of delivery
gravida
microcephaly
multigravida
Nagele's rule
nulligravida
parity
percutaneous umbilical blood sampling
teratogens

Early prenatal care is crucial to the health of the woman and her unborn baby. In fact, the best strategy is for the woman to seek care before she conceives, as was discussed in Chapter 4. In the year 2000, according to the March of Dimes Perinatal Data Center (2002), approximately 83% of pregnant women began prenatal care in the first trimester, 13% in the second trimester, whereas approximately 4% received late or no prenatal care. Although this statistic falls short of the Healthy People 2000 goal that 90% of pregnant women would begin care in the first trimester, it does show a significant increase compared with 1990 statistics, which indicated 75% of women received early prenatal care.

The goal of early prenatal care is to optimize the health of the woman and the fetus and to increase the odds that the fetus will be born healthy to a healthy mother. Early prenatal care allows for the initiation of strategies to promote good health and for early intervention in the event a complication develops. As a trusted health care provider, the nurse has a large role to play in teaching women about the importance of early and continued prenatal care.

Assessment of maternal and fetal well-being during pregnancy is the focus of prenatal care. The nurse has a large role to play with a heavy emphasis on the teaching role throughout the pregnancy. At each prenatal visit the nurse screens the woman, monitors vital signs, performs other assessments as delegated by the primary care provider, answers questions, and provides appropriate teaching.

ASSESSMENT OF MATERNAL WELL-BEING DURING PREGNANCY

First Prenatal Visit

Ideally the first prenatal visit occurs as soon as the woman thinks she might be pregnant. Often the event that signals the woman to seek care is a missed or late menstrual period. She also may be experiencing some of the signs associated with pregnancy, such as nausea, fatigue, frequent urination, or tingling and fullness of the breasts. The utmost question on the woman's mind, regardless of whether the pregnancy was planned or not, is "Am I pregnant?" If the woman obtained a positive pregnancy test at home, she will want to confirm the results. If she did not, then she may feel anxious, nervous, excited, or any number of emotions until the primary care provider confirms the diagnosis of pregnancy.

The first prenatal visit is usually the longest because the baseline data to which all subsequent assessments are compared are obtained at this visit. The woman may not be mentally prepared for all the questions and tests that must be done, particularly because her main goal at the first visit is to determine whether or not she is, in fact, pregnant. The major objectives of this visit are to confirm or rule out a diagnosis of pregnancy, ascertain risk factors, determine the due date, and provide education on maintaining a healthy pregnancy. These objectives are met through history taking, a physical examination, laboratory work, and teaching. Refer to The Nursing Process for Prenatal Care at the end of the chapter for discussion of teaching topics.

History

The history is one of the most important elements of the first prenatal visit. The woman may be asked to fill out a written questionnaire; the nurse or physician will then confirm the answers. Some health care providers may prefer to obtain the history exclusively by face-to-face interview. Whatever method is chosen, review the history thoroughly and call the primary care provider's attention to any abnormal or unusual details. There are several parts to the history, including chief complaint, reproductive history, medical-surgical history, family history, and social history.

Chief Complaint. The chief complaint will be elicited, which is usually a missed menstrual period. Ask the woman about presumptive and probable signs of pregnancy.

Reproductive History. Note the time of menarche, as well as a summary of the characteristics of the woman's normal menstrual cycles. Common questions include, "Are your periods regular?" "How frequently do your periods occur?" The first day of the last menstrual period (LMP) is noted, if the woman knows this information. Details of each pregnancy are reviewed, including history of miscarriages or abortions and the outcome of each pregnancy (i.e., how many weeks the pregnancy lasted and whether or not the pregnancy ended with a living child).

Here's a tip that should increase the accuracy of the history. If a partner or other family members accompany the woman, find a tactful way to separate them for at least part of the history collection. A woman may have a history of a previous pregnancy, an abortion that she may not wish to reveal to her family members, or she may be the victim of domestic violence. In any of these instances, it is necessary to interview the woman alone if truthful answers are to be expected. Assure her that all information is held in strict confidence and shared only with other members of the health care team on a need-to-know basis.

A problem the woman had in a previous pregnancy may manifest itself again in the current pregnancy or increase the chance that she will develop another type of complication.

The obstetric history is a part of the reproductive history and is recorded in a specific format that is a type of medical shorthand. The word "gravid" means pregnant. The number of pregnancies the woman has had (regardless of the outcome) is recorded as the **gravida**. For example, a woman who has had one pregnancy is a gravida 1, whereas a woman who has had five pregnancies is a gravida 5. A woman who has never been pregnant is a **nulligravida**, whereas a woman who has had more than one pregnancy is a **multigravida**.

Once the total number of pregnancies has been determined and recorded, the next part of the obstetric history is parity. **Parity**, or para, communicates the outcome of previous pregnancies. If a gravida 1 delivers a live-born infant, or an infant who is past the age of viability (greater than 20 weeks), she is then referred to as a gravida 1, para 1. Nonviable fetuses that are delivered before the end of 20 weeks' gestation are considered abortions (either spontaneous or induced) and are not counted in the parity. For example, if a woman had a pregnancy that ended at 17 weeks, another at 26 weeks, and another at 40 weeks, and she is currently pregnant, she is a gravida 4 para 2 abortus 1. The parity refers to the outcome of the pregnancy and is counted as 1, even if the woman delivers twins or triplets.

One of the most common methods of recording the obstetric history is to use the acronym GTPAL. "G" stands for gravida, the total number of pregnancies. "T" stands for term, the number of pregnancies that ended at term (at or beyond 38 weeks' gestation); "P" is for preterm, the number of pregnancies that ended after 20 weeks and before the end of 37 weeks' gestation. "A" represents abortions, the number of pregnancies that ended before 20 weeks' gestation. "L" is for living; the number of children delivered who are alive as of the time the history is taken. Some primary care providers further divide abortions into induced and spontaneous and note multiple births and ectopic pregnancies. Box 7-1 defines terms associated with the obstetric history.

It also is important to obtain information regarding complications that may have occurred with other pregnancies. If a woman hemorrhaged after a previous delivery, she has a higher risk of hemorrhaging after subsequent deliveries. If she develops gestational diabetes with a pregnancy, she will likely develop the condition again with subsequent pregnancies. If she has a history of preterm delivery, her risk is increased that she will deliver another baby prematurely. Any abnormality that presented itself in a previous pregnancy must be noted.

BOX 7.1 Obstetric History Terms

- *Gravida*: Total number of pregnancies a woman has had, including the present pregnancy.
- *Para*: The number of fetuses delivered after the point of viability (20 weeks' gestation), whether or not they are born alive.
- *Nulli* (null or none), *primi* (first or one), and *multi* (many): Prefixes used in front of the terms "gravida" and "para" to indicate whether or not the woman has had previous pregnancies and deliveries.
- GTPAL: Acronym that represents the obstetric history.
  - **G**ravida
  - **T**erm deliveries
  - **P**reterm deliveries
  - **A**bortions
  - **L**iving children

Medical–Surgical History. After a thorough reproductive history is elicited, the primary care provider must obtain a detailed medical–surgical history of the woman. If she has any major medical problems, such as heart disease or diabetes, she will require closer surveillance throughout the pregnancy. All medications the woman is taking, including over-the-counter medications and herbal remedies, should be noted in the prenatal record.

The medical history also involves determining if there are risk factors for infectious diseases. Exposure to anyone with tuberculosis indicates the need for further screening to rule out the disease. The immunization status should be assessed. Although most immunizations are contraindicated during pregnancy, the woman who is at risk for an infectious disease can take precautions to decrease the chance she will contract infection during pregnancy. Risk factors for human immunodeficiency virus/acquired immunodeficiency syndrome (HIV/AIDS) and other sexually transmitted infections (STIs) must be determined (Box 7-2).

Family History. A family history also is important because it may highlight the need for genetic testing or

BOX 7.2 Risk Factors for Sexually Transmitted Infections (STIs)

- Sex with multiple partners
- Sex with a partner who has risk factors
- Intravenous drug use (needle sharing)
- Anal intercourse
- Vaginal intercourse with a partner who also engages in anal intercourse
- Unprotected (no condom) intercourse

TABLE 7.1 Genetic Disorder Screening Criteria by Ethnicity

Ethnicity	Genetic Disorders for Which Screening May Be Recommended
African-American, Indian, Middle Eastern	Sickle cell anemia; thalassemia
European Jewish, French Canadian	Tay-Sachs disease
Mediterranean, Southeast Asian	Thalassemia
Caucasian	Cystic fibrosis

counseling. Inquiry will be made regarding the health status of the father of the baby and any close relatives of the woman and her partner. If there is a family history for cystic fibrosis or hearing loss, genetic screening may be indicated. The ethnic background of the woman and relatives of the unborn child are important factors to note. For instance, many people of African-American descent are carriers for sickle cell anemia; people of Mediterranean descent are at increased risk for thalassemia. See Table 7-1 for examples of ethnic-related genetic diseases.

Social History. The social history focuses on environmental factors that may influence the pregnancy. A woman who has strong social support, adequate housing and nutrition, and greater than a high school education is less likely to develop complications of pregnancy than is a woman who lives with inadequate resources. The type of employment may also have a bearing on the health of the pregnancy. A job that requires exposure to harmful chemicals is less safe for the woman and fetus than is a job that does not involve this type of exposure.

Smoking, alcohol, and illicit and over-the-counter drug use can all potentially harm a growing fetus, so it is important to determine the woman's consumption patterns, particularly since conception. If the woman owns a cat or likes to garden, she is at increased risk for contracting toxoplasmosis, an infection that can cause the woman to lose the pregnancy or can result in severe abnormalities in the fetus.

Physical Examination

The physical examination covers all body systems and is completed by the primary care provider. The nurse provides assistance, as needed. The head-to-toe physical is done first. The examiner is looking for signs of disease that may need treatment and for any evidence of previously undetected maternal disease or other signs of ill health. A breast examination is part of the physical. Although it is rare, breast cancer in a young pregnant woman is a possibility.

The head-to-toe physical is followed by a vaginal speculum examination and a bimanual examination of the uterus. During the speculum examination, a Papanicolaou test or Pap smear is done, and some signs of pregnancy, such as Chadwick's sign, can be noted (see Nursing Procedure 7-1). The bimanual examination (Fig. 7-1) allows the practitioner to feel the size of the uterus and to elicit Hegar's sign.

Laboratory Assessment

There are many laboratory tests that will be done during the course of the pregnancy. A complete blood count (CBC) gives the health care provider an indication of the overall health status of the woman. Anemia will be manifested as a low blood count and low hemoglobin and hematocrit. Anemia is one indication of suboptimal nutritional status and is associated with poor pregnancy outcomes, unless it is caught and treated early. A woman who is at risk for sickle cell anemia or thalassemia is given a hemoglobin electrophoresis test.

Other laboratory tests routinely ordered include a blood type and antibody screen. This test helps identify women who are at risk of developing antigen incompatibility with fetal blood cells. A, B, and O incompatibilities can develop, as well as Rh_0(D) incompatibilities. If an

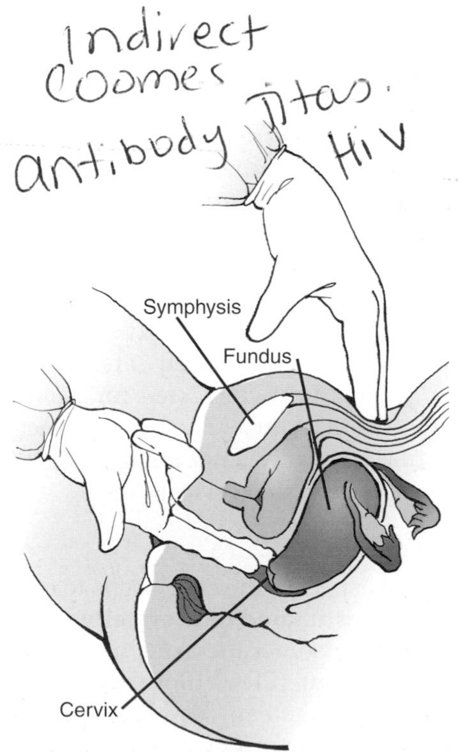

● ***Figure 7.1*** Bimanual examination. The fundus (top portion) of the uterus is palpated through the abdominal wall while the hand in the vagina holds the cervix in place. In this way the examiner can determine the size of the uterus, which helps date the pregnancy.

Nursing Procedure 7.1
Assisting the Practitioner With a Pelvic Examination and Collection of the Pap Smear

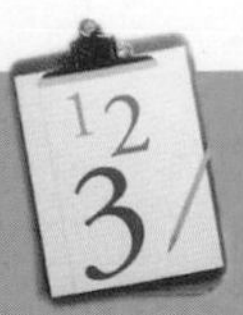

EQUIPMENT

Examination table with stirrups or foot pedals
Drapes
Sterile gloves for the examiner
Speculum
Swab for the Pap test
Glass slide
Fixative
Sterile lubricant (water-soluble)

PROCEDURE

1. Explain procedure to the patient.
2. Instruct the patient to empty her bladder before the procedure.
3. Wash hands thoroughly.
4. Assemble equipment, maintaining the sterility of the equipment.
5. Position patient on stirrups or foot pedals so that her knees fall outward.
6. Drape the patient with a sheet or other draping for privacy, covering the abdomen and legs, leaving the perineal area exposed.
7. Open packages as needed throughout the procedure.
8. After the practitioner obtains the specimen and swipes the slide, spray the fixative on the slide.
9. Place the sterile lubricant on the practitioner's fingertips, when indicated for the bimanual examination.
10. Wash hands thoroughly.
11. Label specimen according to facility policy.
12. Send sample to laboratory with appropriate request form.
13. Rinse reusable instruments and dispose of waste appropriately.
14. Wash hands thoroughly.

Note: A full bladder interferes with the pelvic examination and causes discomfort for the woman.

antigen incompatibility develops, the fetus may suffer from hemolytic anemia as the mother's antibodies cross the placenta and attack his red blood cells (refer to Chapter 20 for further discussion of antigen incompatibilities).

Other tests screen for the presence of infection. The woman will be tested for hepatitis B, HIV, syphilis, gonorrhea, and Chlamydia. Each of these infections can cause serious fetal problems unless they are treated. A rubella titer will be drawn to determine if the woman is immune. If she is not, this fact will be noted in her chart, and she will need a rubella immunization immediately after delivery because the rubella vaccine cannot be given safely during pregnancy. A urine culture will screen for bacteria in the urine, a situation that can lead to urinary tract infection and premature labor if it is not treated. The Pap smear is evaluated to screen for cervical cancer.

Determining the Due Date

One important aspect of the first visit is to calculate the due date, or the **estimated date of delivery** (EDD). An older term that is sometimes still used is **estimated date of confinement** (EDC). Both terms refer to the estimated date that the baby will be born. This is critical information for the primary care provider to know because she will manage problems that may arise during the pregnancy differently, depending on the gestational age of the fetus. Therefore, it is essential to have an accurate due date.

There are several means by which to date a pregnancy. The most common way to calculate the EDD is to use **Nagele's rule.** To determine the due date using Nagele's rule, add 7 days to the date of the first day of the LMP, then subtract 3 months. This is a fairly simple way to estimate the due date, but it is dependent upon knowing when the first day of the LMP was. Sometimes this date is impossible to determine, particularly if the woman experiences irregular menstrual cycles, or if she just cannot remember the date.

During the pelvic examination, the practitioner can feel the size of the uterus to get an idea of how far along the pregnancy is. For instance, a uterus that is the size of a hen's egg is approximately 7 weeks. If the uterus feels to be the size of an orange, the pregnancy is approximately 10 weeks along, and at 12 weeks the uterus is the size of a grapefruit. Other ways to validate the gestational age are to note landmarks in the pregnancy. The fetal heart beat can first be detected by Doppler ultrasound between 10 and 12 weeks. Quickening typically occurs around 16 weeks for multigravidas and 20 weeks for primigravidas.

One of the most common and reliable ways to date the pregnancy is for the practitioner to order an obstetric sonogram. During this procedure, high frequency sound waves reflect off fetal and maternal pelvic structures and allow them to be visualized in real time. Fetal structures, such as the femur and the head, are measured. The measurements allow the practitioner to estimate the gestational age of the fetus, and thereby determine a due date. The earlier in the pregnancy the sonogram is done, the more accurate the due date. If there is a discrepancy between the EDD calculated using Nagele's rule and the EDD determined by sonogram, the results of the sonogram (if it is done early in the pregnancy) will be used to base treatment decisions.

Risk Assessment

The risk assessment is done by taking into account all of the information gathered from the history, physical examination, and laboratory tests. There are many factors that put a pregnancy at risk. These factors include a negative attitude of the woman toward the pregnancy (e.g., an unwanted pregnancy), seeking prenatal care late in the pregnancy, and maternal substance abuse (alcohol, tobacco, or illicit drugs). A history of complications with previous pregnancies or poor outcomes, and the presence of maternal disease also put the current pregnancy at risk. Social factors that increase the risk of poor outcomes include inadequate living conditions and domestic violence or physical abuse. If the woman is unaware of the adverse effects of tobacco and alcohol, the benefits of folic acid, or the risk of HIV, the pregnancy is at increased risk for complications and poor outcomes. Age also plays a factor. Young teens and women older than 35 years of age are at higher risk for a complicated pregnancy. An unplanned pregnancy or a pregnancy when the woman is unsure of her LMP date may also be at risk.

Test Yourself

- What is the obstetric term used to indicate the number of pregnancies a woman has had?
- List four laboratory tests that are routinely ordered during the first prenatal visit.
- State how to calculate the due date using Nagele's rule.

Subsequent Prenatal Visits

Traditionally women are seen once monthly from weeks 1 through 32. Between weeks 32 and 36, prenatal visits are biweekly. From week 36 until delivery the woman is seen weekly in the primary care provider's office. Current research shows that fewer visits for low-risk pregnancies and more visits for at-risk pregnancies may be more beneficial overall than a rigid adherence to the traditional schedule of visits. In any event, the woman needs encouragement to keep her appointments and maintain regular prenatal care throughout the pregnancy.

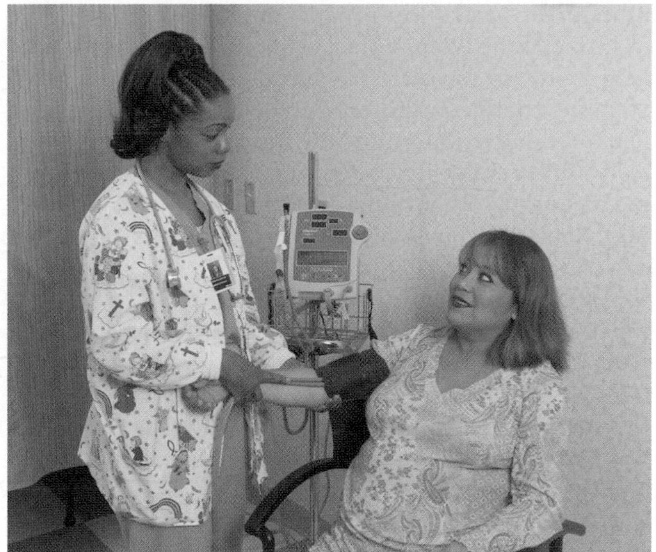

● ***Figure 7.2*** The Practical Nurse measures the blood pressure at a prenatal visit.

Most subsequent visits include specific assessments. Weight, blood pressure (Fig. 7-2), urine protein and glucose, and fetal heart rate are all data that may be collected by the practical nurse. At every visit, inquiry should be made regarding the danger signals of pregnancy (discussed in the The Nursing Process for Prenatal Care). The woman should be asked about fetal movement, contractions, bleeding, and membrane rupture. Normally the pelvic examination is not repeated until late in the pregnancy, close to the expected time of delivery.

At each office visit the practitioner will measure the fundal height in centimeters (Fig. 7-3). This measure provides a confirmation of gestational age between weeks 18 and 32. In other words, between weeks 18 and 32, the fundal height in centimeters should match the

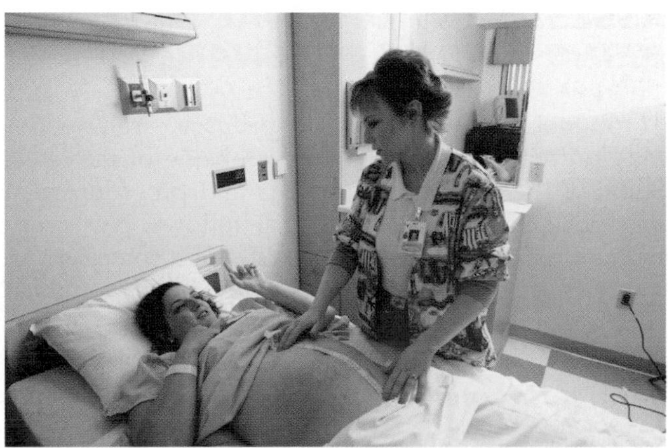

● ***Figure 7.3*** The Certified Nurse Midwife (CNM) measures the fundal height. Between 18 and 32 weeks' gestation there is a good correlation between the gestation in weeks and the fundal height in centimeters.

number of weeks the pregnancy has progressed. For example, if the woman is 18 weeks pregnant, the fundal height should measure 18 centimeters. If there is a discrepancy between the size and dates, a sonogram is usually done to determine the cause of the discrepancy. A fundal height that is larger than expected could mean, among other things, that the original dates were miscalculated, that the woman is carrying twins, or that there is a molar pregnancy (Chapter 17).

The woman undergoes screening at particular times during the pregnancy. Sometime between 15 and 20 weeks' gestation, a maternal serum alpha-fetoprotein (MSAFP) should be drawn (see the discussion in the section on fetal assessment). Between 24 and 28 weeks, all women should be screened for gestational diabetes. At 28 weeks, a woman who is Rh_0(D)-negative should be screened for antibodies and given anti-D immune globulin (RhoGam), if indicated (see Chapter 23 for further discussion of hemolytic disease of the newborn). The woman should be screened for Group B streptococcus (GBS) after 35 weeks and before the end of 37 weeks. Positive cultures indicate the need for antibiotics for the woman during labor and close observation of the newborn for 48 hours after birth.

Test Yourself

- How often is a woman with an uncomplicated pregnancy seen in the office from weeks 1 through 32?
- What purpose does measuring the fundal height serve during prenatal visits?
- List the time during pregnancy when a woman is normally screened for gestational diabetes.

ASSESSMENT OF FETAL WELL-BEING DURING PREGNANCY

Throughout the pregnancy the primary care provider may order tests to assess the well-being of the fetus. Some of the most common tests and procedures are described in the discussion that follows. Not every woman will receive every test, although some screening tests are recommended for all pregnant women at certain points during the pregnancy.

Fetal Kick Counts

A healthy fetus moves and kicks regularly, although the pregnant woman usually cannot perceive the movements until approximately gestational week 16 to 20. The primary care provider or the nurse instructs the woman to monitor her baby's movements on a daily basis. Instruct the woman to choose a time each day in which she can relax and count the baby's movements. Each kick or position change counts as one movement. Using a special form, or a blank sheet of paper, instruct the woman to note the time she starts counting fetal kicks, then she is to keep counting until she counts 10 movements. A healthy fetus will move at least 10 times in 2 hours. If it takes longer than 2 hours for the fetus to move 10 times, or if the woman cannot get her baby to move at all, she should immediately call her health care provider. The primary care provider will want to do additional tests to determine the well-being of the fetus.

Don't forget. "Routine" for the nurse is not at all routine for the woman. She will need careful explanation of all testing that is planned, whether or not it is a normal part of prenatal care or performed for some other reason. If a screening test result is "suspicious," or further testing is indicated, remember that the woman will need emotional support. It is scary not knowing what to expect while waiting for test results. Accept and let her talk through her feelings.

Ultrasonography

Ultrasound has been used for many years in the United States to determine gestational age, observe the fetus, and diagnose complications of pregnancy. Because it appears to be a safe and effective way to monitor fetal well-being, the procedure is performed frequently (Fig. 7-4). One result of monitoring virtually every pregnancy with ultrasound is that most parents know the gender of their child before she is born. Many sonographers take a still picture of the fetus and provide this to the parents, if desired.

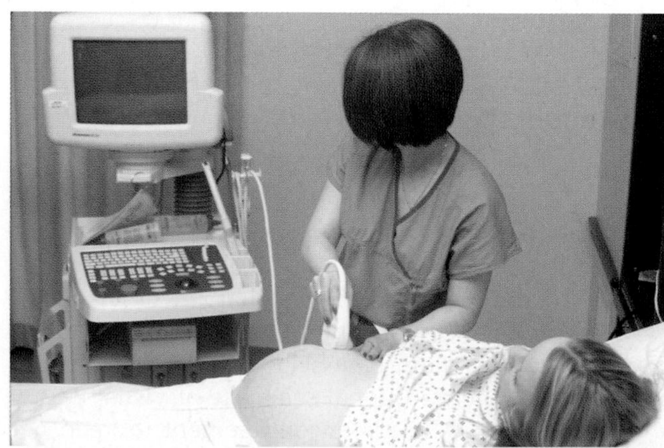

● ***Figure 7.4*** Ultrasound is used to identify fetal and placental structures during pregnancy.

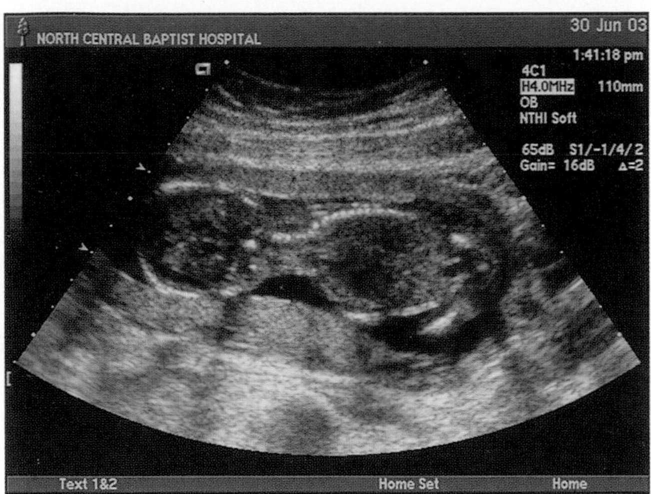

● ***Figure 7.5*** Fetus viewed via ultrasound. The outline of the fetal head and trunk can be clearly seen in the transverse position.

As stated earlier in the chapter, ultrasound uses high frequency sound waves to visualize fetal and maternal structures (Fig. 7-5). The developing embryo can first be visualized at about 6 weeks' gestation. An ultrasound performed at this stage is usually done to diagnose the pregnancy. The fetus is visualized in real time, so that his cardiac activity and body movements can be monitored. Box 7-3 lists ways ultrasound technology is used to monitor the pregnancy and fetal well-being.

BOX 7.3 **Uses for Ultrasound Technology During Pregnancy**

- Diagnose pregnancy: intrauterine and ectopic (outside the uterine cavity).
- Diagnose multifetal pregnancies (twins, triplets).
- Monitor fetal heart beat and breathing movements. The fetus makes "practice" breathing movements in utero as early as 11 weeks gestation.
- Take measurements of the fetal head, femur, and other structures to determine gestational age or diagnose fetal growth restriction.
- Detect fetal anomalies.
- Estimate the amount of amniotic fluid that is present. Either too much (hydramnios) or too little (oligohydramnios) can indicate problems with the pregnancy.
- Identify fetal and placental structures during amniocentesis or umbilical cord sampling.
- Detect placental problems, such as abnormal placement of the placenta in placenta previa or grade the placenta (determine the age and functioning).
- Diagnose fetal demise (death). Absence of cardiac activity is used to diagnose fetal death.
- Verify fetal presentation and position.
- Estimate the birth weight, particularly if the fetus is thought to be abnormally large (macrosomic).

Most abnormalities of the fetus, placenta, and surrounding structures are best detected between 16 and 20 weeks' gestation. Detailed sonograms can diagnose severe congenital heart, spine, brain, and kidney defects. However, ultrasound cannot pick up all abnormalities. Some anomalies, such as Down syndrome, have subtle characteristics that often cannot be picked up until late in the pregnancy. However, a skilled practitioner can detect 70% to 80% of Down syndrome cases when observing for nuchal translucency (fetal neck thickness) on ultrasound between weeks 11 and 14. There are two main ways an ultrasound can be done–the transabdominal approach, in which the transducer is placed on the abdomen to visualize the pregnancy, and the endovaginal approach, in which a specialized probe is inserted into the vagina to visualize the cervix and fetal structures.

Transabdominal Ultrasound

It is important for the woman to have a full bladder for the procedure, particularly during the first trimester. A full bladder pushes the uterus up so that the contents can more easily be seen. Instruct the woman to drink several large glasses of water 2 hours before the procedure and not to empty her bladder.

If you are assisting during the procedure, make certain that a small wedge or sandbag is placed under one hip to prevent vena-caval hypotension. Explain to the woman that a special gel will be used on her abdomen and that it probably will be cold. She should not feel any discomfort during the procedure, other than the discomfort of a full bladder. The procedure is performed in a darkened room. Although the technician performing the sonogram can see fetal structures and obvious defects during the sonogram, it will take several hours to get the official results because the radiologist must review the films and dictate the diagnosis. After the procedure, clean the excess gel off of the woman's abdomen and assist her to the bathroom.

Endovaginal Ultrasound

The endovaginal approach allows for clearer image because the probe is very close to fetal and uterine structures. The pregnancy can usually be visualized sooner than with the transabdominal method. The endovaginal method has been used to predict or diagnose preterm labor because the cervix can be measured and analyzed for changes.

The woman's bladder can be empty for the endovaginal examination. Assist the woman into lithotomy position (as for a pelvic examination) and drape her for privacy. A female attendant must be present in the room at all times during the procedure. The examiner covers the probe (which is smaller than a speculum) with a specialized sheath, a condom, or the finger of a glove; applies ultrasonic transducer gel to the covered probe; and inserts the probe into the vagina. The woman will feel the probe being moved about in different directions during the test. The probe may cause mild discomfort but generally is not painful.

Doppler Flow Studies

Another test that uses ultrasound technology is a Doppler flow study, or Doppler velocimetry. A specialized ultrasound machine is used to measure the flow of blood through fetal vessels. The ultrasound transducer is placed on the woman's abdomen, and blood flow can be assessed in the umbilical vessels, fetal brain, and fetal heart. If the test shows that blood flow through fetal vessels is less than normal, the fetus may not be receiving enough oxygen and nutrients from the placenta, and additional studies will most likely be ordered. Preparation and nursing care for a Doppler flow study are the same as for ultrasonography.

Maternal Serum Alpha-fetoprotein Screening

Alpha-fetoprotein is a protein that is manufactured by the fetus. The protein is found in small amounts in the pregnant woman's bloodstream. Many physicians recommend measuring MSAFP between 16 and 18 weeks' gestation because abnormal levels may indicate a problem and the need for additional testing.

MSAFP levels are elevated in several conditions. Higher-than-expected levels of MSAFP may indicate that the pregnancy is farther along than was predicted initially. When the woman is carrying multiple fetuses, such as twins or triplets, or when the fetus has died, MSAFP levels will be elevated. The main reason physicians screen MSAFP is to check for neural tube defects, such as anencephaly (failure of the brain to develop normally) or spina bifida (failure of the spine to close completely during development). MSAFP levels are usually elevated if the fetus has either of these anomalies or omphalocele or gastroschisis (failure of the abdominal wall to close). Low MSAFP levels may also indicate a problem, in particular Down's syndrome.

It is important for the parents-to-be to understand the reasons for and implications of MSAFP testing. Even when the levels are abnormal, approximately 90% of the time the woman will be delivered of a healthy baby. However, abnormal results increase the likelihood that the fetus has an abnormality, and additional testing with ultrasound and/or amniocentesis is usually indicated. Even when the follow-up ultrasound is normal, there is no guarantee that the fetus will be healthy. An elevated MSAFP in the presence of a normal ultrasound increases the risk that the woman will develop a complication of pregnancy such as preeclampsia or intrauterine growth restriction.

Some women want to have the test done so that they can decide whether or not to end the pregnancy before the age of viability. Other women feel strongly that abortion is not an option, but they may want to know if an anomaly is present so that they can deliver in a hospital with high-level care and have specialists immediately available to resuscitate and care for the baby. Other women may decide against testing because a false-positive test might be needlessly worrisome and lead to more invasive, riskier tests, such as amniocentesis, even though the baby might be healthy. These are issues each woman must consider in consult with her partner and physician. No matter what decision the woman makes regarding testing, it is critical that she be supported in her decision.

Triple-Marker (or Multiple-Marker) Screening

The sensitivity of MSAFP testing is increased when the levels of two other hormones are measured in conjunction with MSAFP. When MSAFP, human chorionic gonadotropin (hCG), and unconjugated estriol (uE3) levels are measured from the same maternal blood sample, the test is called a triple-marker screen. A low MSAFP, low estriol, and elevated hCG suggests that the baby has Down syndrome; whereas low levels of all three hormones increases the risk the fetus has trisomy 18, a more severe and less common chromosomal defect. A fourth biochemical marker in maternal serum, inhibin A, has been found to increase the ability of blood tests to predict chromosomal abnormalities of the fetus, so some practitioners add this fourth screen. The test is then known as a multiple-marker screen.

Sometimes the physician will order serial estriol levels in the third trimester to monitor the well-being of the fetus. Falling estriol levels in the third trimester may indicate that the fetus is in jeopardy, in which case an emergency cesarean delivery may be done to save the fetus' life. Nursing care for MSAFP or triple marker screening is the same as that for any venous blood sampling of the woman.

Amniocentesis

An **amniocentesis** is a diagnostic procedure whereby a needle is inserted into the amniotic sac and a small amount of fluid is withdrawn. A variety of biochemical, chromosomal, and genetic studies can be done using the amniotic fluid sample.

The procedure is usually performed between 15 and 20 weeks' gestation, and genetic studies are done to identify fetal abnormalities. Because early amniocentesis (<14 weeks) is associated with a higher rate of pregnancy loss (abortion) and fetal foot deformities, most practitioners will not perform amniocentesis

BOX 7.4 Selected Indications for Chromosomal Studies by Amniocentesis or Chorionic Villus Sampling

- Advanced maternal age (generally accepted as older than 35)
- Previous offspring with chromosomal anomalies
- History of recurrent pregnancy loss
- Ultrasound diagnosis of fetal anomalies
- Abnormal MSAFP, triple marker screen, or multiple marker screen
- Previous offspring with a neural tube defect
- Both parents known carriers of a recessive genetic trait (such as cystic fibrosis, sickle cell anemia, or Tay-Sachs disease)

14-20

before 14 weeks. Early and second trimester cases are done to determine the genetic makeup of the fetus. This can be done because fetal cells are found within the amniotic fluid. Box 7-4 lists indications for first and second trimester amniocentesis. Third trimester amniocentesis is usually done to determine fetal lung maturity to allow for the earliest possible delivery in certain at-risk pregnancies.

Because amniocentesis is an invasive procedure that carries a small risk of spontaneous abortion, injury to the fetus, and chorioamnionitis (infection of the fetal membranes), informed consent is required. The physician explains the procedure and risks to the woman and answers her questions. If you are asked to witness the consent, be certain that the woman has had all her questions answered before she signs. Explain the procedure to her so that she knows what to expect. Many women are worried that the procedure will be painful. Although pain is a subjective feeling that is experienced differently for each person, most women find that the procedure is much less painful than they anticipated. Usually women report feeling a slight pinching sensation or vague cramping.

Ultrasonography is done before amniocentesis to locate a pocket of amniotic fluid. Without ultrasound to guide the needle, there is a high risk that the needle could puncture the placenta or the fetus. After the pocket of fluid is located (usually on the upper portion of the uterus), the site is prepared with Betadine or alcohol, and sterile drapes are placed on the abdomen around the site. The ultrasound transducer is also covered with sterile drapes. Next the practitioner inserts a 20- to 22-gauge spinal needle into the chosen site. The practitioner watches the ultrasound picture and guides the needle along the chosen path into the pocket of fluid. The first 0.5 cc of fluid is discarded to avoid contamination of the specimen with maternal cells. Then 20 mL of fluid is withdrawn, and the needle is removed. At this point the practitioner monitors the fetal heart rate by ultrasound to ensure fetal well-being. Then the fluid, which is normally straw colored, is placed into sterile tubes, labeled, and sent to the laboratory for analysis. Results are usually available within 2 to 3 weeks and are highly accurate (approximately 99%).

The woman should remain on bed rest the day of the procedure. Attach continuous electronic fetal monitoring to observe the fetal heart rate and contractions, if they should occur. Women who are Rh_0(D)-negative should receive anti-D immunoglobulin (RhoGam) after the procedure. The site should be monitored for leakage of amniotic fluid (a rare complication), and the woman's temperature should be monitored. Any temperature elevation, leaking of fluid from the site or from the vagina, vaginal bleeding, cramps, or contractions should be immediately reported to the RN or the attending practitioner. After several hours of monitoring, the woman may be sent home. Instruct her to remain on bed rest for the rest of the day. The following day she may do light housework chores, and the third day she may resume regular activities. Warning signs that should be reported to the attending practitioner immediately include fever, amniotic fluid leakage, vaginal bleeding, and/or cramping.

As with any medical procedure that carries risk, amniocentesis has advantages and disadvantages that each woman and her partner must consider carefully before submitting to the procedure. The most common reason for undergoing amniocentesis is to determine if there is a fetal abnormality so that the pregnancy might be ended (elective abortion) before the age of viability. Many women will not consider an abortion under any circumstances. In these cases, there are still benefits to amniocentesis. If the fetus does have a chromosomal abnormality, knowing in advance allows for the medical team and the parents to prepare for the birth. It also allows the physician to make better decisions about managing the pregnancy. Every woman who is contemplating amniocentesis should have genetic counseling. Then, no matter what decision the woman makes, it is critical that the health care team be supportive of her decision.

Chorionic Villus Sampling

Chorionic villus sampling (CVS) is a newer procedure that can provide chromosomal studies of fetal cells similar to amniocentesis. Indications for CVS are the same as for amniocentesis (see Box 7-4). One advantage of CVS testing is that it is done earlier in the pregnancy than is amniocentesis, which allows for a decision about elective abortion to be made sooner in the pregnancy. Elective abortions are safer for the woman the earlier they are performed. CVS is typically performed at 10 to 12 weeks' gestation. Because CVS is an invasive procedure, informed consent is required.

Just before the procedure, ultrasonography is performed to confirm fetal well-being, the location of the placenta, and gestational age. For the transcervical approach, the woman is placed in lithotomy position in stirrups, and her vagina and cervix are cleaned with Betadine or other antiseptic fluid. Using ultrasound guidance, a small catheter is inserted into the woman's vagina and through the cervix. Placental tissue is then extracted into a syringe to obtain fetal cells for chromosomal analysis. The procedure can also be done transabdominally with a needle, similar to the procedure for amniocentesis. The woman usually experiences minimal discomfort and may resume normal activities after the test. Anti-D immunoglobulin (RhoGam) should be administered after the procedure to Rh_o(D)-negative women.

One advantage of CVS testing is that the results are available in 7 to 10 days, much faster than with amniocentesis. However, there are disadvantages to this technique. First, some authorities report a higher rate of pregnancy loss[1] with transcervical CVS versus transabdominal CVS and second trimester amniocentesis. Other authorities indicate that the risk for pregnancy loss with CVS is comparable with that of amniocentesis. The risk is lowered for both procedures as the skill level of the practitioner increases. A second potential disadvantage is that because no amniotic fluid is withdrawn in CVS, the amniotic alpha-fetoprotein cannot be evaluated, as it can with amniocentesis. This would mean the woman would need to have MSAFP levels drawn at 16 to 18 weeks' gestation to test for neural tube defects. A woman who has amniocentesis performed does not need the MSAFP test because the fetal alpha-fetoprotein level, which is a more accurate predictor of spinal defects than maternal serum levels, is already known. The third disadvantage of CVS is that there is a small risk that the cells taken from the placenta will be different than fetal cells. If this happens, a situation called "placental mosaicism," the test results would be abnormal, even if the fetus were normal. Some authorities suggest if CVS is performed before 9 weeks' gestation, it can cause fetal limb and digit deformations.

Percutaneous Umbilical Blood Sampling

Percutaneous umbilical blood sampling (PUBS), also known as **cordocentesis**, is a procedure similar to amniocentesis, except that fetal blood is withdrawn, rather than amniotic fluid. The woman is prepared in the same manner as for amniocentesis, informed consent is obtained, and ultrasound is performed to locate the placenta and fetal structures and to confirm gestational age and viability. A thin needle is inserted transabdominally under ultrasound guidance, and blood is withdrawn from the umbilical cord close to its insertion with the placenta. Alternatively blood can be withdrawn from the fetal heart or from the umbilical vein within the liver, although these sites are not commonly chosen. The blood is then sent for testing.

Sometimes PUBS is done specifically to diagnose and treat certain diseases of the blood, such as von Willebrand's disease, alloimmune thrombocytopenia, and hemolytic disease. It is also used to diagnose and treat cases of fetal infection, such as toxoplasmosis, rubella, cytomegalovirus, varicella zoster, human parvovirus, and HIV. Through the technology of cordocentesis, the fetus with thrombocytopenia can receive weekly infusions of platelets until delivery. The fetus with hemolytic disease can receive exchange transfusions (part of the fetus' blood is withdrawn and the same amount replaced with healthy blood). The fetus found to be have an infection can be treated with antibiotics or receive other therapies, depending upon the type of infection. The blood obtained from cordocentesis can also be sent for rapid chromosomal studies. Results are back within 48 to 72 hours. The risks associated with PUBS are approximately the same as those of amniocentesis.

Nonstress Test

The nonstress test (NST) is a noninvasive way to monitor fetal well-being. Usually around 28 weeks and onward, the fetal nervous system is developed enough so that the autonomic nervous system works to periodically accelerate the heart rate. Therefore, the woman can be attached to an electronic fetal monitor (EFM), and the fetal heart can be observed for accelerations.

The woman requires no special preparation other than placement of EFM (refer to Chapter 10 for in-depth discussion of fetal monitoring). She may or may not be given an event marker to hold.[2] If she is given

[1] The latest report available from the Centers for Disease Control (CDC) is 1995. In that report, a pregnancy loss of 0.5% to 1.0% (1/200 to 1/100) was found with transcervical CVS, as compared with a 0.25% to 0.50% (1/400 to 1/200) risk with amniocentesis. These data are probably no longer valid because the technique has been perfected over time.

[2] In the past it was very important to monitor the fetal heart rate in conjunction with fetal movement. Now it is generally felt that spontaneous accelerations with or without fetal movement are indicative of fetal well-being, so it is not necessary to have the woman track fetal movements, although some practitioners may prefer this.

one, she is instructed to push the button every time she feels the fetus move. The fetal monitor strip is evaluated after 20 minutes. If there are at least two accelerations of the fetal heart in a 15×15 window, that is the fetal heart accelerates at least 15 beats above the baseline for at least 15 seconds, the NST is said to be "reactive" provided that the baseline and variability are normal and that there are no decelerations of the fetal heart rate. In the presence of a reactive NST,[3] fetal well-being is assumed for at least the next week.

If, however, there are no accelerations or less than 2 occur within 20 minutes, the strip is said to be "nonreactive." In this case the monitoring would continue for another 20 minutes in the hopes of obtaining a reactive NST. This decision is made based on knowledge of fetal sleep cycles, which last for approximately 20 minutes. During fetal sleep, it is expected that there will be no accelerations, so waiting an additional 20 minutes is indicated. Sometimes the nurse will attempt to stimulate the fetus. She may clap loudly close to the woman's abdomen or may manipulate the fetus through the abdomen with her hands, or she may give the woman something cold to drink. Any of these activities might stimulate a sleeping fetus to wake up, and a reactive tracing may be obtained. If the tracing remains nonreactive or equivocal (results cannot be positively interpreted), additional testing is warranted. In these instances the practitioner will frequently recommend vibroacoustic stimulation or a contraction stress test.

Vibroacoustic Stimulation

Vibroacoustic stimulation of the fetus is obtained with an artificial larynx placed a centimeter from or directly on the maternal abdomen. The sound stimulates the fetus to wake up, and in healthy fetuses a reactive NST will be obtained. Some practitioners use vibroacoustic stimulation for all NSTs because it decreases the length of time needed to obtain a reactive tracing and decreases the number of false-nonreactive tracings. Other practitioners use vibroacoustic stimulation as the second step after obtaining a nonreactive NST.

Contraction Stress Test

Uterine contractions cause a momentary reduction of uteroplacental blood flow. This situation stresses the fetus. A contraction stress test (CST) monitors the fetus' response to contractions to determine his well-being. The woman is placed on EFM as for the NST. There are three ways to obtain uterine contractions for a CST. If the woman is having spontaneous Braxton Hicks contractions, the fetal response to these contractions can be assessed. Another way is to induce uterine contractions through nipple stimulation. Nipple stimulation is thought to cause a release of oxytocin from the posterior pituitary gland. The oxytocin then stimulates the uterus to contract. The third way is to start an intravenous drip of Pitocin (synthetic oxytocin) to induce contractions.

No matter what way is used, the goal is to have three contractions of at least 40 seconds' duration within a 10-minute period of time. Then the fetal monitor strip is reviewed to determine the reaction of the fetus to the stress of the contractions. If there are no late decelerations (decelerations that occur after the contractions—refer to chapter 10 for detailed information on decelerations) after any of the contractions, the CST is said to be negative, which is a reassuring sign. A negative CST indicates that the fetus is not suffering from hypoxia and does not need immediate delivery. An equivocal CST occurs when there are late decelerations after some, but not all, of the uterine contractions. This result is suspicious of fetal hypoxia and may cause the physician to decide to perform a cesarean delivery of the fetus. A positive CST, late decelerations after every contraction, is indicative of fetal hypoxia and requires delivery of the fetus. An unsatisfactory CST occurs when there are insufficient contractions. The test must then be repeated within 24 hours, or a biophysical profile might be ordered.

Biophysical Profile

Biophysical profile (BPP) uses a combination of factors to determine fetal well-being. Five fetal biophysical variables are measured. Fetal heart rate acceleration is measured by performing the NST. Then breathing, body movements, tone, and amniotic fluid volume are measured using ultrasound. Each variable is given a score of 0 or 2 for a maximum score of 10. A score of 8 to 10 indicates fetal well-being. A score of 6 means possible fetal asphyxia, whereas a score of 4 indicates probable fetal asphyxia. Scores of 0 to 2 are ominous and require immediate delivery of the fetus.

Test Yourself

- How many times should the fetus move in a 2-hour period of time?
- What three tests are included in the triple-marker screening test?
- What tissue is extracted for study when chorionic villus sampling is used?

[3] Some authorities define a reactive NST based on the gestational age of the fetus. In these cases, a reactive test is defined as gestational age >34 weeks: ≥15 bpm for ≥15 secs, and gestational age <34 weeks: ≥10 bpm for ≥15 secs.

● The Nursing Process for Prenatal Care

The nurse is in a unique position to positively influence behaviors of the pregnant woman and to increase the chance she and her baby will stay healthy. Through consistent use of the nursing process, the nurse can detect problems early in order to intervene, or assist the primary care provider to intervene, and support the woman through her pregnancy. Of course teaching remains the primary nursing intervention throughout pregnancy.

ASSESSMENT

Ongoing assessment and data collection are essential components of prenatal visits. During the first prenatal visit, pay close attention to cues the woman may give regarding her feelings toward the pregnancy. Ambivalence is normal. The woman may express feelings of doubt about the pregnancy or her ability to be a good parent. These are normal reactions when a woman first finds out she is pregnant, and she needs reassurance that her responses are normal. Withdrawal or consistently negative remarks are warning signs that should be brought to the attention of the registered nurse (RN) or primary care provider.

If you are asked to administer the initial questionnaire, show the woman all the pages and assist her to complete it, if necessary. Review the document carefully when she is done to ensure completeness. Look for answers that indicate the need for further assessment. Alert the RN or the primary care provider when possible risk factors are identified in the history.

Assess for signs of nervousness and anxiety. She may express her nervousness by being restless or tense or by being quiet and withdrawn. Be attuned to signals she is giving regarding her comfort level. Inquire carefully regarding current medications, food supplements, and over-the-counter remedies she is using. This assessment should be done at every visit.

Note if the woman has been experiencing nausea and vomiting. Pay close attention to signs that might indicate poor nutritional status. Weight is an obvious clue. If the woman is overweight or underweight, she will need special assistance with nutritional concerns throughout the pregnancy. Other warning signs of poor nutritional status include dull, brittle hair; poor skin turgor; poor condition of skin and nails; obesity; emaciation; or a low hemoglobin level. Ask the woman to write down a typical day's food consumption pattern, and then compare her normal intake to the food guide pyramid to determine if her diet is adequate for her nutritional needs.

> **Don't make unfounded assumptions.** Teaching is important no matter how many babies the woman has delivered. Don't make the mistake of assuming that just because this is not the woman's first baby, or because she is educated, or even that she is a nurse, that she has the information she needs to maintain a healthy pregnancy. Assess her knowledge level by asking her questions and entertaining her questions.

Determine her education level and knowledge of pregnancy and prenatal care. If she is highly knowledgeable, she may ask high-level questions that indicate an understanding of basic issues. Conversely, she may ask basic questions, or no questions at all, which could indicate a knowledge deficit.

During subsequent visits, you may be asked to assess for signs of fetal well-being. These include obtaining fetal heart tones (FHTs) with an ultrasonic Doppler device (Fig. 7-6) beginning in week 10, and soliciting reports of active fetal movements after quickening. Pay close attention to vital signs, particularly the blood pressure. Monitor for danger signs of pregnancy (Box 7-5).

SELECTED NURSING DIAGNOSES

- Anxiety related to uncertainty regarding pregnancy diagnosis and not knowing what to expect during the office visit

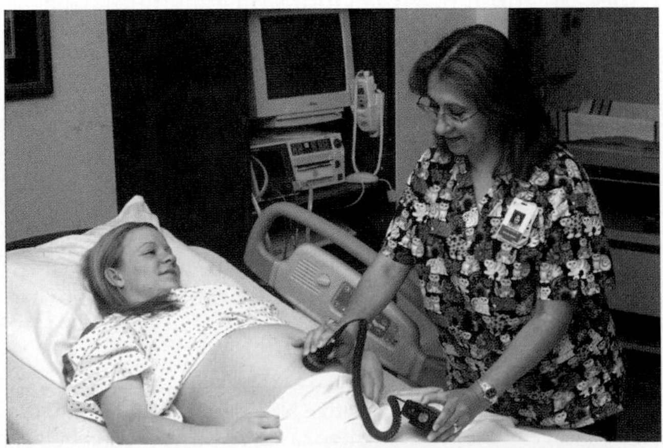

● ***Figure 7.6*** The nurse listens to fetal heart tones with a Doppler device.

BOX 7.5 Danger Signs of Pregnancy

Inquire regarding these warning signals at every visit. Instruct the woman to report any of these signs, if she should experience them, to her health care provider right away.

- Fever or severe vomiting
- Headache, unrelieved by Tylenol or other relief measures
- Blurred vision or spots before the eyes
- Pain in the epigastric region
- Sudden weight gain or sudden onset of edema in the hands and face
- Vaginal bleeding
- Painful urination
- Sudden gush or constant, uncontrollable leaking of fluid from the vagina
- Decreased fetal movement
- Signs of preterm labor
    - Uterine contractions (four or more per hour)
    - Lower, dull backache
    - Pelvic pressure
    - Menstrual-like cramps
    - Increase in vaginal discharge
    - A feeling that something is not right

- Health-seeking behaviors related to maintaining a healthy pregnancy and concerns regarding the common discomforts of pregnancy
- Deficient Knowledge of self-care during pregnancy
- Risk for Injury related to complications of pregnancy
- Fear related to the unknown of childbirth, concerns regarding safe passage of self and infant through the delivery experience, and concerns related to assuming the parenting role

OUTCOME IDENTIFICATION AND PLANNING

Maintaining the health of mother and fetus is the primary goal of nursing care during the prenatal period. Specific goals are that the woman's anxiety will be reduced, she will manage the symptoms and discomforts associated with pregnancy; that she will feel confident in her ability to care for herself throughout the pregnancy; that she nor the fetus will experience injury from complications of pregnancy; that she will have sufficient knowledge to adequately meet her needs and those of the growing fetus throughout the pregnancy; and that she will express confidence in her ability to go through the labor and birth experience and assume the parenting role.

IMPLEMENTATION

Relieving Anxiety

Escort the woman to the examination room and explain the normal procedure and what she can expect during the visit. Much anxiety can be alleviated when the woman knows what to expect. Maintain a calm, confident demeanor while giving care. Protect the woman's privacy during invasive examinations.

Try to understand the woman's perspective. Note if her anxiety level increases. Anticipate concern when fetal testing is planned. Solicit questions and correct misconceptions the woman may have. Provide factual information concerning the treatment plan. Use active listening. Encourage positive coping behaviors.

Relieving the Common Discomforts of Pregnancy

Pregnant women tend to experience similar discomforts because of the significant bodily changes they undergo. Some discomforts tend to occur in early pregnancy, some toward the end, and others continue throughout. Selected discomforts are listed in Table 7-2 along with hints for helping the woman cope with these discomforts.

Nasal Stuffiness and Epistaxis

A pregnant woman is prone to nasal stuffiness and epistaxis (nosebleeds). Estrogen is the hormone most likely culpable for this discomfort because it contributes to vasocongestion and increases the fragility of the nasal mucosa. Sometimes the woman may have symptoms of the common cold that persist throughout pregnancy. Nasal decongestants, other than normal saline nasal sprays, are generally not recommended. In any event, the woman should consult with her primary care provider before taking any medications, including over-the-counter remedies. Menthol applied just below the nostrils before bedtime might help relieve some discomfort from congestion.

Avoiding vigorous nose blowing may prevent nosebleeds. It is also helpful to keep the nasal passages moist. Using a humidifier in the house and staying well hydrated can accomplish this. If a nosebleed occurs despite precautions, instruct the woman to pinch the nostrils and hold pressure for at least 4 minutes until the bleeding stops. Ice may help stop the bleeding. If the bleeding is heavy or does not stop with pressure, instruct the woman to consult with her primary care provider.

Nausea

Morning sickness, or nausea, is a common complaint of early pregnancy. Rising levels of human chorionic gonadotropin (hCG) are thought to be a

TABLE 7.2 Common Discomforts of Pregnancy

Discomfort	Contributing Factor or Cause	Hints for Relieving the Discomfort
Bleeding gums	Stimulating effects of estrogen on the gums	• Visit the dentist • Use rinses and gargles to freshen the oral cavity • Use a soft-bristled toothbrush
Nasal stuffiness	Effects of estrogen on the nasal mucosa cause vasocongestion and stuffiness.	• Use a cool-air vaporizer • Try normal saline nasal sprays • Try to avoid commercial medicated nasal sprays because initial relief may be followed by rebound stuffiness
Nosebleeds	The tiny veins of the nasal lining are prone to breaking and causing nosebleeds. Dry nasal passages increase the risk.	• Avoid vigorous nose blowing • Use a humidifier • Drink plenty of fluids
Breast tenderness	Progesterone and estrogen are thought to contribute to the tingling or heavy sensations in the breasts that come and go throughout pregnancy.	• Wear a well-fitted support bra • Wearing a bra at night might be helpful if breast discomfort is interfering with restful sleep.
Nausea	Rising levels of hCG are thought to contribute to nausea.	• Begin the day with a high-carbohydrate food, such as melba toast, saltines, or other crackers. • Eat small high-carbohydrate meals frequently throughout the day. • Avoid noxious odors. • Take a walk outside in the fresh air. • Delay iron or vitamin supplementation until the second trimester.
Feeling faint	Postural hypotension can easily develop with the hemodynamic changes that occur in a normal pregnancy as the blood vessels in the periphery relax and dilate.	• Change positions slowly. • Avoid abrupt position changes. • Eat small, frequent, high-carbohydrate meals.
Fatigue	Cause is unknown. Progesterone may contribute.	• Plan for daily naps. • Take frequent rest breaks throughout the day. • Go to bed early.
Shortness of breath	In early pregnancy the effects of progesterone can create a sense of shortness of breath. In later pregnancy the uterus pushes on the diaphragm.	• Sit up straight to increase diameter of the chest. • If shortness of breath is interfering with sleep, prop up with pillows.
Heartburn	Relaxation of the LES under the influence of progesterone and increased intra-abdominal pressure due to the growing uterus cause acid reflux into the lower esophagus.	• Eat small, frequent meals • Avoid substances that increase acid production, in particular cigarette smoking. • Avoid substances that cause relaxation of the LES, such as coffee, chocolate, alcohol, and heavy spices. • Avoid lying down after a meal. • Avoid lying flat.
Stretch marks (striae gravidarum)	Stretch marks can occur on the breasts and abdomen. They are thought to be caused by increased levels of glucocorticoids. Stretch marks appear red during pregnancy, then gradually fade to a silvery white color.	• It may help to gain weight gradually over time, sudden bursts of weight may contribute to formation of stretch marks. • Regular exercise may also be helpful in preventing stretch marks.

TABLE 7.2 (continued) Common Discomforts of Pregnancy

Discomfort	Contributing Factor or Cause	Hints for Relieving the Discomfort
Low back pain	Changes in the center of gravity and loosened ligaments	• Avoid gaining too much weight. • Avoid high-heeled shoes. • Always bend at the knees, not the waist. • Avoid standing for too long at one time. • Keep one foot on a stool when standing. Frequently change the foot that is resting on the stool.
Round ligament pain	Sharp, severe pain, usually on the right side brought on by stretching of the round ligaments that support the uterus.	• Avoid sudden changes in positions or sudden movements. • Apply heat. • Lie on the side opposite the pain.
Leg cramps	Imbalanced calcium/phosphorus ratio; pressure of the uterus on the nerves; and circulatory changes in the lower extremities	• Avoid plantar flexion. • Eat foods high in calcium. • Try taking Tums (high in calcium). • Rest frequently with the feet elevated. • When cramps occur, extend the affected leg and dorsiflex the foot.
Varicose veins	Increased pelvic pressure, vasodilation in the lower extremities and vagina, along with pooling of blood in the lower extremities can contribute to varicosities of the legs and vagina.	• Exercise daily. • Rest with the legs elevated several times daily. • Wear compression stockings. Put them on before getting out of bed in the morning. • Avoid prolonged periods of standing or sitting. Move around frequently. Stretch and take small walks. • When you must stand for a time, frequently exercise the leg muscles and change positions frequently. • Keep within the recommended weight range during pregnancy.
Ankle edema	Progesterone effects, increased pressure in the lower extremities, increased capillary permeability	• Avoid prolonged periods of standing. • Rest frequently with the feet elevated. • Soak in a warm pool or bath. • Avoid constrictive garments on the lower extremities.
Flatulence	Relaxation of the gastrointestinal tract under the influence of progesterone, pressure of the uterus on the intestines, air swallowing	• Avoid gas-producing foods. • Chew foods thoroughly. • Get plenty of exercise. • Maintain regular bowel habits.
Constipation and hemorrhoids	Slowing of the gastrointestinal tract under the influence of progesterone and increased blood flow and pressure in the pelvic area	• Drink at least 8 glasses of non-caffeinated beverages per day. • Eat plenty of fiber. • Get adequate exercise. • Use a stool softener, if prescribed by the health care provider. • Use topical anesthetic agents to treat the pain of hemorrhoids.
Trouble sleeping	Many discomforts of pregnancy, as well as the increase in size of the abdomen, can all contribute to sleepless nights in the third trimester.	• Get adequate exercise. • Try different positions and use pillows to support and wedge. • Try sleeping in a sitting position. • Drink a glass of warm milk before retiring. • Have a late-night, high-carbohydrate snack • Try progressive muscle relaxation or guided imagery.

cause. Although "morning sickness" is the lay term for the nausea of pregnancy, many women experience nausea at other times during the day, or even throughout the day.

Fortunately, caloric intake during the first trimester is not as crucial as it is in the second and third trimesters, so the nausea is usually not harmful to the pregnancy. Some helpful suggestions include advising the woman to place a high-carbohydrate snack, such as melba toast or saltine crackers, at the bedside before retiring. In the morning before getting out of bed, she should eat the snack. This can help prevent early morning nausea. Other helpful hints are to encourage the woman to eat small amounts frequently throughout the day, instead of consuming three, heavy meals hours apart, and to never let the stomach become completely empty. It also helps for her to avoid strong odors. Sometimes it is easier for the woman to eat when someone else prepares the meal. Persistent vomiting may be a sign of hyperemesis gravidarum, a complication of pregnancy that can lead to dehydration and electrolyte imbalances. If the vomiting is severe or prolonged, the primary care provider should be consulted. Fortunately, nausea generally subsides by the end of the first trimester.

Feeling Faint

Sometimes women feel faint during the first few weeks of pregnancy. This could be caused by postural hypotension and is aggravated by low blood sugar levels. Advise the woman to change positions slowly and to avoid abrupt position changes. Eating frequent high-carbohydrate meals helps to keep blood sugar levels up. If she feels faint, a walk outside might help. Or she might need to lie down with her feet elevated or sit with her head lower than her knees until the feeling passes.

Frequent Urination

Frequent urination can be bothersome and interfere with sleep. It is thought that frequent urination in the first trimester is caused by the increasing blood volume and increased glomerular filtration rate. Frequency usually diminishes during the second trimester, only to reappear in the third trimester because of pressure of the enlarging uterus on the bladder.

Increased Vaginal Discharge

Leukorrhea, or increased vaginal discharge, is common during pregnancy. Increased production of cervical glands and vasocongestion of the pelvic area contribute to the discharge. If the discharge causes itching or irritation, or if there is a foul smell noted, the health care provider should be contacted because these are signs of infection. Douching should be avoided. Sanitary pads can be worn to absorb the discharge.

Shortness of Breath

Shortness of breath may occur during the first trimester because of the effects of progesterone. The woman may feel an increased sense of the need to breath. This sensation can be uncomfortable and is often perceived as shortness of breath. During the latter half of pregnancy as the uterus pushes upward on the diaphragm, shortness of breath can occur.

Advise the woman to take her time and rest frequently. If shortness of breath occurs during exercise, she may need to decrease the level of intensity. During late pregnancy, shortness of breath may interfere with sleep. Propping up with pillows can help expand the chest and decrease the sensation of being unable to catch her breath. Shortness of breath accompanied by chest pain or coughing up blood or a smothering sensation with fever are danger signs that indicate the need for medical intervention. The former is a sign of pulmonary embolism; the latter is a sign of severe respiratory infection, such as pneumonia.

Heartburn

Heartburn, or pyrosis, is a common complaint during pregnancy. Several factors contribute to this discomfort. Progesterone causes a generalized slowing of the gastrointestinal tract and can cause relaxation of the lower esophageal sphincter (LES). When the LES is relaxed, acid content from the stomach can back up into the lower part of the esophagus and cause a burning sensation, known as heartburn. The increased pressure in the abdomen from the enlarging uterus contributes to the problem.

Prevention is generally the best way to treat heartburn. Several factors aggravate the condition. Smoking increases the acid content of the stomach and should be avoided. Certain foods and beverages, such as coffee, chocolate, peppermint, fatty or fried foods, alcohol, and heavy spices, can contribute to LES relaxation and exacerbate heartburn.

The woman should be advised to eat smaller meals more frequently and to avoid drinking fluids with meals. Filling the stomach with a heavy meal or with food and fluid increases the pressure and contributes to gastric reflux. It is best if the woman avoids lying down after meals. If she must lie down, suggest that she lie on her left side with her head higher than her abdomen. Placing 6-inch blocks under the head of the bed, or propping pillows at night to keep the chest higher than the abdomen can also help prevent heartburn. The physician may prescribe an antacid. If so, vitamins should not be taken within 1 hour of taking antacids. Sodium bicarbonate should not be used as an antacid during pregnancy.

Backaches

About one half of all pregnant women experience low back pain at some point during pregnancy. Obesity and previous history of back pain are risk factors. Softening and loosening of the ligaments supporting the joints of the spine and pelvis can contribute to low back pain, as can the increasing lordosis of pregnancy and the changing center of gravity.

Low back pain is best prevented by advising the woman to use good body mechanics, such as bending the knees to reach something on the floor, rather than stooping over from the waist. She should also avoid high-heeled shoes. Good pelvic support with a girdle might be helpful for some women. Severe back pain is usually associated with some type of pathology and should be investigated.

Round Ligament Pain

The round ligaments support the uterus in the abdomen. As the uterus expands during pregnancy, pressure is applied to the round ligaments and they stretch and thin. Some women experience round ligament pain as a result of this stretching. The pain most frequently occurs on the right side and can be severe. The pain can occur at night and awaken the woman from sleep, or exercise can bring it on.

Helpful hints to treat round ligament pain include the application of heat. A heating pad or warm bath might be soothing. Sometimes lying on the opposite side can relieve some of the pressure on the ligament and reduce the pain. Avoiding sudden movements may help prevent round ligament pain. If fever, chills, painful urination, or vaginal bleeding accompanies the pain, the woman should seek emergency care because the pain is likely caused by a medical condition.

Leg Cramps

Leg cramps are a common occurrence during pregnancy. An imbalanced calcium/phosphorous ratio, pressure of the uterus on nerves, and circulatory changes in the lower extremities can all contribute to leg cramps. Preventive measures include getting enough rest, resting several times per day with the feet elevated, walking, wearing low-heeled shoes, and avoiding constrictive clothing. Another preventive measure is for the woman to avoid plantar flexion (pointing the toes forward). Making certain that the diet includes enough calcium is also important to prevent leg cramps. When cramps occur, the woman's partner can help by assisting her to extend her leg, then dorsiflex the foot so that the toes point toward the woman's head. If she is alone, she can extend her leg and dorsiflex the foot until the cramp resolves.

Constipation and Hemorrhoids

The natural slowing of the gastrointestinal tract under the influence of hormones can lead to constipation during pregnancy, and constipation can lead to hemorrhoids. The best way to treat constipation is to prevent it. The same common sense approaches to preventing constipation that are advisable under normal situations are also helpful during pregnancy. These include drinking at least 8 glasses of noncaffeinated beverages each day. Advise the woman to get adequate exercise. Adding fiber to the diet or a bulk-forming supplement such as Metamucil to the daily routine are also helpful hints.

Hemorrhoids can become a problem during pregnancy because of the increased blood flow in the rectal veins and pressure of the uterus that prevents good venous return. Elevating the legs and hips intermittently throughout the day can help counteract this problem. Constipation aggravates the condition. Pain and swelling can be relieved by applying topical anesthetics, such as Preparation H or Anusol cream, and compresses such as witch hazel pads.

Trouble Sleeping

Many of the discomforts discussed previously, such as heartburn and shortness of breath, can contribute to restlessness at night and trouble sleeping. As the pregnancy progresses, it becomes increasingly difficult to find a position of comfort in bed. Suggest that the woman try lying on her side with plenty of pillows to support her back and legs. If that position doesn't help, she may find it easier to sleep in an armchair. Sleep may be easier in the sitting position. Urinary frequency returns during the third trimester and can contribute to sleeplessness because of frequent trips to the restroom. Drinking the majority of fluids early in the day and limiting fluids in the evening hours can reduce this problem. Heartburn can contribute to reduction in sleep, as can the movements of an active fetus. Some degree of sleeplessness and restlessness at night is to be expected in the third trimester.

Teaching Self-Care During Pregnancy

The woman is usually too distracted during the first visit to absorb and retain much information that is given to her. Keep teaching sessions brief and give her printed materials to read at home. The primary care provider should have a list of resources, such as books and websites, that could be put in a handout format to give to the woman. Teaching topics should be tailored to the individual needs of the woman during subsequent visits. Important self-care topics are discussed below. Family Teaching Tips: Major Topics to Cover During Prenatal Care highlights key topics that should be covered with the pregnant woman during the course of prenatal care.

Maintaining a Balanced Nutritional Intake

During the first trimester the fetus' demands on maternal stores are less than at other times during the pregnancy. This is helpful because sometimes it is difficult for the woman to eat a well-balanced diet when she is coping with nausea. Focus on assessing the adequacy of her diet and answering her questions during the first visit. Emphasize the importance of taking the prenatal vitamins the primary care provider ordered for her. On subsequent visits, assist the woman to assess her own diet for adequacy by using the food guide pyramid (Fig. 7-7). Teach principles of adequate nutritional intake during pregnancy.

The key to healthy nutrition during pregnancy is quality and variety. Some pregnant women may be overwhelmed by detailed nutritional guidelines. In general it is safe to counsel the pregnant woman about the following general strategies. Make certain there is enough food to eat and then advise the woman to eat the amount and type of food that she wants, salting it to taste. The Food Guide Pyramid can assist the pregnant woman achieve a balanced diet. Monitor weight gain throughout pregnancy. There should be a steady increase in weight throughout pregnancy, for a total increase of 25 to 35 pounds. Sudden weight gain often is associated with fluid retention and may be a sign of developing preeclampsia. Periodically assess the diet by asking the woman to do a 1- to 3-day food recall. Encourage the woman to take her iron and folic acid supplement. Monitor the hemoglobin and hematocrit at the 28-week checkup for any decreases.

FAMILY TEACHING TIPS

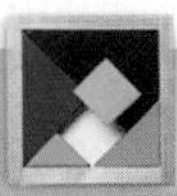

Major Topics to Cover During Prenatal Care

The pregnant woman should be taught to:

- Avoid alcohol. Alcohol harms the fetus; no amount of alcohol is safe during pregnancy.
- Avoid smoking. Smoking harms the fetus. It can lead to lower birth weight and increase the incidence of preterm labor.
- Eat a healthy, well-balanced diet. If you consume a variety of nutritious foods daily, you will likely get the nutrients you need.
- Consume approximately 300 calories more per day than before pregnancy.
- Take an extra 400 micrograms of folic acid per day. If the doctor ordered prenatal vitamins, the recommended dose will be met.
- Avoid dieting during pregnancy. Every pregnant woman with a normal body mass index should gain 25 to 30 pounds during the pregnancy.
- Continue to exercise during pregnancy. However, do not exercise to the point of exhaustion or start a grueling new workout that you were not doing before pregnancy.
- Avoid handling raw meat and cat litter. Wear gloves when gardening to prevent contracting toxoplasmosis from animal droppings, an infection that is very harmful to the baby.
- Handle cold cuts carefully. Heat thin slices of meat in the microwave until steaming hot. Wash hands with hot soapy water after handling deli meats to avoid listeriosis, a bacterial infection that is harmful to the baby.
- Avoid douching. Douching during pregnancy can cause a fatal air embolism.
- Avoid taking any medication (other than Tylenol) or over-the-counter herbal remedy unless your primary care provider has approved it.

Dental Hygiene

A pregnant woman needs to continue regular dental checkups and practice excellent dental hygiene. This includes at least twice daily brushing, once daily flossing, and a nutritious diet. If pregnancy gingivitis is a problem, then regular dental checkups are a must. Untreated gingivitis can damage the gums and result in bone and tooth loss.

Vomiting in association with morning sickness can be hard on teeth. Stomach acids in the vomitus can make the teeth more susceptible to injury from the toothbrush. To reduce the impact of this problem, instruct the woman to rinse with water after vomiting, followed by a fluoride rinse or sugarless chewing gum to help neutralize the stomach acid. She should avoid brushing her teeth for at least 1 hour after vomiting to decrease the risk of enamel loss.

Exercise

Exercise is healthy during pregnancy. A woman may generally maintain her normal exercise routine during pregnancy, as long as she does not become overheated or excessively fatigued. Conditioned women have safely run marathons during pregnancy. In fact, women who exercise during pregnancy experience shorter labors, have fewer cesarean deliveries, and have fetuses that experience fewer episodes of fetal distress.

The American College of Obstetricians and Gynecologists recommends that a well-conditioned

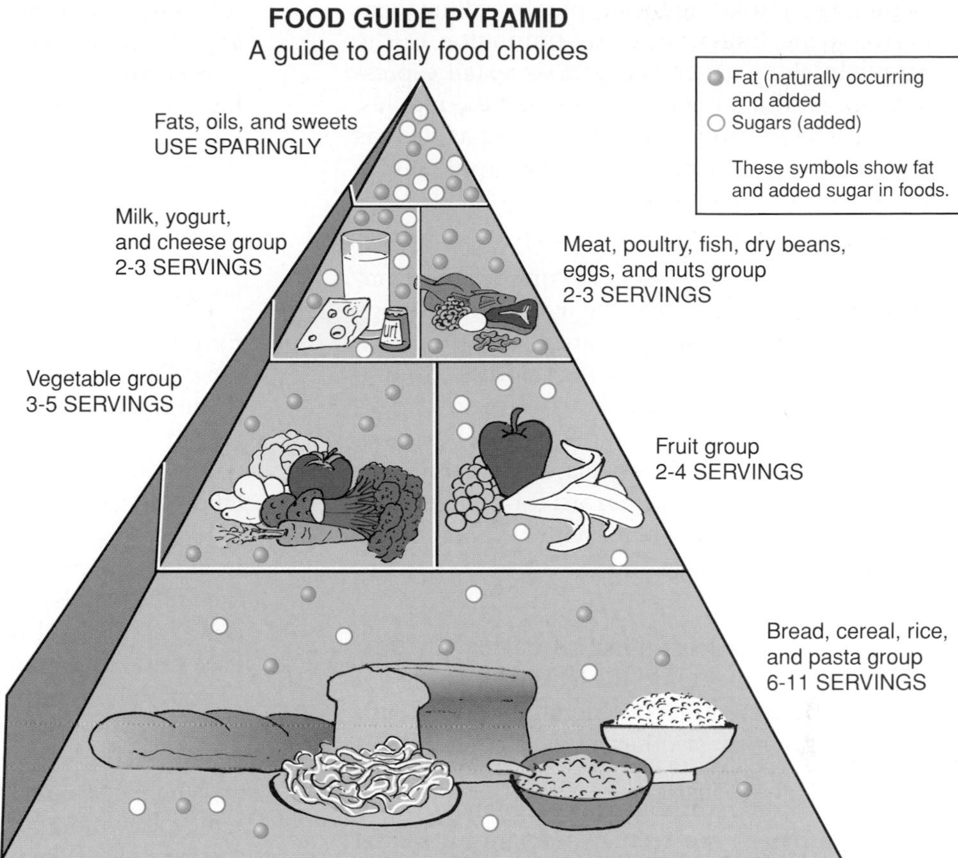

● ***Figure 7.7*** The food guide pyramid.

woman continue her pattern of aerobic exercise during pregnancy. If the woman is sedentary before pregnancy, she should not start a vigorous aerobic routine. In this situation, walking is the preferred exercise. There are some high-risk conditions, such as premature rupture of membranes, pregnancy-induced hypertension, vaginal bleeding, or incompetent cervix, in which exercise is contraindicated.

General common sense guidelines include advising the woman to listen to her body. If she is feeling fatigued, she should slow down or stop. She should not allow her heart rate to exceed 140 beats per minute. In the last trimester as the center of gravity changes, extra care should be taken to avoid injury during exercise.

Hygiene

Perspiration and vaginal discharge increase during pregnancy, making personal hygiene a concern for some pregnant women. In general, tub baths or showers can continue throughout pregnancy with an eye toward safety. The following general considerations should be given to hygiene during pregnancy.

- Bathe in warm, not hot, water. Extreme temperature elevations associated with hot showers, baths, saunas, hot tubs, and fever are dangerous to the developing fetus and should be avoided.
- Take care, particularly in the third trimester, when getting in and out of the tub or shower. Fainting can occur. This situation is enhanced if the water is too hot. Because the center of gravity changes, balancing can become problematic. Handrails in the shower or tub are ideal. Rubber bath mats are also helpful.
- Avoid douching during pregnancy. This practice is dangerous and can result in an air embolism due to the increased vascularity of the genital area. Gentle cleansing of the genital area with warm water and soap are sufficient to control discomfort from increased vaginal secretions.

Breast Care

A pregnant woman is well advised to wear a bra that fits well and supports the breasts. She should be taught to use only clean water to wash the nipples. Soap dries the nipples and can lead to cracking.

Some women wish to condition their nipples for breast-feeding. Exposing the nipples to air and sunlight for a portion of each day is helpful.

Manually stimulating the nipples by rolling them between the fingers or oral stimulation of the nipple by the partner as a part of sexual expression are additional ways to toughen the nipples. These practices are acceptable as long as there is no history of preterm labor because nipple stimulation can stimulate labor.

Clothing

Clothing should be loose and comfortable. Constricting garments around the waist or on the legs should not be worn. If finances are tight, the woman might try borrowing clothes from a friend or relative, rather than investing in expensive maternity clothes. She might also buy used maternity clothes. High heels exacerbate backache and can be a safety hazard for the pregnant woman who has problems with balance. Shoes should fit comfortably.

Sexual Activity

Many couples are fearful that sexual activity during pregnancy might hurt the fetus. Unless there is a history of preterm labor, vaginal bleeding, ruptured membranes, or other medical contraindication, intercourse and other sexual activities can be safely continued throughout pregnancy. Many factors influence the woman's desire for sexual activity. During the first trimester she may feel nauseous and tired, so her interest in sex might be low. During the second trimester, she often feels better and may have a heightened interest in sex. The increased blood flow to the pelvic area can intensify the sexual experience for the pregnant woman. Some women experience orgasm for the first time during pregnancy. During the third trimester, fatigue may reduce her desire. Or she might fear hurting the fetus.

A word of caution: If the couple practices anal intercourse, it is important to warn them not to proceed to vaginal intercourse after engaging in anal intercourse. The danger is that the bacteria *Escherichia coli* will be introduced into the vagina and cause an ascending infection.

The partner's sexual desire is also dependent on several interrelated factors. Some men find the pregnant body sexually appealing and desirable. Others may have trouble adjusting to their partner's changing body shape. Some men are afraid of hurting their partner or the unborn child during intercourse. It may be helpful to have a tactful discussion regarding sexual concerns with the woman and the partner. During the third trimester the male superior position may become difficult to accomplish. A side-lying or woman superior position might be easier.

Sometimes the woman might be content with kissing, cuddling, and caressing as forms of sexual expression. If her partner needs more release, the woman might stimulate him to ejaculation, or he may prefer to masturbate. The essential ingredient is ongoing respectful communication between the partners regarding their sexual needs and desires.

Employment

How long a woman can remain safely employed during pregnancy is dependent on several factors. In general, a woman with a low-risk pregnancy can continue working until she goes into labor, unless there are specific hazards associated with her job. Research demonstrates that women in physically demanding jobs, such as working in the fields (day laborers), experience a higher incidence of low birth-weight infants, preterm delivery, and hypertension during pregnancy. A woman who is required to stand for long periods as part of her job also is at increased risk for preterm delivery.

When a woman chooses to work during pregnancy, it is most helpful if she can take frequent rest periods. If she must stand for prolonged periods, suggest that she shift her weight back and forth, and that she take frequent breaks to walk around and to sit with her feet elevated. Of course she should avoid excessive fatigue.

Exposure to **teratogens**, substances capable of causing birth defects, is always a concern when a woman works during pregnancy. The woman should investigate the type of chemicals or other substances she is exposed to during the course of her work and then work with her employer to limit exposure to harmful substances.

Travel

Travel is generally not limited during the first trimester and can be carried out safely in the second and third trimesters with careful planning. One concern when traveling long distances is the chance that labor will occur while the woman is away from her health care provider. It is advisable for the woman to carry copies of her prenatal records with her when she travels. In this way, appropriate care can be rendered if she must seek health care away from home.

When travel by car is permitted, the woman should be encouraged to make frequent stops (at least every 2 hours) so that she can empty her bladder and walk about. Sitting for prolonged periods in one position can predispose the woman to clot formation. Decreasing fluid intake to avoid having to stop to void is not recommended. Insufficient fluids can lead to dehydration and increase the risk for clot formation, constipation, and hemorrhoids. There is no increased risk with air travel, other than the risk of developing complications in an area remote from the help needed.

The greatest risk to the fetus during an automobile crash is death of the mother. Therefore, it is recommended that all pregnant women use three-point seat belt restraints when traveling in the car. The lap belt should be under her abdomen and over her thighs. The shoulder harness should fit between her breasts. Safety belts should be snugly and comfortably applied. The use of airbags is controversial. Some authorities suggest that airbags are safe to use during pregnancy. Others have encountered stillbirths after airbag deployment in a car crash (Cunningham et al., 2001).

Test Yourself

- List three suggestions for reducing nausea in early pregnancy.
- Name three actions the pregnant woman can take to reduce heartburn.
- Why should the pregnant woman avoid hot showers or baths?

Medication Use

The general principle regarding medication use during pregnancy is that almost all medications cross the placenta and can potentially affect the fetus. No medication, including over-the-counter medications and herbal remedies, should be used during pregnancy without the express approval of the primary care provider. Before any medication is taken, a careful appraisal of risk versus benefit should be made. There are some diseases and conditions for which the pregnant woman must continue to receive treatment, such as epilepsy, asthma, diabetes, and depression.

The problem with most medications is that they are known to cross the placenta, but it is not always known what affect the medication has on the fetus or pregnancy. Because of ethical concerns, controlled trials of medication use during human pregnancy are usually not possible. The little that is known about medication effects during pregnancy comes from animal trials and from experience over the years in treating chronic maternal conditions. The problem with animal studies is that there is no guarantee that human pregnancies or fetuses will respond in the same way as the animal that is being studied responds. Box 7-6 describes the Food and Drug Administration's five pregnancy categories for medications.

Substance Use and Abuse

Substance use is a term that simply refers to use of a substance, whereas the term *substance abuse* specifically identifies that a problem is identified with the use of the substance. Although many substances have the potential for abuse, this

BOX 7.6 FDA Pregnancy Categories of Medications

The Food and Drug Administration (FDA) has delineated five categories for medication use during pregnancy. Each category details the overall threat, if any, the drug in that category might pose to the fetus or pregnancy. The categories are differentiated according to the type and reliability of documentation available and the risk-versus-benefit ratio. The categories are as follows:

Category A: Adequate studies in pregnant women have not demonstrated a risk to the fetus in the first trimester of pregnancy, and there is no evidence of risk in later trimesters.

Category B: Animal studies have not demonstrated a risk to the fetus, but there are no adequate studies in pregnant women. Or animal studies have shown an adverse effect, but adequate studies in pregnant women have not demonstrated a risk to the fetus during the first trimester of pregnancy, and there is no evidence of risk in later trimesters.

Category C: Animal studies have shown an adverse effect on the fetus, but there are no adequate studies in humans; the benefits from the use of the drug in pregnant women may be acceptable despite its potential risks. Or there are no animal reproduction studies and no adequate studies in humans.

Category D: There is evidence of human fetal risk, but the potential benefits from the use of the drug in pregnant women may be acceptable despite its potential risk.

Category X: Studies in animals or humans demonstrate fetal abnormalities or adverse reaction; reports indicate evidence of fetal risk. The risk of use in a pregnant woman clearly outweighs any possible benefit.

In any case, no drug should be given during pregnancy unless there is a clear benefit for its use.

section covers caffeine, tobacco, alcohol, and recreational drug use. More extensive coverage regarding potential fetal effects is given to this topic in Chapter 20.

Caffeine. There is controversy and uncertainty regarding the role of caffeine use during pregnancy. Current recommendations are that coffee and caffeine in moderation may be safely used during pregnancy without risk of adverse effects. Caffeine in large doses, such as that found in 5 cups of coffee or more per day, increases the risk of spontaneous abortion.

Tobacco. Smoking is contraindicated during pregnancy. Smoking increases the risk for low birth weight, preterm delivery, abortions, stillbirths, sudden infant death syndrome (SIDS), birth defects, and neonatal respiratory disorders, including asthma. Smoking poisons the fetus with carbon monoxide and nicotine, leading to fetal hypoxia. It also affects the placenta, causing it to age sooner than normal, a condition that reduces blood flow to the fetus, contributing to hypoxia and stunted growth.

In 1998, 12% of American women smoked during pregnancy. These 12% delivered 20% of the low birth-weight neonates born that year (Cunningham et al., 2001). It is clear that reducing the number of women who smoke during pregnancy will decrease the number of low birth-weight infants. As mentioned, low birth-weight infants are at much higher risk for neonatal morbidity and mortality. Although nicotine gum is classified as a pregnancy Category C (see Box 7-6) drug and the transdermal patch is in pregnancy Category D, the risk of harm caused by smoking may outweigh the risk of harm from these aids to stop smoking.

Alcohol. There is no safe amount of alcohol consumption during pregnancy. A pregnant woman is strongly advised not to drink any alcoholic beverages during pregnancy or when she thinks she might be pregnant because alcohol is a known teratogen. For years, the risk of fetal alcohol syndrome (FAS) has been linked to the use of large amounts of alcohol during pregnancy. This syndrome is characterized by **microcephaly**, a very small cranium, facial deformities, growth restriction, and mental retardation. Although smaller amounts of alcohol may not lead to a full-blown case of FAS, subtle features of the syndrome might present to include milder forms of mental retardation.

Marijuana. There is conflicting data about the effects of marijuana on pregnancy. However, infants born to women who smoke marijuana during pregnancy show evidence of stressed nervous systems. These infants tend to have high-pitched cries, tremulousness, and reduced response to visual stimuli. As they grow, these children tend to have lower IQs, impaired cognitive function, and deficits in language, behavior, and performance of visual-perceptual tasks. One study shows an increased risk of SIDS when the father uses marijuana during and after the pregnancy.

Cocaine. Cocaine has many negative effects on pregnancy. Cocaine use is associated with a higher rate of spontaneous abortion and premature labor. Infants born to women who use cocaine during pregnancy tend to be small and have a higher incidence of low birth weight. Cocaine use during pregnancy can cause the placenta to pull away from the uterine wall prematurely (placental abruption), leading to fetal and maternal hemorrhage. These infants exhibit withdrawal behaviors after birth and must receive special treatment for the withdrawal (refer to Chapter 20).

Maintaining Safety of the Woman and Fetus

Monitor the woman at every visit for warning signs of pregnancy (see Box 7-5). If she reports experiencing any of the warning signs, notify the RN or primary care provider immediately. If at any time during the pregnancy an elevated blood pressure is noted, report this finding immediately to the RN or primary care provider, particularly if it is accompanied by a headache, epigastric pain, or blurred vision.

Preparing the Woman for Labor, Birth, and Parenthood

The woman who is well prepared for labor, birth, and parenting is likely to feel confident and use positive coping measures. There are many ways to prepare for the birth and parenting experience. Many women search the Internet for information and to find resources. There are many books available that address these issues. The primary care provider should provide lists of resources available in the local community.

Packing for the Hospital or Birthing Center

As the woman prepares for the birth of her baby, she will begin to gather items she will need at the hospital or birthing center. She should pack one bag of items she will need for labor and another bag of things for her postpartum stay and the trip home from the hospital (Box 7-7).

Communicating Expectations About Labor and Birth

It is important for the woman to feel comfortable communicating her desires regarding labor and birth. Some women feel very strongly about

BOX 7.7 What to Pack for the Hospital or Birthing Center

Labor Items

- Lotion for massage or effleurage
- Sour lollipops (counteracts nausea, moistens mouth, gives energy)
- Mouth spray or toothbrush and toothpaste
- Chapstick or lip balm
- Socks
- Tennis ball, ice pack, back massager (for pressure for back labor)
- Picture or object for focal point
- Camera with good batteries and plenty of film (check with hospital regarding policies on cameras during delivery)
- CD player and CDs for relaxation music
- Contact lens case and solutions
- Hair brush and hair ribbon or band to get hair off neck
- Hand fan
- Favorite pillows

Postpartum Items

- Nursing gowns
- Robe and slippers
- Nursing bras
- Toilet articles (toothpaste and toothbrush, deodorant, tissues)
- Cosmetics
- Pen and paper
- Baby book
- Personal address book with telephone numbers
- Loose fitting clothes for the trip home
- Socks for baby
- Clothes for baby to wear home
- Baby blankets appropriate for weather

Be careful. It isn't helpful to make promises that you can't keep. If a woman or her partner is communicating unrealistic expectations about the birth process, be honest and tell her that it is unlikely her expectation will be met. The woman will appreciate if you are up-front with her. This will give her the opportunity to decide if her expectation is negotiable or if she needs to go elsewhere to get her needs met.

having natural childbirth or breast-feeding. Others want an epidural as soon as possible after they go into labor. These are only three examples of expectations a woman may have. Encourage the woman to write down her questions and expectations and to communicate these to her primary care provider. Some women develop written birth plans (Box 7-8) to communicate their desires. These can be helpful to the woman and the primary care provider. If the expectations are communicated early, there is time for the woman to find another provider if her current provider cannot or will not meet her expectations.

Choosing the Support Person

The expectant mother may have choices involving her labor support team if she delivers in the hospital or birthing center. Some hospitals limit her to one or two persons for labor support. Other women may have the option of having more support persons for labor. The woman may have the father of the baby as her main support person. In other situations, the primary support person might be her mother, sister, other family member, or friend.

The mother also may choose to have a **doula** with her as a support person. The word "doula" is Greek for servant. DONA, an acronym for Doulas of North America (founded in 1992), is an international association of doulas who are trained "to provide the highest quality emotional, physical and educational support to women and their families during childbirth and postpartum." A doula may be contracted to provide support for labor and birth and help with establishing breast-feeding. Other doulas are contracted to provide support for the postpartum period. Many doulas provide both prenatal and postnatal support. The doula's role may include assisting the woman and her partner in preparing for and carrying out their plans for the birth, providing emotional support, physical comfort measures, and an objective viewpoint, as well as helping the woman get the information she needs to make good decisions. A woman may choose to hire a doula because she wants to decrease the likelihood of needing pharmacologic pain management, Pitocin, forceps, vacuum extraction, or cesarean birth and because she wants an advocate at a time when she feels unable to vocalize her needs adequately.

Childbirth Education Classes

Since the 1970s, many parents have begun to prepare for labor and childbirth by attending classes (Fig. 7-8). Today, classes are offered by childbirth educators in private practice, not-for-profit organizations, and hospitals. Some classes adhere to the philosophy of one method of unmedicated childbirth (Box 7-9). Others combine philosophies of two or more methods of childbirth. Still others tend to teach the woman little about birthing a baby without medical pain management and focus on what medical procedures and routines she can expect

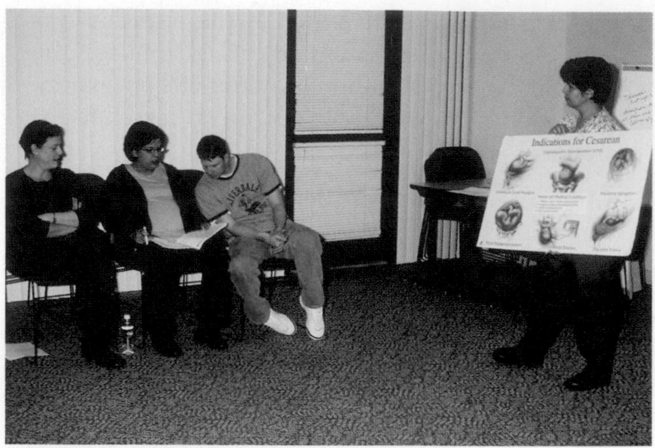

● ***Figure 7.8*** The nurse is teaching couples in a childbirth class.

when she is admitted to the hospital. Some programs combine information about birth, baby care, and breast-feeding in one series of classes. Others offer separate classes for which the woman and her partner can register. Box 7-10 lists common topics included in childbirth education classes.

Other Birth and Parenthood Preparation Classes

In addition to labor and birth preparation, other educational offerings include pregnancy and postpartum exercise classes, baby care classes, breast-feeding classes, and sibling preparation classes. In some communities, childbirth educators in private practice or not-for-profit childbirth education organizations provide classes to clients who seek and pay for these classes. In other communities, hospital-based family education programs dominate the parenting education arena.

Pregnancy and Postpartum Exercise Classes. The purpose of these classes is to enhance endurance, as well as strengthen arms, legs, pelvic floor, back, and abdomen. A certified childbirth educator or a nurse usually offers these classes. Some fitness centers also offer pre- and postnatal exercise classes. Basic pregnancy exercises, such as the pelvic tilt, Kegel, tailor sit and tailor stretch, and stretches as comfort measures for the discomforts of pregnancy, should be included, as well as exercises that allow the woman to be able to utilize beneficial labor positions comfortably. Postnatal exercise classes strengthen muscles affected by the pregnancy. Sometimes, they incorporate the baby as part of the exercise.

Baby Care Classes. These classes are usually offered to the pregnant woman and her partner. Basics such as infant bathing, diapering, and feeding are featured. Parents-to-be are also presented with information on newborn sleeping and waking patterns and infant comforting and rousing techniques. Safety information including proper handling of the baby, car seat safety, and safety proofing the home is included. Signs of illness and guidelines for when to call the pediatrician are an important part of this class. Items needed for the layette are usually discussed or a list of the items needed is provided in handouts (Box 7-11).

Breast-feeding Classes. This class is usually taught by an International Board Certified lactation consultant but also may be conducted by certified breast-feeding educators or specially trained nurses. Usually offered in the last trimester of pregnancy, this class is designed to educate the woman and her partner on the benefits of breast-feeding, signs of good latch and position, and establishing a good milk supply. Selection of and using a breast pump and milk storage are topics of interest in this class as many women plan to return to work and continue to nurse their infants. Attendance of this class by the woman's partner increases his support and ability to provide assistance, thus contributing to the success of breast-feeding. Usually, telephone numbers for community resources for lactation support are offered.

Siblings Classes. Many hospitals provide sibling classes for children who are soon to be big brothers and big sisters. Siblings' class goals include preparing children for the time of separation from mother while she is in the hospital and helping the children accept the changes resulting from the arrival of the new baby in the family. Basic infant care is demonstrated, with emphasis on how the child can be included or help with the tasks related to baby care. Tours of the maternal–child areas of the hospital are usually included. Suggestions are shared with parents on ways to help the older siblings accept changes in the household after the baby arrives.

In hospitals where siblings are allowed to attend births, siblings classes may include information on how to help prepare the older child for being present at delivery. Most hospitals require an adult to be responsible for children at birth, in addition to the partner who is caring for the laboring woman.

EVALUATION: GOALS AND EXPECTED OUTCOMES

- **Goal:** The woman's anxiety is reduced.
  Expected Outcomes: The woman will verbalize a reduction in anxiety and will name at least two outlets for dealing with her anxiety.

(text continues on page 161)

BOX 7.8 Sample Birth Plan

Birth plan for Rachel Thompson
Due date: March 23, 2005
Patient of Dr. Maria Martinez
Scheduled to deliver at Metropolitan Medical Center

January 10, 2005

Dear Dr. Martinez and Staff at Metropolitan Medical Center,

I have chosen you because of your reputations for working with parents who feel strongly about wanting as natural a birth as possible. I understand that sometimes birth becomes a medical situation. The following is what I would prefer as long as medical interventions are not indicated. I would appreciate you working with me to have our baby in the way described in our birth plan, if possible.

Sincerely,

Rachel Thompson

Laboring

I would prefer to avoid an enema and/or shaving of pubic hair.
I would like to be free to walk around during labor.
I prefer to be able to move around and change position at will throughout labor.
I would like to be able to have fluids by mouth throughout the first stage of labor.
I will be bringing my own music to play during labor.
I do not want an IV unless I become dehydrated.
I need to wear contact lenses or glasses at all times when conscious.

Fetal Monitors

I do not want to have continuous fetal monitoring unless it is required by the condition of my baby.

Stimulation of Labor

If labor is not progressing, I would like to have the bag of water ruptured before other methods are used to augment labor.
I would prefer to be allowed to try changing position and other natural methods before oxytocin is administered.

Medication/Anesthesia

I do not want to use drugs if possible. Please do not offer them. I will ask if I want some.

C-section

If a cesarean delivery is indicated, I would like to be fully informed and to participate in the decision-making process.
I would like my husband present at all times if my baby requires a cesarean delivery.
I wish to have regional anesthesia unless the baby must be delivered immediately.

Episiotomy

I am hoping to protect my perineum. I am practicing ahead of time by squatting, doing Kegel exercises, and perineal massage.
If possible, I would like to use perineal massage to help avoid the need for an episiotomy.

Pushing

I would like to be allowed to choose the position in which I give birth, including squatting.
Even if I am fully dilated, and assuming my baby is not in distress, I would like to try to wait until I feel the urge to push before beginning the pushing phase.

Immediately After Delivery

I would like to have my baby placed on my chest.
I would like to have my husband cut the cord.
I would like to hold my baby while I deliver the placenta and any tissue repairs are made.
I plan to keep my baby with me following birth and would appreciate if the evaluation of my baby can be done with my baby on my abdomen unless there is an unusual situation.
I would prefer to hold my baby skin to skin to keep her warm.
I want to delay the eye medication for my baby until a couple hours after birth.
I have made arrangements to donate the umbilical cord blood if possible.

Postpartum

I would like a private room so my husband can stay with me.
Unless required for health reasons, I do not wish to be separated from my baby.

Nursing My Baby

I plan to nurse my baby very shortly after birth if baby and I are OK.
Unless medically necessary, I do not wish to have any formula given to my baby (including glucose water or plain water). If my baby needs to be supplemented, I prefer an alternative method to using a bottle.
I do not want my baby to be given a pacifier.
I would like to meet with a lactation consultant.

Photo/Video

I would like to make a video recording of labor and/or the birth and want pictures of the doctor and the baby.

Labor Support

My support people are my husband, Owen, and friends Judy and Margaret and I would like them to be present during labor and/or delivery.
I would like my other children (ages 4 years and 6 years) to be present at the birth. My physician has approved this. Judy and Margaret will take care of the other children during the birth.

BOX 7.9 Methods of Prepared Childbirth

Dick-Read Method

The work of Dr. Grantly Dick-Read has been recognized as fundamental to most methods of prepared childbirth. Dr. Dick-Read was a British obstetrician who practiced from 1919 to 1940. Dr. Dick-Read regarded fear as the basis of pain in childbirth and believed that civilization had culturally conditioned women to expect childbirth to be painful. He described a fear–tension–pain cycle and was convinced that women expected birth to be painful. Therefore, when labor began, the laboring woman tensed in fear at the beginning of each contraction. This tension resulted in the increase of pain; the pain reinforced the belief that labor was painful; and thus the cycle continued. He believed that pregnant women could interrupt this fear–tension–pain cycle with prenatal education and knowledge to reduce fear of the birth process and conscious relaxation during labor.

Lamaze Method

This method is based on Dick-Read's ideas and Pavlov's experiments with conditioned response. It is named after the French obstetrician Dr. Fernand Lamaze, who studied the Pavlov method in Russia and brought back his newfound knowledge to his patients in Paris. The Lamaze instructor teaches the pregnant woman to rehearse conditioned positive responses (i.e., relaxation, breathing, and attention focusing) to a stimulus (i.e., beginning of a contraction). Then, when she is in labor, the goal is for her to respond with the helpful conditioned responses, instead of natural responses (e.g., panic, breath holding, and increased tension) that can slow the progress of labor and increase the level of pain perceived by the woman. Her partner is trained to respond by supporting the laboring woman with encouragement and praise; providing focus and offering physical comfort measures, such as position changes, controlling the environment, massage, talking her through the contractions, enhancing her relaxation, and instilling confidence (Bing, 1994).

Bradley Method

Dr. Robert Bradley also based his obstetric practice on the work of Dick-Read. Dr. Bradley became convinced that the way to make childbirth an enjoyable experience was to copy what animals do naturally. The Bradley method of childbirth is explained in Dr. Bradley's book *Husband Coached Childbirth*. The principles of the Bradley method include:

- The need for darkness and solitude. Animals usually choose to birth babies in dark secluded places, therefore the room should be darkened.
- The need for quiet. Loud or unexpected noises are disturbing.
- The need for physical comfort. Comfort measures, such as controlling the room temperature, pillows for support, positioning, nonconstricting clothing, and familiar objects, contribute to the laboring woman's needs.
- The need for physical relaxation. Conscious relaxation on the part of the laboring woman increases her comfort and allows her uterus to work more effectively and quickly. Tensing up during contractions produces increased pain.
- The need for controlled breathing. Slow, deep, sleep-like breathing by mouth is encouraged throughout labor.
- The need for closed eyes and the appearance of sleep. Shutting the eyes enhances concentration on deep breathing by shutting out visual stimuli.

Underwater Birth Method

During the 1980s, the concept of giving birth in water began to gain popularity. In written accounts of these births, often published in lay magazines, women read of laboring and delivering in tubs of warm water at home or in birthing centers and also in shallow natural bodies of water, such as seas or bays near a beach. Those who encourage water births cite that humans begin life surrounded by liquid in the womb. Moreover, soaking in a warm bath enhances relaxation. Free from gravity's pull on the body, and with reduced sensory stimulation, the laboring woman's body is less likely to secrete stress-related hormones, thus allowing production of endorphins. As a result, there is believed to be an analgesic effect on the laboring woman. In Belgium, Dr. Serge Weisel studied the effects of laboring in water on hypertension and states that women experience a drop in blood pressure within 10 to 15 minutes after entering the water. An apparent benefit of birthing in water is the increased elasticity of the perineum, reducing the frequency of and severity in tearing of the perineum.

In 1989, Barbara Harper, RN, founded Waterbirth International/GMCHA (Global Maternal Child Health Association). This organization provides information and facilitates networking among those who are interested in learning more about birthing in water.

Hypnotherapy for Birth

Some women use traditional hypnosis with posthypnotic suggestions during labor and delivery. Others use forms of self-hypnosis, incorporating the basics of Drs. Dick-Read and Lamaze, such as deep relaxation and breathing for each phase of labor. A recent article in the *Journal of Family Practice* (Martin, Schauble, Surekha, & Curry, 2001) concludes that using hypnosis to prepare for labor can have positive clinical outcomes by reducing the number of complications, surgical interventions, and length of postpartum stay.

BOX 7.10 Common Topics Included in Childbirth Education Classes

- Psychological and emotional aspects of pregnancy
- Fetal development
- Anatomic and physiologic changes involved in pregnancy and childbirth
- Induction of labor: indications for induction and what to expect
- Stages/phases of labor: physical and emotional changes of each
- Partner's role in providing support for each stage/phase of labor
- Comfort measures for labor: relaxation, movement, breathing, focus, massage, pressure, encouragement, and support
- Medication and anesthesia options for labor and birth
- Back labor: causes, physical signs, and comfort measures
- Communication with obstetrician/pediatrician: verbal and written birth plans
- What to pack for the hospital
- Hospital admission routine
- Medical procedures and interventions, such as vaginal examinations, routine laboratory work, fetal monitoring, artificial rupture of membranes (AROM), IVs, vacuum extraction, and forceps
- Cesarean birth
- Choosing a pediatrician
- Physical and emotional aspects of the postpartum period

- **Goal:** The woman's symptoms and discomforts of pregnancy are manageable.
  Expected Outcomes: Voices feeling relaxed and confident in her ability to deal with the common discomforts of pregnancy, and demonstrates the use of effective strategies for coping with the discomforts of pregnancy.
- **Goal:** The woman will feel confident in her ability to care for herself throughout pregnancy.
  Expected Outcomes: Verbalizes understanding of how to modify lifestyle to accommodate the changing needs of pregnancy; answers questions regarding self-care appropriately; asks informed questions.
- **Goal:** The woman and fetus remain free from preventable injury throughout the pregnancy.
  Expected Outcomes: Schedules and attends prenatal visits; describes warning signs to report; calls with questions and concerns; calls if warning signs are experienced.
- **Goal:** The woman will express confidence in her ability to go through the labor and birth experience and assume the parenting role.

BOX 7.11 Suggested Items for the Layette

Clothes
- 4 to 6 "onesies"
- Gowns
- Sleepers
- 2 to 3 Blanket Sleepers
- 4 to 6 Undershirts
- 4 to 6 Pairs of socks
- 4 to 6 Receiving blankets
- 3 to 4 Hooded towels
- 4 to 6 Washcloths
- 4 to 6 Bibs
- 4 to 6 Burp cloths
- Several packages of newborn size diapers and wipes or washcloths

Baby Supplies
- Baby lotion
- Baby shampoo
- Zinc oxide ointment
- Cotton swabs
- Rubbing alcohol
- Cradle or bassinet
- Crib
- Changing pad or table
- Sling
- Swing
- Stroller
- Baby bathtub

Expected Outcomes: Expresses realistic expectations regarding plans for labor and birth; schedules and attends childbirth education and/or parenting classes; prepares the home for arrival of the baby.

Test Yourself

- Identify at least five ways smoking increases pregnancy risk.
- How much alcohol is it OK for a pregnant woman to drink?
- What is a doula?

KEY POINTS

- The goal of early prenatal care is to increase the chances that the fetus and the mother will remain healthy throughout pregnancy and delivery.

- The first prenatal visit is the longest one. The main goals are to confirm a diagnosis of pregnancy, identify risk factors, determine the due date, and provide education regarding self-care and danger signs of pregnancy.
- The obstetric history looks at previous pregnancies and their outcomes. Determining the gravida and parity of the woman is an important part of the obstetric history. The parity is usually further subdivided into the number of term deliveries, preterm deliveries, abortions (spontaneous or induced), and living children.
- A complete physical examination will be done during the first visit to include a breast exam, a speculum examination with a Pap test, and a bimanual examination of the uterus.
- The most common laboratory assessments (in addition to the Pap test) done on the first visit include a CBC, blood type and screen, hepatitis B, HIV, syphilis, gonorrhea, Chlamydia, rubella titer, and a urine culture.
- Nagele's rule is used to determine the due date. Add 7 days from the first day of the last menstrual period, then subtract 3 months to obtain the due date.
- Any abnormal part of the history, physical examination, or lab work can put the pregnancy at risk. A history of difficult pregnancy or pregnancy complications puts subsequent pregnancies at risk.
- Subsequent prenatal visits are shorter and focus on the weight, blood pressure, urine protein and glucose measurements, fetal heart rate, and fundal height. Inquiry is made regarding the danger signals of pregnancy at each prenatal visit.
- Ultrasonography uses high frequency sound waves to visualize fetal and maternal structures. Ultrasound is done to determine or confirm gestational age, observe the fetus, and diagnose fetal and placental abnormalities.
- Maternal serum alpha-fetoprotein testing is recommended for every pregnant woman between 16 and 18 weeks. Elevated levels are associated with various defects, in particular fetal spinal defects.
- Amniocentesis involves aspiration of amniotic fluid through the abdominal wall to obtain fetal cells for chromosomal analysis. Amniocentesis is usually done between 15 and 20 weeks' gestation.
- Chorionic villus sampling is similar to amniocentesis, but it can be performed earlier, usually at 10 to 12 weeks. Placental tissue is aspirated through a catheter that is introduced into the cervix.
- The nonstress test measures fetal heart rate acceleration patterns. A reactive NST is reassuring. The contraction stress test exposes the fetus to the stress of uterine contractions. A negative CST is reassuring. A positive CST indicates probable hypoxia or fetal asphyxia.
- The biophysical profile combines the NST and several ultrasound measures, breathing, movements, tone, and amniotic fluid volume to predict fetal well-being.
- Common nursing diagnoses during the pregnancy are anxiety, health-seeking behaviors, risk for injury, and deficient knowledge.
- Nursing interventions are tailored to the needs of the individual woman. Nursing care is focused on relieving anxiety and the common discomforts of pregnancy, such as nausea and heartburn. Assisting the woman to maintain a balanced nutritional intake occurs throughout the pregnancy. Maintaining safety is done by monitoring the blood pressure and weight and inquiring regarding the danger signals at each visit. Teaching is ongoing throughout the pregnancy.
- Helping the woman prepare for labor, birth, and parenting is an important nursing task. The nurse can refer the woman to community resources, such as childbirth education or sibling classes.
- Nursing care has been successful if the woman is less anxious, reports that pregnancy discomforts are tolerable, consumes a balanced diet, and verbalizes an understanding of self-care.

REFERENCES AND SELECTED READINGS

Books and Journals

Bing, E. (1994). *Six practical lessons for an easier childbirth* (3rd rev. ed.). New York: Bantam Books.

Brundage, S. C. (2002). Preconception care. *American Family Physician, 65*(12), 2507–2514. Retrieved October 12, 2002, from http://www.aafp.org/afp/20020615/2507.pdf

Cunningham, F. G., Gant, N. F., Leveno, K. J., Gilstrap, L. C. III, Hauth, J. C., & Wenstrom, K. D. (2001). *Williams obstetrics* (21st ed.). New York: McGraw-Hill Medical Publishing Division.

Drugan, A., Feldman, B., Johnson, M. P., & Evans, M. I. (1999). Prenatal diagnosis: Procedures and trends. In Avery, G. B., Fletcher, M. A., & MacDonald, M. G. (Eds.), *Neonatology: Pathophysiology & management of the newborn* (5th ed., pp. 161–171). Philadelphia: Lippincott Williams & Wilkins.

Ferber, A., & Sicherman, N. (2001). The amniocentesis report: A decision guide for expectant parents and health care professionals. Retrieved October 27, 2002, from http://www.amniocentesis.org/1233asdflkjabasopir-woier55876985/thankyoudownload.html

Martin, A. A., Schauble, P. G., Surekha, H. R., & Curry, R. W. (2001). The effects of hypnosis on the labor processes and birth outcomes of pregnant adolescents. *The Journal of Family Practice, 50*(5), 441–443.

North American Nursing Diagnosis Association (NANDA). (2001). *NANDA nursing diagnoses: Definitions & classification 2001–2002*. Philadelphia: Author.

Olney, R. S., Moore, C. A., Khoury, M. J., Erickson, J. D., Edmonds, L. D., & Atash, H. K. (1995). Chorionic villus sampling and amniocentesis: Recommendations for prenatal counseling. *MMWR, 44*(RR-9), 1–12. Retrieved October 27, 2002, from http://aepo-xdv-www.epo.cdc.gov/wonder/prevguid/m0038393/m0038393.asp

Wilkinson, L. D. (2000). Prenatal care for the family physician, Part 1: Preconception and early pregnancy care. *Family Practice Recertification, 22*(10), 37–58.

Websites

Prenatal care

http://www.nlm.nih.gov/medlineplus/prenatalcare.html

Prenatal teaching

http://www.midwife.org/focus/sharewithwomen.cfm
http://www.2bparent.com/pregnancy.htm

Nutrition

http://www.pueblo.gsa.gov/cic_text/food/food-pyramid/main.htm

Doulas

http://dona.org/
http://www.doula.com/

WORKBOOK

NCLEX-STYLE REVIEW QUESTIONS

1. A woman reports that her LMP occurred on January 10, 2005. Using Nagele's rule, what is her due date?
   a. October 17, 2005
   b. October 17, 2006
   c. September 7, 2005
   d. September 7, 2006
2. A woman presents to the clinic in the first trimester of pregnancy. She has three children living at home. One of them was born prematurely at 34 weeks. The other two were full term at birth. She has a history of one miscarriage. How do you record her obstetric history on the chart using GTPAL format?
   a. G3 T2 P1 A1 L3
   b. G4 T3 P0 A1 L3
   c. G4 T2 P1 A1 L3
   d. G5 T2 P1 A1 L3
3. A woman who is 28 weeks' pregnant presents to the clinic for her scheduled prenatal visit. The nurse midwife measures her fundal height at 32 centimeters. What action do you expect the midwife to take regarding this finding? The midwife will
   a. order a multiple marker screening test.
   b. order a sonogram to confirm dates.
   c. schedule more frequent prenatal visits to monitor the pregnancy closely.
   d. take no action. This is a normal finding for a pregnancy at 28 weeks' gestation.
4. A G1 at 20 weeks' gestation is at the clinic for a prenatal visit. She tells the nurse that she has been reading about "group B strep disease" on the Internet. She asks when she can expect to be checked for the bacteria. How does the nurse best reply?
   a. "I'm glad that you asked. You will be getting the culture done today."
   b. "The obstetrician normally cultures for group B strep after 35 weeks and before delivery."
   c. "You are only checked for group B strep if you have risk factors for the infection."
   d. "You were checked during your first prenatal visit. Let me get those results for you."
5. Results of an early CVS test show that a woman's baby has severe chromosomal abnormalities. When the obstetrician explains the findings to her, she becomes tearful. She shares with you that it is against her religious beliefs to have an abortion. How would you best respond to her?
   a. "Abortion is really the best thing for the baby. He has no chance of a normal life."
   b. "I agree with you. It is against my religious beliefs, too."
   c. "It is dangerous to carry a fetus with chromosomal abnormalities to term. You really should consider an abortion to protect your health."
   d. "You don't have to decide what to do today. Take some time to talk this over with your family. I will support you whatever decision you make."

STUDY ACTIVITIES

1. Do an Internet search on "genetic counseling." Make a list of at least three genetic counselors in your area to which a pregnant woman could be referred.
2. Using the following table, fill in key points for each topic regarding self-care during pregnancy. Note any special precautions for that topic that would be important to emphasize to the pregnant woman.

Topic	Key Points	Special Precautions
Nutrition		
Dental hygiene		
Exercise		
Hygiene		
Breast care		
Clothing		
Sexual activity		
Employment		
Travel		
Medication use		

3. Develop a teaching plan for pregnant women who are 20 weeks and greater. Address common discomforts of pregnancy that the women are likely to encounter during the last half of pregnancy.

CRITICAL THINKING: What Would You Do?

Apply your knowledge of the nurse's role during pregnancy to the following situations.

1. Theresa Martinez presents to the clinic because she thinks she might be pregnant.
   a. What nursing assessments should be completed?
   b. During the history, Theresa reports that there is a history of type II diabetes in her family, and that her mother delivered large babies (10 and 11 pounds). What should you do with this information?
   c. The obstetrician asks you to assist her during the physical examination. What equipment and supplies will you gather?
2. Amanda Jones calls the clinic. She is a G2 P1 at 28 weeks' gestation. She is worried because she thinks the baby is moving less than usual.
   a. What should you tell Amanda to do first?
   b. Amanda comes to the office to be checked because she is still worried about the baby. What is the priority nursing assessment that should be completed at this time? Why?
   c. Because Amanda has decreased fetal movement, the physician orders a biophysical profile (BPP). How would you explain this test to Amanda? Which part of this test would you normally expect to be a nursing function?
3. Rebecca Richards is pregnant for the first time. She is 40 years of age. The obstetrician has suggested chromosomal studies.
   a. Explain the advantages and disadvantages of chorionic villus sampling (CVS) versus amniocentesis.
   b. Rebecca tells you that she is opposed to abortion for any reason. She asks why she should go through CVS because she will not accept an abortion. How would you respond to Rebecca?
   c. Halfway through the pregnancy, Rebecca's fetus is diagnosed with thrombocytopenia. What therapy will likely be ordered for the fetus? Explain this therapy to Rebecca.

UNIT 4

Labor and Birth

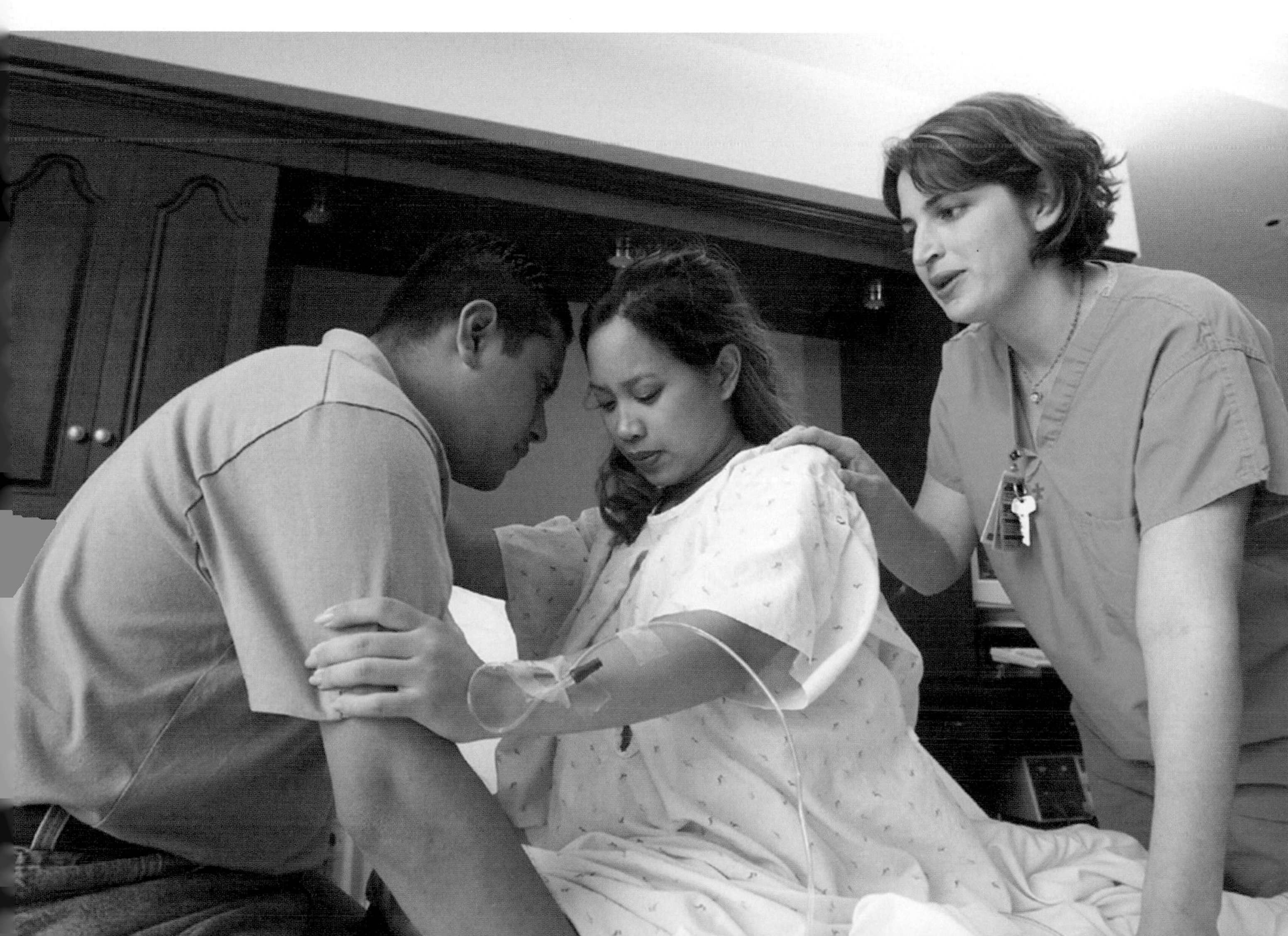

The Labor Process

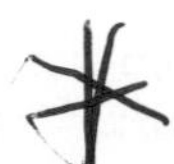

STUDENT OBJECTIVES

On completion of this chapter, the student should be able to

1. Explain the four essential components of the labor process.
2. Illustrate how the four components of labor work together to accomplish birth.
3. Identify three current theories regarding causes of labor onset.
4. Differentiate between Braxton Hicks contractions and true labor contractions.
5. Outline the seven mechanisms of a spontaneous vaginal delivery.
6. Classify the stages and phases of labor.
7. Discuss ways the woman physiologically and psychologically adapts to labor.
8. Describe fetal physiologic responses to labor.

KEY TERMS

android pelvis
anthropoid pelvis
caput succedaneum
cardinal movements
diagonal conjugate
effacement
engagement
false pelvis
fetal attitude
fetal lie
fetal presentation
gynecoid pelvis
molding
obstetric conjugate
platypelloid pelvis
station
true pelvis

It is essential for the nurse to understand the components of labor, how these components work together in the process of labor, and how the woman and fetus adapt to labor (in normal situations). This knowledge allows the nurse to support the laboring woman appropriately and assist her through a safe labor and delivery. In this chapter, each component of labor and birth is explored separately, followed by a discussion of the combined components during the process of labor. Normal maternal and fetal adaptation to labor also are explored.

THE FOUR ESSENTIAL COMPONENTS OF LABOR

Four essential components of labor have been identified. These factors are sometimes referred to as the "four Ps" of labor: passageway, passenger, powers, and psyche. A problem in any of these four areas will negatively influence the labor process.

Passageway

The bony pelvis forms the rigid passageway through which the fetus must navigate to be delivered vaginally. The basic shape and dimensions of the pelvis may favor a vaginal birth or may interfere with the ability of the fetus to descend and be delivered vaginally. The soft tissue of the cervix and vagina form the birth canal and also are part of the passageway.

The flared upper portion of the bony pelvis is referred to as the **false pelvis**. The false pelvis is not considered part of the bony passageway. The portion of the pelvis below the linea terminalis is called the **true pelvis**. The true pelvis is the bony passageway through which the fetus must pass during delivery. Important landmarks of the true pelvis include the inlet (entrance to the true pelvis), midpelvis, and outlet (exit point). Figure 8-1 illustrates important parts of the pelvis.

Pelvic Shape

It is the shape of the inlet that determines the pelvic type. There are four basic pelvic shapes: gynecoid, anthropoid, android, and platypelloid (Fig. 8-2). The **gynecoid pelvis** is most favorable for a vaginal birth. This pelvic type is categorized as a typical female pelvis, although only about half of all women have a gynecoid pelvis. The rounded shape of the gynecoid inlet allows the fetus room to negotiate the dimensions of the bony passageway.

The **anthropoid pelvis** is elongated in its dimensions and is sometimes referred to as apelike. The anterior-posterior diameter is roomy, but the transverse diameter is narrow compared with that of the gynecoid pelvis. However, a vaginal birth often can be accomplished in the approximately 25% of women who have an anthropoid pelvis (Mattson & Smith, 2000).

Take note of this detail. The shape and dimensions of the inlet cannot be determined by the size of the woman. A woman might be small in stature but have a roomy gynecoid pelvis. A larger woman may have a small, contracted platypelloid or android pelvis.

The **android pelvis** is the typical male pelvis. The heart shape of the android pelvis is not favorable to a vaginal delivery. The fetus often gets stuck in this type of pelvis and must be delivered by cesarean section. Approximately 20% of women have an android pelvis.

The least common type is the **platypelloid pelvis**. This pelvis is flat in its dimensions with a very narrow anterior-posterior diameter and a wide transverse diameter. This shape makes it extremely difficult for the fetus to pass through the bony pelvis. Therefore,

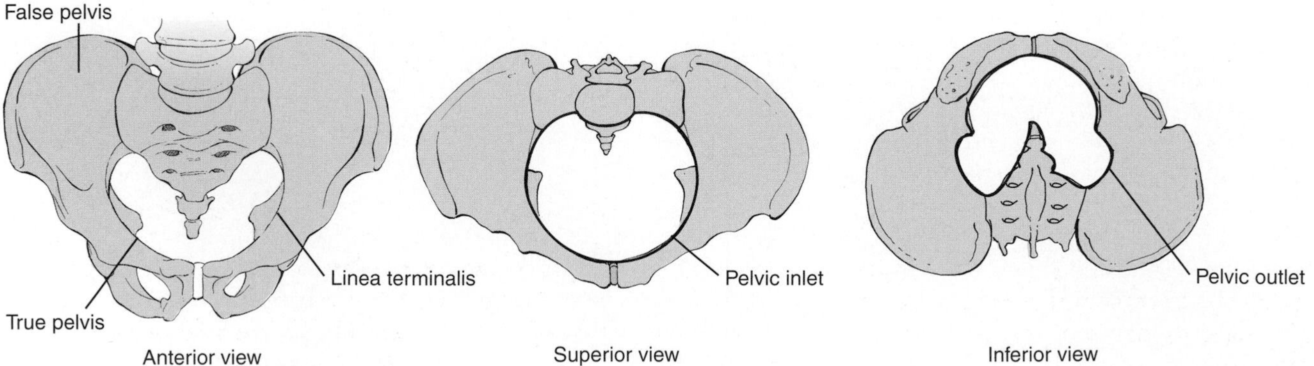

● ***Figure 8.1*** Important landmarks of the pelvis.

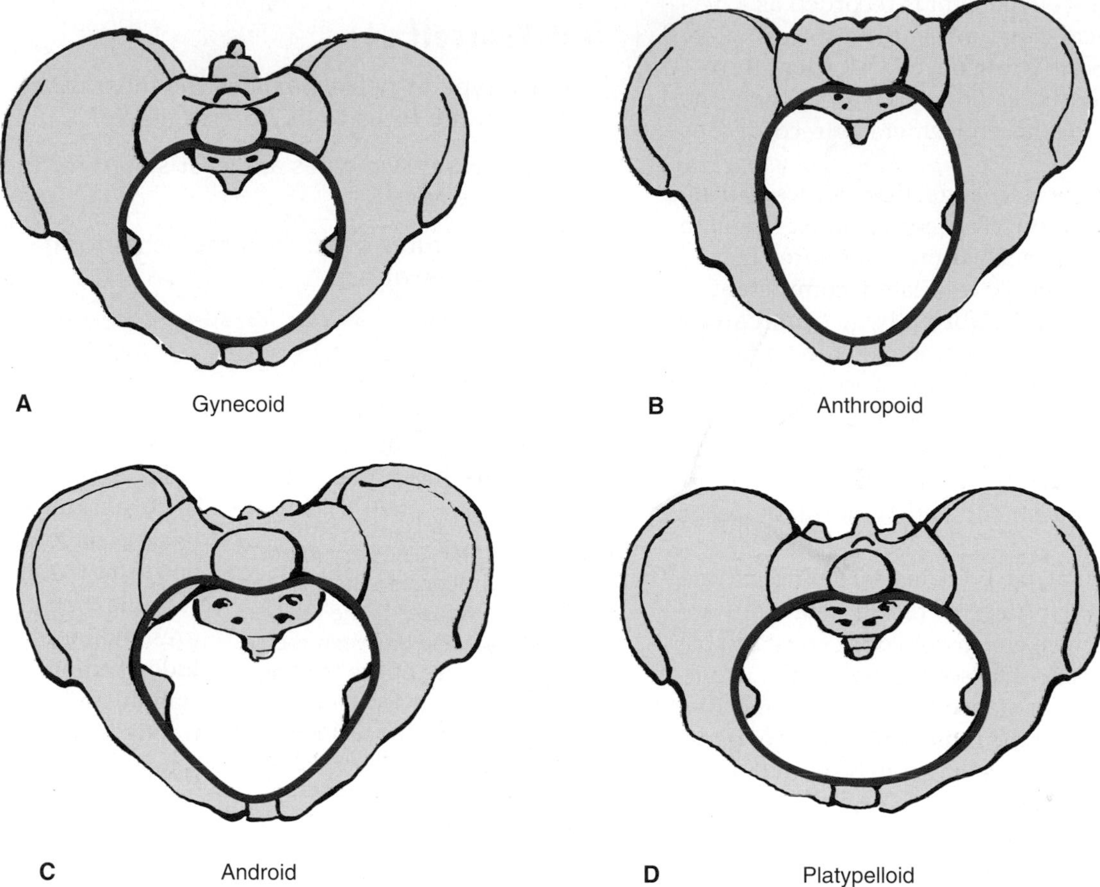

● ***Figure 8.2*** Pelvic shapes. (**A**) Gynecoid, (**B**) anthropoid, (**C**) android, and (**D**) platypelloid.

women with a platypelloid pelvis (about 5% of women) usually must deliver the fetus by cesarean section.

Pelvic Dimensions

Early in the pregnancy, particularly if a woman has never delivered a baby vaginally, the health care provider may take pelvic measurements to estimate the size of the true pelvis. These measurements can help predict if the pelvis is adequate for a vaginal delivery.

The most important measurement of the inlet is the **obstetric conjugate** because this is the smallest diameter of the inlet through which the fetus must pass. However, the obstetric conjugate cannot be measured directly; therefore, the health care provider must estimate the size. The estimate is obtained by measuring the **diagonal conjugate**, which extends from the symphysis pubis to the sacral promontory. Then, 1.5 to 2.0 centimeters are subtracted from the measurement of the diagonal conjugate to approximate the dimensions of the obstetric conjugate. An obstetric conjugate measurement of 11 centimeters is considered to be adequate to accommodate a vaginal delivery.

Measurements of the midpelvis are taken at the level of the ischial spines. If the ischial spines are prominent and extend into the midpelvis, they can reduce the diameter of the midpelvis and might interfere with the journey of the fetus through the passageway during labor. One important measurement of the outlet is the angle of the pubic arch. This angle should be at least 90 degrees.

Here's an interesting fact. A woman's pelvis might be roomy enough for a vaginal delivery in one portion, but too small in another portion. That is to say that just because the inlet and the outlet are adequate for delivery does not mean that the midpelvis is adequate. The midpelvis might be contracted and too small to allow the fetus to pass through that section of the bony passageway.

Soft Tissues

The cervix and vagina are soft tissues that form the part of the passageway known as the birth canal. In early pregnancy, the cervix is firm, long, and closed. As the time for delivery approaches, the cervix usually begins to soften. Then, when labor begins, uterine contractions affect the cervix in two ways. First, the cervix begins to get shorter, a process called effacement. Cervical effacement is recorded as a percentage. The cervical canal measures approximately 2 centimeters when it is uneffaced. At a length of 1 centimeter, the cervix is 50% effaced. When the cervix is paper thin, the effacement is recorded as 100%.

The second cervical change that occurs during normal labor is dilation. The cervix must open to allow the fetus to be born. Dilation is measured in centimeters. When the cervix is dilated completely, it measures 10 centimeters. Normally, a primiparous woman will experience effacement before dilation. For a multiparous woman, both processes usually occur at the same time. Often, the multipara will be dilated 1 to 2 centimeters for several weeks before labor begins. Figure 8-3 illustrates the processes of cervical dilation and effacement as they normally occur for the primipara.

The vaginal canal participates in childbirth via passive distention. The rugae of the vaginal walls are obliterated during birth, which allows for considerable expansion. The muscles and soft tissues of the primipara provide greater resistance to stretching and distending than do those of the multipara. This is one reason the first baby often takes longer to be born than do subsequent babies.

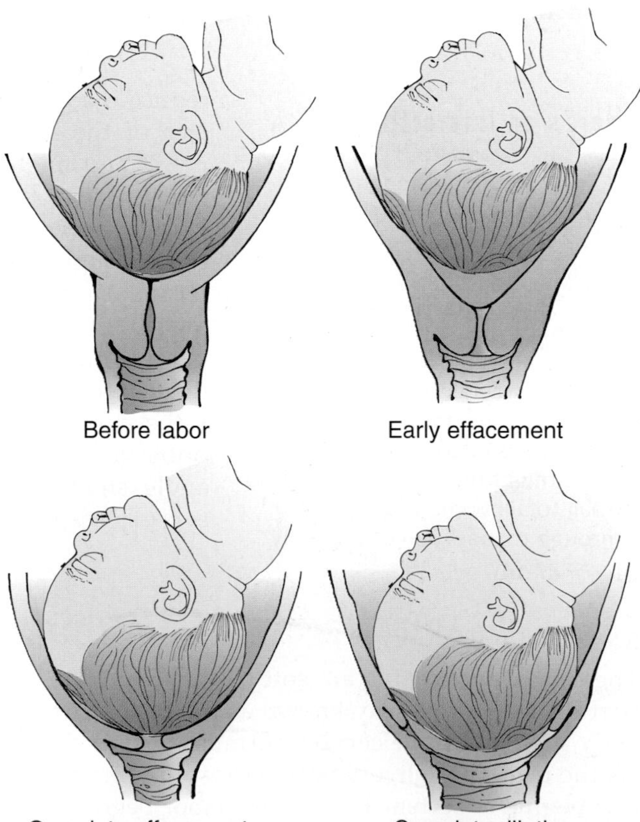

● **Figure 8.3** Cervical dilation and effacement.

Test Yourself

- Which type of pelvis provides the most room to allow the fetus to be born vaginally?
- Which two pelvic types are least suited for a vaginal delivery?
- What structures other than the pelvis form the passageway?

Passenger

The "passenger" refers to the fetus. Although the fetus basically has a passive role to play, the size of the fetal skull and fetal accommodation to the passageway (i.e., fetal lie, presentation, attitude, position, and station) can significantly affect labor progress. Each concept is defined and discussed in relation to its influence on the progression of labor.

Did you know? One very important consideration of the passenger is the relationship between the size of the fetal head and pelvic dimensions. The diameters of the fetal skull, as well as the way the fetus positions himself in relation to the pelvis, have a major impact on the process of labor and the type of delivery that results.

Fetal Skull

The skull is the most important fetal structure in relation to labor and birth because it is the largest and least compressible structure (Fig. 8-4). The diameters of the fetal skull must be small enough to allow the head to travel through the bony pelvis. Fortunately, the fetal skull is not entirely rigid. The cartilage between the bones allows for the bones to overlap during labor, a process that reduces the diameter of the head. **Molding**, or elongation of the fetal skull, is another way that the head accommodates to the birth canal. Molding may be particularly pronounced for the newborn of a primipara.

Fetal Accommodation to the Passageway

Fetal Lie. Fetal lie describes the long axis of the fetus in relation to the long axis of the pregnant woman. Basically, there are three ways that the fetus can situate itself in the uterus: in a longitudinal, transverse, or oblique position (Fig. 8-5). A longitudinal lie, in which the long axis of the fetus is parallel to the long axis of the mother, is the most common. When the fetus is in a transverse lie, the long axis of the fetus is perpendicular to the long axis of the woman. An oblique lie is in between the two.

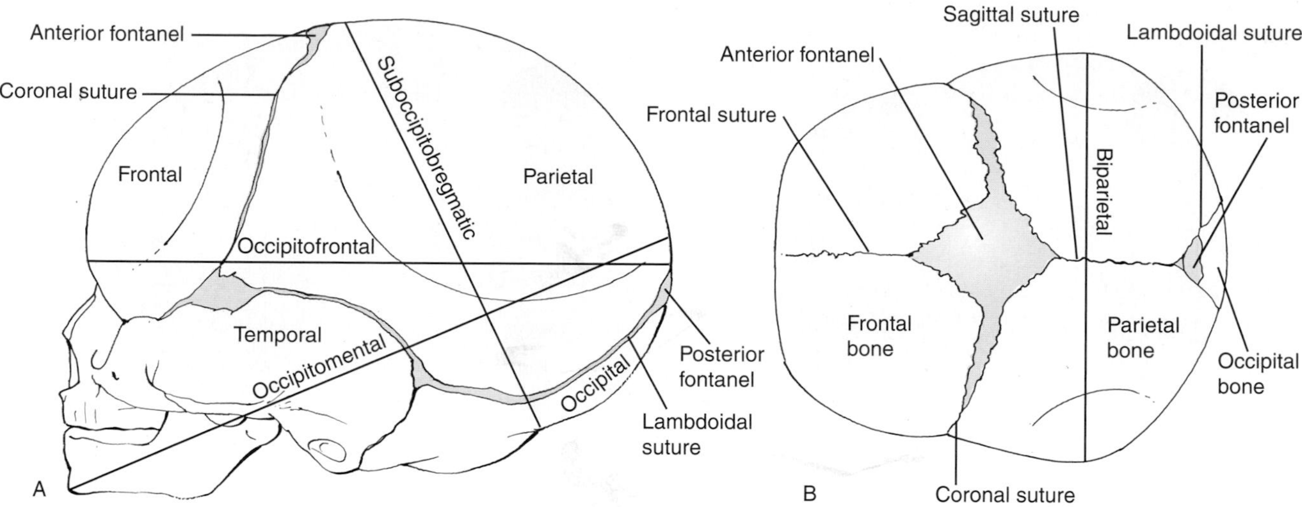

● ***Figure 8.4*** Clinically important landmarks of the fetal skull. (**A**) Side view showing important diameters in a cephalic presentation. (**B**) Top view showing sutures and fontanels.

Fetal Presentation. Fetal presentation refers to the foremost part of the fetus that enters the pelvic inlet. There are three main ways that the fetus can present to the pelvis: head (cephalic presentation), feet or buttocks (breech presentation), or shoulder (shoulder presentation). Approximately 96% of fetuses are in a cephalic presentation at the end of pregnancy (Cunningham et al., 2001).

Breech presentations occur in approximately 3.5% of term pregnancies (Cunningham et al., 2001). Figure 8-6 illustrates different types of breech presentations. Shoulder presentations are the least common, occurring in less than 0.5 % of all term pregnancies (Cunningham et al., 2001). This presentation is associated with a transverse lie.

Fetal Attitude. Fetal attitude refers to the relationship of the fetal parts to one another. In a cephalic presentation, there are several different ways the head can present to the maternal pelvis, depending on fetal attitude. The most common attitude, and the one that is

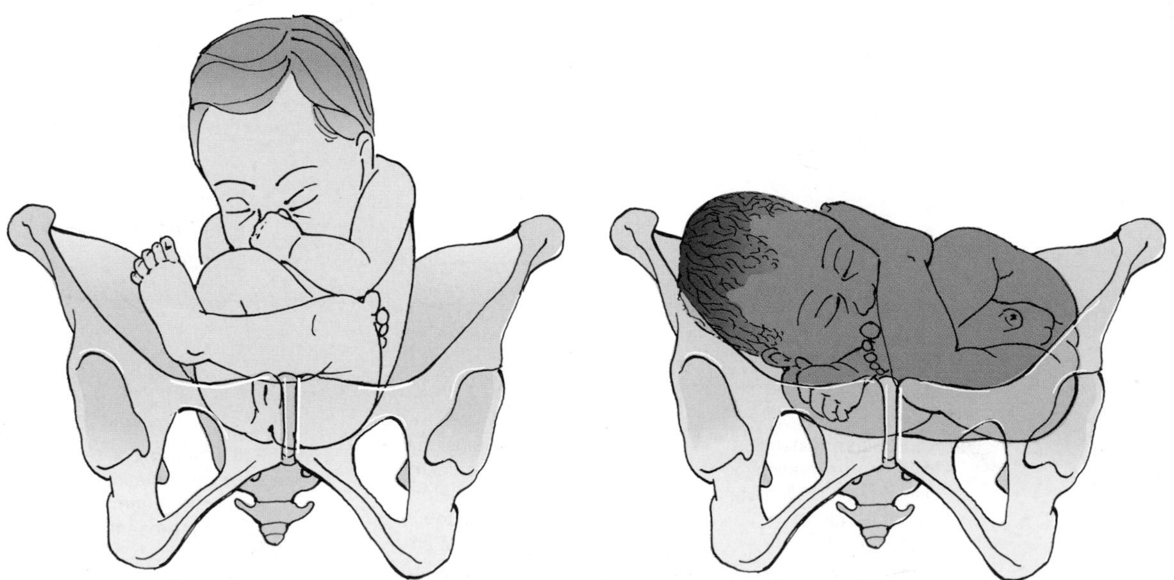

● ***Figure 8.5*** Longitudinal versus transverse lie. The drawing on the left illustrates a breech presentation in a left sacrum posterior (LSP) position. The lie is longitudinal (the fetus lies parallel to the maternal spine). The drawing on the right is a transverse lie (the fetus lies crosswise to the maternal spine).

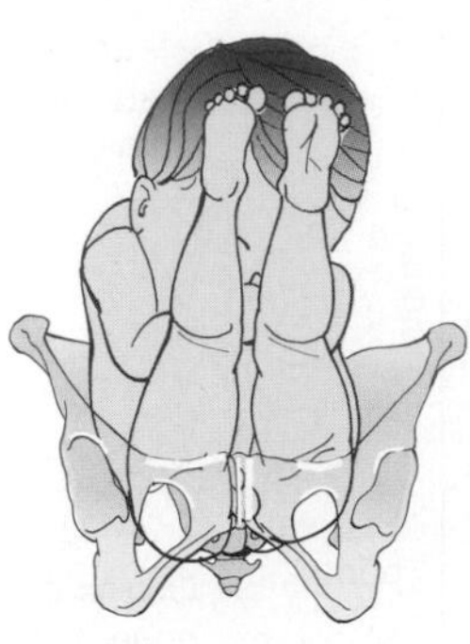

Frank breech presentation. Right sacrum posterior (RSP) position. Well-flexed attitude.

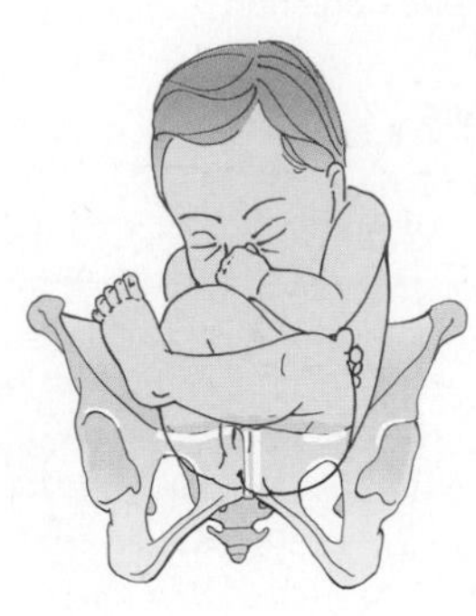

Complete breech presentation. Left sacrum posterior (LSP) position. Well-flexed attitude.

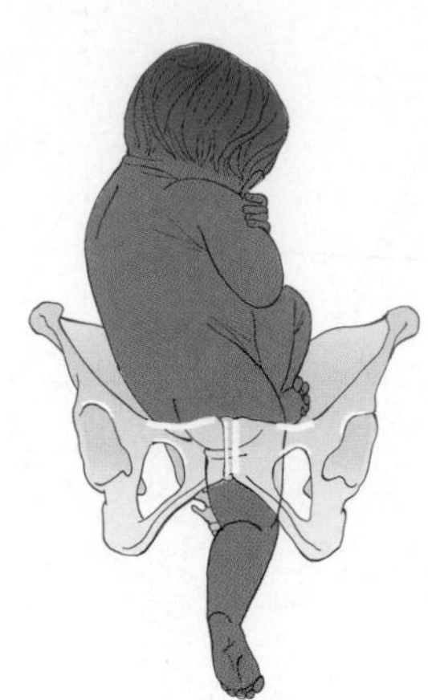

Single footling (incomplete) breech presentation. Presenting part: one foot. Right sacrum anterior (RSA) position. Partially extended attitude.

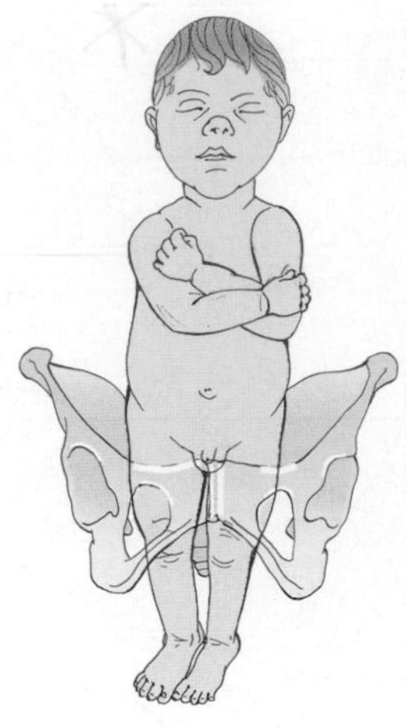

Double footling (incomplete) breech presentation. Presenting part: both feet. Sacrum posterior (SP) position. Attitude of extension.

● ***Figure 8.6*** Types of breech presentations. Each fetus is in a longitudinal lie.

most favorable for a vaginal birth, is an attitude of flexion, also called a vertex presentation. When the fetus curls up into an ovoid shape, she presents the smallest diameters of her skull to the bony pelvis. When the fetus is neither flexed nor extended, she is in a military presentation and a larger head diameter presents. If the fetus demonstrates an attitude of partial extension, the brow (or frontum) becomes the presenting part. In an attitude of full extension the face presents. Figure 8-7 shows variations of cephalic presentation in association with fetal attitude.

Position. The fetal position is determined by comparing the relationship of an arbitrarily determined reference point on the presenting part to the quadrants of the maternal pelvis (Table 8-1). To determine position, the nurse must first establish the presenting part and locate the appropriate reference point. Then a determination is made as to which pelvic quadrant the reference point is facing.

When position is being documented, the side of the maternal pelvis the presenting part is facing is named first, followed by the reference point. The last

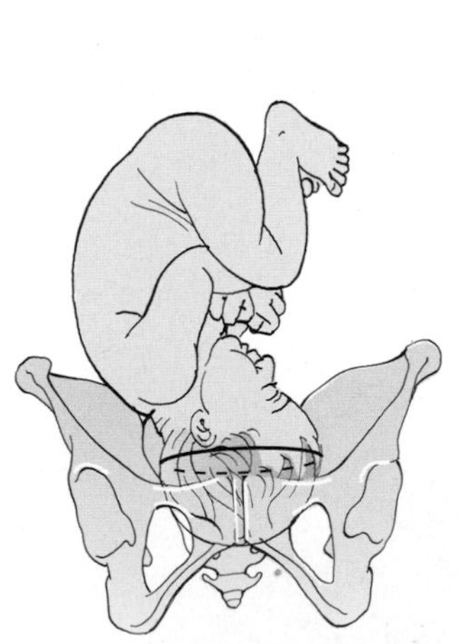

Well-flexed attitude: Vertex presentation Smallest diameter presents–9.5 cm

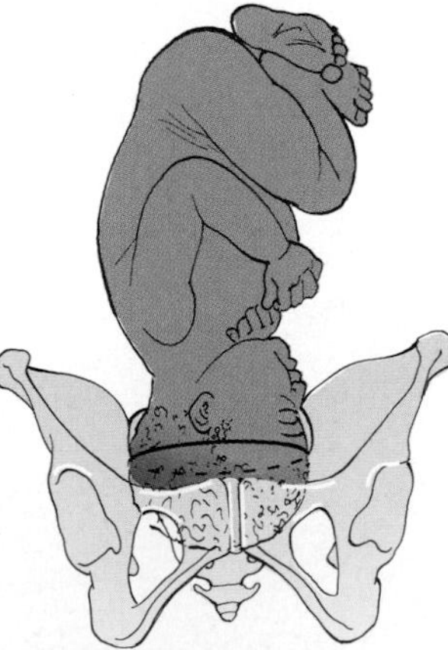

No flexion or extension: Military presentation Occipitofrontal diameter presents–11 cm

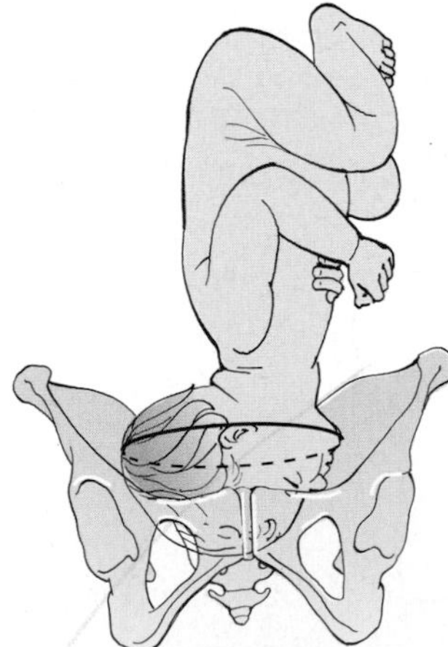

Partial extension: Brow presentation Largest diameter (occipitomental) presents–13.5 cm

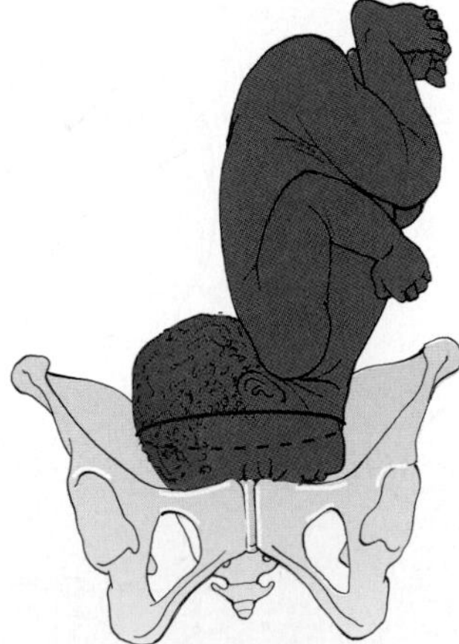

Full extension: Face presentation Submentobregmatic diameter presents–9.5 cm

● ***Figure 8.7*** Relationship of fetal attitude and the diameter of the fetal skull that presents to the maternal pelvis. All of the fetuses are in a cephalic presentation and are exhibiting a longitudinal lie. The presentations can be further differentiated as vertex, military, brow, and face presentations, respectively. Notice the varying degrees of fetal flexion.

TABLE 8.1	Reference Points for Determining Position
Presenting Part	**Reference Point**
Vertex	Occiput
Brow	Frontum (brow)
Face	Mentum (chin)
Breech	Sacrum
Shoulder	Scapula (acromial process)

part of the designation is used to specify whether the presenting part is facing the anterior or the posterior portion of the pelvis or whether it is in a transverse position. For instance, the occipital bone, or occiput, is the reference point in a vertex presentation. If the occiput is facing the right anterior quadrant of the pelvis, the position is recorded as right occiput anterior (ROA). Box 8-1 describes how to determine the abbreviation used to document fetal position in the clinical record. Figure 8-8 illustrates different positions in a vertex presentation. (See Figure 8-6 for examples of different positions in a breech presentation.)

BOX 8.1 Recording Fetal Position

For each presentation there are eight possible positions. Record the notation as an abbreviation using the following criteria:

First Designation
Refers to the side of the maternal pelvis in which the presenting part is found*
Right (R)
Left (L)

Second (Middle) Designation
Reference point on the presenting part
- Occiput (O)—vertex and military presentations
- Frontum or brow (Fr)—brow presentation
- Mentum or chin (M)—face presentation
- Sacrum (S)—breech presentation
- Scapula (Sc)—shoulder presentation

Third (Last) Designation
Refers to the front, back, or side of the maternal pelvis in which the reference point is found
- Anterior (A)—front of the pelvis
- Posterior (P)—back of the pelvis
- Transverse (T)—side of the pelvis

* This designation is not included in the notation if the reference point is exactly in the middle and is turned neither to the left nor to the right.

Be careful! A transverse position is not the same as a transverse lie. The lie refers to the general way the fetus is positioned (lying) in the uterus; whereas, position refers to the way the landmark on the presenting part is facing a specific quadrant of the pelvis. Therefore, in a transverse lie, the shoulder presents to the pelvis; however, a fetus could be in a breech or a cephalic presentation, with the presenting part in a transverse position in reference to the pelvis.

Station. Station refers to the relationship of the presenting part to the ischial spines (Fig. 8-9). When the widest diameter of the presenting part is at the level of the ischial spines, the station is recorded as zero (0). If the presenting part is above the level of the ischial spines, the station is recorded as a negative number and is read "minus." If the presenting part is below the level of the ischial spines, the station is recorded as a positive number and is read "plus." For example, in a cephalic presentation, if the vertex is 1 centimeter above the level of the ischial spines, the station is reported as a minus one and recorded as −1. If, on the other hand, the presenting part is 1 centimeter below the level of the ischial spines, the station is reported as a plus one and recorded as +1.

Think about this. When the fetus is floating, he is said to be high in the pelvis. A high station is recorded as a negative (minus) number. On the other hand, if the fetus has moved deep into the pelvis, his station is low and is recorded as a positive (plus) number. As the fetus is being born, his station is a plus four (+4).

When the station is a minus four (−4) or higher, the fetus is said to be floating and unengaged. When the fetus is floating, the presenting part has not yet entered the true pelvis. When the presenting part has settled into the true pelvis at the level of the ischial spines, the fetus is at a station of zero (0) and engaged.

Test Yourself

- What term is used to describe the fetal part that enters the birth canal first?
- When the nurse describes the relationship of fetal parts to one another, what term does she use?
- How is fetal lie described if the fetus is lying perpendicular to the maternal spine?

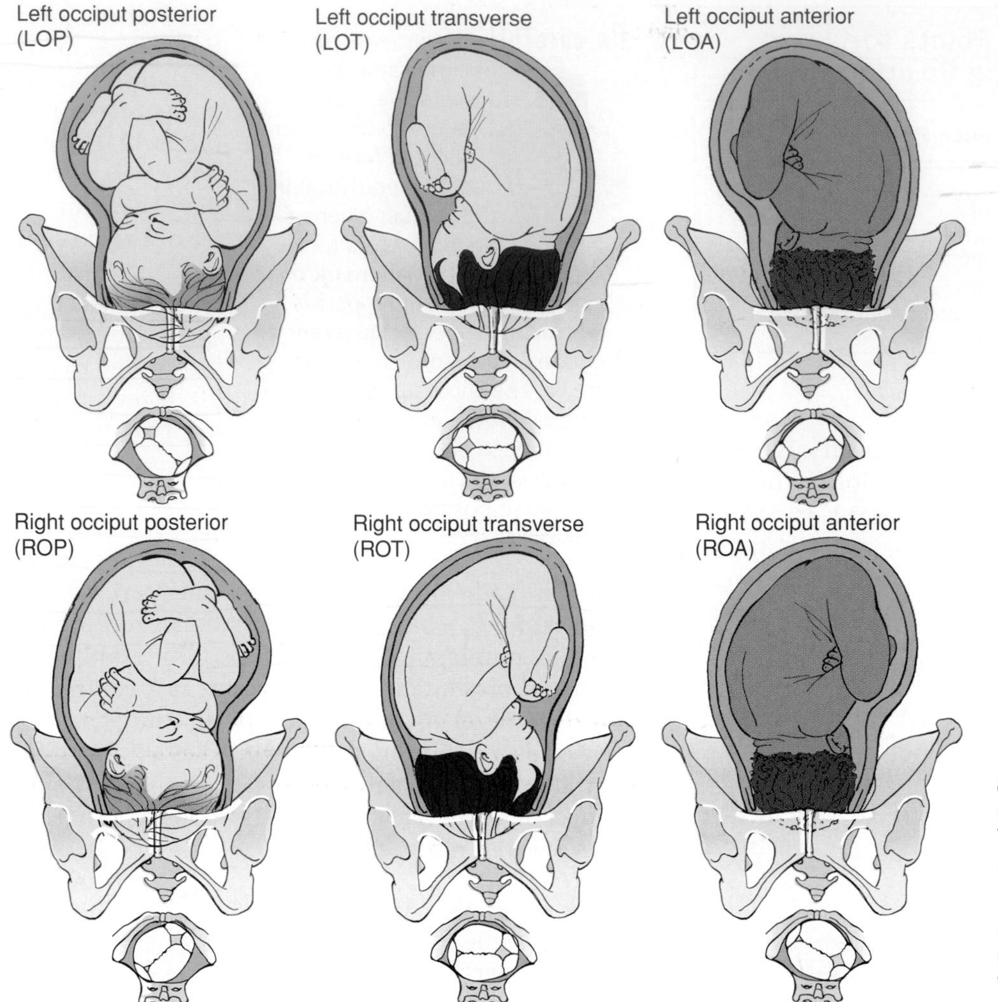

● ***Figure 8.8*** Examples of fetal position in a vertex presentation. The lie is longitudinal for each illustration. The attitude is one of flexion. Notice that the view of the top illustration is seen when facing the pregnant woman. The bottom view is that seen with the woman in a dorsal recumbent position.

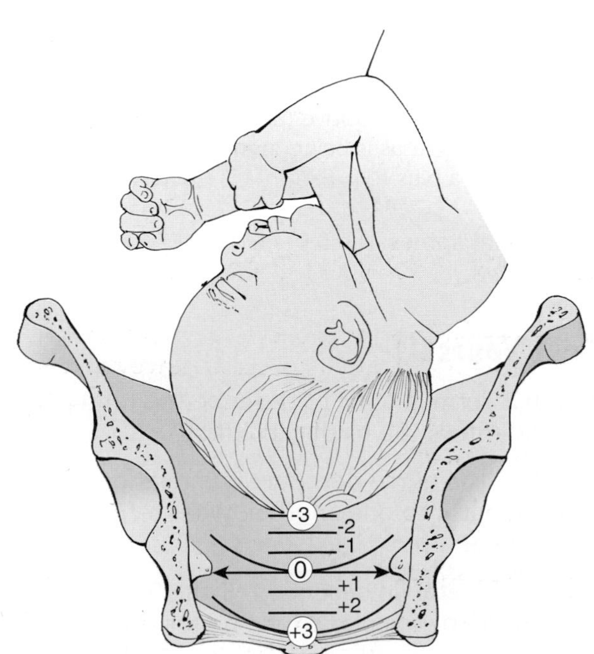

● ***Figure 8.9*** Fetal station.

Powers

The primary force of labor comes from involuntary muscular contractions of the uterus. These labor contractions cause dilation and effacement of the cervix during the first stage of labor. Secondary powers are voluntary muscle contractions of the maternal abdomen during the second stage of labor that help expel the fetus.

Each involuntary uterine contraction is composed of three phases—increment, acme, and decrement—followed by a relaxation period (Fig. 8-10). The increment, or building up of the contraction, is the longest phase. During the increment, the contraction gains strength until the acme, or peak, of the contraction is reached. The decrement is the letting-up phase, as the contraction relaxes gradually to baseline.

The rhythmic, intermittent nature of contractions is documented using three descriptors: frequency, duration, and intensity (see Fig. 8-10). Frequency refers to how often the contractions are occurring and is measured by counting the time interval from the beginning of one contraction to the beginning of the

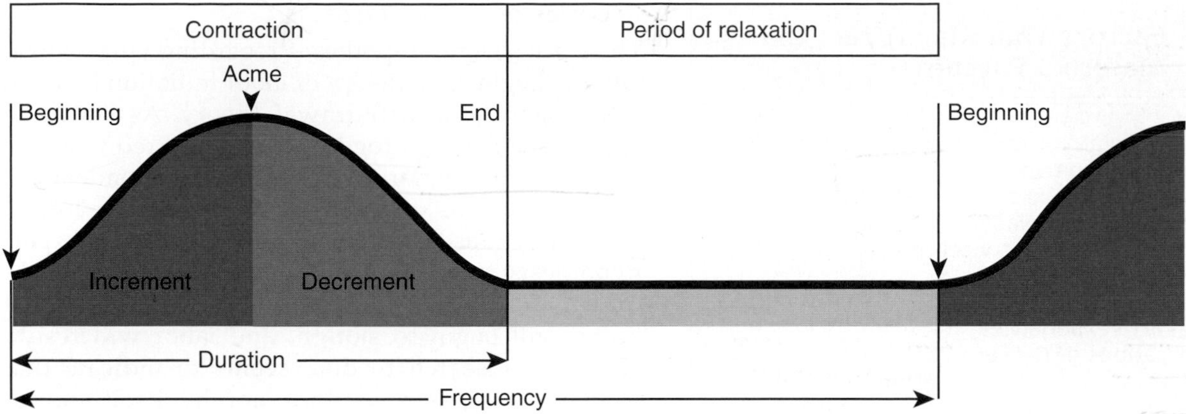

● ***Figure 8.10*** Anatomy of a uterine contraction. The three phases of a contraction are the increment (building up in intensity), acme (peak intensity), and decrement (decreasing intensity). The contraction is normally followed by a period of relaxation. The nurse assesses the contraction pattern by measuring duration (length of time from the beginning to the end of one contraction), intensity (strength of the contraction, measured at the acme, or peak), and frequency (length of time from the beginning of one contraction to the start of the next contraction).

following contraction. Duration is the interval from the beginning of a contraction to its end. Intensity refers to the strength of the contraction. This characteristic is most often estimated by palpating the fundus at the peak of the contraction and is documented as mild, moderate, or strong. Intensity can also be measured directly with an intrauterine pressure transducer, although this technique is not used routinely.

It is extremely important to the well-being of the mother and the fetus that there is a period of relaxation between contractions (see Fig. 8-10). The blood vessels that supply the placenta are compressed with each contraction, thereby decreasing the amount of oxygen that flows to the fetus. The relaxation period allows for the vessels to fill with oxygen-rich blood to supply the uterus and placenta. Relaxation also is necessary so that maternal muscles do not become overly fatigued and to allow the laboring woman momentary relief from the pain of labor.

This is an important point. Because blood flow to the placenta is interrupted temporarily with each contraction, oxygen to the fetus is decreased. It is as if the fetus must hold his breath during each contraction. Obviously, the fetus cannot tolerate contractions that last too long, are too strong, or that have no rest period between them for any prolonged period of time.

Psyche

Many factors affect the psychological state or psyche of the laboring woman (Box 8-2). When the woman feels confident in her ability to cope and finds ways to work with the contractions, the labor process is enhanced. However, if the laboring woman becomes fearful or has intense pain, she may become tense and fight the contractions. This situation often becomes a cycle of fear, tension, and pain that interferes with the progress of labor.

Test Yourself

- From where does the primary force of labor come?
- How is the frequency of uterine contractions measured?
- What is the purpose of the relaxation period between uterine contractions?

THE PROCESS OF LABOR

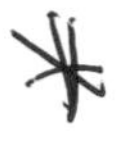

The discussion thus far has centered on the individual components of the labor process. However, it is the interplay between the components that allows for labor to progress so that the fetus can be born. The following section illustrates how the labor process works to accomplish birth.

The Onset of Labor

Scientists often search for reasons why things work as they do. One question that intrigues scientists is, "What is the trigger that causes labor to begin?" As

BOX 8.2 Factors That May Affect the Maternal Psyche

Factors that may affect the woman's psyche during labor include the woman's:

- Current pregnancy experience
  - Unplanned versus planned pregnancy
  - Amount of difficulty conceiving
  - Presence of risk factors
  - Complications of pregnancy
- Previous birth experiences
  - Complications of delivery
  - Mode of delivery (cesarean versus vaginal)
  - Birth outcomes (e.g., fetal demise, birth defects)
- Expectations for current birth experience
  - View of labor as a meaningful or a stressful event
  - Realistic and attainable goals versus idealistic views that conflict with reality (a situation that can lead to disappointment)
- Preparation for birth
  - Type of childbirth preparation
  - Familiarity with institution and its policies and procedures
  - Type of relaxation techniques learned and practiced
- Support system
  - Presence and support of a birth companion
    - Husband
    - Mother
    - Lesbian partner
    - Friend
    - Doula
- Culture
  - A woman's culture influences and defines
    - The childbirth experience
      Shameful versus joyful
      Superstitions and beliefs about pregnancy and birth
      Prescribed behaviors and taboos during the intrapartum period
    - Relationships
      Interpersonal interactions
      Parent–infant interactions
      Role expectations of family members
      Support person involvement
    - Pain
      Meaning and context of pain
      Acceptable responses to pain
    - The significance of touch
      Soothing versus intruding
      May be a symbol of intimacy

Adapted from Mattson, S., & Smith, J. E. (Eds.). (2000). *Core curriculum for maternal–newborn nursing* (2nd ed., pp. 227–229). AWHONN publication. Philadelphia: WB Saunders.

pregnancy nears term, the pregnant woman is more concerned with when labor will begin than with what causes labor to begin. She often asks the physician, "When will I go into labor?" This section explores both sets of questions.

Theories of Labor Onset

There are several hypotheses regarding what causes labor to begin. One theory of labor initiation is called the progesterone-withdrawal theory. As stated in previous chapters, progesterone is referred to as the "hormone of pregnancy" because it has a tendency to relax the uterus and maintain the uterine lining. These functions help to maintain the pregnancy. This hypothesis suggests that if progesterone is withdrawn, the uterus will begin to contract, the uterine lining will begin to slough, and labor will result. However, research to date seems to indicate that blocking progesterone does not by itself induce labor.

Oxytocin theory is another hypothesis regarding the cause of labor. Because the hormone oxytocin causes the uterus to contract, some scientists have proposed that a rise in oxytocin levels may be responsible for initiating labor. However, blood levels of oxytocin do not measurably increase before labor begins; therefore, some researchers have concluded that oxytocin is probably not the main factor that stimulates labor to begin. Finally, much research has been done regarding the prostaglandin theory of labor. It has been determined that prostaglandins influence labor in several ways, which include softening the cervix and stimulating the uterus to contract. However, evidence supporting the theory that prostaglandins are the agents that trigger labor to begin is inconclusive.

Because a single causative factor of labor initiation has not yet been determined, the most likely answer seems to be that labor results from a combination of factors working together that stimulates the onset of labor (Ruiz, 1998).

Anticipatory Signs of Labor

Although it cannot be said with certainty what factors actually initiate labor, nature usually provides clues as to the nearness of labor. Approximately 2 weeks before labor the presenting part may settle into the pelvic cavity, causing the pregnant woman to sense that the baby has "dropped." This subjective feeling is called "lightening." The woman will be able to breathe more easily, and she may need to urinate more frequently because of the pressure of the fetus on the urinary bladder. Not all women experience lightening before the onset of labor. Multiparous women often do not experience lightening until labor begins.

Braxton Hicks contractions occur more frequently and are more noticeable as pregnancy approaches term. These irregular, false labor pains usually decrease in intensity with walking and position changes. The woman may experience gastrointestinal disturbances, such as diarrhea, heartburn, or nausea and vomiting as labor approaches. Sometimes the mucous plug will be expelled a week or two before labor ensues.

Frequently the woman will experience a burst of energy 24 to 48 hours before the onset of labor. She may have the energy and desire to do spring cleaning or some other big project in anticipation of the baby's arrival, a phenomenon known as the nesting urge. The nurse should caution the woman regarding the nesting urge and advise her to conserve her energy for the work of labor.

Clinical signs that labor is approaching include ripening or softening and effacement (thinning) of the cervix. Dilation of the cervix may accompany softening and effacement, particularly in multiparous women. The practitioner will inform the woman of these changes when a pelvic examination is done during a scheduled office visit.

Differences Between False and True Labor

Here's a helpful hint. The definition of true labor contains the core information needed to tell the difference between true and false labor. By definition, true labor results in progressive dilation and effacement of the cervix to bring about the birth of the fetus. If contractions are occurring but the cervix is not getting thinner (effacing) or opening (dilating), the woman is not in true labor.

At the end of pregnancy, Braxton Hicks contractions increase in frequency and become more noticeable. These practice contractions can be quite uncomfortable, making it difficult to distinguish true labor from false labor (Table 8-2). Sometimes a woman presents to the labor suite because she thinks she is in labor. After the initial assessment, the woman may be asked to walk for an hour or two. Then a vaginal examination is performed to determine any cervical changes. If there are changes, true labor is diagnosed and the woman is admitted to the hospital. If there are no changes, she may be sent home with instructions to return if the contractions become stronger, more regular, or if other signs of true labor occur, such as increased bloody show or rupture of the membranes.

Mechanisms of a Spontaneous Vaginal Delivery

For a vaginal birth to occur, the passenger must pass through the passageway. The turns and movements made during the journey are referred to as the mechanisms of delivery or the **cardinal movements**, and include engagement, descent, flexion, internal rotation, extension, external rotation, and finally, expulsion (Fig. 8-11). Although the movements will be discussed separately, it is important to understand that these mechanisms may overlap or occur simultaneously.

You may want to make a note of this! Traditionally it has been said that if the primigravida begins labor before engagement has occurred, she has a higher likelihood of having a cesarean birth. However, a study published in the *Journal of Nurse Midwifery* reports that an unengaged vertex in the nullipara in early labor does not by itself predict whether or not a vaginal birth can be accomplished (Diegmann, Chez, & Danclair, 1995).

Initial descent of the fetal head may result in **engagement** (presenting part descends to the level of the ischial spines). Engagement may occur as much as

TABLE 8.2 Characteristics of False Versus True Labor

	True Labor	False Labor
Cervical changes	Progressive dilation and effacement	No change
Membranes	May bulge or rupture spontaneously	Remain intact
Bloody show	Present	Absent; may have pinkish mucous or may expel mucus plug
Contraction pattern	Regular (may be irregular at first) pattern develops in which contractions become increasingly intense and more frequent	Pattern tends to be irregular, although the contractions may seem to have a regular pattern for a time
Pain characteristics	Often starts in the small of the back and radiates to the lower abdomen; may begin with a cramping sensation	May be described as a tightening sensation; usually the discomfort is confined to the abdomen
Effects of walking	Contractions continue and become stronger	May decrease the frequency or eliminate the contractions altogether

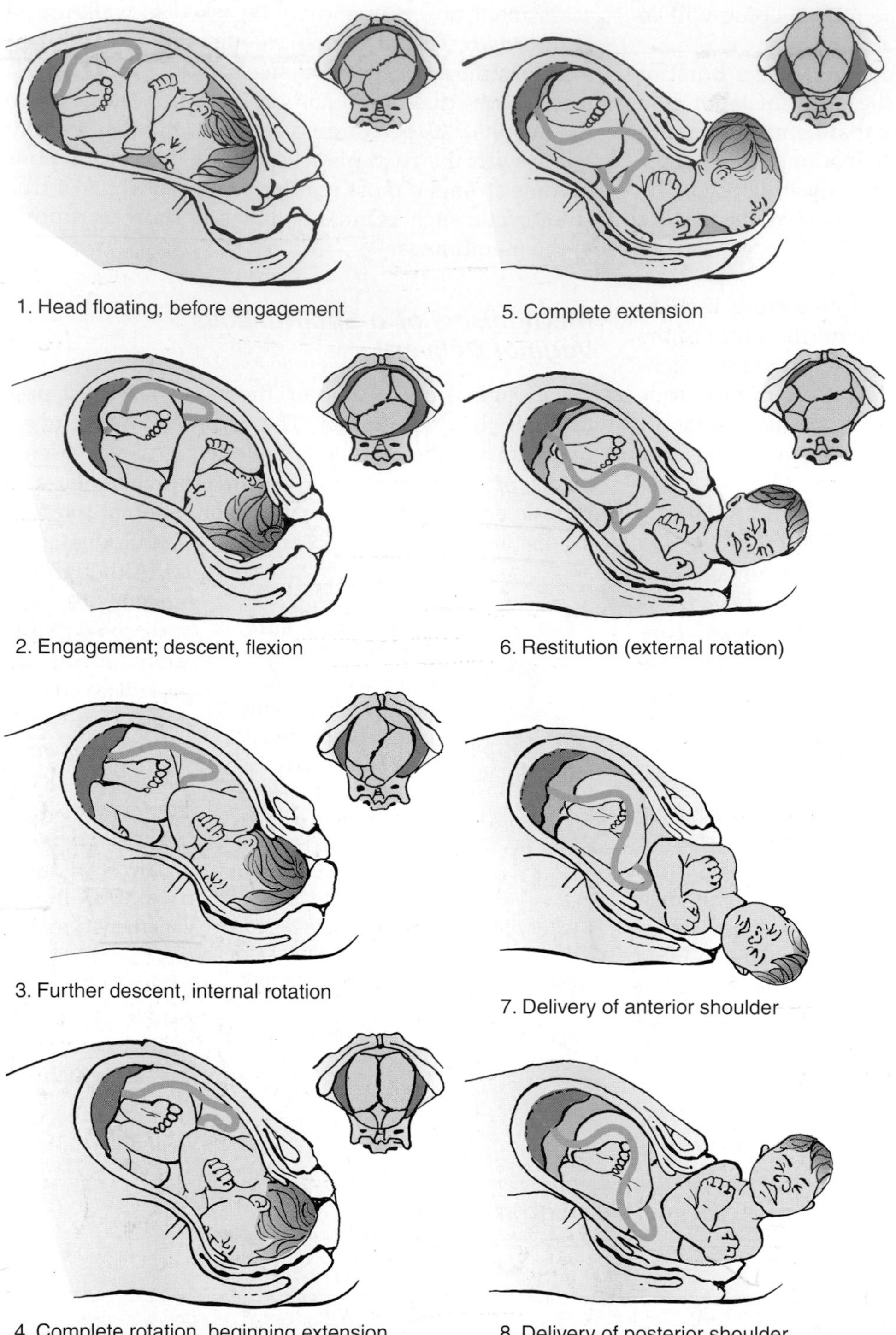

● ***Figure 8.11*** The cardinal movements (or mechanisms) of delivery.

2 weeks before labor or not until after the onset of labor. Engagement is more likely to occur earlier in the primigravida and later in the multigravida.

Flexion is the attitude that presents the smallest diameters of the fetal head to the dimensions of the pelvis. As the head descends during labor, the fetus often is coaxed into and assumes an attitude of flexion as the head encounters resistance from the muscles of the pelvic floor.

Frequently in early labor the fetal head presents to the pelvis in a transverse position because the pelvis is widest from side to side. During active labor, the fetal head typically rotates from a transverse position to an anterior position that is most favorable for a vaginal delivery. This movement is called internal rotation. Labor can be prolonged if the fetus does not rotate because the widest diameters of the fetal head present to the pelvis, resulting in a less than optimal fit

Think this through. If the fetal head enters the pelvis in a transverse position, the fetus has to rotate only 45 degrees to the anterior position. However, if the fetal head enters the pelvis in an occiput posterior position, the fetus must rotate 90 degrees to the preferable anterior position. Several things may happen in this scenario. The labor may be unusually prolonged and painful while the baby rotates, and/or the birth may be painful and traumatic if the fetus delivers face up, a condition referred to as a persistent posterior position. It is typical for a woman to complain of back labor when the fetus is in the posterior position. Sometimes a cesarean delivery is needed if the fetus does not rotate to the anterior position.

between the head and the bony passageway.

Extension must occur for the fetal head to pass under the pubic arch. The head is usually well flexed on the chest as the fetus travels through the birth canal, but when the fetus reaches the pubic arch, it must extend under the symphysis pubis. As the newborn's head is born, external rotation (restitution) lines the head up with the shoulders. Expulsion (birth) occurs after delivery of the anterior and posterior shoulders.

Test Yourself

- List three anticipatory signs of labor.
- What is the main difference between true and false labor?
- List the cardinal movements of labor.

Stages and Duration of Labor

Labor is categorized into four stages, and the first stage is divided further into three phases. Each stage and phase of labor has unique characteristics that help the nurse and physician or midwife determine if labor is progressing as expected. It is important to note that individual labors vary greatly with regard to length. Many factors affect the progress of labor, such as use of agents to soften the cervix, labor induction techniques, and type of anesthesia (if any) used. These factors are discussed in other chapters.

Pay attention! This can be confusing. Although technically a woman who has never delivered a viable child is considered a nullipara, when she goes into labor, she is usually referred to as a primipara.

The following discussion focuses on the physical characteristics of each stage of labor and approximate time periods of each stage. Because parity influences labor progress, typical differences between the primiparous woman and the multiparous woman are noted.

First Stage: Dilation

The first stage of labor begins with the onset of true labor and ends with full dilation of the cervix at 10 centimeters. This stage is subdivided into three phases: latent, active, and transition.

Early Labor (Latent Phase). Early labor begins when the contractions of true labor start and ends when the cervix is dilated 4 centimeters. Contractions during this phase are of mild intensity and may occur as infrequently as every 30 minutes, although the frequency typically ranges between 5 and 10 minutes with a duration of 30 to 45 seconds. In a normal labor, the pattern of contractions during the latent phase becomes increasingly regular with shorter intervals between contractions.

This advice may be helpful on a test! It is easy to confuse phases of the first stage of labor with stages of labor. Be sure you are able to clearly define each stage and phase so that you do not confuse the phases with the stages during an examination.

This phase lasts on average approximately 8 to 9 hours for a primiparous woman but generally does not exceed 20 hours in length. Multiparous women usually experience shorter labors. The average length of the latent phase for a multipara is approximately 5 hours, with an upper limit of 14 hours.

Active Labor (Active Phase). The active phase begins at 4 centimeters cervical dilation and ends when the cervix is dilated 8 centimeters. Contractions typically occur every 2 to 5 minutes, last 45 to 60 seconds, and are of moderate to strong intensity. This stage is characterized normally by progressive cervical dilation and fetal descent.

Here's a tip for encouraging the woman. Sometimes nulliparous women become discouraged during the early phase of labor, particularly if the length approaches the 20-hour mark and the cervix is still dilated less than 3 cm. The woman should be told that the cervix of a woman who has never delivered a child effaces before it dilates. The contractions during early labor thin the cervix, whereas the contractions of active labor tend to cause more rapid dilation.

For primiparas, dilation should occur at approximately 1.2 centimeters/hour. Multiparas progress at a slightly faster pace of 1.5 centimeters/hour. These designations are only approximations and may vary a great deal if the woman receives medication, anesthesia, or other medical intervention during labor. Fetal descent is often slow in the first stage of labor regardless of parity. Occasionally the fetus does not descend during active labor.

Transition (Transition Phase). Transition is considered to be the most difficult part of labor. This phase of the first stage of labor starts when the cervix is dilated 8 centimeters and ends with full cervical dilation. The contractions are of strong intensity, occur every 2 to 3 minutes, and are of 60 to 90 seconds in duration.

Frequently the woman will experience a strong urge to push as the fetus descends. It is important for the woman to resist the urge to push until the cervix is dilated completely. Pushing against a partially dilated cervix can cause swelling, which slows labor, or the cervix can develop lacerations, leading to hemorrhage.

Second Stage: Birth

The second stage begins when the cervix is dilated fully and ends with the birth of the infant. The contractions usually continue at a frequency of every 2 to 3 minutes, last 60 to 90 seconds, and are of strong intensity. The average length of the second stage is 1 hour for primiparas and 20 minutes for multiparas, although it is considered normal for a primipara to be in this stage for 2 hours or longer.

During the second stage, the woman is encouraged to use her abdominal muscles to bear down during contractions while the fetus continues to descend and rotate to the anterior position. Fetal descent is usually slow but steady for the primipara. Frequently the fetus of a multipara, after not making significant downward progress for several hours during active labor, will suddenly descend and be born with one push. When the fetus is at a station of +4, he proceeds to move through the cardinal movements of extension and external rotation, followed by delivery of the shoulders and expulsion of the rest of the body.

Third Stage: Delivery of Placenta

Stage three begins with the birth of the baby and ends with delivery of the placenta. A time frame of 5 to 20 minutes is considered normal for both primiparas and multiparas. Signs that indicate the placenta is separating from the uterine wall consist of a gush of blood, lengthening of the umbilical cord, and a globular shape to the fundus.

The placenta usually delivers spontaneously by one of two mechanisms. Expulsion by Schultze's mechanism indicates that the fetal or shiny side of the placenta delivers first. Delivery by Duncan's mechanism specifies that the maternal or rough side of the placenta presents first.

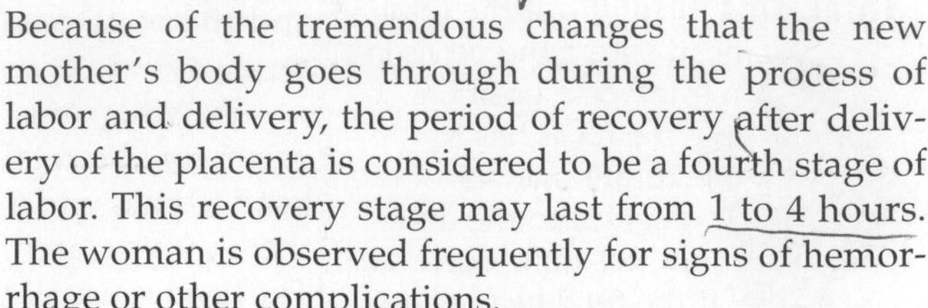

Fourth Stage: Recovery

Because of the tremendous changes that the new mother's body goes through during the process of labor and delivery, the period of recovery after delivery of the placenta is considered to be a fourth stage of labor. This recovery stage may last from 1 to 4 hours. The woman is observed frequently for signs of hemorrhage or other complications.

MATERNAL AND FETAL ADAPTATION TO LABOR

Maternal Physiologic Adaptation

Labor has an effect on the woman as if she were engaged in moderate to vigorous aerobic exercise. There is an increased demand for oxygen during the first stage of labor, attributable in part to the energy used for uterine contractions. To meet the demand, there is a moderate increase in cardiac output throughout the first stage of labor. During pushing (second stage), cardiac output may be increased as much as 40% to 50% above the prelabor level. Immediately after birth, it may peak at 80% above the prelabor level.

The pulse is often at the high end of normal during active labor. These normal increases in the heart rate are accentuated if the woman becomes dehydrated or exhausted with the work of labor. Blood pressure, however, does not change appreciably during normal labor, although the stress of contractions may cause a 15-mm Hg increase in the systolic pressure. The increased demand for oxygen and the pain of uterine contractions cause the respiratory rate to increase, which puts the laboring woman at risk for hyperventilation. Mouth breathing and dehydration contribute to dry lips and mouth.

Labor prolongs the normal gastric-emptying time. This change often leads to nausea and vomiting during active labor and increases the woman's risk for aspiration, particularly if general anesthesia is required. Traditionally, the laboring woman has been given intravenous (IV) fluids while solid food and fluids are withheld. However, research shows that the risk for aspiration remains high, even if the woman is maintained on a nothing by mouth (NPO) status because gastric secretions become more acidic during periods of fasting. The newer recommendations are to allow the laboring woman to have clear liquids, unless there is a high likelihood that she will deliver by cesarean.

Pressure on the urethra from the presenting part may cause overfilling of the bladder, a decreased sensation to void, and edema. A full bladder is uncomfortable and slows the progress of labor. As the bladder fills, it rises upward in the pelvic cavity, which puts pressure on the lower uterine segment and prevents the head from descending. Sometimes the use of an in-and-out (straight) urinary catheter becomes necessary to empty the bladder.

Some laboratory values are affected by labor. The stress of vigorous labor may cause an increase in the white blood cell (WBC) count to as high as 30,000/mm^3. This increase is the body's normal response to inflammation, pain, and stress. Frequently the urine specific gravity is high, indicating concentrated urine, and there may be a trace amount of urinary protein because of increased metabolic activity. Gross proteinuria is never considered normal during labor and is a sign of a developing complication.

Maternal Psychological Adaptation

Labor is hard work that puts a demand on the woman's coping resources. The woman's response changes as labor progresses. During early labor the woman is often excited and talkative, although anxiety and apprehension are common responses. As labor becomes active, the woman becomes more introverted and focuses her energies on coping with the stress of contractions. Women who are unprepared psychologically for labor lose control easily during the active phase and may resort to crying, screaming, or thrashing about during contractions. This response may impede the labor process by causing muscular tension. Tense muscles work against cervical dilation and fetal descent.

Transition is the most intense phase of the first stage of labor, and many women, even ones who have had natural childbirth classes, have a difficult time maintaining positive coping strategies during this phase of labor. Many women describe feeling out of control during this phase of labor. A woman in transition needs support, encouragement, and positive reinforcement. Once pushing efforts begin, the woman usually feels more in control and is better able to cope.

CULTURAL SNAPSHOT

The laboring woman's culture influences her response to pain. In some cultures the woman is expected to accept pain stoically. In other cultures loud expressions of pain are accepted. It is important to perform a careful assessment of a woman's discomfort and to determine measures the laboring woman thinks would be helpful to relieve the pain. Just because the woman is quiet during labor does not mean that she is not experiencing pain. (Refer to Chapter 9 for an in-depth discussion of pain management during labor.)

BOX 8.3 Evaluating Fetal Scalp pH

Fetal pH

- Greater than 7.25
  - Reassuring
  - Associated with normal acid-base balance
- Between 7.20 and 7.25
  - Worrisome
  - May be associated with metabolic acidosis
- Less than 7.20
  - Critical
  - Represents metabolic acidosis
- Less than 7.0
  - Damaging
  - Frequently associated with fetal neurologic damage

Maternal responses to the actual birth vary widely. Many mothers are excited and eager to see and hold the baby. Others are exhausted and may doze intermittently. Most new mothers are anxious about the baby's health. When the woman holds the baby for the first time, it is normal for her to use fingertip touching and for her to explore the infant and count his fingers and toes.

Fetal Adaptation to Labor

Normal labor stresses the fetus in several ways. Intracranial pressure is increased as the fetal head meets resistance from the birth canal. Sometimes this increased pressure results in a slowing of the fetal heart rate at the peak of a contraction—a normal phenomenon described in Chapter 10. Placental blood flow, the source of oxygen for the fetus, is temporarily interrupted at the peak of each contraction. Placental blood flow is interrupted for longer periods during pushing efforts. Because of these changes, even the healthy fetus experiences a slowly decreasing pH throughout labor. Box 8-3 describes normal and abnormal changes in fetal pH. Although the fetal cardiovascular system is stressed, a healthy fetus is able to compensate and maintain the heart rate within normal limits.[1] This ability to compensate demonstrates the presence of a healthy neurologic system.

The act of passing through the birth canal is beneficial to the fetus in two ways. The process of labor stimulates surfactant production to promote respiratory adaptation at birth, and as the fetus descends, maternal tissues compress the body, a process that helps clear the respiratory passageways of mucus.

[1] An in-depth discussion of fetal heart rate changes is presented in Chapter 10.

Infants who are born by cesarean section usually require more frequent suctioning because they have not had the benefit of this "vaginal squeeze."

Pressure on the fetus caused by progress through the birth canal may result in areas of ecchymosis or edema, particularly on the presenting part. Pressure on the vertex may cause formation of a **caput succedaneum**, swelling of the soft tissue of the head, or development of a cephalohematoma, collection of blood under the scalp.

Test Yourself

- How many centimeters must the cervix dilate before a woman is considered to be in active labor?
- Which stage requires the woman to help by pushing?
- In which stage of labor does birth occur?

Review

KEY POINTS

- Four essential components of the labor process are the passageway (maternal pelvis and soft tissues), passenger (fetus), powers (involuntary and voluntary muscle contractions), and psyche (psychological state of the woman).
- The bony pelvis is the rigid passageway through which the fetus must pass. There are four basic pelvic shapes: gynecoid, anthropoid, android, and platypelloid. The gynecoid type is the most favorable for vaginal birth. The diameters of the inlet, midpelvis, and outlet are important in determining the adequacy of the pelvis for vaginal delivery.
- The cervix, part of the soft tissue of the passageway, must completely efface (thin) and dilate (open) for the fetus to be born. Full dilation is equal to 10 centimeters.
- The fetal skull is the most important fetal structure because it is the largest and least compressible. A comparison of the diameters of the true pelvis to the diameters of the fetal skull is important when the physician is attempting to determine if a vaginal delivery is possible.
- Fetal lie refers to the relationship of the long axis of the fetus to the long axis of the mother. A longitudinal lie is the most favorable to a vaginal birth.
- The large majority of fetuses enter the pelvis head first, a condition referred to as a cephalic presentation. When the feet or buttocks present first, it is called a breech presentation. A shoulder presentation is uncommon.
- A flexed fetal attitude presents the smallest diameters of the fetal head to the pelvis.
- The part of the fetus that is closest to the cervix is the presenting part. Presentation and attitude together determine the presenting part.
- To determine fetal position, the nurse must first verify the presenting part and locate the reference point: occiput, frontum, mentum, sacrum, etc. Then the relationship of the reference point to maternal pelvic quadrants is determined to confirm fetal position.
- Station is a determination of the relationship of the presenting part to the ischial spines. Zero station occurs when the presenting part is at the level of the ischial spines. When the fetus is high in the pelvis (above the ischial spines), the station is recorded as a negative number. A low station (below the ischial spines) is recorded as a positive number.
- The primary power of labor comes from involuntary uterine contractions, which serve to efface and dilate the cervix. Secondary powers are supplied by maternal pushing efforts during the second stage of labor.
- The contraction pattern (frequency, duration, and intensity) and the resting interval are important to assess because the fetus can become hypoxic if contractions are too close together, too strong, or do not have a rest period.
- Maternal psyche is an important influence on the labor process. Nursing interventions can help break the cycle of fear, tension, and pain that can interfere with labor.
- Theories of what causes labor to begin include progesterone withdrawal theory and the oxytocin and prostaglandin theories. It is most likely that all three of these influences, along with other factors, work together to initiate labor.
- Anticipatory signs of labor include lightening, Braxton Hicks contractions, a burst of energy, and cervical ripening and dilation.
- True labor results in progressive effacement and dilation. It is characterized by contractions that become progressively stronger and occur more frequently. Walking does not cause true labor contractions to stop.
- Engagement, descent, flexion, internal rotation, extension, and external rotation are the mechanisms of delivery or cardinal movements by which the fetus is born.
- Labor is categorized in four stages: first stage, dilation; second stage, birth; third stage, expulsion of placenta; and fourth stage, recovery. The first stage is composed of three phases: latent, active, and transition. Each phase and stage has unique characteristics that differentiate it from other phases and stages.

- Labor affects the mother in much the same way as vigorous exercise does. The heart rate, cardiac output, and respiratory rate increase to meet the body's increased oxygen need. Other systems, notably the gastrointestinal and urinary, are also affected.
- The healthy fetus is able to withstand the stress that labor makes on the cardiovascular system. A vaginal birth helps mature the respiratory system and clears mucus from the respiratory tract

REFERENCES AND SELECTED READINGS

Books and Journals

Cunningham, F. G., Gant, N. F., Leveno, K. J., Gilstrap, L. C. III, Hauth, J. C., & Wenstrom, K. D. (2001). Section IV: Normal labor and delivery. In *Williams obstetrics* (21st ed., pp. 249–330). New York: McGraw-Hill Medical Publishing Division.

Diegmann, E. K., Chez, R. A., & Danclair, W. G. (1995). Station in early labor in nulliparous women at term. *Journal of Nurse Midwifery, 40*(4), 382–385.

Mattson, S., & Smith, J. E. (Eds.). (2000). *Core curriculum for maternal–newborn nursing* (2nd ed.). AWHONN publication. Philadelphia: WB Saunders.

Ruiz, R. J. (1998). Mechanisms of full-term and preterm labor: Factors influencing uterine activity. *JOGNN: Journal of Obstetric, Gynecologic, & Neonatal Nursing, 27*, 652–660.

Simpson, K. R., & Creehan, P. A. (2001). *AWHONN Association of Women's Health, Obstetric and Neonatal Nurses: Perinatal nursing*. Philadelphia: Lippincott Williams & Wilkins.

Wolcott, H. D., & Conry, J. A. (2000). Normal labor. In A. T. Evans & K. R. Niswander (Eds.), *Manual of obstetrics* (6th ed., pp. 392–424). Philadelphia: Lippincott Williams & Wilkins.

Websites

http://www.emedicine.com/aaem/topic284.htm

http://www.ecc.cc.mo.us/ecc/library/web/reserves/normallabor.htm

http://www.ecc.cc.mo.us/ecc/library/web/reserves/normal_labor2.htm

http://www.methodisthealth.com/pregnancy/labor.htm

http://www.pelvicfloor.com/library/library.html?show=yes&subcategoryid=18

http://www.avc.edu/alliedhealth/documents/LaborandDeliveryII.ppt

* flexed fetal attitude presents smallest diameter of fetal head to pelvis.

WORKBOOK

NCLEX-STYLE REVIEW QUESTIONS

1. A 32-year-old woman is dilated 4 centimeters. The physician states that she has a roomy pelvis and the baby is in a right occiput anterior (ROA) position at a +1 station. Her contractions are occurring every 10 minutes, lasting 30 to 40 seconds, and palpate mild in intensity. She is calm and relaxed. Given these data, which essential component of labor is unexpected and likely to slow the progress of labor at this time?
   a. Passageway
   b. Passenger
   c. Powers
   d. Psyche
2. A woman near the end of pregnancy comments to the nurse, "I'm curious. What causes labor to begin?" Which reply by the nurse is best?
   a. "It is a mystery. No one knows."
   b. "It is believed that several factors work together to stimulate labor to begin."
   c. "The pituitary gland in the brain releases a special hormone that signals labor to begin."
   d. "You don't need to worry about that. The baby will come when he is ready."
3. The fetus is in a cephalic presentation. His occiput is facing toward the front and slightly to the right of the mother's pelvis and he is exhibiting a flexed attitude. How does the nurse document the position of the fetus?
   a. LOA
   b. LOP
   c. ROA
   d. ROP
4. A woman has just delivered a healthy baby girl, but the placenta has not yet been delivered. What stage of labor does this scenario represent?
   a. First
   b. Second
   c. Third
   d. Fourth

STUDY ACTIVITIES

1. Using the table below, write a brief definition or explanation of each of the "four Ps" of labor. List critical nursing observations/assessments that should be made for each area and briefly describe what should be documented.

Four Ps of Labor	Definition or Explanation	Observations (What to Look for)	Documentation
Passageway			
Passenger			
Powers			
Psyche			

2. Develop a teaching aid or poster explaining the stages of labor to a first-time pregnant woman.
3. Have a discussion with your clinical group about the way culture affects behaviors and choices regarding labor and birth. Compare different rituals and taboos of which your classmates are aware that relate to labor and birth.

CRITICAL THINKING: What Would You Do?

Apply your knowledge of the components of labor to the following situation.

1. Anna, a 25-year-old gravida 2, has been in labor for several hours, but her cervix is not dilating. The physician says that Anna's pelvis is roomy and adequate for a vaginal delivery.
   a. In what way do you anticipate the journey of the fetus through the passageway will be affected because Anna's cervix is not dilating?
   b. Discuss two possible causes of the failure of Anna's cervix to dilate.
2. Anna's midwife performs a vaginal examination and states the fetus is "occiput posterior."
   a. Anna asks you, "What does it mean that the baby is occiput posterior?" How would you explain this situation to Anna?
   b. What will you tell Anna's partner regarding the probable progress of labor because the fetus is in a posterior position?

3. Anna has been in active labor for 7 hours. She has been quietly coping with contractions with the help of her partner. Now she begins to cry, "I can't stand it anymore!" She screams at her partner, "This is all your fault. You're not helping me at all!"
   a. The nurse performs a pelvic examination. How far do you expect Anna to be dilated? What stage and phase of labor is most likely represented in this scenario?
   b. How will you advise Anna's partner? How can he continue to be helpful and understanding during this difficult part of labor?

4. Anna progresses to the second stage of labor, but the fetus has not rotated to an anterior position, so the baby is delivered face up.
   a. What does the physician document in the delivery note regarding the position of the baby at birth?
   b. How would you expect the baby's head to look after his long journey through the birth canal?
   c. How do you expect Anna will react to the birth of her baby?

Pain Management During Labor and Birth

STUDENT OBJECTIVES

On completion of this chapter, the student should be able to

1. Describe sources of labor pain.
2. Discuss principles of labor pain management.
3. Explain various relaxation techniques that help a woman cope with labor.
4. Compare nonpharmacologic interventions to manage labor pain.
5. Differentiate analgesia from anesthesia.
6. Describe advantages and disadvantages of opioid administration.
7. Compare methods of regional anesthesia.
8. Explain major complications associated with epidural and spinal anesthesia.
9. Discuss reasons general anesthesia is risky for a pregnant woman and her fetus.
10. List life-threatening complications associated with general anesthesia.

KEY TERMS

analgesia
anesthesia
effleurage
intrathecal
opioids

Pain is an individual, subjective, sensory experience. However, a complex interplay of physiologic, psychological, emotional, environmental, and sociocultural factors influences the way a person perceives and responds to pain. A woman's response to labor pain is influenced by all of the aforementioned factors to include her expectations about labor and her confidence in her ability to cope with labor. The licensed practical nurse (LPN) assists the registered nurse (RN) to manage the pain associated with labor and birth.

THE PAIN OF LABOR AND CHILDBIRTH

Uniqueness of Labor and Birth Pain

The pain of labor and birth is different from other types of pain in several ways. In most instances, pain is a warning sign of injury, but labor pain is associated with a normal physiologic process. In other types of pain, greater intensity is often associated with greater injury. During labor, intensity increases as the woman approaches birth, which is the desirable and positive outcome. Although the pain of labor begins without warning, once it is established it occurs in a predictable pattern with respite from pain between contractions. This characteristic is different than most other types of pain. Because it is predictable, the woman can prepare for and better cope with the pain.

Physiology and Characteristics of Labor Pain

There are two general concepts related to pain that are helpful to understand: threshold and tolerance. The pain threshold is the level of pain necessary for an individual to perceive pain. Pain tolerance refers to the ability of an individual to withstand pain once it is recognized. Each woman has her own pain threshold and tolerance of pain. Each woman responds to labor in a unique way, and the experience of labor is reported differently among women. In addition, each labor is experienced uniquely in a woman who bears more than one child.

Pain sensations associated with labor originate from different places, depending on the stage of labor. During the first stage of labor, stimulation of pain receptors in the cervix and lower uterine segment predominates in response to the stretching required to thin and open the cervix. Some researchers hypothesize that labor pain is associated with ischemia to the uterus, in much the same way that ischemia causes angina. However, this theory is debated because blood flow to the uterine muscle is actually increased during a contraction, whereas blood flow to the placenta is decreased. During the second stage of labor the main source of pain is from pressure on the perineum and birth canal as the fetus descends.

Caution! Don't assume that the woman who reports severe pain has low pain tolerance. Always do a thorough assessment because pain that is not manageable with normal interventions may be a signal that something else, other than labor, is occurring. For instance, severe unrelenting abdominal pain in conjunction with a uterus that does not relax may indicate placental abruption. Severe pain may occur with uterine rupture. Epigastric pain is often present in severe preeclampsia just before a seizure. And don't forget that the pregnant woman may also have an undetected medical condition, such as perforated bowel or appendicitis.

Labor pain in the first stage of labor has characteristics similar to other types of abdominal pain. It is often diffuse in nature, occurs in the lower abdomen, and may be referred to the lower back, buttocks, and thighs. It is often described as occurring in waves, with some "waves" more powerful than others. The contraction begins as a sensation of cramping in the lower abdomen or lower back and gradually increases in strength to the peak of the contraction, and then it slowly abates until pain is no longer perceived.

The pain of birth is sometimes described as the most intense sensation of pain. It is generally experienced as an intense sensation of burning in the perineum as the tissues stretch in response to the fetus pressing against them during descent. Often the sensation is so intense that an episiotomy can be done without anesthesia, and the woman does not perceive it.

Factors Influencing Labor Pain

Many factors influence the pain of labor and birth, making it a multidimensional experience. Examples of psychosocial influences include the level of the woman's fear and anxiety, her culture, and the circumstances surrounding the birth experience, such as whether or not the pregnancy is planned or unplanned, the child is wanted or unwanted, the birth is preterm or term, and the fetus is living or dead.

The perceived intensity of labor pain is affected by many variables. The younger the woman, the more likely she is to report severe pain. Women bearing children for the first time also report more intense levels of pain. High levels of anxiety and fear correlate with high levels of perceived pain. A woman who has experienced significant nonobstetric forms of pain usually reports lower levels of pain during labor than does a woman who does not have prior experience with severe pain.

There also are physiologic variables that affect the experience of labor pain. A woman who is physically conditioned usually reports lower levels of pain during labor and birth. The stress of labor causes the body to release endorphins, natural pain-killing substances similar to morphine. Interestingly, levels of endorphins rise as labor progresses and peak immediately after birth. When pharmacologic methods are used to treat the pain of labor, the levels of endorphins circulating in the woman's bloodstream are decreased.

Physiologic factors directly related to the birthing process also affect the perception of pain. In general, the longer the labor the more likely the woman is to report extreme pain. Obstructed labor is usually perceived as being more painful. Obstructed labor can result from fetopelvic disproportion and abnormal fetal positions. Labor that is induced with oxytocin often is reported to be extremely strong. The contractions may be described as intense and lacking the gradual ebb and flow of naturally occurring contractions. Back labor usually is perceived as being intensely painful, even excruciating. Some women report that back labor feels as if the back is literally breaking in two. In addition, when a woman experiences back labor, her pain may not completely resolve between contractions.

Principles of Pain Relief During Labor

There is no one "perfect way" to control labor pain. Each woman responds to the experience uniquely. Research has shown that women report higher levels of satisfaction with their labor experience when they feel a high degree of control over the experience of pain (McCrea & Wright, 1999). The nurse owes it to the woman to inform her of pain management options and to be supportive of the choices that she makes. It is also important to remember that the woman has the right to change her mind about the acceptability of any particular pain management technique at any time before or during labor.

Sensitivity and understanding go a long way! It is important for the nurse to be nonjudgmental when assisting a woman to cope with pain. Too often, nurses project their own values regarding labor pain onto the woman. Some nurses feel very strongly that a woman should have a "natural" childbirth without pharmacologic intervention. Other nurses don't understand why any woman would want to "suffer" through labor without an epidural. In both situations, the nurse is in danger of not providing the support that the laboring woman needs and deserves.

Rarely is there a completely pain-free labor. Even when a woman receives an epidural, she frequently reports severe pain before the epidural is administered. Caregivers commonly underrate the severity of pain when compared with the woman's ratings (Leeman et al., 2003a). It is important to accept the woman's description of the severity of the pain, even when she may not appear to be in pain.

CULTURAL SNAPSHOT

A woman's cultural values influence the way that she responds to pain. Some women are very vocal. They may cry or moan with pain. Some women display a stoic response to pain. They may be very quiet or appear to be resting. Caregivers frequently underestimate the pain of both types of women. The woman who is vocal may be labeled a "difficult" patient who does not handle pain well. The stoic woman may be labeled a "good" patient. However, neither of them is likely to get the pain control that they need, unless the nurse does a careful pain assessment.

Ideally the woman will discuss labor pain management with her primary care provider during the pregnancy and will attend prenatal classes. The woman who enters labor knowing what to realistically expect usually copes better and reports a more satisfying labor experience than does one who is not as well prepared. However, if the woman is not prepared, the nurse can teach the woman what to expect and assist her to cope when she presents in labor.

PAIN MANAGEMENT TECHNIQUES

Labor pain management techniques can be divided into two major categories: nonpharmacologic interventions and pharmacologic interventions. Safety considerations for the woman and her fetus are an important part of the nursing care plan for both categories.

Nonpharmacologic Interventions

Almost every woman uses some type of nonpharmacologic pain intervention during labor, even when pharmacologic methods are used. Most commonly, a woman uses a combination of techniques to cope with labor. She may need assistance coping before medication is used or in conjunction with medication.

There are numerous methods of nonpharmacologic pain relief. Some interventions have been researched and are known to be effective. Some have not been well

TABLE 9.1 Comparison of Selected Nonpharmacologic Interventions for Relief of Labor Pain

Intervention	Effectiveness to Relieve Labor Pain	Advantages	Disadvantages
Continuous labor support	Highly effective throughout labor. May increase the woman's perception of personal control, a factor that correlates with higher satisfaction with the labor experience.	• Low technological/high-touch intervention • Addresses the emotional and spiritual aspects of labor and birth.	Most busy labor and delivery hospital settings cannot provide this level of support for the laboring woman, so the woman and her husband must usually hire a doula if they desire this level of support.
Patterned breathing	Can be very effective when the woman has practiced before labor and has an attentive labor coach.	• Does not require any special tools. • Promotes relaxation. • Basic patterns can be taught by the nurse when the couple presents in labor.	Requires training and practice before labor to be most effective.
Effleurage	Can be helpful during early labor to decrease the sensation of pain.	• Is easy to learn and simple to perform. • Does not require any special tools.	Is less effective during active labor as the contractions become more intense.
Water therapy	Highly effective to promote relaxation and decrease the sensation of pain, especially during the 1st hour or two of use.	• Many women find water very comforting during labor. • Promotes relaxation.	• Requires availability of a tub—equipment that is not always available in the hospital setting. • May slow labor if used too early. • The woman may notice decreased effectiveness over time.
Imagery	Can be very effective for some women.	• Is noninvasive. • Requires no special tools. • Incorporates spirituality with the birthing process.	• Requires discipline and practice to achieve maximum benefit. • May not be appropriate for individuals with mental illness or history of emotional trauma.
Hypnosis	Carefully selected women can benefit from hypnosis during labor.	• Requires no special tools. • Promotes the woman's sense of control over her pain. • Involves a holistic approach to labor.	• Special training by a therapist is required. • Can be expensive and may not be covered by insurance. • Does not work for all women. • Severe anxiety and psychosis is a possible side effect.
Intradermal water injections	Very effective to relieve back pain during labor.	• Can be administered by the nurse.	• Invasive (requires an injection). • Not effective for abdominal discomfort associated with contractions.
Acupressure and acupuncture	Anecdotal reports suggest that these therapies may be helpful to reduce the pain of labor.	• Addresses the holistic nature of labor and incorporates spiritual and emotional aspects. • Acupressure is noninvasive.	• Requires a trained practitioner to perform. • Acupuncture is invasive and requires special needles.

researched. However, the intervention that works for the woman is frequently the best one to use. Typically a woman will need a variety of interventions throughout labor. As labor becomes more intense, she frequently needs to try different methods. For example, effleurage and distraction are often helpful in early labor, but not as effective in active labor and transition. Table 9-1 compares selected nonpharmacologic interventions.

Continuous Labor Support

Continuous labor support with a trained nurse or doula (trained lay person who supports and coaches a woman during labor) has been shown to be effective to increase the coping ability of the laboring woman. Additional benefits include a decrease in requests for pain medication, fewer obstetric interventions, and a lower cesarean delivery rate. The same benefit is not afforded when nurses provide intermittent labor support, as is typical for busy labor and delivery settings. The nurse can encourage the woman to hire a doula, particularly if childbirth is desired with minimal medical intervention.

Comfort Measures

Don't underestimate the need for comfort measures during labor. Encourage the use of lip balm to keep the lips hydrated during labor. Ice chips, lollipops, and clear liquids (if allowed) can be helpful to moisten the mouth. Mouth breathing during labor can lead to dry mouth.

Change the linens when they become soiled with perspiration or body fluids. Most facilities have pads that are placed under the buttocks to catch bloody show and amniotic fluid during labor. Explain to the woman that it will be impossible to keep her completely dry, but reassure her that you will change the pads frequently. Give perineal care with warm water after she uses the restroom and before changing the linens.

Relaxation Techniques

Relaxation is the objective of almost every nonpharmacologic intervention. When the woman becomes anxious or apprehensive, she tenses her muscles. This action can slow the labor process and decrease the amount of oxygen reaching the uterus and the fetus. When the woman maintains a state of relaxation during and between contractions, she is actually working with her body to facilitate the labor process. The following discussion highlights several techniques that may help the woman to relax during labor. Some of these methods should be learned from a trainer and practiced before labor to be most effective, although the nurse can teach the woman and her partner some of the basic techniques when she presents to the delivery suite.

Patterned Breathing. In times past, very structured breathing techniques were taught during childbirth classes. Now the trend is to teach basic principles of patterned breathing without emphasizing strict patterns. In general the woman begins with a slow-paced breathing pattern. She maintains the slow-paced pattern until it is no longer working to enhance relaxation, and then she switches to a higher level. Table 9-2 describes the basic breathing patterns that are often taught in childbirth preparation classes.

All breathing patterns should begin and end with the woman taking a cleansing breath. A cleansing

TABLE 9.2 Patterned Breathing Techniques for Labor*

Breathing Pattern	Description
Slow-paced breathing	The woman takes slow, deliberate breaths while she focuses on maintaining a relaxed stance. She may use effleurage, music, or any technique that encourages relaxation while using slow-paced breathing. The rate is approximately 6 to 10 breaths per minute.
Modified-paced breathing	The woman begins taking slow, deep breaths at the beginning of the contraction. She then increases the rate while decreasing the depth of respirations as she reaches the contraction peak, after which she slows the rate and increases the depth.
Patterned-paced breathing or the "pant-blow" technique	This technique is similar to modified-paced breathing with the addition of a rhythmic pattern. There are several rhythms that can be taught; however, the 4-to-1 rhythm is a popular one. The woman takes 4 light breaths and then blows out through her lips, as if she is blowing out a candle. Different rhythms can be used, such as 4-to-1, followed by 6-to-1 and repeating through the peak of the contraction.

* Note that each pattern begins and ends with a cleansing breath.

breath is a deep, relaxed breath that signals the woman to relax and provides deep ventilation. Breathing may be done through the nose or through the mouth, whichever is most comfortable and natural for the woman. If she breathes through her mouth, pay particular attention to measures to keep the mouth moist.

Breathing should be comfortable to the woman and should not cause her to hyperventilate. If she feels short of breath, she may need to take deeper breaths. If she begins to tingle in her hands and around her mouth, she is probably hyperventilating. She should slow her breathing and breathe into her cupped hands or a paper bag until the tingling stops.

Attention Focusing. Many childbirth classes teach methods of attention focusing, or concentration. Women attending Lamaze-oriented classes are encouraged to focus internally or externally, whichever is more effective. Bradley classes advocate an internal focus because Dr. Bradley, the method's founder, believed that external focus distracts the woman from the job of "listening to her body" while laboring. Attention focusing, or concentration, helps the woman to work with her body, instead of panicking.

Another name for internal focus is imagery. Imagery is a technique used to help the woman associate positive thoughts with the birth process. The method engages the senses and promotes relaxation. The woman is encouraged to visualize a positive, healing situation during contractions. For example, some childbirth educators encourage the woman to visualize each contraction as a wave. As the contraction strengthens, the tide rises. As the contraction fades away, the tide ebbs. Or the woman may visualize her body opening and allowing the fetus to pass through. Sometimes the woman visualizes herself at a favorite relaxing place, such as the beach or in a comfortable chair at a vacation cabin. Music is sometimes used in association with imagery to help the woman focus and relax.

The woman who focuses externally opens her eyes and focuses on a picture, person, or object that is helpful to her. For example, one woman used a picture of her grandmother as her focus. As she looked into her grandmother's face during her contractions, she drew strength remembering that her grandmother had birthed 11 babies, all at home without drugs. Another used as her focus a picture of a mountain she and her husband had climbed. As she labored, she remembered her feelings as she overcame the challenges of the ascent of the mountain and likened it to the challenge of her labor. Knowing the feeling of accomplishment she felt as she reached the peak of the mountain, she felt strengthened knowing she would have a strong sense of achievement when she felt her baby slide from her body and held him in her arms. Focusing on sounds, music, voices, relaxation, and breathing may also benefit the laboring woman.

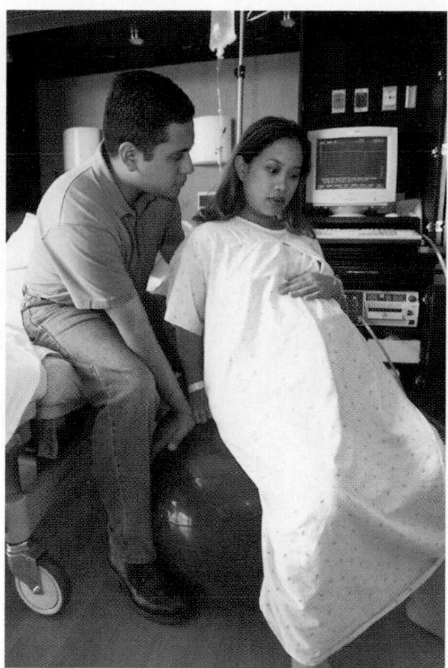

● ***Figure 9.1*** A woman uses a birthing ball to position herself during labor.

Movement and Positioning. Changing positions frequently can be helpful during labor. Any position of comfort is acceptable, as long as the fetal heart rate stays within the normal range. If the woman wants to be on her back, be certain to place a pillow or a wedge under one hip to prevent supine hypotension. The woman may find a birthing ball to be helpful (Fig. 9-1). The ball allows her to rock and move to a position of comfort. Women who are encouraged to ambulate and reposition themselves, as needed, during labor report higher satisfaction levels with the birthing process.

Touch and Massage. Effleurage, a form of touch that involves light circular fingertip movements on the abdomen, is a technique the woman can use in early labor (Fig. 9-2). The theory is that light touch stimulates the nerve pathways to the brain and keeps them busy, thereby blocking the pain sensation. As contractions become stronger during active labor, effleurage becomes less effective. At that point, deeper pressure can be used. Direct pressure may be applied with the hands over the area of greatest pain intensity, often above the pubic bone or on the upper thighs. Abdominal pressure may be applied by the woman or by her partner/coach.

If the woman is experiencing intense back labor, it is often helpful for the nurse or partner to give the woman a massage over the lower back or to use the fists or palms of the hands to apply counter-pressure (Fig. 9-3). Alternately, a tennis ball can be used to massage the lower back.

Water Therapy. Exposure to warm water either by showering or bathing in a tub or whirlpool can signifi-

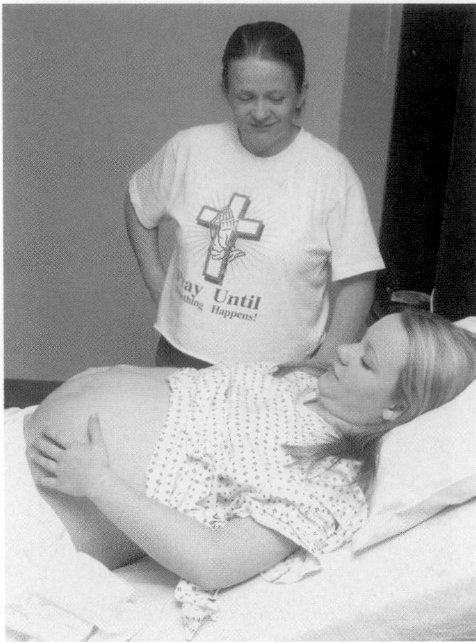

● ***Figure 9.2*** Effleurage. The woman uses her fingertips to lightly touch her abdomen using circular strokes. This form of light touch often decreases the sensation of pain in early labor.

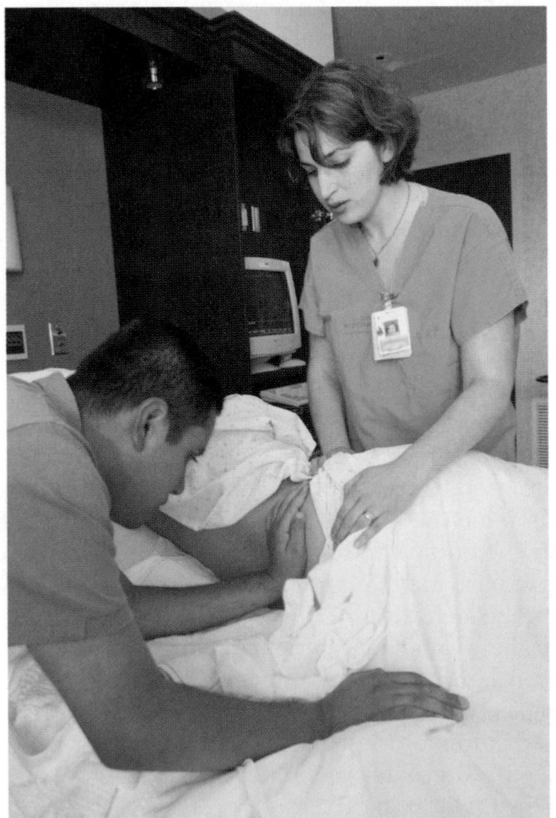

● ***Figure 9.3*** The woman's partner uses the palm of his hand to apply counter-pressure to the woman's lower back.

cantly increase the ability of the laboring woman to cope with uterine contractions. In fact, some women use water not only to provide labor pain relief, but they also deliver in water. Figure 9-4 shows a woman using water to help her relax during labor.

Suggestions for using water safely during labor differ slightly between authors. Leeman et al. (2003a) recommend that the water temperature be maintained at or lower than body temperature, that the woman be in active labor (at 5 centimeters) before using water, and that the bath be limited to 1 to 2 hours in length. Waterbirth International (undated) recommends using a water temperature of 95°F to 100°F (not to exceed 101°F). This organization also suggests that the woman get in the water whenever she chooses to do so, with the caveat that entering water before 5 centimeters of cervical dilation may cause labor to progress more slowly. There is no time limit given for bathing, although the organization does suggest that the 1st hour in the water is usually the most relaxing and helpful for the laboring woman.

There are differing opinions in the medical establishment regarding the safety and advisability of using water during labor and birth. Current research confirms the safety and efficacy of this intervention. However, more research is needed to establish guidelines for practice and to encourage more hospital settings to provide water therapy during labor.

Hypnosis. Hypnosis has been successfully used to help a woman relax and decrease the pain of labor. The woman attends several sessions with a trained therapist during pregnancy. At each session she learns how to induce a trance-like state that she can use during labor. Hypnosis can induce intense states of anxiety or psychosis in certain individuals.

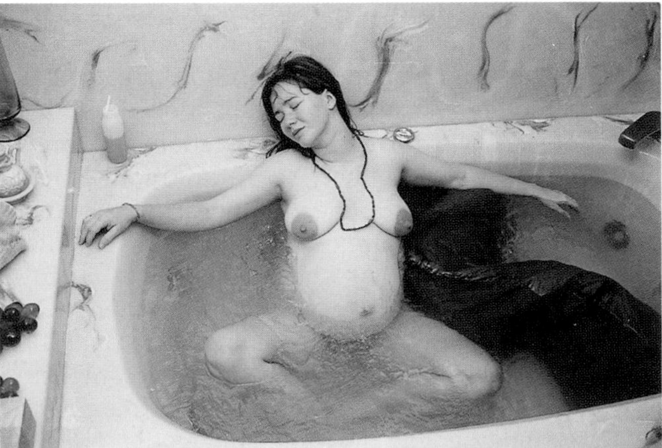

● ***Figure 9.4*** A woman at full dilation waits for the urge to push while relaxing in water at home. The woman reports that although this was her largest child, this labor and birth was the easiest for her. She attributes this to the water therapy. Photo by Kaye Bullock, CPM.

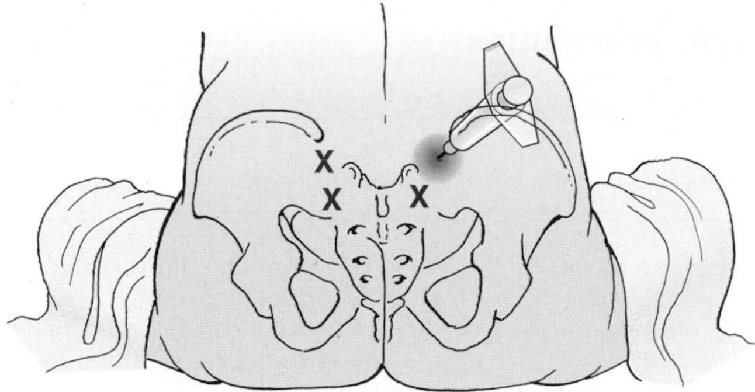

● ***Figure 9.5*** Location of intradermal water injections. The nurse administers four sterile water injections to relieve the pain of back labor.

Intradermal Water Injections

Intradermal injections of sterile water have been found to be effective in relieving the pain of back labor (Leeman et al., 2003a). The technique is most effective when two caregivers administer the injections simultaneously. Four injections of 0.1 mL sterile water are given into the intradermal space in the lower back (Fig. 9-5). The injections significantly reduce back pain for 45 to 90 minutes after they are given.

Acupressure and Acupuncture

Acupressure and acupuncture are two similar techniques used in traditional Chinese medicine. The goal is to restore balance by promoting the flow of energy, which decreases muscle tension, promotes relaxation, and decreases the sensation of pain. Acupuncture involves the use of needles, whereas acupressure is a noninvasive form of massage. Both methods involve stimulating energy points. Research has demonstrated that both forms of treatment can be helpful in the treatment of pain; however, research is limited regarding the usefulness of these methods for treating labor pain (Koehn, 2000).

Test Yourself

- Name two general principles of pain relief during labor.
- List three nonpharmacologic methods of labor pain management.
- Describe three relaxation techniques that help increase the woman's ability to cope with labor pain.

Pharmacologic Interventions

One reason women began to choose the hospital as a place to deliver babies was for the pharmacologic pain relief methods that were available. The pendulum has swung back and forth regarding the favor in which pharmacologic methods are viewed. In the 1950s women were given strong medications that caused them to forget the pain of labor. Beginning in the 1960s and 1970s, women demanded to have more control and more say over the birth process, and natural childbirth came into favor as the "best" way to experience labor and birth. Currently, many women choose to deliver in hospitals so that they can get pain relief from epidural analgesia.

It is important to understand the difference between analgesia and anesthesia, although the terms are sometimes used interchangeably. **Analgesia** is the use of medication to reduce the sensation of pain. **Anesthesia** is the use of medication to partially or totally block all sensation to an area of the body. Anesthesia may or may not involve loss of consciousness. Table 9-3 compares pharmacologic medications used to relieve labor pain.

Analgesia and Sedation

Sedatives are given to promote sedation and relaxation; however, they do not provide direct pain relief (analgesia). Barbiturates, such as secobarbital (Seconal) and pentobarbital (Nembutal), may be given in early labor to promote sleep. These medications can cause respiratory and central nervous system depression in the newborn if given within 12 to 24 hours of birth (Poole, 2003).

Be very careful! Always warn the woman and her support person to call the nurse before she tries to get up after IV sedation has been administered. Women have experienced falls when attempting to ambulate after IV sedation. Women have delivered their babies unattended in the bathroom after being sedated because they mistake the urge to push for the need to have a bowel movement. Physical injury can occur to the newborn when the delivery is unattended. For example, the cord can break, leading to hemorrhage. Or the newborn can be physically injured from falling and hitting the floor.

Opioids, medications with opium-like properties (also known as narcotic analgesics), are the most frequently administered medications to provide analgesia during labor. Opioids, such as meperidine (Demerol) and fentanyl (Sublimaze), blunt the pain sensation but do not completely relieve the pain. These medications frequently assist the woman to better tolerate labor

TABLE 9.3 Comparison of Selected Pharmacologic Interventions for Relief of Labor Pain

Medication Class	Associated Side Effects	Advantages	Disadvantages
Sedatives	• Excessive sedation and/or central nervous system depression • Decreased FHR variability	• Promote sleep in the early stage of labor. • Decrease anxiety. • Promethazine (Phenergan) and hydroxyzine (Vistaril) may be administered with an opioid to decrease nausea and vomiting. • May increase effectiveness of uterine contractions.	• Do not provide pain relief. • Can produce neonatal respiratory depression if given within 12–24 hours of birth.
Opioids (narcotic analgesics)	• Nausea and vomiting • Pruritus • Delayed gastric emptying • Dysphoria • Drowsiness • Hypoventilation • Decreased FHR variability • Neonatal depression (Poole, 2003)	• Increases the woman's ability to cope with uterine contractions. • May be nurse administered.	• Reduces but does not eliminate pain sensations. • Associated with neonatal central nervous system and respiratory depression. • Inhibits neonatal sucking and delays effective feeding. • May decrease neonatal alertness (Leeman et al., 2003b).
Paracervical block	• Fetal bradycardia • Maternal complications are uncommon but include fainting, laceration of the vaginal mucosa, local anesthetic toxicity, hematomas, postpartum neuropathy, paracervical or subgluteal abscesses (Poole, 2003)	• Provides excellent pain relief for the first stage of labor. • Does not interfere with maternal mobility.	• Requires multiple injections because the duration of pain relief is short. • Cannot be used for pain relief in the second stage of labor. • Rapidly crosses the placenta, which can lead to fetal central nervous system depression. • Can cause constriction of the uterine artery, with resultant decrease in blood flow to the placenta. • Is not used frequently because of the association with fetal bradycardia.
Epidural analgesia/ anesthesia	• Hypotension, which often requires administration of medication to raise the blood pressure • Maternal fever • Shivering • Itching (if opioids are used) • Inadvertent injection of anesthetic into the bloodstream • Accidental intrathecal block with possible spinal headache • Inadequate pain relief or failed block • Fetal distress	• Relieves pain better than do opioids. • Often completely eliminates pain sensation. • Anesthesia can be continued indefinitely • If the woman needs a cesarean section, the epidural can be used to provide anesthesia, which saves time in an emergency situation. • Serious side effects are rare.	• Often impairs motor function, which decreases the ability to walk during labor. • Women frequently require urinary catheterization. • Increases the need for labor augmentation with oxytocin, particularly when administered before 5 cm of dilation. • Increases the duration of the second stage of labor. • Vacuum assistance and forceps are more frequently required.

TABLE 9.3 (continued) Comparison of Selected Pharmacologic Interventions for Relief of Labor Pain

Medication Class	Associated Side Effects	Advantages	Disadvantages
			• Increases the likelihood of maternal fever, which increases neonatal sepsis evaluation and antibiotic treatment (Leeman et al., 2003b). • Must be administered by an anesthetist or anesthesiologist. • Requires complex nursing care.
Intrathecal anesthesia (spinal block)	• Hypotension • Shivering • Spinal headache	• Rapid onset of analgesia. • Provides excellent pain relief. • It's the anesthetic method of choice for planned cesarean birth.	• A complete block results in the woman's lower extremities being temporarily paralyzed. • Used alone for labor, the dose might wear off before labor is completed. • Must be administered by an anesthetist or anesthesiologist. • Requires complex nursing care.
General anesthesia	• Hypertension during intubation • Hypotension during maintenance • Difficult or failed intubation • Aspiration of stomach acid/contents • Malignant hypothermia • Uterine atony	• Especially useful in emergency situations because total anesthesia can be accomplished rapidly. • Provides total pain relief.	• Requires intubation, which is more challenging during pregnancy. • All agents used to induce and maintain general anesthesia cross the placenta and can cause severe neonatal depression.

contractions and may induce relaxation and sleep between contractions. Opioids are most frequently given by the intravenous (IV) route because this route provides fast onset and more consistent drug levels than do the subcutaneous or intramuscular routes.

Timing of analgesia administration is important to the safety of the woman and her fetus. If analgesia is given too early in the labor process, the contractions may decrease in frequency and intensity, which can actually prolong labor. If opioids are given too close to delivery, the fetus may be born with respiratory depression, which can interfere with the vital first breaths. Given at the appropriate time, opioids can promote relaxation and cause labor to progress more quickly.

Test Yourself

- What is the difference between analgesia and anesthesia?
- What is another name for opioids?
- What side effect is likely to occur when opioids are given too close to delivery?

Anesthesia

There are three basic types of anesthesia: local, regional, and general. Local anesthesia is used to numb the perineum just before birth to allow for episiotomy and repair.

Keep this tidbit in mind. In general, neonatal respiratory depression is more likely to occur if opioids are administered between 1 and 3 hours before birth occurs. Respiratory depression occurs infrequently when analgesia is timed within 1 hour of birth or at least 4 hours before delivery (Poole, 2003). However, it is not always possible to time medications this precisely. Therefore, be prepared to administer naloxone (Narcan) to the newborn whenever maternal analgesia has been given during labor.

Several types of regional anesthesia are discussed here. In general, regional anesthesia, rather than general anesthesia, is preferred for cesarean births.

Regional Anesthesia. Regional anesthesia involves blocking a group of sensory nerves that supply a particular organ or area of the body. Local anesthetics and opioids are given to induce regional anesthesia/analgesia. The types of regional anesthetics that may be used during labor are pudendal block, paracervical block, epidural anesthesia, combined epidural/spinal anesthesia, and spinal block.

Anytime an anesthetic is administered using any of the techniques described, there is a chance that the local anesthetic agent will inadvertently enter the bloodstream and cause a toxic reaction in the woman. Fortunately, this situation rarely occurs; however, the nurse must be prepared to assist with a full resuscitation, if one is needed. Every facility in which regional anesthetics are administered must have emergency equipment available, including oxygen, oral airway, equipment for emergency intubation and cardiac monitoring, and emergency medications.

It is the nurse's role to assist the anesthesia provider and to closely monitor the woman and her fetus during and after administration of anesthesia. Most of these techniques require IV access. Vital signs must be closely monitored during the procedure and afterward until the vital signs are stable and the effects of the anesthetic have abated.

Pudendal Block. A pudendal block is given just before the baby is born to provide pain relief for the birth. Two injections are given bilaterally into the vaginal wall to block pain sensations to the pudendal nerve. A pudendal block can be helpful when vacuum extraction or forceps are needed to assist the delivery. This method is most effective when administered by an experienced practitioner. If an incomplete block occurs, the practitioner may have to inject additional local anesthesia for episiotomy repair.

Paracervical Block. A paracervical block involves the injection of a local anesthetic in the area close to the cervix. This method provides significant pain relief during the first stage of labor. It cannot be used once complete dilation is attained. The procedure must be repeated frequently because the duration of action is short. One advantage of the technique is that it does not block sensation and movement in the lower extremities, as does epidural anesthesia. Many practitioners do not perform paracervical blocks because of the risk of fetal bradycardia.

Test Yourself

- List three types of regional anesthesia.
- Why is it critical for all facilities in which regional anesthesia is provided to have emergency equipment available?
- Describe a pudendal block.

Epidural Anesthesia. Epidural anesthesia for the management of labor pain has become increasingly popular in the United States. This method usually provides excellent pain relief, often completely blocking pain sensation. The anesthesiologist or nurse anesthetist places a small catheter into the epidural space and then injects the catheter with local anesthetics or opioids to provide pain relief. Sometimes a one-time dose of medication is placed into the spinal fluid (in the subarachnoid space), which is called an **intrathecal** injection, in conjunction with epidural anesthesia. The advantage of the combined epidural/intrathecal technique is that the intrathecal dose is effective almost immediately. It provides pain relief until the epidural begins to work.

Although its use is popular, epidural anesthesia is not without risk. There is significant risk of maternal hypotension that often must be treated with vasopressors (medication to raise the blood pressure). Before a woman receives epidural anesthesia, an IV line must be in place. She must receive 500 to 2,000 mL of IV fluid bolus before medications are administered to reduce the risk of hypotension. Because it is an invasive procedure, informed consent is required.

The anesthetist must evaluate the woman before placing an epidural. The anesthetist reviews the medical history and laboratory results and interviews the woman. The procedure is explained, questions answered, and informed consent obtained. The nurse gives the IV fluid bolus and positions the woman for epidural placement. The woman can be sitting up on the edge of the bed with her feet dangling, or she may be side lying. In either case, it is important for her spine to be arched because this position opens up the spaces between the vertebrae and allows for easier insertion of the catheter. The nurse holds the woman in position or assists the support person to do so (Fig. 9-6). The pulse and oxygen saturation are monitored continuously during the procedure using pulse oximetry. The blood pressure is monitored frequently (sometimes every 3 to 5 minutes) during the procedure.

When the woman is positioned properly, the anesthetist prepares a sterile field with the supplies and medications that will be needed. The woman's back is prepared with alcohol and Betadine. A local anesthetic is used to numb the planned insertion area. A needle is used to enter the epidural space (just outside the dura mater) and a test dose is administered (see Figure 9-6). The anesthetist questions the woman regarding how she feels and what she is experiencing to detect any adverse reaction. If there is none, the anesthetist proceeds to place the epidural catheter, remove the needle, and tape the catheter securely to the woman's back. At this point the nurse assists the woman to a position of comfort. The supine position is avoided, or a wedge is placed under the right hip.

Once the epidural catheter is in place, the anesthetist may intermittently bolus the catheter when the woman begins to feel pain, or a continuous infusion can be set up and connected to the catheter. In either case, it is critical that the epidural catheter be clearly marked so that medications are given by the right route. Management of the epidural is the role of the anesthetist. The nurse monitors for, reports, and treats any untoward effects.

After delivery, the RN stops the continuous infusion and removes the epidural catheter. A sterile pressure dressing is applied to the site. Nursing care during recovery from epidural anesthesia includes assessment of return of sensory and motor function to the lower extremities, and monitoring for urinary retention. The nurse should instruct the woman not to ambulate without assistance. It is a good idea to allow the woman to dangle her legs for a while before she attempts to ambulate. The nurse should be available to provide immediate assistance, if needed, during initial ambulation attempts.

Intrathecal Anesthesia. Intrathecal anesthesia, also known as a spinal block, is similar to epidural anesthesia. The main difference is the location of the anesthetic. Instead of injecting local anesthesia and/or opioids into the epidural space, these medications are placed in the subarachnoid space into the spinal fluid (see Figure 9-6). This type of anesthesia is most frequently used for planned cesarean deliveries. The disadvantage to using

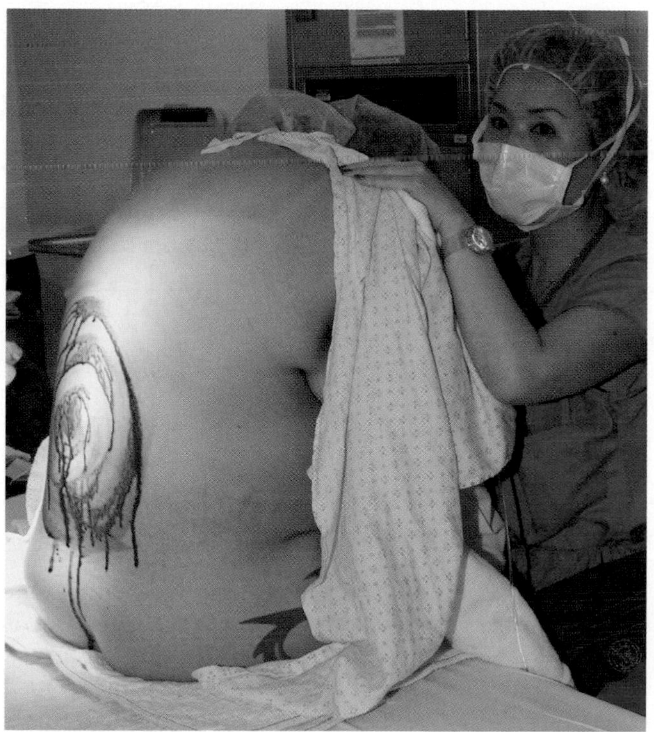

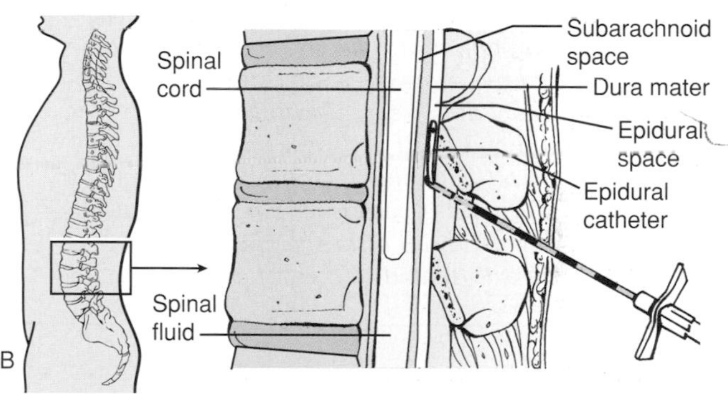

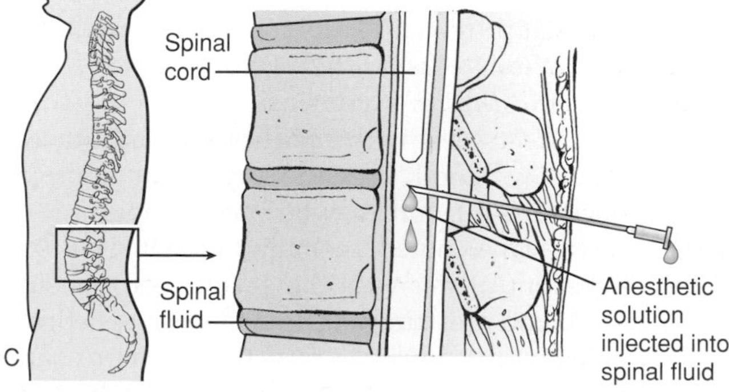

● ***Figure 9.6*** Epidural or intrathecal anesthesia. (**A**) The woman is correctly positioned for epidural anesthesia. (**B**) Location of epidural catheter. Note that the epidural space is located just outside the dura mater. No spinal fluid is present in the epidural space. The epidural catheter is left in place to allow for intermittent or continuous infusion of medications to relieve the pain of labor and birth. (**C**) Location of intrathecal injection. Notice that the needle has a drop of spinal fluid at the hub to indicate the subarachnoid space has been entered. The local anesthetic or narcotic is then injected into this space.

A PERSONAL GLIMPSE

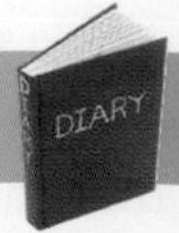

I was 37 weeks' pregnant with my first baby. I started to have some contractions while I was at work. Nothing big; I wasn't even sure they were contractions because they didn't hurt, but I was able to time them at 10 to 15 minutes apart. I went home at lunchtime and called my husband to tell him that I thought I was in labor. He hurried home to be with me. I stayed home the rest of the day and did some light housework. Around 6 p.m. the contractions started to get more intense. I ran some warm water and soaked in the tub. It made me feel better for a while. My husband kept timing the contractions until they were 5 minutes apart. Then I called the hospital, and the nurse told me to come on in. We arrived at the hospital at about 8 p.m. The nurse checked me and said I was at 4 cm and 95% effaced. The nurse suggested that we walk the hallways to speed things along. Sure enough, 45 minutes later, I was a good 5 cm. She asked me if I wanted anything for the pain, and I said no. I was hanging in there just fine. The pain wasn't as bad as I thought it would be. After approximately 45 minutes, the contractions became more intense, and I begged my husband to call the nurse. The nurse checked me and I was 7 cm. By now I was begging for an epidural. The anesthesiologist came in and asked me some questions and told me about some risks. I didn't care. I just wanted the epidural. I had to sit very still through several contractions while the doctor put in the epidural, but it was worth it because the pain went away right away. An hour after the epidural was inserted I was dilated to 8 cm. I was very excited, but then I got stuck at 8 cm for several hours. The doctor thought that the epidural must have slowed down my labor. They were having a hard time monitoring my baby with the external device so they had to insert an internal monitor. Then the nurse started me on Pitocin to help me progress. Sure enough, after an hour of Pitocin I was completely dilated and ready to push. For me, pushing was the hardest part. I still felt no pain because of my epidural, so the nurse had to tell me when I was having a contraction so that I could start pushing. I threw up several times from pushing so hard. However, the baby just didn't come down. After 2 hours, I was totally exhausted. The nurse asked if I wanted her to call the doctor and have her come and use the vacuum to help get the baby out. I was just so tired that I said yes. Elizabeth Michelle was born after just two pushes with the vacuum. She didn't cry at first, so the nurse rushed her to the warming table and gave her some oxygen. Then I heard the most beautiful sound in the world, a cry. My husband and I were thrilled. After the nurse dried the baby, I got to hold her for a while before they took her to the nursery. The baby weighed 7 pounds even, and was 19 1/2 inches long. She was worth everything I went through to have her.

Laura

LEARNING OPPORTUNITY: What questions should the nurse ask the woman about pain relief during labor? What should the nurse tell the woman about pain management options when she presents to the birthing facility in labor?

a spinal block during labor is that the anesthetic might wear off while the woman is still in labor. Nursing care is similar to that provided for epidural anesthesia.

Complications Associated With Epidural and Intrathecal Anesthesia. Hypotension is the most frequent side effect seen with epidurals or intrathecal anesthesia. Low blood pressure occurs in approximately one-third of women who receive epidural or spinal anesthesia. As noted, prehydration with IV fluids helps to prevent or decrease the severity of this side effect. If the blood pressure falls dramatically, ephedrine may be given intravenously to raise the blood pressure.

Spinal headaches occur rarely because of advanced techniques and smaller needle sizes than those used in the past. A spinal headache is suspected when the woman has an intense headache in the upright position that is relieved when she lies still. Treatment involves hydration and having the woman lie flat. Sometimes caffeine is prescribed. Usually the headache will resolve spontaneously in several days. If it does not resolve, an epidural blood patch may be done. In a procedure similar to that used to provide epidural anesthesia, the anesthesia provider injects 20 mL of the woman's blood into the epidural space. The headache is relieved in 95% of women who have the patch.

When narcotics are used in addition to anesthetics, pruritus is a common side effect. Most women tolerate the itching, particularly because the pain relief is generally excellent for the first 24 hours after surgery. Nalbuphine (Nubain), a narcotic agonist-antagonist, and diphenhydramine (Benadryl), an antihistamine, are two medications that may be ordered to treat severe pruritus.

Respiratory depression is another possible side effect when narcotics are used for spinal and/or epidural anesthesia. For this reason, it is recommended that naloxone (Narcan) be readily available to be given intravenously if respiratory depression occurs. Sometimes the anesthesiologist may order continuous pulse oximetry for the first 24 hours. In all cases it is prudent to take vital signs at least every 2 hours and to check on the woman frequently during the first 24 hours after spinal or epidural narcotics have been administered. Nursing Care Plan 9-1: The Woman With Labor Pain describes pain management for a woman in labor.

General Anesthesia. General anesthesia is not used frequently in obstetrics because of the risks involved. The pregnant woman is at higher risk for aspiration. It requires more skill to intubate a pregnant woman because of physiologic changes in the trachea and thorax. In fact, failed intubation is the leading cause of anesthesia-related maternal mortality (Poole, 2003). In addition, general anesthetic agents cross the placenta and can result in the birth of a severely depressed neonate who requires full resuscitation.

When general anesthesia is to be used, the anesthetist usually orders preoperative medications to reduce the risk of aspiration. Bicitra 30 mL may be given orally. Antacids often are ordered to be given intravenously before surgery.

The anesthetist may use an inhalation agent, an IV agent, or more commonly both to induce anesthesia. The woman is preoxygenated with 100% oxygen and then rapidly put to sleep. The RN gives cricoid pressure (pressure with the thumb and forefinger over the cricoid cartilage in the trachea), which closes off the esophagus and decreases the risk of aspiration. Cricoid pressure is maintained until the woman is intubated and the cuff inflated. The anesthetist then manages the airway and continues to administer anesthetic agents and muscle relaxants as needed throughout surgery. Every attempt is made to deliver the baby as quickly as possible after the woman is anesthetized to avoid neonatal depression. The nurse is prepared to resuscitate the newborn, if necessary.

When the surgery is completed, the anesthetist removes the endotracheal tube when the woman is awake and has regained her protective reflexes (swallowing and gagging). The woman is then taken to the postanesthesia care unit (PACU). The RN completes a full assessment; administers oxygen; and monitors oxygen saturation, vital signs, and the continuous electrocardiogram. The RN must be especially vigilant to monitor for hypoventilation after general anesthesia.

Life-threatening complications can occur with general anesthesia. These include failed intubation, aspiration, and malignant hyperthermia. The nurse must be prepared to act quickly in any of these situations.

Because failed intubation is the leading cause of anesthesia-related maternal deaths, the anesthetist must have a variety of tools readily available to use in the event that the woman cannot be intubated quickly. The woman is preoxygenated before every intubation attempt to give the anesthetist time to perform the procedure. If attempts to intubate are unsuccessful, the anesthetist may try to ventilate without intubating the woman. Other options include reversing the anesthesia (i.e., waking the woman) and performing an emergency tracheostomy.

Aspiration is a real threat for the pregnant woman undergoing general anesthesia. Upward pressure of the pregnant uterus on the stomach increases the risk for reflux of stomach contents with subsequent aspiration. Often preoperative medications are ordered to reduce the risk of aspiration. In addition, cricoid pressure by the trained RN during intubation attempts can help prevent this life-threatening complication.

Malignant hyperthermia is a rare, but potentially life-threatening, complication of general anesthesia. It is an inherited condition in which sustained muscle contractions occur when specific anesthetic agents are administered. For this reason, a thorough history is important before general anesthesia is given. Ideally, a pregnant woman with a family history of malignant hyperthermia will be identified in the prenatal period so the health care team can be prepared to care for the woman if general anesthesia becomes necessary. In these cases, it is best for the woman to receive epidural anesthesia during labor. This practice allows for safe anesthesia if a cesarean delivery is performed. If cesarean delivery is planned, the woman usually receives spinal anesthesia.

The nurse must be alert to the development of signs and symptoms of the disorder. Early signs include severe muscle rigidity, tachycardia, irregular heart rhythm, decreased oxygen saturation, and cyanosis. Body temperature can rapidly increase to lethal levels; however, this may be a late sign. Dantrolene sodium is given intravenously to treat malignant hyperthermia. This medication must be readily available in any area in which general anesthesia is administered.

Postoperative nursing care of the woman who receives general anesthesia is similar to that of the woman who receives regional anesthesia. However, careful assessment for hypoventilation and uterine atony are indicated.

Test Yourself

- Describe the procedure for epidural placement.
- List four complications associated with epidural or spinal anesthesia.
- Name two ways to reduce the threat of maternal aspiration when general anesthesia is used.

NURSING CARE PLAN 9.1

The Woman With Labor Pain

CASE SCENARIO:
Patricia (Pattie) Smith is a 29-year-old gravida 1, para 0 at term. She attended childbirth preparation classes with her husband, Ed. Pattie says that she wants to try natural childbirth, but that she might change her mind and request an epidural if the pain becomes unbearable. She is admitted to the hospital in active labor at 4 centimeters dilation. Admitting vital signs are BP 120/76 mm Hg, T 98.7°F, P 70 bpm, R 20 per minute. She describes her pain as starting in the small of her back and then radiating to her lower abdomen with each contraction. She says that the intensity is strong, particularly at the peak of the contraction. Her contractions are occurring every 5 minutes, last 50 to 60 seconds, and palpate moderate intensity. The fetal heart rate is in the 140s to 150s and is reactive.

NURSING DIAGNOSIS
Acute Pain related to uterine contractions.

GOAL: Reports ability to tolerate the pain of labor.

EXPECTED OUTCOMES:
- Uses nonpharmacologic interventions.
- Uses pharmacologic interventions, if desired.
- Expresses satisfaction with pain control.

NURSING INTERVENTIONS	***RATIONALE***
Perform a pain assessment at least every hour during labor to include pain description, location, duration, and intensity (measured by a pain scale).	A thorough pain assessment will reveal the need for more intensive interventions to control the pain of labor.
Note reports of continuous, severe pain. If this occurs, report it to the RN in charge immediately.	Severe, unrelenting pain may be associated with a complication of labor.
Assess general comfort at least every hour. Note the condition of the lips and offer lip balm PRN. Offer ice chips and lollipops to relieve complaints of dry mouth. Give perineal care as indicated, and change the under-buttock pad frequently. Change the linen when it becomes moist with perspiration or other body fluids.	Comfort measures increase the ability of the woman to cope with labor. It is more difficult to cope if the woman has dry, cracked lips, a dry mouth, moist linens, and is in need of perineal care.
Encourage the use of relaxation techniques that are helpful for Pattie.	The more relaxed the woman can remain during labor, the better she will be able to cope with the pain of labor.
Reinforce the use of patterned breathing. Encourage her to switch to a more complex pattern of breathing when simpler patterns are no longer helpful.	Patterned breathing techniques are learned during childbirth classes. Use of these techniques can facilitate relaxation and increase the woman's ability to cope.
Assist Pattie to change positions frequently.	Position changes can help the woman to better cope. If she remains "frozen" in one position, she is more likely to become tense, which increases the perception of pain.
Encourage the use of effleurage, for as long as it is helpful. Encourage the use of pressure when effleurage is no longer helpful.	The use of touch, such as effleurage and pressure, can interrupt the sensation of pain.

Pattie progresses to 8 centimeters dilation. At this point she is having difficulty maintaining control. She thrashes about at the peak of contractions and says that nothing is helping the pain. She begs for an epidural. The obstetrician agrees, and the anesthesiologist is called.

NURSING DIAGNOSIS
Acute Pain related to advanced progress of labor.

GOAL: Ability to cope with labor.

NURSING CARE PLAN 9.1 continued

The Woman With Labor Pain

EXPECTED OUTCOMES:
- Uses nonpharmacologic and pharmacologic interventions.
- Expresses satisfaction with pain control.

NURSING INTERVENTIONS	*RATIONALE*
Remain supportive of Pattie's decision to use an epidural for pain relief.	The woman has the right to change her mind about pain relief interventions and to choose interventions that will best help her to cope.
Reassure Ed that this is a normal response to this phase of the labor process, and that Pattie's request does not represent a failure on his part as her coach.	There is a danger that the coach may feel that he has somehow "failed" when pharmacologic interventions are requested.
Continue to perform a pain assessment every 30 minutes after the epidural is placed.	Frequent assessment of pain will allow for rapid detection of the onset of pain.
Report new complaints of pain to the anesthesiologist.	New reports of pain may signal the need for a bolus of medication through the epidural catheter.

NURSING DIAGNOSIS
Risk for Injury related to possibility of hypotension associated with epidural anesthesia.

GOAL: Maintenance of adequate blood pressure to support perfusion to vital organs, including the placenta.

EXPECTED OUTCOMES:
- Blood pressure will not drop below 90/60 mm Hg.
- Oxygen saturation will remain above 96%.
- Fetal monitor strip baseline will remain above 120 with reactive patterns noted.

NURSING INTERVENTIONS	*RATIONALE*
Prehydrate Pattie with 1,000 cc of lactated Ringer's solution, as ordered.	Prehydration with IV fluid will decrease the risk of hypotension.
Monitor oxygen saturation with pulse oximetry.	A decrease in oxygen saturation can be quickly detected and treated, which will help prevent adverse fetal affects.
Monitor fetal heart tones and reactivity.	Monitoring is done to detect decreases in the fetal heart rate, which may indicate inadequate placental perfusion.
Assist Pattie to a sitting position with her feet dangling over the side of the bed. Demonstrate to Ed how to hold Pattie in the proper position for catheter insertion.	When the woman is in the proper position, the epidural is placed more easily.
Monitor the blood pressure, pulse, and oxygen saturation every 3 to 5 minutes during the procedure.	Frequent monitoring allows for early detection of changes that may indicate the development of a complication.
Once the epidural catheter is taped in place, assist Pattie to a side-lying position.	The side-lying position enhances blood pressure and placental perfusion.
Monitor for signs of urinary retention and insert a Foley catheter, as ordered, if needed.	Epidural anesthesia frequently causes urinary retention, which may interfere with the progress of labor.
Check for progress of labor shortly after the epidural takes effect.	Rapid progress of labor sometimes occurs because the woman relaxes after the pain is relieved.
Monitor for ability to push effectively in the second stage of labor. Report this finding to the anesthesiologist.	Sometimes, epidural anesthesia can interfere with the ability to push effectively. The anesthesiologist may decrease the amount of medication given to allow for partial return of sensation with an increased ability to push.

EVALUATION:
Pattie pushes well and delivers a healthy baby boy 3 hours after she receives her epidural. Her blood pressure remains above 90/60 mm Hg. She reports that she is very satisfied with her labor experience and does not regret getting the epidural.

KEY POINTS

- Sources of pain during the first stage of labor are the thinning and stretching of the cervix in response to uterine contractions. Sources of pain during the second stage of labor are the stretching of tissues in the perineum as the fetus descends.
- Major principles of labor pain management include that women are more satisfied when they have control over the pain experience; caregivers commonly underrate the severity of pain; and women who are prepared for labor usually report a more satisfying experience than do women who are not prepared.
- Nonpharmacologic interventions to relieve labor pain include continuous labor support, comfort measures, various relaxation techniques, intradermal water injections, and acupressure and acupuncture.
- Relaxation techniques that help a woman cope with labor include patterned breathing, attention focusing, movement and positioning, touch and massage, water therapy, and hypnosis.
- Most nonpharmacologic interventions are noninvasive, address emotional and spiritual aspects of birth, and promote the woman's sense of control over her pain. Disadvantages include that many of the interventions require special training and/or practice before birth, and these methods are not effective for every woman.
- Analgesia reduces the sensation of pain. Anesthesia partially or totally blocks all sensation to an area of the body.
- Advantages of opioid administration during labor include an increased ability for the woman to cope with labor, and the medications may be nurse administered. Disadvantages include frequent occurrence of uncomfortable side effects, such as nausea and vomiting, pruritus, drowsiness, and neonatal depression; and pain is not eliminated completely.
- Types of regional anesthesia include pudendal block, paracervical block, epidural anesthesia, combined epidural/spinal anesthesia, and spinal block. A pudendal block provides pain relief for the birth. Paracervical blocks and epidurals provide pain relief during labor.
- Complications associated with epidural and spinal anesthesia include hypotension, maternal fever, shivering, pruritus, inadvertent injection into the bloodstream, spinal headache, and fetal distress.
- General anesthesia is risky for the pregnant woman because of the increased risk for aspiration. It is risky for the fetus because the medications cross the placenta and may result in severe neonatal depression that requires intensive resuscitation.
- Life-threatening complications associated with general anesthesia include failed intubation, aspiration, and malignant hyperthermia. Preoperative antacids and cricoid pressure reduce the incidence of aspiration. Dantrolene sodium is used to treat malignant hyperthermia.

REFERENCES AND SELECTED READINGS

Books and Journals

Cunningham, F. G., Gant, N. F., Leveno, K. J., Gilstrap, L. C. III, Hauth, J. C., & Wenstrom, K. D. (2001). *Williams obstetrics* (21st ed.). New York: McGraw-Hill Medical Publishing Division.

Hawkins, R. M. F. (2001). A systematic meta-review of hypnosis as an empirically supported treatment for pain. *Pain Reviews, 8*, 47–73.

Koehn, M. L. (2000). Alternative and complementary therapies for labor and birth: An application of Kolcaba's theory of holistic comfort. *Holistic Nursing Practice, 15*(1), 66–77.

Leeman, L., Fontaine, P., King, V., Klein, M. C., & Ratcliffe, S. (2003a). The nature and management of labor pain: Part I. Nonpharmacologic pain relief. *American Family Physician, 68*(6), 1109–1112.

Leeman, L., Fontaine, P., King, V., Klein, M. C., & Ratcliffe, S. (2003b). The nature and management of labor pain: Part II. Pharmacologic pain relief. *American Family Physician, 68*(6), 1115–1120.

Mattson, S., & Smith, J. E. (Eds.). (2000). *Core curriculum for maternal–newborn nursing*. AWHONN publication (2nd ed.). Philadelphia: WB Saunders.

McCrea, B. H., & Wright, M. E. (1999). Satisfaction in childbirth and perceptions of personal control in pain relief during labour. *Journal of Advanced Nursing, 29*(4), 877–884.

Poole, J. (2003). Analgesia and anesthesia during labor and birth: Implications for mother and fetus. *JOGNN, 32*(6), 780–793.

Vincent, R. D., & Chestnut, D. H. (1998). Epidural analgesia during labor. *American Family Physician, 58*(8), 1785–1792.

Waterbirth International. (Undated). FAQs: All about Waterbirth. Retrieved March 6, 2004, from http://www.waterbirth.org/spa/content/category/5/65/40/

Websites

http://www.childbirth.org/articles/labor/painrelief.html
http://www.reddinganesthesia.com/labor.htm
http://www.painfreebirthing.com/anatomy.htm

WORKBOOK

NCLEX-STYLE REVIEW QUESTIONS

1. A 22-year-old gravida 2 para 0 is in the doctor's office for a checkup at 36 weeks' gestation. Which comment by the woman indicates that she needs additional information about pain relief during labor?

   a. "I have discussed pain relief options with the doctor and my childbirth educator."

   b. "I'm so glad that I won't have any pain because I'm going to have an epidural."

   c. "I've been practicing the relaxation exercises I learned in my childbirth class."

   d. "I want to have medications through the IV if the pain gets so bad that I can't handle it."

2. The labor nurse reports to the nurse on the on-coming shift, "The woman in labor room 2 is handling her pain very well. She smiles whenever I go in to talk to her, and she doesn't complain at all!" What assessments by the on-coming labor nurse would best reveal if the off-going labor nurse's observations were correct?

   a. Asking the woman to describe her pain and rate it on a scale of 0 to 10.

   b. Observing for grimacing, moaning, and other nonverbal indicators of pain.

   c. Taking the woman's vital signs and observing her interactions with visitors.

   d. No additional assessments are indicated until the woman begins to report pain.

3. A woman asks the nurse during a doctor's visit, "What pain relief method is best?" What answer by the nurse best answers the question?

   a. "Epidurals are best because they provide complete pain relief."

   b. "Most women need IV pain medications at some point during labor."

   c. "It is best to learn and use several methods of pain relief to find the one that works best for you."

   d. "There is no one best way. However, natural childbirth is best for the baby."

4. A 34-year-old gravida 3 para 2 is experiencing severe back pain with each contraction. She is extremely uncomfortable and upset because she never had this type of pain with her other labors. What interventions are most likely to help in this situation?

   a. Comfort measures, intermittent labor support by the nurse, and reassurance that the pain is temporary

   b. Counter-pressure with a fist or tennis ball to the lower back and intradermal water injections

   c. Effleurage, ambulation, and frequent position changes

   d. Hypnosis, imagery, and slow chest breathing

5. The nurse is preparing a woman for epidural anesthesia. The woman asks, "Why is my IV running so fast? It feels cold!" What reply by the nurse is best?

   a. "Don't worry. This is a routine procedure in preparation for an epidural."

   b. "I'll slow the IV down so you won't feel so cold."

   c. "IV fluids help prevent spinal headaches."

   d. "IV hydration helps prevent the blood pressure from dropping too low."

STUDY ACTIVITIES

1. Use the following table to compare advantages and disadvantages of pain relief methods for labor.

Method	Advantages	Disadvantages
Natural childbirth		
IV analgesia		
Epidural anesthesia		
General anesthesia		

2. Develop a teaching plan on the advantages and disadvantages of epidural anesthesia to present to a childbirth education class.
3. Interview the following caregivers in the community regarding their recommendations for pain relief during labor: a doula, a nurse-midwife, a family practice physician, and an

obstetrician. What similarities did you find in their answers? In what ways did they disagree? Which argument did you find most convincing? Share your findings with your clinical group.

CRITICAL THINKING: What Would You Do?

Apply your knowledge of pain management during labor to the following situation.

1. Betty, a 30-year-old gravida 1, reports that she wants to try natural childbirth.
   a. What recommendations will you make to increase the chances that she will be able to experience natural childbirth?
   b. About what will you caution her to decrease the likelihood that she will have unrealistic expectations about pain relief during labor?
2. Betty presents to the labor suite in labor. She is 3 cm dilated, 90% effaced, and at a -1 station. Her contractions are every 3 to 5 minutes apart and of moderate intensity.
   a. What nonpharmacologic pain interventions are most helpful at this point in Betty's labor?
   b. Several hours later, Betty is 5 cm dilated, 100% effaced, at a 0 station. She is requesting IV analgesia. How will you reply?
   c. When Betty reaches 8 cm, she is screaming at the peak of contractions. She says, "I can't stand the pain anymore. I want an epidural." How will you reply?

Nursing Care During Labor and Birth

10

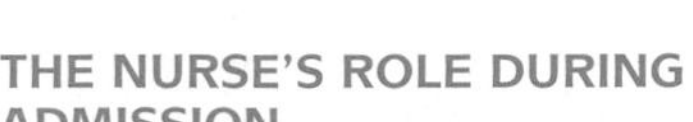

THE NURSE'S ROLE DURING ADMISSION

Immediate Assessments
- *Birth Imminence*
- *Fetal Status*
- *Risk Assessment*
- *Maternal Status*

Additional Assessments
- *Maternal Health History and Physical Assessment*
- *Labor Status*
- *Labor and Birth Preferences*

Performing Routine Admission Orders

THE NURSE'S ROLE: ONGOING ASSESSMENT OF UTERINE CONTRACTIONS AND FHR

Monitoring Uterine Contractions
- *External Methods*
- *Internal Method*

Monitoring FHR
- *Intermittent Auscultation of FHR*
- *Continuous EFM*
- *Evaluating FHR Patterns*
- *Measures Used to Clarify Nonreassuring FHR Patterns*

THE NURSE'S ROLE DURING EACH STAGE OF LABOR

The Nursing Process During the First Stage of Labor (Dilation)

Latent Phase (Early Labor)
- *Assessment*
- *Selected Nursing Diagnoses*
- *Outcome Identification and Planning*
- *Implementation*
- *Evaluation: Goals and Expected Outcomes*

Active Phase (Active Labor)
- *Assessment*
- *Selected Nursing Diagnoses*
- *Outcome Identification and Planning*
- *Implementation*
- *Evaluation: Goals and Expected Outcomes*

Transition Phase
- *Assessment*
- *Selected Nursing Diagnoses*
- *Outcome Identification and Planning*
- *Implementation*
- *Evaluation: Goals and Expected Outcomes*

The Nursing Process During the Second Stage of Labor: Expulsion of the Fetus
- *Assessment*
- *Selected Nursing Diagnoses*
- *Outcome Identification and Planning*
- *Implementation*
- *Evaluation: Goals and Expected Outcomes*

The Nursing Process During the Third Stage of Labor: Delivery of Placenta
- *Assessment*
- *Selected Nursing Diagnoses*
- *Outcome Identification and Planning*
- *Implementation*
- *Evaluation: Goals and Expected Outcomes*

The Nursing Process During the Fourth Stage of Labor
- *Assessment*
- *Selected Nursing Diagnoses*
- *Outcome Identification and Planning*
- *Implementation*
- *Evaluation: Goals and Expected Outcomes*

STUDENT OBJECTIVES

On completion of this chapter, the student should be able to

1. Discuss the assessments and procedures the nurse performs during the woman's admission to the hospital.
2. Illustrate how to apply the external fetal monitor.
3. Compare and contrast advantages and disadvantages of external fetal monitoring with that of internal fetal monitoring.
4. Identify the role of the practical (vocational) nurse in the interpretation of fetal heart rate patterns.
5. Define three major deviations from the normal fetal heart rate baseline.
6. Differentiate between early, variable, and late decelerations with regard to appearance, occurrence in relation to uterine

KEY TERMS

acceleration
amnioinfusion
early deceleration
late deceleration
lochia
long-term variability
nadir
open-glottis pushing

STUDENT OBJECTIVES

contractions, causes, and whether or not the pattern is reassuring or nonreassuring.
7. Outline appropriate nursing interventions for each major periodic change: early, variable, and late deceleration patterns.
8. Discuss advantages and disadvantages of intermittent auscultation, fetal stimulation, fetal scalp sampling, fetal pulse oximetry, and continuous electronic fetal monitoring for monitoring fetal status.
9. Assess a laboring woman for progress of labor and birth throughout each stage and phase of labor.
10. Identify common nursing diagnoses associated with each stage of labor and birth.
11. Choose appropriate nursing interventions for each stage of labor and birth to facilitate safe passage of the mother and fetus.
12. Evaluate the effectiveness of care given during labor and birth.

KEY TERMS

periodic changes
ritual
short-term variability
urge-to-push method
uteroplacental insufficiency
variability
variable deceleration
vigorous pushing

The onset of labor heralds the transition from pregnancy to motherhood, and the transformation of the fetus to a newborn. The process is experienced on many dimensions, including physiologic, psychological, social, and spiritual. When the powers, passageway, passenger, and psyche work together harmoniously, the miracle of birth progresses in an orderly and predictable sequence.

The practical nurse's role in labor and delivery is to provide care to the laboring woman under the supervision of a registered nurse (RN). The licensed practical nurse (LPN) must have a basic understanding of the processes of labor and birth to provide care to the woman and her family. It is important for the LPN to be able to recognize deviations from the "normal" or expected sequence of labor and birth and to report deviations immediately. The LPN is expected to answer the woman's and her support person's questions regarding labor and birth. Although the LPN does not independently perform many of the procedures and assessments described in this chapter, a basic understanding of these procedures and assessments is necessary for the LPN to effectively assist the RN or physician.

The role of the obstetric nurse is central to the care of the laboring woman and her family. The nurse facilitates the labor process and ensures safe passage of the laboring woman and fetus through this critical life event. The effective obstetric nurse has an attitude of acceptance of the mother's preferences during labor and birth, utilizes supportive actions, and develops keen assessment skills to detect subtle changes in maternal or fetal status.

Although labor and birth are normal physiologic events, the nurse must be prepared to recognize and manage complications that may arise during the process. It also is critical that the nurse be prepared to give intensive support to the laboring woman and her partner or coach. Assisting the family during the miracle of labor and birth is a challenging but ultimately satisfying and rewarding experience.

Every woman's labor is unique, and if a woman bears more than one child, each birth is experienced differently. This chapter focuses on the nursing care of a first-time mother undergoing normal progression of labor and birth who does not experience complications. Common deviations associated with the nursing care of the multiparous woman are noted. For purposes of this chapter, it is assumed that the delivery environment is a labor, delivery, and recovery room (LDR) in a hospital setting. Similar nursing interventions apply to other settings, and the labor process is the same regardless of the environment in which birth occurs.

THE NURSE'S ROLE DURING ADMISSION

The woman may present to the birthing suite at any phase of the first stage of labor. Therefore, it is important for the nurse to immediately assess birth imminence, fetal status, risk factors, and maternal status. If birth is not imminent and the fetal and maternal conditions are stable, the nurse performs additional admission assessments, including the status of labor, the full admission health history, and a complete maternal physical assessment.

IMMEDIATE ASSESSMENTS

Birth Imminence

Nursing assessment for signs that birth is imminent begins from the moment the woman arrives in the labor and delivery unit. If the woman is introverted and stops to breathe or pant with each contraction, the nurse infers that she is in an advanced stage of labor. In addition, if the woman makes statements such as, "I feel a lot of pressure," or "The baby is coming," or "I want to have a bowel movement," it is likely the woman is in the second stage of labor, and the baby will be born directly. Other signs that birth is imminent include sitting on one buttock (if the woman is brought to the unit in a wheelchair) and bearing down or grunting with contractions. When any of these signs is present, it is prudent to quickly move the woman to a labor bed, perform a vaginal examination if the presenting part is not yet visible, and be prepared to assist with the birth.

Nursing judgment is in order. If the woman presents to the hospital in an advanced stage of labor, and it appears that delivery is imminent, the admission history and physical is abbreviated to focus on current status. The history can be completed later, even after delivery, if necessary.

Occasionally the nurse is the only person available to deliver the baby. Figure 10-1 illustrates the steps to follow for an emergency birth. You may not have time to perform all the steps listed. Do the best you can with the time and equipment there is available to you. It is helpful to instruct the woman to remain calm and reassure her that you know what to do to assist with the delivery. Instruct her to blow out through her lips in little puffs (as if she were blowing out candles) so that she won't forcefully expel the baby in an uncontrolled manner. Then follow the steps in Figure 10-1 to assist with the birth.

Once the baby is delivered it is not necessary to cut the cord immediately. However, in most facilities the protocol is to double clamp the cord and cut between the clamps. Dry the infant thoroughly to prevent heat loss and place him under a radiant warmer for resuscitation, or place the newborn in skin-to-skin contact with his mother and cover them both with a blanket.

The birth attendant usually arrives before delivery of the placenta. However, if signs of placental separation occur (a gush of blood, lengthening of the cord at the introitus), allow the placenta to deliver, and then massage the uterus to help it contract. Another way to prevent excessive blood loss immediately after delivery of the placenta is to place the infant to the woman's breast. The suckling action of the newborn will stimulate the woman's body to release oxytocin, which helps her uterus to contract and control bleeding.

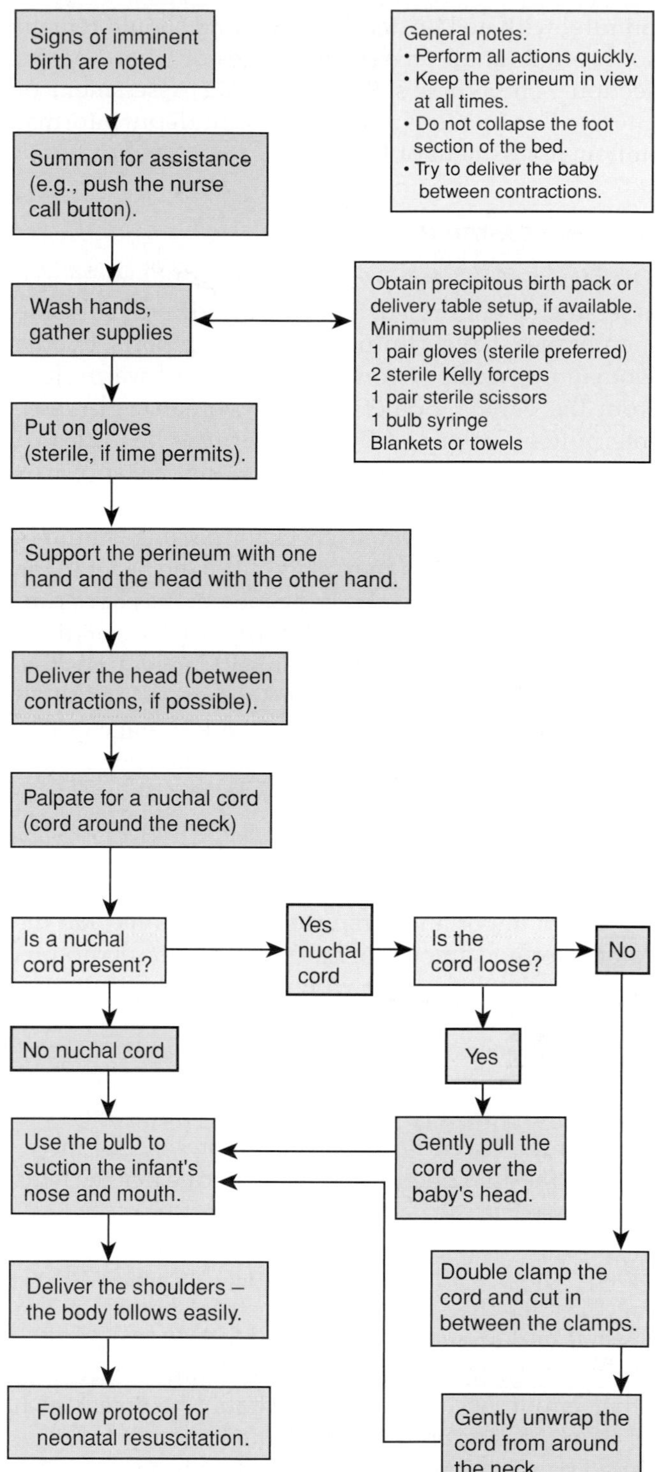

● ***Figure 10.1*** Emergency delivery by the nurse.

Fetal Status

When the woman arrives at the hospital, perform an immediate assessment of fetal status. In most delivery suites the woman is placed on the fetal monitor for continuous monitoring, but it is within accepted standards of care to check the fetal heart rate (FHR) by fetoscope or by Doppler ultrasonography for the low-risk woman. The FHR should be strong and regular, with a baseline between 110 and 160 beats per minute[1] with no late decelerations and should remain so throughout all phases and stages of labor. See the section "The Nurse's Role: Ongoing Assessment of Uterine Contractions and FHR" for in-depth information on assessment of FHR.

Risk Assessment

The status of the membranes is one of the initial risk assessments performed. Symptoms indicating that the membranes have ruptured include reports by the woman of a gush or continual leaking of warm fluid from the vagina. Sometimes the woman will report intermittent leaking of fluid, and it may be unclear if the membranes have ruptured. In this instance it is important to look for objective signs of rupture. The RN may use a speculum to check for pooling of fluid in the vagina. Or the RN may place nitrazine paper in the fluid to determine the pH. If the membranes have ruptured, the nitrazine paper will turn dark blue, indicating that the fluid is alkaline. This is called a positive nitrazine test. If the status of the membranes is still in doubt, a fern test may be done. The RN will collect a fluid sample and smear it on a slide. The slide is then taken to the laboratory or given to the physician to observe under a microscope. If a ferning pattern is seen, the fern test is positive, and a diagnosis of membrane rupture is made.

Other important parameters to assess include the color, odor, and amount of fluid and the time of rupture. The fluid should be clear with specks of vernix caseosa and no foul odor. If the membranes have been ruptured for several hours, the woman should be assessed carefully for signs of infection, such as elevated maternal temperature, cloudy or foul-smelling fluid, and fetal tachycardia. Green fluid signals the presence of meconium in the amniotic sac and may indicate that the fetus is distressed.

Assess for vaginal bleeding. The presence of bloody show is an expected finding, but heavy bleeding (heavier than a normal menstrual period) is not normal and should be reported to the charge nurse immediately. In addition to the amount of bleeding, other important characteristics should be noted, such as color (dark or bright red), amount and type of associated pain, and time that the bleeding began.

When delivery is imminent, it is important to ask the woman if she experienced any problems with this pregnancy, such as bleeding, high blood pressure, or diabetes. Determine if any prenatal fetal assessment tests were done and if any complications were diagnosed. Verify the expected due date. Ask if any complications were experienced with previous pregnancies. Establish the approximate number of times the woman saw the health care provider for prenatal care and during what month of pregnancy prenatal care began. Each of these assessments is important to determine if risk factors are present that might require a specialist to be present at the delivery.

Some nurses find this approach helpful. If the woman presents to the labor unit complaining of "bleeding," ask her how many times she has changed sanitary napkins. Her answer will guide your determination of the approximate amount of bleeding and allow you to teach the woman about expected versus abnormal amounts of bleeding during labor.

Maternal Status

A quick physical assessment of the woman's status upon admission to the hospital is crucial. Assess the woman's vital signs, including temperature, pulse, respiration, and blood pressure, for signs of infection, hypertension, or shock. If there is not enough time before delivery to do a full assessment of vital signs, the blood pressure is the most critical immediate measurement.

ADDITIONAL ASSESSMENTS

Maternal Health History and Physical Assessment

The admission health history is taken as part of the initial assessment and includes an obstetric history, determination of current status, a medical–surgical history, social history, desired plans for labor and birth, and desires/plans for the newborn. Box 10-1 lists examples of data that are obtained routinely for each category in the admission health history. Review the prenatal record to obtain baseline vital signs

This is critical to remember. Monitoring for the development of pregnancy-induced hypertension (PIH) is an important nursing function throughout pregnancy and childbirth. Signs of PIH that should be reported immediately include elevated blood pressure (greater than 140/90 mm Hg), brisk DTRs or presence of clonus, protein in the urine, edema of the hands or face, sudden weight gain, and reports of headache or blurred vision.

[1]In the past the baseline FHR was expected to be between 120 and 160 beats per minute. Newer standards list 110 as the lower acceptable limit of normal.

BOX 10.1 Components of the Admission Health History

- Obstetric history
  - Number and outcomes of previous pregnancies in GTPAL (gravida, term, preterm, abortions, living) format (refer to Chapter 9 for a detailed explanation of using these terms to describe an obstetric history)
  - Estimated delivery date (EDD)
  - History of prenatal care for current pregnancy
  - Complications during pregnancy
  - Dates and results of fetal surveillance studies, such as ultrasound or nonstress test (NST)
  - Childbirth preparation classes
  - Previous labor and birth experiences
- Current status
  - Time of contraction onset
  - Contraction pattern
  - Status of membranes
  - Description of bloody show or bleeding
  - Current fetal movements
- Medical–surgical history
  - Chronic illnesses
  - Current medications
    - Prescribed
    - Over-the-counter
    - Herbal remedies
- Social history
  - Drug and alcohol use during pregnancy
  - Amount of smoking during pregnancy
  - Marital status
  - Support system
  - Domestic violence screen
  - Cultural/religious considerations that affect care
- Desires/plans for labor and birth
  - Presence of a partner, coach, and/or doula (refer to Chapter 8 for discussion of doulas)
  - Pain management preferences
  - Other personal preferences affecting intrapartum nursing care
- Desires/plans for newborn
  - Plans for feeding—breast or formula
  - Choice of pediatrician
  - Circumcision preference, if the infant is male
  - Rooming-in preference

and weight and to identify other pertinent information.

Obtain the woman's current weight and compare it with her weight at her most recent prenatal visit (Fig. 10-2). Sudden weight gain indicates fluid retention and may signal the onset of pregnancy-induced hypertension (PIH). Measure vital signs, which should be similar to the woman's baseline. It is normal for the pulse to increase slightly during labor, but the blood pressure, measured during the relaxation phase of a contraction, should not be elevated. Collect a urine specimen to screen for the presence of protein, ketones, glucose, blood cells, or bacteria.

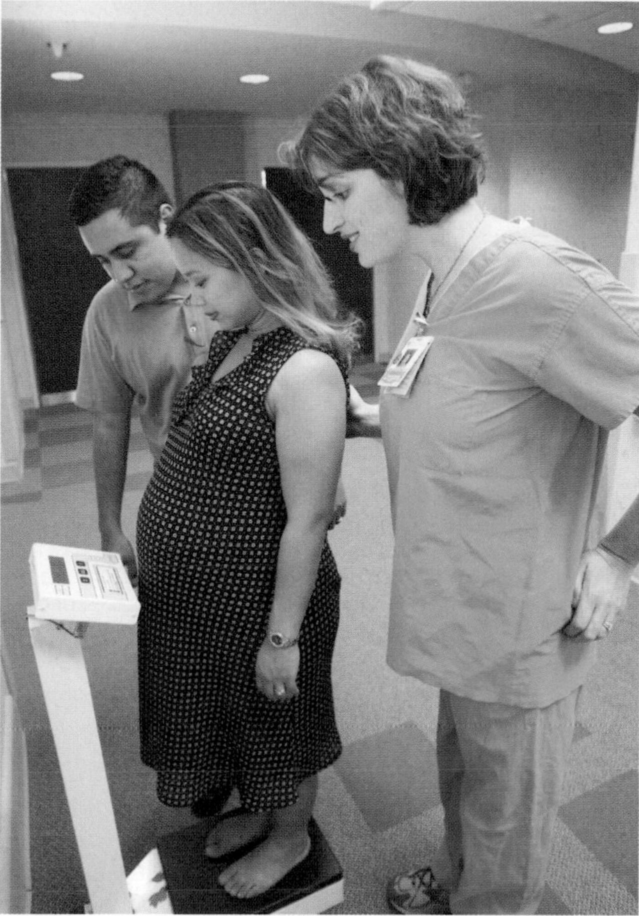

● ***Figure 10.2*** The nurse measures the woman's weight during the admission process to labor and delivery. Photo by Joe Mitchell.

Assist the RN to perform a head-to-toe physical assessment. Critical measurements include lung sounds, the presence or absence of right upper quadrant (RUQ) pain or tenderness, deep tendon reflexes (DTRs), clonus, and amount and location of any edema.

Labor Status

Assess the woman's contraction pattern to include frequency, duration, and intensity (see the section "The Nurse's Role: Ongoing Assessment of Uterine Contractions and FHR" for in-depth information on monitoring uterine activity).

It also is important to determine fetal lie, presentation, attitude, position, and station when the laboring woman first presents to a birthing facility. This process begins through the use of Leopold's maneuvers. Fetal presentation, position, and attitude often can be determined using this technique. The four steps are outlined and illustrated in Nursing Procedure 10-1.

The initial vaginal examination is done to assess dilation and effacement of the cervix and allows for specific information to be gathered regarding the

Nursing Procedure 10.1 Leopold's Maneuvers

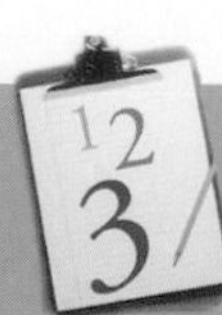

Leopold's maneuvers are a noninvasive method of assessing fetal presentation, position, and attitude. This technique can also be used to locate the fetal back before applying the fetal monitor.

EQUIPMENT

Warm, clean hands

PROCEDURE

1. Determine presentation.
   Stand beside the woman, facing her. Place both hands on the uterine fundus and palpate the contents of the fundus. If the buttocks are in the fundus indicating a vertex presentation (which is true 96% of the time), you will feel a soft, irregular object that does not move easily. However, if the head is in the fundus indicating a breech presentation, you will palpate a smooth, hard, round, mobile object.

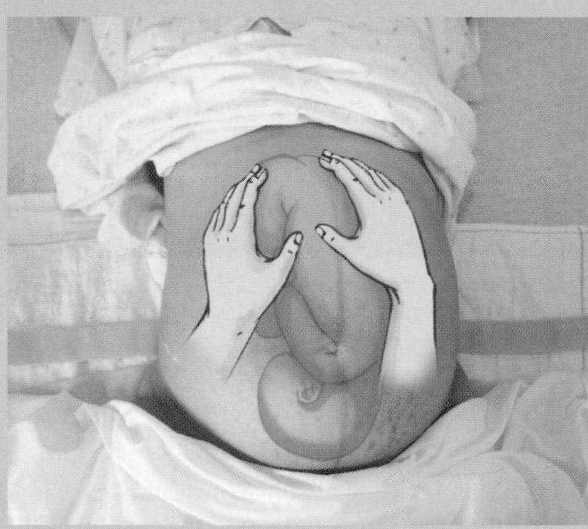

2. Determine position.
   Place both hands on the maternal abdomen, one on each side. Use one hand to support the abdomen while you palpate the opposite side with the other hand. Repeat the procedure so that both sides of the abdomen are palpated. Try to determine the location of the fetal back and extremities in relationship to the maternal pelvis. The back will feel hard and smooth and the extremities will be irregular and knobby.

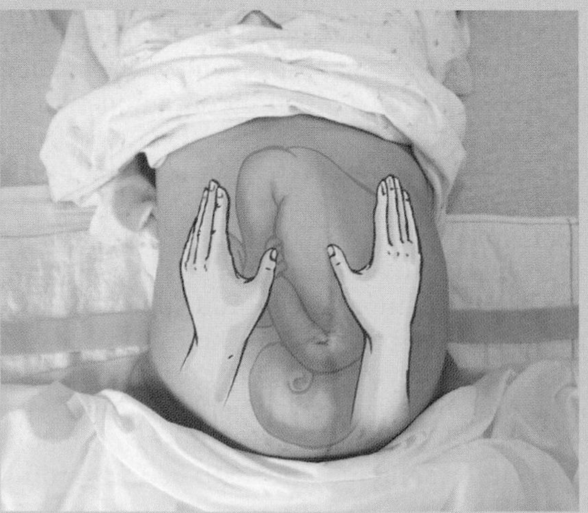

3. Confirm presentation.
   Place one hand over the symphysis pubis and attempt to grasp the part that is presenting to the pelvis between your thumb and fingers of one hand. In the vast majority of cases you will feel a hard, round fetal head. If the part moves easily, it is unengaged. If the part is not movable, engagement probably has occurred. If the breech is presenting, you will feel a soft, irregular object.

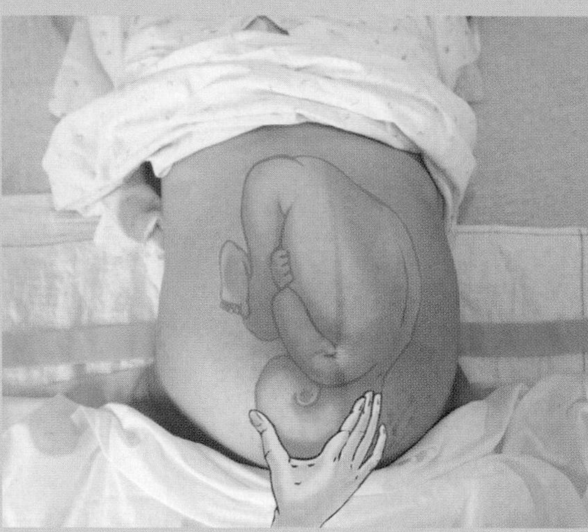

4. Determine attitude.
   Begin the last step by turning to face the woman's feet. Using the finger pads of the first three fingers of each hand, palpate in a downward motion in the direction of the symphysis pubis. If a hard bony prominence is felt on the side opposite the fetal back, you have located the fetal brow, and the fetus is in an attitude of flexion. If the bony prominence is found on the same side as the fetal back, you are palpating the occiput, and the fetus is in an attitude of extension.

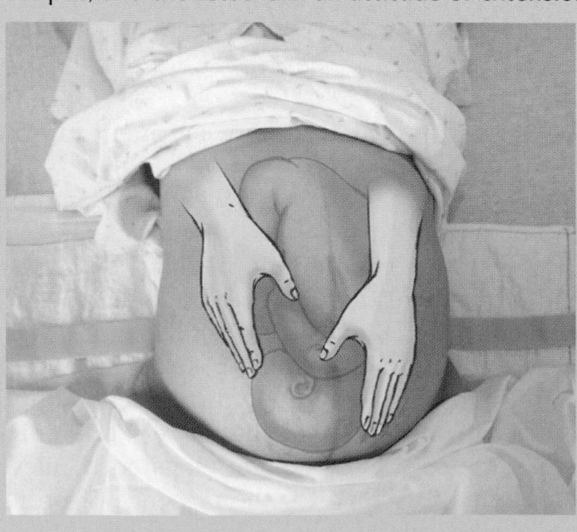

passenger's progress through the birth canal. In addition to confirming presentation, position, and attitude, fetal station can be established. In the full-term primigravida, the fetus is usually engaged, although it is not uncommon for the fetus to be unengaged and ballottable for the multipara during early labor.

As the LPN, it is your role to assist with vaginal examinations. There is no firm rule that establishes how frequently vaginal examinations should be performed during labor. The RN observes for cues that labor is advancing, so that vaginal examinations will only be done as frequently as is necessary to evaluate labor progress. Because vaginal examinations are invasive, performing them too frequently increases the risk for infection. Vaginal examinations are done when other labor assessments indicate labor is advancing, before administering pain medications, when the water bag breaks, or for the sudden onset of deep variable decelerations. Vaginal examinations should never be done if the woman presents with bright red painless bleeding until placenta previa is ruled out (see Chapter 17 for a description of placenta previa).

Balance is the order of the day. Vaginal examinations should be done frequently enough to adequately assess labor progress but not frequently enough as to cause infection. Usually the practitioner or RN does not perform a vaginal examination unless there are indications that labor progress has been made (e.g., increased bloody show, increased restlessness and introversion of the laboring woman, or a desire to push) or there are signs of umbilical cord compression. In this instance a vaginal examination is done to check for a prolapsed cord.

Record the results of the initial vaginal examination in the woman's clinical record. These results can then be compared with the results of subsequent examinations to demonstrate progress of labor or to diagnose arrest of dilation or descent. One example of a form used to graph results of cervical examinations is the partograph (Fig. 10-3). This graph gives a visual representation of the progress of labor and allows for documentation of parameters indicating maternal and fetal status. Each time a vaginal examination is done, the cervical dilatation and location of the fetal head is plotted on the graph. The "alert" line on the graph allows for the nurse or physician to quickly determine if labor is not progressing as expected. No cervical change in 2 hours when the woman is in active labor is called "arrest of dilatation." Failure of the fetus to descend (the station does not change) in a primigravida is a sign that labor is not progressing as expected, even if cervical dilation is occurring. The fetus of a multigravida may not descend until full dilation has occurred and then may move down the birth canal rapidly. The physician or nurse midwife should be notified when labor does not progress as expected.

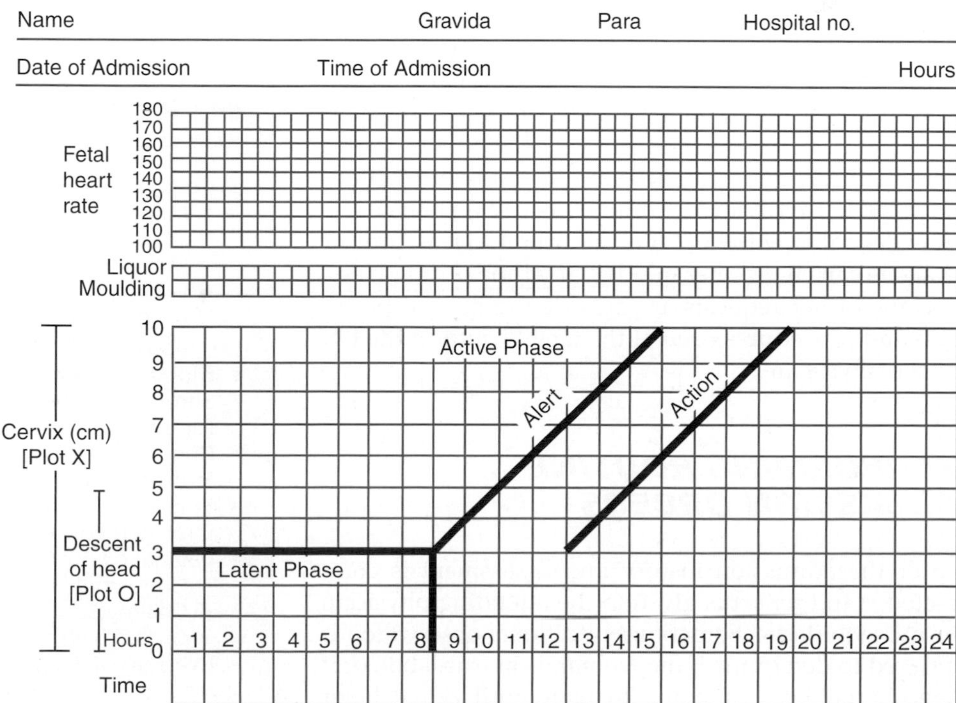

● ***Figure 10.3*** Partograph for recording labor progress.

CULTURAL SNAPSHOT

A woman's culture has a tremendous impact on the type and quantity of support she needs and on her methods of coping with the stress of labor. Some cultures frown on the presence of men during the labor and birth process. In these cases, it would be counterproductive for the nurse to pressure the man to be the support person.

Ask the woman to identify who should provide support. Inquire regarding the relationship of the support person to the woman. Ask the woman to identify any special methods that might help her cope with labor. This information will help you to individualize care while taking into account the woman's culture.

Labor and Birth Preferences

One very important part of the assessment is to determine if the woman and her partner have special requests for labor and birth. Some women go to great lengths to plan the birth. Ask if the woman has a written birth plan. It is hoped she has reviewed the plan with her physician well ahead of time and the physician has approved the document. Read through the plan and notify the RN of the contents. Birth plans often contain preferences regarding such things as mobility during labor, intravenous (IV) fluids during labor, episiotomy, presence of friends and family at the birth, fetal monitoring, pain management, and food and fluids during labor.

Many women do not have birth plans. However, it is very important to ask the woman specific questions regarding her preferences and needs. What expectations does she have about the labor process? How does she expect her pain to be managed? Did she attend childbirth class? Does she want to try natural childbirth? What individuals, if any, does she want in the delivery room with her? It is important to reassure her that she can change her mind at any time during labor. If some of her requests are outside the normal protocols and procedures used at the facility, inform the RN or the physician.

PERFORMING ROUTINE ADMISSION ORDERS

After the admission history and assessment is completed, a full report is given to the attending physician or nurse midwife. Sometimes additional observation is ordered to determine if the woman is in true labor, or if she should be sent home to wait until active labor ensues. If the woman is to be admitted, the nurse carries out routine admission orders, which may include a perineal shave preparation or clip or Fleet enema if the membranes are intact. However, these procedures are no longer considered to be a routine part of labor care. In most facilities, some type of IV access is started. Usually a liter of the ordered IV solution is hung and titrated to the specified rate. Alternatively, a saline lock may be inserted to allow for IV access if needed for medication administration or fluid bolus. Some practitioners and facilities do not routinely insert an IV as part of the admission procedure.

A little sensitivity is in order. If the woman is not in true labor and is to be discharged, she may feel embarrassed. Reassurance and acceptance can help relieve her anxiety. Instruct the woman regarding when to return to the hospital. It is a good idea to provide the telephone number to the delivery suite. This may be comforting for the woman, particularly if she is encouraged to call with concerns or questions.

Laboratory studies are part of the routine admission orders. The results are compared with the prenatal record to determine if changes have occurred during pregnancy. For example, a VDRL or RPR serology test is drawn to determine if the woman has developed a syphilis infection during pregnancy so that mother and baby can be treated, if necessary. Box 10-2 lists laboratory work that is ordered routinely when a woman is admitted to the delivery suite.

BOX 10.2 Admission Laboratory Studies

- Complete blood count (CBC)
  - Monitor hemoglobin and hematocrit for signs of iron-deficiency anemia (hemoglobin levels below 11 g/dL).
  - White blood cell count (WBC) may increase to 20,000/mm^3 with the stress of labor. Levels above 20,000/mm^3 may indicate infection.
- Blood type and Rh factor
- Serologic studies, such as VDRL or RPR, to test for syphilis
- Rubella titer (not done if prenatal record indicates the woman is immune)
- ELISA to detect HIV antibodies (requires informed consent)
- Vaginal or cervical cultures
  - Gonorrhea
  - Chlamydia
  - Group B streptococcus
- Urinalysis (clean-catch specimen)

THE NURSE'S ROLE: ONGOING ASSESSMENT OF UTERINE CONTRACTIONS AND FHR

The nurse makes frequent assessments of uterine activity and FHR during labor. These assessments are necessary to determine adequacy of the labor pattern and to detect signs of fetal well-being or distress. Table 10-1 compares the advantages and disadvantages of each of the methods discussed in the text for monitoring uterine and fetal status during labor.

MONITORING UTERINE CONTRACTIONS

The uterine contraction pattern should be evaluated every time the FHR is assessed (see Box 10-5 for frequency of assessment). The contraction pattern can be evaluated using external or internal methods.

External Methods

If intermittent assessment techniques are used, the pattern is evaluated by palpation. If electronic fetal monitoring (EFM) is used, a tocodynamometer (toco) is used to measure contraction frequency and duration. The toco is a transducer with a sensor that works like a moveable button. It is placed on the fundus with the sensor facing down and then strapped securely to the abdomen with a belt (see Nursing Procedure 10-3). As the uterus contracts, the sensor is displaced; an action that sends a signal to the microprocessor. The signal is converted by the microprocessor into a graphic representation of the uterine contraction on the video display and printout along with the FHR pattern tracing. In this way the health care provider can monitor the FHR pattern in conjunction with the uterine contraction pattern.

Here's a helpful hint. It is difficult for inexperienced nurses to determine the intensity of uterine contractions by palpation. One suggestion is to touch the tip of your nose, if the fundus can be indented as far as the tip of your nose at the peak of a contraction, the contraction can be recorded as mild. If the fundus feels firmer, as when you touch your chin, the contraction is of moderate intensity. A fundus that cannot be indented, one that feels like you are pushing on your forehead, is indicative of a strong contraction.

Contraction frequency and duration are determined by evaluating the EFM tracing. However, unless the woman has an internal uterine pressure catheter, the contractions must be palpated manually to evaluate intensity. As you will recall from Chapter 8, the height of the contraction is an estimate of its intensity. However, many factors affect the height of the contraction on an external tracing. For example, a small woman with minimal adipose tissue may be having mild contractions, but on the monitor strip the contractions appear tall and pronounced. On the other hand, an obese woman may be having strong contractions that barely register on the tracing. For these reasons, palpation is the most accurate way to estimate intensity when using external monitoring. Nursing Procedure 10-2 describes how to palpate uterine contractions.

Internal Method

Infrequently, an intrauterine pressure catheter is used. The physician places the catheter tip above the presenting part in a pocket of amniotic fluid, and then the catheter is connected to the fetal monitor. In addition to recording the frequency and duration of contractions, the internal catheter accurately measures the intensity of uterine activity. This information is particularly useful when the woman is undergoing labor after a previous cesarean delivery or when she is receiving oxytocics to induce labor.

Test Yourself

- Name three signs that indicate that birth is imminent.
- List the four parameters that must be charted regarding ruptured membranes.
- How do you evaluate the uterine contraction pattern when external EFM is used?

MONITORING FHR

Labor is not only stressful for the woman, but it stresses the fetus as well. If there is decreased blood flow to the placenta, or the fetus is subjected to chronic hypoxia, the fetus may not be able to withstand the stress of labor. General characteristics of the FHR and any changes that occur with uterine contractions give clues as to fetal status. For these reasons the fetal heart rate is monitored in relation to the contraction pattern.

TABLE 10.1 Comparison of Monitoring Techniques During Labor

Technique	Description	Advantages	Disadvantages
Intermittent FHR auscultation	Fetoscope, Doppler, or EFM used to periodically check FHR	• Noninvasive • Increases maternal comfort and mobility • Focus of health care provider is the laboring woman, rather than technology	• Requires one-to-one nurse-to-patient staffing ratios • Subtle signs of distress may be overlooked
Continuous external EFM	External transducer placed on maternal abdomen with straps to detect the FHR via ultrasound technology	• Noninvasive • Provides a continuous tracing of FHR • Allows for detection of signs of fetal compromise	• Cannot accurately detect short-term variability • An active fetus or maternal movement can interfere with the continuity of the tracing • Generally confines the laboring woman to bed, unless telemetry unit is used
Continuous external monitoring of uterine contractions	External toco placed on maternal abdomen with straps to detect uterine contraction	• Noninvasive • Shows the frequency and duration of uterine contractions • Allows for comparison of FHR pattern with uterine contraction pattern	• Does not accurately depict the intensity of uterine contractions • Tends to be confining and limits maternal movement
Continuous internal EFM	Electrode is placed on the fetal scalp and connected to a reference electrode on the maternal thigh to record electrical activity of the fetal heart	• Yields accurate information regarding variability • Allows for continuous monitoring of active fetus • Allows for continuous monitoring even if laboring woman is restless and changes positions frequently	• Invasive; requires that the membranes be ruptured and the cervix be at least partially dilated • Requires a specially trained practitioner for insertion • Increased risk for complications, such as chorioamnionitis, fetal scalp cellulites, or osteomyelitis (rare)
Continuous internal monitoring of uterine contractions	Intrauterine pressure catheter inserted into a pocket of amniotic fluid to detect pressure changes within the uterus and record the contraction pattern	• Allows for more accurate determination of contraction intensity than external techniques • Useful for labors in which there is a risk for uterine rupture (e.g., previous uterine incision or induction with oxytocics)	• Invasive; requires that the membranes be ruptured and the cervix be at least partially dilated • Requires a specially trained practitioner for insertion • Increased risk for complications, such as chorioamnionitis
Fetal scalp sampling	Small sample of fetal scalp blood is taken during a special vaginal examination and tested for pH level	• Gives direct evidence of fetal status • Allows for better practitioner decisions regarding continuation of labor	• Invasive; requires that the membranes be ruptured and the cervix be at least partially dilated • Requires a specially trained examiner to collect the specimen • Increased risk for infection, blood incompatibilities, and fetal anemia
Fetal scalp pulse oximetry	Sensor placed on the fetus' cheek or brow to detect oxygen saturation	• Does not require a blood sample to be taken • Allows for continuous reading of fetal oxygenation status • Gives direct evidence of fetal status	• Invasive; requires that the membranes be ruptured and the cervix be at least partially dilated • Requires a specially trained practitioner for insertion • Fetal oximetry is fairly new technology; equipment expense may prohibit its use.

Nursing Procedure 10.2
Palpation of Uterine Contractions

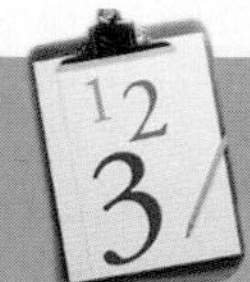

EQUIPMENT

Warm, clean hands

PROCEDURE

1. Explain procedure to the woman and her partner.
2. Wash hands thoroughly.
3. Locate and place one hand on the uterine fundus.
4. Use the tips of your fingers to feel changes in the uterus as it contracts.
5. At the beginning of the contraction you will feel the muscle begin to tighten.
6. Note the time the contraction begins.
7. Use your fingertips to evaluate how strong the contraction gets before the muscle begins to relax. Intensity is measured at the strongest point (the acme) of the contraction.
8. Note the time the contraction ends to determine duration.
9. Continue with your hand on the fundus through the next three contractions. Note if the uterus completely relaxes by becoming soft between contractions.
10. Note the time from the beginning of one contraction to the beginning of the following contraction to determine frequency. Frequency is documented as a range when appropriate (e.g., every 3–5 minutes, or every 2–3 minutes), unless they are occurring regularly (e.g., every 2 minutes, every 5 minutes).
11. Wash hands.
12. Chart the contraction pattern (frequency, duration, and intensity) in the labor record. Document whether or not the uterus is fully relaxing between contractions.

Note: It is best to time several contractions consecutively before charting frequency because it is rare for contractions to be exactly "x" minutes apart. It is more common that the contraction pattern occurs every "x" to "y" minutes apart (e.g., every 3 to 5 minutes). Palpation is a method that takes practice. It is best to learn to palpate contractions in conjunction with the use of EFM. In this way, you can see the contraction begin and concentrate on perceiving the tightening of the uterus with your fingertips. You can also see the acme, which lets you know when to evaluate intensity.

Intermittent Auscultation of FHR

An acceptable method for monitoring FHR in a low-risk pregnancy is to use intermittent auscultation. Usually the woman is placed on external EFM for 20 minutes to get a baseline evaluation of the FHR. If the pattern is reassuring, then a fetoscope, hand-held Doppler device, or the external EFM is used to monitor the FHR at intermittent intervals. The FHR is auscultated with the same frequency as is recommended for continuous monitoring methods (see Box 10-5). The FHR is monitored for at least 1 full minute and is auscultated throughout at least one uterine contraction. If any abnormalities are noted, or if there is slowing of the FHR with or after contractions, the woman is placed on a fetal monitor for continuous monitoring.

There are several advantages to the use of intermittent auscultation. The woman has more freedom to move about than when she is strapped continuously to a fetal monitoring device, and nurses are encouraged to focus on the laboring woman and her support person, rather than on the technology.

There are also disadvantages to the use of intermittent auscultation. This approach takes more of the nurse's time than does continuous EFM, a situation that requires higher staffing levels. Therefore, intermittent auscultation may not be practical in a busy labor and delivery unit. Another drawback is the potential that an ominous FHR pattern might be missed. Although intermittent auscultation is recommended only for low-risk pregnancies, it is possible for a complication to develop during labor in a heretofore low-risk pregnancy. A nonreassuring FHR pattern might be the only indication that a complication has developed. If this pattern is not recognized quickly, the fetus could become severely compromised before interventions are initiated.

Continuous EFM

As with monitoring uterine contractions, there are two ways the FHR can be monitored using a continuous fetal monitoring device. Continuous EFM can be accomplished using external (indirect) methods or through the use of internal (direct) monitoring techniques.

External EFM

The most common way to assess fetal status during labor is with the use of an external EFM. Although fetal monitors are manufactured by several companies and vary in shape and size, the basic components are the same and include a microprocessor, transducer, tocodynamometer (toco), audio capability, and graphic printout. The external monitor works on the principle of ultrasound. The transducer releases ultrasonic waves that are intercepted by the movement of fetal heart valves as the heart beats. The signal is then interpreted by the microprocessor, with results sent to the recording units. Characteristics of the fetal heart rate pattern can then be monitored continuously via a video display

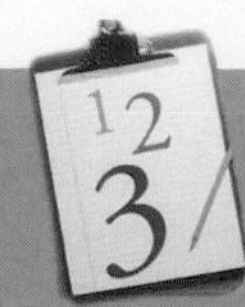

Nursing Procedure 10.3
Application of External Fetal Monitors

EQUIPMENT

Electronic fetal monitor
Tocodynamometer (toco)
Transducer
Two belts
Ultrasonic gel
Monitor paper

PROCEDURE

1. Thoroughly wash your hands.
2. Locate the fetal back through the use of Leopold's maneuvers (see Nursing Procedure 10-1).
3. Assist the woman to a position of comfort. If she wishes to be on her back, a wedge should be placed under one hip to tilt the uterus off of the great vessels.
4. Place ultrasonic gel on the transducer and turn on the power to the fetal monitor.
5. Place the transducer on the woman's abdomen over the fetal back.
6. Turn up the volume and move the transducer over the abdominal wall until the heartbeat is clearly heard.
7. When the monitor is consistently recording the FHR, secure the transducer in place with a belt.

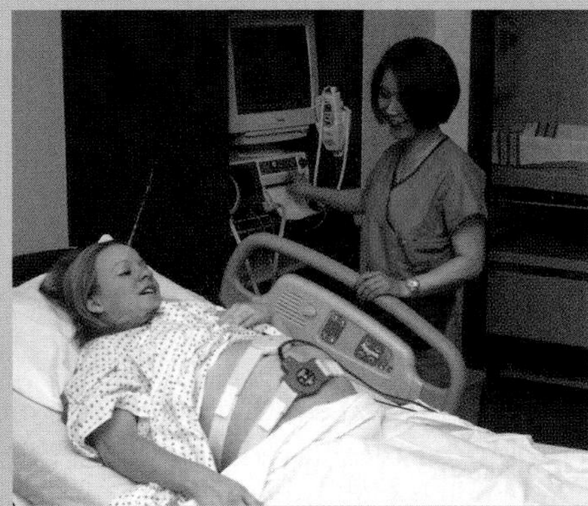

8. Next locate the hardest part of the uterine fundus.
9. Place the toco over the fundus and secure it to the maternal abdomen with a belt (see figure).
10. Check to make sure the paper is recording the FHR and uterine contraction pattern.

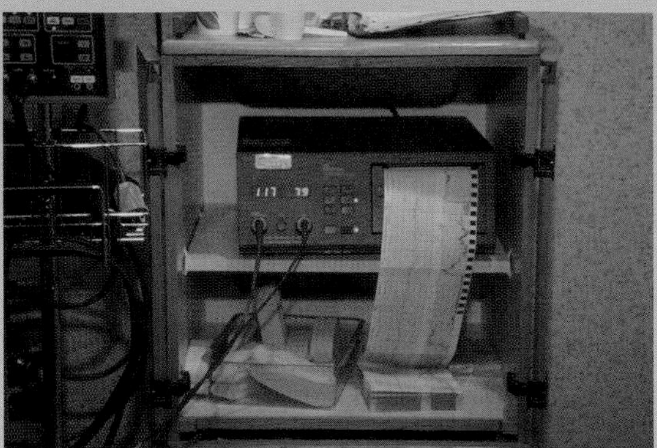

11. Label the EFM strip with the laboring woman's identification data, the date and time the EFM was applied, and maternal vital signs and position.
12. Be sure the call light is within reach before you leave the room.
13. Thoroughly wash your hands.

Note: It is important to position the woman comfortably before attempting to locate the fetal heart. If you wait until after you locate the FHR to reposition, you may lose the FHR and need to relocate the transducer.

and/or a continuous printout. As stated, the toco is used to monitor the contraction pattern, which allows for monitoring of the FHR pattern in conjunction with the uterine contraction pattern. See Nursing Procedure 10-3: Application of External Fetal Monitors.

External EFM is used to screen for signs of fetal compromise. It is noninvasive and used widely. However, the information gleaned from external monitoring is less precise than that of internal monitoring. Sometimes it is difficult to get a consistent tracing if the fetus is small or extremely active or if the woman is obese. Maternal positioning can adversely affect the quality of the tracing, and many women find external monitoring uncomfortable and confining.

Some EFM manufacturers have developed telemetry units, which provide wireless transmission of FHR patterns and uterine activity to the monitoring device so that the woman is not attached by cables to the EFM. These units allow for continuous EFM while the woman ambulates, alternates her position, or uses a birthing ball. Telemetry units have even been developed that allow for the woman to submerse her body in water to soothe the discomfort of labor.

Internal EFM

Internal EFM is an invasive procedure in which a spiral electrode is attached to the presenting part just under the skin (Fig. 10-4). A wire that extends from the

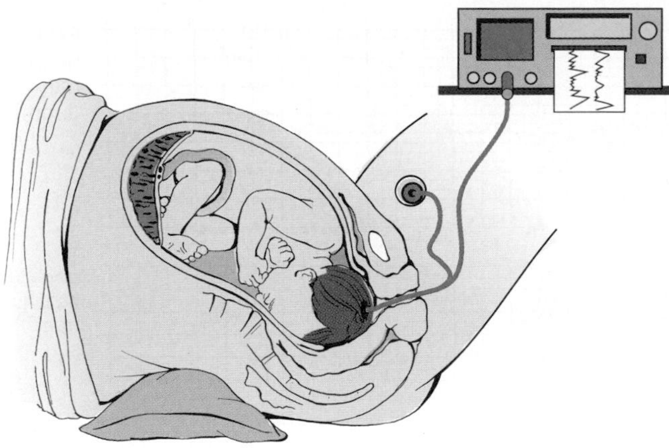

● ***Figure 10.4*** Internal fetal scalp electrode in place on the fetal scalp, connected to the reference electrode on the maternal thigh and to the EFM. Internal monitoring techniques allow for more precise measurement of the electrical activity of the fetal heart.

spiral electrode is connected to a reference electrode that is placed on the laboring woman's inner thigh. The signal is interpreted by the microprocessor, and a graphic representation of the electrical activity of the fetal heart is recorded. This method gives more precise results than does external monitoring and is more reliable for detecting signs of fetal compromise. It is easier to obtain a consistent tracing regardless of fetal activity and is not usually affected by maternal position changes. When internal techniques are used, the most frequent combination is that of internal fetal scalp electrode with an external toco to record the contraction pattern. Infrequently, an intrauterine pressure catheter is used (refer to the previous discussion). Because internal techniques are invasive, the fetal membranes must be ruptured and the cervix must be adequately dilated to use them. Accordingly, these procedures increase the risk of maternal and fetal infection and injury.

This is important! All invasive procedures carry risks, particularly increased risk for infection. In this instance, both the woman and the fetus can become ill with infection because of the use of the internal monitor. Chorioamnionitis is a serious uterine infection that requires intravenous antibiotics and a lengthened hospital stay. Newborns have experienced cellulitis of the scalp and even the dangerous bone infection osteomyelitis after internal scalp monitoring was used during labor. Fortunately this situation rarely occurs (Wolcott & Conry, 2000).

Evaluating FHR Patterns

Baseline FHR

The obstetric nurse is responsible for monitoring FHR patterns. Not only must the pattern be assessed and interpreted accurately, but the nurse also must know how to intervene and when to notify the physician or certified nurse midwife (CNM). The LPN is not expected to make a final decision about an FHR pattern; that is the responsibility of the trained RN. However, the LPN must be able to differentiate reassuring and nonreassuring signs in order to get help when it is indicated.

When you are asked to interpret a fetal monitor tracing, the first element that must be evaluated is the baseline FHR. The baseline rate is measured between uterine contractions during a 10-minute period. The normally accepted baseline rate is between 120 beats per minute (bpm) and 160 bpm, although the lower limit is considered to be 110 bpm by some researchers. Rates between 110 and 120 bpm are usually acceptable if all other signs are reassuring.

The baseline **variability**, fluctuations in FHR, also is evaluated. There are two types of variability: **short-term variability** (STV) and **long-term variability** (LTV). STV (sometimes called "beat-to-beat" variability) refers to the moment-to-moment changes in FHR that result in roughness of the EFM tracing. LTV refers to the wider fluctuations that make the EFM tracing look wavy over time. LTV is considered to be normal if the fluctuations are greater than 6 bpm and less than 25 bpm (Fig. 10-5). Box 10-3 gives definitions of LTV.

A word of caution is in order. Make certain that a nonreassuring pattern is not attributable to medical intervention. For example, fetal bradycardia may result from maternal hypotension that arises when the woman receives epidural anesthesia. Or a narcotic analgesic administered to the woman may cause decreased variability. In these examples, correcting the maternal condition may be all that is needed to correct the nonreassuring pattern.

BOX 10.3 Fetal Heart Rate (FHR) Long-Term Variability (LTV) Definitions

- Absent: No fluctuations of FHR
- Minimal: Less than or equal to 5 bpm
- Moderate: 6 to 25 bpm (normal)
- Marked: Greater than 25 bpm

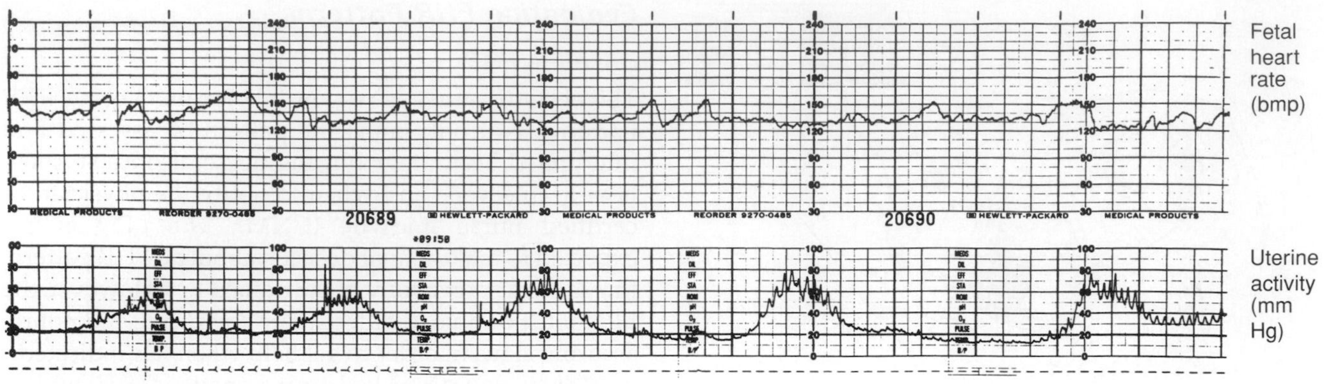

● ***Figure 10.5*** The EFM tracing shows moderate (normal) LTV.

FHR variability results from the interplay between the sympathetic and parasympathetic branches of the autonomic nervous system. The sympathetic division nudges the FHR higher, whereas the parasympathetic division tugs the FHR downward. Therefore, variability in the tracing is a reassuring sign that the fetal nervous system is intact.

There are three major deviations from a normal FHR baseline: tachycardia, bradycardia, and absent or minimal variability. Fetal tachycardia is defined as a baseline rate of greater than 160 bpm. When the baseline FHR falls below 110 bpm, the condition is identified as fetal bradycardia. Tachycardias and bradycardias are diagnosed if the abnormal rate continues for at least 3 minutes. The absence of variability also is a nonreassuring sign. Examples of conditions that can cause fetal tachycardia, bradycardia, and absent variability are listed in Table 10-2.

Periodic Changes

The next step after evaluating the baseline is to check for **periodic changes**, variations in the FHR pattern that occur in conjunction with uterine contractions. Periodic changes are designated as reassuring, benign, or nonreassuring. Figure 10-6 illustrates the appearance and causes of certain periodic changes.

TABLE 10.2 Conditions That Can Influence the FHR Baseline

Baseline FHR Deviation	Possible Causes
Tachycardia (>160 bpm) Mild 161–180 bpm Severe >180 bpm	• Maternal or fetal infection • Dehydration • Fever • Hyperthyroidism • Fetal hypoxemia (acute or chronic) or anemia • Premature fetus • Fetus with congenital anomalies • Certain medications given to the woman in labor, particularly tocolytics (medications used to stop preterm labor), and any drug that causes maternal tachycardia (e.g., caffeine, epinephrine, or theophylline) • Street drugs
Bradycardia (<110 bpm) Moderate 80–100 bpm Severe < 80 bpm	• Maternal hypotension • Supine hypotensive syndrome • Vagal stimulation • Fetal decompensation

Decreased or absent variability	• Medications
	  • Narcotics
	  • Magnesium sulfate (to treat preterm labor or PIH)
	  • Tocolytics (medications to stop labor)
	• Fetal sleep (normal fetal sleep cycle is 20 minutes)
	• Prematurity
	• Fetal hypoxemia

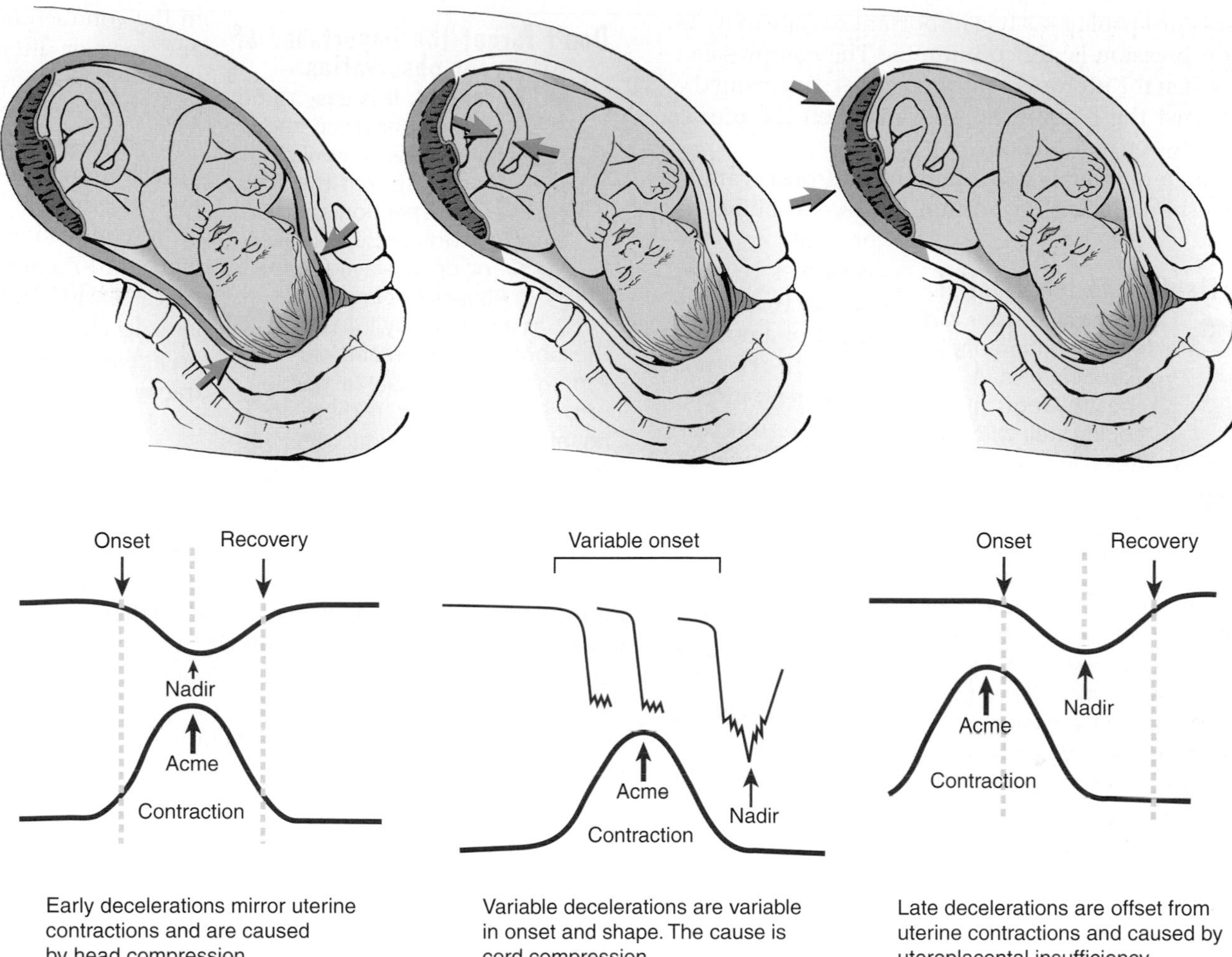
Onset
Recovery
Nadir
Acme
Contraction
Variable onset
Acme
Contraction
Nadir
Onset
Recovery
Acme
Nadir
Contraction
Early decelerations mirror uterine contractions and are caused by head compression.
Variable decelerations are variable in onset and shape. The cause is cord compression.
Late decelerations are offset from uterine contractions and caused by uteroplacental insufficiency.

● ***Figure 10.6*** Appearance and causes of periodic changes: early, variable, and late decelerations.

Reassuring Periodic Changes. Spontaneous elevations of the FHR, **accelerations**, above the baseline by at least 15 bpm for at least 15 seconds (15 × 15 window) are considered to be reassuring. In fact, as stated in Chapter 7, accelerations are the basis for the nonstress test (NST).

Benign Periodic Changes. Sometimes instead of accelerations, you will notice slowing of the FHR. If the dip in the FHR tracing occurs in conjunction with and mirrors a uterine contraction, it is called an **early deceleration**. This type of deceleration is shaped like a U on the EFM tracing, like that of a contraction. Three criteria must be met for the deceleration to be classified as early. The FHR begins to slow as the contraction starts. The lowest point of the deceleration, the **nadir**, coincides with the acme (highest point) of the contraction. The deceleration ends by the end of the contraction.

Current scientific evidence indicates that early decelerations are caused by pressure on the fetal head as it meets resistance from the structures of the birth canal. The contraction pushes the fetal head downward, causing pressure, which in turn leads to a slowing of the FHR. As long as the baseline remains within normal limits and the variability is good, early decelerations are considered benign. Therefore, no specific nursing intervention is indicated other than to continue to monitor the tracing and observe closely for the development of nonreassuring patterns.

Nonreassuring Periodic Changes. A **variable deceleration** is so named because it may occur at any point during a contraction, and it has a jagged, erratic shape on the EFM tracing. The FHR suddenly drops from the baseline and then recovers. A variable deceleration may be shaped like a U, V, or W.

The presence of variable decelerations, or *variables*, as labor and delivery personnel commonly call them, indicates some type of acute umbilical cord compression. Often it will be found at delivery that the umbilical cord is wrapped around a body part, such as the neck (nuchal cord) or foot. At other times the cause of compression is oligohydramnios (decreased amount of amniotic fluid), or it occurs as the result of an occult (hidden) cord prolapse.[2] It is important to note that the cord compression is not continuous. The compression occurs when the uterus is contracting and squeezing the cord against the fetus. It is relieved when the uterus relaxes between contractions.

Variable decelerations require careful observation. If the baseline is within normal limits, variability is present, and the variables recover quickly (within the space of a normal contraction), there is no immediate cause for alarm. However, you should be aware that the fetus is being stressed whenever the cord is compressed because the umbilical cord is his lifeline to oxygen. It is as if he must hold his breath while the cord is being compressed during the contraction. Therefore, nursing interventions are aimed at relieving the compression.

Pay attention to the details! Here's how to tell if variable decelerations indicate distress. A healthy fetus that is coping well with the stress of cord compression will show small "shoulders" (accelerations) on either side of the deceleration. As hypoxia develops, the shoulder on the recovery side will get larger (this is called "overshoot"), followed by loss of shoulders altogether and loss of variability. Finally, the variable deceleration will develop a late component, seen as a slow recovery to baseline. Any variable deceleration that lasts longer than 1 minute or dips deeper than 60 bpm below the baseline is worrisome.

First assist the woman to change positions. Try to find a position that is comfortable for the woman that relieves the compression. If the variables stop after the position change, you will know that the compression has been relieved. However, if the variables continue, try a variety of position changes, including the knee-chest position.

Other interventions for persistent or prolonged variables include stopping any oxytocic infusion, increasing the rate of IV fluids (if they are infusing), starting oxygen via face mask at 10 to 12 liters per minute, and notifying the charge nurse and physician. The charge nurse may perform a vaginal examination to rule out a prolapsed cord. Sometimes the physician will order an **amnioinfusion**, infusion of normal saline into the uterus, to cushion the umbilical cord and relieve compression.

The most ominous type of periodic change is a pattern of **late decelerations**. Like early decelerations, these decelerations appear smooth and U shaped on the EFM tracing, but unlike early decelerations, they are offset from the contraction. Late decelerations begin late in the contraction and recover after the contraction has ended. The slope and size of the deceleration mirrors the intensity of the contraction. Figure 10-7 compares early and late decelerations on a fetal monitor tracing.

Don't forget the importance of your observation skills. It is easy to be so concerned about the fetal monitor tracing that the skills of inspection and palpation are overlooked or downplayed. Always begin your assessment by looking at the laboring woman and performing a quick visual inspection of the environment. If there are no immediate problems, then you may turn your focus to reading the EFM strip. Technology does not replace the need for your assessment skills.

Late decelerations are associated with **uteroplacental insufficiency**, diminished or deficient blood flow to the uterus and placenta. This pattern occurs when the blood supply is interrupted chronically, rather than acutely, as is the case with variable decelerations. This is a grave situation because the placenta is the fetus' sole source of oxygen. Interventions are aimed at improving blood flow to the placenta.

When late decelerations are detected on the monitor, the following interventions are indicated. Position the woman on her right or left side[3] to relieve compression on the maternal great vessels. Discontinue the infusion of oxytocics (if present). Apply oxygen via a face mask at 10 to 12 liters per minute. Immediately notify the charge nurse and physician. Sometimes the physician will order tocolytics (medications to relax the uterus) in an attempt to improve blood flow to the placenta. Box 10-4 lists signs of an increasingly distressed fetus.

Test Yourself

- What are the components of the electronic fetal monitor?
- What is the baseline fetal heart rate?
- How does a late deceleration appear on the fetal monitor tracing?
- What interventions should be taken when a pattern of late decelerations is detected?

[2]A cord prolapse is an obstetric emergency that is discussed in Chapter 18.

[3] Research shows that positioning the woman on either side relieves pressure on the abdominal aorta and inferior vena cava and improves blood flow to the placenta. Previously it was thought that positioning on the left side afforded the best blood flow. Some health care providers may still prefer to use the left side when late decelerations are detected.

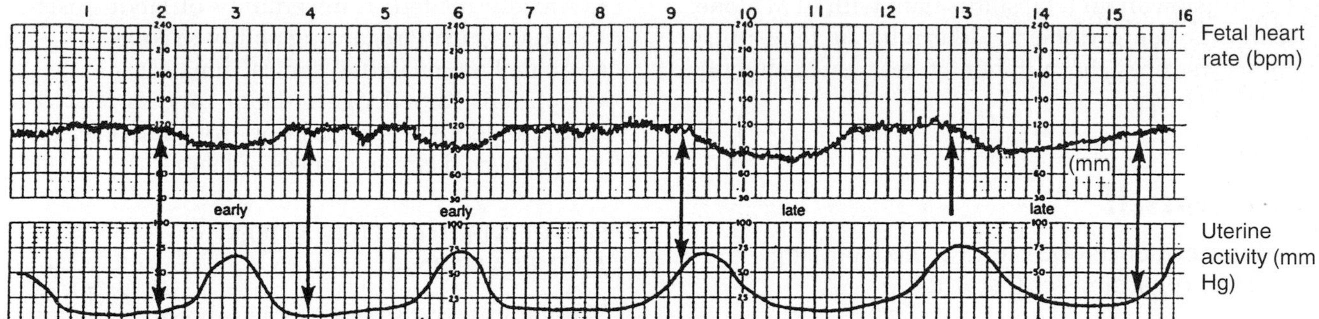

● ***Figure 10.7*** An early deceleration mirrors the contraction, is caused by head compression, and is benign, requiring no intervention. A late deceleration mirrors the contraction but is offset because a late deceleration begins after the contraction has started and ends after the contraction has ended. The cause is uteroplacental insufficiency, and interventions are aimed at improving blood flow to the placenta.

Measures Used to Clarify Nonreassuring FHR Patterns

When a nonreassuring FHR pattern is detected with EFM, more accurate methods for determining fetal hypoxia and acidosis are sometimes necessary. Some techniques currently in use include fetal stimulation, fetal scalp sampling, and fetal scalp pulse oximetry.

Fetal Stimulation

Because the presence of a nonreassuring pattern does not always correlate with fetal compromise, the physician or CNM may elect to try fetal stimulation. For this procedure the fetus is stimulated indirectly with an acoustic vibrator through the abdominal wall or is stimulated directly on the scalp by the gloved fingers of the examiner's hand during a vaginal examination. If the fetus responds by accelerating the heart rate, fetal acidosis is not present. If FHR accelerations do not occur after stimulation, fetal acidosis is a strong possibility.

BOX 10.4 Signs of an Increasingly Distressed Fetus

As the fetus becomes hypoxic, certain physiologic signs can be noted. These signs are listed in order of least distress to most distress. As you move down the list, the signs are indicative of ever-worsening hypoxia.

1. Absent accelerations
2. Gradual increase in FHR baseline
3. Loss of baseline variability
4. Late deceleration pattern develops
5. Decelerations gradually increase in length and take longer to recover to baseline
6. Persistent bradycardia
7. Death

Fetal Scalp Sampling

Fetal scalp sampling, a technique for checking fetal status, was developed in the late 1960s to verify fetal distress. Many physicians continue to use fetal scalp sampling to determine fetal pH when nonreassuring FHR patterns are detected with EFM.

For this procedure the physician places a cone-like device into the vagina through the dilated cervix and holds it on the fetal scalp. The scalp is cleaned; a tiny cut is made (like a finger stick to check for blood sugar); a small amount of blood is collected in a tube; and pressure is placed on the fetal head wound until the bleeding stops. The blood sample is tested immediately to determine the pH. A fetal pH within the normal range (between 7.20 and 7.25) is reassuring. If, however, the pH is abnormally low (less than 7.20), the fetus is acidotic. Fetal acidosis indicates that the fetus is truly in distress and needs to be delivered quickly so that the newborn can be resuscitated outside of the womb.

Although the risk is low, complications can result from fetal scalp sampling. The fetus can get an infection from the cut on the scalp; fetal and maternal blood may intermingle, potentially leading to blood incompatibilities; and the fetus can experience anemia from blood loss.

Fetal Scalp Pulse Oximetry

Because of the possibility of complications associated with fetal scalp sampling, a newer technique is sometimes used to monitor fetal oxygenation: fetal scalp pulse oximetry. This technology uses the same principles of pulse oximetry as those used to measure oxygen saturation in adult patients. In this instance, the sensor must be inserted into the uterus and placed next to the fetal cheek or temple. The sensor detects fetal oxygen saturation levels. The signal is then interpreted by a microprocessor, which sends the information to a monitor that gives a continuous readout. In this way, the physician or nurse midwife can make a better decision about fetal status than with EFM alone. Research is being done to determine if fetal pulse oximetry reduces the number of cesarean deliveries for fetal distress.

Test Yourself

- What evidence does fetal scalp sampling reveal regarding fetal status?
- What is fetal scalp pulse oximetry?

THE NURSE'S ROLE DURING EACH STAGE OF LABOR

● The Nursing Process During the First Stage of Labor (Dilation)

The first stage of labor is traditionally divided into three phases: latent, active, and transition. The first stage begins with the onset of labor and ends when the cervix is 10 cm dilated and 100% effaced. The nurse's role during this stage of labor focuses on assessment, providing physical care to the mother and fetus, providing psychological care to the mother, and keeping the physician informed about labor progress (Box 10-5).

Latent Phase (Early Labor)

ASSESSMENT

During the latent phase of labor, assess fetal status at least once every hour. Evaluate labor status every 60 minutes. Contractions during early labor are typically 5 to 10 minutes apart, last 30 to 45 seconds, and are of mild intensity. The cervix is dilated from 1 to 3 cm, and effacement has begun. Additional assessment parameters include maternal status and the status of the membranes.

It is also important to assess the woman's psychosocial state during the latent phase of labor. She may be talkative and express feelings of confidence and excitement. Conversely, she may be fearful, particularly if she is not prepared for the event; or she may experience anticipatory anxiety.

SELECTED NURSING DIAGNOSES

- Risk for Injury (fetal and maternal) related to possible complications of labor
- Anxiety related to uncertainty of labor onset and insecurity regarding ability to cope
- Acute Pain related to contractions
- Deficient Knowledge of labor process related to inadequate preparation for delivery or unexpected circumstances of labor

OUTCOME IDENTIFICATION AND PLANNING

Maintaining the safety of the laboring woman and her fetus throughout the latent phase of the first stage of labor are primary goals when planning care. Other goals and interventions are planned according to the individual needs of the laboring woman and her partner. Appropriate goals may include that fetal and maternal injury will be avoided; that the laboring woman's anxiety will be reduced and her pain will be manageable; and that the woman and her partner will have adequate knowledge of the labor process.

IMPLEMENTATION

Preventing Fetal and Maternal Injury

Monitor the woman's vital signs every hour. The temperature may be taken every 4 hours unless the water bag is not intact, which requires hourly monitoring. Mild tachycardia may be associated with anxiety or the stress of labor contractions. Immediately report elevations in the blood pressure or temperature.

Check the fetal monitor tracing frequently. Record FHR and uterine contraction pattern at least hourly during the latent stage of labor. Report extended periods of reduced variability, FHR decelerations, or other signs of fetal distress.

Relieving Anxiety

Encourage the woman to verbalize her fears and uncertainties. It may be helpful to ask what most concerns her about labor. Often anxiety is measurably decreased once fears are verbalized. When the source of anxiety is determined, specific measures can be implemented to decrease the anxiety. For example, if the woman is unsure she will be able to withstand the pain of labor, a discussion of pain relief options may be helpful. If she does not know what to expect, she may benefit from a brief explanation of the normal process of labor.

The woman also may fear losing control. In this instance, it may be appropriate to involve the partner in developing a plan to assist her if she starts to lose control. Verbal cues and position changes can be suggested as part of the plan. It is always advisable to inquire regarding coping behaviors that have been helpful to her

BOX 10.5 Nursing Care for the First Stage of Labor

Caring for the Woman

Assess the woman's vital signs.

- Temperature
  - If membranes are intact, monitor and record every 4 hours.
  - If membranes are ruptured, measure every 2 hours.
  - An elevated temperature may be associated with dehydration or infection.
- Blood pressure, pulse, and respirations
  - Measure every 60 minutes during the latent phase of labor.
  - Measure every 30 minutes during active labor and transition.
  - Measure every 15 minutes during the second stage of labor.
  - When certain procedures are done, such as induction of labor or placement of epidural anesthesia, the vital signs will be taken more frequently.

Monitor hydration status.

- Maintain strict intake and output.
- Maintain and monitor IV fluids, if present.
- Offer ointment for dry lips.
- Provide frequent mouth care.
- Offer fluids and ice chips if allowed/desired.
- Encourage voiding every 2 hours.
- Check for the presence of glucose or protein in the urine.

Remain attuned to the maternal psyche.

- Provide ongoing assessment of maternal coping status.
- Assess effectiveness of partner coach, or doula in supporting and comforting the woman.
- Promote positive coping.
  - Teach/reinforce patterned breathing techniques (Chapter 9).
  - Encourage frequent position changes.
  - Encourage rituals and creative approaches to dealing with contractions.
  - Administer analgesia appropriately, if desired by the woman.
  - Assist with the administration of anesthesia as ordered, if desired by the woman.
- Provide supportive care.
  - Provide privacy.
  - Provide a relaxing environment.
    - A fan may helpful if the woman is hot.
    - Soft lighting or darkening the room promotes relaxation.
    - Keep noise to a minimum.
      - Some women need absolute quiet during a contraction.
      - Some women find music to be soothing.
  - Provide for personal hygiene needs.
    - Absorbent pads are placed under the hips and buttocks to catch the continual drainage associated with labor.
    - Frequent perineal care and pad changes promote comfort.
    - Some women find a shower comforting.
  - Keep the woman and her partner or coach informed of labor progress and purpose of procedures.
- Be a role model for the support person.
  - Actively involve the partner or coach, if so desired by the laboring woman. Remember some cultures discourage participation by the father in the birthing process.
  - Encourage the support person to take breaks as needed.

Caring for the Fetus

Assess FHR* (*Note:* The recommendations apply to both intermittent and continuous monitoring techniques):

FHR of the low-risk laboring woman should be evaluated every

- 1 hour during latent phase of the first stage of labor
- 30 minutes during active phase of the first stage of labor
- 15 minutes during the second stage of labor

FHR of the at-risk laboring woman should be evaluated every

- 30 minutes during latent phase of the first stage of labor
- 15 minutes during the active phase of the first stage of labor
- 5 minutes during the second stage of labor

Additional times for monitoring and documenting the FHR pattern

- Immediately after artificial or spontaneous rupture of the membranes
- Before and after medication administration during labor and at time of peak medication action
- Before and after any invasive procedure (e.g., vaginal exam, enema expulsion, urinary catheterization, amnioinfusion)
- Before and after ambulation
- After any increase in frequency, duration, or intensity of uterine contractions

Management of the Labor Process

Observe for spontaneous rupture of the membranes, or assist when the birth attendant performs an artificial rupture of the membranes.

- Observe the color of the fluid (should be clear); green or cloudy fluid should be reported.
- Record the time of rupture, the characteristics and amount of fluid, and an assessment of the FHR.

Monitor for signs of umbilical cord prolapse (this labor complication is discussed in Chapter 18).

- Immediately after the membranes rupture, when the risk for prolapse is greatest, assess the FHR for 1 full minute.
- If fetal bradycardia is present, perform a vaginal examination to check for a prolapsed cord.
- Continue ongoing fetal assessments because prolapse can occur anytime after the membranes rupture.

(box continues on page 226)

BOX 10.5 (continued) Nursing Care for the First Stage of Labor

Assess uterine contraction pattern each time the FHR is assessed.
- Pattern should generally correlate with the phase of labor.
- Uterus should relax completely between contractions.
- Tetanic contractions (lasting longer than 90 seconds and of strong intensity) or failure of the uterus to relax should be reported.

Assess bloody show.
- An increase may be a sign of advancing labor.
- Heavy bleeding is a sign that a complication of labor is developing.

Assist the RN or childbirth attendant with vaginal examinations to determine progress of dilatation, effacement, and descent. To decrease the risk of infection:
- Sterile technique should be used.
- The number of examinations should be kept to a minimum.

Note maternal and fetal response to interventions.
Document all assessments and procedures.

* Recommendations of the American College of Obstetrics and Gynecology (ACOG) and Association of Women's Health, Obstetric, and Neonatal Nurses (AWHONN).

during other stressful situations. In this way, the couple can be assisted to adapt successful coping strategies to assist coping efforts during labor.

Promoting Comfort

It is important to support the woman and her partner in their attempts to cope with the discomfort and stress of labor. If the membranes are intact, encourage the woman to ambulate. Even if the membranes are ruptured, she may ambulate with a support person or nurse, if the fetus is engaged and well applied to the cervix. If the membranes are ruptured she should not ambulate alone or leave the nursing unit. Ambulation and upright positions are frequently helpful throughout the labor process. If the woman chooses not to ambulate, assist with comfort measures and position changes. However, at no time should the woman be allowed to remain flat on her back.

If the woman and her coach are well prepared for labor, they may decide to stay at home during the latent phase. This practice is permissible as long as the membranes are intact, and some nurses encourage it to allow the woman more control over the early labor process. Encourage distraction techniques. Engaging in conversation, watching television, and shopping are examples of diversionary activities that may be helpful during the latent phase of labor. Food and beverage intake during labor is a subject of debate (Box 10-6).

Providing Patient Teaching

The latent phase of labor is an excellent time to teach the woman and her partner or coach about the process of labor. Important teaching points include what the woman and her coach can expect to experience during each phase and stage of labor. Pain relief options and appropriate timing of analgesia and anesthesia should be explained and discussed. Briefly describe the frequency and purpose of nursing assessments and interventions common to each stage of labor.

It is important that the woman and her partner understand how to work with the labor

BOX 10.6 Food and Fluid Intake During Labor

For the past 50 decades in the United States the normal practice has been to withhold food and fluids from the laboring woman. This practice was recommended to prevent the woman from aspirating in the event that anesthesia would be needed for a cesarean delivery. Now there are a wide range of practices and opinions on the issue.

Nurse midwives who deliver patients at home or in birthing centers often allow food and fluid intake during the latent phase of labor and then restrict the woman to clear fluids during active labor. Fluids are needed during labor to prevent dehydration. Because the woman who delivers at home rarely has an IV, she is usually encouraged to take fluids by mouth. Many midwives who deliver in birthing centers give IV fluids to the woman in active labor. In this instance the woman is usually allowed clear liquids as a comfort measure.

Practices regarding food and drink during labor vary widely at hospitals across the country. Many physicians prefer to give IV fluids to every woman in active labor and allow only ice chips, while others allow clear liquids. Currently, more research is needed before updated recommendations can be made. The nurse is well advised to follow the practitioner's recommendations regarding food and fluid intake during labor.

process and how to avoid fighting against it. If the woman has not attended childbirth preparation classes, use this time to quickly teach basic relaxation techniques. Otherwise, review and reinforce breathing and relaxation techniques that the couple learned in class (refer to Chapter 9 for discussion of breathing and relaxation techniques).

The partner or coach needs encouragement regarding the importance of his or her role during labor. Give information regarding measures the woman may find comforting during each stage of labor, and encourage the partner to take breaks periodically to conserve energy for the duration of labor. Explain the importance of using the nurse as a resource and source of support for the partner and the woman throughout labor. Anxiety and fear are reduced and the labor process is enhanced if the woman knows what to expect and is supported during labor.

Evaluation: Goals and Expected Outcomes

- **Goal:** Fetal and maternal injury is avoided.
  Expected Outcomes: Maternal vital signs are stable.
  - Blood pressure is not elevated above baseline levels.
  - The woman is afebrile.
  - Fetal heart tones are within the expected range without decelerations or other signs of distress.
- **Goal:** The woman's anxiety is reduced.
  Expected Outcomes: She verbalizes confidence in her ability to cope with labor.
- **Goal:** The woman's pain is manageable.
  Expected Outcomes: She is relaxed and coping with contractions.
  - Demonstrates the use of effective strategies for coping with labor.
  - Expresses the ability to cope with her pain.
- **Goal:** The woman and her partner have adequate knowledge of the labor process.
  Expected Outcomes: The woman and her partner express realistic expectations regarding the duration, intensity, and process of labor.

Test Yourself

- What assessment findings would lead the nurse to keep the low-risk laboring woman on bed rest?
- Describe four important nursing interventions during the latent phase of labor.

Active Phase (Active Labor)

ASSESSMENT

Assess the woman's psychosocial state. Note if the woman is becoming more introverted, restless, or anxious; if she is feeling helpless or fears losing control; or if distraction techniques are failing to promote coping. These behaviors signal that the woman is moving into the active phase of labor.

Assessment of Labor Progress

During the active phase, evaluate the contraction pattern every 30 minutes. Typically, contractions occur every 2 to 5 minutes, last 45 to 60 seconds, and are of moderate to strong intensity. The cervix should dilate progressively from 4 to 8 cm. The fetus should descend steadily, although descent does not typically progress as rapidly as does cervical dilation. As the fetus descends below the level of the ischial spines, station is described in positive numbers. Plot cervical changes and fetal descent on a labor graph to evaluate labor progress. It is also critical to assess whether the uterus is relaxing completely between contractions. An adequate relaxation period allows for sufficient blood flow to the placenta and promotes oxygenation of the fetus.

Assessment of Fetal Status

Fetal status must be assessed and documented at least every 30 minutes. Record the baseline FHR every 30 minutes, and evaluate the strip for signs of distress. Variability should be present, except for brief periods of fetal sleep or when narcotics or other medications are administered, and no late decelerations should be present. Accelerations of the FHR are reassuring.

Assessment of Maternal Status

Maternal status should be assessed with the same frequency as fetal status. The woman becomes more introverted during active labor because the contractions are closer together, of a stronger intensity, and last longer than during early labor. Blood pressure may rise slightly but should be lower than 140/90 mm Hg. It is important to take the blood pressure between contractions because the stress of a uterine contraction can cause the blood pressure to rise briefly, resulting in an inaccurate measurement.

Pulse and respirations may also increase with the work of labor. Monitor for signs of tachycardia and hyperventilation. A falling blood pressure and a rising pulse could indicate the onset of shock and must be reported immediately. There are several labor complications that can cause shock, including hemorrhage or uterine rupture.

Assess the presence and character of pain at least hourly during active labor. Ask the woman to rate her pain on a standardized pain scale to make pain assessments measurable. Anxiety and tension often decrease the woman's ability to cope with contractions; therefore, it is important to document how the woman and her partner are coping and to determine if the coping strategies are helpful. For example, if the woman is using patterned breathing techniques to manage contractions, she may hyperventilate and need assistance to regain control of her breathing technique.

Evaluate breathing patterns frequently. Assess for signs of hyperventilation, which include tachypnea, feelings of lightheadedness or dizziness, complaints of tingling around the mouth or in the fingers, and carpopedal spasms (Fig. 10-8).

Exercise caution! When the membranes rupture, whether it be spontaneously or artificially, check the FHR for 1 full minute immediately afterward. If fetal bradycardia occurs, or deep variable decelerations are noted on the EFM tracing, assist the woman to the knee-chest position and call the RN immediately to perform a vaginal examination to check for a prolapsed cord.

Check for dry cracked lips, thick saliva, and a coating on the tongue that may be caused by mouth breathing and lack of oral intake (if restricted). Measure the temperature every 4 hours if the water bag is intact and hourly after the membranes have ruptured. Monitor for signs of infection, such as elevated temperature, fetal and maternal tachycardia, and cloudy, foul-smelling amniotic fluid. Box 10-7 lists danger signs to watch for during labor.

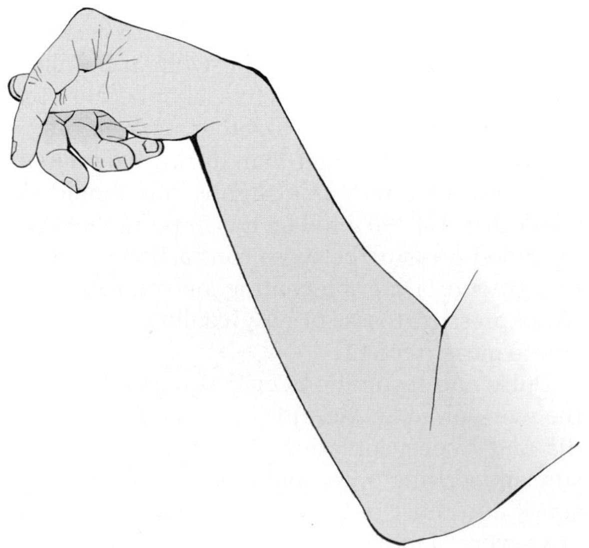

● ***Figure 10.8*** Carpopedal spasms.

BOX 10.7 Danger Signs During Labor

If any of the following signs occur during labor, immediately notify the RN, physician, or nurse midwife.

- Elevated maternal blood pressure (BP) (≥140/90 mm Hg)
- Low or suddenly decreased maternal BP (≤90/50 mm Hg)
- Elevated maternal temperature (>100.4°F)
- Amniotic fluid that is green, cloudy, or foul smelling
- Nonreassuring FHR patterns
- Prolonged uterine contractions (>90 seconds duration)
- Failure of the uterus to relax between contractions
- Heavy or bright red bleeding
- Maternal reports of unrelenting pain, right upper quadrant pain, or visual changes

SELECTED NURSING DIAGNOSES

- Risk for Trauma to the woman or fetus related to intrapartum complications or an undetected full bladder
- Acute Pain related to the process of labor
- Anxiety related to fear of losing control
- Ineffective Coping related to situational crisis of labor
- Ineffective Breathing Pattern: hyperventilation related to anxiety and/or inappropriate application of breathing techniques
- Impaired Oral Mucous Membrane related to dehydration and/or mouth breathing
- Risk for Infection related to invasive procedures (e.g., vaginal examinations) and/or rupture of amniotic membranes

OUTCOME IDENTIFICATION AND PLANNING

In addition to maintaining maternal and fetal safety during the active phase of the first stage of labor, appropriate goals may include that the laboring woman will verbalize her ability to cope with pain; exhibit lessened anxiety; demonstrate effective strategies for coping with labor; display effective breathing patterns; maintain an intact oral mucosa; and remain free of signs of infection.

IMPLEMENTATION

Preventing Trauma During Labor

It is important to continue to closely monitor the fetus during active labor. Any signs of fetal distress that do not respond to position changes should be reported immediately. Abnormal vital signs should also be reported. Immediately report heavy bleeding or failure of the uterus to relax well between contractions.

Another source of trauma that can interfere with the progress of labor is a full bladder. Every 2 hours palpate the area just above the symphysis pubis feeling for a rounded area of distention, which indicates the bladder is full. Failure of the fetus to descend is another sign that the bladder might be full. Offer the bedpan every 2 hours or assist the woman to the restroom, if allowed. If the woman is unable to void, perform a sterile in-and-out catheterization procedure.

Providing Pain Management

The active phase of labor is the time when pain relief measures are most often implemented. Epidural anesthesia may be initiated, or narcotic analgesia may be administered (pain relief options are discussed in greater detail in Chapter 9); however, it is critical to respect the woman's preferences for pain control. If the woman desires a natural childbirth, you will be challenged to provide intensive support throughout the active phase of labor.

Implementing general comfort measures can help to manage the pain and discomfort of labor. Work closely with the coach to demonstrate distraction and relaxation techniques, such as effleurage, back rubs, or application of pressure to the lower back during contractions, as discussed in Chapter 9. A cool, damp washcloth to the forehead is often comforting.

Linens and gowns are soiled frequently during active labor with perspiration, amniotic fluid, and bloody show. Linen savers, such as chucks or other under-buttocks pads, should be placed under the hips and replaced as needed. Provide frequent perineal care. At a minimum, perineal care should be done after any invasive procedure involving the vagina and after elimination.

Reducing Anxiety

During active labor, assist the woman and her partner to implement the anxiety reduction plan that was agreed upon during early labor. Continue to encourage the woman to verbalize her concerns. If her chosen method of pain relief is not working, remind her that she can change her mind about pain relief options. You may need to repeat earlier instruction and reassure the couple that it does not represent a failure on the woman's part if she chooses an alternate method of pain management. If she starts to lose control, assist the labor coach to use verbal cues and position changes to help the laboring woman regain control.

Promoting Effective Coping Strategies

It is important to support the woman and her partner in their attempts to cope. Some women do not benefit from the use of patterned breathing techniques. Frequently these women will develop personalized "rituals" to help them cope with contractions.

A **ritual** is a routine; a repeated series of actions that the woman uses as an individualized way of dealing with the discomfort of labor. For example, one woman might find it helpful to close her eyes and attempt to visualize a peaceful scene during contractions. Another woman might involve her partner by squeezing his hands throughout each contraction. Still another woman might assume a particular position during contractions. As long as these creative approaches to coping are helpful, encourage and support their use. When the ritual is not working to promote adaptation, assist the woman in trying other approaches.

Here's a helpful hint. Vigorous application of breathing techniques can lead to hyperventilation. Hyperventilation can cause respiratory alkalosis. Breathing into a paper bag retains CO_2, reverses alkalosis, and relieves associated symptoms.

Promoting Effective Breathing Patterns

Frequently reinforce breathing techniques appropriate to the active phase of labor (see Chapter 9). Often it helps to make eye contact and perform the breathing patterns with the woman during her contraction to help keep her focused (Fig. 10-9). If hyperventilation occurs, breathing into cupped hands or a paper bag usually relieves the problem.

Maintaining Integrity of the Oral Mucosa

Frequent mouth care stimulates saliva production, which helps to keep the oral mucosa moist. Suggest that the woman brush her teeth or gargle with normal saline when her mouth feels dry. Chewing gum also stimulates saliva production and leaves a pleasant taste in the mouth. Providing ice chips, sips of clear liquids, flavored ice, or hard candy (if allowed) can be soothing. Lip balm is comforting if the lips are dry or chapped. If the

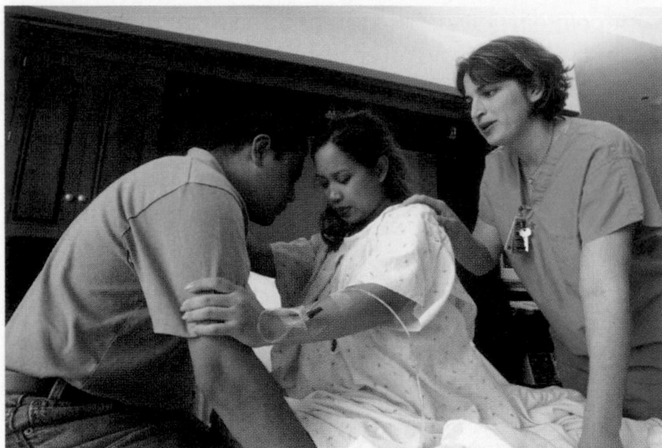

● ***Figure 10.9*** The nurse instructs the labor coach to maintain eye contact and breathe with his partner during contractions to help keep her focused. Photo by Joe Mitchell.

woman does not have lip balm, the water-soluble lubricant available in most labor rooms can be used to moisten the lips.

Preventing Infection

Handwashing remains the number one way to prevent the spread of infection. Wash your hands thoroughly be- fore and after providing care. Encourage the woman and her partner to wash their hands before and after any contact with the perineum and after using the restroom.

Frequent vaginal examinations are discouraged, particularly if the membranes are ruptured. Nursing judgment is indicated to determine frequency. Usually it is best not to examine the cervix unless there is a clear indication that labor is progressing. Assist the examiner to maintain sterile technique when it becomes necessary to perform a vaginal examination.

Invasive procedures, such as the application of an internal fetal monitor or insertion of a urinary catheter, should be kept to a minimum and done only if there are clear indications for their use. Strict adherence to sterile technique when performing an invasive procedure is critical.

Check out this tip. A full bladder may interfere with fetal descent. Encourage the woman to void at least every 2 hours during labor.

EVALUATION: GOALS AND EXPECTED OUTCOMES

- **Goal:** Fetal and maternal trauma is avoided.
  Expected Outcomes: Maternal vital signs are stable.
  - Blood pressure is not elevated above baseline levels.
  - The woman is afebrile.
  - Bladder distention does not occur.
  - The uterus is relaxing well between contractions.
  - Fetal heart tones are within the expected range without decelerations or other signs of distress.
- **Goal:** Pain is manageable.
  Expected Outcomes: The woman is relaxed and coping with contractions.
  - States that the pain of labor is tolerable.
  - States pain relief techniques are effective.
- **Goal:** Anxiety is reduced.
  Expected Outcomes: The woman reports decreased anxiety.
- **Goal:** Coping is effective.
  Expected Outcomes: The woman demonstrates individualized rituals to cope with labor.
  - Uses social supports (partner, coach, relative, or doula) to help cope with labor.
- **Goal:** Breathing techniques are effective.
  Expected Outcomes: The woman uses slow and accelerated breathing techniques during contractions.
  - Does not hyperventilate.
- **Goal:** Oral mucosa remains intact.
  Expected Outcomes: Lips and mucous membranes remain moist and intact.
- **Goal:** Exhibits no signs of infection.
  Expected Outcomes: The woman remains afebrile.
  - White blood cell count remains within expected limits.
  - Amniotic fluid remains clear and odorless.
  - No foul-smelling drainage.
  - No fetal tachycardia.

Test Yourself

- Why is it important for the laboring woman to void frequently?
- What assessment findings are associated with the nursing diagnosis Ineffective Breathing Pattern: hyperventilation?
- List five nursing interventions appropriate for the active phase of labor.

Transition Phase

ASSESSMENT

Assess for signs that the woman has reached the transition phase of the first stage of labor. Look for an increase in the amount of bloody show and a strong urge to push if fetal station is low. It is important to assess the woman's ability to cope. She will often express irritability, restlessness, and will feel out of control. She may tremble, vomit, or cry. It is important to assess for hyperventilation during this phase.

Do you know the why of it? Nausea and vomiting are common occurrences during labor because of decreased gut peristalsis and delayed gastric emptying time. If vomiting occurs, assist the woman to turn to her side to help prevent aspiration.

Check the contraction pattern at least once every 30 minutes; contractions should occur every 2 to 3 minutes, last 60 to 90 seconds, and be of strong intensity. The uterus should relax completely between uterine contractions. Cervical examination during transition re-veals dilation between 8 and 10 cm.

It is important to continue to evaluate fetal status at least every 30 minutes. The FHR baseline should remain between 110 and 160 bpm and should not significantly increase or decrease. It may be normal to see variable decelerations as the fetal head descends. Variability should be present. There should be no late decelerations or other signs of fetal distress.

SELECTED NURSING DIAGNOSES

- Acute Pain related to intense uterine contractions and pressure of the descending fetal head
- Ineffective Breathing Pattern: hyperventilation related to intense uterine contractions and loss of control of breathing techniques
- Powerlessness related to intensity of the labor process
- Fatigue related to energy expended coping with the intensity of labor

OUTCOME IDENTIFICATION AND PLANNING

Major goals for the transition phase of the first stage of labor include that the woman's pain will be manageable; she will exhibit effective breathing patterns; she will maintain a sense of control; and she will rest between uterine contractions.

IMPLEMENTATION

Managing Pain

The woman should be assured that although this period of labor is the most intense, it is usually short in duration. Narcotics are not given at this advanced stage of labor to prevent delivery of a neonate who is too sleepy to take his first breath. Continue to assist the coach to provide comfort and support during uterine contractions. Frequent position changes, breathing with the woman during contractions, and providing other comfort measures may help decrease the intensity of the pain stimulus.

Promoting Effective Breathing Patterns

If the woman has been trained in patterned breathing techniques, encourage her to switch to a more advanced technique when the pattern she is using is no longer working. Assist the coach to breathe with her and to assess for signs of hyperventilation. She may feel the urge to push. Explain the importance of resisting the urge to push until the cervix is fully dilated.

This advice could save the day. If the woman is feeling a strong urge to push, assist her to blow at the peak of the contraction when the urge is most intense. Pushing efforts before the cervix is fully dilated can result in cervical lacerations or can cause edema of the cervix and slow dilatation.

Promoting a Sense of Control

Accepting behavioral changes of the laboring woman is an important nursing intervention during this forceful period of labor. You will need to provide intensive psychological support. If the woman falls asleep between contractions, awaken her at the beginning of a contraction so that she can begin her coping strategy before the contraction reaches full intensity.

Supporting the Woman Through Fatigue

Relaxing with contractions may be almost impossible; assist the woman to achieve relaxation or even sleep between contractions. Help her to find a position that is comfortable. Support her position with pillows. Placing a cool cloth to her forehead or giving her a back rub may help her relax between contractions (Fig. 10-10). Some women find music to be soothing. When she is able to relax between contractions she conserves energy that she will need during the next stage in order to push effectively. The partner/coach is often fatigued as well; encourage him or her to take breaks as necessary.

Preparing the Room for Delivery

Often the nurse prepares the room for delivery during the transition phase (Fig. 10-11). Many delivery units have physician preference cards so that the nurse can prepare the equipment and

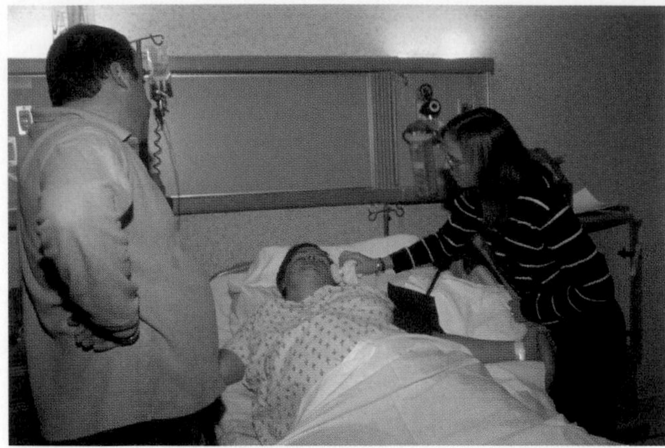

● ***Figure 10.10*** The labor coach provides comfort measures, such as a cool washcloth to the face and forehead, to help the woman relax as much as possible during the transition phase of labor. © B. Proud.

supplies most often needed by the attending physician. Prepare the table maintaining surgical asepsis so that a sterile field is available during delivery. It is important to ensure that supplies and medications needed for the birth are readily available. Check the infant resuscitation area and replace any missing supplies or malfunctioning equipment.

EVALUATION: GOALS AND EXPECTED OUTCOMES

- **Goal:** The woman's pain is manageable.
  Expected Outcomes: She tolerates the pain of contractions and pressure from the fetal head without pushing.
- **Goal:** The woman's breathing pattern is effective.
  Expected Outcomes: She uses accelerated breathing techniques during contractions.
  - Does not hyperventilate.
- **Goal:** The woman maintains a sense of control.
  Expected Outcomes: She expresses ability to deal with contractions.
- **Goal:** The woman rests between uterine contractions.
  Expected Outcomes: She sleeps or rests with eyes closed between uterine contractions.
  - Remains quiet and calm between uterine contractions.

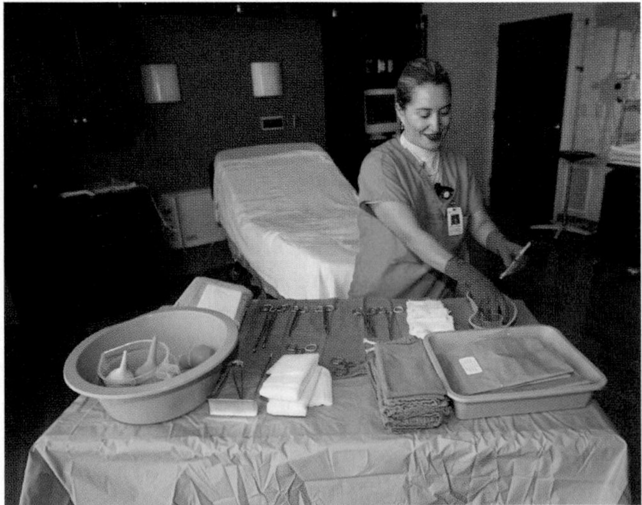

● ***Figure 10.11*** The nurse prepares the labor room for delivery. Photo by Joe Mitchell.

Test Yourself

- Discuss the five signs associated with the transition phase of labor.
- What responsibilities does the nurse have for supporting the partner or coach?
- Why is it important that the woman refrain from pushing until the cervix is completely dilated?

● The Nursing Process During the Second Stage of Labor: Expulsion of the Fetus

The second stage of labor begins when the cervix is 10 cm dilated and 100% effaced and ends with the birth of the newborn. Nursing care during this stage of labor focuses on providing physical and psychological support to the woman while she pushes the fetus through the birth canal. Assessment of maternal and fetal well-being during this stage is crucial.

ASSESSMENT

During the second stage of labor, close observation of the laboring woman and her fetus is indicated. Monitor the blood pressure, pulse, and respirations every 15 to 30 minutes. Cervical examination reveals that the cervix is fully dilated (10 cm) and completely effaced. The fetal station is usually 0 to + 2.

Assess the contraction pattern every 15 minutes. The pattern will be similar to that found in the transition phase (i.e., contractions occur every 2 to 3 minutes, last 60 to 90 seconds, and are of strong intensity). Assess for the woman's report of an uncontrollable urge to push, which is caused by pressure from the descending fetal head.

Assessment of the fetus during the second stage is essential. As the fetus descends into the pelvis, the pressure on his head is very intense. There may also be pressure on the cord during contractions. It is not uncommon for the fetal monitor strip to reveal early or variable decelerations. Variables are usually not ominous at this stage as long as the FHR returns quickly to baseline as the contraction relaxes, the baseline remains between 110 and 160 bpm, and variability is present. Check the FHR every 15 minutes for low-risk women and every 5 minutes for women determined to be at risk for labor complications.

Evaluate the woman's psychosocial status; the laboring woman may find it less difficult to cope with the contractions now that she can push. Often she is less irritable and more cooperative. Assess the woman's level of fatigue. If the second stage is prolonged, she may become extremely fatigued and experience difficulty finding the energy to push.

SELECTED NURSING DIAGNOSES

- Fatigue related to pushing efforts
- Risk for Trauma related to pushing techniques and positioning for delivery.

OUTCOME IDENTIFICATION AND PLANNING

Appropriate goals for the second stage of labor include that the woman will push effectively despite fatigue and that she will give birth with minimal or no trauma to the fetus and herself.

IMPLEMENTATION

Promoting Effective Pushing Despite Fatigue

All of the comfort measures appropriate to active labor continue to apply during the second stage, particularly while the woman is pushing. Using comfort measures such as applying a cool cloth to the forehead and offering ice chips and mouth care can promote relaxation between contractions, which helps to conserve energy and prevent exhaustion.

Assist the woman to the chosen position for pushing and provide support throughout each pushing effort. For instance, if the woman is using the sitting position to push, the nurse and coach can assist her to the sitting position when the contraction starts and support her back while she pushes.

If the woman has experienced a prolonged labor and is having a difficult time pushing effectively, it may be appropriate to position her on her side for comfort and allow her to rest for 30 minutes to an hour in order to regain her strength. As long as there is no evidence of fetal distress on the monitor tracing, allowing for a break from pushing is acceptable. In fact, if the woman is able to push more effectively after the break, often the fetus will descend and birth will occur soon afterward.

Reducing the Risk for Trauma: Using Effective Pushing Techniques and Positions

The LPN assists the RN to ensure the safety of mother and baby during the second stage by promoting effective pushing techniques and positions for pushing.

Effective Pushing Techniques. Once the cervix is fully dilated, the woman can begin pushing

A PERSONAL GLIMPSE

After 2 days of doctors trying to induce labor, I was about ready to request a cesarean section. Although I truly desired a vaginal birth, my husband and I were at our wits' end after having tried every measure available to start labor. During those frustrating days, the nurses I had were so supportive. They encouraged me to think positively and hold onto hope that I would eventually have a vaginal birth. When I was finally able to push, my labor and delivery nurse, Mary Ellen, was so supportive. Somehow, she convinced me that every push was the first one. With her gentle guidance, I believed I could get my baby out, even when it seemed it would never happen. I will never forget how helpful and tender she was. She told me time and again that I was "almost there" while my doctor shook his head in disagreement. Having spent more time with Mary Ellen than with the doctor who would eventually deliver my child, I believed her assessment far more than his! I don't think I even remember his name, but I will always remember Mary Ellen for her reassurance and gentle care.

Sara

LEARNING OPPORTUNITY: Describe three supportive nursing behaviors that can encourage a woman to not give up when labor seems overwhelming.

Why do you think the nurse's support is beneficial to prevent unnecessary cesarean deliveries?

efforts. Traditionally, obstetric nurses have taught women to use vigorous pushing techniques. When **vigorous pushing** is used, the woman is told to take a deep breath, hold the breath and push while counting to 10. She is encouraged to complete three "good" pushes in this manner with each contraction. However, recent research has revealed that vigorous pushing techniques that employ the Valsalva maneuver are associated with changes in the mother's heart rate and blood pressure, and the FHR may be adversely affected.

Based on research, two natural forms of pushing are advocated: open-glottis pushing and the urge-to-push method. Encourage the woman to use **open-glottis pushing,** which is characterized by pushing with contractions using an open glottis so that air is released during the pushing effort. The nurse also may encourage the woman to use the **urge-to-push method,** in which the woman bears down only when she feels the urge to do so using any technique that feels right for her. No matter what pushing technique is used, never leave the woman alone during pushing efforts.

Watch out! When the mother is pushing effectively, delivery can occur rapidly. Monitor for signs of imminent delivery, which include grunting, bulging of the perineum, crowning of the fetal head, and exclamation that "the baby is coming!"

Positions for Pushing. There are many different positions that are acceptable for pushing and for delivering the baby. However, in this country most deliveries are accomplished in a modified dorsal recumbent position in which the woman's legs are on foot pedals and the head of the bed is elevated approximately 45 degrees. Occasionally the practitioner will ask for the legs to be positioned in stirrups (lithotomy position). The nurse removes the bottom part of the bed to allow easy access to the perineum. Dorsal recumbent and lithotomy positions allow for greater control by the attendant but are not necessarily the most comfortable or effective positions for enhancing delivery.

Don't forget! Prevention of supine hypotension remains a priority during delivery. If a lithotomy position is used, place a wedge under the woman's hip to tilt the uterus away from the major vessels.

One major disadvantage of the lithotomy position is that gravity is not used to assist the birth.

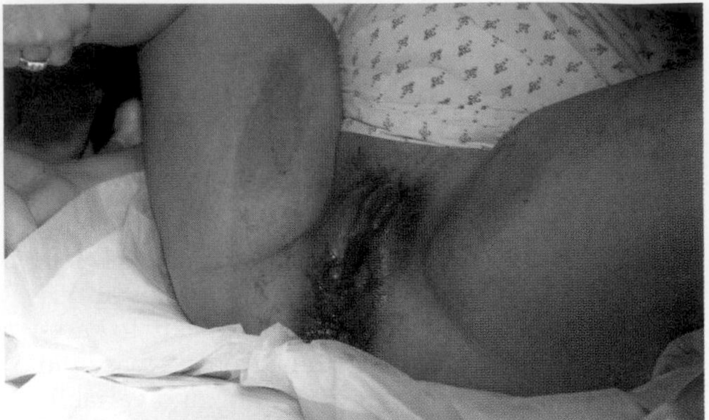

● ***Figure 10.12*** Bulging of the perineum is an indicator of imminent delivery. © B. Proud.

Other positions use gravity to aid in the pushing process, which conserves energy during the second stage of labor. Some positions, such as hands and knees, encourage rotation of the fetus, which shortens the second stage of labor. The hands and knees position enhances blood flow to the placenta, resulting in less fetal distress. Table 10-3 illustrates and compares positions used for pushing and delivery of the baby.

Preparing for Delivery of the Newborn

Nursing judgment is necessary to decide when to prepare the woman for delivery. The nurse may observe bulging of the perineum or crowning of the fetal head, which indicate imminent delivery (Fig. 10-12). Preparation of the primipara is typically done when the fetus is crowning, whereas preparation of the multipara may be done when the fetus reaches a +2 or +3 station. However, preparation may be done sooner in both cases if the fetus is descending rapidly.

If the woman has been laboring in a birthing bed and the semisitting or lithotomy position is to be used for delivery, the bed is "broken"—the lower part of the bed is removed to allow room for the birth attendant to control the delivery. Often the woman's feet are placed on foot pedals. If stirrups are used, take care to position the stirrups properly, then lift both legs together and place them in the stirrups. Clean the woman's perineum with an antiseptic solution (Fig. 10-13, p. 243); often a Betadine scrub is used. Position the instrument table close to the birthing bed and uncover it. If necessary, an in-and-out catheterization of the urinary bladder is done.

Prepare the equipment necessary to receive the baby in anticipation of the birth. This preparation involves turning on the radiant warmer and placing a warm blanket under the warmer. Be sure that the forms to begin the baby's chart

TABLE 10.3 Comparison of Positions for Pushing and Delivery

Position	Advantages	Disadvantages
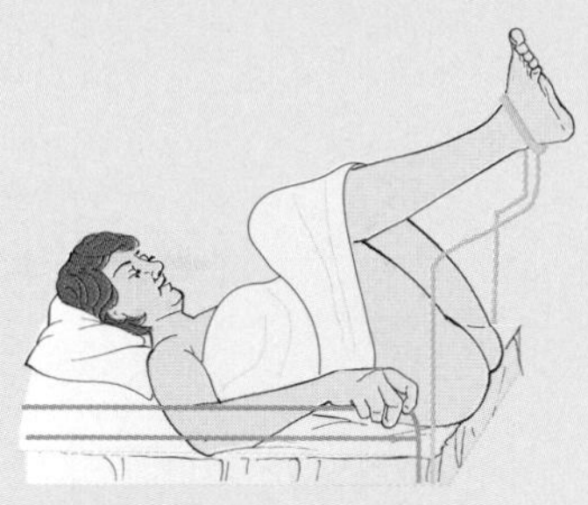 Lithotomy: This was the position used by the majority of physicians in the 1960s to 1980s. It is still used occasionally. The woman is positioned on a flat delivery bed with her legs in stirrups.	Easy access to the perineum and greater control of delivery by birth attendant	Greater risk of supine hypotensive syndrome and positioning injuries (e.g., clot formation from compression or muscle strain from improper placement in stirrups)
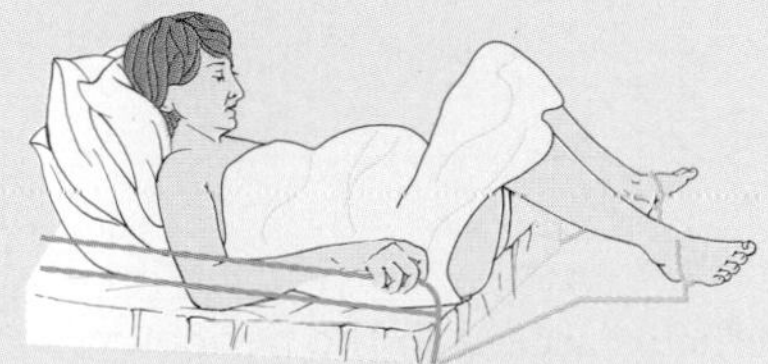 Modified dorsal recumbent or semi-sitting: This is a common pushing position. When it is time for delivery, the woman's feet are placed on foot pedals and the birthing bed is "broken" in preparation for delivery.	Easy access to the perineum and good control of delivery by birth attendant	May be uncomfortable for the woman. May not be the best position to facilitate expulsion of the baby.
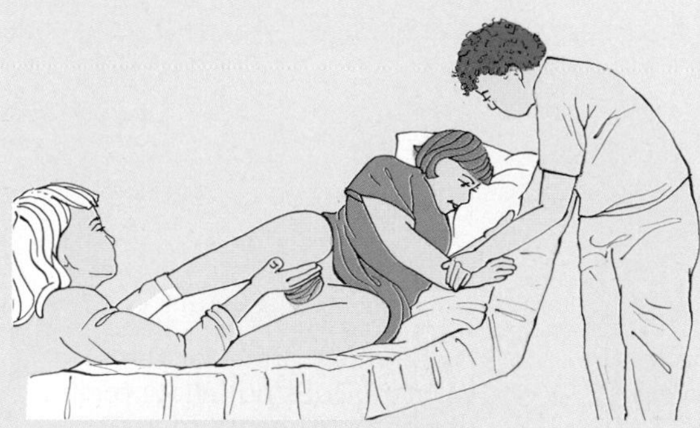 Side-lying	May increase comfort of the woman.	Decreases access to the perineum by the birth attendant. Requires high degree of cooperation from the woman and possible assistance of the nurse or support person to hold the upper leg during delivery.

(table continues on page 236)

TABLE 10.3 (continued) Comparison of Positions for Pushing and Delivery

Position	Advantages	Disadvantages
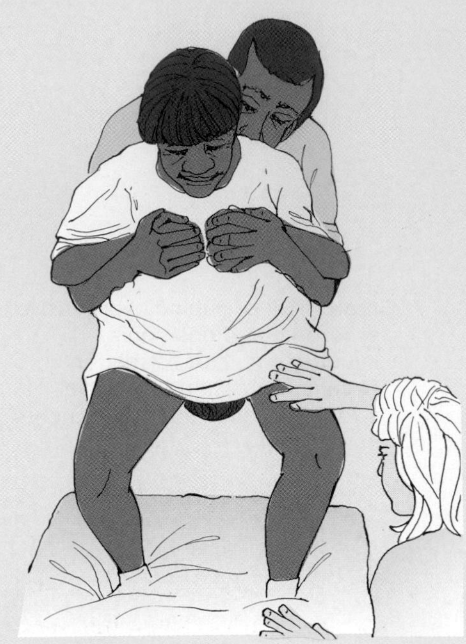 Squatting	Highly likely to increase the comfort of the woman. Uses gravity to facilitate expulsion of the baby.	Difficult access to the perineum. Requires a birth attendant who is flexible and willing to use this approach. The woman may lose her balance in this position. A pushing bar can help maintain balance, or a birthing stool may be used.
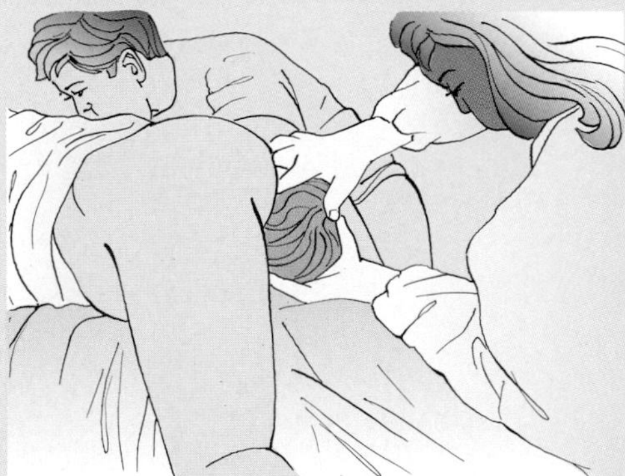 Hands and knees: The woman is assisted to her hands and knees on the birthing bed to push and deliver the baby.	Encourages rotation of the fetal head, which hastens delivery. Enhances placental blood flow, which decreases fetal stress. Allows for the perineum to stretch better than other positions so that an episiotomy is less often required. Allows for greater access to the perineum by the birth attendant than some of the other alternative positions.	May be more tiring for the woman. Does not allow for the use of instruments to assist delivery.

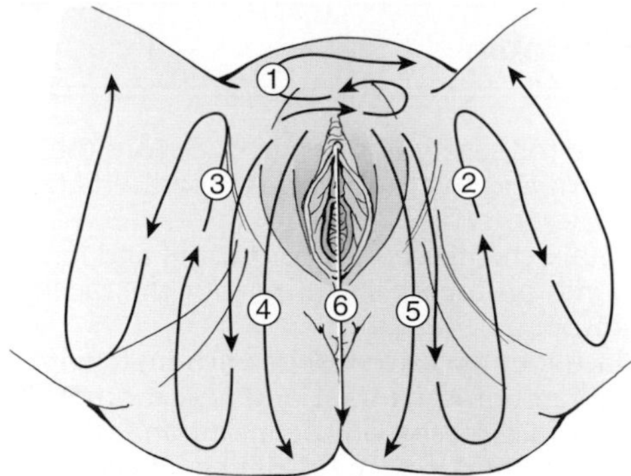

● *Figure 10.13* Perineal scrub in preparation for delivery. An antiseptic solution is used to clean the perineum just before delivery. The numbers represent the order in which each stroke is completed. The arrows represent the direction of the scrub. A new sponge is used for each stroke.

are in the room, and check the resuscitation equipment once more before delivery.

The RN is responsible for overseeing events in the delivery room. Surgical terms are used to describe the role of the RN; therefore, she is referred to as the circulator. The RN should remain in the delivery room until after the infant is born, the placenta is delivered, and mother and baby are stable. Box 10-8 lists the major responsibilities of the nurse in the delivery room, including immediate care of the newborn (see Chapters 13 and 15 for comprehensive coverage of newborn care). Figure 10-14 (pp. 246–247) shows a delivery sequence from crowning through birth of the newborn.

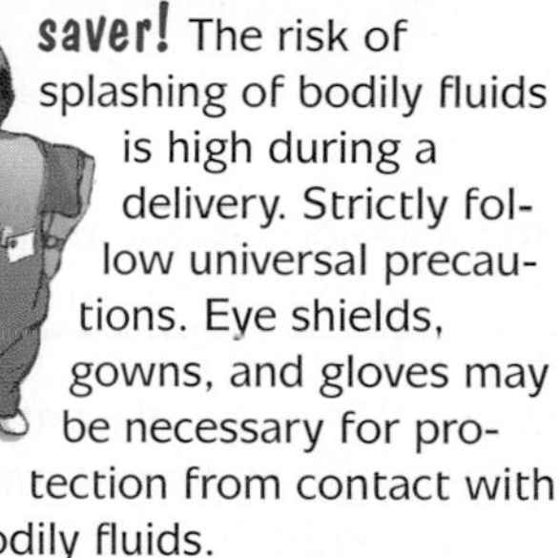

This advice could be a life-saver! The risk of splashing of bodily fluids is high during a delivery. Strictly follow universal precautions. Eye shields, gowns, and gloves may be necessary for protection from contact with bodily fluids.

EVALUATION: GOALS AND EXPECTED OUTCOMES

- **Goal:** The woman will push effectively despite fatigue.
  Expected Outcomes: She maintains the energy to push effectively with contractions.
  - The partner or coach retains a supportive, active participant role.
- **Goal:** Trauma to the woman and her fetus are avoided.
  Expected Outcomes: Maternal vital signs remain stable.
  - Fetal heart rate remains within acceptable limits.

Test Yourself

- What instructions should be given to the laboring woman regarding pushing?
- What are the major responsibilities of the nurse in the delivery room?

● The Nursing Process During the Third Stage of Labor: Delivery of Placenta

The third stage of labor begins with the birth of the newborn and ends with delivery of the placenta. Nursing care during this stage of labor focuses on monitoring for placental separation and providing physical and psychological care to the woman.

ASSESSMENT

Assess the woman's psychosocial state after she gives birth. Immediately after birth the new mother often experiences a sense of relief that the birth has been accomplished and contractions have ceased. Monitor for signs of placental separation, which generally occur within 5 to 20 minutes of delivery. These signs begin with a uterine contraction, then the fundus rises in the abdomen, the uterus takes on a globular shape, blood begins to steadily trickle from the vagina, and the umbilical cord lengthens as the placenta separates from the uterine wall.

The placenta may deliver in one of two ways (Fig. 10-15, p. 246). The most common way is for the smooth, shiny fetal side to deliver first (Schultze's mechanism). Sometimes the edge of the placenta appears at the introitus, revealing the rough maternal surface (Duncan's mechanism). The latter mechanism of delivery is more frequently associated with retained placental fragments. After the placenta is delivered, the birth attendant inspects it for completeness. Palpate the fundus to make certain the uterus is well contracted, and monitor the perineum for excess bleeding.

SELECTED NURSING DIAGNOSES

- Risk for Deficient Fluid Volume related to blood loss in the intrapartum period
- Risk for Trauma: Hemorrhage, amniotic fluid embolism, or uterine inversion related to separation of the placenta during the third stage of labor

BOX 10.8 Responsibilities of the Nurse in the Delivery Room

Closely monitor the laboring woman.
- Record vital signs and status assessments per facility protocol.
- Assess for maternal response to anesthesia.

Closely monitor the fetus. Assess FHR
- Every 15 minutes for low-risk labors.
- Every 5 minutes for at-risk labors.

Maintain accurate delivery room records.
- Note and record the time of delivery.
- Record all nursing procedures performed and maternal/newborn response.

Provide immediate newborn care (refer to Chapters 13 and 15 for in-depth discussion of newborn adaptation and care).
- Maintain warmth.
  - Immediately dry the newborn on the woman's abdomen or under the radiant warmer.
  - Wrap the newborn snugly and place a cap on the head when not in skin-to-skin contact with the woman or when not under a warmer.
- Assess adaptation to extrauterine life.
  - Assess and record Apgar scores (see Chapter 15 for a discussion of Apgar scoring).
- Maintain a patent airway.
  - Position the newborn to facilitate drainage.
  - Suction secretions with a bulb suction device or with wall suction.
- Provide for safety and security. Before the newborn and the mother are separated after delivery
  - Obtain the newborn's footprints and mother's thumb or fingerprint (if part of the facility protocol).
  - Place identification bands with matching numbers on the infant and new mother. Two bands are placed on the infant and one on the new mother. In some facilities a band is also placed on the new father or support person.

Promote parental-newborn bonding.
- Allow/encourage the woman and her partner to hold the newborn.
- Allow/encourage breast-feeding immediately after delivery.
- Encourage skin-to-skin contact with the newborn.
- Point out positive characteristics of the newborn.

Assist the birth attendant.
- Perform sponge and instrument counts.
- Ensure that supplies are available for episiotomy and repair, if needed.
- Obtain additional supplies as needed, such as forceps or vacuum extractor for difficult deliveries, or extra suturing material.

OUTCOME IDENTIFICATION AND PLANNING

The major goals during the third stage of labor are that the new mother will maintain adequate fluid volume and that she will remain free of trauma.

IMPLEMENTATION

Preventing Fluid Loss

Monitor the woman's vital signs at least every 15 minutes during the third stage of labor to detect signs of dehydration. Tachycardia and a falling blood pressure are signs of impending shock and should be reported immediately. Note how much time has passed since the birth of the newborn. The placenta normally separates within 20 minutes of delivery. If a longer period of time has passed, the woman may be experiencing retained placenta, which can lead to acute fluid loss from hemorrhage. Monitor intravenous fluids to ensure patency and prevent the development of dehydration.

Maintaining Safety and Preventing Trauma

Monitor the woman for any sudden change in status. Complaints of shortness of breath, chest pain, or tachypnea may indicate the development of an amniotic fluid embolism (a discussion of this complication is found in Chapter 18).

Administer oxytocin as soon as the placenta is delivered. Oxytocin causes the uterus to contract, which puts pressure on the open blood vessels at the former placenta site. When the placenta separates from the uterine wall, it leaves an open wound that is subject to hemorrhage if the uterus does not contract effectively. Oxytocin is most frequently added to the IV fluids, but some physicians and midwives prefer that it be given using the intramuscular method. It is important not to give an oxytocic medication before the placenta is delivered because the drug given at this time will increase the risk of a retained placenta.

EVALUATION: GOALS AND EXPECTED OUTCOMES

- **Goal:** The woman will maintain an adequate fluid volume.
  Expected Outcomes: Blood pressure does not fall and the pulse does not rise.
- **Goal:** The woman remains free of trauma.
  Expected Outcomes: The placenta is delivered intact with less than 500 milliliters of blood loss.
  - Respirations remain unlabored.
  - Lung sounds are clear.
  - Fundus remains firm.

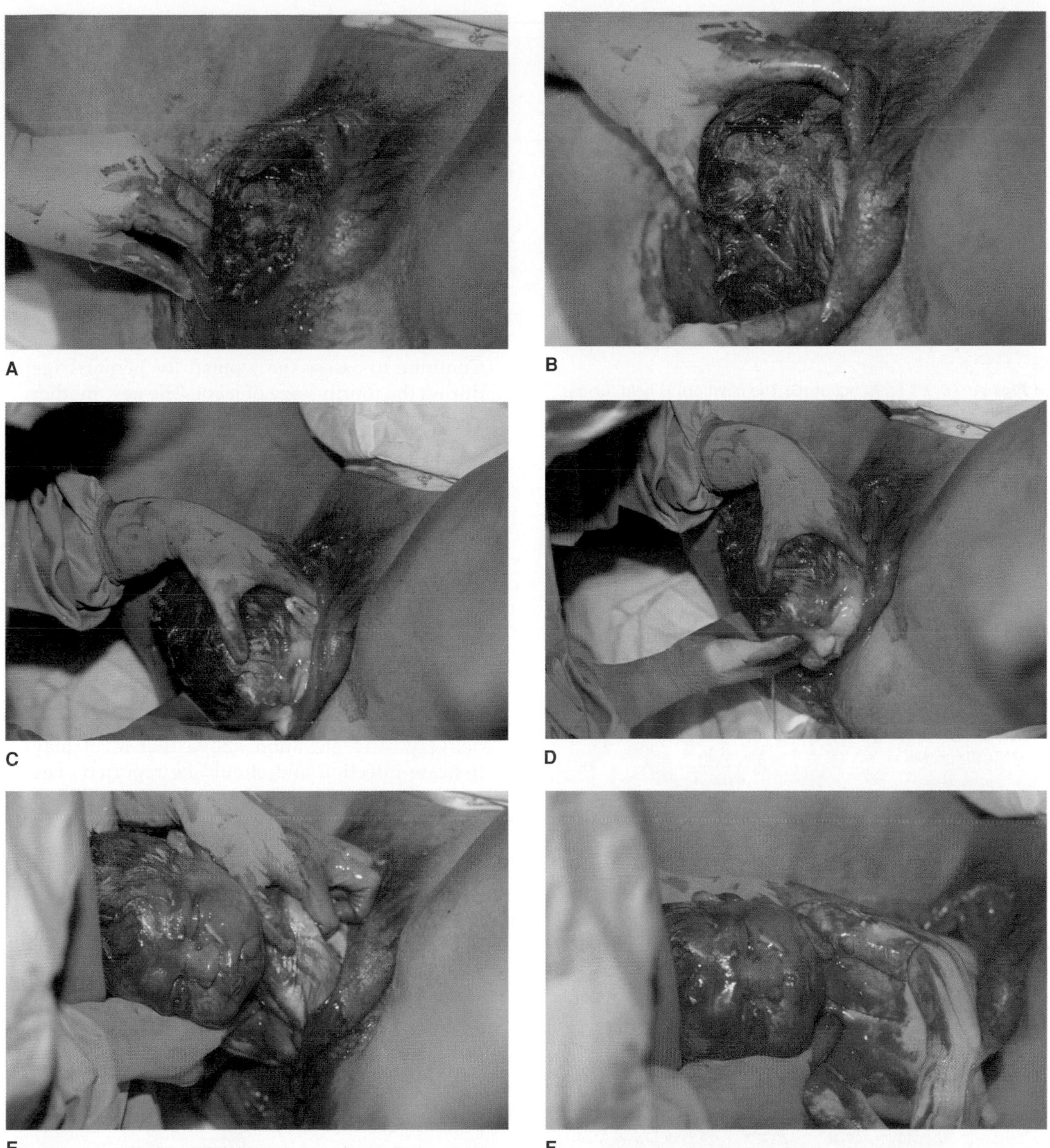

● ***Figure 10.14*** Delivery sequence from crowning through birth of the newborn. (**A**) Early crowning of the fetal head. Notice the bulging of the perineum. (**B**) Late crowning. Notice that the fetal head is appearing face down. This is the normal OA position. (**C**) As the head extends, you can see that the occiput is to the mother's right side—ROA position. (**D**) The cardinal movement of extension. (**E**) The shoulders are born. Notice how the head has turned to line up with the shoulders—the cardinal movement of external rotation. (**F**) The body easily follows the shoulders.

(figure continues on page 240)

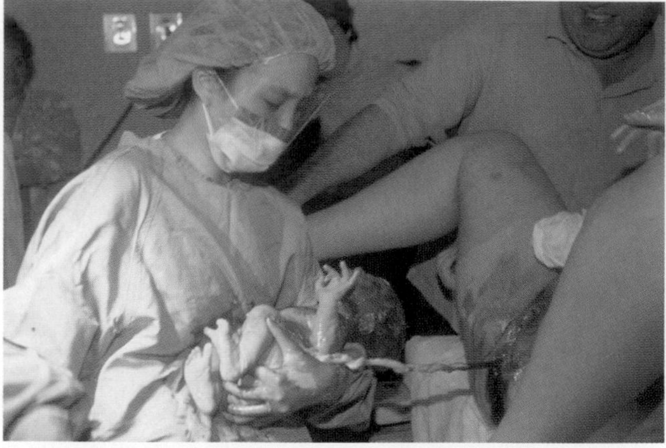

G

● ***Figure 10.14*** (continued) (**G**) The newborn is held for the first time! © B. Proud.

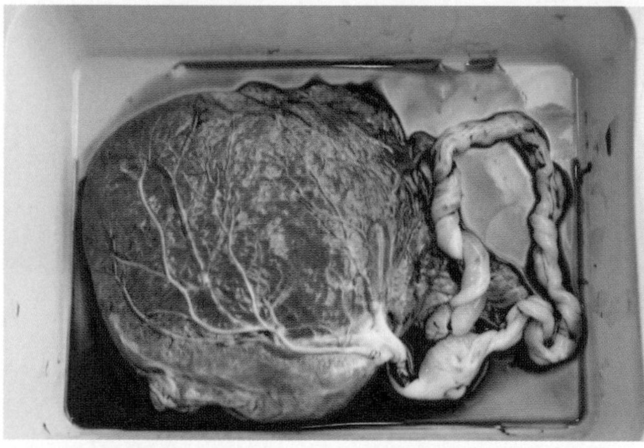

A

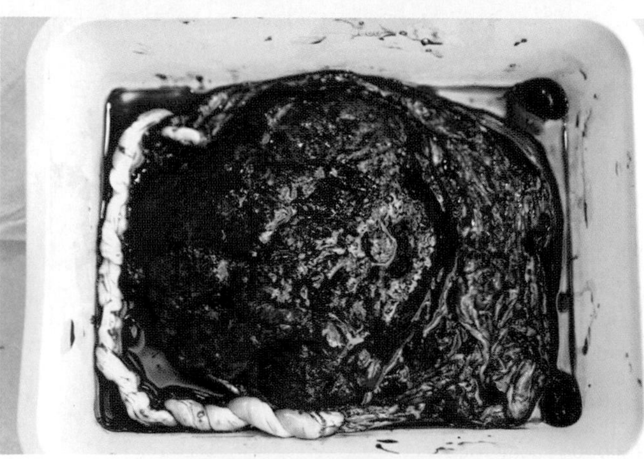

B

● ***Figure 10.15*** A healthy placenta after delivery. (**A**). Notice the shiny surface of the fetal side. The umbilical cord is inserted in the center of the fetal surface. (**B**). The maternal side is rough and divided into segments (cotyledons). Photos by Joe Mitchell.

● The Nursing Process During the Fourth Stage of Labor

The fourth stage of labor begins with delivery of the placenta and ends when the woman's physical condition has stabilized (usually within 2 hours). Nursing care during this stage focuses on continued assessment and care of the woman and promoting parental–newborn bonding.

ASSESSMENT

Continue to assess the woman for hemorrhage during the fourth stage of labor. The new mother is at highest risk for hemorrhage during the first 2 to 4 hours of the postpartum period. Monitor the woman's vital signs, and palpate the fundus for position and firmness. The fundus should be well contracted, at the midline, and approximately one fingerbreadth below the umbilicus immediately after delivery. Assess the **lochia** (vaginal discharge after birth) for color and quantity. The lochia should be dark red and of a small to moderate amount.

Monitor for signs of infection. The temperature may be elevated slightly, as great as 100.4°F, because of mild dehydration and the stress of delivery. Any elevation above that level may indicate infection and should be reported. The lochia should have a fleshy odor but should not be foul smelling.

The woman should void within 6 hours after delivery. Trauma from the birth may have caused edema in the perineal area or anesthesia may persist, leading to an inability to sense a full bladder. Both conditions can lead to urinary retention. Monitor for suprapubic distention and a high fundus that is displaced to the right. These signs indicate that the urinary bladder is full.

Assess the woman's comfort level. There are many sources of pain during the immediate postpartum period. Cramping from uterine contractions and perineal pain from edema or episiotomy repair are common sources of pain for the new mother. Ask the woman to describe the location of the pain and to rate it on a standardized pain scale.

Assess the mother's psychosocial state during the fourth stage. Typically, the mother is fatigued and ravenously hungry. It is normal for her to be self-absorbed and demonstrate dependent behaviors. She also has an intense need to talk about the labor and delivery experience.

Assess initial bonding behaviors of the new family. It is normal for parents to want to hold and touch the newborn as soon as it is born. You may notice that the parent begins initial inspection of the newborn with the fingertips; this is normal behavior and indicates positive beginning attachment.

Perhaps this advice will be useful. Many nurses use a numbered scale from 0 to 10 to assess their patients for pain. Explain that "0" indicates no pain, whereas "10" indicates the worst pain imaginable, and then ask the woman to choose a number that most closely matches her pain level. In this way you can easily evaluate the effectiveness of your interventions by asking her to rate her pain again on the same scale after intervening.

Be careful not to be too hasty to diagnose inadequate bonding. Some mothers are so fatigued that they may not desire prolonged interaction with the newborn beyond the initial inspection. Behaviors that indicate a risk for inadequate attachment include turning away from the newborn or making disparaging comments about the newborn.

SELECTED NURSING DIAGNOSES

- Risk for Impaired Parent–Infant Attachment related to disappointment regarding the gender of the newborn or an unwanted pregnancy
- Risk for Deficient Fluid Volume related to possibility of hemorrhage from the former site of placenta attachment
- Risk for Infection related to invasive procedures and vaginal examinations during labor
- Impaired Urinary Elimination related to perineal trauma during delivery
- Acute Pain related to episiotomy, birth trauma, and/or afterpains
- Fatigue related to energy expended during labor

OUTCOME IDENTIFICATION AND PLANNING

Appropriate goals for the new mother during the fourth stage of labor (recovery) are that the parents will begin a positive bonding process with their newborn, and that the woman will maintain adequate fluid volume, remain without signs of infection, fully empty the bladder at the first voiding, report a tolerable pain level, and report the ability to rest and sleep during the immediate postpartum period.

IMPLEMENTATION

Providing Care Immediately After Delivery

After the birth attendant has completed his or her duties, inspect and cleanse the perineum. Remove the soiled drapes and linen and place an absorbent pad under the buttocks with two sterile perineal pads against the perineum. Place a warm blanket over the new mother. Reassemble the birthing bed. If stirrups were used, remove both legs from the stirrups at the same time.

Promoting Parent–Newborn Attachment

While the birth attendant is suturing any lacerations or episiotomy and making a final inspection of maternal tissues, it is important to promote parental bonding with the newborn. Hand the newborn to the woman as soon as it is determined that he does not need extraordinary resuscitation. If the father is present at the delivery, encourage him to hold and interact with the newborn (Fig. 10-16). This is a good time for the new mother to attempt breast-feeding for the first time. If the woman permits it, place the newborn skin-to-skin against her body and place several blankets over them. This technique (called kangaroo care) keeps the infant warm and promotes bonding.

Maintaining Adequate Fluid Volume

Continue to monitor the woman for signs of fluid volume deficit or hemorrhage. Take vital signs every 15 minutes during the fourth stage of labor. Falling blood pressure and tachycardia may indicate fluid volume deficit or hemorrhage and should be reported. Massage the fundus

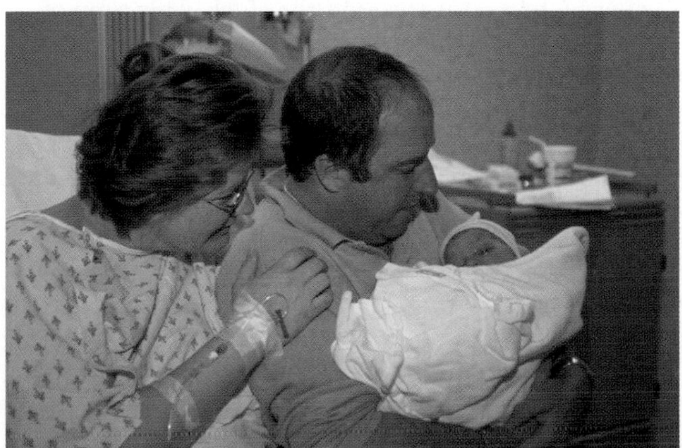

● ***Figure 10.16*** The father and mother bond with their newborn son soon after birth.

every 15 minutes and inspect the lochia for amount and color. The fundus should be firm or should quickly become firm when gently massaged. Continue to monitor IV fluids and offer food and fluids to the new mother.

Preventing Infection
Continue to use excellent handwashing technique. Hands should be washed before and after care, between patients, and any time bodily fluids are contacted. Of course, it is critical to use standard precautions. Wear gloves at all times when you perform procedures anywhere near the perineum or dirty linens. Anything that comes in direct contact with the perineum should be sterile. The perineal pads should be handled from the ends and not touched in the middle area.

Promoting Urinary Elimination
If the woman has the urge to void, assist her to the bathroom unless she is still under the effects of anesthesia and does not have complete control of her legs. It is much easier for her to void sitting on a toilet than it is on a bedpan. Have her dangle her feet at the bedside for several minutes before assisting her to a standing position. Once she is safely in the bathroom, run water or let her soak her hands in warm water if she is having difficulty getting the stream of urine started. An in-and-out catheterization is usually not done unless there is significant suprapubic distention or discomfort from the full bladder or until 6 hours have passed without voiding.

Minimizing Pain
Nonsteroidal anti-inflammatory drugs (NSAIDs) and oral narcotic analgesics, such as codeine, often are prescribed for pain after delivery. The NSAIDs are quite effective at reducing painful uterine cramping. Many providers order large doses (600 to 800 mg) of ibuprofen to be given every 6 to 8 hours around the clock. This type of dosing is often more effective at keeping pain under control than is an "as needed" schedule, in which the woman must ask for the medication before it is given.

Combination medications consisting of a mild analgesic, such as acetaminophen, with a narcotic such as codeine, may be ordered on an as-needed basis for breakthrough pain. Sometimes codeine is ordered for perineal pain, and the NSAIDs are given to control cramping. Assess the woman's pain frequently and administer medications before the pain becomes intolerable.

Warmth to the abdomen may be helpful in reducing the discomfort of uterine cramping. Position changes may also be helpful. If the pain is from an episiotomy or edema of the perineum, it is helpful to apply ice packs. Most labor units have combination perineal pads/ice packs. These are convenient for the nurse, but a clean glove filled with ice also works as an ice pack. If used, it should be applied between the two perineal pads so that a nonsterile object does not come in direct contact with the perineum.

Watch out! Extreme perineal pain may indicate the development of a perineal hematoma. Inspect the perineum with each vital sign check. Inquire further regarding perineal pain if the new mother becomes restless, is unable to find a comfortable position, tilts to one side when sitting, or reports unbearable pain in the perineum. The RN in charge should be notified immediately if any of these signs is present.

Reducing Fatigue
After the initial bonding period, it may be helpful to discourage visitors and promote rest for the new mother. Her partner can stay with her to care for the newborn if the newborn is rooming-in or if the hospital provides couplet care. If the newborn is to be stabilized in a newborn nursery, this is a good time for both the new mother and her partner to get some much-needed rest and sleep, if possible.

EVALUATION: GOALS AND EXPECTED OUTCOMES

- **Goal:** The parents begin a positive bonding process.
  Expected Outcomes: They inspect the newborn immediately after birth.
  - They make positive comments about the newborn.
- **Goal:** The woman maintains an adequate fluid volume.
  Expected Outcomes: Blood pressure and pulse remain within expected limits.
  - Fundus remains firm.
  - Vaginal bleeding remains small.
- **Goal:** The woman remains free of signs of infection.
  Expected Outcomes: She remains afebrile.
  - Lochia has a normal fleshy odor and is not malodorous.
- **Goal:** The woman empties her bladder effectively.
  Expected Outcomes: She expresses the ability to void without difficulty.
  - No suprapubic distention.

- **Goal:** The woman expresses a tolerable pain level.
  Expected Outcomes: She reports that interventions are effective at relieving pain.
- **Goal:** The woman avoids extreme fatigue.
  Expected Outcomes: She reports the ability to rest and sleep in the immediate postpartum period.

Test Yourself

- Identify four signs of placental separation.
- How often are vital signs checked during the fourth stage of labor?
- Name three parameters that should be assessed with each vital sign check during the fourth stage of labor.

KEY POINTS

- Continuous support of a skilled obstetric nurse facilitates the labor process and the woman's satisfaction with the birth experience.
- Throughout the labor process, the nurse is responsible for monitoring maternal and fetal status and labor progress. Frequent assessment of vital signs and FHR are critical nursing functions.
- When a woman arrives at the labor unit, immediate assessment involves observing for signs that birth is imminent, in which case admission procedures are abbreviated until after delivery.
- If the birth is not imminent, admission assessment includes a thorough obstetric, medical–surgical, and social history and a complete physical assessment. Fetal, maternal, and labor statuses are determined, and a report is made to the birth attendant.
- Intermittent auscultation of FHR allows for freedom of maternal movement and focuses the nurse's attention on the woman, rather than the technology. Disadvantages are that subtle signs of fetal distress may be missed.
- External fetal monitoring is noninvasive and allows for evaluation of baseline FHR and long-term variability. However, it is less precise than internal monitoring, which can detect short-term variability and provides a more consistent tracing. Internal monitoring requires that the membranes be ruptured and the cervix be at least partially dilated.
- To apply the fetal monitor, first locate the fetal back, and then apply the transducer using ultrasonic jelly. Next locate the fundus and place the toco on the firmest part of the fundus. Both the toco and transducer are secured to the abdomen with straps.
- The LPN must be able to detect nonreassuring FHR patterns so that he can notify the charge nurse and/or the primary health care provider, who then makes a final decision regarding care of the patient.
- No intervention is required for early decelerations, other than continued monitoring. Nursing interventions for variable decelerations are aimed at relieving cord compression and include maternal position change or amnioinfusion. Late decelerations require aggressive management. The woman is positioned on either side, oxygen is started via face mask, and any oxytocin infusion is discontinued. Sometimes tocolytics are prescribed to decrease the frequency and duration of uterine contractions, which improves blood flow to the placenta.
- Fetal stimulation is another way to measure how well the fetus is tolerating the stress of labor. It can be done noninvasively with an acoustic vibrator or invasively during a vaginal examination. An increase in the FHR with stimulation is reassuring.
- Fetal scalp sampling is an invasive procedure that provides direct evidence of fetal status via the pH. Disadvantages include that it requires that the membranes be ruptured and there is a small chance that fetal and maternal blood will intermingle and lead to incompatibilities. Fetal pulse oximetry gives direct evidence of fetal oxygenation without being directly invasive to the fetus. It does, however, require that the membranes be ruptured.
- The latent phase of the first stage of labor is marked by feelings of excitement and also by anticipatory anxiety and fear. Teaching about the labor process can help reduce anxiety. Distraction techniques are helpful in facilitating coping.
- Contractions become more frequent and stronger during the active phase of labor. Distraction techniques typically do not help during active labor. Support of the woman and her partner include encouragement to continue behaviors that promote coping and assistance in finding alternative approaches when coping is ineffective. Reinforcing breathing techniques and rituals can be helpful.
- The transition phase is the most intense phase of labor. The woman becomes irritable and less cooperative. The challenge for the nurse is to assist the woman to rest between contractions and to avoid pushing efforts until the cervix is fully dilated.
- Full dilation of the cervix marks the beginning of the second stage of labor. Because the woman can now participate actively by pushing, she often feels re-energized to deal effectively with the labor. The open-glottis method of pushing is

recommended. Encouragement and reinforcement of pushing techniques are helpful nursing interventions.

- The placenta is delivered in the third stage of labor. The nurse monitors for signs of placental separation and ensures that the fundus remains contracted after the placenta delivers. Risk for trauma from birth-related complications is an appropriate nursing diagnosis.
- During the fourth stage of labor, or the recovery period, the risk for hemorrhage is high. Close monitoring of the fundus, lochia, and vital signs is warranted. Risk for deficient fluid volume and risk for birth-related trauma are priority nursing diagnoses.

REFERENCES AND SELECTED READINGS

Books and Journals

Association of Women's Health, Obstetric and Neonatal Nurses (AWHONN). (2000). *Fetal assessment. AWHONN Position Statement*. Retrieved September 14, 2001, from http://www.awhonn.org/resour/POSITION/psresp.html

Association of Women's Health, Obstetric and Neonatal Nurses (AWHONN), Mattson, S., & Smith, J. E. (Eds.). (2000). *Core curriculum for maternal–newborn nursing* (2nd ed.). Philadelphia: W. B. Saunders Company.

Berkowitz, K., & Nageotte, M. P. (2000). Intrapartum fetal monitoring. In A. T. Evans & K. R. Niswander (Eds.), *Manual of obstetrics* (6th ed., pp. 313–329). Philadelphia: Lippincott Williams & Wilkins.

California College of Midwives. (1999). *Intermittent auscultation augmented with episodic electronic fetal monitoring (EEFM) for community-based midwives. Technical Bulletin No.* 2. Retrieved January 20, 2002, from http://www.goodnewsnet.org/college99/efm99bb.htm

Cuervo, L. G., Rodriguez, M. N., & Delgado, M. B. (1998). Enemas during labor. *Cochrane Review Abstract*. Retrieved September 14, 2001 from http://www.medscape.com/cochrane/abstracts/ab000330.html

Cunningham, F. G., Gant, N. F., Leveno, K. J., Gilstrap, L.C. III, Hauth, J. C. & Wenstrom, K. D. (2001). *Williams obstetrics* (21st ed.). New York: McGraw Hill Medical Publishing Division.

Hodnett, E. (1996). Nursing support of the laboring woman. *Journal of Obstetric, Gynecologic, and Neonatal Nursing (JOGNN), 25*(3), 257–264.

Mozurkewich, E., & Wolf, F. M. (2000). Near-infrared spectroscopy for fetal assessment during labour. From *Cochrane Abstracts*. Retrieved January 20, 2002, from http://search.medscape.com/Cochrane/abstracts/ab002254.html

Nettina, S. M. (2001). Nursing management during labor and delivery. In *The Lippincott Manual of Nursing Practice* (7th ed., pp. 1124–1151). Philadelphia: Lippincott Williams & Wilkins.

University of Pennsylvania Health System. (Undated). A century of obstetrics. Retrieved January 20, 2002, from http://www.obgyn.upenn.edu/History/clinobhis.html

Wolcott, H. D., & Conry, J. A. (2000). Normal labor. In A. T. Evans & K. R. Niswander (Eds.), *Manual of obstetrics* (6th ed., pp. 392–424). Philadelphia: Lippincott Williams & Wilkins.

Websites

http://www.childbirth.org/
http://www.childbirth.org/articles/labor.html
http://www.thebabycorner.com/pregnancy/labor.html

Doulas

http://doulanetwork.com/

WORKBOOK

NCLEX-STYLE REVIEW QUESTIONS

1. A woman presents to the labor suite and states, "I have water leaking down my legs." What assessment is most appropriate in this situation?
   a. DTRs
   b. Fern test
   c. Blood pressure check
   d. Urine test for protein
2. A primipara is dilated 8 cm and is completely effaced at a +1 station. She tells the nurse, "I can't keep myself from pushing when I have a contraction." What intervention is most appropriate in this situation?
   a. Offer comfort measures.
   b. Reapply the fetal monitor.
   c. Assist the woman to blow at the peak of contractions.
   d. Tell the coach that it is not good for the baby if she pushes right now.
3. A G1 P0 is in the active phase of labor. She is a low-risk patient. You evaluate the fetal monitor strip at 10:00 a.m. Moderate variability is present. The FHR is in the 130s with occasional accelerations, no decelerations. At what time do you need to re-evaluate the FHR?
   a. 10:05 a.m.
   b. 10:15 a.m.
   c. 10:30 a.m.
   d. 11:00 a.m.
4. A G3 P2 with no apparent risk factors presents to the labor and delivery suite in early labor. She refuses the fetal monitor. She says that she delivered her second baby at home without a monitor and everything went well. How do you plan to handle this situation?
   a. Explain that she will need to be on the monitor for a few minutes to be certain this baby is doing well. After this initial assessment the baby can then be monitored intermittently.
   b. Insist that the fetal monitor be used because there are not enough staff members to adequately monitor her using any other method.
   c. Request that the charge nurse reassign you to another patient because you do not want to be responsible if anything were to happen to her baby during labor.
   d. Tell her that it is her decision, but continuous EFM is the only recommended way to monitor how well her baby is doing during labor.
5. In which situation is it most likely that the physician would consider performing an amnioinfusion? The EFM tracing shows
   a. consistent early decelerations, variability present, and occasional accelerations.
   b. flat line without variability and no decelerations.
   c. occasional mild variable decelerations and moderate variability present.
   d. deep variable decelerations with every contraction.

STUDY ACTIVITIES

1. Choose what you think are the three most important nursing assessments and interventions during labor. Using the table below, compare your top three picks for the laboring woman during the active phase, transition phase, and the second stage of labor. Include the frequency of the interventions. What similarities do you see? What differences are apparent?

	Active Phase	Transition	Second Stage
Major nursing assessments			
Major nursing interventions			

2. Run a search on the Internet using the key words "birth plans." How many sites returned? After exploring some of the sites, what are the main issues covered in a birth plan? Does a birth plan seem realistic to use if the woman intends to deliver in the hospital? Why or why not?
3. Interview a labor and delivery nurse. Ask her how her facility handles birth plans. Does she recall a time when parts of the birth plan could

not be honored? How was the situation handled? What was the outcome?

CRITICAL THINKING: What Would You Do?

Apply your knowledge of the labor process and the nurse's role during labor and birth to the following situation.

1. Priscilla, a 26-year-old G1 P0, presents to the birthing center because her "labor pains" have begun. She talks excitedly with her husband, who is to be her coach. She says that she is pleased that the happy day is finally here, but she is afraid that she will "lose it" when the contractions get stronger. She and her husband have attended childbirth preparation classes.
   a. What nursing assessments should be completed?
   b. What phase/stage of labor do you suspect Priscilla is in?
   c. What do you expect the vaginal examination will reveal?
   d. What nursing interventions will you implement for Priscilla and her husband?
   e. How would your care be different if the couple had not attended childbirth classes?
2. Several hours after admission to the birthing center, Priscilla is dilated 5 cm and the cervix is completely effaced. When a contraction begins, Priscilla kneels on the bed, rests her upper body against her husband, closes her eyes and sways slowly while humming softly. At the end of the contraction her husband gently places her on her side and she rests with her eyes closed until the next contraction begins.
   a. What phase/stage of labor is Priscilla in?
   b. What nursing assessments need to be completed at this time?
   c. What is your assessment of Priscilla's coping technique?
   d. What nursing actions are appropriate for Priscilla and her partner at this point in her labor?
3. Three hours later, Priscilla becomes agitated and snaps at her husband and the nurse. She exclaims, "I can't stand this anymore! I want to go *home*!"
   a. What nursing assessments should be completed at this time? Why?
   b. What nursing interventions are appropriate for Priscilla and her husband now?
   c. How would you decide whether or not your interventions had been effective?
4. It is the beginning of your shift. The charge nurse gives you report on Martha Brown, a 29-year-old G2 P1. The fetus is in a vertex presentation and the water bag is intact. A vaginal examination was done 1 hour previously. At that time her cervix was 4 cm dilated and 80% effaced. The station was +1 and the position was LOT. Continuous EFM is ordered, and IV fluids are infusing into her left arm.
   a. What assessments do you make, in what order, when you enter Martha's room?
   b. How do you evaluate the contraction pattern?
5. A few hours later, you go to check on Martha. You notice that she is much more restless than she has been. The fetal monitor tracing shows the FHR baseline in the 140s. Moderate variability is present. During each contraction the FHR dips into the 120s. The dip is smooth with a gentle slope on both sides, like a contraction, only upside down. The FHR is back to 140 by the end of the contraction. You do perineal care because Martha has a lot of bloody show.
   a. How do you interpret the FHR pattern? Is the pattern reassuring or nonreassuring? Defend your answer.
   b. What should your next action be? Why?

Assisted Delivery and Cesarean Birth

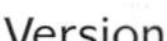

Version
- *External Version*
- *Internal Version*

Induction of Labor
- *Indications*
- *Contraindications*
- *Labor Readiness*
- *Cervical Ripening*
- *Artificial Rupture of Membranes*
- *Oxytocin Induction*
- *Nursing Care*

Amnioinfusion
- *Contraindications and Possible Complications*
- *Nursing Care*

Assisted Delivery
- *Episiotomy*
- *Vacuum-Assisted Delivery*
- *Forceps-Assisted Delivery*
- *Nursing Care*

Cesarean Birth
- *Indications*
- *Incidence*
- *Risks*
- *Incision Types*
- *Steps of a Cesarean Delivery*
- *Nursing Care*

Vaginal Birth After Cesarean
- *Prerequisites*
- *Contraindications*
- *Procedure*
- *Nursing Care*

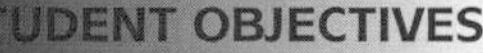

STUDENT OBJECTIVES

On completion of this chapter, the student will be able to

1. Describe external version to a patient who is scheduled for the procedure.
2. Identify at least four medical indications for induction of labor.
3. Explain the Bishop score and its usefulness in predicting the likelihood of induction success.
4. Contrast mechanical methods for hastening cervical readiness with pharmacologic methods.
5. Outline essential steps and possible complications associated with oxytocin induction.
6. Describe the procedure of amnioinfusion.
7. Compare mediolateral and midline episiotomies.
8. Differentiate between vacuum extraction and forceps-assisted delivery.
9. Explain maternal and fetal complications of cesarean delivery.
10. Name two of the most common and three less common indications for cesarean birth.
11. Differentiate between vertical and transverse skin and uterine incisions.
12. Compare nursing interventions needed to prepare a family for a planned cesarean birth with those for a family who is to undergo emergency cesarean delivery.
13. Explain important aspects involved with attempted VBAC.

KEY TERMS

amnioinfusion
amniotomy
Bishop score
cesarean birth
chorioamnionitis
elective induction
episiotomy
fetal fibronectin
forceps
laminaria
version

There are many tools and techniques available to the birth attendant to decrease the risk of labor and/or birth to the woman and her fetus.[1] Some procedures, such as repositioning the fetus, are done before labor. Induction techniques are used to initiate labor, if delivery is indicated. Some tools allow the primary care provider to intervene during labor when conditions arise that threaten the safety of the woman or her fetus. The birth attendant also has tools that are used to assist the delivery. Many of these options help avoid cesarean delivery, which subjects the woman and her fetus to all the hazards of major surgery.

Before the advent of surgical asepsis and antibiotics, if a laboring woman could not deliver a child vaginally, there were few options available to the physician or midwife. Sometimes the woman died. Other times extreme measures were taken and the unborn child's life was sacrificed to save the life of the mother (*Encyclopaedia Britannica,* 2002). Today, cesarean birth is frequently done if other options do not work or the risk of vaginal delivery outweighs the risk of surgical intervention.

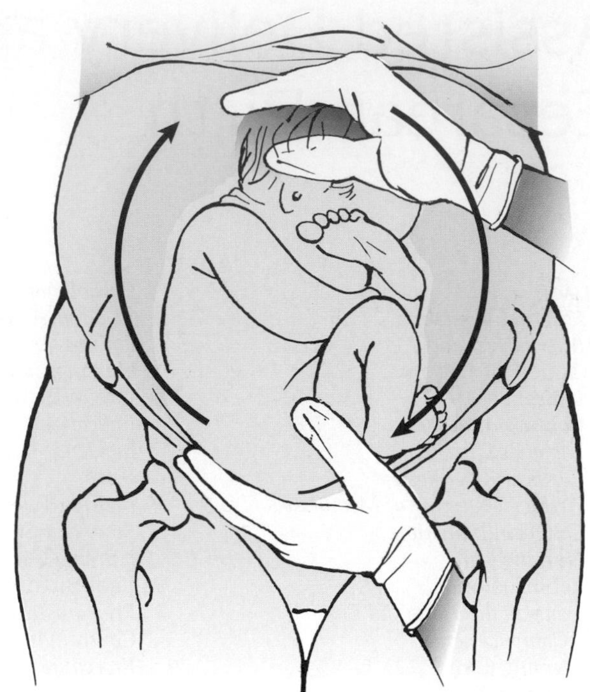

● ***Figure 11.1*** External version. One or two physicians manipulate the fetus through the abdominal wall to coax the fetus to turn to a vertex presentation.

VERSION

Version is a process of manipulating the position of the fetus while in utero. There are two types of version: external and internal.

External Version

External version is a procedure that is most frequently done to reposition a fetus that is breech or shoulder presentation near term (37 weeks and beyond). It must be done in a facility that has full capacity to perform an emergency cesarean delivery, if one should become necessary. The procedure is uncomfortable and occasionally has to be stopped because of discomfort of the woman.

The fetal monitor is connected, and a nonstress test (NST) performed by the registered nurse (RN). If the NST is reactive, the process can begin. An intravenous (IV) line is started, and laboratory work drawn in the event an emergency cesarean delivery becomes necessary. An ultrasound examination is performed to confirm the presentation and lie of the fetus, note placental location, determine if enough amniotic fluid is present, and rule out congenital anomalies and nuchal cord (umbilical cord around the fetus' neck). Some physicians have better success when a tocolytic, such as SQ terbutaline, is given to relax the uterus. The physician's hands are then placed on the abdomen in an attempt to manipulate the fetus to turn to a vertex presentation (Fig. 11-1). Often (approximately 65% of the time) the maneuvers are effective, and the fetus turns. Occasionally, the fetus will turn around again (revert) to a breech position, although this is more likely to occur if the fetus is premature. The ultrasound examination is repeated afterward to determine if the maneuvers were successful.

Nursing care includes assisting the woman to empty her bladder just before the procedure. Position the woman supine with a pillow or wedge under the right hip. If ordered, the RN administers tocolytics. Take and record vital signs before and after the procedure. Afterward the RN monitors the fetus for 30 minutes to an hour. You may be instructed to administer Rho (D) immune globulin (RhoGAM) to the Rh-negative woman.

Internal Version

Internal version is done infrequently and is usually reserved to turn a second twin when she is breech. The physician inserts his fingers through the cervix (which must be sufficiently dilated to allow the procedure) and manipulates the fetus to turn. Alternatively, the

[1] The student should be aware that all of the procedures discussed in this chapter carry risk. Many of these procedures are done to correct problems discussed in Chapter 18. Although many of these techniques are frequently used, they should not be considered routine.

physician may do an internal podalic version by bringing down the fetal legs into the maternal pelvis.

INDUCTION OF LABOR

When a condition exists that could endanger the life of the woman or the fetus, the physician may elect to induce labor, rather than wait for nature to take its course. The rate of induced labors has risen dramatically over the past few years (Martin et al., 2003). There are many reasons for this rise, although one contributing factor seems to be an increase in the number of elective inductions. An **elective induction** is one in which the physician and woman decide to end the pregnancy in the absence of a medical reason to do so. Simpson and Atterbury (2003) caution against elective induction unless the woman understands that elective inductions often result in more interventions, longer labors, higher costs, and possible cesarean birth.

There are several ways to induce labor. Stripping the membranes and cervical ripening procedures may be used to encourage the onset of labor or to prepare the cervix for oxytocin-induced labor. Artificial rupture of membranes is a common practice used to induce labor or to augment a naturally occurring labor. Pitocin, a synthetic form of oxytocin, given intravenously is another common method used to induce or augment labor.

Indications

Any condition that endangers the life of the woman or the fetus if the pregnancy were to continue is considered a medical indication for induction of labor. There are many such conditions. Postdate pregnancy, a pregnancy that persists beyond the expected due date, is probably the most common reason that labor is induced. Premature rupture of membranes (PROM); spontaneous rupture of membranes (SROM) without the onset of spontaneous labor; **chorioamnionitis**, infection of the fetal membranes; pregnancy-induced hypertension; and preeclampsia are obstetric complications that often require labor induction. Other examples include severe intrauterine fetal growth restriction or maternal medical conditions such as diabetes mellitus or gestational diabetes. Sometimes labor is induced in an attempt to avoid an unattended delivery. For example, a woman who has a history of rapid labors and who lives far away from the hospital or birthing center may have labor induced at or near term. In any case, the risks of allowing the pregnancy to continue are weighed against the risks of labor induction before a decision is made to induce labor.

Contraindications

Conditions in which spontaneous labor is contraindicated are also contraindications for the induction of labor. For example, complete placenta previa, history of a classical uterine incision, or more than two previous low transverse uterine incisions are contraindications for both spontaneous and induced labor. Fetal contraindications include certain anomalies, such as hydrocephalus, fetal malpresentations, and fetal compromise. Structural abnormalities of the pelvis and invasive cervical cancer are maternal contraindications. Certain medical conditions that necessitate a cesarean delivery, such as active genital herpes, preclude labor induction.

Labor Readiness

Cervical readiness is generally a prerequisite for successful labor induction. A cervix that is favorable for induction is called a "ripe" cervix. One commonly used scoring method to determine cervical readiness is the **Bishop score** (Table 11-1). Five factors are evaluated: cervical consistency, position, dilation, effacement, and

TABLE 11.1 Bishop Scoring System

	Factor				
Score	Dilatation (cm)	Effacement (%)	Station*	Cervical Consistency	Cervical Position
0	Closed	0–30	−3	Firm	Posterior
1	1–2	40–50	−2	Medium	Midposition
2	3–4	60–70	−1.0	Soft	Anterior
3	≥5	≥80	+1, +2		

*Station reflects a −3 to +3 scale.

Adapted with permission from Bishop, E. H. (1964). Pelvic scoring for elective induction. *Obstet Gynecol, (24)*, 266–268.

fetal station. Each factor is given a score of 0 to 3: the higher the score, the greater the chance that induction will be successful. In general, a score of 9 or greater is associated with a favorable response to oxytocin-induced labor; that is the cervix is soft, in an anterior position, partially dilated and effaced, with an engaged fetus. A Bishop score of 5 or less indicates an unripe or unfavorable cervix, and labor induction is less likely to be successful.

One relatively new method for predicting labor readiness is determination of cervical length by endovaginal ultrasound. A cervix that measures 28 millimeters in length (or less) is associated with a favorable induction rate, even in the presence of a low Bishop score. Refer to Chapter 7 for a description of this diagnostic procedure.

Another newer method for determining labor readiness is measurement of fetal fibronectin levels. **Fetal fibronectin** is a protein found in fetal membranes and amniotic fluid. Its presence in cervical secretions is associated with labor readiness. The test consists of swabbing the cervical area during a speculum examination to obtain a secretion sample. The sample is then sent to a laboratory to test for fetal fibronectin levels. However, this test is not done widely to determine labor readiness at term; it is more often used as a predictor of preterm labor risk.

In addition to cervical readiness, the fetus should be mature before labor is induced, unless a condition exists in which the risks of prematurity are outweighed by the risks of continued pregnancy. Maturity can be assessed in several ways. If the pregnancy has completed at least 38 weeks' gestation (as determined by reliable dating methods), the fetus is considered to be mature. Fetal lung maturity is the most important factor to be considered. Measuring the lecithin/sphingomyelin (L/S) ratio via amniocentesis assesses lung maturity. An L/S ratio greater than 2.0 or a positive phosphatidyl glycerol test indicates fetal lung maturity.

Cervical Ripening

Frequently labor induction is indicated, but the cervix is not ready. In this situation a procedure to ripen the cervix may be used before induction with oxytocin is started. The following discussion explores mechanical and pharmacologic methods used to ripen a cervix in preparation for labor induction.

Mechanical Methods

One of the most common mechanical methods used to hasten cervical readiness is a procedure called "membrane stripping." The primary care provider inserts a gloved finger through the internal cervical os and sweeps the finger 360 degrees to separate the membranes from the lower uterine segment. Plasma levels of prostaglandins (one substance associated with the onset of labor) are measurably higher after membrane stripping. Several research studies support the efficacy of membrane stripping to initiate spontaneous labor and decrease the use of oxytocin without increasing the risk of maternal infection or likelihood of cesarean birth (Cunningham et al., 2001, p. 474).

Mechanical dilation of the cervix is sometimes attempted by inserting a catheter into the cervix and inflating the balloon. Mechanical dilation can be accomplished with or without infusion of normal saline, a procedure known as extra-amnionic saline infusion, although the addition of saline does not increase the likelihood of success. The risk of uterine hyperstimulation and the risk for cesarean birth are both reduced with the use of mechanical dilation as compared with the use of pharmacologic methods to induce labor (Boulvain, Kelly, Lohse, Stan, & Irion, 2003).

Laminaria, or cervical dilators, are sometimes used to soften and dilate the cervix. Laminaria are made from the root of seaweed. The cylindrical material is placed in the cervix and works by absorbing moisture, which causes it to expand slowly. As the material expands, it dilates the cervix gradually. Laminaria are most frequently used to induce abortion for therapeutic and elective reasons, or to induce labor when the fetus has died in utero. Few scientific studies have been done to evaluate their use for induction of labor at term, although some practitioners use them for this purpose.

Pharmacologic Methods

Locally applied prostaglandins have been found to be effective in preparing an unripe cervix for labor. There are two main preparations, although the only substance approved by the United States Food and Drug Administration (FDA) for this purpose is prostaglandin E_2 gel or vaginal inserts (dinoprostone). Prostaglandin E_1 (misoprostol) is used frequently for cervical ripening, although it is not approved for this use.

Prostaglandin E_2 (Dinoprostone)

There are two preparations of prostaglandin E_2 available for use: prostaglandin E_2 gel (Prepidil) and prostaglandin E_2 vaginal inserts (Cervidil). Prepidil comes in a 2.5-mL syringe that dispenses 0.5 mg of dinoprostone. The practitioner injects this preparation into the cervix. Cervidil is available as a 10-mg vaginal insert that is placed into the posterior fornix during a vaginal examination. If uterine hyperstimulation occurs, Cervidil can be removed by pulling on the string that is left in the vagina.

The woman receiving dinoprostone should be in a facility that has continuous fetal monitoring capabilities. Assist the RN to place the fetal monitor and run a tracing for at least 20 minutes to obtain a reactive NST.

When the practitioner is ready, bring the medication to the bedside and assist with a vaginal examination. Instruct the woman about the importance of lying in a recumbent position (do not forget to put a wedge under one hip) for at least 30 minutes. Continue the fetal monitor tracing, as ordered (usually for 30 minutes to 2 hours), and monitor for signs of uterine hyperstimulation or fetal distress.

Prostaglandin E_2 is usually administered in the evening. Sometimes the woman is allowed to go home and return when labor ensues. However, some physicians prefer to keep the woman in the delivery suite overnight and begin oxytocin induction of labor in the morning (6 to 12 hours after dinoprostone is applied).

Prostaglandin E_1 (Misoprostol)
The synthetic prostaglandin E_1 analog misoprostol (Cytotec) is an antiulcer agent whose properties promote cervical ripening. It is available in a 100-microgram tablet that is usually divided. The practitioner or a specially trained nurse places one quarter of the tablet (25 micrograms) in the posterior vaginal fornix. The dose can be repeated every 4 to 6 hours (Goldberg & Wing, 2003). Sometimes a higher dosing protocol (1/2 tablet or 50 micrograms) is used. However, the higher dose is associated with more cases of uterine hyperstimulation and fetal distress and is not recommended. Misoprostol (Cytotec) can be given orally. Results similar to the 25-microgram vaginal dose are obtained when one tablet (100 micrograms) is given by mouth. Nursing care for the woman receiving misoprostol is similar to that described for dinoprostone.

Artificial Rupture of Membranes

Artificial rupture of membranes (AROM), also known as an **amniotomy**, can be done to induce labor or to augment labor that has already begun. A hard plastic instrument with a hook on the end, an Amnihook, is introduced into the vagina during a digital examination. The practitioner then guides the instrument through the cervix with two fingers and uses the hook to snag a hole in the membranes. At this point amniotic fluid is usually expelled. This process causes the body to release prostaglandins, which enhances labor.

Oxytocin Induction

Labor is often induced through the use of intravenous oxytocin (Pitocin), a synthetic form of the posterior pituitary hormone that causes the uterus to contract. The woman is admitted to a labor and delivery suite and the external fetal monitor is attached. After at least 20 minutes of fetal monitoring to obtain a baseline fetal heart assessment, a mainline IV is started. Then a secondary IV line that contains oxytocin is started via an infusion pump so that the dose of the medication can be controlled carefully. One common protocol is to place 10 units of oxytocin in 1,000 mL of IV fluid. Using this protocol, 6 mL/hour is equal to a dose of 1 milliunit/minute. The dose is usually titrated up by 1 to 2 milliunits every 15 to 20 minutes until an adequate contraction pattern is obtained.

Several potential complications are associated with the use of oxytocin for inducing labor. There is a higher risk that a cesarean birth will become necessary whenever labor is induced. This is particularly true for primigravidas (Simpson & Atterbury, 2003). There is also a risk that the uterus will be hyperstimulated. Hyperstimulation leads to contractions that occur one after the other without a sufficient rest period in between. This can lead to fetal distress and even uterine rupture. Another potential complication is water intoxication. Because oxytocin is a posterior pituitary hormone, it is chemically related to antidiuretic hormone. Therefore, oxytocin can have an antidiuretic effect, causing the kidneys to retain water. Symptoms of water intoxication include hyponatremia, confusion, convulsions, or coma. Congestive heart failure and death also can occur.

Nursing Care

The licensed practical nurse's (LPN's) role during induction depends upon the procedure. The RN maintains responsibility for monitoring the woman and her fetus during pharmacologic cervical ripening procedures and oxytocin induction and augmentation. However, the LPN may be asked to assist the birth attendant during a pelvic examination in which mechanical methods of cervical ripening are used (i.e., membrane stripping and laminaria insertion) or during amniotomy. When amniotomy is done, document the fetal heart rate before and after the procedure. Notify the RN or birth attendant if the rate drops precipitously. Sometimes the birth attendant will ask for suprapubic or fundal pressure during the procedure. It is permissible to give this assistance, if you have been properly trained to do so.

Test Yourself

- True or false: External version always requires the use of a tocolytic to relax the uterus.
- Name two medical indications for the induction of labor.
- Which locally applied prostaglandin is approved by the FDA to be used for cervical ripening?

AMNIOINFUSION

Amnioinfusion is infusion of sterile fluid into the uterine cavity during labor. This procedure is done to relieve persistent deep variable decelerations associated with cord compression. It is also done to dilute thick meconium-stained amniotic fluid in an effort to decrease morbidity and mortality from meconium aspiration syndrome. Prerequisites for this procedure include ruptured membranes and adequate cervical dilation to allow introduction of the intrauterine pressure catheter (IUPC) into the uterus. Only physiologically compatible fluid is to be used. Lactated Ringer's and 0.9% normal saline are suitable. Never use a dextrose solution. It is recommended that the fluid be warmed using a blood warmer when the fetus is preterm. Term fetuses can tolerate room temperature fluids.

Exercise caution! Fluids should never be placed in a baby blanket warmer or in the microwave. Doing so is against manufacturer's recommendations and could result in serious burns.

Contraindications and Possible Complications

Contraindications include any situation in which placement of the IUPC is inadvisable, such as placenta previa, abruptio placenta, and so on. Other contraindications include multiple gestation, malpresentation of the fetus, absent/diminished fetal heart rate variability or other signs of fetal distress, fetal anomalies incompatible with life, uterine anomalies, and chorioamnionitis.

Possible complications of this procedure include polyhydramnios from trapped amniotic fluid, high intrauterine pressure readings, placental abruption, chorioamnionitis, and problems caused by solution temperature issues, e.g., maternal chilling from fluid that is too cold or fetal tachycardia from fluid that is too warm.

Nursing Care

The RN is responsible for monitoring the woman who receives an amnioinfusion. The solution is connected to IV tubing and primed. The RN will assist the physician or nurse midwife to insert the IUPC according to manufacturer's guidelines. After the IUPC is in place, the IV tubing is attached to the infusion port. A fluid bolus of 250 mL (or the amount ordered) is given. Then the tubing is connected to an IV pump and the rate decreased to approximately 150 mL/hour or as ordered.

The RN will monitor the resting tone of the uterus at least every 30 minutes. The resting tone should not exceed 25 mm Hg. You may be asked to assist the woman with perineal care. Assess and record the amount, color, and odor of the fluid that is being expelled onto the under-buttocks pad. If no fluid is returning at all, notify the RN immediately.

ASSISTED DELIVERY

Sometimes a problem develops in one of the essential components toward the end of labor. The fetus may descend to the pelvic floor without rotating to the anterior position. Or the mother may become tired and stop pushing effectively. In cases such as these, the birth attendant may elect to use an operative technique or device to hasten the delivery. Types of assisted delivery include episiotomy, vacuum-assisted delivery, and forceps delivery.

Episiotomy

An **episiotomy** is a surgical incision made into the perineum to enlarge the vaginal opening just before the baby is born. In the recent past, physicians performed episiotomies on virtually all primigravidas delivered in the United States. This procedure is no longer considered to be routine, although episiotomies are still performed in approximately 40% of all deliveries (Simpson & Creehan, 2001, p. 326).

It was commonly believed that an episiotomy was less painful and healed faster than a jagged tear that might result if an episiotomy were not performed. However, research has not validated these assumptions. In fact, research studies demonstrate that an episiotomy increases the risk that the perineum will tear into the anal sphincter (Carroli & Belizan, 2004), a condition that increases maternal discomfort as well as the risk of infection and long-term consequences, such as anal incontinence. In addition, women on whom an episiotomy is performed may lose more blood than women who are delivered over an intact perineum (Simpson & Creehan, 2001, p. 326). Box 11-1 lists several measures that can reduce the need for episiotomy.

There are, however, situations in which an episiotomy may be indicated. These include:

- The baby's shoulders are stuck in the birth canal after the head is born (shoulder dystocia).
- The head will not rotate from an occiput-posterior position (persistent occiput-posterior).
- The fetus is in a breech presentation.
- Forceps or vacuum-assisted delivery is used to shorten the second stage of labor.

BOX 11.1 Methods to Minimize the Need for Episiotomy

- Kegel exercises during pregnancy to strengthen perineal muscles
- Using natural pushing techniques, particularly in the side-lying position
- Patience with the delivery process
- Protection of the perineum immediately before birth (by the birth attendant) to avoid uncontrolled delivery of the fetal head

There are two basic types of episiotomies (Fig. 11-2). A median or midline episiotomy extends from the fourchette straight down into the true perineum. This type of episiotomy increases the risk for extension into the anal sphincter but is easier for the physician to repair and causes less discomfort for the woman than a mediolateral episiotomy, which is angled to the right or left of the perineum.

Repair of the perineum is needed if an episiotomy is performed. If the woman had epidural anesthesia, she may not need additional anesthesia for repair. Often, local anesthesia is used to numb the perineum for repair. Have suture readily available according to the physician or nurse midwife preference. Reassure the woman that the sutures are absorbable and do not need to be removed.

Vacuum-Assisted Delivery

A device sometimes used to hasten delivery is the vacuum extractor. In this procedure the birth attendant places a suction cup (some are soft silicone cups and others are hard metal cups) on the fetal head; then suction is applied, and the device is used to gently guide the delivery of the infant (Fig. 11-3). The nurse provides

A PERSONAL GLIMPSE

When I was pregnant with my second child, I re-read everything about the experience: the pregnancy, the delivery, the recovery, and nursing. Having had one healthy baby before this one, I felt like I was prepared for what was going to happen in the whole process of delivering a baby.

When my water broke at 4 a.m. on a Saturday, my husband and I rushed to the hospital. The vaginal delivery went well and quickly. However, after our little girl was born, I was told that I had been given an "episiotomy." Of course during the delivery, I was numb from the epidural, and I really had no idea what had gone on other than being told to push numerous times. The nurse left me some cotton pads, and told me to keep myself clean until the stitches "melted."

The area of the episiotomy caused me a lot of pain. Every time I sat on the toilet to urinate, my vaginal area would hurt. I would avoid having bowel movements, as those were very painful as well. When I told the nurses about how much it hurt, they would tell me to clean myself better after urinating, and got a doctor to prescribe me a stool softener to take home.

It wasn't until I was discharged and my mother was staying at home with me to help out, that we figured out what the problem was. I asked my mother to look at my vaginal area, and she saw that one of the stitches had a knot that had irritated the skin around it and caused a sore.

It would have been better if one of the nurses had looked for me (with my giant belly after the delivery, I couldn't see a thing) and figured out what the problem was before I had left the hospital.

Shelly

LEARNING OPPORTUNITY: Discuss two actions the nurse could take to better prepare this new mother to understand how to take care of her episiotomy. What assessments do you think the nurse should make for a patient with an episiotomy?

A

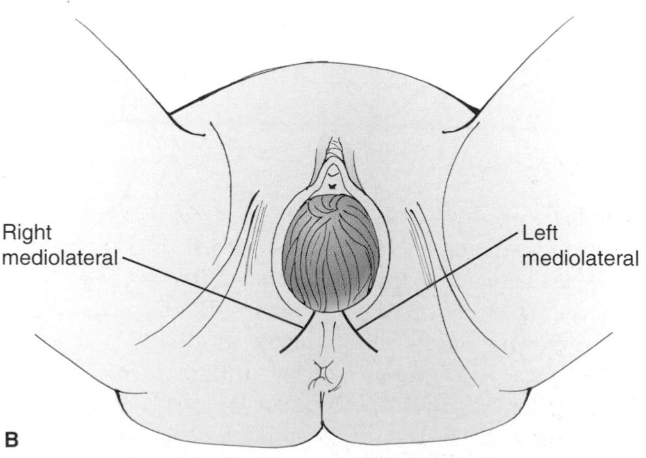

B

● ***Figure 11.2*** Two basic types of episiotomy. (**A**) Midline episiotomy extends straight down into the true perineum. (**B**) Mediolateral episiotomy angles to the right or the left of the perineum.

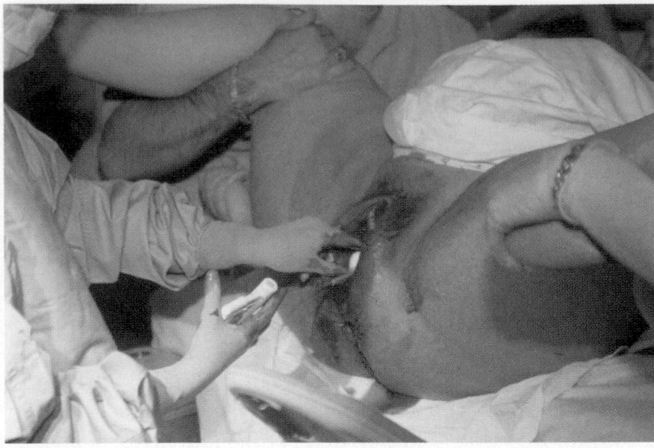

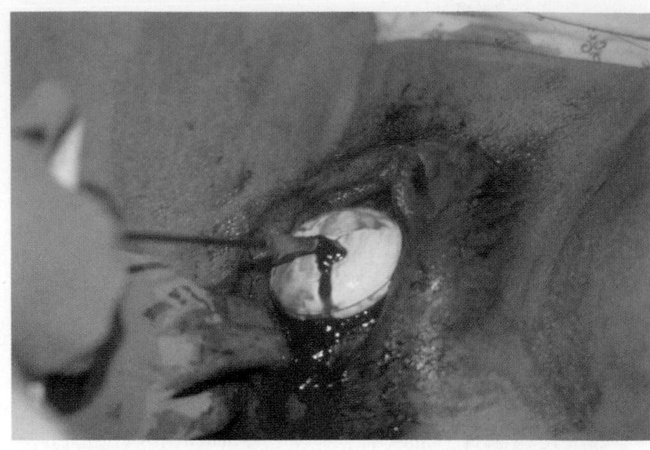

A B

● ***Figure 11.3*** Delivery assisted by vacuum extraction. (**A**) The birth attendant has just placed the suction cup on the fetal head and is using the hand pump to increase the pressure. (**B**) Gentle traction is placed on the fetal head to assist it through the last maneuvers of delivery.

the necessary equipment, connects and regulates the suction as instructed by the birth attendant, monitors fetal status, and supports the laboring woman during the procedure by keeping her informed of the procedure and progress.

Forceps-Assisted Delivery

Forceps are metal instruments with curved, blunted blades (somewhat like large hollowed-out spoons) that are placed around the head of the fetus by the birth attendant to facilitate delivery (Fig. 11-4). Low and outlet forceps are used more frequently than are midforceps. Outlet forceps are applied when the fetal head can be seen at the introitus; low forceps are used when the station is equal to or greater than + 2, but the head is not yet showing on the perineum; whereas, midforceps are used when the fetal head is well engaged but still relatively high in the pelvis (higher than +2). Midforceps are most often used to assist the fetus to rotate to an anterior position.

Indications and prerequisites for use of forceps and the vacuum extractor are similar. Any problem that causes the second stage of delivery to be prolonged or any situation of concern that is likely to be relieved by delivery of the infant may be an indication for assisted delivery. Maternal indications include fatigue (the woman may become exhausted while pushing), certain chronic conditions such as heart or lung disease, and prolonged second stage of labor. If fetal distress is evident and the criteria for forceps delivery are met, then forceps may be used to rapidly deliver the infant and relieve the cause of distress.

Nursing Care

During an assisted delivery the nurse obtains needed equipment and supplies; monitors maternal and fetal

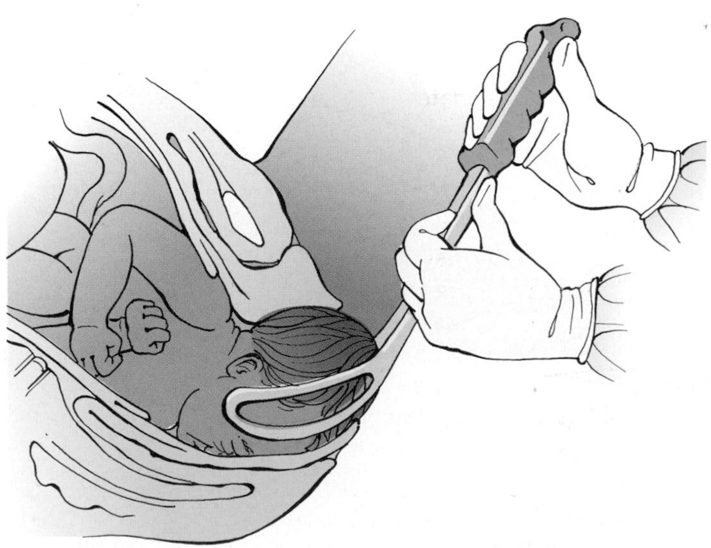

● ***Figure 11.4*** Forceps-assisted delivery.

status before, during, and after the procedure; assists the birth attendant; provides support for the woman; and documents the type of procedure, as well as maternal and fetal response. The nurse is aware that use of a technique to assist vaginal delivery may not work and anticipates the possibility of cesarean delivery. Episiotomy care after delivery is discussed in Chapter 12.

For both vacuum-assisted and forceps-assisted deliveries (operative vaginal deliveries), inspect the infant carefully for signs of trauma. This could include cephalhematoma, retinal hemorrhage, bruising, edema, exaggerated caput (chignon), forceps mark, and transient facial paralysis. Reassure the parents that forceps marks and exaggerated caput from vacuum-assisted deliveries will subside in a few days.

Maternal soft tissue trauma may also result from an operative vaginal delivery. Inspect the perineum for bruising and edema. Monitor closely for excessive bleeding or development of a hematoma. (Refer to Chapter 19 for nursing care of the woman with postpartum hemorrhage.)

Test Yourself

- Name two indications for amnioinfusion.
- Name two situations in which an episiotomy is helpful.
- List at least two fetal complications and one maternal complication of forceps or vacuum-assisted delivery.

CESAREAN BIRTH 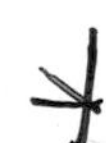

A **cesarean birth** is the delivery of a fetus through abdominal and uterine incisions: laparotomy and hysterotomy, respectively. Cesarean comes from the Latin word "caedere," meaning, "to cut." Sometimes the term "cesarean section" is used. This discussion uses the terms "cesarean birth" and "cesarean delivery" because the focus for the nurse and the woman is the birth experience.

Indications

There are many indications for cesarean birth. The majority (more than 85%) are done for the following four reasons:

1. History of previous cesarean
2. Labor dystocia (difficult labor)
3. Fetal distress
4. Breech (buttocks or feet first) presentation (Cunningham et al., 2001)

Other less common obstetric indications include placenta previa (placenta covers the cervix), abruptio placentae (placenta separates from the uterus before birth), cephalopelvic disproportion (fetal head cannot fit through the pelvis), active vaginal herpes lesions, prolapse of the umbilical cord, and ruptured uterus. Sometimes medical and obstetric conditions necessitate early delivery of the fetus and require cesarean delivery. Examples include maternal diabetes mellitus, pregnancy-induced hypertension, and erythroblastosis fetalis.

Incidence

Cesarean birth was rarely done before the development of antibiotics and antiseptic surgical techniques because of high maternal mortality rates from infection. This method of delivery has become increasingly accepted in modern times. The rate of cesarean deliveries quadrupled (from 4.5% to 22.8%) between 1965 and 1988 (Cunningham et al., 2001). There are multiple contributing factors to this dramatic increase, which include an increase in the percentage of pregnant women who are carrying their first child,[2] a rise in the number of older pregnant women, almost universal use of continuous electronic fetal monitoring, a trend toward delivering breech presentation through the abdomen, and an increasing concern regarding malpractice litigation. From 1988 to 1996 the rate fell, attributable in large part to a decrease in the rate of primary cesarean births and an increase in the number of vaginal births after cesarean (VBAC). From 1996 through the year 2000, overall cesarean rates steadily rose from 14.6% to 16.1% (Joseph et al., 2003). In 2002, the rate rose to 26.1%, the highest cesarean delivery rate ever reported in the United States. Much of this overall increase is probably related to a dramatic decrease in the rate of VBACs, from 23% in 2001 to 12.6% in 2002 (Martin et al., 2003).

Risks

Cesarean birth is a major surgery and carries with it all the risks associated with surgery combined with the risks of birth itself. A woman who is delivered by cesarean is up to four times more likely to die than is a woman who delivers vaginally (*ACOG News Release*, 2003), although death is a rare occurrence in obstetrics. Some surgical risk factors are increased because of the normal physiologic changes of pregnancy. For example, thrombophlebitis is a complication of both surgery and pregnancy, so the risk is compounded during cesarean delivery. There are risks to the fetus, as well. A fetus delivered by cesarean may inadvertently be delivered

[2] A primigravida is more likely to experience cesarean delivery than a multigravida.

prematurely, and he is more likely to have respiratory distress. For these reasons the American College of Obstetricians and Gynecologists (ACOG) recommends that cesarean delivery be performed only when the risks of vaginal delivery clearly outweigh the risks of surgery.

Because of the higher morbidity and mortality rates associated with cesarean delivery versus vaginal delivery, attempts have been made to decrease the cesarean delivery rate. Much research has focused on determining ways to safely deliver a woman vaginally after a previous cesarean birth and on methods to treat labor dystocia. These treatment modalities are discussed elsewhere in this chapter.

Maternal Complications

Maternal complications that can occur during the operation include laceration of the uterine artery, bladder, ureter, or bowel; hemorrhage requiring blood transfusion; and hysterectomy. The most common postoperative complication associated with cesarean birth is infection. Two common infection sites are the uterus and the surgical wound, although sepsis, urinary tract infection, and other infections also can occur. Pneumonia, postpartum hemorrhage, thrombophlebitis, and other surgical-related complications may be experienced during the postoperative period.

Fetal Complications

The most common fetal complications are unintended delivery of an immature fetus because of miscalculation of dates and respiratory distress because of retained lung fluid. Because a fetus delivered by scheduled cesarean birth does not go through labor, he does not have the chance to get most of the amniotic fluid squeezed out of his lungs, as does a baby born vaginally. Therefore, respiratory distress is seen more frequently in these newborns. In addition, the fetus' respiratory drive can be depressed if the mother is given general anesthesia, making it difficult for the newborn to take her first breath. Less commonly, the fetus can be injured, that is, the scalpel cutting through the uterine wall can nick the baby. Usually these wounds are superficial and require minimal intervention.

Incision Types

There are two major incisions made during cesarean birth: one through the abdominal wall and the other into the uterus.

Abdominal Incisions

Abdominal incisions can be done using a vertical approach. These are done in the midline of the lower abdomen. A low transverse incision also can be performed. This type is called *Pfannenstiel's* incision, commonly known as a "bikini cut." Although a low transverse incision slightly increases the risk for bleeding, this is usually the preferred method for cosmetic reasons.

Uterine Incisions

Uterine incisions can be vertical or low transverse (Fig. 11-5). There are two types of vertical uterine incisions: classical and low cervical. The classical incision extends through the body of the uterus to the fundus. This incision is used only in severe emergencies, when it is critical to deliver the fetus immediately or when the fetus is unusually large. Bleeding during surgery is more likely with a classical uterine incision. It carries a higher risk for abdominal infection and the highest risk for uterine rupture in subsequent pregnancies. The low

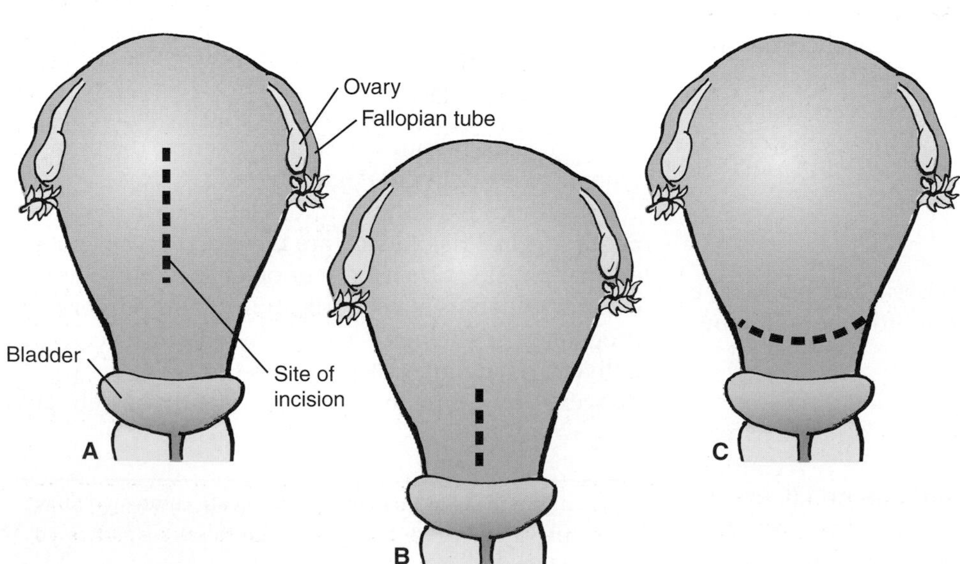

● ***Figure 11.5*** Types of uterine incisions used for cesarean delivery. (**A**) Classical approach. This incision is only used in extreme emergencies when it is critical to deliver the fetus, or when the fetus is too large to use a smaller incision. (**B**) Low (cervical) vertical approach. This incision is used infrequently. It has the advantage of allowing for extension of the incision into the body of the uterus, if the surgeon has difficulty extracting the fetus. (**C**) Low (cervical) transverse approach. This incision is used most frequently. The scar has a lower risk of rupturing during subsequent pregnancies and is associated with fewer complications.

cervical vertical incision is smaller and carries a lower risk for uterine rupture than does the classical approach, but it is infrequently used because it is more complicated to perform, carries higher risk of maternal injury, and is associated with a higher risk of uterine rupture than is the low cervical transverse incision. The low cervical transverse incision is the preferred method. This incision is associated with the least risk of uterine rupture, is easier to repair, and is least likely to cause adhesions.

Don't get confused. The type of skin incision does not indicate the type of incision used on the uterus. If the woman is not known by the surgeon, he will ask for the previous surgical record, if it is available, to determine the type of uterine incision.

Test Yourself

- Cesarean delivery involves incisions into what two structures?
- Name three possible complications of cesarean birth.
- What is Pfannenstiel's incision?

Steps of a Cesarean Delivery

Because cesarean delivery involves major surgery, the time period encompassing the procedure is referred to as the perioperative period, which is divided into three phases: preoperative, intraoperative, and postoperative. Care of the woman during the preoperative and intraoperative phases is completed using a team approach, sometimes referred to as collaborative management. The LPN is frequently involved in some of the preoperative care to prepare the woman for surgery. The LPN may also be a part of the intraoperative care by functioning in the scrub nurse role. The immediate postoperative care in the postanesthesia care unit (PACU) is usually carried out by the RN. The LPN may assume care of the woman during the postoperative phase, after she has sufficiently recovered from anesthesia. The major steps of a cesarean delivery are delineated in the following sections and Figures 11-6, 11-7, and 11-8.

Preoperative Phase

Preparing the woman for the cesarean birth is the focus of preoperative care. Nursing duties during the preoperative phase are discussed in the Nursing Care section. The anesthesiologist interviews the woman; explains the planned anesthesia to include risks; obtains verbal consent; reviews laboratory results; and orders preoperative medications, such as antacids and, less frequently, a sedative.

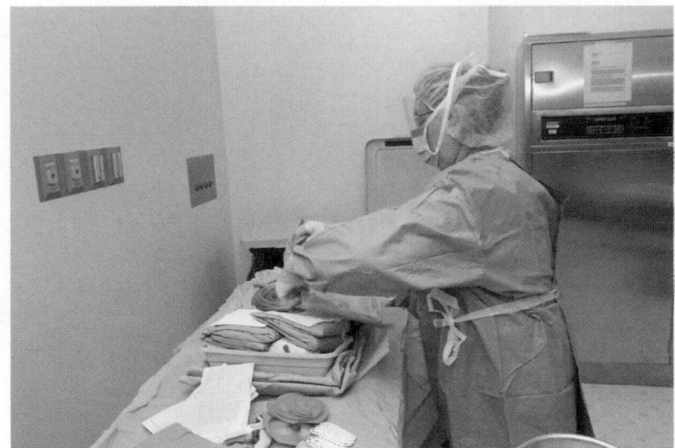

● ***Figure 11.6*** The scrub nurse sets up the back table in preparation for cesarean delivery.

The scrub technician or nurse opens the sterile cesarean delivery pack and instruments, puts on a sterile gown and gloves, and proceeds to prepare the back table and mayo instrument stand (Fig. 11-6). The circulating RN fastens the back of the scrub nurse's gown, and together the circulating RN and scrub nurse perform an initial instrument, sponge, and sharp count.

The support person changes into attire (usually disposable scrub suit or a disposable gown that covers the clothes) appropriate for the operating room (OR). A surgical cap and mask are also provided. The preoperative checklist and chart are reviewed for completeness. A surgical cap is placed on the woman's head to cover her hair, and she is transported to the OR suite by wheelchair or stretcher, or she may ambulate to the OR.

Intraoperative Phase

The intraoperative phase begins once the woman enters the OR. The woman is positioned on the operating table for regional anesthesia.[3] She may be placed in the sitting position with her legs dangling to one side, or she may be placed in the side-lying position. The nurse supports the woman so that her back remains in a C-shaped curve during placement of regional anesthesia by the anesthesiologist (Fig. 11-7*A*).

The nurse and anesthesiologist assist the woman to the supine position on the OR table. At this point, the Foley catheter is inserted, if not already placed in the preoperative area. The nurse places a wedge under one hip, and then places a warm blanket and a safety strap on the woman's legs. The fetal heart rate is checked for at least 1 minute. A grounding pad is placed

[3] It is uncommon for general anesthesia to be performed. Nursing care variations for this type of anesthesia are addressed in Chapter 9.

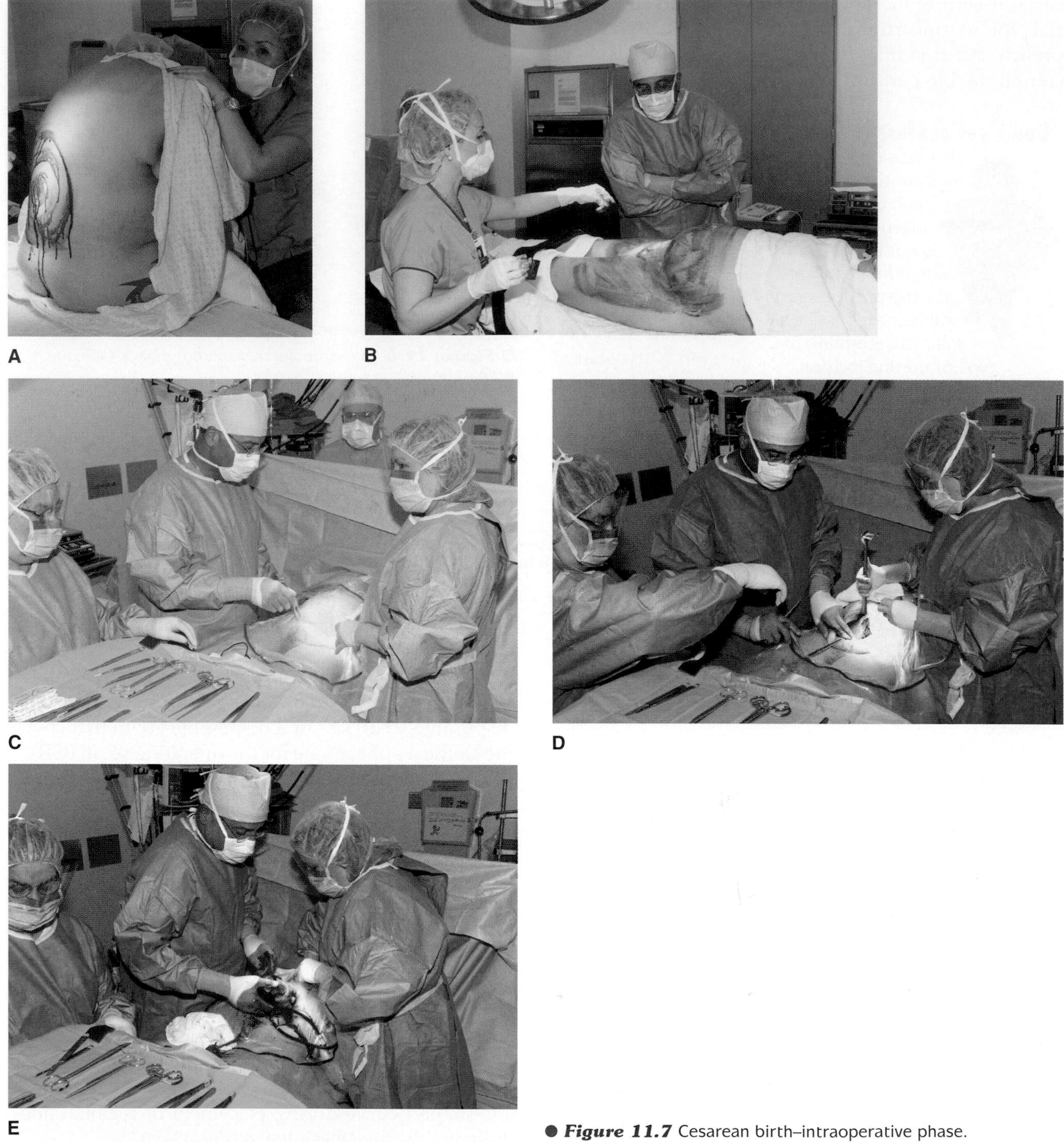

● *Figure 11.7* Cesarean birth–intraoperative phase.

on the woman's thigh. The anesthesiologist places electrocardiogram leads, a blood pressure cuff, and pulse oximeter device and connects them to the monitoring equipment. The woman's arms are positioned on arm boards and gently restrained with soft restraints.

Meanwhile, the surgeon and the assistant perform a surgical scrub. The circulating RN performs a sterile abdominal preparation with alcohol, or Betadine, as per facility policy (Fig. 11-7*B*). Then, the surgeon and assistant place sterile drapes on the woman. During the draping procedure, the RN calls for the individuals who will be attending the newborn. The RN also calls for the support person, who is seated at the woman's head behind the surgical drapes.

The surgeon uses small pickup forceps to test the level of anesthesia before proceeding (Fig. 11-7*C*). Once the surgeon is satisfied that the anesthesia level is sufficient, the surgeon makes the initial cut and proceeds to cut through the layers of skin, fascia, and muscle until the lower segment of the uterus is exposed (Fig. 11-7*D*).

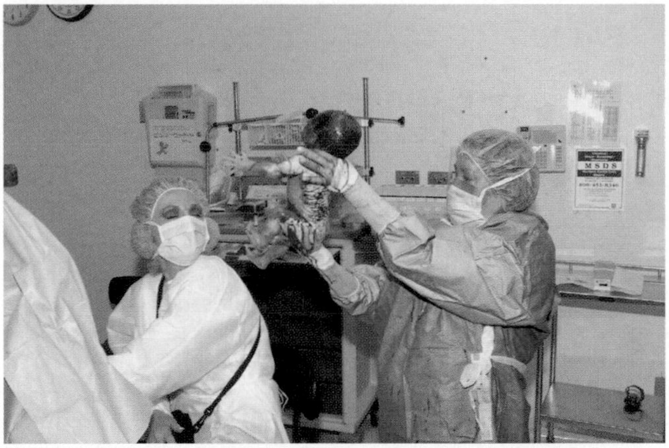

F

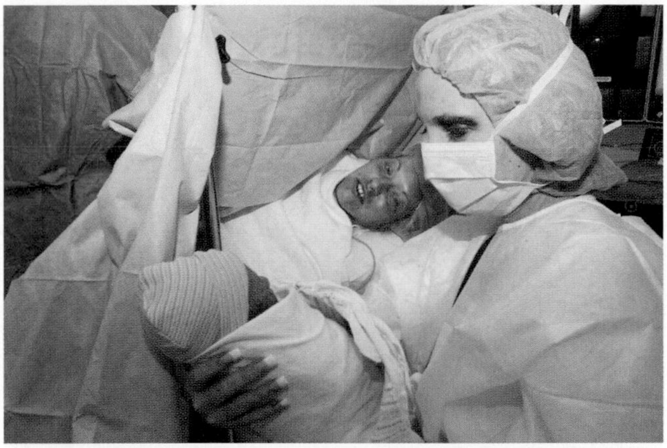

G

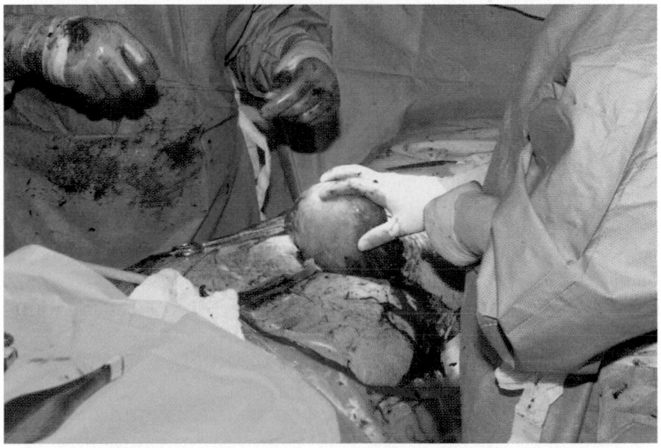

H

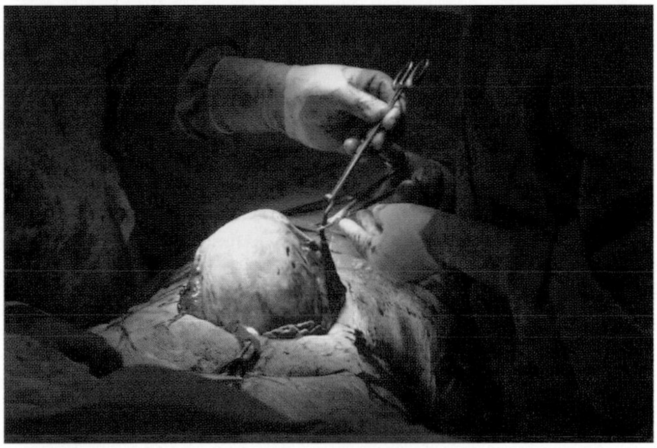

I

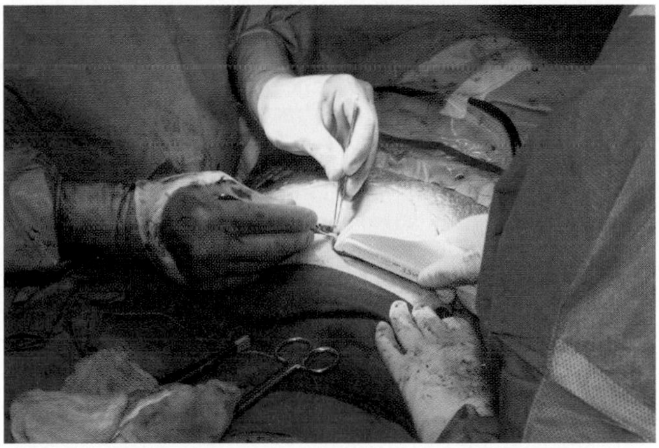

J

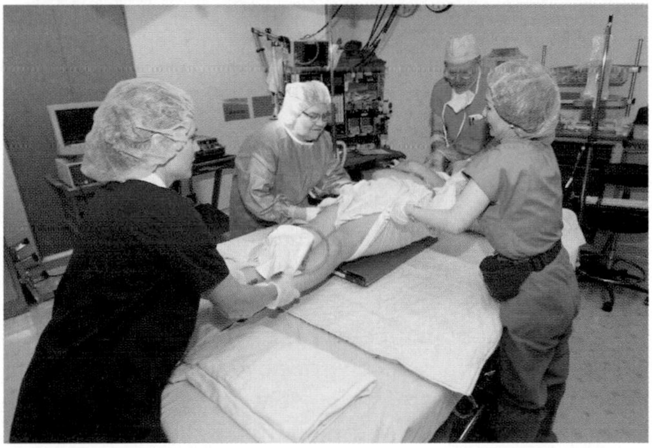

K

● *Figure 11.7* Continued

Then the surgeon makes the incision into the uterus. The newborn's head is delivered (Fig. 11-7*E*), followed by the body. The umbilical cord is double clamped and cut, and the newborn is briefly shown to the mother and support person (Fig. 11-7*F*) before being taken to the warmer for assessment and resuscitation, as needed. The placenta is delivered manually shortly after the baby is born.

When the newborn is breathing well and the skin color is pink, he is double-wrapped in prewarmed blankets, a cap is placed on his head, and he is taken to the woman and support person for initial bonding (Fig. 11-7*G*).

The fundus and body of the uterus are brought through the incision (Fig. 11-7*H*), and the inside is cleaned thoroughly by the surgeon; then the uterine incision is sutured close. The circulating RN and scrub technician perform the second OR count. If the woman desires a tubal ligation, it is performed at this time. The tubes are tied and ligated (Fig. 11-7*I*), and the specimens handed to the circulating RN, who labels them to

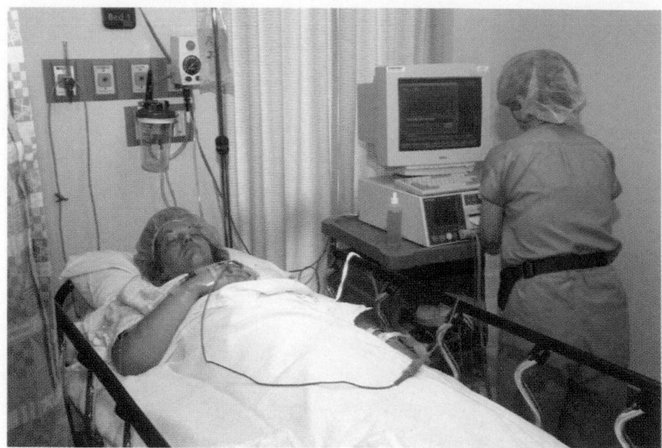

● *Figure 11.8* Cesarean birth—postoperative phase.

be sent to the laboratory. The uterus is then placed back in the pelvic cavity.

Repair of muscle and fascia layers is done with absorbable suture while the third OR count is done. The skin is closed with staples (Fig. 11-7*J*) or suture. A sterile dressing is placed, the drapes are removed, the uterine fundus is massaged, and a sterile perineal pad is placed. The woman is then moved from the OR table to a stretcher (Fig. 11-7*K*), and she is transported to the PACU for initial recovery from anesthesia.

Postoperative Phase

The woman is placed in the PACU, where the PACU RN receives report from the circulating RN (in labor and delivery units, the PACU RN and circulating RN may be the same individual). The RN places the woman on a cardiac monitor, an automatic blood pressure device, and a pulse oximeter (Fig. 11-8). A thorough assessment is done to include level of consciousness, cardiac and respiratory status, condition of the dressing, fundal and lochia status, urinary output, condition and patency of IV site, and a full set of vital signs. This assessment is completed at least every 15 minutes for 1 hour or until the woman meets PACU discharge criteria, which varies by facility and anesthesiologist. The anesthesiologist writes orders for pain control in the PACU and usually for the first 24 hours after surgery.

FAMILY TEACHING TIPS

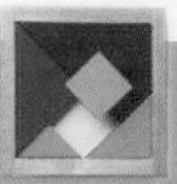

Preparing for a Planned Cesarean Birth

Explain or demonstrate to the pregnant woman and partner

- How and where to preregister and have blood work drawn.*
- Where and when to meet the anesthesiologist for preoperative evaluation.
- Date, time, and location to which to present before the surgery.
- The amount of time she is to remain NPO before surgery.
- Procedures for partner participation in the birth process.
- That an IV will be placed in the preoperative holding area and will remain in place for approximately 24 hours after the procedure, when she is tolerating liquids by mouth.
- That regional anesthesia (epidural or spinal) is usually performed to decrease the risk to mother and baby associated with general anesthesia.
- That a Foley catheter will be inserted into her urinary bladder and will remain in place for approximately 24 hours after surgery.
- How long after the surgery until she will likely be transferred to her postpartum room.
- How to turn, cough, and deep breathe every 1 to 2 hours after surgery.
- The importance of early and frequent ambulation to decrease the pain and distention of gas and to decrease risks associated with major surgery, such as respiratory complications, infection, thrombophlebitis, and so on.
- Methods of pain control most frequently ordered and the importance of requesting pain medications before pain becomes severe.
- Likely sources of pain and the appropriate type of pain control for each (e.g., gas build-up responds best to ambulation and simethicone; incisional pain is usually best treated with narcotics; and uterine cramping often responds well to nonsteroidal anti-inflammatory drugs).
- Nursery procedures, including when she and her partner may reasonably expect to interact with their newborn.
- Ways to cope with breast-feeding after cesarean, such as use of the football hold to decrease pressure on the incision.

* Some of these procedures will be done the morning of surgery, depending upon the protocols of the facility at which the woman has chosen to deliver.

Nursing Care

Providing Family Teaching for a Planned Cesarean Birth

The focus of nursing intervention for a planned cesarean is family education (see Family Teaching Tips: Preparing for a Planned Cesarean Birth). Each time you encounter the woman before surgery is an opportunity to explore with the woman and her partner what they know about cesarean delivery. Do they know the procedural steps to take, such as where to preregister, when and where to have laboratory work drawn, and when and where to present for surgery? Do they know what to expect during the surgical experience? Does the woman know how to help avoid complications in the postoperative period, such as the how and why of taking deep breaths and turning frequently while in bed, and why it is important to ambulate as soon as possible after surgery? Does she know the principles of postoperative pain control and what options are available to her for pain relief? Teaching is more effective when it occurs over time, is repeated, and focuses on topics in which the family is interested.

Providing Preoperative Care

Nursing interventions to help the woman and her partner prepare for cesarean birth depend on many factors, including whether or not the procedure was planned and whether or not the woman has experienced cesarean delivery in the past. Ideally, the woman and her partner will have attended childbirth classes. Part of class discussion centers on the possibility of cesarean birth. When a woman is prepared psychologically for the experience, coping is enhanced.

Whether the cesarean is planned or emergent, several preparations are critical. Always check to see if informed consent has been given and that a signed consent form documents it (Fig. 11-9). Ask the woman when she last had anything to eat or drink. She should have nothing by mouth (NPO) for at least 8 hours before surgery. Frequently an antacid, such as Bicitra 30 mL, is given before surgery to reduce the risk of aspiration while the woman is under the effects of anesthesia. An IV must be in place with a large-bore (generally 18-gauge or lower) catheter. Lactated Ringer's is a commonly ordered IV fluid. Sometimes an abdominal shave preparation is done immediately before surgery, although it is becoming more common to use clippers to remove hair from the abdomen and perineal area. Clippers do not cause skin nicks like razors can, so clippers are the preferred tool to use. A Foley catheter must be in place before the surgery begins to decrease the risk that the surgeon might inadvertently cut or puncture a full bladder during surgery. Sometimes the catheter is placed in the preoperative area. Alternately, the circulating nurse may place it after anesthesia has been administered, which is more comfortable for the woman.

Remember: A patient can always change her mind. If she signed an informed consent but then states she has changed her mind, she's not sure, or she needs more information, alert the charge nurse or physician immediately so that her concerns can be addressed.

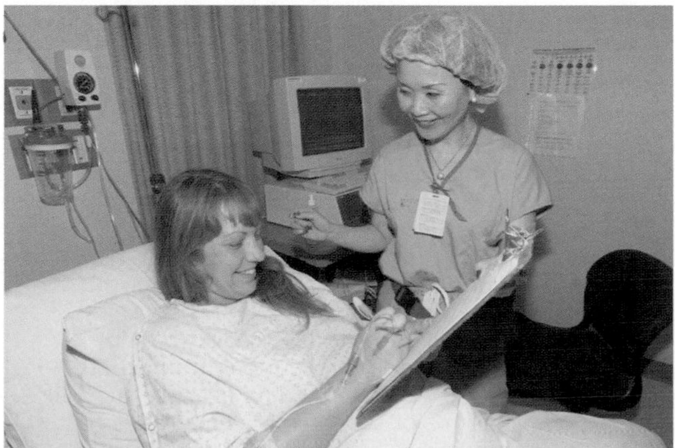

● ***Figure 11.9*** The nurse witnesses signing of the informed consent form.

Certain laboratory studies must be done. The routine complete blood count is important, as is the blood type and screen. When a type and screen is done, the laboratory holds at least 2 units of blood that matches the woman's blood type. In the event of an emergency, the final steps of cross matching are done, so that the appropriate blood can be transfused. Most physicians also order other laboratory studies, such as electrolytes. When the woman is ready for surgery, assist the RN to transfer her to the operating suite and then to the operating table.

Providing Support During an Unplanned or Emergency Cesarean Birth

When a cesarean birth becomes necessary because of an unplanned or emergency situation, the nurse must move quickly to prepare the patient for surgery. The woman and her family are often anxious and worried about the baby. She may be fearful of the surgery or anesthesia, particularly if she has never had surgery before. There is usually not much time for education; therefore, support of the woman and her family becomes paramount (Nursing Care Plan 11-1).

Support is shown in many ways. Explain procedures as you are doing them. If the RN or physician says the fetal monitor tracing is reassuring, reinforce this important fact to the woman and her partner. Explain what sensations she can expect to experience and what to expect next. Be empathic. Acknowledge her feelings and let her know that these feelings are normal considering the situation with which she must cope.

Providing Care in the Immediate Recovery Phase

Nursing care in the postoperative period is influenced by many factors. Some of these are the type of anesthesia that was given, complications that occurred during surgery, the outcome and condition of the neonate, and stability of maternal condition.

Assist the RN to transfer the woman from the operative suite to the PACU. The RN will connect her

NURSING CARE PLAN 11.1

The Woman Undergoing an Unplanned (Emergency) Cesarean Delivery*

CASE SCENARIO

Rene Truitt is a 28-year-old primigravida who went into spontaneous labor at 40 weeks' gestation. She received an epidural when her cervix progressed to 4 centimeters dilation and reported adequate pain relief. She progressed to full dilation and pushed for 2 hours, but the fetal head did not descend below 0 station. The fetal monitor tracing is now showing occasional late decelerations. The physician has ordered a primary cesarean delivery. Rene is voicing concern over the welfare of her baby and is crying softly. Her husband is attempting to comfort her.

NURSING DIAGNOSIS

Anxiety related to fetal status and unexpected surgical procedure.

GOAL: Rene will demonstrate positive coping behaviors to deal with her anxiety.

EXPECTED OUTCOMES:

- Seeks information to reduce anxiety.
- Accepts her husband's offered support.
- Voices acceptance of the situation.

NURSING INTERVENTIONS	*RATIONALE*
Remain with Rene while preparing her for surgery.	Presence of the nurse can be reassuring in a stressful situation.
Display a calm and confident manner.	Promotes trust.
Explain procedures as you perform them.	Understanding what is happening helps decrease anxiety.
Emphasize the qualifications of the surgical team (i.e., surgeon, circulating nurse, anesthesiologist).	Promotes trust and confidence.
Briefly describe what Rene and her husband will experience throughout the procedure.	Understanding what to expect helps decrease anxiety.
Encourage Rene's husband to participate throughout (e.g., holding her hand, remaining with her whenever possible).	The presence of a support person can be comforting.

NURSING DIAGNOSIS

Risk for injury related to major surgical procedure.

GOAL: Rene will not experience preventable injury throughout the perioperative period.

EXPECTED OUTCOMES:

- Gives informed consent for cesarean delivery.
- Urinary output remains at least 30 cc/hour.
- Urine color remains clear yellow.
- Maintains adequate fluid volume.

NURSING INTERVENTIONS	*RATIONALE*
Check the chart for signed informed consent for cesarean delivery. Obtain signed consent, if not already completed.	Although it is primarily the physician's responsibility to obtain informed consent, the signed form is evidence that Rene has consented.
Make certain that Rene and her husband have had any questions or concerns they have about the procedure addressed. If there are additional questions, notify the RN or physician immediately.	It is imperative that Rene understand the risks involved for cesarean delivery, as well as the risks involved for continuing to attempt vaginal birth.
Check the chart for laboratory results. If they are not on the chart, place them in the chart before surgery.	The surgical team will refer to lab results to help determine if extra safety precautions are needed.
Make certain that at least 2 units of packed red blood cells are on hold in the lab, as ordered. Alternatively, the blood should at least be typed and screened.	Rene is at increased risk for bleeding because she will be experiencing major surgery. It is imperative that blood be immediately available, in the event hemorrhage should occur.

NURSING CARE PLAN 11.1 continued

The Woman Undergoing an Unplanned (Emergency) Cesarean Delivery*

NURSING INTERVENTIONS	*RATIONALE*
Check the IV line for patency before surgery. Inform the RN immediately if the IV needs to be restarted.	A patent IV line with a large-bore needle must be in place before Rene can go to surgery.
Check to see if a Foley catheter is in place. If not, insert the catheter before transporting Rene to the OR suite.	A urinary catheter is necessary to keep the bladder drained. This will decrease the chance of bladder injury during surgery.

NURSING DIAGNOSIS

Risk for aspiration (maternal) related to gravid uterus pressing upward on the stomach and anesthesia for cesarean delivery.

GOAL: Rene will not experience respiratory compromise.

EXPECTED OUTCOMES:
- Maintains a respiratory rate between 16 and 22 breaths/minute
- Maintains a regular respiratory rhythm
- Remains free from adventitious breath sounds

NURSING INTERVENTIONS	*RATIONALE*
Report to anesthesiologist the date and time of last oral intake (solid and liquid).	This information allows the anesthesiologist to plan how to best protect the airway during surgery.
Administer IV or PO antacids, as ordered before surgery.	Antacids decrease the acidity of stomach contents, which reduces the potential for injury from aspiration.
Assess respiratory status before and after surgery.	Preoperative assessment will determine baseline respiratory status. Postoperative assessment is done to detect changes that might be associated with aspiration.

* *Note:* This care plan addresses preoperative care of a woman who experiences an unplanned cesarean delivery. Postoperative nursing care is addressed in Chapter 12.

to monitoring devices that will record the electrocardiogram, blood pressure, pulse, and oxygen saturation of the blood. The RN will also take vital sign and pulse oximetry readings every 5 minutes until the readings are stable, and then every 15 to 30 minutes until the patient has met predetermined criteria. The RN will monitor the patient's urinary output to make certain it is at least 30 cc/hour.

In addition to normal PACU activities, postpartum assessments must be done. The condition of the fundus must be evaluated and recorded along with vital signs. The nurse's hand or a pillow can support the incision while the fundus is gently massaged to determine if it is firm. A firmly contracted uterus will minimize bleeding. In conjunction with the fundal check, an assessment of the amount and type of lochia flow is made. These assessments are performed and recorded at the same time interval as the vital signs. (Refer to Chapter 12 for a full discussion of postpartum assessment and nursing care.)

The timing and process of recovery is influenced in large part by the type of anesthesia given. Chapter 9 discusses the different types of anesthesia, including recovery considerations.

A word of caution is in order. During cesarean birth the surgeon is able to thoroughly clean the inside of the uterus. Therefore, there should be less lochia flow than is present after a vaginal delivery. Moderate amounts of lochia after a cesarean delivery should alert the nurse to the possibility of postpartum hemorrhage.

VAGINAL BIRTH AFTER CESAREAN

In times past the adage "once a cesarean, always a cesarean" guided the practice of obstetricians, and most women who had experienced a primary cesarean birth were scheduled for repeat cesareans. During the 1980s, a push was made to decrease the number of cesarean births in the United States by reducing the number of repeat cesarean births. Many obstetricians encouraged their patients to attempt a vaginal birth after one or more cesarean births (VBAC). However, recent studies and experience have shown that the risk for uterine rupture during VBAC often outweighs the benefits of a vaginal birth, and many obstetricians no longer offer this procedure for their patients. However, there are women who may be potential candidates for VBAC. These women are counseled by their physician regarding the benefits and risks.

Prerequisites

ACOG recommendations regarding trial of labor for a woman who has previously delivered by cesarean include an adequate pelvis, no previous uterine ruptures, personnel and facilities available to perform an immediate cesarean delivery, and no more than two previous low transverse uterine scars (Cunningham et al., 2001, p. 542). In 2002, ACOG added stipulations to include signed informed consent that lists benefits and risks; surgeon, anesthesia provider, and operating room personnel in the hospital; ability to perform a cesarean delivery in less than 18 minutes after the order is given; sufficient blood in the hospital; and a practitioner (this is often the RN) at the bedside who can read and interpret EFM tracings and who can recognize the signs and symptoms of uterine rupture (Dauphinee, 2004).

Contraindications

The risk for uterine rupture during VBAC is much higher when a classical incision was previously done on the uterus; therefore, VBAC is contraindicated when this type of scar is present. It is also contraindicated if the woman has a history of previous uterine rupture.

Procedure

If VBAC is determined to be a valid option, the woman is given what is called a "trial of labor." Generally she is allowed to go into labor on her own. Then her progress is monitored carefully. The woman is attached to continuous EFM throughout labor, and the nurse must be vigilant to monitor for signs of uterine rupture (Box 11-2). The use of oxytocin during labor is not contraindicated absolutely, but its use requires monitoring that is even closer than usual.

BOX 11.2 Signs of Uterine Rupture

- Dramatic onset of fetal bradycardia or deep variable decelerations
- Reports by the woman of a "popping" sensation in her abdomen
- Excessive maternal pain (can be referred pain, such as to the chest)
- Unrelenting uterine contraction followed by a disorganized uterine pattern
- Increased fetal station felt upon vaginal examination (e.g., station is now −3 when it has been −1)
- Easily palpable fetal parts through the abdominal wall
- Signs of maternal shock

Nursing Care

It is outside the scope of the LPN to care for a laboring woman who has a history of a previous cesarean delivery. An experienced RN will manage the labor. Special written informed consent that outlines the risks and benefits of VBAC is required. The woman may verbally withdraw her consent at any time during the course of labor. At the time she withdraws her consent, the trial of labor is discontinued, and the woman is prepared for a cesarean delivery (Dauphinee, 2004).

During the labor the RN continuously monitors the EFM tracing. Any nonreassuring patterns are immediately reported because a nonreassuring pattern is the most significant sign of a ruptured uterus. The specially trained LPN may function as the scrub nurse if a cesarean is indicated during trial of labor.

Test Yourself

- What is the primary focus of nursing intervention when a cesarean delivery is planned?
- What is the primary focus of nursing intervention when a cesarean birth is emergent?
- What is one contraindication for a trial of labor after previous cesarean delivery?

KEY POINTS

- External version is done in an attempt to reposition a fetus in a breech or shoulder presentation to a more favorable vertex presentation.
- Medical indications for the induction of labor include postdate pregnancy, PROM, chorioamnionitis, pregnancy-induced hypertension, intrauterine fetal growth restriction, or certain medical conditions such as maternal diabetes.
- The Bishop score is used to help determine cervical readiness for labor. Five factors are evaluated: cervical consistency, position, dilatation, effacement, and fetal station.
- Mechanical methods to enhance ripening of the cervix include membrane stripping and mechanical dilation of the cervix with either a catheter or laminaria.
- Pharmacologic methods to ripen the cervix require closer monitoring of the woman and include local application of prostaglandin gel or vaginal inserts, or insertion of a prostaglandin tablet.
- Oxytocin induction requires continuous fetal monitoring, a mainline IV, and a secondary IV line that contains the oxytocin, which is connected to an IV pump. Oxytocin is titrated up until an adequate contraction pattern is obtained.
- Complications associated with the use of oxytocin include higher risk for cesarean delivery, hyperstimulation of the uterus with possible fetal distress, and uterine rupture. Water intoxication is another potential complication.
- Amnioinfusion involves infusing fluid via an IUPC into the uterine cavity after the membranes have ruptured and the cervix is at least partially dilated. This procedure is done to relieve signs of cord compression and to dilute thick meconium-stained fluid.
- An episiotomy is a surgical incision made in the perineum to enlarge the vaginal opening just before delivery. A midline episiotomy extends straight downward into the true perineum. A mediolateral episiotomy is angled to the right or the left of the perineum.
- Vacuum extraction uses a suction cup that is attached to the fetal head, which allows the physician to provide gentle downward traction to assist delivery.
- In a forceps-assisted delivery, hard metal tools shaped something like large hollowed-out spoons are applied to the fetal head. Midforceps are used to rotate the fetus to an anterior position. Low and outlet forceps are more frequently used to shorten the second stage of labor.
- Cesarean delivery is a major surgical procedure. It carries with it all the risks and complications associated with abdominal surgery in addition to those associated with normal birth.
- The four most common indications for cesarean delivery are history of previous cesarean, labor dystocia, fetal distress, and breech presentation. Other less common indications include placenta previa, abruptio placentae, cephalopelvic disproportion, active vaginal herpes lesions, prolapse of the umbilical cord, ruptured uterus, and certain medical and obstetric conditions.
- Both skin and uterine incisions can be vertical or transverse. The uterine incision is the most important of the two. The classical uterine incision is associated with the highest risk for rupture in subsequent pregnancies. The low cervical transverse uterine incision is the preferred method.
- Nursing interventions for a planned cesarean birth are focused on education to prepare the family for the birth. Interventions for an emergency cesarean include mostly supportive behaviors, such as explaining procedures as they are done and providing appropriate reassurance.
- A woman who wishes to experience VBAC must be given a trial of labor. Because of the risk for uterine rupture, the woman is carefully screened for this procedure. History of a classical uterine incision or a previous uterine rupture is a contraindication for VBAC.

REFERENCES AND SELECTED READINGS

Books and Journals

ACOG News Release. (2003). Weighing the pros and cons of cesarean delivery. The American College of Obstetricians and Gynecologists (ACOG). Retrieved March 20, 2004, from http://www.acog.org/from_home/newsrel.cfm (Scroll down and click on the article).

Boulvain, M., Kelly, A., Lohse, C., Stan, C., & Irion, O. (2003). Mechanical methods for induction of labour (Cochrane Review). *The Cochran Library, Issue 1*(2003). [Abstract]. Retrieved April 6, 2003, from http://www.cochrane.org/cochrane/revabstr/ab001233.htm

Carroli, G., & Belizan, J. (2004). Episiotomy for vaginal birth (Cochrane Review). *The Cochrane Library, Issue 1*(2004). [Abstract]. Retrieved March 7, 2004, from http://212.49.218.202/abstracts/ab000081.htm

Caughey, A. B., & Mann, S. (2002). Vaginal birth after cesarean delivery. In: S. D. Spandorfer, F. Talavera, C. V. Smith, F. B. Gaupp, & L. P. Shulman (Eds.). *eMedicine*. Retrieved April 24, 2003, from http://www.emedicine.com/med/topic3434.htm

Coco, A. S., & Silverman, S. D. (1998). External cephalic version. *American Family Physician*. Retrieved April 24, 2003, from http://www.aafp.org/afp/980901ap/coco.html

Cunningham, F. G., Gant, N. F., Leveno, K. J., Gilstrap L. C. III, Hauth, J. C., & Wenstrom, K. D. (2001). *Williams obstet-*

rics (21st ed.). New York: McGraw Hill Medical Publishing Division.

Dauphinee, J. D. (2004). VBAC: Safety for the patient and the nurse. *Journal of Obstetric, Gynecologic, and Neonatal Nursing (JOGNN), 33*(1), 105–115.

Encyclopaedia Britannica (Eds.). (2002). Cesarean section. Retrieved January 28, 2002, from http://www. britannica. com/eb/article?eu=22509

Goldberg, A. B., & Wing, D. A. (2003). Induction of labor: The misoprostol controversy [Abstract]. *Journal of Midwifery & Women's Health, 48*(4), 244–248.

Harman, J. H., & Kim, A. (1999). Current trends in cervical ripening and labor induction. *American Family Physician, 61*(August), 477–488. Retrieved April 5, 2003, from http://www.aafp.org/afp/990800ap/477.html

Joseph, K. S., Young, D. C., Dodds, L., O'Connell, C. M., Allen, V. M., Chandra, S., & Allen, A. C. (2003). Changes in maternal characteristics and obstetric practice and recent increases in primary cesarean delivery. *Obstetrics & Gynecology: Original Research, 102*(4), 791–800. Retrieved March 7, 2004, from http://www.acog.org/from_home/publications/green_journal/wrapper.cfm?document=2003/ong14583fla.htm

Martin, J. A., Hamilton, B. E., Sutton, P. D., Ventura, S. J., Menacker, F., & Munson, M. L. (2003). Births: Final data for 2002. *National Vital Statistics Reports, 52*(10), 1–114. Retrieved March 7, 2004, from http://www.cdc.gov/nchs/data/nvsr/nvsr52/nvsr52_10.pdf

Simpson, K. R., & Atterbury, J. (2003). Trends and issues in labor induction in the United States: Implications for clinical practice. *Journal of Obstetric, Gynecologic, and Neonatal Nursing (JOGNN), 32*(6), 767–779.

Simpson, K. R., & Creehan, P. A. (2001). *Perinatal nursing* (2nd ed.). Philadelphia: Lippincott Williams & Wilkins.

Weismiller, D. G. (1998). Transcervical amnioinfusion. *American Family Physician, 57*(3), 504–512. Retrieved April 26, 2003, from http://www.aafp.org/afp/980201ap/articles.html

Wilk, P. R., & Galan, H. (2002). Postdate pregnancy. In B. D. Cowan, F. Talavera, R. S. Legro, F. B. Gaupp, & L. P. Shulman (Eds.), *eMedicine*. Retrieved April 5, 2003, from http://www.emedicine.com/med/topic3248.htm

Websites

Labor Induction

http://www.hattiesburgclinic.com/front/61801/inside/show. asp?durki=634

http://www.parents.com/articles/pregnancy/1014.jsp?page=1

Cesarean Birth

http://www.noah-health.org/english/pregnancy/pregnancy.html (Scroll down to the "Delivery" section on the page. Click on the link "Cesarean Birth." When you are done exploring that section, click on the link "Vaginal Birth After Cesarean.")

Photos

http://pregnancy.about.com/library/blsection.htm

WORKBOOK

NCLEX-STYLE REVIEW QUESTIONS

1. A woman who has an episiotomy asks the nurse, "When will I get my stitches taken out?" How should the nurse best reply?
   a. "I don't know. Ask the doctor."
   b. "It depends on the type of episiotomy. A mediolateral episiotomy requires that the stitches be removed, while a midline does not."
   c. "The doctor will remove the stitches when the perineum stops hurting."
   d. "The stitches will be absorbed on their own. They do not need to be removed."
2. A primigravida is tired of being pregnant. She asks the nurse, "Why can't my doctor just schedule a cesarean delivery? My friend had a cesarean and everything went very well." What is the best reply by the nurse?
   a. "A cesarean birth involves major surgery, which puts you and your baby at higher risk for complications. Your physician will discuss the options with you."
   b. "I will ask your doctor. Sometimes he will allow a first-time mother to have a cesarean birth if she wants to do so."
   c. "Oh no. This would not be good for the baby. Try not to think too much about it. It is always better to have a vaginal delivery."
   d. "Why do you want to do that? Don't you know a vaginal delivery is the preferred way to have a baby?"
3. A woman whose fetus is breech is scheduled for external version. She says to the nurse, "I'm really scared of the procedure. Will it hurt badly?" What is the best reply by the nurse?
   a. "Don't worry. An external version procedure is not painful."
   b. "Sometimes the procedure is uncomfortable. If it becomes too painful, let the doctor know and she will stop the procedure."
   c. "The procedure can be quite uncomfortable, but it is best for your baby. You want to do what's best for the baby, right?"
   d. "You can do it. I'll hold your hand throughout the procedure and you should be just fine."
4. A woman is dilated 9 centimeters and the fetus is in an anterior position at a +1 station. The bag of waters is ruptured. She has been in labor for several hours and is exhausted, so she asks the nurse, "My friend was tired at the end of her labor, and the doctor used forceps to help deliver the baby. Could the doctor pull the baby out with forceps so I can get this over with?" What response by the nurse is best?
   a. "I don't know. Let me ask the doctor."
   b. "The cervix must be completely dilated before forceps can be applied safely."
   c. "No. Once the water bag ruptures, the doctor cannot apply forceps."
   d. "Forceps are too dangerous. I'll get a vacuum extractor ready for your delivery."

STUDY ACTIVITIES

1. Develop a 15-minute presentation on cesarean delivery to give to a group of first-time mothers at a prenatal education class.
2. Discuss how care of the newborn during cesarean delivery is different from care of the newborn after vaginal delivery. What additional risk factors does the newborn delivered by cesarean have?
3. Using the table below, compare methods of cervical ripening.

Method	How it Works to Ripen the Cervix	Special Nursing Considerations

CRITICAL THINKING: What Would You Do?

Apply your knowledge of cesarean birth and assisted deliveries to the following situations.

1. Amy Jones is a 21-year-old gravida 1 who is attending a prenatal childbirth education class. She comments that she thinks she will not attend next week's class because cesarean delivery is going to be discussed, and she does not plan to have a cesarean. How would you reply to Amy's comment?
2. A woman who is close to term asks the nurse at a normal obstetric visit, "My doctor says I have a Bishop score of 4. What does that mean?"
   a. How would you reply?
   b. If the physician felt that the woman's labor needed to be induced, what recommendation would she likely make to the woman? Why?
3. You are going to assist the physician to perform a fetal fibronectin test. What equipment do you need?
4. Ellen Hess, a 30-year-old gravida 2, has chosen to attempt a VBAC. After 4 hours of labor, she reports to you severe pain and a "popping" sensation in her abdomen. What would you do?

UNIT 5

Postpartum and Newborn

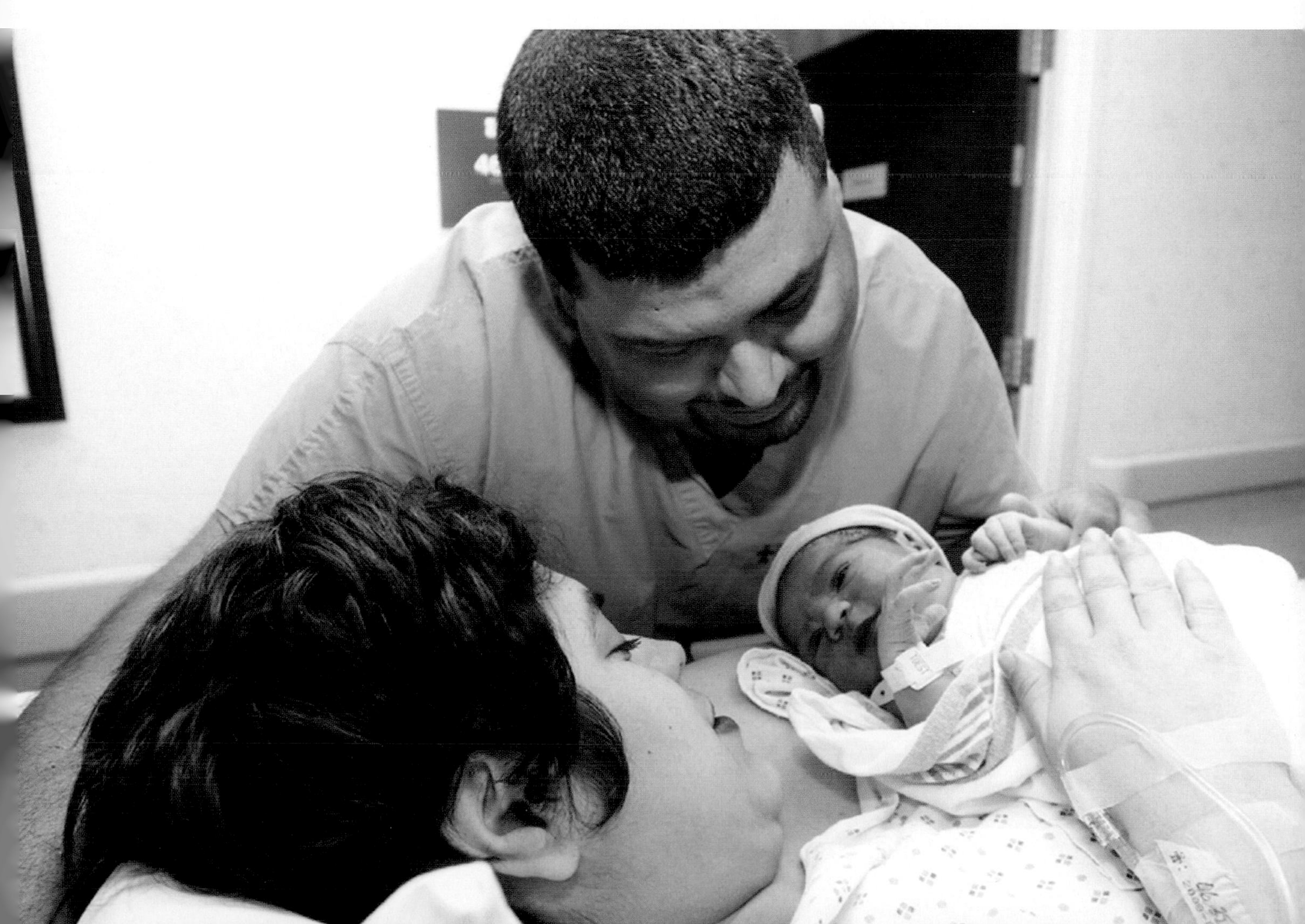

The Postpartum Woman

here

12

STUDENT OBJECTIVES

On completion of this chapter, the student will be able to

1. Describe the physiologic adaptation of the woman during the postpartum period.
2. Discuss major points related to psychological adaptation during the postpartum period.
3. Describe a postpartum assessment.
4. Discuss the responsibilities of the practical (vocational) nurse in caring for the woman in the early postpartum period.
5. Compare and contrast the nursing care of the woman who delivers vaginally with that of the one who delivers by cesarean.
6. Outline the nurse's role in preparing the woman for discharge.

KEY TERMS

attachment
boggy uterus
bonding
breakthrough pain
colostrum
diastasis recti abdominis
dyspareunia
en face
grand multiparity
involution
lochia
postpartum blues
puerperium

The processes of pregnancy and birth challenge the woman's psychological and physiologic coping mechanisms. It is during the postpartum period, sometimes referred to as the 4th trimester of pregnancy, that the woman must adjust to the reality of her new role as mother. This is also the period during which her body must return to the nonpregnant state. The postpartum period, or **puerperium**, encompasses the 6 weeks after birth. For ease of discussion, the puerperium can be subdivided into three categories: the immediate postpartum period, which covers the first 24 hours; the early postpartum period or 1st week; and late postpartum period, which refers to weeks 2 through 6. This chapter discusses the adaptations a low-risk woman makes during the puerperium and the nursing care that promotes healing and wellness.

MATERNAL ADAPTATION DURING THE POSTPARTUM PERIOD

Physiologic Adaptation

The woman's body undergoes tremendous changes to accommodate pregnancy. Every body system and organ is affected. It is during the weeks after pregnancy that the body recovers from the stress of pregnancy and returns to its normal prepregnancy state.

Reproductive System

The organs and hormones of the reproductive system must gradually return to their nonpregnant size and function. The shrinking or returning to normal size of the uterus, cervix, and vagina is called the process of **involution**.

Uterus

Uterine Contraction and Involution. Immediately after the placenta delivers, the uterus contracts inward, a process that seals off the open blood vessels at the former site of the placenta. If the uterus does not contract effectively, the woman will hemorrhage. The clotting cascade also is initiated, a process that causes clot formation to control bleeding. Large blood vessels at the former placental site degenerate and are replaced by smaller ones. Gradually the decidua is shed, new endometrial tissue forms, and the placental area heals without leaving fibrous scar tissue.

Uterine contraction also leads to uterine involution. Involution is assessed by measuring fundal height. Immediately after delivery the fundus is firm and located in the midline halfway between the umbilicus and symphysis pubis. One hour after delivery the uterus should be contracted firmly, with the fundus midline at the level of the umbilicus. The day after delivery the fundus is found 1 cm below the umbilicus. The normal process of involution thereafter is for the uterus to descend approximately 1 fingerbreadth (1 cm) per day until it has descended below the level of the pubic bone and can no longer be palpated. This occurs by the 10th postpartum day (Fig. 12-1).

There are several factors that promote uterine contraction and involution. Breast-feeding stimulates oxytocin release from the woman's posterior pituitary gland. Oxytocin stimulates the uterus to contract. Early ambulation and proper nourishment also foster normal involution.

In addition, there are factors that can inhibit or delay uterine involution. A full bladder impedes uterine contraction by pushing upward on the uterus and displacing it. Any condition that overdistends the uterus during pregnancy can lead to ineffective uterine contraction after delivery. Examples include a multifetal pregnancy and hydramnios. Maternal exhaustion and excessive analgesia during labor and delivery also can hinder contraction of the uterus. Other factors include retained placental fragments, infection, and **grand multiparity**, five or more pregnancies. When the uterus does not contract effectively, blood and clots collect in the uterus, which makes it even more difficult for the uterus to contract. This leads to a **boggy uterus** and hemorrhage if the condition is not arrested. A boggy uterus feels soft and spongy, rather than firm and well contracted.

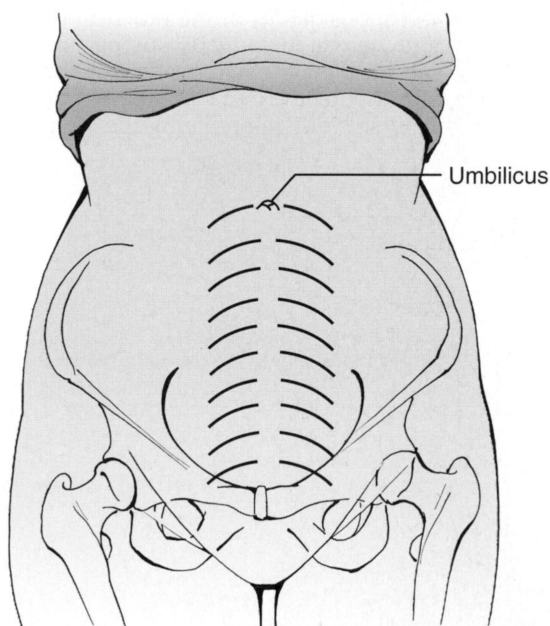

● ***Figure 12.1*** Normal uterine involution occurs at a predictable rate. One hour after childbirth the fundus is at the level of the umbilicus. On the first postpartum day the fundus is approximately 1 fingerbreadth or 1 cm below the level of the umbilicus. Thereafter, it descends downward at the rate of 1 fingerbreadth per day until it becomes a pelvic organ again on the 10th day postpartum.

Afterpains. After a multipara delivers, the uterus contracts and relaxes at intervals. This leads to afterpains, which can be quite severe. For the primipara, the uterus normally remains contracted, and afterpains are less severe than that of the multipara. However, breast-feeding, because it causes the release of oxytocin, increases the duration and intensity of afterpains for both the primipara and multipara.

Lochia. The uterine lining that helped nourish the pregnancy must be shed. Blood, mucus, tissue, and white blood cells are cast away from the uterus during the postpartum period. This discharge is called **lochia**. Lochia discharge progresses through three stages:

- Lochia rubra: Occurs during the first 3 to 4 days; is of small to moderate amount; is composed mostly of blood; is dark red in color; and has a fleshy odor.
- Lochia serosa: Occurs during days 4 to 10; decreases to a small amount; and takes on a brownish or pinkish color.
- Lochia alba: Occurs after day 10; and becomes white or pale yellow because the bleeding has stopped and the discharge is now composed mostly of white blood cells.

Lochia may persist for the entire 6 weeks after delivery but often subsides by the end of the 2nd or 3rd week. The lochia should never contain large clots. Other abnormal findings include reversal of the pattern (e.g., the lochia has been serosa, then goes back to rubra); lochia that fails to decrease in amount or actually increases versus gradually decreasing; or a malodorous lochia.

Warning! Normal lochia has a fleshy, but not offensive, odor. If the lochia is malodorous or smells rotten, infection is most likely present. This finding must be reported immediately to the RN or the practitioner.

Ovaries

Ovulation can occur as soon as 3 weeks after delivery. Menstrual periods usually begin within 6 to 8 weeks for the woman who is not breastfeeding. However, the lactating woman may not resume menses for as long 18 months after giving birth. Although lactation may suppress ovulation, it is not a dependable form of birth control. It is wise for the woman to use some type of birth control when she resumes sexual activity, unless she wishes to immediately become pregnant again.

Did you know? Ovulation can occur without return of the menstrual period. Conversely, the woman can have menstrual bleeding without ovulating. Explain to the woman that she may be able to conceive even if the menses does not resume immediately.

Cervix

During labor the cervix thins and dilates. This process does not occur without some trauma. Directly after delivery the cervix is still partially open and contains soft, small tears. It may also appear bruised. Although abnormal, large tears may be an uncommon cause of postpartum hemorrhage. The internal os closes after a few days. Gradually the muscle cells regenerate, and the cervix recovers by the end of the 6-week puerperium. The external os, however, remains slightly open and has a slit-like appearance, in comparison with the dimple-like appearance of the cervix of a nulliparous woman (Fig. 12-2).

Vagina and Perineum

The vagina may have small tears that will heal without intervention. Immediately after delivery, the walls of the vagina are smooth. Rugae begin to return to the vaginal walls after approximately 3 weeks. The diameter of the introitus gradually becomes smaller by contraction but rarely returns to its prepregnant size. Muscle tone is never fully restored to the pregravid state; however, Kegel exercises may help increase the tone and enhance sexual enjoyment. Because breast-feeding suppresses ovulation, estrogen levels remain lower in the lactating woman, which can lead to vaginal dryness and **dyspareunia**, painful intercourse.

The labia and perineum may be edematous after delivery and may appear bruised, particularly after a difficult delivery. If an episiotomy was done or a perineal tear repaired, absorbable stitches will be in place. The edges of the episiotomy or repair should be well approximated. The episiotomy takes several weeks to fully heal. The labia tend to be flaccid after childbirth.

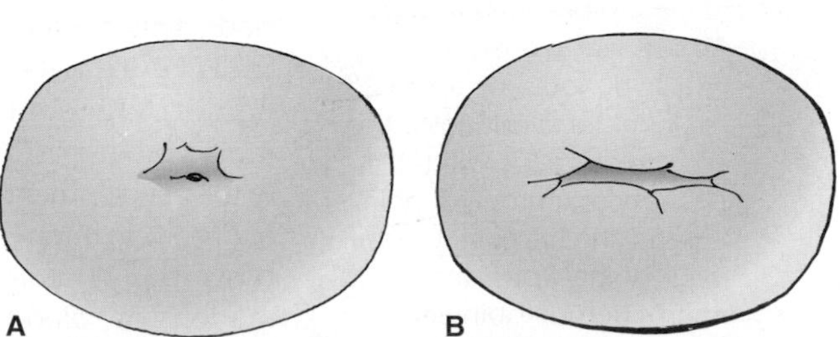

● ***Figure 12.2*** Appearance of the cervix in nulliparous and multiparous women. **(A)** This drawing represents the cervix of a nulliparous woman. Notice the dimple-like structure of the external os. **(B)** This is a representation of the cervix of a multiparous woman. The external os of the multiparous cervix is slit-like in appearance.

Tone may improve over time but never completely returns to the prepregnant state.

Breasts

Colostrum, the antibody-rich breast secretion that is the precursor to breast milk, is normally excreted by the breasts in the last weeks of pregnancy and continues to be excreted in the first few postpartum days. Prolactin levels rise when estrogen and progesterone levels fall after delivery of the placenta. Suckling at the breast also causes prolactin levels to rise. Prolactin stimulates milk production by the breasts, and the milk normally comes in on the 3rd day. See Chapter 14 for a detailed discussion of breast physiology, milk production, and breast-feeding.

Test Yourself

- Where is the fundus normally located on the day after delivery?
- Name three factors that can inhibit or delay uterine involution.
- Name the three stages, in order, through which lochia passes.

Cardiovascular System

The additional fluid volume that is present during the pregnancy is eliminated in the early postpartum period via the skin and urinary routes and through blood loss. The woman who experiences a normal vaginal delivery loses approximately 300 to 500 mL of blood during delivery. If she has a cesarean delivery, normal blood loss is between 500 and 1,000 mL. As the blood volume returns to normal, some hemoconcentration occurs that causes an increase in the hematocrit.

If you can remember this, you'll be able to approximately determine the amount of blood loss in the early postpartum period. For every 250 mL of blood loss, the hematocrit will fall approximately 2 points, and the hemoglobin will fall 1 point. For example, if the woman's hemoglobin and hematocrit were 12.0 and 34, respectively, before delivery, then fall to 10.0 and 30 the day after, she has lost approximately 500 mL of blood.

High plasma fibrinogen levels and other coagulation factors mark the postpartum period. This is protective against hemorrhage, but it also predisposes to the development of deep vein thrombosis (DVT), formation of blood clots in the deep veins of the legs. Dehydration, immobility, and trauma can add to the risk for DVT. Refer to Chapter 19 for discussion of DVT in the postpartum period.

The white blood cell count is elevated to approximately 15,000 to 20,000/ mL, and may reach as high as 30,000/mL. Leukocytosis helps protect the woman from infection, as there are multiple routes for infection to occur in the early postpartum period.

Immediately after delivery, the woman may experience a shaking postpartum chill. This is thought to be caused by hormonal and physiologic changes and is not harmful, unless accompanied by fever greater than 100.4°F or other signs of infection. The shivering normally resolves within minutes, especially if a prewarmed blanket is placed over the woman.

Vital Signs

The temperature may be elevated slightly during the first 24 hours because of the exertion and dehydration of labor. After the first 24 hours, a temperature of 100.4°F or greater is abnormal and may indicate infection.

Here's a tip to help you get accurate blood pressure readings. Take the woman's blood pressure with the woman in the same position each time. The preferred position is supine because orthostatic hypotension is common immediately after delivery. If you take the blood pressure immediately after the woman sits up from a lying position, the reading may be falsely low.

The blood pressure should remain at the woman's baseline level. An elevated blood pressure could be a sign of developing preeclampsia and should be reported. (See Chapter 17.) A falling blood pressure, particularly in the presence of a rising pulse is suggestive of hemorrhage. The woman should be assessed carefully for a source of blood loss if her blood pressure drops.

It is normal for the pulse to be slow in the 1st week after delivery. A heart rate as low as 50 beats per minute is considered normal. Occasionally the woman may experience tachycardia. This is more likely to occur after a difficult labor and delivery, or it may indicate excess blood loss.

Musculoskeletal System

The most pronounced changes are found in the abdominal muscles, although other muscles may be weak because of the exertion of labor. The abdomen is soft and sagging in the immediate postpartum period. Often the woman has to wear loose clothing for the first few weeks. The abdomen usually regains its tone with exercise. However, in some women the abdomen remains slack. In this situation if another pregnancy occurs, the abdomen will be pendulous and the woman will have more problems with backache. **Diastasis recti abdominis** is a condition in which the abdominal muscles separate during the pregnancy, leaving part of the abdominal wall without muscular support. Exercise can improve muscle tone, if diastasis recti abdominis occurs. A woman is predisposed for poor muscle tone and diastasis if she has poor muscle tone or is obese before the pregnancy, her abdomen is overdistended during the pregnancy, or she is a grand multipara.

Gastrointestinal System

Immediately after delivery the postpartum woman often is very hungry. The energy expended during labor uses up glucose stores, and food has generally been restricted. Restriction of fluids and loss of fluids in labor, in the urine, and via diaphoresis often lead to increased thirst.

The postpartum woman may be troubled by constipation. Intra-abdominal pressure decreases rapidly after childbirth, and peristalsis is diminished. These factors make it more difficult for feces to travel down the gastrointestinal tract. The woman may be afraid to defecate in the early postpartum period because of hemorrhoidal discomfort and perineal pain. Suppressing the urge to defecate complicates the problem of constipation and may actually cause increased pain when defecation finally occurs. Iron supplementation adds to the problem. However, by the end of the 1st postpartum week, bowel function has usually returned to normal.

Urinary System

The urinary system must handle an increased load in the early postpartum period as the body excretes excess plasma volume. Healthy kidneys are able to adjust to the increased demands. Urinary output exceeds intake. Transient glycosuria, proteinuria, and ketonuria are normal in the immediate postpartum period.

During the process of labor and delivery trauma can occur to the lower urinary system. Pressure of the descending fetal head on the ureters, bladder, and urethra can lead to transient loss of bladder tone and urethral edema. Trauma, certain medications, and anesthesia given during labor can also lead to a temporary loss of bladder sensation. The result can be urinary retention. Sometimes the woman voids small amounts but does not completely empty the bladder. Or she may not be able to void at all. If the urethra has been traumatized, voiding may be painful.

Here's an assessment tip! A full bladder can push up on the uterus, which displaces it (usually to the right side) and interferes with effective uterine contraction. If you palpate the fundus and find that it is above the umbilicus, deviated to the right side, and boggy, the most likely cause is a full bladder. Assist the woman to void, and then re-evaluate the fundus.

The urinary system is more susceptible to infection during the postpartum period. Hydronephrosis, dilation of the renal pelves and ureters, is a normal change that occurs during pregnancy because of hormonal influences. This condition persists for approximately 4 weeks after delivery. Hydronephrosis and urinary stasis predispose the woman to urinary tract infection (UTI).

Integumentary System

Copious diaphoresis occurs in the first few days after childbirth as the body rids itself of excess water and waste via the skin. The perspiration is noticed particularly at night. The woman may wake up and be drenched in sweat. This is a normal finding and is not a cause for concern.

Striae, stretch marks, are found on the abdomen and sometimes on the breasts. Immediately after birth they appear red or purplish. Over time they fade to a light silvery color and remain faintly visible.

Weight Loss

Immediately after delivery approximately 10 to 12 pounds are lost with expulsion of the fetus, placenta, and amniotic fluid. The woman loses an additional 5 pounds in the early postpartum period because of fluid loss from diaphoresis and urinary excretion. The average woman will have returned to her prepregnant weight 6 months after childbirth, if she was within the recommended weight gain of 25 to 30 pounds during pregnancy. Some women take longer to lose the additional pounds. In general, the breastfeeding woman tends to lose weight faster than the woman who does not breast-feed because of increased caloric demands.

Test Yourself

- A falling blood pressure and rising pulse in the early postpartum period is suggestive of ____________.
- Name two factors that contribute to constipation in the postpartum period.
- How long does it take for the average woman to return to her prepregnant weight after delivery?

Psychological Adaptation

Role change is the most significant psychological adaptation the woman must make. This process may be especially pronounced for first-time mothers, but it occurs with each new addition to the family. Each child is a unique being with her own temperament and needs. In fact, the whole family must adapt to the addition of a new member.

Maternal role development begins during pregnancy as the expectant mother anticipates the birth of the baby. She fantasizes about and prepares for her newborn's arrival. After the birth, the woman must take on the role of mother to the baby. This is a continuous process that occurs over the months and years as the child grows and changes.

The nurse can influence the development of positive family relationships in many ways. Careful assessment of maternal psychological adaptation and anticipatory guidance regarding postpartum blues and expected psychological adjustments can go a long way toward fostering positive transition for the woman and the new family.

Maternal Role Development

The adjustment of the woman to her new role as mother occurs through a series of developmental stages. Although each woman takes on her role as mother in her own way, influenced by her culture, upbringing, and role models, there are patterns of behavior that can be noted. One nurse researcher, Reva Rubin, observed that women go through three general phases in the first few days and continuing through the first year after delivery. These phases are taking in, taking hold, and letting go.

Taking In Phase

In the early puerperium the new mother demonstrates dependent behaviors. She has difficulty making decisions and needs assistance with self-care needs. She tends to be inwardly focused and concerned about her own physical needs, such as food, rest, and elimination. She relives the delivery experience, and has a great need to talk about the details. This process is important for her to integrate the experience into her concept of self. She may remain in this dependent, reintegration phase for several hours or days. This is not an optimum time to teach detailed newborn care because the new mother is not readily receptive to instruction. Listen with an attitude of acceptance. No feeling the woman expresses is "wrong." Help her interpret the events of her birth experience.

Taking Hold Phase

Most women move quickly from the dependent stage to increasing independence in self and newborn care. After she has rested and recovered somewhat from the stress of the delivery, the new mother has more energy to concentrate on her infant. At this point she becomes receptive to infant care instruction. The first-time mother in particular needs reassurance that she is capable of providing care for her newborn. She may feel that the nurse is more adept than she is at meeting the newborn's needs. Therefore, it is important to encourage her to perform care for her newborn while you provide gentle guidance and support. She responds well to praise for her early attempts at child care during this phase. This phase lasts anywhere from 2 days to several weeks.

Don't yield to temptation!
Sometimes it may seem easier to do the infant care yourself, rather than observe and support the woman as she cares for the newborn. However, it is important for you not to assume the mothering role. The new mother needs practice and praise to begin to feel confident in her new role. Otherwise she may feel incompetent to carry out her parenting role when she goes home.

Letting Go Phase

Most nurses do not witness the transition into the third postpartum phase of psychological adjustment because this phase occurs in the late puerperium. Letting go of previous roles and defining her new parenting role requires grief work. It is normal for the woman to experience a wide range of emotions as she gives up her fantasy child and gets to know the real child. She begins to see her infant as separate from herself. It is during this phase that family relationships are adjusted to accommodate the infant.

Development of Positive Family Relationships

The enduring emotional bond that develops between the parent and infant is called **attachment**. However, this process does not happen automatically. Attachment occurs as parents interact with and respond to their infant. In the early postpartum period, the woman may have a wide range of emotions and responses to her newborn. Humans seem to respond to gains and losses in similar ways. Disbelief and shock are often the initial reactions. You may hear the mother say over and over, "I can't believe I just had a baby." Ambivalence also is a normal response. The new parents may communicate uncertainty over their readiness to take on the parent role. Frequently the new mother may experience negative feelings about the baby in the first few days after birth. However, she may not express these feelings because of the cultural expectation that "mothers always love their babies." If she does express negativity, such as "I'm

A PERSONAL GLIMPSE

I delivered my first child after 14 hours of intense labor. I went through my labor naturally without an epidural with the help of my doula. I pushed for 2 hours, so I was pretty exhausted after delivery. The midwife had to cut an episiotomy because she said it was a tight fit. My baby weighed 9 pounds! The next day while the baby was in the room I remember that everything felt so unreal. I kept telling myself that I should feel happy. But all I really wanted to do was to cry. The nurse came in and told me what a beautiful baby I had and asked me her name. I started to cry and said that I wasn't sure that I could be a good mother. I felt scared and confused and unready to take care of a baby. The nurse told me that the feelings I was having were very normal. She said that this was a huge change for me and that it takes time to get adjusted to the new mother role. She asked me if I had someone to help me at home. I told her that my sister was going to stay with me for several weeks. The nurse gave me a card with the phone number for the hospital. She wrote her name on it and told me that she would be happy to answer any questions I had after I went home. She said that I could talk to any of the nurses, if she wasn't on duty when I called. I felt relieved. The nurse then stayed with me a while and watched while I changed the baby's diaper. She told me that I was a quick learner and that I was very gentle with the baby. I felt so much better. I knew that it was going to be ok.

Holly

LEARNING OPPORTUNITY: Why do you think this new mother felt better after her interaction with the nurse? In what ways can you in your role as a nurse support the new mother when she expresses negative feelings about her baby or her abilities as a mother?

not sure that I like my baby," the nurse or family members may reply in a way that denies or dismisses the emotion. "Oh, I'm sure you don't mean that," is one such dismissive response. It is important to remember that negative feelings are part of the process as mother and baby adjust to each other and become acquainted.

The initial component of healthy attachment is a process called **bonding**. This is the way the new mother and father become acquainted with their newborn (Fig. 12-3). The process begins with a predictable pattern of parental behavior. Initial inspection of the newborn begins with fingertip touching. The new mother explores her newborn's extremities, counting his fingers and toes. She then advances to using the palms of her hands to touch the newborn and begins to explore larger body areas. Eventually she enfolds the newborn with her hands and arms and holds her close. As bonding continues she begins to spend more time holding the newborn in the **en face** position in which she interacts face-to-face with the newborn. She places the baby's face within her direct line of vision and makes full eye contact with the newborn. The new mother often will talk to the baby in high-pitched tones and smile and laugh while she continues the en face posture. Box 12-1 lists the sequence of initial attachment.

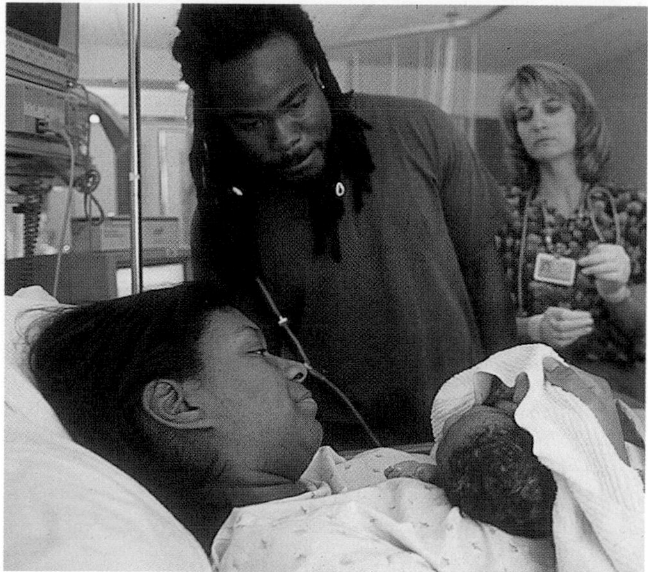

● ***Figure 12.3*** A mom and dad bond with their newborn immediately after birth. At first some parents are tentative, but gradually they will bond.

Acceptance is not as hard as you think. If the new mother makes a negative comment, you can respond in a way that is accepting and supportive. You might reply, "It is natural to have feelings of uncertainty as you adjust to having a new baby." Or, "Having a new baby can seem a bit overwhelming at first. Take your time as you get to know your baby." Be creative. I'm sure you can come up with some great supportive phrases.

One important component in the development of healthy attachment between the new parents and their baby is the amount and type of social support the new family has available to them. If supportive friends and relatives surround them, attachment is enhanced. When a new mother is isolated and without adequate social support, attachment is threatened. If you encounter this situation, it is important to assist the woman to find sources of support. Perhaps there is someone she can call who might be willing to provide

BOX 12.1 Progression of Initial Attachment Behaviors

The new mother and father both begin their interaction with the new baby in a fairly predictable sequence. Note that this process may take anywhere from hours to days.

1. Exploration begins with fingertip touching.
2. Next the new parent explores the infant's extremities.
3. Fingertip touching gives way to touching with the palmar surface of the hands.
4. Then larger body surfaces are touched and caressed.
5. Soon the infant is enfolded with the hands and arms and cuddled closely to the parent.
6. Progressively more time is spent in the en face position talking to and smiling at the new baby.

support. Discuss the situation with the RN in charge. A referral to social services may be in order.

Healthy bonding behaviors include naming the newborn and calling the newborn by name. Making eye contact and talking to the newborn are other indicators that healthy attachment is occurring. It is important to differentiate between a new parent who is nervous and anxious about her new role and one who is rejecting her parenting role. Warning signals of poor attachment include turning away from the newborn, refusing or neglecting to provide for the care of the newborn, and disengagement from the newborn.

It was once thought that the mother was the first and most important person to bond with the new baby. It is now accepted that the baby can make many bonds (Fig. 12-4). The father benefits from early contact with the newborn immediately after delivery. It is common for the father to describe strong emotions of pride, joy, and other positive emotions when he first holds his newborn. The father may be engrossed with the newborn. He progresses through a pattern of touching similar to that of the mother.

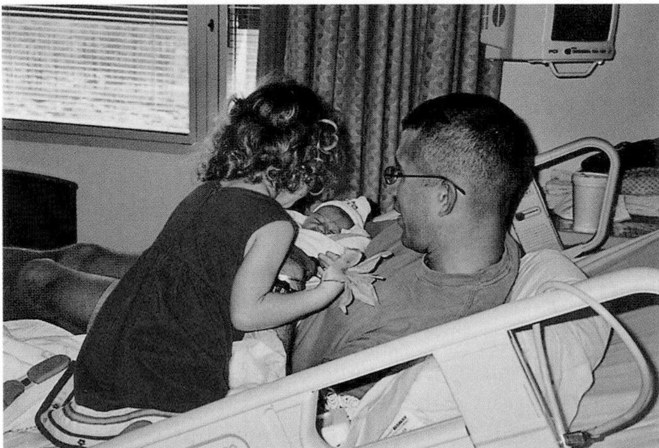

● ***Figure 12.4*** The proud father snuggles with his newborn son and introduces big sister to her new baby brother.

Siblings can also bond with the new baby. There are special considerations that the parents need to make for older siblings of a new baby. The birth of a new baby requires a role change for the sibling. Sometimes the new baby does not meet the sibling's expectations. For instance, the baby might be a boy, but the sibling wanted a sister. It is common for the sibling to regress for a few days after the birth.

Postpartum Blues

Approximately 50% to 70% of postpartum women will experience the **postpartum blues**, sometimes called the "baby blues." The postpartum blues is a temporary depression that usually begins on the 3rd day and lasts for 2 or 3 days. The woman may be tearful, have difficulty sleeping and eating, and feel generally let down. It is thought that a combination of factors contributes to the baby blues. Psychological adjustment along with a physiologic decrease in estrogen and progesterone are thought to be the greatest contributors. In addition, too much activity, fatigue, disturbed sleep patterns, and discomfort also may contribute. It is important for the woman and her family to know that this is a normal reaction; however, if the depression lasts for more than several days, or if the symptoms become severe, further psychological evaluation is needed. (See Chapter 19 for a discussion of postpartum depression.)

Test Yourself

- Name two characteristics of women who are in the taking in phase of psychological adjustment after delivery.
- Define attachment.
- List the normal progression of interaction that occurs during the initial bonding experience between a new parent and the newborn.

● Nursing Process for the Early Postpartum Period

Most women who deliver vaginally go home within 24 to 48 hours after delivery. This challenges the nurse caring for the woman in the early postpartum period to do thorough assessments to pick up on any complications that might be developing, and to use every available opportunity to do teaching regarding self- and newborn care.

ASSESSMENT

After the initial recovery period, the woman may be transferred to a postpartum room. If she delivered in a labor, delivery, recovery, and postpartum (LDRP) setting, she will stay in the room in which she delivered. Whatever the setting, the postpartum nurse must do a thorough initial assessment.

Data Collection

Much of the data collection is done before the woman delivers and can be found on the initial admission assessment done in the labor and delivery unit (L&D). It is important to check the initial assessment and the prenatal record as part of the initial data collection. The L&D nurse gives report when the woman is transferred to the postpartum nurse. The report should include significant medical history, pregnancy history, labor and birth history, newborn data, and initial postpartum recovery data.

The medical and pregnancy histories are important because they alert the postpartum nurse to risk factors that might lead to postpartum hemorrhage or other complications and give clues as to bonding potential. The report includes the gravida and para, the estimated date of delivery (EDD), blood type and Rh, complications experienced during the pregnancy, group B streptococcus (GBS) culture status, and any medical problems, including sexually transmitted infections (STIs).

The labor and birth history includes the length of labor, type and time of birth, type and timing of analgesia or anesthesia administered, type and timing of any IV medications given, and any complications experienced during labor. Important information regarding the newborn includes sex, Apgar scores, resuscitation efforts, congenital anomalies, current status, the mother's plans for feeding, and whether or not feeding was initiated in the delivery room. Initial postpartum recovery data that should be reported includes status of the fundus, lochia, and perineum; type of pain, if any, and success of analgesics and comfort measures to control the pain; whether or not the woman ambulated after delivery and how she tolerated it; type and amount of IV fluids infusing, if any; status of the bladder; and response of the woman and her partner to the newborn.

Physical Assessment

Initial Assessment in the First Hour After Delivery

If the woman is going to hemorrhage, she is most likely to do so within the 1st postpartum hour. For this reason, she is monitored closely during this time period. Her vital signs are monitored every 15 minutes during the 1st hour. With each vital sign check, determine the position and firmness of the uterine fundus, the amount and character of lochia, the status of the perineum, and monitor for signs of bladder distention. If the woman had a cesarean delivery, also check the incisional dressing for intactness and determine if any incisional bleeding is occurring. Measure the temperature and determine the status of the breasts once immediately after delivery and then again just before transfer to postpartum. Some institutions continue monitoring as above every 30 minutes for the 2nd hour, then every 4 hours during the first 24 hours after delivery.

Complete Postpartum Assessment

At least once per shift a complete head-to-toe assessment should be completed. A quick visual survey and speaking to the woman reveals her level of consciousness and affect. Assist her to empty her bladder, if necessary, before commencing the full assessment. First, take the vital signs. Respirations should be even and unlabored. Be sure to rule out shortness of breath and chest pain. The heart rate should be regular without murmurs and may be as slow as 50 beats per minute. The lungs should be clear in all five lobes (Fig. 12-5). After the vital signs assessment, there are 11 main areas that must be assessed and monitored in the postpartum period. These areas are

- breasts
- uterus

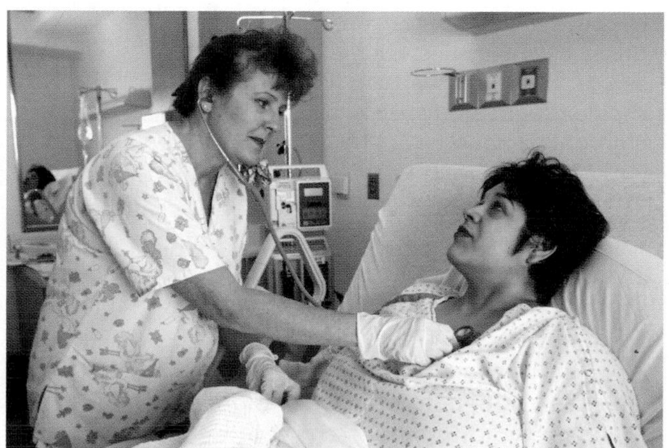

● ***Figure 12.5*** The nurse auscultates the lungs as part of a complete postpartum assessment.

- lochia
- bladder
- bowel
- perineum
- lower extremities
- pain
- laboratory studies
- maternal–newborn bonding
- maternal emotional status

Breasts. Inspect the breasts and nipples for signs of engorgement, redness, or cracks. Palpate the breasts gently to determine if they are soft, filling, or engorged with milk. Note if there are any painful areas. With a gloved hand palpate the nipples to determine if they are erect or inverted. The breasts should be soft during the 1st postpartum day, and begin filling on the 2nd and 3rd days. Engorgement may occur on the 3rd day. There should be no reddened areas on the breasts, and the nipples should be intact without cracks or fissures.

Uterus. With the woman lying supine, palpate the fundus (Nursing Procedure 12-1). Note the position of the uterus and palpate the uterus to determine consistency, tone, position, and size. It should be firm, not boggy, located in the midline, and at the appropriate height in relation to the umbilicus, depending on what hour/day it is after delivery.

Notice this difference. When a woman has had a cesarean delivery, she usually has less lochia than a woman who delivers vaginally. This occurs because the surgeon thoroughly wipes out the uterine cavity before suturing it closed, which removes much of the blood and debris. However, she should still progress through the same stages (i.e., rubra, serosa, then alba), and the flow should progressively become smaller in amount.

Lochia. Determine the amount and character of the lochia. Is it scant, small, moderate, or heavy? Is it rubra or serosa? Is there a foul smell? Be sure to check under her buttocks for pooling. Ask her how many times she has changed her sanitary napkins/pads since the previous assessment and determine if she is saturating pads. The lochia should be rubra of small to moderate amount without large clots and no foul odor.

Bladder and Bowel. The woman should be voiding adequate amounts (more than 100 mL per each voiding) regularly. Voiding frequently in amounts smaller than 100 mL with associated suprapubic distention (a rounded area just above

Nursing Procedure 12.1 Fundal Palpation and Massage

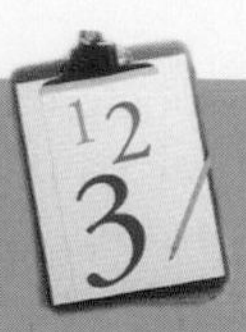

EQUIPMENT

Warm, clean hands
Clean gloves

PROCEDURE

1. Explain procedure to the woman.
2. Instruct her to empty her bladder, if necessary.
3. Wash hands thoroughly.
4. Position her supine with the head of the bed flat.
5. Locate and place one hand on the uterine fundus. It should feel hard and rounded—something like a melon.
6. Place the other hand in a cupped position just above the symphysis pubis, as in the picture. Use this hand to gently support the uterus.

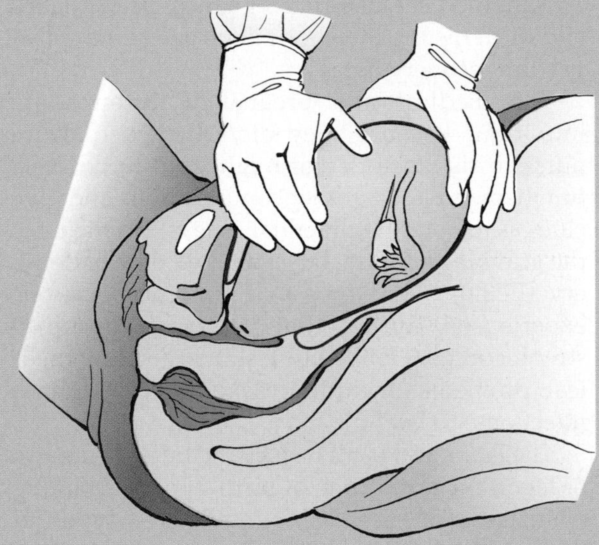

7. Gently massage the fundus, if it is soft or boggy.
8. Notice the location, height, and position of the uterus.
9. Wash hands.
10. Document the tone (soft, boggy, or firm) and the location of the fundus in finger breadths above or below or at the level of the umbilicus. Note whether or not the fundus is midline or deviated to one side.

Note: Vigorous fundal massage or overstimulation can cause the uterus to become flaccid, rather than helping it to contract. Take measures to avoid overmassaging the fundus.

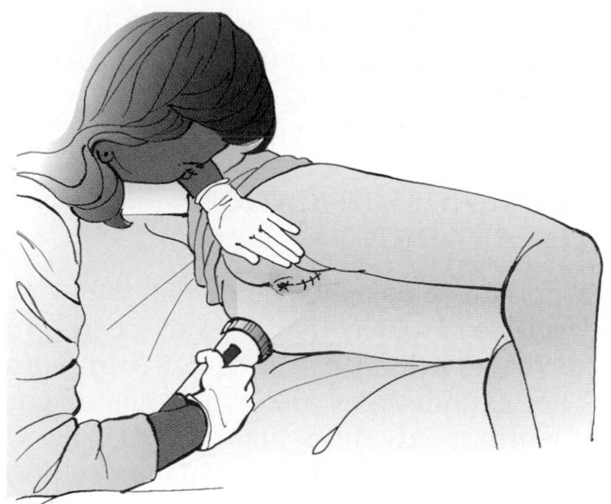

● ***Figure 12.6*** Notice that the woman is in the Sims' position. The nurse lifts the upper buttock and inspects the perineum.

the symphysis pubis) is indicative of urinary retention. Next, visually inspect the abdomen and auscultate for bowel sounds. Bowel sounds should be present in all four quadrants. Ask the woman if she has had a bowel movement after delivery.

Perineum. Assist the woman to the Sims' position. Lift the top buttock, and with a good light source (such as a penlight or flashlight) inspect the perineum for redness, edema and ecchymosis. If an episiotomy was done or a tear occurred, check the sutures and be certain the edges are well approximated. Determine if there is any drainage from the stitches. Palpate gently with a gloved hand to determine if there are any hematomas forming in the area. Note any hemorrhoids. The perineum should be intact, with only minimal swelling and no hematomas. Figure 12-6 depicts a nurse performing an assessment of the perineum.

Lower Extremities. Inspect the extremities for edema (Fig. 12-7*A*), equality of pulses, and capillary refill. Check for Homans' sign (Fig. 12-7*B*). Feel along the calf area for any warmth or redness. The calves should be of equal size and warmth bilaterally. There should be no reddened, painful areas, and there should be no pain in the calves when the feet are dorsiflexed (negative Homans' sign), or when the woman is walking.

Pain. Determine if the woman is experiencing any pain. If so, investigate the source (e.g., afterpains, episiotomy, painful urination, pain in the calves). Determine the characteristics, quality, timing, and relief after comfort measures.

Laboratory Studies. Monitor the hemoglobin and hematocrit (H&H). Note the H&H before delivery. Most practitioners order a postpartum H&H on the morning after delivery. If the values drop significantly, the woman may have experienced postpartum hemorrhage. Note the blood type and Rh. If the woman is Rh-negative, she will need a RhoGAM workup. Determine the woman's rubella status. If she is nonimmune, she will need a rubella immunization before she is discharged home.

Maternal–Newborn Bonding and Maternal Emotional Status. Anytime the newborn is in the room, note maternal–newborn interactions.

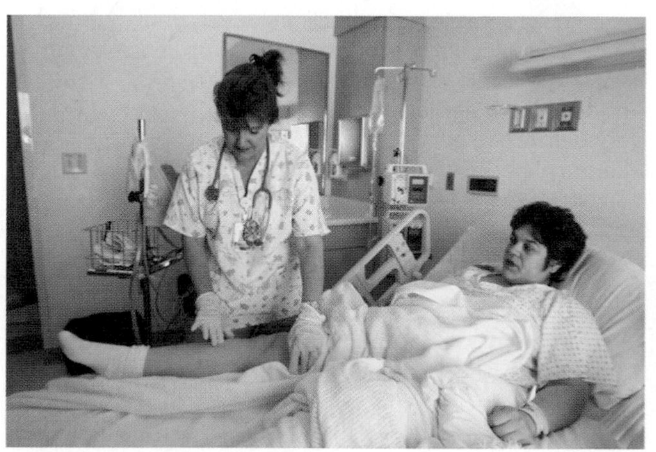

A

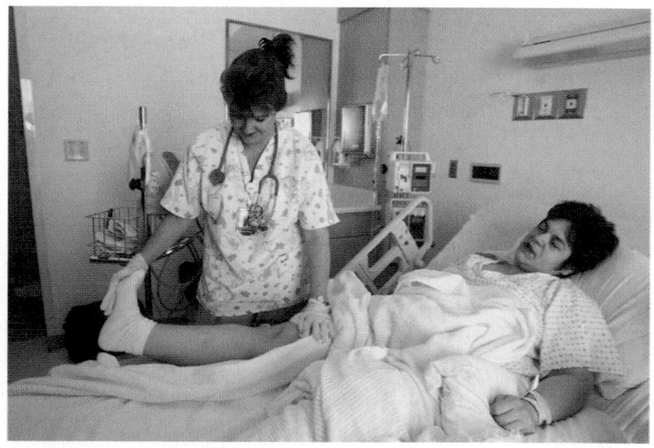

B

● ***Figure 12.7*** Assessment of the lower extremities. **(A)** The nurse checks the right lower extremity for edema. **(B)** The nurse dorsiflexes the foot and asks the woman if she feels pain in the calf of her leg. No pain is recorded as a negative Homans' sign. If pain is present, a positive Homans' sign is recorded and the RN or physician is notified. A positive Homans' sign may indicate the presence of deep vein thrombosis. Homans' sign is recorded and the RN or physician is notified. A positive Homans' sign may indicate the presence of deep vein thrombosis.

BOX 12.2 Warning Signs of Poor Attachment

- Making negative statements about the baby
- Turning away from the baby
- Refusing to name the baby
- Refusing to care for the baby
- Withdrawing
- Verbalizing disappointment with the sex of the baby
- Failing to touch the baby
- Limited handling of the baby

Assess successfulness of breast-feeding attempts. Notice the quantity and quality of social support available to the woman. Monitor her mood and affect. Box 12-2 lists warning signs of poor attachment.

Test Yourself

- List five major components of the woman's history that are important for the postpartum nurse to know when assuming care of the woman after delivery.
- Describe the appropriate way to perform an assessment of the episiotomy.
- Name three important laboratory studies to which the nurse should pay attention after delivery.

SELECTED NURSING DIAGNOSES

- Risk for Injury: Postpartum hemorrhage related to uterine atony, undetected lacerations, or hematoma formation
- Acute Pain related to sore nipples, afterpains, or episiotomy discomfort
- Risk for Infection related to multiple portals of entry for pathogens, including the former site of the placenta, episiotomy, bladder, and breasts
- Risk for Injury: Falls related to postural hypotension and fainting
- Urinary Retention related to periurethral edema, injury to the bladder during birth, or lingering effects of anesthesia
- Risk for Constipation related to slowed peristalsis, inadequate fluid or fiber intake, and fear of pain during defecation
- Risk for Injury: Thrombus formation related to increased coagulation factors and inadequate fluid intake
- Disturbed Sleep Pattern related to excess fatigue, overstimulation, or adjusting to newborn's frequent feeding needs
- Risk for Impaired Parent–Newborn Attachment

OUTCOME IDENTIFICATION AND PLANNING

Appropriate goals may include that the woman will not experience injury from postpartum hemorrhage; will express adequate pain control; will not exhibit signs and symptoms of infection; will not experience injury from falls; will have adequate urinary elimination without retention; will experience adequate bowel elimination; will not experience injury from DVT; will verbalize feeling rested after sleeping; and will exhibit behaviors that indicate the beginning of a healthy attachment with the newborn. Other goals and interventions are planned according to the individual needs of the woman and her partner.

IMPLEMENTATION

Promoting Hemostasis

As discussed earlier in the chapter the postpartum woman is subject to hemorrhage from several sources. The most common type of hemorrhage is related to uterine atony. If the uterus feels boggy or soft to palpation, massage it until it tones up beneath your fingers. Monitor IV fluids and administer oxytocics, such as Pitocin, to prevent uterine atony. Teach the woman to perform periodic self-fundal massage.

Be prepared. Anytime the woman has been in bed for a length of time, the lochia will pool in the vagina. Therefore, when she gets up for the first time after delivery, or in the morning after reclining all night, it is normal for the lochia to seem heavy and to flow down her legs. Reassure her before she gets up that this is a normal occurrence and does not signify that she is hemorrhaging.

Bright red bleeding that occurs in a steady stream in the presence of a firm fundus is most likely caused by a vaginal or cervical laceration that was not repaired. Report this finding to the RN or the primary care provider immediately. Also report bleeding from or separation of the edges of the episiotomy. Monitor for and report any very painful, soft, and possibly pulsing, masses palpable in the perineal area. These are signs of hematoma formation.

Providing Pain Management

There are several possible sources of pain that can occur during the postpartum period. To manage the pain adequately, you must first determine the source of pain.

Managing Breast Pain. Breast pain should be investigated to determine if it is unilateral and associated with increased warmth and redness. This could be a sign of mastitis, a postpartum complication that is discussed in Chapter 19. If the breasts are painful bilaterally because of engorgement, interventions chosen will be dependent on whether or not the woman is breast-feeding. If she is breast-feeding, warmth seems to help the most. Have her run warm water over her breasts in the shower, or place a warm washcloth as a compress on the breasts. If the engorgement is preventing the baby from latching on, assist the woman to express some milk before attempting to breast-feed.

If the breasts are engorged and the woman is bottle-feeding her newborn, instruct her to keep a support bra on 24 hours per day. Cool compresses, or an ice pack wrapped in a towel, will usually be soothing and help to suppress milk production.

If the nipples are painful during breast-feeding attempts, examine the nipples for cracks or fissures. Observe the woman when she puts her newborn to the breast and ensure that she is positioning the newborn properly to prevent sore, cracked nipples. Encourage the use of a lanolin-based cream to keep the nipples soft and promote healing. A mild analgesic may be helpful. (See Chapter 14 for additional breast-feeding interventions.)

Managing Afterpains. If the source of pain is afterpains, ibuprofen or other nonsteroidal anti-inflammatory drugs (NSAIDs) are usually helpful. The primary care provider often will order 600 to 800 mg of ibuprofen every 6 to 8 hours as needed for pain. For multiparas, it may be appropriate to schedule the medication around the clock, rather than waiting for the woman to ask for it. Timing administration of the drug so that it is given 30 to 45 minutes before breast-feeding is also helpful because breast-feeding intensifies uterine cramping and associated afterpains. Nonpharmacologic methods that might be helpful include warm compresses to the abdomen, positioning for comfort, adequate rest and nutrition, and early ambulation.

Managing Perineal Pain. If the pain is arising from the perineum, the perineum should be visualized before taking measures to control the pain to rule out development of a hematoma and to make certain the episiotomy is well approximated. Early interventions within the first 24 hours include ice packs to the perineum (Nursing Procedure 12-2). Ice will help reduce swelling and ease painful sensations. Most institutions use special perineal ice packs that incorporate the cold source into the perineal pad. The ice pack should be on for 20 minutes, then off for 20 minutes to be most effective.

After the first 24 hours, warm sitz baths can be especially comforting to a sore perineum (Nursing Procedure 12-3). Throughout the first few postpartum days, mild analgesics combined with a narcotic are usually most helpful for perineal pain. Examples of combination products include acetaminophen with codeine (Tylenol No. 3) and hydrocodone with

Nursing Procedure 12.2 Application of Perineal Ice Packs

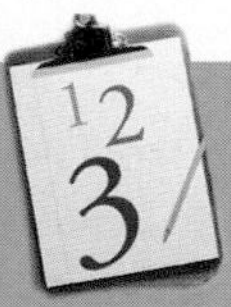

EQUIPMENT

A commercial ice pack or a clean glove and ice
Clean gloves

PROCEDURE

1. Explain procedure to the woman.
2. Wash hands thoroughly.
3. Position her in dorsal recumbent position.
4. Activate the commercial pack as instructed in the directions for use, or fill a clean glove with crushed ice and tie a knot at the opening at the top of the glove.
5. Cover the pack or the glove with a thin covering, such as a towel.
6. Place the pack on the perineum.
7. Assist her to a position of comfort.
8. Wash hands.
9. Leave in place for 20 minutes then remove for 10 minutes. Repeat as necessary for comfort during the first 24 hours postpartum.

Note: If the ice pack is allowed to stay next to the perineum continuously for prolonged periods, tissue damage could result.

Be careful. When administering combination products for pain, be certain you know the dose of each product in the combination. Be particularly watchful that you do not exceed the maximum daily-recommended dosage of acetaminophen when giving products that contain this medication.

Nursing Procedure 12.3 Assisting the Postpartum Woman With a Sitz Bath

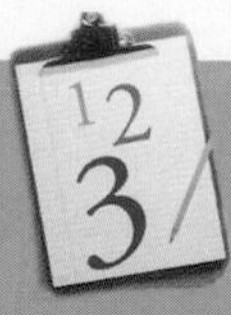

EQUIPMENT

New sitz bath in manufacturer's packaging with directions
Clean gloves

PROCEDURE

1. Explain procedure to the woman.
2. Instruct her to empty her bladder, if necessary.
3. Wash hands thoroughly.
4. Place the sitz bath in the toilet as per the manufacturer's instructions.
5. Place the tubing in the allotted slot and clamp the tubing.
6. Fill the bag with warm (102°F to 105°F) water and hang it at a level of a few feet above the toilet.
7. Unclamp the tubing and allow the warm water to fill the basin.
8. Reclamp the tubing and refill the bag with warm water. Seal the bag with the locking mechanism provided.
9. Assist the woman to sit on the basin so that her perineum is submerged in the water.
10. Ensure that she can reach the emergency call bell.
11. Instruct her to unclamp the tubing periodically to allow water to run over the perineum and into the toilet.
12. Encourage the woman to stay on the sitz bath for at least 20 minutes.
13. Provide a clean towel with which to pat dry and clean sanitary napkins to apply when she is finished.
14. With clean-gloved hands, assist her to rinse out the basin, dry it and store it for the next use.
15. Wash hands.

Note: Encourage the woman to use the sitz bath three times per day for at least 20 minutes per session, or as needed for comfort. Some women may prefer cooler water temperatures, which is an acceptable practice.

acetaminophen (Lortab, Vicodin). Local anesthetics, such as witch hazel pads or benzocaine sprays, may be helpful. The pain of hemorrhoids can be reduced by use of sitz baths, witch hazel pads, and/or products that contain hydrocortisone.

Preventing Infection

There are multiple portals of entry for infection in the postpartum period. However, the number one way of preventing infection continues to be handwashing. Wash your hands before and after caring for the patient, even if you will be wearing gloves. It is also important to teach the woman to wash her hands before touching her breasts or feeding the baby; before and after using the restroom or performing perineal care; and before eating. Early ambulation, adequate fluid intake, and good nutrition strengthen the immune system and help to prevent infection.

The best way to prevent mastitis (infection in the breast), in addition to frequent handwashing, is to avoid cracked nipples. Assist the woman to properly position the infant at the breast to prevent this complication. Other measures that help prevent cracked nipples are to rub the nipples with a few drops of expressed milk after breast-feeding and allow the nipples to air dry. Lanolin cream may also be a helpful measure. The woman should breast-feed at regular, frequent intervals. Milk stasis can lead to obstruction of a duct, which can lead to inflammation and then infection.

Endometritis, or infection of the uterine lining, is another type of infection that can occur in the postpartum period. Handwashing before and after using the bathroom and performing perineal care are the best ways to prevent this infection. In addition, have the woman use a peribottle to perform perineal care and change her sanitary napkins/pads at least every 4 hours. Instruct her to fill the peribottle with warm water (a gentle soap can be added, if desired). After using the restroom, she should squeeze the bottle while aiming at the perineum so that the water flows from front to back. She can then use a washcloth or tissue to gently pat and dry the perineum from front to back. Instruct the woman to avoid touching the center part of the sanitary napkins/pads; she should handle the pads only by the ends. The part of the peripad that touches her perineum should be sterile. These measures can also help prevent infections of the episiotomy.

The postpartum woman is prone to bladder infections because of urethral trauma and perhaps from stasis related to incomplete bladder emptying. Urinary catheterization may be necessary to treat urinary retention; however, this invasive procedure increases the risk for urinary tract infection (UTI). Taking steps to avoid urinary catheterization, when possible, is helpful in decreasing the risk for UTI. Adequate fluid intake and measures to prevent retention are also helpful.

Preventing Injury from Falls

The first time the woman gets up, she is at risk for fainting and falling because of postural hypotension. When the woman is going to get out of bed for the first time after delivery, assist her to dangle her legs at the side of the bed for 5 minutes. If she is not feeling dizzy, assist her to the bathroom. Remain with her until she returns to bed. If she begins to feel dizzy at anytime, help her to sit down with her head forward for a few minutes. If she begins to black out, gently support her to the floor until she comes to. Another time she is at increased risk for fainting is the first time she is in the shower. The warm water may cause peripheral dilation of blood vessels, which leads to hypotension and fainting. Stay in the woman's room while she is showering for the first time. Have a shower chair available for her to sit on if she begins to feel faint.

Promoting Urinary Elimination
The best way to assist the woman to empty her bladder is to help her up to the restroom to void. However, sometimes this is not possible because of incomplete recovery from regional anesthesia. In this instance, assist the woman to sit up on the bedpan, a position that may promote emptying of the bladder. Be certain that the woman has privacy. If she is having difficulty voiding, running water in the sink, or using the peribottle to run warm water over the perineum may help. It also helps to give her plenty of time in which to void. If she feels rushed, this may contribute to urinary retention. If the woman cannot void on her first trip to the bathroom after delivery, it may be appropriate to allow her to wait for a while longer. If she is still unable to void and it has been longer than 6 hours, or there are signs of bladder distention, you may need to perform an in-and-out urinary catheterization to empty her bladder. Likewise, catheterization may be necessary if she is voiding small amounts (less than 100 cc) in frequent intervals.

Promoting Bowel Elimination
All of the normal measures that help prevent constipation are helpful in the postpartum period. Adequate fluid intake keeps the feces soft, facilitating passage. Early ambulation stimulates normal bowel peristalsis. Adding plenty of fruits, vegetables, and fiber to the diet also helps to prevent constipation. A bulk-forming agent, such as Metamucil, may also be helpful. Sometimes the primary care provider orders a stool softener for the first few days after birth. Encourage the woman not to suppress the urge to defecate.

Preventing Injury From Thrombus Formation
Assist the woman to ambulate as soon as possible after delivery. Early ambulation decreases the chance of thrombus formation by promoting venous return. Encourage liberal fluid intake. Dehydration contributes to the risk of thrombus formation.

Promoting Restful Sleep
Monitor the woman's sleep–wake cycle. Encourage her to continue presleep routines she normally uses at home. Promote a relaxing, low-stress environment before sleep. Dim the lights and monitor noise and traffic near the woman's room during sleep time. Medicate for pain, if needed, at bedtime. Plan care activities so that sleep is disturbed as infrequently as possible. For instance, if the postpartum recovery is going well, and vital signs have been stable, consult with the RN about waiting until the 6 a.m. laboratory draw to obtain vital signs, rather than awaking the patient at 2 a.m. Or instruct the woman to call you if she awakens in the night to use the restroom; you can perform the vital signs at this time.

Of course it is challenging for a new mother to get enough sleep because newborns may awaken to feed every 2 to 3 hours. Encourage the woman to rest when the baby is sleeping. She may also wish to get in the habit of maintaining a quiet atmosphere and keeping the lights low when feeding the baby during the night. This practice helps to develop the baby's sleep–wake pattern so that it coincides with light and dark periods of the day. If the lights are turned on, and the parents talk loudly and play with the baby in the middle of the night, he will think it is playtime and stay awake longer.

Promoting Parent–Newborn Attachment
It is important to allow as much parent–newborn contact as possible during the early postpartum period. Encourage the parents to cuddle the newborn closely. Role model attachment behavior by talking to the newborn and calling the newborn by name. Point out positive features of the baby. Encourage the parents to participate in the care of the newborn. Provide privacy for the family to interact with the newborn. Assist the parents to be attuned to the baby's cues that he is ready for interaction, that he is overstimulated, or that he is ready for sleep. Encourage the parents to interact with the newborn while she is in the alert state. Meet the woman's needs for pain relief, rest, and self-care so that she will have the energy to care for and interact with her newborn.

EVALUATION: GOALS AND EXPECTED OUTCOMES

- **Goal:** Maternal injury from postpartum hemorrhage is avoided.

Expected Outcomes:
- Fundus is firm and in the midline.
- Lochia flow is rubra (dark red in color) and small to moderate in amount.
- There is no bright red bleeding from any source.

- **Goal:** The woman's pain is manageable.
Expected Outcomes:
  - The woman reports pain before it becomes severe.
  - The woman verbalizes a tolerable pain level and a decrease in pain level after interventions.
- **Goal:** The woman remains free from the signs and symptoms of infection.
Expected Outcomes:
  - The woman remains afebrile (temperature less than 100.4°F).
  - There is no redness or heat in localized areas of the breast.
  - Lochia has a normal fleshy scent without a foul odor.
  - Episiotomy remains well approximated without purulent discharge.
  - There is no severe pain when voiding.
- **Goal:** No injury is experienced because of fainting/falling.
Expected Outcomes:
  - If the woman faints, she is gently guided to the floor.
  - There is no evidence of head injury, bruises, or lacerations from a fall.
- **Goal:** Urinary retention is avoided.
Expected Outcomes:
  - Voids spontaneously within 6 hours of delivery.
  - Urinary output is greater than 100 cc per episode every 3 to 4 hours.
- **Goal:** Normal bowel elimination occurs without constipation.
Expected Outcome:
  - Passes a soft, formed stool within the first 3 days after birth.
- **Goal:** Deep vein thrombosis is avoided.
Expected Outcomes:
  - Homans' sign is negative.
  - There is no unilateral swelling of the lower extremities.
  - There is no redness or heat in the calf area.
- **Goal:** Experiences adequate amounts of restful sleep.
Expected Outcome:
  - Verbalizes feeling rested with adequate energy to care for self and infant.
- **Goal:** Demonstrates signs of healthy attachment to the newborn.
Expected Outcomes:
  - Calls the newborn by name.
  - Interacts with the newborn in the en face position.
  - Talks to the newborn lovingly.
  - Makes positive comments about the newborn.

Test Yourself

- Name two ways the nurse can promote hemostasis for the postpartum woman.
- List three nursing actions that can help a new mother avoid endometritis.
- What are three things a nurse can do to help promote rest and sleep for a new mother?

Nursing Process for Postpartum Care After Cesarean Birth

The woman who has a cesarean birth faces the major postpartum challenges; however, she has also undergone major surgery. This section discusses how postpartum nursing care differs for the woman who has a cesarean birth. Remember that most of the nursing considerations discussed above for the postpartum woman also apply to the woman who delivers by cesarean section.

ASSESSMENT

In addition to the normal postpartum assessment, the woman who has experienced a cesarean delivery requires close monitoring. Auscultate lung sounds at least every 4 hours in the first 24 hours and at least every 8 hours thereafter. The lungs should be clear without adventitious sounds and not diminished in any lobe.

If a narcotic, such as Duramorph, was used in conjunction with the spinal or epidural anesthesia, the woman must be monitored closely for signs of respiratory depression. Many anesthesiologists have preprinted orders that include how often the respirations should be monitored after this type of anesthesia. Usually the respiratory rate is counted every 1 to 2 hours for the first 24 hours. Report respiratory rates of 12 per minute or less. Pulse oximetry, either continuous or intermittent, is often ordered. The oxygen saturation should remain above 95%.

Monitor the IV for rate of flow and correct solution. Check the IV site at least every 2 hours for redness, swelling, and pain. The IV usually remains in place for the first 24 hours after delivery. At that time, it may be removed or a saline lock may be put in place.

The sources of pain and discomfort for the woman who delivers by cesarean are similar to those of a woman who has delivered vaginally. Usually a woman who experiences cesarean birth does not have an episiotomy, although rarely this may be the case. However, she does have an abdominal incision that is an additional source of pain. The buildup of intestinal gas and referred shoulder pain are other sources of pain. Pruritus, itching, is a common side effect of narcotic administration during regional anesthesia. This can be a source of discomfort for the woman who had a cesarean birth.

The abdominal incision is a site for possible hemorrhage and infection. Monitor for drainage on the dressing in the first 24 hours. Assess the incision at least once every 8 hours after the dressing is removed. The incision should be well approximated with sutures or staples. A small amount of redness is normal. An increase in the amount of redness, edema, or drainage from the site is an abnormal finding.

Monitor bowel sounds at least every 4 hours. Check closely for abdominal distention and pain associated with gas formation. It may be difficult for the woman to pass flatus after cesarean delivery because of decreased peristalsis. Ask the woman if she is passing gas. Instruct her to report bowel movements.

Observe the Foley catheter for urinary output. The catheter usually remains in place for the first 24 hours after cesarean birth. Output should be at least 30 mL per hour. The urine should be clear yellow or a light straw color. Cloudy urine is associated with infection. After the Foley catheter is removed, observe the woman for the first few voids to make certain she is voiding adequately without retention.

Assess for signs of thrombus formation. The calves should be of equal size without redness, warmth, or pain. The woman who delivers by cesarean is at even higher risk for thrombus formation than is the woman who delivers vaginally.

SELECTED NURSING DIAGNOSES

- Ineffective Breathing Pattern related to respiratory depression from narcotics
- Risk for Injury: Hemorrhage from the normal postpartum routes and from the incision
- Risk for Infection related to postpartum status, stasis of secretions in the lungs, abdominal incision, and presence of the Foley catheter
- Acute Pain related to incision, discomfort from pruritus, or inability to pass flatus
- Risk for Injury: Thrombus formation related to postpartum status, bed rest, and lowered activity levels

OUTCOME IDENTIFICATION AND PLANNING

Appropriate goals include that the woman will maintain an adequate respiratory rate; will not experience injury from hemorrhage; will remain free from signs of infection; will verbalize a tolerable pain level; and will remain free of injury from thrombus formation.

IMPLEMENTATION

Monitoring for an Adequate Respiratory Pattern

If the woman has had narcotics administered via the spinal or epidural routes, monitor her closely for respiratory depression. The respirations should be monitored at least every 2 hours for the first 24 hours after spinal narcotics are administered. Have naloxone (Narcan) readily available. The anesthesiologist writes orders for naloxone administration if the respiratory rate falls below 10 to 12 per minute. Monitor oxygen saturation, as ordered. Report continuous levels below 95%.

Preventing Injury From Hemorrhage

Do not forget to check the fundus. It is not necessary to massage the fundus unless it is soft and the woman is bleeding vaginally. Any manipulation of the fundus increases pain. However, it is important to note the position and height of the fundus and whether or not it is well contracted.

Assess the dressing for drainage. Mark any areas of drainage so that you can tell if the area is increasing during subsequent assessments. If the dressing becomes saturated, reinforce it and apply pressure to the site. Notify the RN or primary care provider for further orders.

Preventing Infection

One major difference between care of the woman who has delivered vaginally and one who has had a cesarean is that of lung status. The lungs of a woman who has experienced cesarean birth must be assessed carefully at least every 4 hours during the first 24 hours. You must also assist the woman to turn, cough, and deep breathe at least every 2 hours. It will not be easy for her to take deep breaths or to cough. Assist her to splint her incision with a pillow while she coughs. This stabilizes the area and reduces pain. An incentive spirometer will be ordered. Assist the woman to use it hourly for the first 24 hours when she is awake.

The incision is another possible site for infection. During the first 24 hours the original dressing usually covers the incision. After the physician has removed the dressing, assess the incision for increasing redness, edema, or drainage. Proper incision care includes washing the hands thoroughly before touching the incision for any reason. Instruct the woman to wash the incision with soap and water, and then pat it dry thoroughly. Nothing wet should remain against the incision.

The continuous Foley catheter that is in place during the first 24 hours is another potential source of infection. Provide frequent perineal and Foley care. Monitor IV fluids to ensure adequate infusion of fluids. When the woman is well hydrated, her kidneys will produce enough urine to keep a steady flow going. The flow helps to wash out bacteria. When the catheter is removed, assist the woman to void within 6 hours of removal.

Providing Pain Management

Pain management for the woman after cesarean birth is an area that challenges the postpartum nurse. During the first 24 hours, the anesthesiologist usually manages the pain. Generally, if the woman had a spinal narcotic administered, she will have orders for a PRN medication for **breakthrough pain**. Breakthrough pain occurs when the basal dose of analgesia does not control the pain adequately.

Another form of pain control that may be ordered is patient-controlled analgesia (PCA). This type of analgesia allows the woman to control how often she receives pain medication. A narcotic (usually morphine) is given via a pump into the IV line. The pump is locked to prevent tampering. The pump is set per physician orders so that the patient can receive a prescribed amount of narcotic each time she pushes a button. A lockout interval is also prescribed so that the woman cannot accidentally overdose herself. Many women require reassurance that they cannot administer too much medication when PCA is used.

Infrequently, narcotics will be ordered at PRN intervals after cesarean birth. In this instance, plan to administer the narcotic around the clock for the first 24 hours. Research has shown that it is easier to control pain before it becomes severe and that adequate pain control in the first 24 hours reduces the total amount of pain medication needed by the woman. Adequate pain control is necessary for the woman to ambulate well and for her to provide self- and newborn care.

Pruritus is a common side effect of narcotics given by the spinal or epidural routes. This side effect can become quite uncomfortable for the woman and can lead to scratching and excoriation. An antipruritic, usually diphenhydramine (Benadryl), is frequently ordered to help control this side effect. If nothing is ordered, notify the anesthesiologist. Other comfort measures include applying lotion, administering a back rub, and using cool compresses or diversion to help control the itching. In some cases it becomes necessary to administer naloxone (Narcan). It is best to avoid this if possible because naloxone reverses the effect of the narcotic and can lead to increased pain sensation.

Another common source of pain for the woman who delivers by cesarean is gas pain. Because peristalsis is naturally slowed in the postpartum period and because of the lingering effects of anesthesia and analgesia, and manipulation of the intestines during surgery, the woman is at increased risk for gas formation. If it builds up and cannot be released, the woman becomes bloated and can experience severe pain.

This pain is usually not relieved by analgesics. Many surgeons order simethicone (Mylicon) prophylactically. If this is the case, simethicone will be given around the clock. It may also be ordered PRN. Frequent and early ambulation stimulates peristalsis and passing of flatus. Instruct the woman to avoid very hot or very cold beverages, carbonated beverages, and drinking through straws. All of these things can increase the formation and discomfort of gas. Other medical interventions may become necessary, such as rectal suppositories or enemas. Encourage the woman to lie on her left side. This position allows the gas to be expelled more easily.

Preventing Injury From Thrombus Formation

Many women come back from surgery with thromboembolic disease stockings (TEDS) already in place. If not, there will be an order to apply them. Pneumatic compression devices also may be ordered during the first 24 hours. These devices stimulate venous return to the heart, an action that helps prevent pooling and thrombus formation. Once the woman can get out of bed and ambulate, frequent ambulation is advised. This is the best way to prevent a thrombus from forming. Another important nursing action is to ensure adequate fluid intake.

EVALUATION: GOALS AND EXPECTED OUTCOMES

- **Goal:** The respiratory pattern is not compromised.

Expected Outcomes:
- Maintains an adequate respiratory pattern (16 to 20 breaths per minute).
- Oxygen saturation remains above 95%.

- **Goal:** Injury from hemorrhage is avoided.
  Expected Outcomes:
  - Fundus remains firm in the midline.
  - Lochia flow remains scant to small.
  - There is no drainage or bleeding from the incision.
- **Goal:** Remains free from signs and symptoms of infection.
  Expected Outcomes:
  - Temperature remains below 100.4°F.
  - Lungs remain clear to auscultation.
  - Incision is clean, dry, well-approximated without redness or drainage.
  - Lochia does not have a foul odor.
  - Urine remains clear.
- **Goal:** Pain is manageable.
  Expected Outcomes:
  - Reports pain before it becomes severe.
  - Uses PCA, as ordered.
  - Voices adequate pain relief after interventions.
  - States pruritus is at a tolerable level.
- **Goal:** Remains free from thrombus formation.
  Expected Outcomes:
  - Negative Homans' sign.
  - No unilateral swelling, redness, or warmth in the lower extremities.
  - No shortness of breath or chest pain.

● Nursing Process for Preparing the Postpartum Woman for Discharge

Discharge planning for the new mother begins upon admission and continues until she is dismissed home. Most interventions related to discharge focus on teaching the woman to care for herself and the baby when she goes home. It is also important to observe how the woman and her partner are adapting to their new role as parents and to support healthy adaptation behaviors.

ASSESSMENT

Bearing a child is a life-changing event. Observe how the parents interact with each other and with the baby. Watch for interactions between other members of the family, such as grandparents and siblings of the new baby. Determine what behaviors are helping the new family adjust and note if any actions are getting in the way of positive adjustment.

Because teaching is the focus of most nursing interventions when planning for discharge, it is important to determine the woman's knowledge base. It is important not to assume that a woman knows certain things just because she may be educated, or she is a nurse, or she has other children, and so on. The only way to know what a woman knows about self-care and baby care is to ask and to observe. This section focuses on maternal self-care at home. Newborn care is discussed in Chapter 15.

SELECTED NURSING DIAGNOSES

- Health-Seeking Behaviors
- Risk for Injury related to Rh negative blood type and/or nonimmunity to rubella
- Deficient Knowledge of self care

OUTCOME IDENTIFICATION AND PLANNING

Appropriate goals include that the woman and her partner will demonstrate positive adjustment to the parental role; no injury will occur related to Rh status or rubella nonimmunity; and the woman will verbalize danger signs that should be reported immediately. Another goal is that the woman will demonstrate the ability to perform self-care to include breast care, fundal checks and massage, care of lochia and the perineum, pain management, and prevention of constipation and fatigue.

IMPLEMENTATION

Supporting Health-Seeking Behaviors

Reinforce positive family behaviors. Take particular care to praise the woman and her partner for positive parenting skills. When assistance is needed as the parents learn new skills, provide positive verbal support. If the woman makes a mistake, don't focus on the mistake in a negative way. For instance, it is not helpful to tell the mother, "No. That's not the way to do it. Do it like this." Instead focus on the things she is doing right and use positive language to guide her when she is having difficulty with the task. Use words that convey acceptance, such as, "Some women find it helpful to do it this way." Or "the baby might find this to be soothing."

Anticipatory guidance is helpful when siblings are involved. Explain to the parents that it is normal for the older sibling to regress in the first few days after the birth of the baby. Tell them it helps if they do not focus undue attention on regressive behaviors, such as a return to bedwetting, sucking the thumb, or clinging to a favorite toy or blanket. It is particularly important for the parents not to criticize or belittle the older child for regressive behaviors. Explain that the behavior is temporary and will pass as the child adjusts to his new role in the family. Suggest that the parents set aside time every day that is just "big brother or sister" time. The sibling will find it easier to adjust if he is assured that his parents still care for and value him. Another helpful suggestion is to provide the older child with a doll and allow the child to take care of the doll, as the parent is caring for the baby. This activity helps the older child to feel included and can help to develop nurturing skills.

Preventing Injury From Rh-Negative Blood Type or Nonimmunity to Rubella

Before the woman is discharged, it is important to check to see if the woman who is Rh negative is a candidate for RhoGAM. If the woman is Rh-negative and the baby is Rh-positive, the woman will need an injection of RhoGAM to prevent the development of antibodies to Rh-positive blood. The RhoGAM must be given within 72 hours of delivery to be most effective. If the baby is Rh negative, the woman will not need RhoGAM. Box 12-3 highlights nursing considerations for administering RhoGAM.

You must also determine the woman's rubella status. If she is nonimmune to rubella, the rubella titer is less than 1:8, she will need to receive the rubella vaccine before she is discharged. It is important for her to know that she should not get pregnant for at least 3 months after receiving the vaccine. Box 12-4 discusses nursing considerations for giving the rubella vaccine.

BOX 12.3 Pharmacology Focus: Prevention of Antibody Development

Medication: Rh immune globulin (RhoGAM)
Method of action: Prevents development of antibodies to Rh D-positive blood, if given to the Rh-D negative woman within 72 hours of abortion, invasive procedure such as amniocentesis, or delivery of an Rh D-positive infant.
Usual dosage and administration: One vial given via the IM route
Antidote: None
Nursing interventions:

1. Ensure that the woman is a candidate for RhoGAM. She
   a. Is Rh D-negative
   b. Has never been sensitized to Rh D-positive blood
   c. Has had an abortion, ectopic pregnancy, or delivered an Rh D-positive infant within the past 72 hours
2. Explain that the woman is receiving RhoGAM to prevent her from being sensitized to Rh-positive blood. This will prevent hemolytic disease of the newborn in subsequent pregnancies.
3. Inform the woman that RhoGAM is a blood product.
4. Ensure that you are administering the correct vial to the woman. RhoGAM is cross-matched to each specific woman. The lot number should be checked by two nurses before RhoGAM is administered.
5. Explain that there may be soreness at the site.
6. Ask the woman which site she prefers for the IM injection. The deltoid and gluteal muscles are both acceptable sites.
7. Give the woman a card indicating her Rh status and the date of RhoGAM administration. Instruct her to carry the card with her at all times.

Providing Patient Teaching

Because the postpartum stay is very short, it is important to grab every available opportunity for teaching. On the day of discharge, give the woman written self-care instructions. It is best to ask her questions regarding how she plans to care for her breasts, perineum, pain, and so on; to determine how much information she has retained; and to reinforce areas she may not have absorbed. Instruct the woman that she needs to make an appointment with her primary care provider for a 6-week postpartum checkup. It is important for the woman to know danger signs that should be reported to the primary care provider. Box 12-5 lists these danger signs.

Breast Care

Teach breast care as you are assisting the woman to breast-feed or when she takes a shower. Explain that plain water is sufficient to clean the nipples because soap is drying and can contribute to sore, cracked nipples. Encourage the use of lanolin cream on the nipples. After a feeding, teach the woman to express a drop of breast milk, rub it into each nipple, and allow the nipples to air dry. She should wear a good support bra at all times.

Fundal Massage

Teach self-fundal massage when you are assessing the fundus. Assist her to touch the top of the uterus and to gently massage it as she makes certain it stays firmly contracted. Explain to her that the uterus should no longer be palpable by the 10th day.

Perineum and Vaginal Care

Instruct the woman on proper perineal care the first time she gets up to use the bathroom. Help her fill the peribottle with warm water, and

BOX 12.4 Pharmacology Focus: Development of Immunity to Rubella

Medication: Live rubella vaccine
Method of action: Causes the body to produce antibodies against the rubella virus, thereby stimulating the development of immunity to rubella.
Usual dosage and administration: One vial given subcutaneously in the upper, outer aspect of the arm.
Antidote: None
Nursing interventions:

1. Determine whether there are any contraindications for administering the vaccine. The woman
   a. Is sensitive to neomycin
   b. Is immunosuppressed
   c. Has received a blood product within the past 3 months
2. Explain possible adverse reactions.
   a. Discomfort at the injection site.
   b. Development of rash, sore throat, headache, and general malaise within 2 to 4 weeks of the injection.
3. Obtain informed consent before administering the vaccine.
4. Instruct the woman on the importance of avoiding pregnancy for at least 3 months. Because the rubella vaccine is a live virus, it could be teratogenic to the fetus.
5. Inform the breast-feeding woman that the rubella vaccine crosses over into the breast milk. The newborn benefits from short-term immunity but may become flushed, fussy, or develop a slight rash. Suggest that the woman speak to the pediatrician if she has concerns.

BOX 12.5 Postpartum Danger Signs

- Fever greater than or equal to 100.4°F
- Shaking chills
- Localized reddened, painful area on one breast
- Frequency, urgency, and painful urination
- Sudden onset of shortness of breath and/or chest pain
- Severe unremitting abdominal or back pain that is unrelieved by normal pain measures
- Foul smelling lochia
- Increased or heavy lochia flow or passage of clots
- Return to lochia rubra after it has been serosa or alba
- Severe pain, redness, or swelling in the episiotomy or cesarean incision
- Swollen, reddened, painful area on the calf
- Prolonged or severe depression
- Thoughts of harming the baby or self (suicidal thoughts)

instruct her to squirt the water over her perineum to wash away lochia. Watch as she pats dry. Be certain that she pats from front to back. Explain the importance of this action to help prevent bladder and episiotomy infections. Show her how to open the sanitary napkins and how to handle them to avoid contaminating the center of the pad. Explain that she will need to continue to use sanitary napkins until the lochia stops. Tampons are not used because they contribute to uterine infection until the placental site has healed. Reinforce that she should continue perineal care after every voiding and defecation until the lochia stops. Encourage handwashing before and after performing perineal care.

Remind the woman that lochia flow should become progressively lighter. Lochia rubra generally lasts for approximately 2 to 3 days. This is followed by lochia serosa for the remainder of the 1st week after delivery. After the 1st week, the flow should be lochia alba. She shouldn't saturate peripads, and there shouldn't be any large clots.

Here's a good teaching tip. If the woman engages in vigorous exercise during the postpartum period, the amount of lochia will temporarily increase. This is a normal finding.

Teach the woman to avoid sexual intercourse, tampons, or introduction of any substance into the vagina until the placental site and episiotomy or tear have healed to prevent additional trauma and infection. Healing is indicated when the lochia flow stops and there is no discomfort when two fingers are placed inside the vaginal opening. Hormonal changes associated with breast-feeding sometimes contribute to vaginal dryness and associated dyspareunia. For this reason breast-feeding mothers may find it helpful to use a water-soluble jelly (e.g., KY jelly) for lubrication during sexual intercourse.

Pain Management

Teach the woman about pain management as you provide pain management for her. Explain that it is more effective to control pain before it becomes severe. Many women are afraid to take pain medication when they are breast-feeding. Reassure her that the analgesics the primary care provider has ordered will not harm her baby. Clarify that breast-feeding is promoted when the mother is comfortable and pain free. Tell her the name of the medication that you are giving her and briefly describe its benefit. For instance, when the woman complains of afterpains, administer the ordered ibuprofen, and explain that ibuprofen is usually very effective in controlling the pain of cramping. If she complains of her stitches hurting, administer the ordered analgesic-narcotic combination and make clear that this medication is most effective at controlling episiotomy pain. Tell her how frequently she can have each medication and why it is important not to take pain medication more frequently or at higher dosages than what is ordered.

Explain the benefits of using nonmedicinal ways of easing pain, such as applying warmth to the abdomen to help soothe afterpains. When you assist her with the sitz bath, encourage her to continue using it at home until the episiotomy has healed. Some women worry that the stitches will have to be removed and anticipate that this will be painful. Reassure her that the stitches will be absorbed by the body and do not need to be removed.

Nutrition

Nutrition is an important aspect of self-care. Meal times are a good time to discuss nutrition with the woman. Determine what her normal pattern of intake is. Give her brochures that explain the food pyramid. Discuss with her how to use the food pyramid to plan meals. Instruct the woman who is not breast-feeding to decrease her caloric intake by approximately 300 kcal per day (i.e., she should reduce her intake to prepregnancy levels). Because the lactating woman was using 300 kcal extra per day during the pregnancy, she will need to add an additional 200 kcal, for a total of 500 kcal above prepregnancy requirements.

Constipation

As you are caring for the woman, explain how different activities contribute to or prevent constipation. Describe how activity helps the bowel to regain its tone, which helps prevent constipation. When you fill her water pitcher, explain that she needs to drink liberally of noncaffeinated fluids to help keep the stool soft. Explain that caffeine is a diuretic, so it is best to limit caffeinated fluids. Encourage her to drink fluids that she enjoys. If she does not like water, explore alternatives with her, such as noncaffeinated herbal tea, juice, and sugar-free gelatin. Explain to her the importance of heeding the urge to defecate. Ignoring the urge can contribute to constipation. Teach her about high fiber foods when you serve her a meal or bring her a snack. If the primary care provider has prescribed a stool softener, tell her the name of the medication and its intended effect when you administer it. Offer her a large glass of water when she takes the stool softener and emphasize the importance of adequate hydration when taking a stool softener.

Proper Rest

It is important for the woman to know that it is easy to over-do it in the first few days after having a baby. Explore the possibility of asking a friend or relative to help out for the first few days. Reassure her that her health and that of her baby are the most important concerns while she is recovering from childbirth. Give her hints such as, "When you are tired, rest. If you are exhausted, you will not have the energy to care for your baby." It might be helpful to suggest that she rest with her feet up when the baby is napping during the day. Reassure her that housecleaning chores can wait, if she is too tired to do them. Also, the woman should not do heavy lifting. Teach the woman the good rule of thumb not to lift anything heavier than the baby for the first 6 weeks after delivery.

When the father is present, explain to him how much energy it takes for the body to repair itself after childbirth. If he was present at the birth, he probably readily understands this concept. If appropriate, encourage him to help out with household chores and older sibling care while the woman recuperates.

EVALUATION: GOALS AND EXPECTED OUTCOMES

- **Goal:** Both parents demonstrate positive adjustment to the parental role.
  Expected Outcomes:
  - Cares for her newborn with confidence.
  - Demonstrates positive attachment behaviors with her newborn.
- **Goal:** No injury will occur related to Rh type or rubella nonimmunity.
  Expected Outcomes:
  - Receives RhoGAM within 72 hours after delivery, if eligible.
  - Receives rubella vaccine (or instructions as to where to obtain the vaccine) if nonimmune.
- **Goal:** Demonstrates adequate self-care behaviors.
  Expected Outcomes:
  - Explains danger signals that need to be reported.
  - Demonstrates the ability to perform self-care to include
    - Breast care
    - Fundal checks and massage
    - Perineal care

- Pain management
- Constipation prevention
- Avoidance of fatigue and sleep deprivation

Test Yourself

- Describe four major ways that assessment of the woman after cesarean delivery is different from that for a woman who delivers vaginally.
- Explain the proper way to perform perineal care.
- List four signs of infection that the new mother should report.

KEY POINTS

- The organs of the reproductive system gradually return to the nonpregnant size and function in the process of involution.
- Fundal height decreases at a rate of 1 fingerbreadth (1 cm) per day until the uterus is no longer palpable on the 10th postpartum day.
- Multiparas more frequently experience afterpains than do primiparas.
- Lochia progresses from rubra to serosa to alba as the uterine lining and other cells are cast away from the uterus.
- Kegel exercises can help the postpartum woman regain tone in the perineal area, although the size and tone of the introitus never fully return to the prepregnant state.
- The extra fluid volume that built up during the pregnancy is eliminated in the early postpartum period, leading to high urinary output and diaphoresis.
- The woman's temperature may be slightly elevated during the first 24 hours after delivery because of dehydration and exhaustion. After that it should be under 100.4°F. The blood pressure should remain at the level it was during labor. It is normal for bradycardia to be found in the early postpartum period.
- The woman is often very hungry and thirsty after delivering a baby. She should be allowed to eat and drink unless there are medical contraindications for doing so.
- Trauma to the lower urinary tract can lead to urinary retention in the postpartum period.
- The woman must adapt to her new role as mother. She usually does this in three stages: taking in, taking hold, and letting go.
- Bonding is the initial component of healthy attachment between a parent and the newborn. Healthy bonding generally occurs in a predictable sequence.
- Postpartum blues is a temporary mood disorder that manifests itself through tearfulness and other signs of mild depression.
- Postpartum assessment involves data collection to include pregnancy history, medical history, and labor and birth history. It also involves a thorough head-to-toe physical assessment with focus on expected postpartum changes.
- The focus of nursing interventions in the early postpartum period is on preventing and detecting hemorrhage, treating pain, preventing infection, preventing falls, detecting and treating urinary retention, preventing constipation, preventing and detecting thrombus formation, promoting sleep, and promoting healthy parental–newborn attachment.
- Additional nursing considerations for the woman who has a cesarean birth involve the surgical status of the woman. Respiratory compromise is a possible complication that requires monitoring and nursing intervention.
- The woman who delivers by cesarean has an abdominal incision that can be an additional source of pain, infection, and hemorrhage.
- Helping the woman to turn, cough, and deep breath and encouraging early and frequent ambulation after cesarean delivery are necessary measures to help prevent respiratory compromise and thrombus formation.
- The focus of nursing interventions when assisting the woman to prepare for discharge is teaching the woman to perform self- and infant care.
- Self-care includes breast care, fundal massage, assessment of lochia, perineal care, pain management, prevention of constipation, and prevention of fatigue.

REFERENCES AND SELECTED READINGS

Books and Journals

Bukowski, R., & Silver, H. (2000). The puerperium. In A. T. Evans & K. R. Niswander (Eds.), *Manual of obstetrics* (6th ed., pp. 479–495). Philadelphia: Lippincott Williams & Wilkins.

Cunningham, F. G., Gant, N. F., Leveno, K. J., Gilstrap, L. C. III, Hauth, J. C., & Wenstrom, K. D. (2001). The puerperium. In *Williams obstetrics* (21st ed., pp. 403–421). New York: McGraw-Hill Medical Publishing Division.

Franzblau, N., & Witt, K. (2002). Normal and abnormal puerperium. In R. Levine, F. Talavera, G. F. Whitman-Elia, F. B. Gaupp, & L. P. Shulman (Eds.), *eMedicine*. Retrieved

February 2, 2003, from http://www.emedicine.com/med/topic3240.htm

Ladewig, P. W., London, M. L., Moberly, S., & Olds, S. B. (2002) *Contemporary maternal–newborn nursing care* (5th ed.). Upper Saddle River, NJ: Prentice Hall.

Martell, L. K. (2003). Postpartum women's perceptions of the hospital environment. *Journal of Obstetric, Gynecologic, & Neonatal Nursing (JOGNN), 32*(4), 478–485.

Scoggin, J. (2000). Physical and psychological changes. In S. Mattson & J. E. Smith (Eds.), *Core curriculum for maternal–newborn nursing*. AWHONN publication (2nd ed., pp. 302–313). Philadelphia: WB Saunders.

Websites

Postpartum Resources

http://www.childbirth.org/articles/postpartum.html
http://www.sbpep.org/

Helping Dads Support the New Mom

http://www.dona.org/PDF/DadsandPostpartum-Doulas.pdf

WORKBOOK

NCLEX-STYLE REVIEW QUESTIONS

1. An 18-year-old primipara is getting ready to go home. She had a third degree episiotomy with repair. She confides in the nurse that she is afraid to go to her postpartum checkup because she is afraid to have the stitches removed. Which reply by the nurse is best?

   a. "It doesn't hurt when the midwife takes out the stitches. You will only feel a little tugging and pulling sensation."

   b. "It is very important for you to go to your checkup visit. Besides, the stitches do not have to be removed."

   c. "Many women have that fear after having an episiotomy. The stitches do not need to be removed because the suture will be gradually absorbed."

   d. "Oh, you mustn't miss your follow-up appointment. Don't worry. Your midwife will be very gentle."

2. A woman has just delivered her third baby. Everything has progressed normally up to this point. When the nurse tries to take the woman's blood pressure, she notices that the woman is shaking and that her teeth are chattering. Which action should the nurse take first?

   a. Finish taking the vital signs, and then decide what to do

   b. Notify the RN immediately

   c. Place two prewarmed blankets on the woman

   d. Put on the call bell to summon for help

3. The night shift LPN is checking on a woman who had a cesarean delivery with spinal Duramorph anesthesia several hours earlier. The nurse counts a respiratory rate of 8 in 1 minute. What should the nurse do first?

   a. Administer naloxone (Narcan), per the preprinted orders

   b. Awaken the woman and instruct her to breathe more rapidly

   c. Call the anesthesiologist from the room for orders

   d. Perform bag-to-mouth rescue breathing at a rate of 12 per minute

4. The nurse is performing the initial postpartum assessment for her shift on a woman who had a cesarean delivery the day before. The nurse notices that the woman is scratching her face and her arms. What action by the nurse is indicated?

   a. Administer naloxone (Narcan) immediately, per the preprinted orders

   b. Ask the woman if she wants something for the itching, and then call the anesthesiologist for orders

   c. Determine the severity of the itching and offer to give diphenhydramine (Benadryl), as ordered

   d. Observe and wait until the woman complains about the itching before treating it

5. A woman who has chosen to bottle-feed says that her breasts are painfully engorged. Which nursing intervention is appropriate?

   a. Assist the woman into the shower and have her run warm water over her breasts

   b. Assist the woman to place ice packs on her breasts

   c. Encourage the woman to breast-feed because she is producing so much milk

   d. Provide a breast pump and assist the woman in emptying her breasts

STUDY ACTIVITIES

1. With your clinical group, develop a one-page postpartum instruction sheet to send home with the new mother that covers all of the essential information she needs for self-care at home.
2. Explain how nursing care of a woman after cesarean birth differs from that of a woman who delivers vaginally. What additional risk factors does the woman have after cesarean?
3. Using the table below, compare the different sources of postpartum pain.

Pain Source	Possible Causes	Nursing Care to Prevent and Treat
Breast		
Afterpains		
Perineal pain		
Gas pain and distention after cesarean		
Cesarean incision		

CRITICAL THINKING: What Would You Do?

1. You enter the room of Heather, a 22-year-old primipara, and find her on the floor looking a little dazed. When you ask her what happened, she tells you that she remembers trying to get up to go the restroom and that she started feeling a bit dizzy and faint. The next thing she knew she was on the floor.
   a. What is the likely cause of Heather's fall? What nursing actions could have prevented this occurrence?
   b. Later that day, Heather reports that she feels like she just "dribbles" when she tries to urinate and she feels like she is bleeding too much. What assessments should you make first? What do you expect to find?
   c. What measures can the nurse take to help relieve Heather's urinary retention?
   d. On the 3rd postpartum day Heather says that she is experiencing chills and thinks she is coming down with a fever. In addition to taking the temperature, what other assessments should the nurse make? Why?
2. Marla delivered her fifth child yesterday after a difficult labor that lasted almost 24 hours. The baby weighed 7 pounds 6 ounces, and she is breast-feeding.
   a. What factors put Marla at risk for postpartum hemorrhage?
   b. While you are checking Marla's lochia, you notice that her lochia has saturated through two sanitary napkins/pads since you last checked on her an hour ago. What do you think is causing the bleeding? What is your first action and why? What would you do next? Justify your answer.
3. Mindy had a cesarean delivery. This is her 2nd postoperative day. She is in her bed when you come in to take vital signs. She looks miserable and she says that she just can't get comfortable.
   a. What assessments should you make first?
   b. You determine that Mindy is suffering from incisional pain and gas pain. What remedies should you offer for these two sources of pain?
   c. You perform a complete assessment and discover that Mindy has a positive Homans' sign. What action should you take?

Nursing Assessment of Newborn Transition

13

STUDENT OBJECTIVES

On completion of this chapter, the student should be able to:

1. Identify respiratory adaptations that occur as the newborn makes the transition to life outside the womb.
2. Outline cardiovascular changes that occur immediately after birth.
3. Explain thermoregulatory capabilities of the newborn and why he has a difficult time maintaining body heat.
4. Discuss the role of the liver in the newborn's adaptation to extrauterine life.
5. Describe expected behavioral characteristics of the newborn.
6. Illustrate the major steps of the initial nursing assessment of the newborn.
7. Define expected weights and measures of the newborn.
8. Compare and contrast expected versus unexpected assessment parameters of the newborn.
9. Outline how each newborn reflex is elicited.

KEY TERMS

brown fat
caput succedaneum
cephalhematoma
epispadias
Epstein's pearls
Harlequin sign
hypospadias
jaundice
lanugo
meconium
molding
mottling
phimosis
physiologic jaundice
pseudomenstruation
simian crease
smegma
surfactant
thermoregulation
thrush
vernix caseosa

The newborn is a unique individual different than the fetus, older infant, child, and adult. The newborn's anatomy and physiology change immediately after birth and continue to change as he or she grows. It is essential for the nurse to be aware of adjustments the newborn must make as he transitions to life outside the womb. It also is important for the nurse to know the characteristics of a normal newborn in order to make accurate assessments. In addition, this knowledge will enable the nurse to appropriately answer parents' questions and concerns about their newborn. This chapter explores the immediate and ongoing adaptation of the normal newborn to life outside the womb and describes initial nursing assessments.

PHYSIOLOGIC ADAPTATION

The fetus is fully dependent upon the mother for all vital needs, such as oxygen, nutrition, and waste removal. At birth, the body systems must immediately undergo tremendous changes so that the newborn can exist outside the womb. Table 13-1 compares the anatomy and physiology of the fetus and newborn.

Respiratory Adaptation

Fetal lungs are uninflated and full of amniotic fluid because they are not needed for oxygen exchange. Immediately after birth, the newborn's lungs must inflate, the remaining fluid must be absorbed, and oxygen exchange must begin.

One factor that helps the newborn clear fluid from the lungs begins during labor. Much of the fetal lung fluid is squeezed out as the fetus moves down the birth canal. This so-called vaginal squeeze is an important way nature helps to clear the airway in preparation for the first breath. The vaginal squeeze also plays a role in stimulating lung expansion. The pressure of the birth canal on the fetal chest is released immediately when the infant is born. The lowered pressure from chest expansion draws air into the lungs.

Think about this. An infant who is born by cesarean delivery does not have the same benefit of the vaginal squeeze as does the infant born vaginally. Closely monitor the respirations of the newborn after cesarean delivery. She usually has more fluid in her lungs that must be absorbed after birth, which makes respiratory adaptation more challenging for this newborn.

Chemical changes stimulate respiratory centers in the brain. The newborn's lifeline to oxygen is cut off when the umbilical cord is clamped. Oxygen levels fall and carbon dioxide levels rise causing the newborn's pH to fall. The resulting acidosis stimulates the respiratory centers of the brain to begin their lifelong function of regulating respiration.

It is critical for the newborn to make strong respiratory efforts during the first few moments of life. This effort is best demonstrated and stimulated by a vigorous cry because crying helps to open the small air sacs (alveoli) in the lungs. Immediate sensory and thermal changes stimulate the newborn to cry. It is warm and dark inside the uterus; sounds are muffled; and the fetus is cradled by the confines of the womb. The

TABLE 13.1 Anatomic and Physiologic Comparison of the Fetus and Newborn

Comparison	Fetus	Newborn
Respiratory system	Fluid-filled, high-pressure system causes blood to be shunted from the lungs through the ductus arteriosus to the rest of body	Air-filled, low-pressure system encourages blood flow through the lungs for gas exchange; increased oxygen content of blood in the lungs contributes to the closing of the ductus arteriosus (becomes a ligament)
Site of gas exchange	Placenta	Lungs
Circulation through the heart	Pressures in the right atrium greater than in the left; encourages blood flow through the foreman ovale	Pressures in the left atrium greater than in the right; causes the foreman ovale to close
Hepatic portal circulation	Ductus venosus bypasses; maternal liver performs filtering functions	Ductus venosus closes (becomes a ligament); hepatic portal circulation begins
Thermoregulation	Body temperature maintained by maternal body temperature and warmth of the intrauterine environment	Body temperature maintained through a flexed posture and brown fat

environment changes drastically at the moment of birth. The temperature is colder; it is brighter and louder; the security of the uterus is lost; and the newborn is touched directly for the first time.

Another important factor in the newborn's respiratory adaptation is **surfactant**. Surfactant, a substance found in the lungs of mature fetuses, keeps the alveoli from collapsing after they first expand. The work of breathing is increased greatly when the lungs lack surfactant. The newborn without enough surfactant expends large amounts of energy to breathe and quickly becomes exhausted without medical intervention. By the end of 35 weeks' gestation, the fetus usually has enough surfactant to breathe without lung collapse. Maturity of the respiratory system can be determined prenatally by measuring the lecithin/sphingomyelin (L/S) ratio of amniotic fluid. Box 13-1 lists signs of respiratory distress in the newborn; if seen, such signs must be reported promptly.

Cardiovascular Adaptation

The cardiovascular system also must make rapid adjustments immediately after birth. Fetal circulation differs from newborn circulation in several important ways. As you will recall from Chapter 5, only a small amount of blood flows to the fetal lungs. The rest is shunted away from the lungs. Remember, fetal blood that circulates to the heart has already been oxygenated through the placenta, so only the blood that is needed to supply oxygen to the lung tissue goes to the lungs. The lungs are small and noncompliant in utero; the respiratory system is a resistant, high-pressure system; and pressures in the right atrium are higher than in the left. These pressures help route blood through the foreman ovale and ductus arteriosus, away from the nonfunctioning lungs, back into the general circulation. The ductus venosus shunts fetal blood away from the liver because the woman's liver provides most of the filtering and metabolic functions necessary for fetal life.

Newborn circulation is similar to adult circulation. Deoxygenated blood that enters the heart after birth must go to the lungs for gas exchange; therefore, the fetal shunts must close. Several factors contribute to their closing. The lungs fill with air, causing the pressure to drop in the chest as soon as the newborn takes his first breath. This change results in a reversal of pressures in the right and left atria, causing the foreman ovale to close so that blood is redirected to the lungs. The oxygen content of blood circulating through the lungs increases with the first few breaths. This chemical change contributes to the closing of the ductus arteriosus, which eventually becomes a ligament. The ductus venosus also closes, allowing nutrient-rich blood from the gut to circulate through the newborn's liver.

BOX 13.1 Signs of Respiratory Distress in the Newborn

- Tachypnea (sustained respiratory rate greater than 60 breaths per minute)
- Nasal flaring
- Grunting (noted by stethoscope or audible to the ear)
- Intercostal or xiphoid retractions
- Unequal movements of the chest and abdomen during breathing efforts
- Central cyanosis

Thermoregulatory Adaptation

The newborn is challenged to maintain an adequate body temperature by producing as much heat as is lost. The process by which heat production is balanced with heat loss is called **thermoregulation**. This process is developed poorly in the newborn because of two key factors. First, the newborn is prone to heat loss. The newborn's ratio of body mass to body surface area is much smaller than that of an adult. In other words, the amount of heat-producing tissue, such as muscle and adipose tissue, is small in relation to the amount of skin that is exposed to the environment. Second, the newborn is not readily able to produce heat by muscle movement and shivering.

There are four main ways that a newborn loses heat—conduction, convection, radiation, and evaporation (Fig. 13-1). Conductive heat loss occurs when the newborn is placed on a cold surface, causing body heat to be transferred to the colder object. Heat is lost by convection when air currents blow over the newborn's body. Heat can also be lost to a cold object that is close to, but not touching, the newborn. This radiation heat loss can occur if the newborn is placed close to a cold windowpane, causing body heat to radiate toward the window and be lost. Evaporative heat loss happens when the newborn's skin is wet. As the moisture evaporates from the body surface, heat is taken with the moisture.

A word of caution is in order. It takes oxygen to produce heat. If the newborn is allowed to become cold stressed, he will eventually develop respiratory distress. This is one important reason to protect the newborn from unnecessary heat loss.

The normal newborn is not entirely without protection from heat loss. The newborn naturally assumes a flexed, fetal position that conserves body heat by reducing the amount of skin exposed to the surface and conserving core heat. The newborn can also

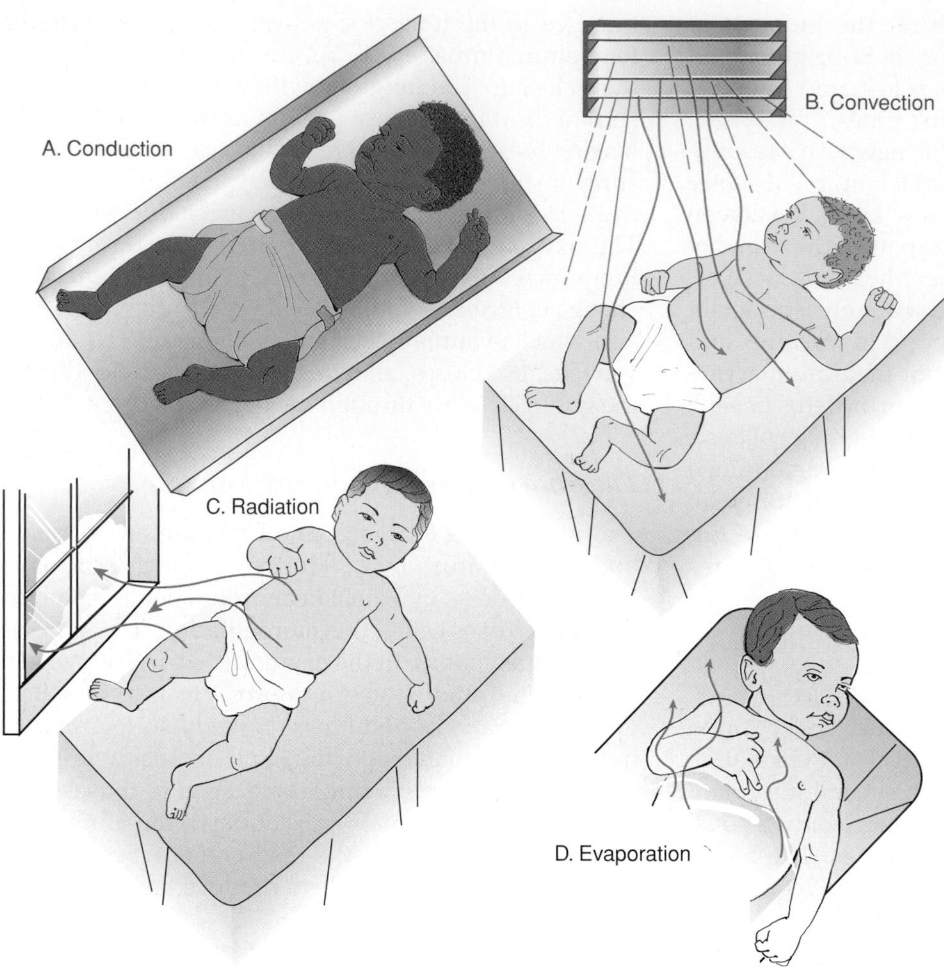

● ***Figure 13.1*** Mechanisms of heat loss. (**A**) Conduction—heat is lost to a cold surface, such as a cold scale or circumcision board, touching the newborn's skin. (**B**) Convection—heat is lost to air currents that flow over the newborn (e.g., from a fan, air conditioner, or movement around the crib). (**C**) Radiation—heat moves away from the newborn's body toward a colder object that is close by, such as a cold window or the sides of the crib. (**D**) Evaporation—heat is lost along with the moisture that evaporates from the newborn's wet skin, if he is not dried immediately after birth or if damp clothes or blankets are left next to his skin.

produce heat by burning **brown fat,** a specialized form of heat-producing tissue found only in fetuses and newborns. Deposits of brown fat are located at the nape of the neck, in the armpits, between the shoulder blades, along the abdominal aorta, and around the kidneys and sternum. Unfortunately, brown fat is not renewable; once stores are depleted, the newborn can no longer use this form of heat production.

Test Yourself

- Name two ways a vaginal birth assists the newborn's respiratory adaptation.
- What is the function of surfactant?
- Describe two factors that make it difficult for a newborn to maintain his body temperature.

Metabolic Adaptation

Throughout life a steady supply of blood glucose is necessary to carry out metabolic processes and produce energy. Glucose is also an essential nutrient for brain tissue. Neonatal hypoglycemia is defined as a blood glucose level of less than 40 mg/dL. The newborn is highly susceptible to hypoglycemia if he is excessively stressed during labor or during the transition period immediately after birth. Respiratory distress and cold stress are two stressors that often lead to neonatal hypoglycemia. Early signs of hypoglycemia in the newborn include jitteriness, poor feeding, listlessness, irritability, low temperature, weak or high-pitched cry, and hypotonia. Respiratory distress, apnea, seizures, and coma are late signs.

Hepatic Adaptation

Although immature, the newborn's liver must handle a heavy task. The fetus has a high percentage of circulating red blood cells to make use of all available oxygen in a low-oxygen environment. After birth, the newborn's lungs begin to function, and more oxygen is available immediately. Therefore, the "extra" red blood cells gradually die and must be broken down by the liver.

Bilirubin (a yellow pigment) is released as the blood cells are broken down. Normally the liver conjugates bilirubin (i.e., makes it water soluble), and then bilirubin is excreted in the feces. However, in the newborn's case, the liver is immature and overwhelmed easily by the large volume of red blood cells. Unconjugated bilirubin is fat soluble. As it builds up in the bloodstream, it crosses into the cells and stains them yellow. If a large amount of unconjugated bilirubin is present (serum levels of 4 to 6 mg/dL and greater), a yellow staining of the skin occurs, which is called **jaundice**. Jaundice is first seen on the head and face; as bilirubin levels rise, it progresses to the trunk and then to the extremities in a cephalocaudal manner.

In approximately one-half of all term newborns a condition known as **physiologic jaundice** will occur. Physiologic jaundice is characterized by jaundice that occurs after the first 24 hours of life (usually on day 2 or 3 after birth); bilirubin levels that peak between days 3 and 5; and bilirubin levels that do not rise rapidly (greater than 5 mg/dL per day). Jaundice that occurs within the first 24 hours is considered pathologic. However, when jaundice is noted, it must be recorded and reported. A more in-depth discussion of jaundice and its treatment can be found in Chapter 20. Breast-feeding jaundice is covered in Chapter 14.

The liver manufactures clotting factors necessary for normal blood coagulation. Several of the factors require vitamin K in their production. Bacteria that produce vitamin K normally are found in the gastrointestinal tract. However, the newborn's gut is sterile because normal flora have not yet taken up residence. Therefore, the newborn cannot produce vitamin K, which in turn causes the liver to be unable to produce some clotting factors. This situation could lead to bleeding problems, so newborns are given vitamin K (AquaMEPHYTON) intramuscularly shortly after birth to prevent hemorrhage (see Chapter 15 for discussion of the vitamin K administration procedure).

Behavioral and Social Adaptation

Each newborn has a unique temperament and personality that becomes apparent readily. Some newborns are quiet, rarely cry, and are consoled easily. Other newborns are frequently fussy or fretful and are more difficult to console. There are as many variations and characteristics as there are newborns.

In 1973 Dr. T. Berry Brazelton developed the Neonatal Behavioral Assessment Scale based on research he had done on the newborn's personality, individuality, and ability to communicate. Dr. Brazelton's key assumptions include that the newborn is a social organism capable of communicating through behavior and controlling his or her responses to the environment.

Dr. Brazelton identified six sleep and activity patterns that are characteristic of newborns. It is important to remember that individual infants display uniqueness in their sleep–wake cycles. Brazelton's states of reactivity are as follows:

1. Deep sleep: quiet, nonrestless sleep state; newborn is hard to awaken
2. Light sleep: eyes are closed, but more activity is noted; newborn moves actively and may show sucking behavior
3. Drowsy: eyes open and close and the eyelids look heavy; body activity is present with intermittent periods of fussiness
4. Quiet alert: quiet state with little body movement, but the newborn's eyes are open and she is attentive to people and things that are in close proximity to her; this is a good time for the parents to interact with their newborn
5. Active alert: eyes are open and active body movements are present; newborn responds to stimuli with activity
6. Crying: eyes may be tightly closed, thrashing movements are made in conjunction with active crying (Adapted from Howard-Glen, 2000, p. 364).

Test Yourself

- Define neonatal hypoglycemia.
- What pigment causes jaundice?
- Describe the quiet alert state of the newborn.

NURSING ASSESSMENT OF THE NORMAL NEWBORN

The initial nursing assessment (sometimes called the admissions assessment) is usually completed within the first few hours after birth. (APGAR scoring and other newborn assessments and care performed in the delivery room are discussed in Chapter 15.) The registered nurse (RN), nurse practitioner, or pediatrician is responsible for the full assessment, but the LPN may be asked to assist with portions of the examination. Therefore, you should be familiar with the procedure and expected findings to assist the practitioner and to be able to promptly report unexpected deviations from normal.

The examination should be conducted in a warm area that is free from drafts to protect the newborn from chilling. There should be plenty of light available to facilitate visual inspection. Indirect lighting works best. All equipment should be checked for proper functioning and should be readily available to allow for economy of motion. An experienced practitioner can complete a thorough examination in a short period of time, which is ideal because newborns become easily fatigued when overstimulated by prolonged examination.

The general order of progression is from general observations to specific measurements. Least disturbing aspects of the examination should be completed before more intrusive techniques are used. It is generally advisable to proceed using a head-to-toe approach. The overall physical appearance of the newborn is evaluated first, followed by measurement of vital signs, weight, and length. Then a thorough head-to-toe assessment is done, ending with assessment of neurologic reflexes and the gestational age assessment. The behavioral assessment is integrated throughout the examination as the practitioner notes how the newborn responds to sensory stimulation.

General Body Proportions and Posture

A typical newborn has a head that is large in proportion to the rest of his body. The newborn's neck is short, and the chin rests on the chest. The newborn maintains a flexed position with tightly clenched fists. The newborn's abdomen is protuberant and his chest is rounded. Note the newborn's sloping shoulders and rounded hips. The newborn's body appears long with short extremities.

Vital Signs

Vital signs are of particular interest to the nurse because they yield clues as to how well the newborn is adapting to extrauterine life. Determine respiratory effort and character at the beginning of the examination while the newborn is quiet. Respirations are activity dependent. The respiratory rhythm is often irregular, a characteristic known as episodic breathing. Momentary cessation of breathing interspersed with rapid breathing movements is typical of an episodic breathing pattern. Extended periods of apnea are not normal. The abdomen and chest rise and fall together with breathing movements. The normal respiratory rate is 30 to 60 breaths per minute and should be counted for a full minute when the infant is quiet.

Here's an interesting way to remember normal heart rate and blood pressure for the newborn. A newborn starts with a low blood pressure (60/40 mm Hg) and a high pulse (120 to 160 bpm). By the time she grows up, the opposite is true: her blood pressure is high (120/80 mm Hg) and her pulse is low (60 to 80 bpm).

The heart rate is taken apically for a full minute. The normal heart rate is the same for the newborn as it is for the fetus, ranging between 110 and 160 beats per minute (bpm), depending upon activity level. When the newborn is sleeping the heart tends to beat in the lower range of normal, and is not considered problematic as long as it stays above 100 bpm. The newborn's heart rate increases with activity and may increase to the 180s for short periods of time with vigorous activity and crying. The rhythm should be regular.

The newborn's temperature is measured in the axilla; the axillary temperature is considered to be reflective of the newborn's core body temperature (Fig. 13-2). Normal temperature range is between 97.7°F and 98.6°F (36.5°C and 37°C). Blood pressures are not taken routinely. If they are measured, the cuff must be an appropriate size, and the pressure may be measured on an arm or leg. Table 13-2 delineates the expected vital signs of the term newborn.

Physical Measurements

Weight and length of a newborn are dependent on several factors, including ethnicity, gender, genetics, and maternal nutrition and smoking behaviors. Generally speaking, the normal weight range for a full-term newborn is between 5 pounds 8 ounces and 8 pounds 13 ounces (2500 to 4000 grams). Nursing Procedure 13-1 lists the steps for obtaining the newborn's weight and length.

It is normal for the newborn to lose 5% to 10% of his birth weight in the first few days. For the average newborn, this physiologic weight loss amounts to a total loss of 6 to 10 ounces, and the cause is a loss of excess fluid combined with a low fluid intake during the first few days of life. The newborn should regain the weight within 7 to 10 days, after which he or she begins to gain approximately 2 pounds every month until 6 months of age.

Length can be difficult to measure accurately because of the newborn's flexed posture and resistance to stretching. The newborn should be placed on his back with his legs extended completely. Experienced nurses can hold

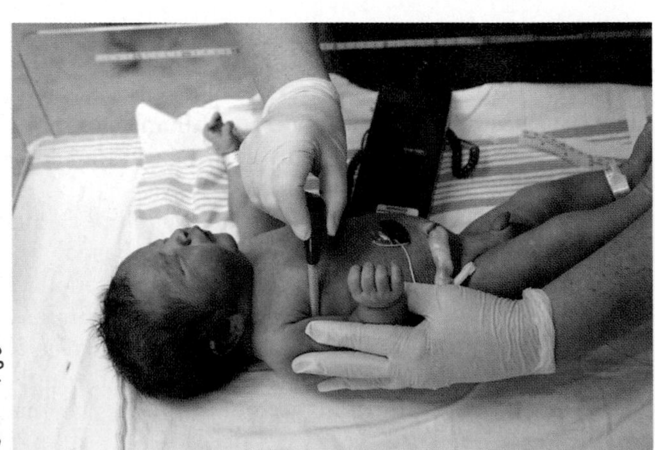

● **Figure 13.2** The nurse measures the newborn's axillary temperature.

TABLE 13.2 Expected Vital Signs of the Term Newborn

Vital Sign	Expected Range	Characteristics
Heart rate	110–160 beats per minute (bpm); during sleep as low as 100 bpm and as high as 180 bpm when crying	Rhythm regular; murmurs may be normal, but all murmurs require medical evaluation
Respiratory rate	30–60 breaths per minute	Episodic breathing is normal; chest and abdomen should move synchronously
Axillary temerature	97.7°F–98.6°F (36.5°C–37°C)	Temperature stabilizes within 8–10 hours after delivery
Blood pressure	60–80/40–45 mm Hg	Not normally recorded for the normal newborn

Nursing Procedure 13.1
Obtaining Initial Weight and Measuring Length

EQUIPMENT

Calibrated scale
Paper to place on the scale
Tape measure
Marker or pen
Clean gloves

PROCEDURE

Weighing the Newborn

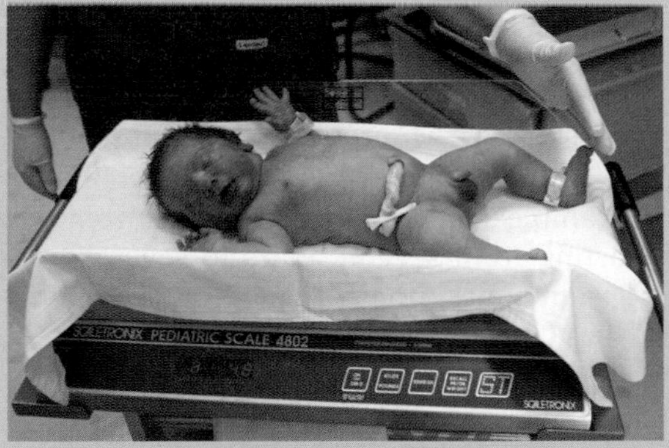

1. Thoroughly wash your hands.
2. Don a pair of clean gloves.
3. Place a paper or other designated covering on the scale to prevent direct contact of the newborn's skin with the scale.
4. Set the scale to zero.
5. Remove the newborn's clothes, including diapers, and blankets and place the newborn on the scale.
6. Hold one hand just above the newborn's body. Avoid actually touching the newborn.
7. Note the weight, in pounds and ounces and in grams.

Measuring the Newborn

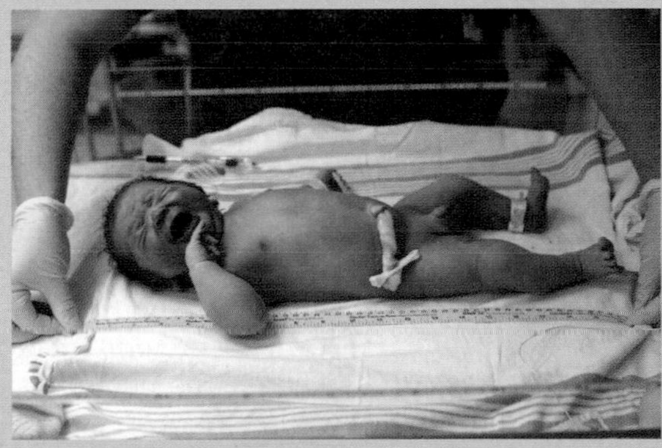

8. Use the marker to place a mark on the paper at the top of the newborn's head.
9. Use one hand to firmly hold the newborn's heels together and straighten the legs.
10. Place a second mark on the paper at the newborn's heel.
11. Measure the area between the two marks with a tape measure. This is the newborn's length.
12. Remove your gloves and thoroughly wash your hands.
13. Record the newborn's weight and length in the designated area of the chart.
14. Be sure to report your findings to the mother, her partner, and other family members, as appropriate.

Note: Gloves are only necessary when handling the newborn before the first bath because of traces of blood, mucus, vernix, and other secretions on the body. Use universal precautions to protect yourself from blood-borne pathogens. To avoid inaccurate results, do not leave clothes, including diapers, on the newborn when he is weighed.

the tape measure and extend the newborn's legs simultaneously to obtain a crown-to-heel measurement. However, it is acceptable to use a writing instrument to make a mark where the crown of the head falls on a paper placed under the newborn and another mark at the heel with the leg extended. Then the length can be measured between the two marks. The average length is 20 inches, with the range between 19 and 21 inches (48 to 53 centimeters[cm]).

Head and chest circumference are two additional important newborn measurements. The head circumference (Fig. 13-3) is obtained by placing a paper tape measure around the widest circumference of the head (i.e., from the occipital prominence around to just above the eyebrows). To measure the chest circumference, place the infant on his back with the tape measure under the lower edge of the scapulae posteriorly and then bring the tape forward over the nipple line (Fig. 13-3). The average head circumference is between 13 and 14 inches (33 and 35.5), approximately 1 to 2 inches larger than that of the chest. Normal ranges for physical measurements of the term newborn are summarized in Table 13-3.

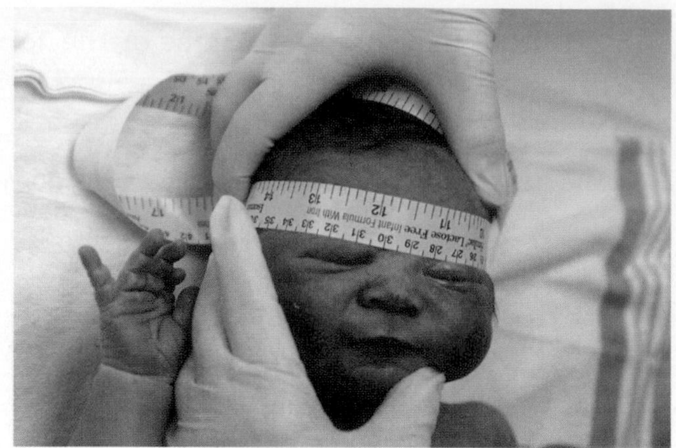

A

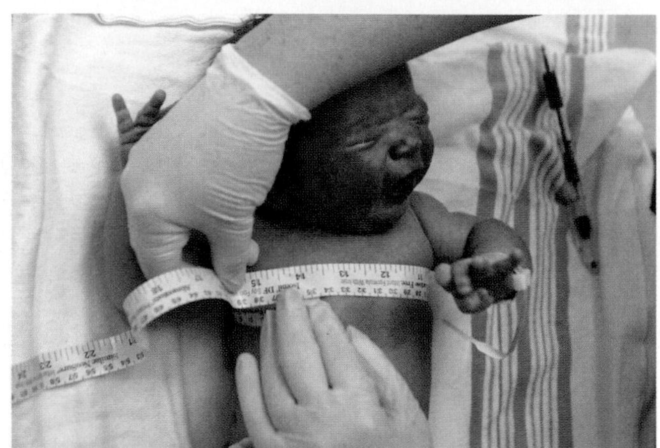

B

● ***Figure 13.3*** (**A**) The nurse obtains the head circumference. (**B**) The nurse obtains the chest circumference.

Head-to-Toe Assessment

Skin

The normal newborn's skin is supple with good turgor, reddish at birth (turning pink within a few hours), and flaky and dry. **Vernix caseosa**, a white cheese-like substance that covers the body of the fetus during the second trimester and protects the skin from the drying effects of amniotic fluid, is normally found only in creases of the term newborn. **Lanugo** is a fine downy hair that is present in abundance on the preterm infant but is found in thinning patches on the shoulders, arms, and back of the term newborn. The hair should be silky and soft. Fingernails are present and extend to the end of the fingertips or slightly beyond.

Common newborn skin manifestations are described in Table 13-4. Milia may be noted on the face. These tiny white papules resemble pimples in appearance. Reassure parents that these are harmless and will subside spontaneously. Acrocyanosis results from poor peripheral circulation and is not a good indicator of oxygenation status. The mucous membranes should be pink, and there should be no central cyanosis. Birthmarks and skin tags may be present. These are not a cause for concern and can generally be removed easily if the parents desire. **Mottling** is a red and white lacy pattern sometimes seen on the skin of newborns who have fair complexions. It is variable in occurrence and length, lasting from several hours to several weeks. Mottling sometimes occurs when the newborn is exposed to cool temperatures. **Harlequin sign**, also referred to as Harlequin coloring, is characterized by a clown-suit like appearance of the newborn. The newborn's skin is dark red on one side of the body while the other side of the body is pale. The dark red color is

TABLE 13.3 Average Physical Measurement Ranges of the Term Newborn

Measurement	Average Range Metric System	Average Range US Customary System
Weight	2,500–4,000 grams	5 pounds 8 ounces–8 pounds 13 ounces
Length (head-to-heel)	48–53 centimeters	19–21 inches
Head circumference	33–35.5 centimeters	13–14 inches
Chest circumference	30.5–33 centimeters	12–13 inches

TABLE 13.4 Common Skin Manifestations of the Normal Newborn

Skin Manifestation	Family Teaching Tips
Acrocyanosis	A bluish color to the hands and feet of the newborn is normal in the first 6 to 12 hours after birth. Acrocyanosis results from slow circulation in the extremities.
Milia 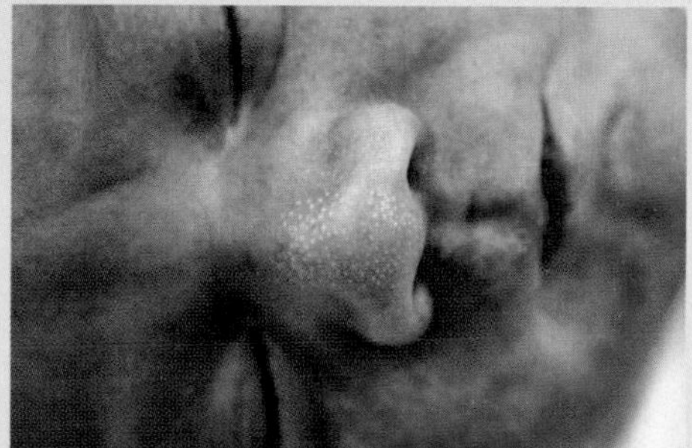	Small white spots on the newborn's face, nose, and chin that resemble pimples are an expected observation. Do not attempt to pick or squeeze them. They will subside spontaneously in a few days.
Erythema toxicum 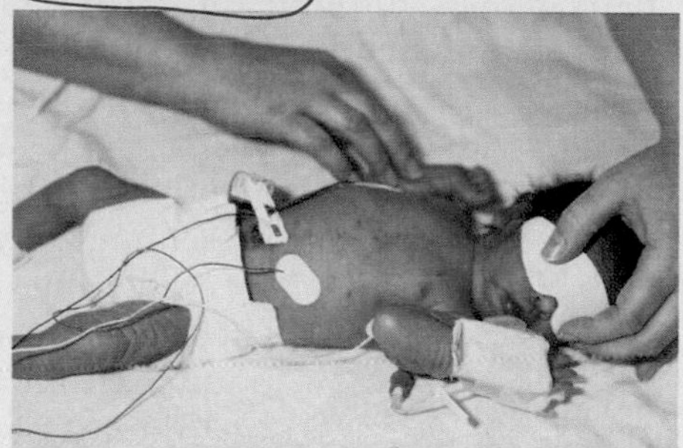	The so-called newborn rash commonly appears on the chest, abdomen, back, and buttocks of the newborn. It is harmless and will disappear.
Mongolian spot 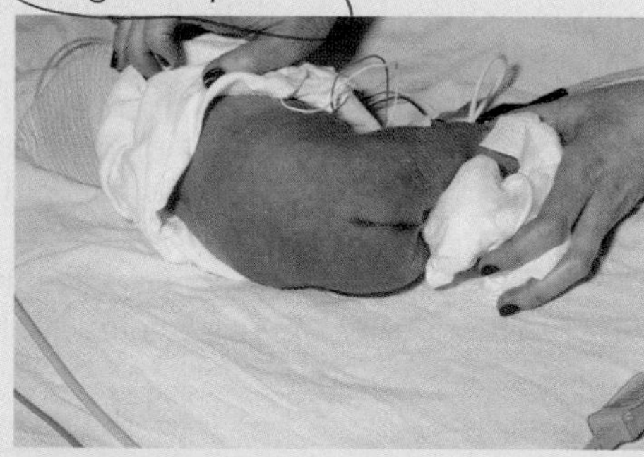	These bluish-black areas of discoloration are commonly seen on the back, buttocks, or extremities of African-American, Hispanic, Mediterranean, or other dark-skinned newborns. These spots should not be mistaken for bruises or mistreatment and gradually fade during the first year or two of life.
Telangiectatic nevi 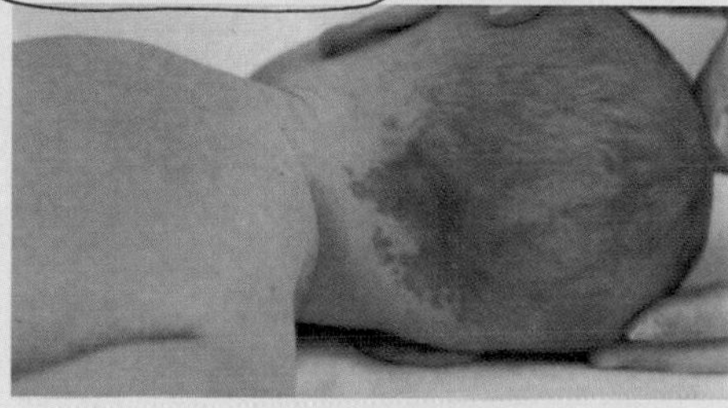	These pale pink or red marks ("stork bites") are sometimes found on the nape of the neck, eyelids, or nose of fair-skinned newborns. Stork bites blanch when pressed and generally fade as the child grows.

(*table continues on page 306*)

TABLE 13.4 (continued)	Common Skin Manifestations of the Normal Newborn
Skin Manifestation	**Family Teaching Tips**
Nevus flammeus or port-wine stain 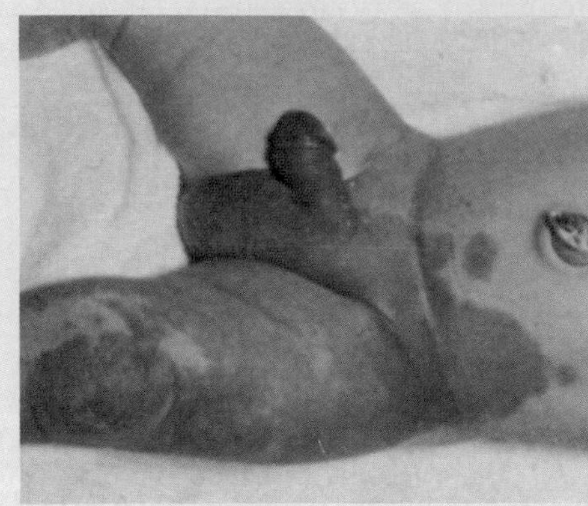	A port-wine stain is a dark reddish purple birthmark that most commonly appears on the face. It is caused by a group of dilated blood vessels. It does not blanch with pressure or fade with time. There are cosmetics available that help cover the stain if it is disfiguring. Laser therapy has been successfully used to fade port-wine stains.

caused by dilation of blood vessels, and the pallor is caused by constriction of blood vessels. This harmless condition occurs most frequently with vigorous crying.

It is important to evaluate the newborn's skin for signs of jaundice. Natural sunlight is the best environment in which to assess for jaundice. If sunlight is not easily available inside the nursery, indirect lighting should be used. Press the newborn's skin over the forehead or nose with your finger and note if the blanched area appears yellow. It is also helpful to evaluate the sclera of the eyes, particularly in dark-skinned newborns. A yellow-tinge to the sclera indicates the presence of jaundice.

Some skin characteristics are attributable to birth trauma or operative intervention. Bruising may be noted over the presenting part or on the face if the labor or delivery was unusually short or prolonged. Forceps marks may be seen on the face. Occasionally there will be a nick or cut on the infant born by cesarean delivery, particularly if the cesarean was done rapidly under emergency conditions.

Test Yourself

- Name the major nursing actions to take while weighing and measuring a newborn.
- What is the significance of acrocyanosis?
- How would you explain the presence of milia to the parents?

Head and Face

The head may be misshapen because of **molding,** an elongated shape caused by overlapping of the cranial bones as the fetus moves through the birth canal (Fig. 13-4), or **caput succedaneum** (caput), swelling of the soft tissue of the scalp caused by pressure of the presenting part on a partially dilated cervix or trauma from a vacuum-assisted delivery. These conditions are often of concern to new parents. Reassure them that the molding or caput will decrease in a few days without treatment.

You may notice this relationship. Molding and caput are more common or more pronounced in first-born babies than in the newborns of multiparas. In addition, many newborns delivered by cesarean do not experience molding or caput unless the fetus is in the birth canal for a prolonged period of time before delivery.

A **cephalhematoma** may be noted. This is swelling that occurs from bleeding under the periosteum of the

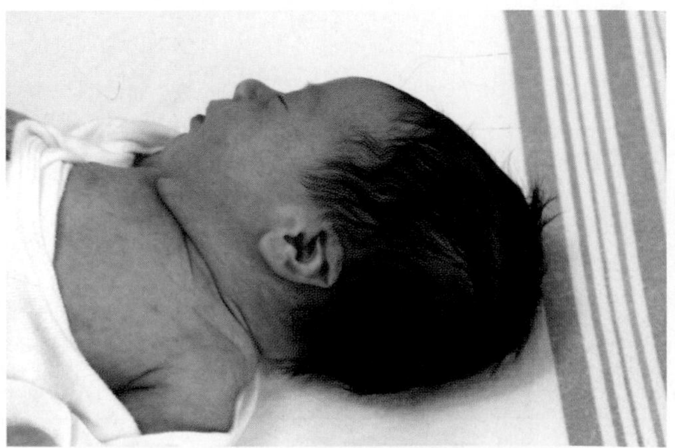

● ***Figure 13.4*** Molding.

A PERSONAL GLIMPSE

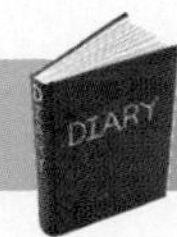

The doctor was just about to use the vacuum extractor because I had been pushing for 3 hours. I gave one additional strong push and felt the absolute relief of my baby sliding out of my body. The doctor said, "It's a girl." My husband was crying, and I couldn't wait to see our little girl. I wanted to examine her, touch her, feed her, and look into her eyes. They laid our tiny baby girl on my chest, and the first thing I noticed was her very long, pointy head. "Oh, my poor little girl," I thought, "that looks so painful and awful." I had heard and read about molding but had no idea it would be so pronounced. I must have had a look of serious concern on my face because the nurse touched my arm and said, "don't worry, her head will be back to a normal size and shape in just a day or two." The nurse then covered my sweet baby's pointy head with a soft pink cap, and my baby and I began to get to know each other.

Isabel

LEARNING OPPORTUNITY: How can nurses' knowledge of normal newborn assessment findings provide assurance to new parents?

Describe how a nurse's reaction to a common newborn finding could encourage or discourage parents.

skull, usually over one of the parietal bones. A cephalhematoma is caused by birth trauma, usually requires no treatment, and will spontaneously resolve. However, the newborn should be evaluated carefully for signs of anemia (pallor) or shock from acute blood loss. It also is important to make certain the cephalhematoma does not cross over suture lines. If it does, a skull fracture is suspected. Sometimes it is difficult for the inexperienced practitioner to tell the difference between a cephalhematoma and caput. Figure 13-5 compares features of these conditions.

Sutures occur in the place where two cranial bones meet. The normal newborn's sutures are palpable with a small space between them. It may be difficult to palpate sutures in the first 24 hours if significant molding is present. However, it is important to determine that the sutures are present. Rarely sutures will fuse prematurely (craniostenosis). It is important to detect this condition because it will require surgery to allow the brain to grow.

Fontanels occur at the junction of cranial bones where two or more sutures meet. The anterior and posterior fontanels are palpable. The anterior fontanel is diamond shaped and larger than the posterior fontanel, which has a triangular shape. The posterior fontanel closes within the first 3 months of life, whereas the anterior fontanel does not close until 12 to 18 months of life. When the newborn is in a sitting position, the anterior fontanel should be flat, neither depressed nor bulging. It is normal to feel pulsations that correlate with the newborn's heart rate over the anterior fontanel. Bulging fontanels may indicate hydrocephalus or increased intracranial pressure, and sunken fontanels are a sign of severe dehydration.

Facial movements should be symmetrical. Facial paralysis can occur from a forceps delivery or from pressure on the facial nerve as the fetus travels down the birth canal. It is easiest to assess for facial paralysis when the newborn is crying. The affected side will not

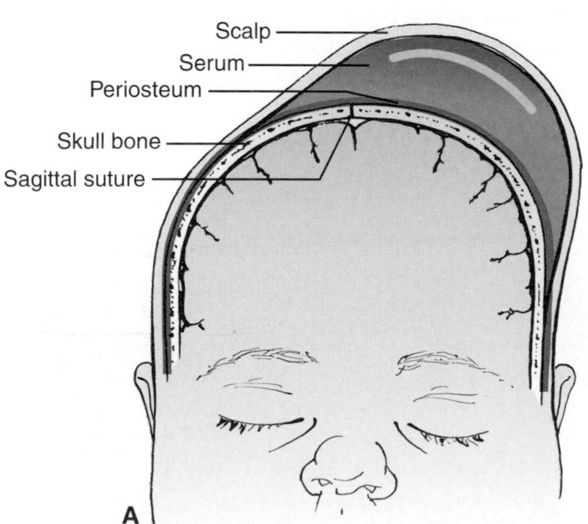

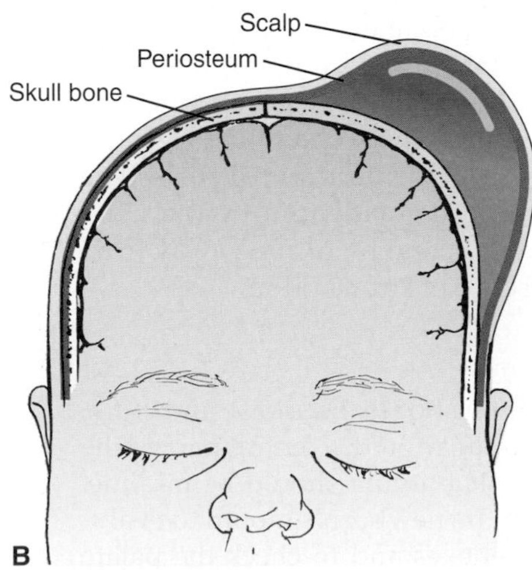

● ***Figure 13.5*** Comparison of caput succedaneum and cephalhematoma. (**A**) Caput is a collection of serous fluid between the periosteum and the scalp. It is found on the area that was pressing against the cervix during labor, or the area to which the vacuum cup was attached. Caput often crosses suture lines. (**B**) Cephalhematoma is a collection of blood between the periosteum and the skull. It does not cross suture lines, unless there is a skull fracture, which is a rare occurrence.

move, and the space between the eyelids will widen. Facial paralysis is usually temporary, but occasionally the deficit is permanent.

Eyes

The eye color of a newborn with light skinned parents is usually blue-gray, whereas a darker skinned infant usually has a dark eye color. It is normal for the eyelids to be swollen from pressure during birth. A chemical conjunctivitis may develop after instillation of eye prophylaxis in the delivery room (see Chapter 15 for discussion of eye prophylaxis).

The sclera should be clear and white, not blue. The pupils should be equal and reactive to light. A red reflex should be present. The red reflex is elicited by shining an ophthalmoscope onto the retina of the eye. The normal response is to see a red reflection from the retina. Absence of the red reflex is associated with congenital cataracts. Small subconjunctival hemorrhages may be present. These usually disappear within a week or two and are not harmful.

Eye movements are usually uncoordinated, and some strabismus (crossed eyes) is expected. A "doll's eye" reflex is normal for the first few days: that is, when the newborn's head is turned, the eyes travel to the opposite side. Persistence of this reflex after the second week should be evaluated.

The newborn is able to perceive light and can track objects held close to the face. He or she likes shapes and colors and shows a definite preference for the human face. Crying is usually tearless because the lacrimal apparatus is underdeveloped.

Nose

The newborn's nose is flat, and the bridge may appear to be absent. The nostrils should be bilaterally patent because the newborn is an obligate nose breather. Nostril patency is presumed if the newborn breathes easily with a closed mouth. The newborn clears obstructions from the nose by sneezing. There should be no nasal flaring, which is a sign of respiratory distress. The sense of smell is present, as evidenced by the newborn's turning toward milk and by turning away from or blinking in the presence of strong odors.

Mouth

The mucous membranes should be moist and pink. Sucking calluses may appear on the central part of the lips shortly after birth. The uvula should be midline. Place a gloved finger in the newborn's mouth to evaluate the suck and gag reflexes and to check the palate for intactness. The suck reflex should be strong, the gag reflex present, and both the hard and soft palates should be intact. Well-developed fat pads are present bilaterally on the cheeks.

Epstein's pearls are small white cysts found on the midline portion of the hard palate of some newborns. They feel hard to the touch and are harmless. Precocious teeth may be present on the lower central portion of the gum. The teeth will need to be removed if they are loose to prevent the infant from aspirating them.

Don't forget! A cleft palate can be present even in the absence of a cleft lip. Check the roof of the mouth carefully to be sure it is intact.

A fungal infection (caused by *Candida albicans*) in the oral cavity, called **thrush,** may be seen in the newborn. The newborn can contract the infection while passing through the birth canal. The fungus causes white patches on the oral mucosa, particularly the tongue, which resemble milk curds. It is important not to remove the patches because doing so will cause bleeding in the underlying tissue. Thrush is treated with an oral solution of nystatin (Mycostatin, Nilstat).

Ears

The pinna should be flexible with quick recoil, indicating the presence of cartilage. The top of the pinna should be even with, or above, an imaginary horizontal line drawn from the inner to the outer canthus of the eye and continuing past the ear (Fig. 13-6). Low-set ears are associated with congenital defects, including those that cause mental retardation and internal organ defects.

In recent years most hospitals have developed newborn hearing screening programs in accordance with recommendations of the American Academy of Pediatrics (AAP) for universal screening. There are two main ways that a newborn's hearing can be tested satisfactorily using current technology: evoked otoacoustic emissions (EOAE) and auditory brain-stem

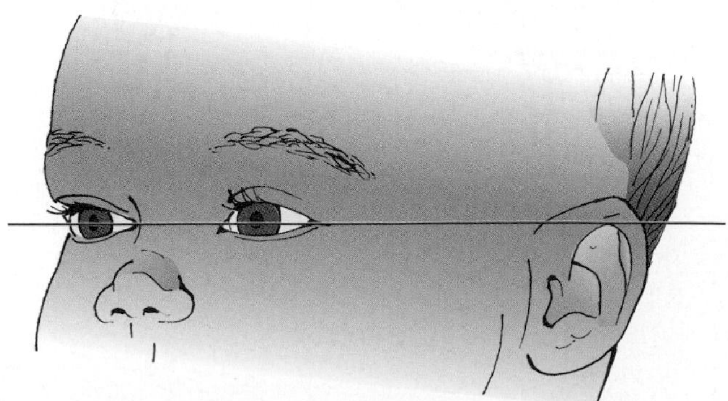

● ***Figure 13.6*** Determining placement of the ears. The top of the pinna should lie above an imaginary line drawn from the inner to the outer canthus of the eye continuing past the ear on either side. Note the line in the drawing.

response (ABR). Both methodologies are noninvasive and easy to perform. Each test takes less than 5 minutes to perform. Each method assesses hearing differently, and each has unique advantages and disadvantages. The important task for the nursery nurse is to make certain that each newborn is screened adequately before he or she is discharged from the hospital.

Neck

The newborn's neck is short and thick. The head should move freely and have full range of motion. Significant head lag is present when the newborn is pulled to a sitting position from a supine one (Fig. 13-7). Newborns can hold up their heads slightly when placed on their abdomens. There should be no masses or webbing.

The clavicles should be intact. Occasionally a clavicle is fractured during a difficult delivery. Signs of a fractured clavicle include a lump along one clavicle accompanied by crepitus (a grating sensation) at the site. An asymmetrical Moro reflex is another indication (refer to the discussion of the Moro reflex later in the chapter).

Chest

The anteroposterior and lateral diameters of the chest are equal, making the chest appear barrel-shaped. The xiphoid process is prominent. Chest movements should be equal bilaterally and synchronous with the abdomen.

Breast enlargement and breast engorgement is normal for both sexes. A thin milky secretion, sometimes called "witch's milk," may be secreted from the nipples. The breasts should not be squeezed in an attempt to express the liquid. Assess for supernumerary (accessory) nipples below and medial to the true nipples.

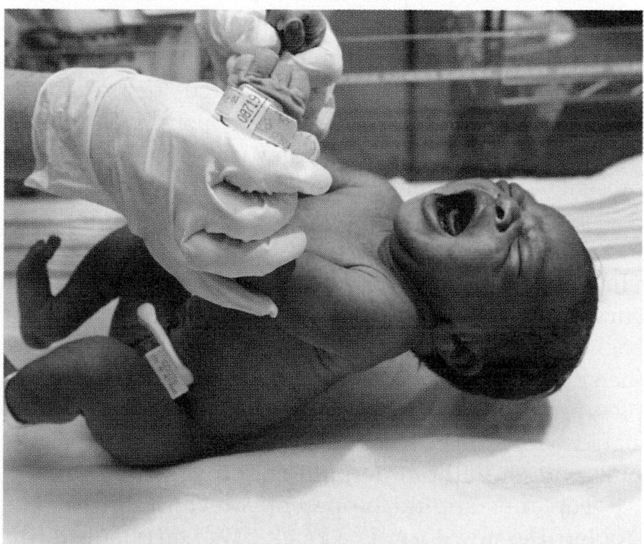

● ***Figure 13.7*** The newborn exhibits significant head lag when pulled to a sitting position from lying on his back.

Abdomen

The newborn's abdomen is dome shaped and protuberant. Respirations are typically diaphragmatic, which make them appear abdominal in nature. Peristaltic waves should not be visible. Bowel sounds should be audible within 2 hours of birth. The abdomen should be soft to palpation without palpable masses. The umbilical cord should be well formed, with three vessels present. The base of the cord should be dry without redness or drainage, and the umbilical clamp should be fastened securely.

Genitourinary

The newborn should void within the first 24 hours of life. Vigorous newborns may urinate for the first time in the delivery room minutes after birth. The stream of a male newborn should be strong enough to cause a steady arch during voiding, and the female should be able to produce a steady stream. The kidneys are not able to concentrate urine well during the first few days, so the color is light, and there is no odor. It is normal to find a small amount of pink or light orange color in the diaper for the first few voidings. This so-called brick dust in the diaper is caused by excess uric acid in the urine.

Both male and female genitalia may be swollen. **Smegma**, a cheesy white sebaceous gland secretion, is often found within the folds of the labia of the female and under the foreskin of the male. It is best to allow the secretion to gradually wear away because vigorous attempts at removal can irritate the tender mucosa. Immediately report the presence of ambiguous genitalia (i.e., it is difficult to tell if the newborn has male or female genitalia).

Female. The labia and clitoris may be edematous. In the term newborn, the labia majora cover the labia minora. A hymenal tag may be present. An imperforate hymen (a hymen that completely covers the vaginal opening) should be reported. A blood-tinged mucous secretion may be discharged from the vagina in response to the sudden withdrawal of maternal hormones. This secretion is called **pseudomenstruation**. Reassure the parents this condition is not cause for alarm.

Male. The urinary meatus should be positioned at the tip of the penis. If the opening is located abnormally on the dorsal (upper) surface of the glans penis, the condition is called **epispadias**. **Hypospadias** occurs when the opening to the urethra is on the ventral (under) surface of the glans. **Phimosis**, tightly adherent foreskin, is a normal condition in the term newborn. The tissue should not be forced over the glans penis. Monitor the adequacy of the urinary stream. If phimosis interferes with urination, intervention will be needed. Spontaneous erections are a common finding.

The male scrotum is pendulous, edematous, and covered with rugae (deep creases). Dark-skinned newborns have deeply pigmented scrotum. Both testes should be descended. Use your thumb and forefinger to gently palpate the scrotal sac while gently pressing down on the inguinal canal with the opposite hand. Repeat the procedure on the opposite side. Failure of the testes to descend (undescended testicles) is a condition called *cryptorchidism*. This condition requires medical evaluation. A hydrocele, fluid within the scrotal sac, may be present and should be noted.

You can diagnose a hydrocele quite easily. Take a penlight and hold it against the scrotal sac. If fluid is present (hydrocele), the light will transilluminate the scrotum. If there is no hydrocele, the light will not shine through solid structures.

Extremities

The term newborn maintains a posture of flexion. He has good muscle tone, and his extremities return quickly to an attitude of flexion after they are extended. The extremities are short in relation to the body and without deformities. Full range of motion is present in all joints, and movements are bilateral and equal.

Count the fingers and toes. Syndactyly refers to fusing or webbing of the toes or fingers, and polydactyly is the term used when extra digits are present. The palms of the hands should have creases. A single straight palmar crease, a **simian crease**, is an abnormal finding that is associated with Down's syndrome. Brachial pulses should be present and equal.

The legs are bowed and the feet flat because of a fatty pad in the arch of the foot. Creases should cover at least two thirds of the bottom of the feet. Palpate the femoral and brachial pulses on each side of the body. The pulses should be equal and strong. A strong brachial pulse with a weak femoral pulse is abnormal and should be reported (Fig. 13-8).

Here's a helpful hint. It takes practice to learn how to palpate the femoral pulses, but this is an important assessment skill to develop. Practice on a newborn who is resting quietly. Leave your fingers in one place long enough to adequately determine if the pulse is present. You will gain confidence as you are consistently able to find the pulses.

You may be asked to assist the RN while she attempts to elicit Ortolani's maneuver and Barlow's sign (Nursing Procedure 13-2) to evaluate the hip for signs of dislocation or subluxation (partial dislocation). A positive sign is associated with subluxation. Other signs of a dislocated hip included uneven gluteal folds and one knee that is lower than the other when the newborn is supine with both knees flexed.

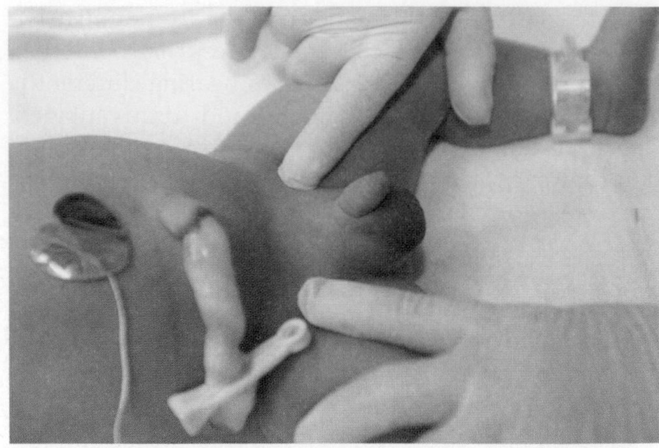

A

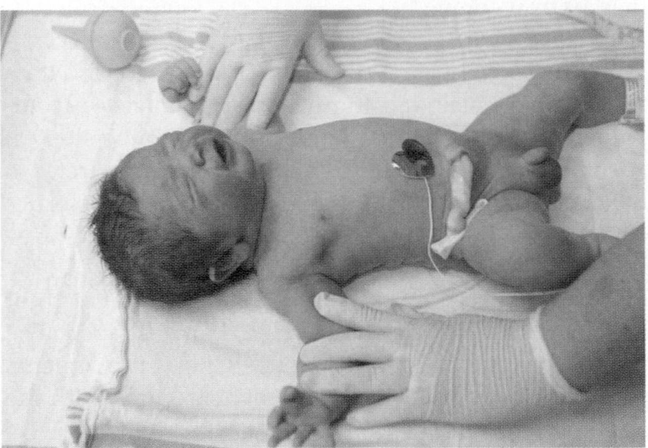

B

● ***Figure 13.8*** **(A)** Palpating the femoral pulse **(B)** Palpating the brachial pulse.

The feet may appear to turn inward because of the way the fetus was positioned in the womb or birth canal. If the feet are easily reducible, that is they can be easily moved to a normal position, the "deformity" is positional and will resolve spontaneously. If the feet do not move to a normal position, true clubfoot may be present. A specialist should evaluate this condition.

Back and Rectum

The spine is straight and flat. The lumbar and sacral curves do not appear until the infant begins to use his back to sit and stand upright. Feel along the length of the spine. There should be no masses, openings, dimples, or tufts of hair. Any of these findings may be associated with spina bifida (an opening in the spinal column with or without herniation of the meninges).

The anus should be patent. **Meconium,** the first stool of the newborn, is a thick black tarry substance composed of dead cells, mucus, and bile that collects in the rectum of the fetus. Passage of meconium should

Nursing Procedure 13.2
Ortolani's Maneuver and Barlow's Sign

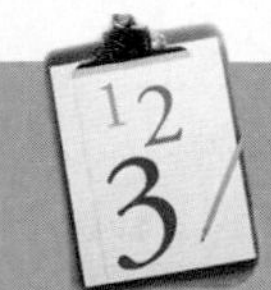

EQUIPMENT

Warm, clean hands
Flat surface

PROCEDURE

1. Wash hands thoroughly.
2. Position the newborn flat on his back on a firm surface.
3. Position the knees together and flex the knees and hips 90 degrees.
4. Place your middle fingers over the greater trochanter of the femur and your thumbs on the inner aspect of the thigh.
5. Apply upward pressure and abduct the hips. A clicking or a clunking sound is a positive Ortolani's sign and is associated with dislocation of the hip.

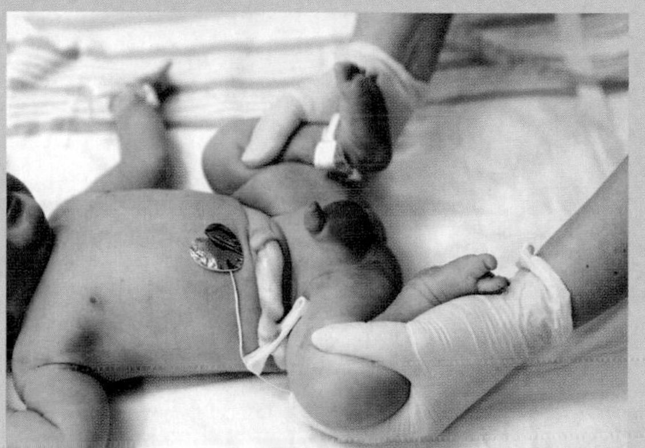

6. Next apply downward pressure and adduct the hips. Continue to maintain 90 degrees flexion. If you feel the head of the femur slip out of the acetabulum, the joint is unstable, and Barlow's sign is positive.

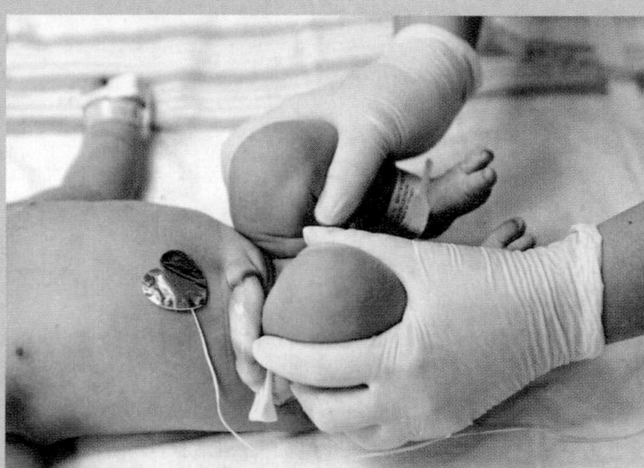

7. Position the newborn comfortably on the back or side.
8. Wash hands thoroughly.
9. Document your findings.

Note: In this instance, a positive Ortolani's or Barlow's sign is not wanted. It is not normal to hear clicking or clunking or to feel the femoral head slip out of the hip socket.

occur within the first 24 to 48 hours and confirms the presence of a patent anus.

Test Yourself

- Name two differences between caput succedaneum and cephalhematoma.
- What is pseudomenstruation?
- Define subluxation of the hip.

Neurologic Assessment

General Appearance and Behavior

The first part of the neurologic examination involves quiet observation of the general appearance and behavior of the newborn. The newborn should maintain an attitude of flexion. Hypotonus (decreased tone) is an abnormal finding, as is hypertonus, distinct tremors, jitteriness, or seizure activity. Any of these states may be associated with neurologic dysfunction, hypoglycemia, hypocalcemia, or neonatal drug withdrawal. The cry should be vigorous and of medium pitch. A high-pitched, shrill cry is associated with neurologic dysfunction.

Reflexes

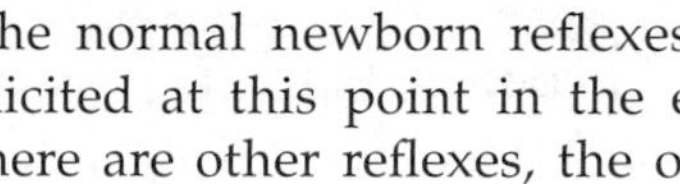

The normal newborn reflexes (Fig. 13-9) should be elicited at this point in the examination. Although there are other reflexes, the ones discussed here are generally the most common reflexes to be assessed. In addition, the newborn should demonstrate the protective reflexes of sneezing, coughing, blinking, and withdrawing from painful stimuli.

Rooting, sucking, and swallowing reflexes are important to the newborn's nutritional intake. The

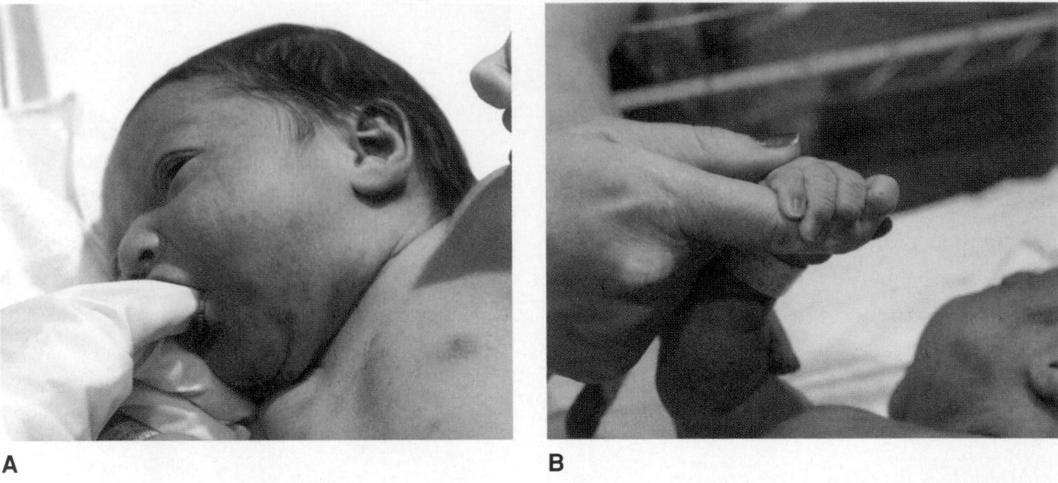

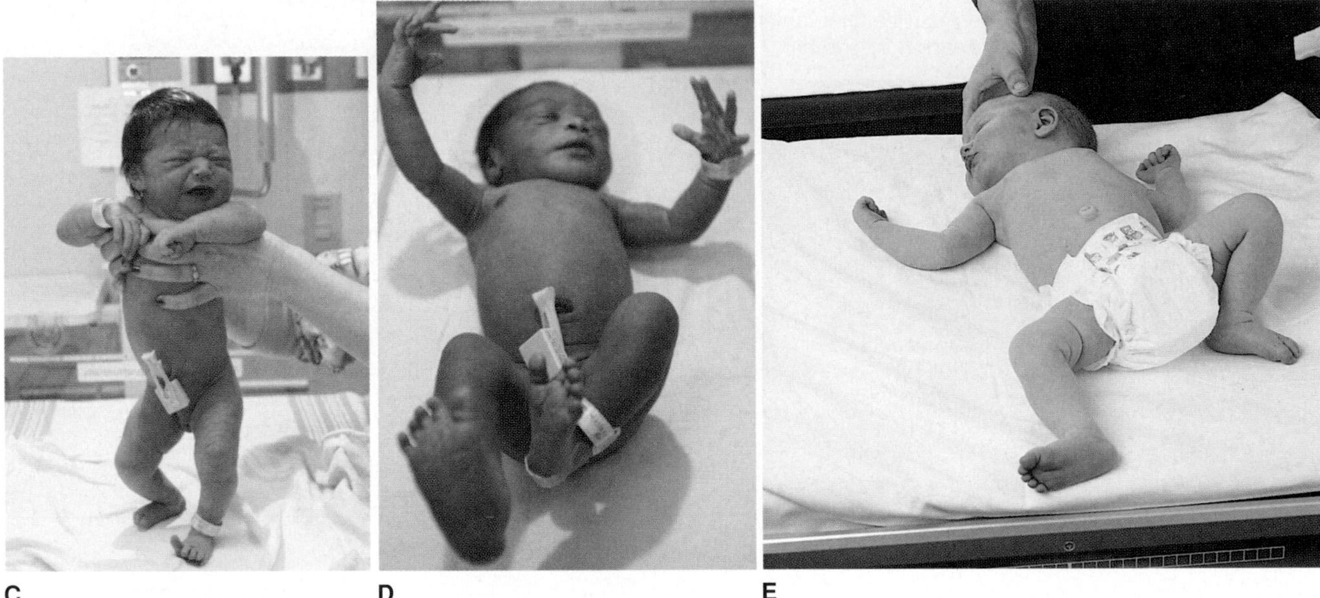

● ***Figure 13.9*** Normal newborn reflexes. (**A**) The nurse elicits the suck reflex in the newborn (**B**) Palmar grasp. The newborn curls her fingers tightly around the nurse's fingers. (**C**) The nurse elicits the stepping reflex. (**D**) The newborn is exhibiting the Moro reflex. Notice the "C" shape of the arms. (**E**) Tonic neck reflex (fencer's position). Notice how the extremities on the side he is facing are extended while the opposite extremities are flexed.

rooting reflex is elicited by gently stroking the newborn's cheek. If the reflex is present she will turn toward the touch with an open mouth looking for food. The new mother can be taught to use this reflex to help the newborn begin breast-feeding (see Chapter 14). Place a gloved finger in the newborn's mouth to test the sucking reflex. The suck should be strong. Swallowing is evaluated when the infant eats. Listen and watch for coordinated swallowing efforts.

The plantar and palmar grasp reflexes are evaluated by placing a finger in the palm or parallel to the toes. The digits will wrap around the finger and hold on. The grasp should be equal and strong bilaterally. The stepping reflex is checked by supporting the newborn in a standing position on a hard surface. He will lift his legs up and down in a stepping motion. Babinski's sign is positive if the newborn's toes fan out and hyperextend and dorsiflexion of the foot occurs in response to a hard object (such as the blunt end of a writing pen) being traced from the heel along the lateral aspect of the foot up and across the ball of the foot. After the infant starts walking, this reflex should disappear and the toes will curl inward, rather than fanning outward.

The Moro reflex is also known as the *startle reflex*. When the newborn is startled, he will extend his arms and legs away from his body and to the side. Then his arms will come back toward each other with the fingers spread in a "C" shape. His arms look as if he is trying to embrace something. The Moro reflex should be symmetrical and can be elicited until approximately 6 months of age. The tonic neck reflex is another total body reflex. With the infant lying quietly on his back, turn his head to one side without moving the rest of his body. He will extend the arm and leg on the side he is facing and flex the opposite arm and leg. This position has been called the "fencer's position" because it looks as if the newborn is poised to begin fencing.

Behavioral Assessment

It is important to note how the parents react to the newborn's behavior states and how the parents talk about the newborn. Newborns who demonstrate self-quieting behaviors are usually considered to be "good" babies. Parents respond positively to newborns who are cuddly and sociable. When a newborn resists cuddling or is difficult to console, the parents may feel rejected, and bonding can be affected adversely.

Teach the parents to watch the newborn for cues as to when he wants to interact. The quiet alert state is a good time for focused interaction with the newborn. When the newborn is in the active alert stage, he likes to play. The drowsy state lets the parents know the newborn needs rest. Crying signals that the newborn has a need. Teach the parents to check for physical problems first, such as a wet diaper, hunger, or need to burp. If the newborn is still crying, the parents can try soothing actions, such as walking, rocking, or riding in the car. Reassure the parents that, contrary to popular opinion, you cannot spoil a newborn by picking him up when he is crying. Being held is reassuring and comforting to the newborn.

This is vital! Teach the parents to NEVER shake an infant. Shaking an infant can cause permanent brain damage. If the parent is frustrated because the crying does not stop no matter what has been tried, encourage the parent to take a minute to stop and count to 10 or ask a friend for help.

Gestational Age Assessment

The gestational age assessment is a critical evaluation. The RN is ultimately responsible for performing the gestational age assessment; however, the LPN should be familiar with the instruments used and be able to differentiate characteristics of the full-term newborn from those of the premature newborn. Chapter 20 details gestational age assessment and compares the preterm with the full-term newborn.

KEY POINTS

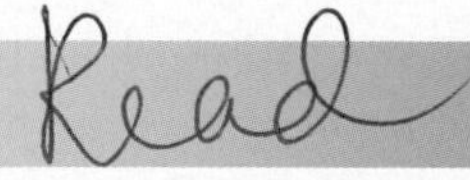

- The newborn must adapt rapidly to life outside the womb and without the placenta that supplies every need in utero.
- In order to adjust to life outside the uterus, the newborn must fill his lungs with air, absorb remaining fluid in his lungs, and begin oxygen exchange.
- All the fetal shunts (foramen ovale, ductus arteriosus, and ductus venosus) must close so that blood will travel to the lungs for gas exchange and so that blood will pass through the liver.
- The newborn exhibits poor thermoregulation because he is prone to heat loss through the skin and because he cannot produce heat through muscle movement and shivering. He loses heat through the processes of convection, conduction, radiation, and evaporation. However, the newborn conserves heat by maintaining a flexed position and produces heat by metabolizing brown fat.
- The newborn's liver is immature. Sometimes it cannot handle the heavy load from the breakdown of red blood cells, and physiologic jaundice appears. This condition is harmless if bilirubin levels do not rise dramatically and if jaundice is not present before the newborn is 24 hours old. Not all of the necessary blood coagulation factors are manufactured directly after birth and the gut is sterile, so vitamin K is given intramuscularly to stimulate appropriate clotting.
- Each infant is unique, but all infants have similar sleep and activity patterns. These include deep sleep, light sleep, drowsiness, quiet alert state, active alert state, and crying.
- The nursing assessment of newborn characteristics is an important way the nurse determines how well the newborn is adapting to life outside the womb. In general, the least disturbing aspects of the examination are done first, such as general observation regarding the newborn's posture. In addition, the respiratory rate and heart rate are taken early in the examination while the newborn is quiet. Then the examination proceeds in a head-to-toe manner, covering vital signs, physical measurements, and assessment of each body part.
- The expected weight range is 5 pounds 8 ounces to 8 pounds 13 ounces (2,500 to 4,000 grams). Length is 19 to 21 inches (48 to 53 cm). Head circumference is 13 to 14 inches (33 to 33.5 cm) and chest circumference is 12 to 13 inches (30.5 to 33 cm).
- The skin should be supple with good turgor and have a pink color to it. There are many variations that are normally present on newborn skin.

- Head and face: Molding may be present. The newborn is an obligate nose breather. The hard and soft palates should be intact.
- Neck and chest: The neck is short and thick. Webbing should not be present. Periodic breathing episodes are normal.
- Abdomen: The abdomen is protuberant. The cord should be clamped and drying at the base with three vessels present.
- Genitourinary: The newborn should void within the first 24 hours. Genitalia of both sexes may be swollen.
- The back should be straight and free of hairy tufts, dimples, or tumors. Meconium, the first stool, should be passed in the first 24 hours.
- The main reflexes elicited to determine neurologic status are rooting, sucking, swallowing, grasping, Moro, Babinski's, and tonic neck or the fencer's position.

REFERENCES AND SELECTED READINGS

Books and Journals

American Academy of Pediatrics Task Force on Newborn and Infant Hearing. (1999). Newborn and infant hearing loss: Detection and intervention (RE9846). *Pediatrics, 103*(2), 527–530. Retrieved July 14, 2002, from http://www.aap.org/policy/re9846.html.

Cunningham, F. G., Gant, N. F., Leveno, K. J., Gilstrap, L. C., III, Hauth, J. C. & Wenstrom, K. D. (2001). The newborn infant. In *Williams Obstetrics* (21st ed., pp. 385–402). New York: McGraw-Hill Medical Publishing Division.

DeMichele, A. M., & Ruth, R. A. (2003). Newborn hearing screening. In R. A. Faust, F. Talavera, P. S. Roland, C. L. Slack, & A. D. Meyers (Eds.), *eMedicine*. Retrieved January 8, 2004, from http://www.emedicine.com/ent/topic576.htm.

Hansen, R. W. R. (2002). Neonatal jaundice. In I. Oussama, R. Konop, B. S. Carter, C. L. Wagner, & N. N. Finer (Eds.), *eMedicine*. Retrieved January 15, 2004, from http://www.emedicine.com/ped/topic1061.htm..

Howard-Glen, L. (2000). Adaptation to extrauterine life and immediate nursing care. In S. Mattson & J. E. Smith (Eds.), *Core Curriculum for Maternal–ewborn Nursing* (2nd ed., pp. 346–359). AWHONN publication. Philadelphia: WB Saunders.

Howard-Glen, L. (2000). Newborn biological/behavioral characteristics and psychosocial adaptations. In S. Mattson & J. E. Smith (Eds.), *Core Curriculum for Maternal–Newborn Nursing* (2nd ed., pp. 360–373). AWHONN publication. Philadelphia: WB Saunders.

St. John, E. B. (2002). Hemorrhagic disease of newborn. In O. Itani, R. Konop, D. A. Clark, C. L. Wagner, & N. N. Finer (Eds.), *eMedicine*. Retrieved January 8, 2004, from http://www.emedicine.com/ped/topic966.htm.

Yan, A. C. (2002). Erythema toxicum. In K. P. Connelly, R. Konop, R. A. Schwartz, M. Poth, & D. M. Elston (Eds.), *eMedicine*. Retrieved January 15, 2003, from http://www.emedicine.com/ped/topic697.htm.

Websites

Newborn Appearance and Behavior

http://www.beryl.net/HTL/NewBaby/22917.htm

http://www.childrenshospitaloakland.org/health_library/pa/hhg/newbappe.htm

Newborn Guidelines

http://www.rcp.gov.bc.ca/Guidelines/Newborn

Newborn skin characteristics

http://www.umm.edu/ency/article/002301.htm

WORKBOOK

NCLEX-STYLE REVIEW QUESTIONS

1. An infant is born by cesarean delivery. In what way is respiratory adaptation more difficult for this infant than the one who is born by vaginal delivery?
   a. More fluid is present in the lungs at birth.
   b. Surfactant is missing from the lungs.
   c. The respiratory centers in the brain are not stimulated.
   d. There is less sensory stimulation to breathe.
2. A new mother says, "I think something is wrong with my baby. She has a milky fluid leaking from her nipples!" What is the nurse's best response?
   a. "I don't know. Let me have the charge nurse check the baby."
   b. "It's nothing to worry about. That's a normal finding."
   c. "This is a normal occurrence. You may clean her with a damp washcloth, but be careful not to squeeze the nipples."
   d. "This means the baby was exposed to an infection during birth. I'll notify the doctor at once!"
3. You are assessing a newborn that is 1 day old. You notice a small amount of white drainage and redness at the base of the umbilical cord. How should you respond?
   a. Call the doctor immediately to ask for intravenous antibiotics.
   b. Carefully clean the area with a damp washcloth and cover it with an absorbent dressing.
   c. Notify the charge nurse because this finding represents a possible complication.
   d. Show the mother how to clean the area with soap and water.
4. A newborn's axillary temperature is 97.4°F. His T-shirt is damp with spit-up milk. His blanket is loosely applied, and several children are in the room running around his crib. The room is comfortably warm, and the bassinet is beside the mother's bed away from the window and doors. What are the most likely mechanisms of heat loss for this newborn?
   a. Conduction and evaporation
   b. Conduction and radiation
   c. Convection and radiation
   d. Convection and evaporation

STUDY ACTIVITIES

1. Do an Internet search using the key words "newborn crying." How many Internet sites returned? List three to four that would be good references for new parents. Compare your list to that of your clinical group.
2. Use the table below to describe important newborn assessments for each body system.

Body System	Critical Parameters to Assess	Expected Findings and Deviation From Normal
Respiratory		
Cardiovascular		
Gastrointestinal		
Metabolic		
Hepatic		
Skin		

3. Research resources in your community designed to help first-time parents in their new role. How many sources did you find? Were you surprised? Share your findings with your clinical group. Discuss ways the community might be more supportive of new parents.

Critical Thinking: What Would You Do?

Apply your knowledge of normal newborn adaptation to the following situation.

1. Mary, a 28-year-old woman, delivered her first baby several hours ago. She and the father of the baby had joyful interaction with the baby immediately after delivery. The newborn breast-fed well with assistance from the delivery room nurse. You are coming on duty for the evening shift and have just entered the room to assess the baby.
   a. You find the baby sleeping with only a diaper on in an open bassinet. It appears the bassinet has been moved against the wall under a window. The baby's skin is mottled, and her extremities feel cool to the touch. What is your initial assessment of the situation? What actions should you take first?

   b. What instructions should you give to the parents?

2. On day 3 of life, you notice that the skin of Mary's baby is a light yellow color.

   a. What is the likely cause of the yellow color?

   b. Mary asks you if the yellow color indicates illness. How do you reply?

3. Mary says she is frustrated. She has been trying to "play" with the baby, but he keeps looking away and yawning. She is worried that her baby doesn't "like" her.

   a. How should you reply to Mary?

   b. Mary expresses concern about a blue-black spot she found on the baby's back. She is worried that he received a bruise in the nursery. How do you explain this finding to Mary?

Newborn Nutrition

14

STUDENT OBJECTIVES

On completion of this chapter, the student should be able to

1. Describe factors that influence the woman's choice of feeding method.
2. Identify advantages of breast-feeding for both the woman and the newborn.
3. Discuss situations for which breast-feeding would not be recommended.
4. Discuss the physical and hormonal control of the breast during lactation.
5. Describe the role of the nurse when assisting a woman to breast-feed.
6. Outline appropriate nursing interventions for three common problems the breast-feeding woman might encounter.
7. List signs that a newborn is not breast-feeding well.
8. Differentiate between breast milk and formula.
9. Compare the various types of formulas available to feed newborns and infants.
10. Name situations in which formula feeding would be beneficial.
11. Outline appropriate teaching topics for the bottle-feeding woman.
12. List several questions the nurse should ask the parents of a newborn who is not tolerating formula.

KEY TERMS

amenorrhea
artificial nutrition
colostrum
engorgement
foremilk
hind milk
immunologic
lactation consultant
mastitis

In utero the fetus obtains all of its nutrition in a passive manner. The nutrients cross from the maternal circulation, across the placenta, and enter the fetus' circulation. From there the nutrients are taken directly to the tissues and used at the cellular level. At birth, this passive intake of nutrition ends, and the newborn must actively consume and digest food.

The newborn has specific nutritional needs. The healthy term newborn needs 108 kcal/kg/day and 160 to 180 mL/kg/day. Breast milk, or an iron-fortified infant formula, will provide the newborn with all the calories and fluids necessary. In addition, breast milk and infant formulas are balanced to meet the carbohydrate, protein, and fat needs of the newborn. Table 14-1 summarizes some of the specific nutritional needs of the newborn.

CHOOSING A FEEDING METHOD

The healthy term newborn can be fed one of two ways. The woman can choose to either breast-feed or bottle-feed her newborn. The choice is ultimately the woman's to make. The nurse has a clear role in providing the woman with enough information for her to make an informed decision. In addition, the nurse has a supportive and teaching role after the woman has made her decision.

There are many factors that influence the woman's decision about whether to breast-feed or bottle-feed. Some of these factors are culture, age, prior experience with or exposure to breast-feeding, and her intent or need to return to work or school.

Culture

Each culture has its own viewpoint on feeding the newborn. Most cultures support breast-feeding. In some situations, such as immigration to a new country, formula feeding is seen as more desirable, and the woman may choose to formula feed, even if she previously breast-fed in her native country. In some cultures the desire is for a strong or large baby, and formula is seen as the way to achieve these desired goals (Riordan & Auerbach, 1998). In some cultures the woman will feed her newborn formula until her milk comes in and then she will breast-feed. In the United States, breast-feeding tends to be more predominant in whites, with 59.7% breast-feeding in the hospital after birth. African-American women have the lowest rate, with 27.2% breast-feeding after birth in the hospital. Hispanics have a 51.7% in-hospital breast-feeding rate (Lawrence & Lawrence, 1999).

Age and Education

Breast-feeding is highest in women older than 35 years of age. Younger women tend to choose bottle-feeding; fewer than 44% of women younger than 20 years of age breast-feed their newborns. This may be attributable to a lack of knowledge regarding the benefits of breast-feeding for the woman and the newborn; a lack of a role model for breast-feeding; or the woman's viewpoint that her breasts are only sexual in nature. Level of education also has an impact on the newborn feeding choice; 73.8% of women with a college degree breast-feed, whereas 46.8% of women with less than a high school education breast-feed (Lawrence & Lawrence, 1999).

Past Experience

A woman's past experience with or exposure to breast-feeding has a great impact on her decision whether or not to breast-feed this newborn. If the woman has previously breast-fed an infant, that experience will affect her decision on how to feed this newborn. The feeding experiences of the woman's support systems also play an important part in assisting the woman in her feeding choice. Their past or current experiences, whether positive or negative, regarding either type of feeding, will influence the woman's current choice of feeding.

Intent to Return to Work or School

The need to return to work or school soon after the newborn's birth plays an important role in the woman's feeding choice. Women who have chosen to breast-feed in the hospital can continue to breast-feed and pump while at work or school or breast-feed when the infant is present and offer formula while she is away, or she can elect to stop breast-feeding. Some women prefer not to begin breast-feeding because of

TABLE 14.1 Daily Nutritional Needs of the Newborn

Protein	Vitamin A	Vitamin C	Vitamin D	Vitamin E	Vitamin K	Calcium
2.2 g/kg	400 μg/day	40 mg/day	5 μg/day	4 mg/day	2.0 μg/day	210 mg/day

their work or school obligations and choose to feed formula from the newborn's birth.

BREAST-FEEDING

Breast-feeding is the recommended method for feeding newborns. The American Academy of Pediatrics (AAP) advocates exclusive breast-feeding until 6 months of age and continuation of breast-feeding until at least 12 months of age. The infant does not have to be weaned at 12 months; the benefits of breast-feeding for both the woman and the infant continue as long as the woman is nursing.

Breast milk is superior nutritionally to **artificial nutrition,** that is, infant formula. Breast-feeding is recommended and encouraged by organizations such as the AAP, World Health Organization (WHO), and the Association of Women's Health, Obstetric, and Neonatal Nurses (AWHONN). Each of these organizations has a policy statement that defines their position on breast-feeding and their recommendations for infant feeding.

Advantages and Disadvantages of Breast-feeding

Advantages

The advantages for the woman include more rapid uterine involution and less bleeding in the postpartum period, a quicker return to her prepregnancy weight level, and decreased incidence of ovarian and premenopausal breast cancers (Riordan & Auerbach, 1998).

The advantages for the newborn are numerous. Breast milk provides **immunologic** properties from the woman that help protect the newborn from infections and strengthen the newborn's immune system. Breast-feeding also provides a unique experience for maternal–newborn bonding. There is a decreased risk in overfeeding of the breast-fed newborn, which results in a lower incidence of overweight infants. Breast-fed infants tend to have lower incidences of otitis media, diarrhea, and lower respiratory tract infections. Breast-feeding also provides a possible protective effect against certain conditions or diseases, such as sudden infant death syndrome, insulin dependent diabetes, and allergic diseases. Finally, there is a possible correlation between enhanced cognitive development and breast-feeding (Riordan & Auerbach, 1998).

There also are several benefits that affect not only the woman and newborn, but also the community at large. Breast-feeding is more economic. The breast-feeding woman does not need to purchase formula, bottles, or nipples. Breast milk is always available, needs no preparation or storage, and no cleanup of utensils or dishes after the feeding is required. When away from home, the woman does not need to carry extra equipment or supplies to feed her newborn. Breast-feeding reduces health care costs because breast-fed infants are healthier and have less illness than do formula-fed infants (Riordan & Auerbach, 1998).

Disadvantages

There is no disadvantage to either the woman or the newborn during breast-feeding. What can be claimed as a disadvantage is actually a circumstance or condition in which breast-feeding is deemed inappropriate. However, there are certain maternal conditions or situations that would contraindicate breast-feeding. Examples of these conditions include:

- Illegal drug use
- Active untreated tuberculosis
- Human immunodeficiency virus (HIV) infection
- Chemotherapy treatment (See Appendix E.)
- Herpetic lesions on the breast

In addition, there are certain conditions the newborn may have that would contraindicate breast-feeding. Galactosemia, an inborn error of metabolism, requires a specialty formula for the newborn because breast milk is high in lactose. With phenylketonuria, another inborn error of metabolism, the newborn may require partial to complete feedings of a specialty infant formula. There are other medical conditions that may necessitate the newborn receiving formula. In some situations, the woman may produce little to no breast milk. In these situations, the infant's diet should be supplemented with or switched over completely to formula.

In addition to reasons that would contraindicate breast-feeding, there are also perceived disadvantages to breast-feeding. Some women feel that breast-feeding would exclude others from caring for or feeding the newborn. Some fathers express an interest in wanting to feed the newborn and feel that breast-feeding would take away this opportunity. In these circumstances the woman can pump her breast milk, and the father or other caregiver could feed the newborn. This way the newborn still receives the superior nutrition that only breast milk can provide and the father or other caregiver can have the feeding time with the newborn. This also gives the woman a respite from feeding the newborn.

There are other perceived disadvantages to breast-feeding. Some women feel that they will be unable to return to work or school if they breast-feed. Others feel that breast-feeding is too difficult or uncomfortable. Breast-feeding may be perceived as sexual in nature, or some women may feel it may detract from the woman's sexuality. Some women feel restrained by breast-feeding in that it ties them to the baby, or they think it will make the baby "too clingy."

Test Yourself

- Name four factors that influence a woman's decision to breast-feed.
- List three advantages to the woman during breast-feeding.
- List four advantages to the newborn during breast-feeding.
- What are the advantages to the community when a woman breast-feeds?

Physiology of Breast-feeding

Newborn Features That Facilitate Breast-feeding

The newborn possesses several unique characteristics that make breast-feeding physiologically possible. These characteristics are found only in the newborn and infant and disappear as the infant gets older. Specifically, the newborn is born with a uniquely shaped nose and mouth, the rooting reflex, and the innate ability to suck.

Newborn Facial Anatomy. The newborn is designed uniquely for breast-feeding. The nose, which looks flattened after birth, is designed to create air pockets when up against the breast. This allows the newborn to breathe without obscuring the nasal opening. Newborns are nose breathers, which allows them to breathe while their mouth is full, without having to release the breast to take a breath. The newborn's mouth is designed to compress the milk ducts located behind the nipple under the areola. The tongue, pharynx, and lower jaw are unique in their shape when these structures are compared with those of the older child or adult. The newborn also has fat pads on each cheek that aid in the sucking process.

Rooting and Sucking Reflex. In addition to these unique anatomical findings, the newborn has a set of reflexes that assist in breast-feeding. The rooting reflex is seen when the newborn's cheek is brushed lightly and the newborn turns toward the stimulation. When the newborn feels the woman's breast touching his face, he turns toward the breast and opens his mouth. This is a feeding cue the woman can observe and know that her newborn is ready to nurse. When the newborn's lips are lightly touched, the newborn will respond by opening his mouth.

The sucking reflex is seen when the nipple is placed into the newborn's mouth and the newborn begins to suck. The term newborn has the ability to coordinate her sucking, swallowing, and breathing in a manner that facilitates nursing and prevents choking, while giving the infant breaks during nursing to rest. The newborn sucks in a burst pattern; sucking several times and then pausing. The length of the pause should be equal to the time the newborn sucks. The type of sucking also changes during the feeding. At the beginning of the feeding, the newborn nurses with rapid, short sucks. These sucks stimulate the breast to release the milk. When the milk is freely flowing, the newborn nurses with longer, slower sucks.

The Breast

The breast is a unique organ that is designed for the purpose of providing the newborn with nourishment. The anatomy of the breast, and the way it makes milk, are unique to the female. The breast makes milk in response to several different stimuli. These include the physical emptying of the breast, hormonal stimulation, and sensory stimulation that the woman's brain receives from her newborn.

Breast Anatomy. The breast is very vascular, with a rich lymphatic and nervous supply. The breast is made up of 15 to 20 lobes containing the milk-producing alveoli. The alveoli are clustered together and empty into ducts. The alveoli produce the milk. The alveoli are surrounded by smooth muscle cells, which help to eject the milk into the ducts. The ducts lead to the nipple, where the milk is released.

Physical Control of Lactation. When the breast is emptied, either by the newborn sucking or by use of a breast pump, the breast responds by replenishing the milk supply. If the breast is not emptied completely, it will not make as much milk the next time. This is why it is important for the newborn to nurse long enough to establish a good milk supply. If the woman is pumping, she should allow sufficient time for the pump to drain both breasts and not stop pumping until the flow of milk has stopped. If the newborn completely empties the breast and then nurses again shortly after the feeding, it will cause the breast to increase its milk supply.

Hormonal Control of Lactation. The breast also is under hormonal control. When the newborn sucks on the breast, the anterior pituitary gland releases prolactin, which causes milk production and milk release in the breast. The newborn's sucking also causes the pituitary to release oxytocin. Oxytocin causes contractions of the muscles in the uterus and also in the myoepithelial cells that surround the alveoli in the breast. Figure 14-1 shows how the hormones respond to the stimulation of the newborn sucking on the breast.

During the first few days, the more often the newborn nurses, the more lactogen receptor sites in

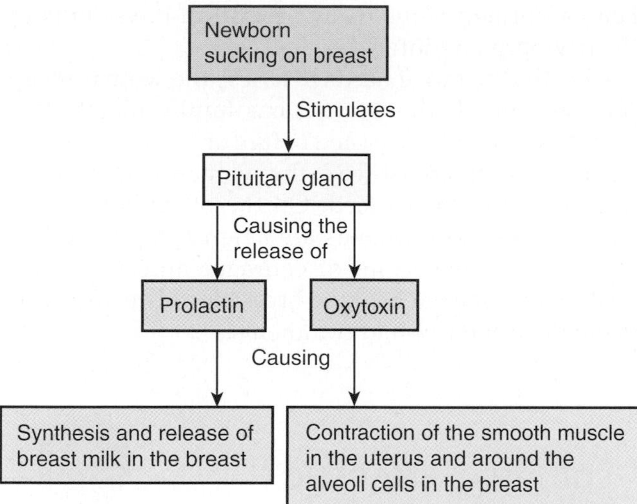

● ***Figure 14.1*** Diagram of the hormonal effect on lactation.

the breast are activated to respond to lactogen, which will aid in the production of milk. If the breast is not stimulated, either by the newborn's sucking or by a breast pump, the number of sites is reduced, which can affect the quantity of the woman's milk supply. The nurse should encourage the woman to feed her newborn every 1½ to 3 hours until her milk supply is established. If she is unable to nurse her newborn, she should pump at least every 3 hours around the clock.

Sensory Stimulation. In addition to hormones and the physical emptying of the breast, the woman's body responds to the sensory information her brain picks up from her newborn. As the woman holds her newborn and the newborn touches her breast or grasps her finger with his hand, the woman's skin is stimulated. These tactile sensations are sent to her brain. As the woman sees her baby, these visual images are also sent to her brain. As the woman hears her baby cry or coo, her brain is also picking up these sounds and processing them. Finally, the olfactory sensations of the smell of a woman's baby are also sent to the woman's brain. These sensory sensations aid the woman's body in having a let-down reflex. This is why some women will report a let-down reflex when hearing another baby cry in public. The let-down reflex can be inhibited by maternal alcohol consumption, so the breast-feeding woman should avoid drinking alcoholic beverages.

Composition of Breast Milk

Breast milk is a unique substance that is unable to be duplicated because of the immunologic factors present. Breast milk is not produced until approximately 3 days after birth. Until this time, the newborn receives a substance called colostrum during the nursing sessions. The breast starts to produce **colostrum,** a thick, and yellowish gold substance during the 2nd trimester. Colostrum is higher in antibodies than breast milk and has a lower fat and higher protein content than what is found in breast milk. There is between 2 and 20 mL of colostrum present for each feeding until the woman's milk comes in about the 3rd day.

CULTURAL SNAPSHOT

Some cultures feel that the colostrum is "old" or "dirty" milk; women from such cultures may not want to breast-feed until the milk comes in.

The woman's milk usually comes in between 3 and 5 days. Breast milk has 20 calories per ounce on the average. Breast milk has two different compositions: foremilk and hind milk. **Foremilk** is very watery and thin and may have a bluish tint. This is what the infant first receives during the nursing session. As the session progresses, the milk changes to hind milk. **Hind milk** is thicker and whiter. It contains a higher quantity of fat than foremilk and therefore has a higher caloric content than foremilk. The hind milk will satiate the infant longer between feedings. If the infant is thirsty and not very hungry, he or she will not nurse very long and will receive only the foremilk. The hungry infant nurses longer to get the hind milk.

It's OK to reassure the woman. Until her milk comes in, the woman may feel that her newborn is not getting enough to eat. Assure the woman that her newborn is getting enough calories and that the frequent nursing will aid in establishing an ample milk supply.

When the woman's milk comes in, she will notice her breasts feel fuller and heavier. A quality nursing bra will help her with supporting her breasts during this time. Many women experience leaking of breast milk or engorgement at this time (see "Teaching About Breast-feeding Special Concerns").

Nutritional Needs of the Breast-feeding Woman

The breast-feeding woman does not need to consume a large diet to produce milk for her infant. A well-balanced nutritious diet and drinking enough fluids to satisfy her thirst will provide her with the nutrition needed to lactate. A woman does not have to consume milk to make milk, but she does need fluids. If the woman does not consume enough fluids to satisfy her thirst or does not rest and eat a balanced diet, she may notice that she stops producing breast milk or that the quantity of her breast milk is diminished. A multivitamin will not make her breast milk more nutritious but will help ensure she obtains her daily required vitamins and minerals for her own body.

Nursing Care of the Breast-feeding Woman

The nurse has several roles when assisting a woman who is breast-feeding. These roles include assessing breast-feeding readiness, assisting with breast-feeding technique, assessing newborn fluid intake, and providing teaching about special breast-feeding topics.

Assessing Breast-feeding Readiness

Ideally, during the prenatal period the caregiver has introduced the question of whether or not the woman wants to breast-feed. At this time the woman should have been given information regarding the benefits of breast-feeding for both her and her newborn. In addition, the caregiver should have assessed the woman's breasts for any problems that might affect breast-feeding. If the woman has flat or inverted nipples, she still can breast-feed. A woman who has these types of nipples needs extra support in the beginning of breast-feeding, until she and the newborn become comfortable with nursing. A woman with flat or inverted nipples may need to use a breast pump for a few minutes before nursing the newborn to help pull out and harden the nipples so the newborn can make a good latch. She may also need to use a nipple shield to assist the newborn in latching on. The sooner women with problematic nipples are identified, the sooner the nurse can assist the woman with interventions and support from a **lactation consultant** (a nurse or layperson who has received special training to assist and support the breast-feeding woman). It is hoped this will minimize any discouragement and/or discomfort the woman may experience during the breast-feeding session and maximize the positive experience of the session.

Women who have had breast augmentation or reduction surgery can still breast-feed, as long as the surgeon left the milk ducts intact. Discuss with the woman who has had breast surgery what her surgeon told her regarding breast-feeding.

Some women are opposed to or repulsed by the thought of the newborn sucking on her breast. Women who are opposed to the newborn nursing on the breast may be willing to pump their breast milk and feed their newborn expressed breast milk from a bottle after being informed of the many benefits of breast milk for the newborn and infant.

Lastly, the nurse needs to assess the woman's support systems. If the woman has family members or friends who have breast-fed before or are supportive of her decision to breast-feed, the woman is more likely to continue to breast-feed. On the other hand, if the woman's support systems are against breast-feeding, the woman may become discouraged and stop breast-feeding or not even begin to breast-feed because of the negative influences and comments.

CULTURAL SNAPSHOT

There are many culturally specific practices associated with breast-feeding. It is important to know the woman's cultural practices regarding modesty, breast-feeding in public or in front of others, the uses of a breast pump, or rituals for the purpose of bringing in good milk or a bountiful supply.

Assisting With Breast-feeding Technique

While assisting the woman, provide support and encouragement; many breast-feeding women are unsure of their ability to nurse their newborn. If the newborn will not nurse after you have provided assistance, contact the registered nurse in charge and take steps to contact the hospital lactation consultant for additional help.

Beginning the Breast-feeding Session. The first breast-feeding ideally should be in the delivery room within an hour after birth, unless the newborn's or woman's condition prevents this. Thereafter, the newborn should be nursed on demand at least every 1½ to 3 hours. If the newborn does not wake up by 3 hours, the woman should wake the newborn and encourage him or her to feed. Supplemental bottles

Here are some breast-feeding hints. Some women may become discouraged if their newborn is sleepy, will not latch immediately, or is crying vigorously and will not latch. Reassure the woman that the newborn will nurse. Take steps to rouse a sleepy newborn: changing the diaper, gentle rubbing of the back or head, and washing the newborn's face with a wet washcloth. If the newborn is crying and not exhibiting signs of hunger, check for other causes of crying, such as a wet or dirty diaper or constricting clothing. Try to calm the newborn before attempting to put the newborn to the breast.

of sterilized water or glucose solutions are discouraged because these will give the new-born a feeling of fullness and space out the feedings longer, which may in turn decrease the woman's milk supply.

CULTURAL SNAPSHOT

Some cultures place a high importance on privacy and/or modesty. The breast-feeding woman may not want to expose herself completely to breast-feed or may not want to breast-feed in the presence of the nurse. Some women may be uncomfortable breast-feeding in front of a male nurse.

A PERSONAL GLIMPSE

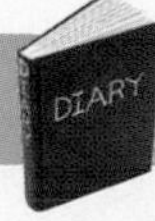

Todd is my second baby. My husband and I hadn't been planning for another child when I found out that I was pregnant. The pregnancy was completely normal with a few more aches and pains than I remembered with my first child, Richard. Right after the delivery I felt completely exhausted and ravenous. The nurse was insisting that I breast-feed and kept giving me a lot of information. I just couldn't deal with it. It seems like such a blur. I feel guilty that I didn't listen more. They whisked the baby away an hour after he was born. I was kind of relieved because I was so tired. But then when they brought him back to my room the nurse said, "They told me that you breast-fed in the delivery room. And since this is your second child, I'm sure you remember how to do it. He should feed for 5 to 10 minutes on each breast." I just looked at her. She handed me the baby and told me to call if I needed anything. Todd was fussy. I kept trying to get him to latch on but couldn't seem to figure out how to do it. I was sitting up in bed and having trouble getting comfortable. My stitches were hurting. But I didn't want to ask the nurse for help because I was afraid she would think I was dumb for not remembering how to get started with breast-feeding. The truth is I was very sick with my first child, so I only breast-fed for a couple of weeks, and it seemed so long ago. I finally gave up and called the nursery for a bottle. Todd immediately gulped down an ounce and a half. After that he didn't seem interested in breast-feeding. Now that he is a year old, I sometimes wish I had tried a little harder to breast-feed. I feel that somehow I missed out on a very special experience.

Rowena

LEARNING OPPORTUNITY: What assumptions did the nurse make that discouraged the mother from asking for help? How could the nurse have approached this situation to give the new mother the help that she needed?

When the nurse brings the newborn to the woman in the hospital for feedings, the first step is to check the newborn's and the woman's identification (ID) bands and make sure they match. After identity is confirmed, the nurse should provide the woman privacy by pulling a curtain around the bed or closing the door. Then assist the woman into a comfortable position. The woman should sit up in bed or a chair or lie on her side in bed. Use pillows as needed to support the woman's back and arms. Make sure there is nothing constricting or obstructing the breast, such as a too-tight bra or a cumbersome hospital gown that is in the woman's line of sight or falling between her and the newborn.

Positioning the Newborn. There are three basic positions for a woman to hold her newborn in while nursing. These are the cradle hold, football hold, and side-lying position (Fig. 14-2). Women who have breast-fed before may already know these three basic holds. However, a woman who has not breast-fed before or who has just had surgery needs more help with positioning her baby correctly. Correct positioning and latching on of the newborn will avoid nipple tissue trauma and sore nipples.

Cradle Hold. In the cradle hold, the newborn's abdomen is facing and touching the woman's abdomen. Make sure the newborn is not being held on his back and turning his head over his shoulder to reach the breast. In this position, the newborn's lower arm should be tucked between the woman's arm and breast and not between the newborn and the breast. The woman supports the breast being offered to the newborn with her free hand (see Fig. 14-2*A*).

Football Hold. In the football hold, the newborn is held with her head under the woman's breast. The newborn's head is supported under the woman's breast by the palm of the woman's hand while a pillow underneath the newborn supports her body. The woman's arm rests along the side of the newborn's body resting on the pillow. This is a good position for women who have undergone surgery or women with large breasts. It also facilitates the newborn and woman being able to see each other with an unobstructed view (see Fig. 14-2*B*).

Side-Lying Position. The side-lying position is with both the woman and the newborn on their sides facing each other while lying in bed. This position facilitates maternal rest and is good for a woman who has undergone surgery. The newborn should be supported with a blanket roll behind his back so he does not roll backward during the feeding. As with the cradle hold, the woman's and newborn's abdomens should be touching and the newborn should not be resting

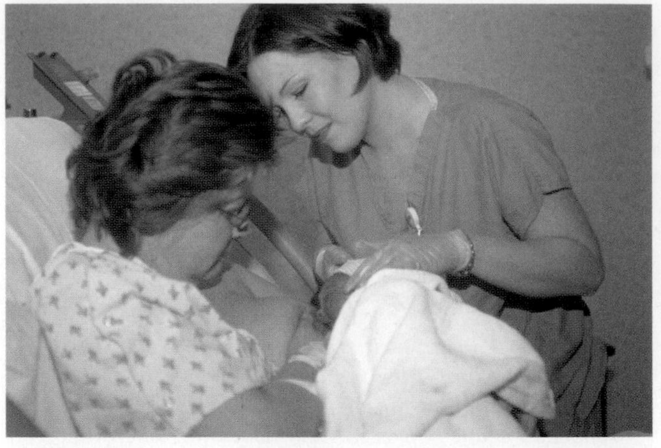
A

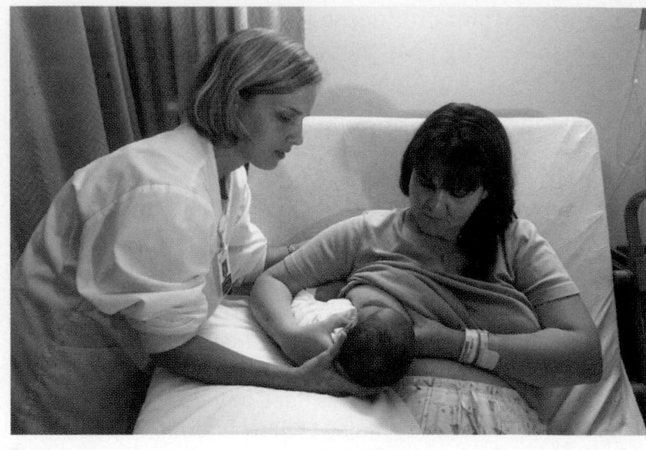
B

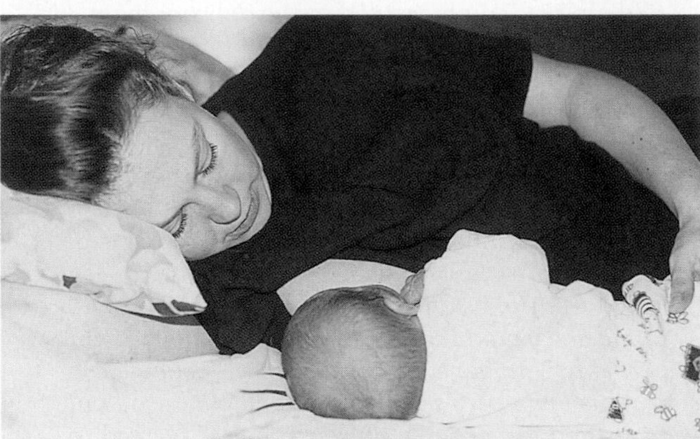
C

● ***Figure 14.2*** (**A**). The nurse is teaching the woman to use the cradle hold to breast-feed her newborn (photo © B. Proud). (**B**). The nurse is teaching the woman to use the football hold to breast-feed her newborn. Note how the woman's arm supports the newborn's body while the newborn's head rests in the palm of the woman's hand. (**C**). In the side-lying position, the woman can rest while feeding her newborn.

on his back during the nursing session or stretching his head over his shoulder to reach the breast (see Fig. 14-2C).

Latching On. After correct positioning, the next step is for the newborn to latch onto the breast. The newborn's mouth needs to be wide open with the tongue down at the floor of the mouth. When the newborn latches onto the breast he or she must take the entire nipple and part of the areola into the mouth. If the newborn takes only the nipple, the milk ducts will not be compressed sufficiently to empty the breast. It will also cause the woman's nipple to become sore and/or cracked and bleeding.

Have the woman make a "c" shape with her free hand and grasp the breast. Make sure that the woman's hand that is supporting the breast being offered does not bump into the newborn's jaw or prevent the jaw from making a good latch. The woman may need to reposition her hand so that it is closer to the chest wall and further from the newborn's jaw. Figure 14-3*A* shows the newborn positioned correctly on the breast, and Figure 14-3*B* shows how the newborn's mouth compresses the milk ducts.

When the newborn is latched onto the breast, make sure the woman does not dimple the breast near the newborn's mouth and nose. Many women will do this thinking they are providing breathing space for the newborn. This action can cause the nipple to be pulled out of the mouth completely, or it can cause the nipple to be pulled to the front of the mouth. If the nipple is toward the front of the newborn's mouth, the newborn's gums will compress it and cause sore nipples. This action can put pressure on the milk ducts, thereby reducing the flow of milk to the newborn, and also can prevent the breast from emptying completely.

Assessing the Breast-feeding Session. After the newborn has latched on and is nursing, the nurse needs to evaluate the effectiveness of the latch and sucking. A newborn who is correctly latched onto the breast will resist being pulled off of the breast. Audible swallowing, rhythmic jaw gliding, and seeing the areola dimple slightly near the newborn's mouth with sucking are positive signs that the newborn is latched on properly and sucking effectively.

In the postpartum period after the newborn has been nursing for a few minutes, many women report an increase in the flow of lochia or uterine cramping. This is a good indication that the newborn is nursing well. With effective sucking at the breast, the hormone

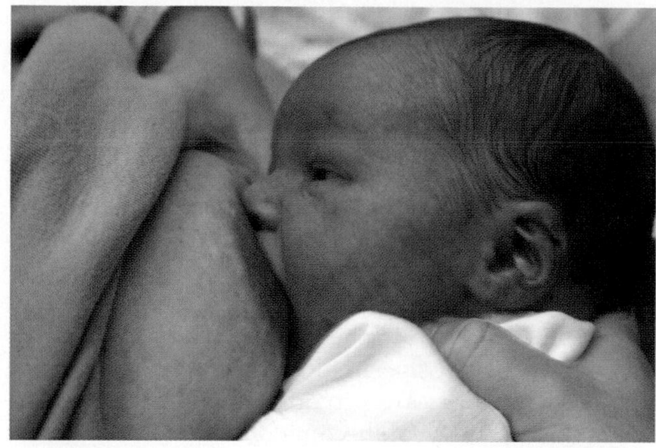

A

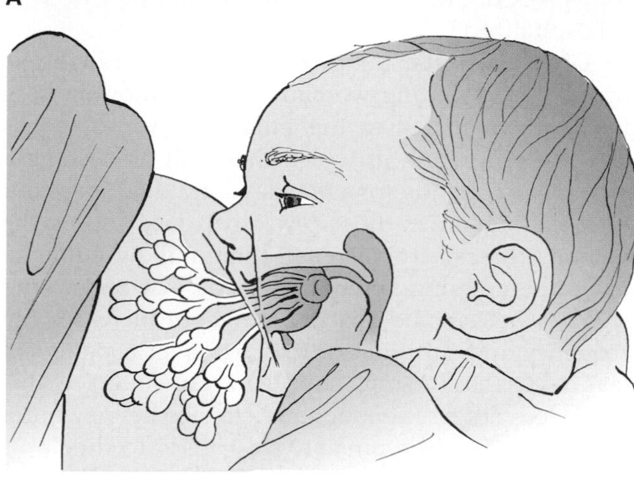

B

● ***Figure 14.3*** (**A**). Newborn with all of nipple and areola in mouth. (**B**). Diagram of newborn on breast correctly compressing milk ducts.

oxytocin is released, which causes uterine contractions. After her milk has come in, the woman may report leaking from the opposite breast or a let-down reflex. This is another good indication that the newborn is latched on and sucking well at the breast.

Ending the Breast-feeding Session. The nursing session should last approximately 10 to 20 minutes per breast. When the newborn is finished, the woman should remove the newborn from the breast. To do so, she should place her finger in the newborn's mouth, between the gums and cheek, to break the suction, and then gently pull the newborn away from the breast. It is important for her to break the suction first if the newborn is still latched on, or it might cause tissue damage to the breast.

After the feeding session, the woman may wish to burp her newborn. Because the newborn swallows less air during a breast-feeding session than in a bottle-feeding one, the newborn may not always burp. Three ways the woman may hold the newborn to burp is over the shoulder, sitting upright, or lying across her lap with the newborn's head elevated slightly above the level of its stomach.

After nursing, the woman should leave the flaps of her nursing bra open to allow her nipples to air dry. Some women express a few drops of colostrum or breast milk onto their nipples before letting them air dry to help with soreness or cracking of the nipples. If the woman has sore nipples, she can apply a purified lanolin ointment (Lansinoh) to her nipples after the nursing session.

Assessing Newborn Fluid Intake

The nurse should assess the newborn's fluid intake. A small bit of milk left in the mouth after the feeding is a good indication the newborn is sucking well. The newborn should be satiated between feedings and after nursing appear to be drowsy or asleep. By the end of the 3rd day of life, the newborn should have at least six very wet diapers and about three bowel movements per day. Newborns who are breast-fed exclusively will have a yellow or mustard colored seedy type of bowel movement that is very loose and not formed. The nurse should explain to the woman that this is normal for the breast-fed newborn. Many breast-fed newborns will have a bowel movement during the nursing session.

The newborn's weight should be monitored daily. The breast-feeding newborn should lose no more than 10% of his birth weight and should return to birth weight by 7 to 14 days of age. The nurse should evaluate the newborn's weight with regards to his feeding status and notify the registered nurse and the primary care provider if problems exist.

Teaching About Breast-feeding Special Concerns

The nurse has a very large role in teaching the breast-feeding woman. Items to be covered include tips on relieving common maternal breast-feeding problems; signs that the newborn is not feeding well; normal increases in the newborn's feeding schedule to accommodate for growth spurts; available resources for the breast-feeding woman; using supplements; breast-feeding amenorrhea; contraception while breast-feeding; and pumping and storing breast milk.

Relieving Common Maternal Breast-feeding Problems. The breast-feeding woman needs information regarding problems she may encounter at home. Some of the most commonly reported problems include sore nipples, engorgement, a plugged milk duct, or mastitis.

Sore Nipples. The newborn latching onto the breast incorrectly generally causes sore nipples. If the woman reports sore nipples or cracked and bleeding nipples, observe how the newborn latches on. The newborn's mouth must open wide, and she must take all of the nipple and part of the areola into the mouth. Other reasons for sore nipples are that the newborn may be a vigorous breast-feeder or the woman may have sensitive or tender skin.

Some women find rubbing a few drops of expressed breast milk onto their nipples after the nursing session helpful. A purified lanolin ointment (Lansinoh) may help other women. Contact the lactation consultant if the woman continues to have sore nipples and the newborn is latched on and positioned correctly.

Engorgement. **Engorgement** occurs when the milk comes in and the woman's body responds with increasing the blood supply to the breast tissues. The woman may have pain in her breasts because of swelling. Cold packs to the breast or warm showers; pumping a small amount of milk; and taking acetaminophen (Tylenol) will help alleviate the discomfort. Reassure the woman that this is temporary and will go away within a few days. Tell the woman not to completely empty her breasts between feedings, as this will increase her milk supply beyond the newborn's needs.

This is helpful advice. Many women with engorgement experience milk leaking from the breasts. Breast pads in the bra will help to absorb the leaking milk. Encourage the woman to change the bra pads as they become damp to avoid maceration or possible infection of the nipple and/or areola.

Plugged Milk Ducts. A common problem encountered during the nursing period is a plugged duct. This happens when one of the milk ducts becomes obstructed, causing a backup of the milk. The woman usually notices a sore, reddened, hard lump in one area of her breast. The woman should be taught to continue nursing; take acetaminophen (Tylenol); apply warm compresses and massage the site; nurse in different positions, including on her hands and knees to facilitate drainage of the breast; and to avoid constricting clothing or bras, including underwire bras. If the site does not improve within a few days, she should contact her health care provider.

Mastitis. Another common problem associated with breast-feeding is **mastitis.** Mastitis is an infection of the breast tissue. Women with mastitis usually describe having a run-down feeling or flu-like symptoms and a low-grade fever. Tell the woman not to ignore these signs and symptoms but to immediately report to her health care provider that she feels these symptoms and is breast-feeding. Treatment consists of antibiotics, analgesics, bed rest, and fluids. The woman needs to know that she can continue to breast-feed during this time. Mastitis will not affect her milk quality, and the antibiotics prescribed usually do not affect the newborn or infant. If the health care provider does prescribe medication that is contraindicated for breast-feeding and there is no alternative medication, the woman can pump and dump her breast milk and resume breast-feeding when the medication course is completed.

Signs the Newborn Is Not Feeding Well. The woman also needs to be taught to evaluate how well her newborn is nursing and when to call for help. Dry mouth, not enough wet diapers per day, difficulty rousing the newborn for a feeding, not enough feedings per day, or difficulty with latching on or sucking are signs that the newborn is not receiving enough breast milk. Explain to the woman that if she notices any of these signs, she should immediately contact the newborn's health care provider and a lactation consultant. Newborns can become dehydrated and suffer from a lack of nutrition very quickly and may need to be hospitalized.

Growth Spurts. Another important teaching topic for the breast-feeding woman is information on how the newborn increases the milk supply. Newborns have growth spurts in which they will nurse longer and more frequently for a few days and then space out their feedings after those few days. This causes the woman's breasts to increase their milk volume to match the growing newborn's needs. A woman who does not understand that the newborn increases the frequency and duration of feedings over a period of days to increase the milk supply may misinterpret this as she does not have enough milk to feed her newborn. This may cause the woman to stop breast-feeding.

Available Resources for the Breast-feeding Woman. The breast-feeding woman needs to be made aware of the many resources available to assist her and her newborn with breast-feeding. Lactation consultants, the La Leche League, and breast-feeding support groups in the community can give both practical and emotional support to the breast-feeding woman.

Lactation consultants are found in the hospital, in the community, and sometimes in the primary care provider's office. In the hospital, lactation consultants can help the woman with positioning and getting the newborn latched on and sucking. After discharge, the hospital may provide follow-up visits or telephone calls to the woman to help ensure that the newborn is breast-feeding as expected. The newborn's pediatrician may have an agreement with a lactation consultant who can provide assistance to the breast-feeding woman.

The La Leche League is a national organization that provides support, education, and literature to the breast-feeding woman. The woman can find the League listed in the telephone book, or the hospital may provide the woman with the telephone number of the local chapter. In addition, the hospital may have a list of breast-feeding support groups the woman can join; these groups can provide both breast-feeding support and socialization.

Using Supplements. Many women have questions about supplements for their nursing newborn. The newborn who is being breast-fed does not need supplemental bottles of water. The foremilk is watery, and the newborn will nurse only a little if thirsty. This will provide the newborn with all fluid needs. In the hospital, newborns are not started on any vitamin or iron supplements. The follow-up health care provider will instruct the woman on when and what types, if any, of supplements the newborn may need.

The woman should be informed that her breast milk is nutritionally superior to any other newborn food and that the newborn should not be started on any solids, including rice cereal, until at least 6 months of age. If there is a family history of allergies, solids should be delayed even longer. Breast milk will exclusively provide the newborn with all of her nutritional needs for the first 12 months.

Breast-feeding Amenorrhea. A very important topic of which the breast-feeding woman should be aware is breast-feeding amenorrhea. The return of the woman's menstrual cycle occurs between 6 to 10 weeks after delivery. The first postpartum menstrual cycle is anovulatory in 75% of women. The woman who is breast-feeding exclusively (i.e., without providing any supplemental bottles or solids) may experience breast-feeding **amenorrhea.** Some women who exclusively breast-feed may not have a return of their menstrual cycle for several months. The woman needs to know that ovulation can happen in the absence of a menstrual period, and she can become pregnant. It is important for her to use contraception during this time.

Contraception While Breast-feeding. The breast-feeding woman needs information about her choices in contraception. Contraception that contains hormones, especially estrogen, can lead to a decrease in the milk supply in the breast-feeding woman. The woman should be informed of this and make alternative contraceptive choices if breast-feeding is to continue. The first choice of contraception for the breast-feeding woman should be nonhormonal. If she chooses a hormonal type of contraception, a nonestrogen type, such as the mini-pill, should be offered before one that contains estrogen. Table 14-2 summarizes different contraceptive choices for the breast-feeding woman.

Pumping and Storing Breast Milk. The breast-feeding woman should be taught about pumping and storing her expressed breast milk. The woman who will be returning to work or school after giving birth can still breast-feed exclusively. The woman should breast-feed exclusively for at least 6 weeks before introducing the bottle. After 6 weeks, she should introduce one feeding per day of expressed breast milk. She also should pump her breasts during this bottle-feeding so her milk supply is not reduced. The bottle should be introduced only after she has established a good milk supply and the newborn is nursing well.

TABLE 14.2 Contraceptive Choices for the Breast-feeding Woman

Nonhormonal		Hormonal	
Permanent	Temporary	Nonestrogen	Estrogen
Tubal ligation Vasectomy	Abstinence Condom Diaphragm Spermicide	Mini-pill Depo-Provera	Birth control pill

Pumping. The woman should wash her hands before pumping her breasts and should use clean equipment. It is recommended the woman use a hospital-grade, dual electric breast pump, which pumps both breasts at the same time (Fig. 14-4). It may be necessary for the woman to use techniques to aid the let-down reflex. Bilaterally massaging the breasts and applying warm packs aids in the let-down of the milk. The woman may also find that looking at a picture of her infant and mentally thinking about her infant's smell, texture, and sounds aids in having a let-down reflex. At home, the woman may want to pump one breast while having the infant nurse on the opposite breast because this will aid her in having a let-down reflex and allow her to collect more breast milk.

Pumping of both breasts at the same time has been shown to increase the quantity of milk expressed at one sitting. The woman should be encouraged to pump until the flow of milk has stopped, usually about 15 to 20 minutes. When she is done pumping, she can refrigerate, freeze, or feed her infant the expressed

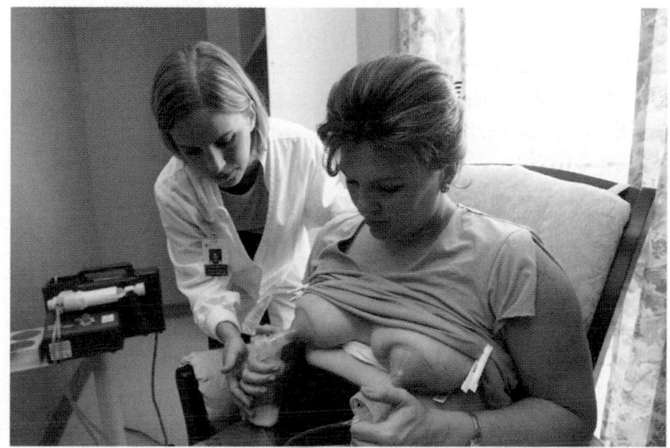

● ***Figure 14.4*** The nurse is assisting the woman to use a hospital pump to pump milk from both breasts at the same time.

breast milk immediately. She also needs to clean her equipment right after pumping. Tap water and a small amount of dish soap are usually sufficient to clean the equipment.

After pumping, she may want to rub a small amount of breast milk onto her nipples and allow them to air dry before covering them with a bra. If the woman experiences soreness with the breast pump, check to make sure she is using it properly and starting the pumping session at the lowest suction necessary.

Storing Breast Milk. Breast milk should be stored in hard plastic bottles or breast milk bags but not in glass containers. There are bags made especially for breast milk storage, and these should be used and not plastic bottle liners. The leukocytes in breast milk adhere to the glass, and this decreases the bacteriostatic properties of the milk. Breast milk should be reheated by placing the bottle/bag into a pan of hot water. It should not be heated in the microwave because this kills the antibodies in breast milk. In addition, milk reheated in the microwave may have hot spots that could burn the newborn's mouth and esophagus. See Table 14-3 provides a timetable for breast milk storage.

Test Yourself

- In what three positions can a woman hold her newborn to breast-feed?
- How can the nurse assess the effectiveness of the newborn's breast-feeding?
- What common problems might a breast-feeding woman encounter?

TABLE 14.3 Breast Milk Storage

Location of Storage	Duration of Storage
Room temperature (19°C–22°C)	Up to 10 hours
Refrigerator (0°C–4°C)	Up to 8 days
Freezer with door opening frequently	2 weeks
Separate freezer compartment with door opening frequently	4 months
Separate deep freeze	6 months
Thawed after being frozen	24 hours

FORMULA FEEDING

Artificial nutrition, that is infant formula or another type of animal milk, has been given to infants since ancient times. In the United States, commercially prepared infant formula has been around since the early 1900s. Today there are several brands available to women who choose not to breast-feed or who need a supplemental formula. There are differences in the composition of formulas available in the hospital. There are also alternative formulas to meet specific infant needs.

Advantages and Disadvantages of Formula Feeding

Infant formulas are helpful in certain circumstances. Many women choose to forgo breast-feeding and feed their infant only formula. The woman who chooses to do so should not be made to feel guilty regarding her decision. However, the nurse should make sure that the woman has made an informed decision and has heard the advantages of breast-feeding before feeding her infant formula.

Advantages

There are specific circumstances in which formula feeding is necessary. These include infants who are adopted or cases in which breast-feeding would be harmful to the infant. In some cases the woman may need to temporarily stop breast-feeding, such as for surgery or while taking a medication that can pass to the infant through the breast milk. For many women, it is easier to quantify how much the infant has consumed with formula feeding than with breast-feeding, which reduces their worries about the infant getting enough to eat. Some women feel it is easier to formula feed than to breast-feed their infant. Formula feeding also allows others to be involved in the infant's care by feeding the infant and preparing the formula and bottles for feeding.

There are certain maternal circumstances in which breast-feeding is discouraged and the newborn should be fed formula. These include maternal illicit drug use, the woman who is receiving chemotherapy, the woman who has HIV or one who has herpetic lesions on her breast.

If the newborn has an inborn error of metabolism, such as phenylketonuria, maple sugar urine disease, or galactosemia, the newborn needs a specific formula that the newborn can digest to avoid or minimize the problems associated with such diseases.

There are women who are opposed to or repulsed by the thought of breast-feeding. For these women, formula feeding gives them an alternative to nursing their newborn. For some women, the breast milk supply dries up sooner than expected. These women may need to formula feed until their newborn is old enough to wean. Some women do not make enough milk to supply the newborn's needs. These women may need to offer supplemental formula.

Disadvantages

Formula feeding has several disadvantages. It is inferior nutrition and has none of the immunologic properties provided by breast milk. Formula is harder for the newborn to digest than breast milk. There is a higher correlation between infants who are formula fed and some illnesses, such as otitis media and allergies.

Make sure the woman is informed! If the woman is on the Women, Infants, and Children's (WIC) program, the woman will need to purchase 25% of the formula because WIC is only a supplemental program.

Infant formula also is expensive. If the family is on a limited budget, formula feeding will create additional financial needs. In addition to buying the formula, the family will need to purchase bottles, nipples, and the equipment needed to clean these items.

There are more steps involved in formula feeding the newborn than in breast-feeding. With formula feeding, the woman or caregiver must mix the right amount of powder or formula concentrate to water; store the mixed preparation; warm it when the newborn is ready to eat; and then wash all of the utensils afterward. Formula can be purchased in three forms: ready to feed, concentrate, and powder. Because of the differences in formulation, there can be errors with the proper dilution of the formula. Errors in preparation can lead to under- and overnutrition in the newborn. These errors can result in serious illness and even death.

Composition of Formula

There are three main types of formula: milk-based, soy-based, and hypoallergenic formulas. Most term newborn formulas are derived from cow's milk and the main carbohydrate source is lactose or corn syrup solids. The protein used is a whey-casein blend to simulate what is found in breast milk. The iron composition in infant formula is defined as either high or low. Iron-fortified formulas contain 1.2 mg of iron per 100 mL. Iron-fortified, or high-iron formula, is the preferred formula to give to the healthy term newborn. Some women are reluctant to feed their newborn iron-fortified formula, thinking it will cause constipation. Studies have shown that there is no significant difference in constipation rates between infants fed iron-fortified and low-iron formulas.

Warn the woman that the newborn may be injured if formula is not properly mixed. Some women may be unable to afford formula and try to make the formula last longer by adding more water than the directions specify. This will cause malnutrition in the newborn. If too much powder is added to the water, the newborn will receive more calories per ounce. This can lead to an overweight infant or formula intolerance, with resulting diarrhea or emesis.

Alternative formulas are available for newborns with special medical needs. Soy-based infant formulas are for newborns who are allergic to cow's milk or when there is a strong family history of cow's milk allergies. Hypoallergenic formulas are for newborns with allergy or malabsorption problems. These formulas have the proteins partially or completely broken down in them. There are also a variety of formulas specially designed for specific medical conditions the newborn may have, including carbohydrate intolerance, impaired fat absorption, cystic fibrosis, congestive heart failure, and intestinal resection or short gut problems. These formulas should be given to the newborn only under a primary care provider's order. Some pediatricians will treat esophageal reflux with a formula thickened with some rice cereal or a specialized formula that already has rice cereal added to it.

There are many different compositions of formulas in the hospital. Formulas vary based on the needs of the newborn. Preterm formulas differ from term formulas in the amounts of vitamins and minerals and caloric and iron content. Preterm formulas have higher levels of sodium, potassium, calcium, and iron than do term infant formulas. Term formula, like breast milk, has 20 calories per ounce, whereas preterm formulas have 22 or 24 calories per ounce. See Table 14-4 for a comparison of different brands of formulas.

Nursing Care of the Formula Feeding Woman

The nurse in the hospital has three major roles when assisting the bottle-feeding woman. These are assisting with formula-feeding technique, assessing the formula-feeding woman and newborn, and teaching about special concerns of formula feeding.

Assisting With Formula-Feeding Technique

In the hospital, standard infant formula comes ready to feed. This means that the nurse does not need to mix or add any additives to the formula before feeding the newborn. The first step in feeding the formula-fed newborn

TABLE 14.4 Comparison of Common Formulas

Category	Formulas (Manufacturer's Name)	Newborn Population/Medical Condition for which Formula Designed
Milk-based formulas	Enfamil (Mead-Johnson), Good Start (Nestle), Similac (Ross)	For full-term healthy newborns
Soy-based formulas	Isomil (Ross), ProSobee (Mead Johnson), Soyalac (Loma Linda)	Milk protein allergy, lactose intolerance, lactase deficiency, or galactosemia
	Lactofree (Mead Johnson)	Lactose intolerance, lactase deficiency
Specific medical conditions	RCF (Ross Carbohydrate Free) (Ross)	Carbohydrate intolerance
	Portagen (Mead Johnson)	Impaired fat absorption, intestinal resection, lymphatic anomalies
	Nutramigen (Mead Johnson)	Protein sensitivity, galactosemia, malabsorption problems
	Pregestimil (Mead Johnson)	Malabsorption syndromes, cystic fibrosis, intestinal resection, short gut syndrome
	Alimentum (Ross)	Food protein sensitivity, cystic fibrosis
	Lonalac (Mead Johnson)	Congestive heart failure, reduced sodium intake
	Similac PM 60/40 (Ross)	Infants predisposed to hypocalcemia and infants with impaired renal, digestive, and cardiovascular functions
	Lofenalac (Mead Johnson), Phenyl-free (Mead Johnson), Phenex-1 (Ross), Phenex-2 (Ross), Pro-Phree (Ross)	Phenylketonuria
	Similac Special Care (Ross), Premature Enfamil (Mead Johnson), Neosure (Ross)	Premature infants

Note: This is not an exhaustive list of all of the types of formulas available or conditions for which formulas may be used.

is to check the primary care provider's order. Many primary care providers have a preference regarding which formula the woman should feed her newborn. Check the label on the formula bottle before taking it to the woman to feed her newborn. Make sure the brand, caloric content, and iron composition matches that of the primary care provider's order.

Compare the newborn's and woman's ID bands to ensure a match. Use pillows as needed to ensure the woman is in a comfortable position and can hold and see her newborn easily. Make sure the woman is in a comfortable position sitting upright. The formula-feeding woman should not feed her newborn in a lying down position. The newborn should be in a semireclined position in the woman's arms. An angle of at least 45 degrees is preferred (Fig. 14-5).

This tip could save a life! It is easier for the newborn to aspirate while sucking from a bottle. Instruct the woman to keep the light on in the room so that she can observe her newborn during the whole feeding.

Teach the woman to assess her newborn's hunger cues and her newborn's ability to suck, swallow, and breathe during the feeding. The woman should also observe her newborn's color while eating. Instruct the woman on what to do if the newborn starts to choke during the feeding. Make sure the nasal aspirator and a burp cloth are within the woman's reach.

Teach the woman not to prop! Sometimes the woman will prop the bottle against a surface so that she does not have to hold the bottle while the newborn sucks. This practice increases the newborn's risk of aspiration and can lead to overfeeding and baby bottle syndrome. Propping the bottle also decreases opportunities for positive bonding with the baby.

Gently shake the bottle of formula because some settling of contents may occur. Attach a sterile nipple and ring unit to the

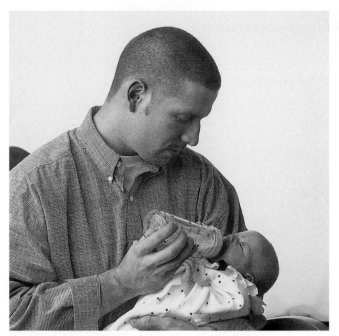

● ***Figure 14.5*** A newborn receives a formula feeding from her father. Notice the correct positioning.

bottle. The woman should feed 1 to 2 ounces at a feeding in the immediate newborn period. She should burp her newborn after every ½ ounce is consumed. As the newborn grows, she should advance the feeding amount slowly, no more than ½ to 1 ounce per feeding. Instruct the woman regarding cues that the newborn is satiated and finished eating. If the newborn consumes too much formula at one time, emesis or diarrhea may result.

The nurse can assist the bottle-feeding woman by feeding the newborn if the woman is unable to (e.g., she is having surgery) or if she is sleeping and requests her newborn to be fed in the nursery during the night.

Assessing the Formula-Feeding Woman and Newborn

The nurse should assess the newborn's feeding ability, amount of formula consumed at each feeding, tolerance of the infant formula, and the woman's comfort level with formula feeding her newborn. Any signs that the newborn is not sucking well, has difficulty swallowing and breathing, or is not tolerating the formula should be reported to the nurse in charge immediately. Signs the newborn is not tolerating the formula include emesis and diarrhea. These assessments should be reported to the nurse in charge. Also assess the newborn's bowel movements. Explain to the woman that her newborn's stool should progress from meconium to transitional and then to a pasty yellow solid consistency (see Chapter 15).

Teaching About Formula Feeding Special Concerns

The nurse has a large role in teaching the formula-feeding woman. Teaching topics include how to prepare bottles of formula, adding supplements to the bottle, maternal breast care, and managing common problems in the formula-fed newborn.

Preparing Bottles of Formula. Teach the woman about the different forms of formula and how to mix each type. Powder formula is the least expensive and requires the addition of water. Concentrate also requires the addition of water but is more costly than the powder form. Ready-to-feed formula is the most expensive but does not require the addition of any water to the formula before feeding. Explain the importance of preparing the formula according to the package directions because malnutrition or dehydration can result from adding too much or too little water to the formula.

The woman will need to know what type of water to add to the powder or concentrate type of formula. This depends on what type of water she has available (e.g., city tap, well, or purified bottled water). She should be taught to mix only as much formula as the newborn needs in 24 hours. After mixing, the formula needs to be refrigerated. After 24 hours, unused formula should be discarded.

Teach the woman how to warm cold formula. The bottle containing the formula should be placed in a pan of hot water until the formula is warm. The bottle should be shaken before feeding the newborn. The microwave should never be used to warm the formula because it can create hot spots that could burn the newborn. When the newborn has finished eating, any remaining formula should be discarded. This is because as the newborn sucks, saliva mixes with the formula and remains in the bottle, and then digestive enzymes in the saliva begin to break down the remaining formula.

Teach the woman to wash the feeding utensils in hot soapy water or in the dishwasher after every feeding. Sterilizing the bottles and nipples is not necessary after each feeding.

Adding Supplements. The newborn's primary care provider will determine if and when the newborn needs any type of supplementation, such as multivitamins or fluoride. Teach the woman that the newborn does not need any other type of nutrition.

Contradict a wives' tale! Some women add rice cereal to the formula because they have heard that doing so will make the newborn sleep longer. This should not be done unless recommended by a primary care provider for a specific reason, such as reflux.

TABLE 14.5 Amount of Formula and Other Foods the Newborn and Infant Should Be Receiving

Age	Amount of Formula	Other Foods
Birth to 4 months	2–6 ounces per feeding 20–24 ounces per day	None
4–6 months	4–6 ounces per feeding 24–32 ounces per day	Infant cereal mixed with formula
6–8 months	6 8 ounces per feeding 24–32 ounces per day	Baby cereal, soft mashed fruits and vegetables, no more than 3–4 ounces of fruit juice
8–10 months	7–8 ounces per feeding 21–32 ounces per day	Same as 6–8 months and begin to add pureed meats
10–12 months	16–32 ounces per day	Same as 8–10 months but consistency may be firmer and portions may be slightly bigger

Instruct her not to add anything to the formula. Some pediatricians tell parents to offer infant cereal mixed with formula, but not juice, around 4 to 6 months. The woman should not begin to feed solid foods until the infant's primary care provider has recommended it, usually around 6 to 8 months of age. Around 12 months of age, the infant's primary care provider will discuss weaning the infant from the formula.

Maternal Breast Care. Women who choose to formula feed exclusively need to know how to care for their breasts in the immediate postpartum period. Explain to the woman that she will produce milk, even though she is not nursing, and that this is a normal physiologic process in response to giving birth. The woman will experience engorgement when her milk comes in. She should be taught not to express any milk because this will continue the milk production process. She should wear a tight bra; the constriction will help prevent leaking and aid in the drying up of the milk supply. In addition, a tight bra will help lessen discomfort from the full breasts. Some women benefit from having their breasts bound tightly with an elastic-type bandage. In the past, some primary care providers prescribed medications that would aid in the drying up of the woman's milk supply. However, it was determined that the benefit of their use did not outweigh the associated risks.

Common Problems in the Formula-Fed Newborn. The woman needs to be taught to monitor for problems in the formula-fed newborn. These include the newborn not wanting to eat, not tolerating the formula, and dental caries.

The woman who is formula feeding is able to accurately determine how many ounces per feeding and per day the newborn is receiving. Table 14-5 lists the amount of formula and other foods the newborn and infant should be receiving at different ages. If the newborn or infant is not taking in enough formula for his age and weight, dehydration may result, and the infant may not gain sufficient weight to develop appropriately and be healthy. If a newborn or infant is refusing to eat, the woman should contact the pediatrician because there may be an underlying medical condition.

Some newborns take in the recommended amount of formula and then have large amounts of emesis after or during feedings. This also needs to be brought to the attention of the newborn's primary care provider because this is not an acceptable situation for growth and nutrition. This may be a symptom of overfeeding, gastroesophageal reflux, formula intolerance, or an underlying medical condition. The nurse should ask the woman the following questions: How much formula is the newborn taking per feeding and per day? When does emesis occur (during or after the feeding, with burps, or with repositioning)? How much emesis does the newborn have per episode? What is the consistency of the emesis? Which formula is being fed, and how is it prepared? What other foods are being fed? The answers to these questions will assist the nurse and the primary care provider to determine the probable cause of the emesis.

If the newborn has diarrhea, this also needs to be investigated. Again, the nurse needs to ask specific questions: How much and what type of formula is the newborn being fed, and how is it prepared? How many episodes of diarrhea has the newborn had in the past 24 hours? What is the consistency of the bowel movement, and is there blood present in the stool? It is important to assess the newborn's intake and output to check for dehydration, as well as to physically examine the child. Possible causes are overfeeding, illness, formula intolerance, or an underlying medical condition.

Inform the parents that newborns and infants can become dehydrated much more quickly than adults can, and that any cases of emesis or diarrhea should be quickly reported to the nurse in the hospital or the primary care provider if the newborn or infant is at home.

Infants can develop dental caries from frequent sucking on a bottle that is filled with milk or juice. This situation has been referred to as "baby bottle syndrome" or "bottle-mouth caries." Often this happens when parents give the infant a bottle at bedtime and the infant sucks on the bottle throughout the night. The frequent exposure of the immature teeth to high levels of sugars found in the milk or juice leads to dental caries. The parents should be informed not to give the infant a bottle when he or she is in the crib. They also should not allow the toddler to carry a bottle around; this practice of continual drinking of formula increases the risk of damage to the infant's teeth and is associated with a higher incidence of aspiration and otitis media.

Test Yourself

- What different types of formula are there?
- When is formula feeding an advantage?
- What topics should the nurse cover when teaching a woman to formula feed?

KEY POINTS

- The woman's decision to breast-feed is influenced by several factors. Some of these factors include culture, age, education, past experience with breast-feeding, and the woman's intent to return to work or school.
- Maternal advantages of breast-feeding include more rapid uterine involution, less bleeding in the postpartum period, and less ovarian and premenopausal breast cancers. Newborn advantages to breast-feeding include a strengthened immune system, fewer overweight infants, and lower incidences of certain infections, such as otitis media, diarrhea, and lower respiratory tract infections.
- There are certain situations in which breast-feeding is not recommended. Maternal situations include a woman actively using illegal drugs, one who has untreated tuberculosis, one with HIV, or a woman receiving chemotherapy medications. Newborn conditions that would exclude breast-feeding include the newborn with galactosemia.
- The breast is under both physical and chemical control to stimulate lactation. The hormones prolactin and oxytocin stimulate milk production and release from the breast. The newborn sucking on and emptying the breast also leads to milk production.
- When assisting a woman to breast-feed, the nurse should provide for privacy, help the woman into a comfortable position, help the woman to hold her newborn correctly, and assess the newborn for a correct latching on and positioning on the breast. The nurse should assess the woman's breasts and nipples, her comfort level with breast-feeding, her support systems, and the newborn's feeding ability.
- When caring for a woman with sore nipples, the nurse should observe the latching on and the positioning of the newborn during nursing. A few drops of expressed breast milk or a purified lanolin treatment applied to the nipples after breast-feeding may help with the soreness.
- When caring for a woman with a plugged milk duct, the nurse should advise the breast-feeding woman to apply warm packs to the site, take a warm shower, take acetaminophen (Tylenol), nurse in different positions, avoid constrictive clothing or bras, and massage the site.
- When caring for a woman with mastitis, the nurse should advise the breast-feeding woman to contact her health care provider, take the antibiotics as prescribed, and continue to breast-feed even on the affected side. If breast-feeding is too uncomfortable on the affected side, she should pump the milk at each feeding so her milk supply does not diminish.
- Signs that a newborn is not breast-feeding well include dry mouth, fewer than expected wet or dirty diapers, difficulty rousing the newborn for feedings, and not enough feedings per day.
- Breast milk is superior to formula because it is easier to digest and has immunologic, bacteriocidal, and fungicidal properties that cannot be duplicated in artificial nutrition. Breast milk is economical and ready to feed and requires no special preparation or storage.
- There are many types of formulas available. The type of formula offered depends upon the newborn's gestational age and medical needs. The formulas for healthy term infants differ from the formula made for specific medical conditions. The formulas vary in types of protein sources, caloric content, and mineral and electrolyte concentrations.
- The formula-feeding woman needs education in the areas of preparation and storage of formula,

care of feeding utensils, how formula is available in the store, and the WIC program.

- Formula feeding would be beneficial in cases in which the woman is unavailable to breast-feed, such as adoption, surgery, or taking a medication that passes through the breast milk and would be harmful to the newborn. Formula feeding also is beneficial when the newborn has a specific medical condition, such as galactosemia.
- The formula-feeding woman should be taught how to feed her newborn and how much and when to increase feedings, how to prepare and store the formula and care for the equipment, how to care for her breasts after delivery, and when to notify the nurse or pediatrician.
- For the formula-fed newborn who is having emesis or diarrhea, the nurse should ask: What type of formula is the newborn on and how is it prepared? How much is the newborn eating per session and per day? What does the emesis/bowel movement look like? What other foods are being consumed by the newborn? How much emesis is there per episode? How many episodes has the newborn had in the last 24 hours?

REFERENCES AND SELECTED READINGS

Books and Journals

Blackburn, S. T., & Loper, D. L. (1992). *Maternal, fetal, and neonatal physiology*. Philadelphia: WB Saunders.

Conkin, C., Campbell, J., Montgomery, C. E., & Phillips, S. (Eds.). (2002). *Pediatric nutrition reference guide*. Houston, TX: Texas Children's Hospital.

Lawrence, R. A., & Lawrence, R. M. (1999). *Breastfeeding: A guide for the medical profession* (5th ed.). St. Louis: Mosby.

Riordan, J., & Auerbach, K. G. (1998). *Breastfeeding and human lactation* (2nd ed.). Sudbury: Jones and Bartlett Publishers.

Websites

American Academy of Pediatrics
http://aappolicy.aappublications.org

National Guideline Clearinghouse
http://www.guideline.gov

La Leche League International
http://www.lalecheleague.org

World Health Organization
http://www.who.int/nut/inf.htm

WORKBOOK

NCLEX-STYLE REVIEW QUESTIONS

1. A woman tells the nurse, "I don't need to use any contraception because I plan on breast-feeding exclusively." Upon which fact should the nurse base her response?
   a. Women who exclusively breast-feed do not ovulate.
   b. Ovulation can occur even in the absence of menstruation.
   c. The birth control pill is the best form of contraception for breast-feeding women.
   d. Breast-feeding women should not use contraception because it will decrease their milk supply.
2. During a prenatal visit an 18-year-old G 1 P 0 in her 36th week says to the nurse, "I don't know if I should breast-feed or not. Isn't formula just as good for the baby?" Upon what information should the nurse base her response?
   a. The benefits of breast-feeding are equal to those of formula feeding.
   b. It is ultimately the woman's choice whether she wants to breast-feed or not.
   c. The immunologic properties in breast milk cannot be duplicated in formula.
   d. The economic status of the woman is an important breast-feeding consideration.
3. The nurse is assessing the breast-feeding woman during a feeding session. What assessment has priority during the feeding session?
   a. Assess the position, latching on, and sucking of the newborn.
   b. Assess the woman's visitors and their opinions regarding breast-feeding.
   c. Check the woman's perineal pad for increased lochia flow.
   d. Determine if the woman needs a visit from the lactation consultant.

STUDY ACTIVITIES

1. Use the following table to compare information contained in your nursing pharmacology reference with information the hospital lactation specialist has on medications and their use during breast-feeding. If the two references disagree, from where did the lactation specialist get her information? Which information do you think is more accurate? Why?

Medication	Pharmacology Reference	Lactation Specialist
Magnesium sulfate		
Phenobarbital		
Depo-Provera		
Vicodin		
Coumadin		

2. Call your local WIC clinic. Interview the nurse to determine what she does to encourage the woman to breast-feed the newborn.
3. Interview the lactation consultant at the local hospital. What foods does she tell the woman to avoid when she is breast-feeding, and why? How many calories should the woman consume? How much liquid should she drink? Share your findings with your clinical group.

CRITICAL THINKING: What Would You Do?

Apply your knowledge of newborn nutrition to the following situations.

1. You are working in the prenatal clinic. Here is a list of several of the patients you encounter and the questions they ask you.
   a. Sally is a 20-year-old G 1 P 0. She tells you she is unsure about feeding her baby and asks you if she should breast-feed or bottle-feed. How would you respond?
   b. Betsy, a G 3 P 1, states she needs to return to work 6 weeks after the baby is born. "I don't know if it's even worth it to begin to breast-feed when I know I'll just have to stop in 6 weeks. It seems like a lot of work." How would you respond?
   c. Elizabeth is a 15-year-old G 1 P 0. She asks you, "I don't want to breast-feed, but I heard you still make milk after the baby is born. How do you stop it from happening?" How would you respond to Elizabeth's question?

2. You are working the mother–baby unit at the hospital. Here are some of your patients for the day and the questions they ask you.

   a. Susan is a 24-year-old G 3 P 1. She delivered 1 day ago and wants to breast-feed. When you examine her newborn, she tells you that she thinks she doesn't have enough milk to feed her baby and asks you to give her baby a bottle so he doesn't starve. How would you respond?

   b. It has been 3 days since Alicia's cesarean delivery, and she is formula feeding her newborn a milk-based formula. She tells you her baby spits up with every feeding. What questions would you ask her and why?

   c. Lanya is a 30-year-old G 2 P 2 who had a postpartum tubal ligation earlier today. It is time to breast-feed her baby, but her abdomen is sore. How would you suggest Lanya feed her newborn and why?

   d. Tricia is a 28-year-old G 1 P 1 who is formula-feeding. She asks you how to mix formula and how she should care for the bottles and nipples. What information would you give her and why?

   e. Maria is a 24-year-old G 1 P 1. She has some questions for you about how long her breast milk is good for after she pumps it. How would you respond?

The Normal Newborn

15

STUDENT OBJECTIVES

On completion of this chapter, the student should be able to

1. Explain how to support immediate transition from fetal to extrauterine life.
2. Illustrate how to assign an Apgar score to a newborn.
3. Outline principles of thermoregulation for the newborn.
4. Describe immediate care of the newborn to include eye prophylaxis and administration of vitamin K.
5. Explain the nurse's role in protecting the infant from misidentification in the hospital.
6. Intervene appropriately with the newborn who has hypoglycemia.
7. Institute effective infection control procedures in the nursery.
8. Protect the newborn from abduction.
9. Recognize signs of pain in the newborn.
10. Compare and contrast the care of the newborn male who is uncircumcised with that of one who is circumcised.
11. Explain what immunizations should be given and what newborn screening tests should be done before the newborn is discharged home.
12. Teach the parents normal newborn care.

KEY TERMS

circumcision
cold stress
kangaroo care
ophthalmia neonatorum
thermoneutral environment

As you learned in Chapter 13, the newborn must make rapid adjustments to successfully adapt to life outside of the womb. The nurse's role is to support the newborn as he adapts to these changes and quickly recognize the development of complications so that intervention can be initiated immediately. Teaching the parents the skills needed to care for their newborn is another critical role of the nurse. This chapter discusses the basic care that must be given when caring for newborns and their families.

● The Nursing Process in Immediate Stabilization and Transition of the Newborn

The current standard of care for resuscitation of the newborn immediately after birth is outlined in the Neonatal Resuscitation Program (NRP) (American Academy of Pediatrics NRP Steering Committee, 2000).[1] The basic principles of newborn resuscitation are reviewed here. Refer to an NRP textbook for detailed guidelines on newborn resuscitation. The licensed practical nurse (LPN) normally is not responsible for a complete resuscitation; however, an ability to initiate resuscitation and assist throughout the process is essential.

The first 6 to 12 hours after birth are a critical transition period for the newborn. The healthy newborn may stay with the mother immediately after delivery and be cared for by the same nurse who is overseeing the mother's recovery. In some facilities the newborn is taken to a transition nursery after a short initial bonding period with his parents. In either case, the nurse caring for the newborn during the transition period must be alert to early signs of distress and be ready to intervene quickly to prevent complications and poor outcomes.

ASSESSMENT

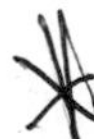

Immediate assessments of the newborn are concerned with the success of cardiopulmonary adaptation. A strong, healthy cry is usually the first response of the neonate to external stimuli, as discussed in Chapter 13. A vigorous or lusty cry, heart rate greater than 100 beats per minute (bpm), and pink color are associated with effective cardiopulmonary adaptation. These assessments are made rapidly during the first seconds after birth. If the newborn does not immediately cry, the cry is weak, or he does not meet the heart rate or color criteria, it is critical for the nurse to act quickly during the first minute after birth (see interventions in the following text).

A traditional immediate assessment of cardiopulmonary adaptation is the Apgar score. The Apgar score was developed by Dr. Virginia Apgar as a means of quickly assessing the success of the newborn's transition to extrauterine life. The score is no longer used as a guide to resuscitation, but it continues to be used to evaluate the effectiveness of resuscitation efforts and to help determine the intensity of care the newborn will require in the first few days of life.

Five parameters are used to determine the total Apgar score: heart rate, respiratory effort, muscle tone, reflex irritability, and color. Each factor receives a score of 0 to 2 points, for a maximum total score of 10 (Table 15-1). Apgar scoring is performed by the nurse and recorded in the delivery room record at 1 and 5 minutes after birth. If the newborn receives a score of less than 7 at 5 minutes, scoring is continued every 5 minutes until the score is 7 or above, the newborn is intubated, or until the newborn is transferred to the nursery.

Scores of 7 to 10 at 5 minutes are indicative of a healthy baby who is adapting well to the extrauterine environment. These newborns typically do well and can be cared for in the regular newborn nursery or can room-in with their mothers. Scores between 4 and 6 at 5 minutes after birth indicate that the newborn is having some difficulty in adjusting to life outside the womb and needs close observation. These newborns are usually taken to a special nursery where they may receive oxygen and other special monitoring until their condition improves. Newborns who receive a score of 0 to 3 at 5 minutes are experiencing severe difficulty in making the transition to extrauterine life. These infants usually require observation and care in a neonatal intensive care unit (NICU).

During the transition period, continue to observe the newborn for signs of respiratory distress or cardiovascular compromise. As you will recall from Chapter 13, signs of respiratory distress include nasal flaring, tachypnea, grunting, sternal retractions, and seesaw respirations. Observe for excess mucus, which could obstruct the airway. Measure the heart and respiratory rates at least every 30 minutes during the first 2 hours of transition.

Observe the newborn closely for **cold stress,** which is a body temperature of less than 97.6°F

[1] Developed and maintained by the American Heart Association (AHA) and the American Academy of Pediatrics (AAP).

TABLE 15.1 Apgar Scoring

Apgar scoring is done at 1 and 5 minutes after birth. The newborn is considered to be "vigorous" if the initial scores are 7 and above. If the 5-minute score is less than 7, scoring is done every 5 minutes thereafter until the score reaches 7. The numbers in the left-hand column represent the number of points that are assigned to each parameter when the criteria in the corresponding column are met.

	Heart Rate	Respiratory Effort	Muscle Tone	Reflex Irritability	Color
2	Heart rate above 100 beats per minutes (bpm)	Strong, vigorous cry	Maintains a position of flexion with brisk movements	Cries or sneezes when stimulated*	Body and extremities pink
1	Heart rate present, but less than 100 bpm	Weak cry, slow or difficult respirations	Minimal flexion of extremities	Grimaces when stimulated	Body pink, extremities blue (acrocyanosis)
0	No heart rate	No respiratory effort	Limp and flaccid	No response to stimulation	Body and extremities blue (cyanosis) or completely pale (pallor)

* Stimulation is provided by suctioning the infant or by gently flicking the sole of the foot.

(36.5°C). Use a thermal skin probe for continuous temperature assessment while the newborn is under the radiant warmer. Measure the axillary temperature at least every 30 minutes until the temperature stabilizes. Then check the temperature again at 4 hours and at 8 hours. If the temperature remains stable, it may be assessed every 8 hours until discharge.

Hypoglycemia is a potential problem that can, if prolonged, have devastating effects on the newborn. Therefore, it is critical for the nurse to know signs and symptoms of hypoglycemia in the newborn, which include:

- Jitteriness or tremors
- Exaggerated Moro reflex
- Irritability
- Lethargy
- Poor feeding
- Listlessness
- Apnea or respiratory distress
- High-pitched cry

The main sign of hypoglycemia is jitteriness, which can be exhibited as an exaggerated Moro reflex. Conversely, the hypoglycemic newborn may have no symptoms. If hypoglycemia is prolonged without treatment, the newborn may have seizures or lapse into a coma. Permanent brain damage can result, leading to lifelong disability.

The nurse must be familiar with factors that increase the risk for hypoglycemia in the newborn (Box 15-1). Any condition that adversely affects blood flow to the placenta during pregnancy puts the newborn at risk for hypoglycemia. If the mother's blood sugar was elevated during the latter part of the pregnancy, such as in maternal diabetes, or if she received medications that elevate her blood sugar, the newborn also is at risk for hypoglycemia. Any condition that puts physiologic stress on the fetus, such as prolonged labor or maternal infection, may deplete glycogen stores, putting the newborn at risk for low blood sugar.

BOX 15.1 Risk Factors for Hypoglycemia

History of any of the following during the pregnancy increases the risk that the newborn will develop hypoglycemia.

- Gestational hypertension
- Maternal diabetes (pre-existing or gestational)
- Prolonged labor
- Fetal distress during labor
- Ritodrine or terbutaline administered to mother

Newborn characteristics that increase the risk for hypoglycemia. Note that many of these conditions result from an at-risk pregnancy.

- Intrauterine growth restriction (IUGR)
- Macrosomia (a very large baby)
- Large-for-gestational age
- Small-for-gestational age
- Prematurity
- Postmaturity
- Respiratory or cardiovascular depression requiring resuscitation

This is a critical point. Never mistake jitteriness in the newborn for "shivering." If the newborn has shaky movements or startles easily, the first thing you should check is the blood sugar. This is particularly important because newborns can develop hypoglycemia even though there are no recognizable risk factors for its development.

If a newborn is exhibiting signs of, or is at risk for, hypoglycemia, check the glucose level using a heel stick to obtain a blood sample for testing (Nursing Procedure 15-1). Blood levels between 40 and 60 mg/dL during the first 24 hours of life are considered normal. Levels less than 40 mg/dL are indicative of hypoglycemia in the newborn.

A full physical assessment, including gestational age assessment as discussed in Chapter 13, is completed within the first few hours of life.

SELECTED NURSING DIAGNOSES

- Impaired spontaneous ventilation related to ineffective transition to newborn life
- Risk for injury: hypoglycemia related to immature metabolism and/or presence of risk factors
- Ineffective thermoregulation related to immature heat-regulating mechanisms
- Risk for infection related to immature immune system, possible exposure to pathogens in the birth canal or in the nursery, and umbilical cord wound
- Risk for imbalanced fluid volume related to immature blood clotting mechanisms
- Risk for injury: misidentification related to failure of delivery room personnel to adequately identify the newborn before separation from the parents

PLANNING AND GOALS

Maintaining the safety of the newborn during transition from intrauterine to extrauterine life is the primary goal when planning care immediately after delivery and in the first 6 to 12 hours of life. Appropriate patient goals include that the newborn will experience adequate cardiovascular, respiratory, thermoregulatory, and metabolic transitions to extrauterine life, and that he will remain free from signs and symptoms of infection, maintain hemostasis, and will be adequately identified before separation from the parents.

IMPLEMENTATION

Supporting Cardiovascular and Respiratory Transition

Nursing interventions to support newborn vital functions begin before the birth occurs. If you will be assisting in the immediate care of the newborn, ensure that adequate supplies are present for a full resuscitation and that all equipment is functioning properly. Most delivery settings have a newborn resuscitation board that is stocked with needed supplies. Check that oxygen is readily available and that there is a functioning suction source. Ensure that a warmer is in the delivery area, and turn it on several minutes before the delivery is expected.

Observe the newborn carefully at birth. The delivery attendant will usually suction the mouth and nose with a bulb syringe and clamp and cut the umbilical cord. If the newborn cries vigorously, you may drape a blanket over the mother's abdomen and support the infant there when the birth attendant hands the newborn to you. Quickly palpate the base of the umbilical cord and count the pulse for 6 seconds. Multiply that number by 10 to calculate the heart rate. A pulse above 100 bpm and a vigorous cry are reassuring signs that indicate the newborn is making a successful transition.

If the newborn does not cry immediately, he must be transported to a preheated radiant warmer for prompt resuscitation. He should be dried quickly to prevent heat loss from evaporation and to provide stimulation to encourage a first breath. If the newborn still does not make adequate breathing efforts, a bag and mask connected to 100% oxygen are used to provide respiratory support until spontaneous breathing occurs.

Most newborns do not need to be resuscitated, and the ones who do generally respond well to a short period of positive-pressure ventilation with a bag and mask. However, a very small number of infants also require chest compressions, intubation, and medications. Refer to the NRP for complete resuscitation guidelines.

Give constant attention to the airway. Newborns often have abundant secretions. The initial intervention is to position the newborn on the side or with the head in a slightly lower position than the body to help prevent aspiration

Nursing Procedure 15.1 Performing a Heel Stick

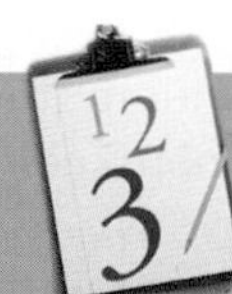

EQUIPMENT

Alcohol wipe
2 × 2 square gauze
Tape
Adhesive bandage
Warm pack
Lancet or other puncturing device
Device to read the glucose level and all supplies needed for its use
Clean gloves

PROCEDURE

1. Thoroughly wash your hands.
2. Place a warm pack on the newborn's heel for several minutes before attempting to obtain specimen.

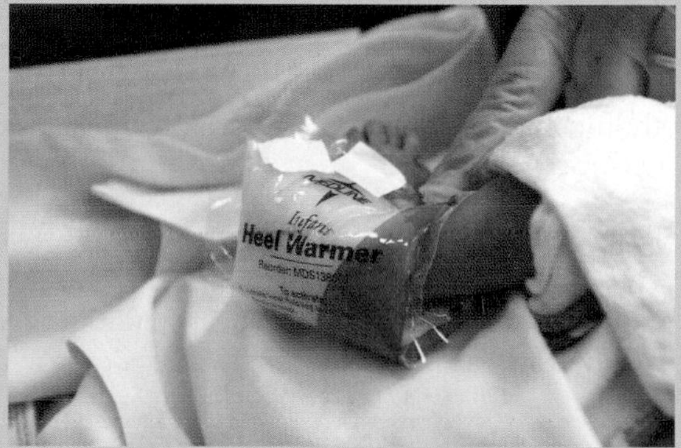

3. Don a pair of clean gloves.
4. Hold the foot so that it is well supported with your thumb or finger covering the flat surfaces of the foot to avoid puncturing this area and causing damage to nerves or blood vessels. The highlighted areas on the lateral aspects of the foot in the illustration are appropriate areas from which to perform a heel stick.

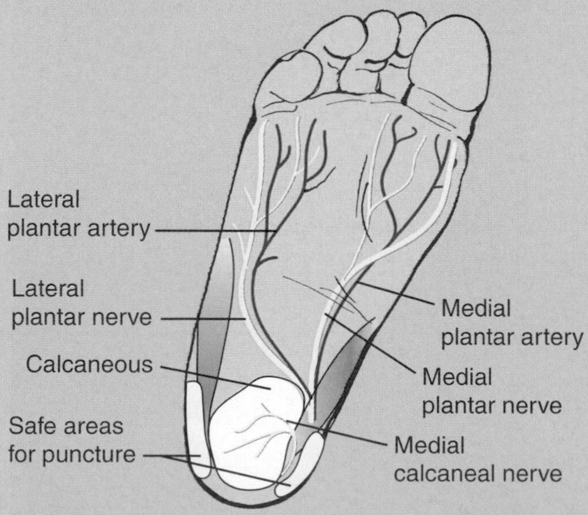

5. Locate a fat pad on either side of the foot. Palpate the chosen site to ensure there is enough padding to avoid puncturing the bone, which could lead to infection.
6. Clean the site with alcohol and allow to air dry.
7. Using the lancet, puncture the site to a depth of no greater than 2 mm. If using a commercial puncturing device, follow the manufacturer's guidelines for use. Place the lancet in a sharps container.

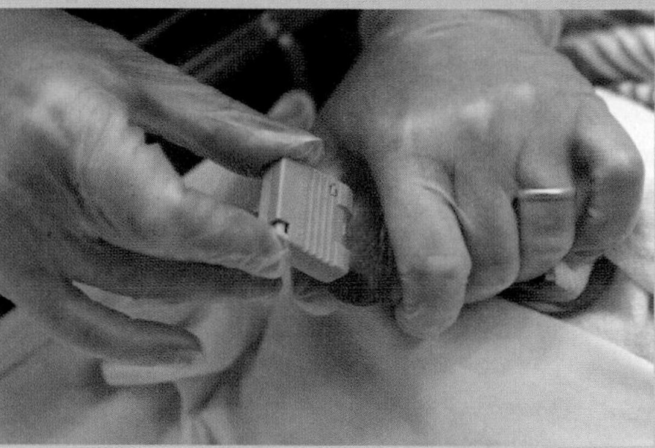

8. Wipe away the first drop of blood. Do not squeeze the tissue close to the puncture site or the reading may not be accurate.
9. Collect the specimen from the second drop of blood. Follow the manufacturer's instructions regarding processing the specimen.

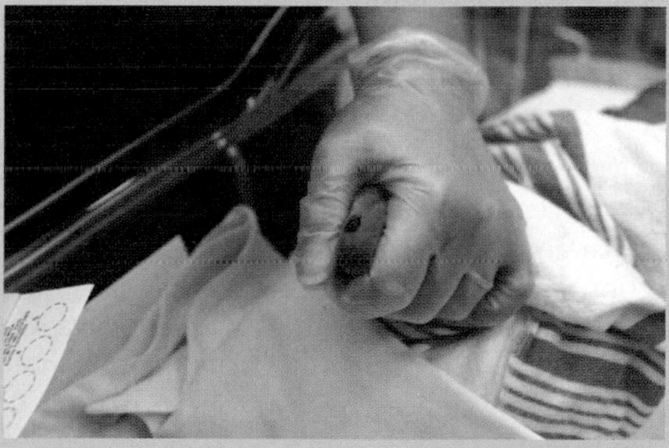

10. Make a pressure dressing from the gauze and tape it over the puncture site. An alternative is to hold pressure for a few moments and then apply an adhesive bandage when the bleeding stops.
11. Remove the gloves and thoroughly wash your hands.
12. Record the glucose level in the designated area of the chart.

Note: Warmth causes vasodilation and draws blood to the surface, making it easier to obtain a specimen. Many facilities have commercial warm packs available for this purpose, such as the one used in the photograph. If a commercial pack is not available, a washcloth dampened with warm (not hot) water may be placed on the heel and covered with a towel or blue pad, or a diaper dampened with warm water may be used. Always check the temperature of the washcloth or diaper with the inside of your wrist before placing it on the newborn's heel. Burns can easily result if the temperature is too hot.

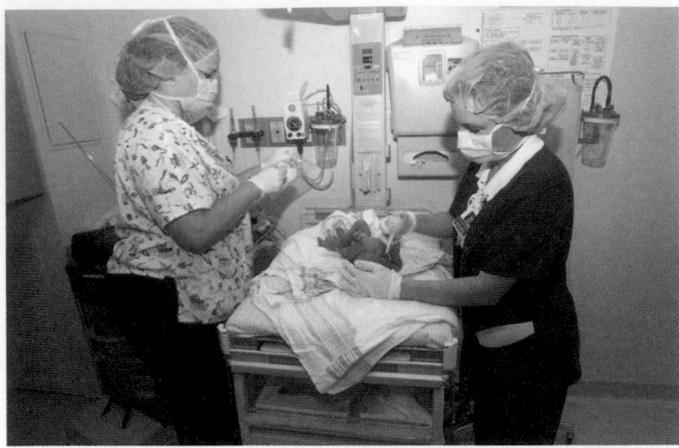

● ***Figure 15.1*** The nurse uses a bulb syringe to suction the mouth of the newborn before suctioning the nares. The bulb is depressed first and then placed in the newborn's oral cavity. Secretions are suctioned into the bulb of the syringe when pressure is released from the bulb. The bulb is then squeezed several times to empty it of secretions before subsequent attempts to suction the newborn.

of secretions. A bulb syringe is used to suction the mouth first and then the nose (Fig. 15-1). Keep the bulb syringe with the newborn and teach the parents how and when to suction the baby. If copious secretions are present that do not resolve with a bulb syringe, a small suction catheter connected to a suction source may be used. Be careful not to apply suction for longer than 5 seconds at a time and to minimize suction pressures to avoid damaging the delicate respiratory structures.

Did you know? It is important to suction the mouth of a newborn before the nose. If the nose is suctioned first, the newborn may gasp or cry and aspirate secretions in the mouth.

Maintaining Thermoregulation

It is critical to protect the newborn from chilling. Cold stress increases the amount of oxygen and glucose needed by the newborn. She can quickly deplete glucose stores and develop hypoglycemia. She can also develop respiratory distress and metabolic acidosis if chilling is prolonged. As stated in the previous section, if the newborn cries vigorously and has an adequate heart rate, he may stay with his mother. Quickly dry the newborn on the mother's abdomen, swaddle him snugly, and apply a cap to prevent heat loss. Another way to maintain the newborn's temperature and promote early bonding is to dry the newborn quickly, place a diaper or blanket over the genital area and a cap on the head, then place the newborn skin-to-skin with the mother or father and cover them both with blankets. This method of keeping the newborn warm is called **kangaroo care** (Fig. 15-2). Kangaroo care is an excellent way to meet the needs of the newborn and provide family-centered care.

It is important to support thermoregulation in the newborn, particularly in the first 24 hours of life. The environmental temperature necessary to maintain a **thermoneutral environment**, an environment in which heat is neither lost nor gained, is slightly higher for the newborn than that required for an older child or adult. Take care to prevent unnecessary heat loss in the nursery. For example, drafts of air can cause convective heat loss, and placing a newborn on a cold surface can lead to conductive heat loss. Conversely, do not allow the newborn to become overheated. Hyperthermia can be just as harmful as hypothermia. A skin temperature probe should be in place on the skin anytime the newborn is under the radiant warmer, and alarms should be set to signal if the skin temperature becomes too hot.

Preventing Injury from Hypoglycemia

The best way to prevent injury from hypoglycemia is to prevent the condition altogether. If the mother is breast-feeding, encourage early

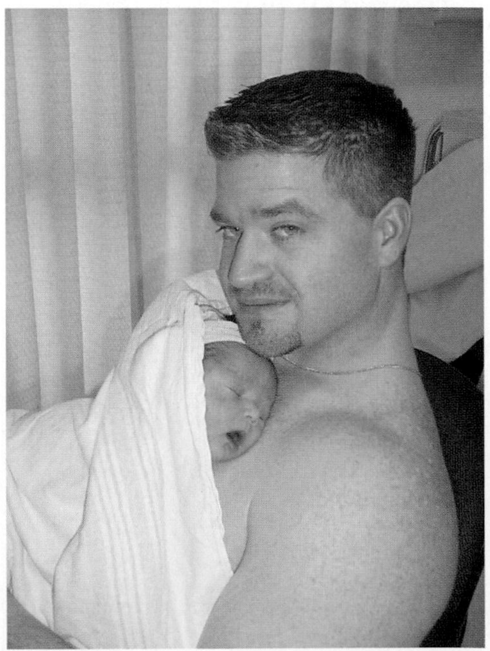

● ***Figure 15.2*** Kangaroo care. A new father keeps his newborn warm using skin-to-skin contact. This method of warming a newborn is called kangaroo care. It is also an excellent way for parents to bond with their newborn.

and frequent feedings. If she is experiencing difficulty, it may be necessary to have a lactation consultant assist the mother. Refer to Chapter 14 for detailed information on breast-feeding and nutrition. If the newborn is to be bottle-fed, early feedings should be initiated.

Asymptomatic newborns at risk for hypoglycemia should be tested at 2, 4, 6, 12, 24, and 48 hours after delivery (Kauffman & Word, 1997). When a newborn displays signs of hypoglycemia, she should be tested. If a heel stick specimen reveals a glucose level of less than 40 mg/dL, it is important to have the results confirmed by laboratory analysis before treatment is initiated. It is common for bedside glucose analyzers to under-read glucose results.

Most facilities have protocols to guide the nurse in the treatment of hypoglycemia. Many pediatricians have preprinted orders that can be initiated if the glucose level falls below a predetermined level (usually 40 mg/dL). In the past, glucose water was used to treat low blood glucose levels, but most authorities now recommend feeding breast milk or formula to the alert newborn. If the infant's symptoms are severe enough to interfere with regular feeding, intravenous dextrose solutions are administered.

Preventing Infection

Within the first hour after birth, an antibiotic ointment must be placed in the newborn's eyes (Fig. 15-3) to prevent **opthalmia neonatorum**, a severe eye infection contracted in the birth canal of a woman with gonorrhea or chlamydia. There are three ophthalmic agents that have been approved for eye prophylaxis: 1% silver nitrate, 0.5% erythromycin, and 1% tetracycline. Silver nitrate is used infrequently because it is irritating to the eyes. In some facilities it is the practice to instill the eye drops in the delivery area immediately after birth, but it is recommended that the instillation be delayed up to 1 hour to allow the newborn and parents to bond while the infant is in a quiet alert state.

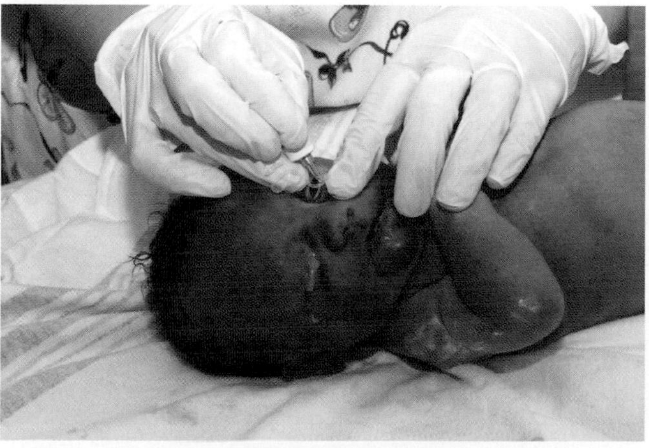

● ***Figure 15.3*** The nurse administers antibiotic ointment to the eyes of the newborn to prevent opthalmia neonatorum.

Another possible infection site is the umbilical cord stump. Careful handwashing and strict aseptic technique should be used when caring for the cord. Often an antiseptic solution such as triple dye, bacitracin ointment, or povidone-iodine is used initially to paint the cord to help prevent the development of infection.

Preventing Imbalanced Fluid Volume

One possible cause of hemorrhage and fluid volume loss is an immature clotting mechanism. Vitamin K is necessary in the formation of certain clotting factors. In the adult, vitamin K is manufactured in the gut by normal flora, but the gut of the newborn is sterile; it has not yet been colonized with symbiotic bacteria. Therefore, it is necessary to supply the newborn with vitamin K to prevent possible bleeding episodes. Within the first hour after birth 0.5 to 1 mg of vitamin K (AquaMEPHYTON) is given intramuscularly (IM). Refer to Nursing Procedure 15-2.

One potential source of hemorrhage is the clamped umbilical cord. An unusually large cord may have large amounts of Wharton's jelly, which may disintegrate faster than the cord vessels and cause the clamp to become loose. This situation could lead to blood loss from the cord. Another cause could be an improperly applied or defective cord clamp. Inspect the umbilical cord for signs of bleeding.

Preventing Misidentification of a Newborn

Fortunately it is a rare occurrence for newborns to be switched in the hospital and go home with the wrong parents, but it has happened. When the mistake is uncovered years later, the situation often results in heartache and heart-wrenching choices for all parties involved. Because of the serious consequences of mistaken identity, the delivery room nurse must take the utmost care to positively identify the newborn before he is separated from his parents.

Many facilities footprint the newborn and fingerprint the mother, but this practice is in decline because footprints are not considered a valid way to identify someone. Most hospitals use some form of bracelet system. Three to four bracelets with identical numbers on the bands are prepared immediately after delivery and before the newborn is separated from his parents. Information

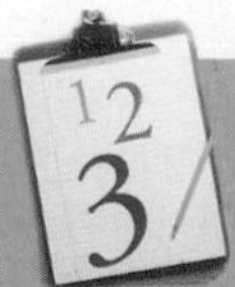

Nursing Procedure 15.2
Administering an Intramuscular Injection to the Newborn

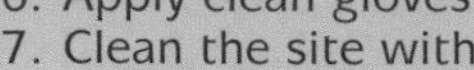

EQUIPMENT

Warm, clean hands
Clean (nonsterile) exam gloves
Syringe
0.5-inch 23- to 25-gauge safety needle
Alcohol pad
Flat surface

PROCEDURE

1. Wash hands thoroughly.
2. Check physician order for medication and dose.
3. Follow normal nursing procedure for drawing medications from a vial or ampule. Do not draw more than 0.5 mL for intramuscular (IM) injection to a newborn.
4. Identify the newborn by identity band. Place the newborn on a flat surface with good lighting.
5. Select an injection site on the vastus lateralis (anterior lateral aspect of the thigh) or rectus femoris (midanterior aspect of the thigh) muscle.

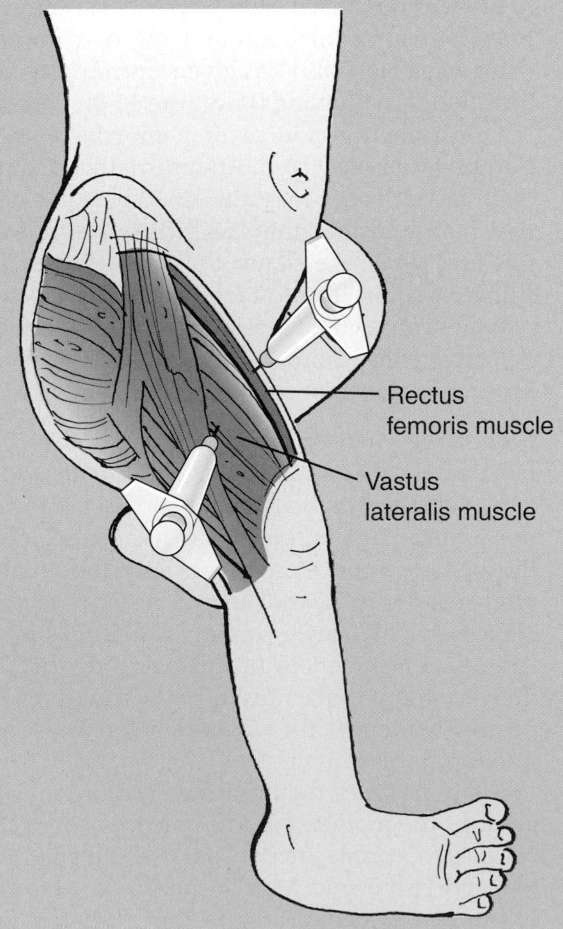

6. Apply clean gloves.
7. Clean the site with an alcohol pad. Use a circular motion from the center of the chosen site outward in ever-widening circles. Hold the alcohol pad between two of your fingers.
8. With your nondominant hand, hold the leg in place.
9. Using your dominant hand, insert the needle at a 90-degree angle with a quick darting motion.
10. Stabilize the needle with your nondominant hand and pull back gently on the plunger to aspirate for blood.
11. If no blood is noted, slowly inject the medication.
12. Use the alcohol pad to stabilize the skin as you withdraw the needle.
13. Discard the syringe and needle in a sharps container. Discard the gloves in a trash receptacle.
14. Wash hands thoroughly.
15. Document on the medication administration record.

Note: If blood is aspirated in step 10, withdraw the needle to avoid intravenous (IV) injection. Discard the syringe, needle, and medication in a sharps container. Go back to step 1 and begin again.

included on the bands is the mother's name, hospital number, and physician, and the newborn's sex, and date and time of birth. Two bands are placed on the newborn, one on the arm and one on the leg. A matching band is placed on the mother and another band may be placed on the father or other designated adult. Instruct the parents to always check the bands when the newborn is brought to them to ensure they are receiving their newborn.

EVALUATION: GOALS AND EXPECTED OUTCOMES

- **Goal:** The newborn will experience adequate cardiovascular and respiratory transition.
  Expected Outcomes: The newborn sustains a heart rate above 100 bpm, maintains a respiratory rate between 30 and 60 breaths per minute without signs of distress, and retains a patent airway.
- **Goal:** The newborn will experience thermoregulatory transition.
  Expected Outcome: The newborn's body temperature stays between 36.5°C and 37.5°C (97.7°F and 99.5°F).
- **Goal:** The newborn will experience adequate metabolic transition.
  Expected Outcome: The newborn's blood glucose level is between 40 and 60 mg/dL.
- **Goal:** The newborn remains free from the signs and symptoms of infection.
  Expected Outcomes: The newborn does not experience purulent conjunctivitis, purulent drainage from the umbilical cord, and has no other signs of sepsis, such as poor suck reflex and lethargy.
- **Goal:** The newborn maintains adequate hemostasis.
  Expected Outcomes: The newborn has no bleeding episodes.
- **Goal:** The newborn will be adequately identified before separation from the parents.
  Expected Outcomes: The newborn possesses a permanent form of identification before he is separated from his parents and can be positively identified by his parents.

Test Yourself

- List the five parameters measured by the Apgar score.
- What is cold stress?
- Describe kangaroo care. List two purposes that it serves.

● The Nursing Process in Providing Care to the Normal Newborn

ASSESSMENT

Nursing care of the normal, stabilized newborn is directed toward controlling risk and early detection of developing complications. The nurse who is responsible for the care of newborns must be familiar with signs that indicate the newborn needs special care.

One common problem is the potential for aspiration from secretions and mucus that are present in the airways during the first few days of life. Monitor the newborn closely for excessive secretions. Gagging and frequent regurgitation are normal in the first few hours of birth. Signs of respiratory distress or central cyanosis should not be present.

Another potential problem is that of infection. Carefully monitor the newborn for signs of infection. An infected umbilical cord will show signs of redness and edema at the base and may have purulent discharge. Early signs of sepsis in the newborn include poor feeding, irritability, lethargy, apnea, and temperature instability. Late signs are an enlarged spleen and liver, jaundice, and petechiae.

Perform a thorough skin assessment. Turgor should be present, and the skin should be intact. Inspect the diaper area for signs of rash or breakdown. Assess for signs of jaundice. As you will recall from Chapter 13, jaundice that occurs within the first 24 hours of life is associated with abnormal lysis of red blood cells and is pathologic in nature.

Between 1983 and 2002, 217 cases of infant abduction by a nonfamily member were reported in the United States (Burgess & Lanning, 2003). Although infant abduction is a rare event, it has devastating effects on hospital personnel and family members of the victim. Studies of the problem have led to a "typical abductor" profile, which is outlined in Box 15-2. When taking care of newborns, be especially alert to any suspicious activity by visitors or persons unknown to you.

The newborn is subjected to numerous startling and noxious stimuli at birth. The womb is dark, confined, and warm. Sounds are muffled through the abdominal and uterine walls. During labor and delivery this situation is reversed. Suddenly the newborn is exposed to a world that is bright, cold, and loud. His extremities flail out when he is startled with seemingly nothing to

BOX 15.2 Profile of a Typical Infant Abductor

- Overweight female of childbearing age
- Has no prior criminal record
- Suffers from low self-esteem and is emotionally immature
- Uses manipulation and deceit within interpersonal relationships
- May be cohabitating or married, but the relationship is often strained
- Often indicates that she has lost a baby or cannot have one
- May announce a false pregnancy and prepare for the arrival of a newborn
- Usually plans the abduction by visiting several hospitals and asking detailed questions regarding nursery routines and exit routes
- Although the abduction is planned, a specific infant is not usually targeted; the abductor strikes when opportunity presents itself
- Frequently poses as a nurse or other health care personnel during the abduction
- Usually demonstrates the ability to take good care of the infant
- Often stays in the community from which the infant was taken

Note: The typical abductor profile was developed from an analysis of 119 cases occurring between 1983 and 1992 (Burgess & Lanning, 2003).

stop them. He does not know his boundaries. In addition the newborn is exposed to invasive and sometimes painful procedures. These early experiences have the potential to cause the newborn to respond to the environment in a disorganized way.

SELECTED NURSING DIAGNOSES

- Ineffective airway clearance related to mucus and secretions
- Risk for infection related to cross-contamination of equipment, poor handwashing, poor hygienic practices, transmission from mother to baby
- Risk for impaired skin integrity
- Risk for injury: newborn abduction
- Risk for disorganized infant behavior related to pain, invasive procedures, or environmental overstimulation

PLANNING AND GOALS

Most continuing newborn care is aimed at monitoring for and preventing complications. After the newborn has had a successful transition, appropriate goals include that the newborn will maintain a clear airway; be free of infection; have clean intact skin; not be abducted from the hospital; and respond to the environment in an organized way. The goal of maintaining an adequate body temperature continues to be addressed throughout the hospital stay. Interventions to meet that goal are interwoven throughout the following implementation section. The goal of maintaining adequate nutrition and hydration is covered in detail in Chapter 14.

IMPLEMENTATION

Keeping the Airway Clear

Keep the bulb syringe in the bassinet with the newborn at all times. Turn the newborn on the side and suction frequently as secretions and mucus accumulate. Teach both parents how to use the bulb syringe. Position the newborn on the side or back to sleep, as recommended by the American Academy of Pediatrics (2003), to decrease the risk of sudden infant death syndrome (SIDS).

Preventing Transmission of Infection

A newborn may contract infection from his mother, visitors, nursery personnel, or the environment. Infection can be particularly devastating for a newborn because the immune system is immature and the newborn has not yet developed effective defenses against invading pathogens. Therefore, it is essential to practice good infection control techniques when caring for newborns.

Handwashing remains the mainstay of infection control, even in newborn nurseries. Many nurseries require a 3-minute surgical-type scrub at the beginning of the shift. Follow the protocol of the facility in which you are working. Of course the hands should be washed thoroughly before and after caring for a newborn. In no instance should a nurse care for a newborn and then proceed to handle or give care to another newborn without washing hands in between. Many newborn nurseries have waterless hand sanitizer available. Hand sanitizer is acceptable to use between newborns when visible soiling of the hands has not occurred.

Other methods for reducing the transmission of infection include keeping all of the newborn's belongings together in the bassinet and not sharing items between newborns. This practice reduces the possibility of cross-contamination. Equipment that is used on multiple newborns, such as a stethoscope, is usually wiped down with alcohol between uses. Rooming-in also reduces the likelihood of cross-contamination. It is no longer considered necessary for nursery personnel to have special scrub suits laundered by the hospital, or for them to wear cover gowns when leaving the nursery. This traditional practice was not found to reduce the incidence of infection in nurseries and has been abandoned.

It is necessary, for the nurse's protection, to use universal precautions. A newborn should not be handled without gloves until after the bath. After this time the newborn may be cared for without gloves unless contact with bodily fluids is likely, such as during diaper changes and when drawing blood for testing.

Providing Skin Care

The first bath (Nursing Procedure 15-3) is delayed until the newborn's temperature is stable. Warm water is usually sufficient for bathing; however, a mild soap can be used. The sponge bath is given under a radiant warmer to minimize heat loss. If a radiant warmer is not used, it is important to keep the infant wrapped and expose only the body part being washed.

Be careful to wash off all traces of blood to minimize transmission of infection from maternal blood-borne pathogens to the newborn or to health care providers. A mild shampoo may be

Nursing Procedure 15.3 Giving the First Bath

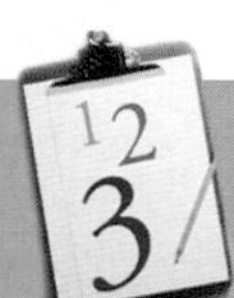

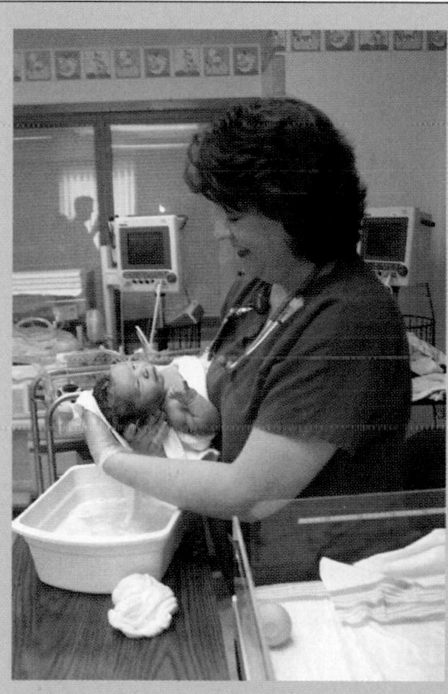

EQUIPMENT

Clean exam gloves
Basin of warm water (98°F to 100°F)
Mild soap and shampoo
Washcloth
Towel
Comb
Cap
Clean diaper
Shirt
Two receiving blankets

PROCEDURE

1. Assemble equipment.
2. Wash hands.
3. Use only clear water (no soap) on the eyes first (proceeding from inner canthus to outer canthus), then the rest of the face.
4. Hold the newborn with your nondominant arm using the football hold. Use the washcloth with the other hand to wipe off visible blood.
5. Lather the hair with shampoo and rinse thoroughly.

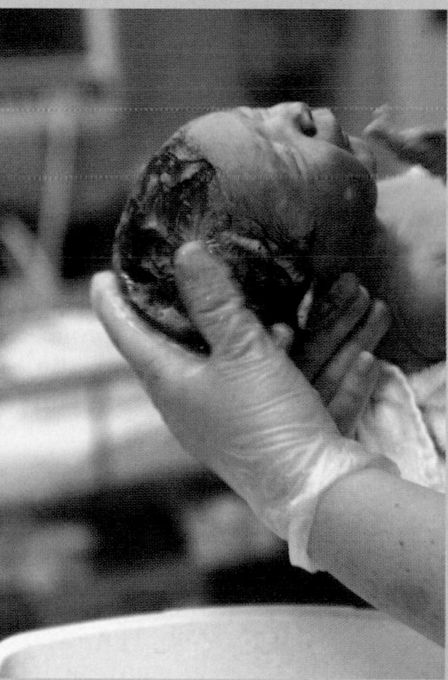

6. Comb through the hair to remove dried blood and to facilitate drying.
7. Place the infant back in the crib or under the radiant warmer (per the facility policy).
8. Bathe and rinse the neck and chest. Be sure to remove blood from the creases of the neck and armpits.

(procedure box continues on page 348)

Nursing Procedure 15.3 (continued) Giving the First Bath

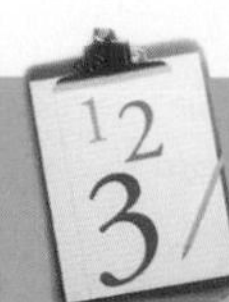

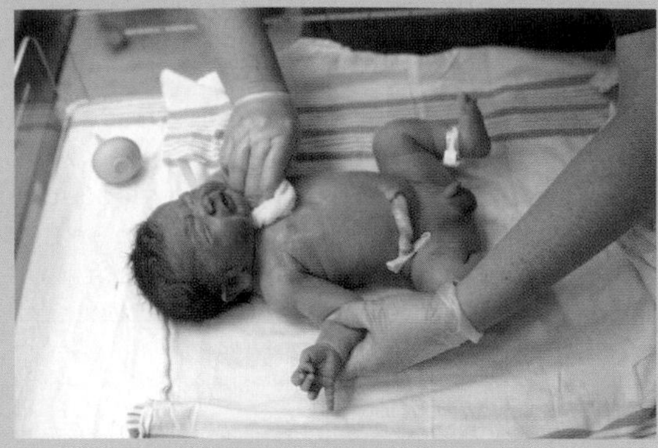

9. Proceed to the abdomen. Take care not to soak the cord in water (a wet cord increases the risk for infection).
10. Wash the extremities, then the back.

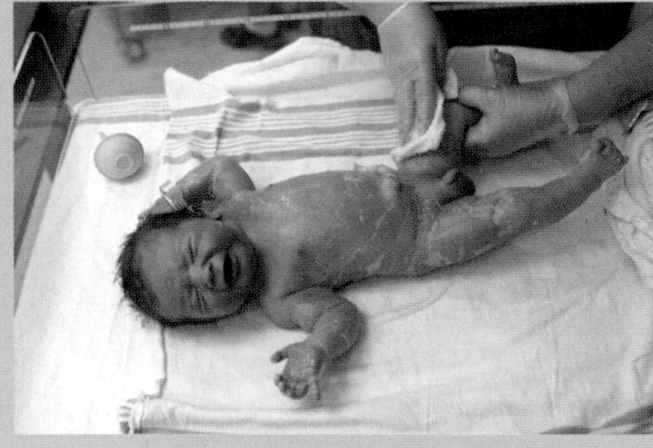

11. Next bathe the genital region. For boys, do not force the foreskin over the glans. For girls, wash from front to back, avoiding contamination of the urethral and vaginal areas with bacteria from the rectum.
12. Last, bathe the anal region.
13. Apply a clean cap, t-shirt, and diaper.
14. Double wrap the newborn with two receiving blankets.
15. Rinse and dry the basin. Store unused soap and shampoo containers and comb in the basin in the storage area of the bassinet.
16. Place the towel and washcloth in the dirty linen hamper.
17. Remove gloves.
18. Wash hands.

Note: The room should be warm, approximately 75°F (24°C) to prevent chilling. In many facilities the first bath is given under the radiant warmer. Bathing should proceed from the cleanest part of the body (face) and end with the dirtiest areas (diaper area). Each body area should be washed, rinsed, and then dried before proceeding to the next area to prevent heat loss from evaporation.

used on the head. Combing the hair helps to remove dried blood. Vernix serves as a lubricant and is protective against infections; therefore, it is best to gently massage the vernix into the skin and allow it to wear off naturally. However, in many facilities vernix is wiped away completely at the first bath to make the baby more presentable.

Be careful. It is important that harsh soaps not be used when bathing newborns. These soaps can irritate the skin. Hexachlorophene in particular is not recommended for bathing because it can be absorbed through the skin and cause central nervous system damage.

Encourage the parents to participate in the bath (Fig. 15-4). This is an excellent time to allow them to interact with their baby and help them gain confidence in parenting skills. When the bath is finished, check the axillary temperature. If it is

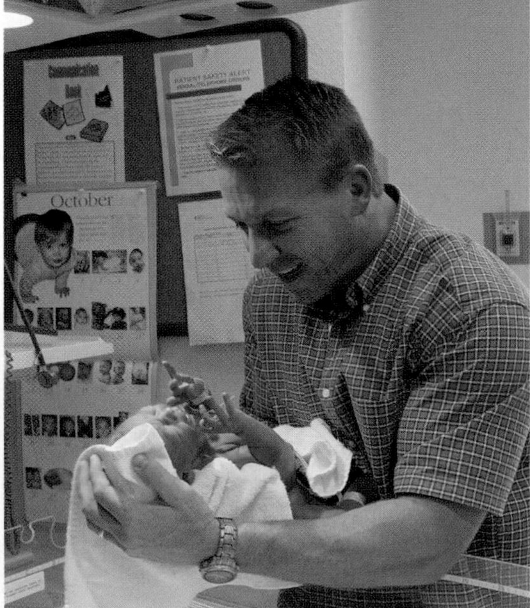

● ***Figure 15.4*** The new father dries his newborn son after giving him his first bath.

within the expected range (see Chapter 13), dress the newborn in a shirt, diaper, and cap. Swaddle the newborn in a blanket and place him in an open crib. If the temperature is below 36.4°C (97.5°F), return the newborn to the radiant warmer.

Warm water can be used to clean the perineal area and buttocks at diaper changes. Frequent diaper changes will help prevent diaper rash and skin breakdown. No special oils or ointments are necessary on clean, intact skin. Talc powders are not recommended because they can cause respiratory irritation when particles are inhaled. Fold the diaper down in the front so that the cord is left open to air (Fig. 15-5). This action protects the cord area from irritation when the diaper is wet and promotes drying of the cord.

Providing Safety

Education and watchful vigilance are the keys to preventing infant abductions. Each facility that cares for newborns should have specific policies and procedures in place that address this problem. Review these policies and know the protocols for the facility in which you will be working.

Most nurseries and mother–baby units are in a part of the hospital that has some security features to discourage abductions. Most nurseries are locked from the outside, and a security code is necessary to gain entrance. Security cameras are usually placed strategically near entrances and exits. Some facilities use security bracelets that set off an alarm if someone attempts to remove it, or it may trip an alarm when a person exits the unit with a newborn. The matching identification bands for newborns and parents also are part of the security plan. In many facilities, identification photos are taken of each newborn. Cooperation of the parents is essential to the effectiveness of any security plan, especially because most infants who are abducted are taken from the mother's room. Family Teaching Tips: Keeping the Newborn Safe lists key points to discuss with parents regarding the safety and security of their newborn while in the hospital.

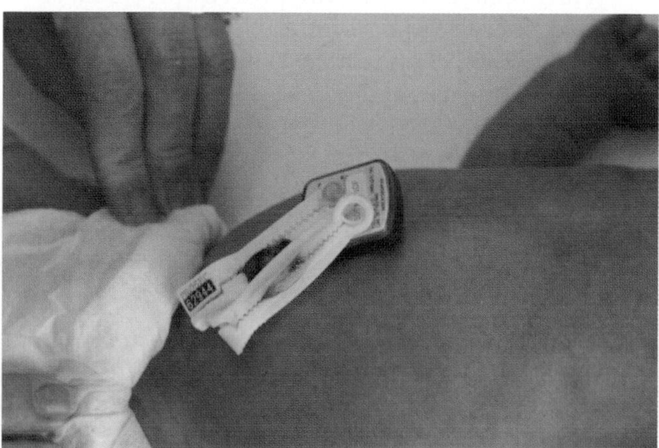

● ***Figure 15.5*** The diaper is folded down so that it does not cover the drying cord.

FAMILY TEACHING TIPS

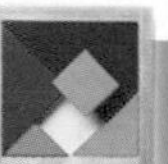

Keeping the Newborn Safe

Review the following points with parents of newborns frequently throughout their hospital stay. Instruct the parents to:

- Never leave their newborn unattended.
- Not remove the identification bands on the newborn until he is discharged from the hospital and to alert the nurses if an identification band falls off or becomes illegible for any reason.
- Not release their newborn to anyone who does not have a hospital picture ID that matches the specific security color or code chosen by the facility to identify personnel authorized to transport and handle newborns.
- Question anyone who does not have the proper identification, or whose picture does not match the identification tag she is wearing, even if she is dressed in hospital attire.
- Alert the nurses immediately if they are suspicious of any person or activity.
- Know the nurses caring for them and their newborn.
- Know when the newborn will be taken for tests, what health care provider authorized the test, and how long the procedure is expected to last.

Enhancing Organized Infant Behavioral Responses

Newborns respond to the environment in more predictable and organized ways when their needs are anticipated. The psychosocial task of infants is developing a sense of trust. Newborns begin to develop trust when the adults around them consistently meet their needs. Feeding the newborn, keeping him dry and comfortable, and holding him are actions that promote trust. Kangaroo care with either parent provides comfort and encourages attachment. Swaddling a newborn snugly is comforting and promotes sleep. Nonnutritive sucking on a gloved finger or pacifier can also be comforting.

EVALUATION: GOALS AND EXPECTED OUTCOMES

- **Goal:** The newborn will maintain a patent airway.

  Expected Outcomes: The newborn's respiratory rate remains between 30 and 60 breaths per minute while at rest, and there are no signs of respiratory distress.

- **Goal:** The newborn will maintain a normal body temperature.
  Expected outcomes: The newborn maintains axillary temperature above 36.4°C (97.5°F) and below 37.5°C (99.5°F)
- **Goal:** The newborn will remain free of the signs and symptoms of infection.
  Expected Outcomes: The newborn has strong, coordinated suck and swallow reflexes, vigorous feeding behaviors, and a drying umbilical cord without purulent drainage or foul odor.
- **Goal:** The newborn will maintain skin integrity.
  Expected Outcomes: The newborn has clean, intact skin.
- **Goal:** The newborn will not be abducted from the hospital.
  Expected Outcomes: The newborn remains safely in the company of family members and/or nursery personnel at all times.
- **Goal:** The newborn will respond to the environment in an organized way.
  Expected Outcomes: The newborn begins to develop predictable sleep/wake patterns, and interacts with caregivers with sustained alertness during interaction.

Test Yourself

- Name three characteristics of a "typical" infant abductor.
- List four things the nurse can do to decrease the spread of infection to newborns.
- Describe three steps parents can take to reduce the risk of infant abduction while in the hospital.

● The Nursing Process in Preparing the Newborn for Discharge

ASSESSMENT

Risk management and promoting healthy adaptation to newborn life continue to guide the nurse when planning for discharge of a healthy newborn. Continue to assess respiratory, cardiovascular, thermoregulatory, nutritional, and hydration status. Monitor for signs of infection. Check vigilantly for developing jaundice.

Watch for signs of pain in the newborn, particularly if he is scheduled for a painful procedure such as circumcision. Until recently, it was not clearly understood how newborns perceive pain and what, if any, long-term effects there might be if pain is prolonged or untreated. Many research studies now support the real physiologic pain responses experienced by the newborn. It appears that untreated pain in the newborn can lead to increased sensitivity to painful experiences later or result in more immediate consequences, such as illness during the neonatal period.

The newborn may experience pain and discomfort from any number of routine procedures carried out in a newborn nursery. Injections and heel sticks are two such sources of painful stimuli. One common procedure that causes pain is **circumcision**, surgical removal of the foreskin of the penis. Because the newborn cannot express pain verbally, other measures must be used to evaluate pain. Pain can be assessed in the newborn by paying attention to behavior, such as crying, sleeplessness, facial expression, and body movements. Changes in heart and respiratory rates, blood pressure, and oxygen saturation can also be used to determine physiologic responses to pain.

It also is important to assess the adaptation of the mother and father to the parenting role. Experienced parents may feel very comfortable in their role and carry out newborn care without difficulty. New parents may ask lots of questions, or may appear afraid to handle the newborn. Assess for signs of positive bonding with the newborn. Refer to Chapter 12 for an in-depth discussion of bonding.

SELECTED NURSING DIAGNOSES

- Pain related to painful procedures such as injections, heel sticks, and circumcision
- Risk for infection related to inadequate immunity in the neonatal period
- Risk for injury from undetected metabolic and hearing disorders
- Deficient knowledge (parental) related to normal newborn care

PLANNING AND GOALS

Prevention of, and relief from, pain are applicable goals throughout the newborn's stay in the hospital; however, these goals become particularly important when the newborn is scheduled for an invasive procedure such as circumcision. Protection from infection and injury from preventable diseases by immunizing against and screening for hepatitis B, phenylketonuria, and other metabolic disorders is a critical goal during this time period. It also is important to evaluate parental knowledge and ability to care for the newborn throughout the hospital stay, but as the time draws near for discharge, this task becomes particularly important.

IMPLEMENTATION

Preventing and Treating Pain

It is the ethical responsibility of the nurse to prevent and treat pain. Enough research exists to document the adverse effects of unnecessary and untreated pain in the neonate. The best treatment is prevention. When possible, avoid situations that may be painful or distressing to the newborn. If there is a choice between an invasive versus noninvasive procedure, choose the noninvasive procedure whenever practical. Use common sense and make suggestions to the charge nurse or physician as appropriate. For instance, it may be less painful to insert an intravenous device than to give multiple intramuscular injections. Or it might be more tolerable for the newborn to have laboratory specimens drawn by venipuncture than to undergo numerous heel sticks.

Provide for a quiet, soothing environment as often as possible. Simple comfort measures can be initiated that decrease the amount of pain perceived by the newborn. Swaddling and holding the infant securely are soothing measures. Nonnutritive sucking on a pacifier can be comforting. Placing sucrose on the pacifier, if allowed by hospital policy, adds the benefit of analgesia suitable for minor pain stimulus.

Assisting With Circumcision

There has been much debate concerning whether or not circumcision should be routinely performed. In the 1970s and 1980s, the American Academy of Pediatrics (AAP) held to a strict policy of strongly discouraging circumcisions based on the rationale that there were no valid medical indications for the procedure. Since that time, the AAP has softened its stance, currently stating, "Existing scientific evidence demonstrates potential medical benefits of newborn male circumcision; however, these data are not sufficient to recommend routine neonatal circumcision." The procedure is contraindicated in newborns who:

- Are still in the transition period
- Are preterm or sick
- Have a family history of bleeding disorder until the disorder is ruled out in the newborn
- Have received a diagnosis of a bleeding disorder
- Have a congenital genitourinary disorder, such as epispadias or hypospadias

The AAP advises that parents should be given enough information to make an informed choice and that pain relief measures should be provided if the procedure is done. Refer to Box 15-3 for a comparison of the advantages and disadvantages of male circumcision. Whatever the parents decide, the nurse must be supportive of their decision.

If the parents decide to have their male newborn circumcised, informed consent is necessary. It is the physician's responsibility to obtain informed consent, although the nurse is usually responsible for witnessing the parents' signatures to a written documentation of that consent. If the parents have unanswered questions, the physician must be notified before the procedure is done. Because of the overwhelming evidence regarding the adverse effects of pain on the newborn, many physicians recommend that language be put into the written consents informing the parents that anesthesia will not be used (if the physician does not use anesthesia) and listing the possible harmful effects of doing the procedure without anesthesia.

After the written consent is signed, prepare for the procedure by gathering all necessary supplies and equipment. Check the physician preference card to determine what procedure the physician

BOX 15.3 Advantages and Disadvantages of Male Circumcision

Advantages

- There is a possible reduction in sexually transmitted infections and urinary tract infections.
- Risk of penile cancer is reduced (it is thought that careful attention to hygiene in uncircumcised males can mitigate the slight increase in risk).
- Neonatal circumcision has fewer complications than adult circumcision (medical necessity for adult circumcision is rare).

Disadvantages

- Neonates experience pain during circumcision.
- All anesthetic methods to block or reduce the pain of circumcision have side effects and possible complications.
- Circumcision can lead to the complications of hemorrhage and infection (infrequent occurrences, but potentially life-threatening), and genital mutilation (extremely rare).

Note: The religious and cultural values of the parents may play a large role in the decision on whether or not to circumcise. These values must be respected.

A PERSONAL GLIMPSE

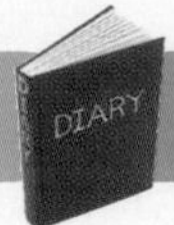

The nurse walked into my room and found me crying and holding my newborn son. She asked me if I was in pain or if something was wrong with the baby. I said, No. She asked if I needed to talk and I nodded my head. I blurted out, "I just don't know if I should circumcise my son or not. My husband thinks we should, but I don't want my baby to be in pain. I just don't know that it is a necessary procedure."

She sat down on the side of my bed and calmly explained that there was no right or wrong decision. She assured me that she and the other nurses and doctors would support us in any decision that we made for our son. Then she gave me several pamphlets to read explaining the pros and cons of circumcision, the pros and cons of choosing not to circumcise, and the latest recommendations from the American Academy of Pediatrics. I felt much better after our talk, and my husband and I were able to make an informed decision about whether or not our son would have this procedure.

Heather

LEARNING OPPORTUNITY: What things can the nurse tell parents about pain control for painful procedures?

In what ways can the nurse act as an advocate for parents when they are trying to decide on whether or not to allow procedures on their newborn?

uses and what special materials are required. The newborn will usually be strapped to a padded circumcision board. If the board is not padded, add blankets or other soft material to the board. Swaddle the infant's upper body during the circumcision.

Check the orders for preprocedure pain relief methods. Acetaminophen may be given within 1 hour before the procedure and then every 4 to 6 hours afterward during the first 24 hours per physician orders or facility protocol. If an anesthetic cream, such as EMLA, is to be used for the procedure, it must be applied approximately 1 hour before the procedure to adequately numb the area. The type of anesthesia that provides the best pain relief appears to be a dorsal penile nerve block. The physician performs the nerve block with buffered lidocaine at least 5 minutes before the circumcision to allow for complete anesthesia in the area. Other methods that can decrease the pain sensation include dimming the lights during circumcision, playing soft music or prerecorded intrauterine sounds for the newborn, and offering a sucrose-dipped pacifier to the infant before and throughout the procedure.

There are several acceptable methods for performing circumcision. Two of the most common are the Gomco (Yellen) clamp (Fig. 15-6) and the Plastibell procedures. Both methods require that the prepuce (foreskin) be separated from the glans penis and incised before the clamp is applied.

Care immediately after the procedure involves holding and comforting the newborn. If the parents are not readily available or cannot perform this action, the nurse must step in to soothe the newborn. Position the newborn on the back or side to avoid excess pressure and pain on the circumcision site. Administer analgesics as ordered on a schedule for pain. Monitor the newborn for signs of unrelieved pain.

Assess the newborn every hour for the first 12 hours after circumcision for evidence of bleeding. If bleeding occurs, apply gentle pressure as needed. Carefully observe for return of voiding and observe the urine stream. Failure to void indicates a complication of circumcision and must be reported to the charge nurse and physician. If a Plastibell was not used, A&D ointment or petroleum jelly must be applied to the site to prevent it from sticking to the diaper. Refer to Family Teaching Tips: Uncircumcised and Circumcised Penis Care for important teaching points to discuss with parents after circumcision or, if circumcision was not done, how to care for the uncircumcised penis.

Preventing Infection Through Neonatal Immunization

Hepatitis B vaccination is recommended by the Centers for Disease Control (CDC) for all newborns before they leave the hospital, regardless of the mother's HBsAg status (all pregnant women who receive prenatal care are tested for hepatitis B surface antigen [HBsAg]). Hepatitis B vaccine requires parental consent. Be sure the parents' written consent is obtained before injecting the vaccine. Instruct the parents to follow up with the recommended vaccination schedule for all immunizations, starting at 2 months and continuing throughout infancy.

The hepatitis B vaccination is especially important in newborns of mothers who are infected with hepatitis B or in whom infection is suspected. Many newborns who contract hepatitis B virus (HBV) from their mothers become chronic carriers of the disease. In some cases the

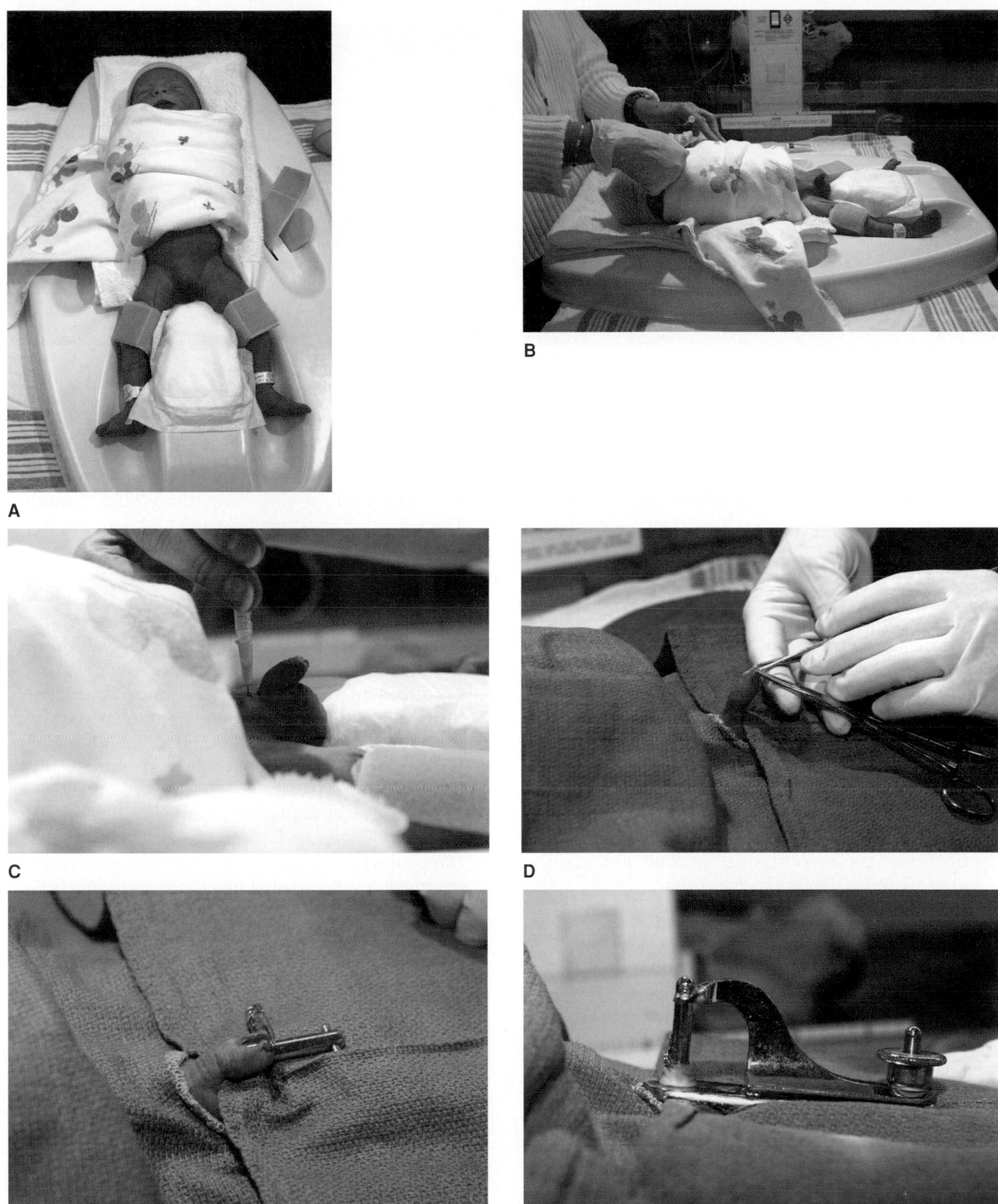

● ***Figure 15.6*** Circumcision using the Gomco (Yellen) clamp. (**A**) The newborn's upper body is swaddled, and his legs are strapped to the circumcision board. (**B**) The nurse injects a small amount of sucrose into the newborn's mouth and allows the newborn to suck on her gloved finger as a method of nonpharmacologic pain relief. (**C**) The physician injects a local anesthetic to numb the area in preparation for the procedure. (**D**) The penis and scrotum are prepped with povidone-iodine and the area draped with sterile towels. Forceps are used to pull the foreskin (prepuce) forward, and an incision is made into the prepuce. (**E**) The prepuce is drawn over the cone. (**F**) The clamp is applied.

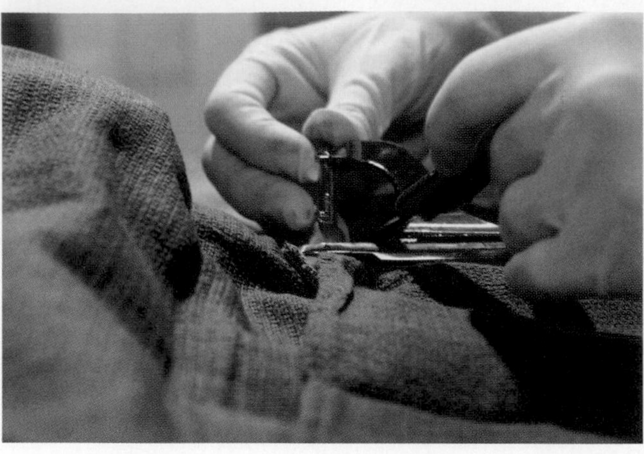

G

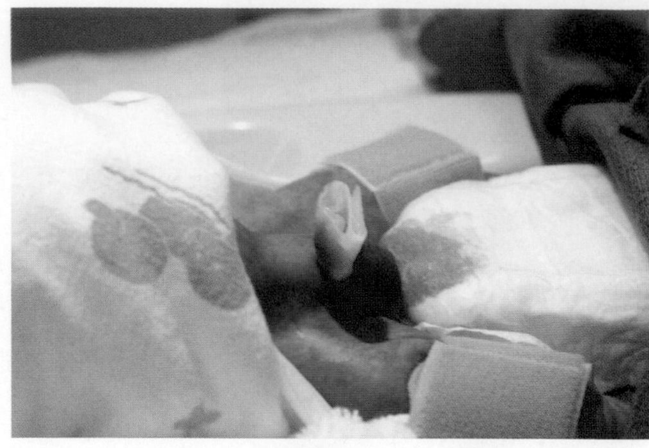

H

● ***Figure 15.6*** (continued) (**G**) Pressure is maintained for 3 to 4 minutes, then a scalpel is used to cut away excess foreskin. (**H**) The clamp is removed and a petrolatum gauze dressing applied.

newborn develops an acute case of hepatitis B and dies of the infection. In other cases the newborn has no symptoms but has an increased risk for developing cirrhosis or hepatocellular carcinoma later in life. If the woman is HBsAg positive, the newborn is bathed thoroughly after birth (to remove traces of blood and decrease the risk of transmission from the mother's blood on his skin when he receives his vaccination). In addition, the newborn is given the hepatitis vaccination and one dose of hepatitis B immune globulin (HBIG) within 12 hours of birth. This dosing schedule is 98% to 99% effective in preventing transmission of HBV from an infected mother to her newborn. If the mother's HBsAg status is unknown, the HBV vaccine is given, and the HBIG dose can be postponed as long as 1 week while awaiting the mother's results.

Preventing Injury Through Neonatal Screening

It is crucial that newborns be screened for several disorders that have the potential to cause lifelong disability if diagnosis and treatment are delayed (Box 15-4). The laws in most states require this initial screening, which is done within 72 hours of birth. The ideal time to collect the specimen is after the newborn is 36 hours old and 24 hours after he has his first protein feeding. Use a heel stick to draw blood from the newborn and collect a specimen on a special collection card. The card has five rings, and each ring must be filled with the newborn's blood (Fig. 15-7). The specimen is then labeled and sent to a special laboratory for testing. A second test is performed at 1 to 2 weeks of age. The mother must be instructed on where and when to take her newborn for the follow-up screening test.

A hearing screen is now encouraged for all newborns before they are discharged home. There are two tests that are used to screen a newborn's hearing: the Auditory Brainstem Response (ABR) and Otoacoustic Emissions (OAE). Both tests use clicks or tones played into the newborn's ear. The ABR measures how the brain responds to sound through electrodes placed on the newborn's head. OAE measures sound waves produced in the inner ear. A probe is placed inside the newborn's ear canal, and the response or echo is measured. Both tests are effective screening devices. An abnormal screening result is followed-up with more extensive testing.

Because significant costs are involved for equipment and follow-up, it is mandated that insurance companies pay for this service. Early diagnosis and treatment results in better outcomes, including better chances for healthy attachment with parents, for newborns who have hearing disorders.

BOX 15.4 Newborn Screening

Disorders for which newborn screening is commonly done:

- Phenylketonuria (PKU)
- Congenital hypothyroidism
- Galactosemia
- Maple syrup urine disease
- Homocystinuria
- Biotinidase
- Sickle cell disease
- Congenital adrenal hypoplasia
- Cystic fibrosis

Note: According to the National Newborn Screening and Genetics Resource Center, all 50 states mandate screening for PKU, congenital hypothyroidism, and galactosemia.

FAMILY TEACHING TIPS

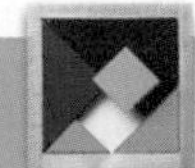

Uncircumcised and Circumcised Penis Care

Review the following points with parents of newborn boys before discharge.

For the uncircumcised newborn, instruct the parents to:

- Wash the penis with each diaper change.
- Not force the foreskin to retract. Bleeding, infection, and scarring can result.
- Teach the child, when he is old enough, to wash under the foreskin daily by gently retracting the foreskin as far as it will go (without using forcible retraction).

For the circumcised newborn, instruct the parents to:

- Inspect the circumcision site each time the diaper is changed. Call the doctor if more than a few drops of blood are present in the diaper.
- Wash the penis with warm water dribbled gently from a washcloth at each diaper change.
- Reapply petroleum jelly at each diaper change for the first 24 to 48 hours unless a Plastibell was used.
- Fasten the diaper loosely to prevent unnecessary friction and irritation.
- Remember that yellow crusting over the area indicates normal healing. The crust should not be removed.
- Hold and comfort your baby frequently while the site is healing. Nonnutritive sucking with a pacifier may be soothing.
- Call the physician if a Plastibell does not fall off within 5 to 8 days.
- Report the following warning signs after circumcision:
  - Bleeding spot larger than a quarter in the diaper.
  - No wet diapers within 6 to 8 hours after circumcision.
  - Fever, low-grade temperature, bad smell to the drainage, pus at the site.
  - Plastibell falls off before 5 days or is displaced.
  - Scarring after the area has healed.

Supporting the Parent's Role through Discharge Teaching

Parent education is an essential part of normal newborn care. There are many things the parents need to know to effectively meet the needs of their infant. Because hospital stays are short, it is difficult to adequately teach parents everything they need to know and to give them time to absorb the information and ask questions. At the very least, instructions should be written so that the parents can refer to them as needed. Family Teaching Tips: General Tips for Newborn Care at Home provides helpful information for new parents.

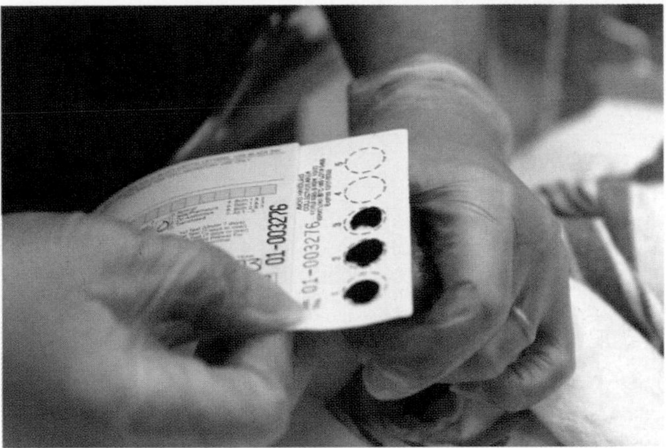

● ***Figure 15.7*** The nurse collects a blood specimen on a special card to screen the newborn for treatable disorders that otherwise might cause mental retardation, disability, or even death.

Some hospitals have newborn teaching videos that can be sent home with the parents. Newborn care classes often are available that can be started before discharge and continued for several weeks or months afterward. Some hospitals have home visitation programs in which a nurse or clinical nurse specialist follows up with the new family at home. All of these are ways to extend the teaching time and allow for parents to absorb the material and formulate questions. Return demonstrations and home visits allow for direct observation of the parents' ability to care for their child. Several important topics that need to be discussed with parents are covered in this section.

Pay close attention. It is important that teaching be individualized to the needs of the parents. If the parents are inexperienced, it is important that they feel confident in their ability to care for their child. Tactfully role model care of the newborn, then give them the chance to develop their skills while you are available to assist. Sincerely compliment them when they do well.

Handling the Newborn. New parents are often anxious about picking up their newborn for the first time. Assist them to slide one hand under the neck and shoulders and place the other hand under the buttocks or between the legs before gently lifting the newborn. Because newborns cannot support their head for the first few months, it is necessary for parents to provide this support when holding the baby.

Demonstrate different ways to hold the newborn (Fig. 15-8). The football hold is one position that allows the parent to support the head and

FAMILY TEACHING TIPS

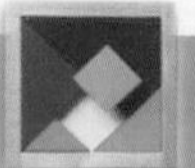

General Tips for Newborn Care at Home

FEEDING

- Most newborns eat every 2 to 4 hours. Feeding patterns become fairly regular in approximately 2 weeks.
- Regurgitation ("spitting up") is expected. Vomiting should be reported to the pediatrician. Frequent vomiting can quickly lead to dehydration. Projectile vomiting may indicate an obstruction.

SLEEPING

- Newborns sleep approximately 16 to 20 hours per day.
- It is a good idea for the caregiver to rest frequently throughout the day and sleep when the baby sleeps.
- For the first 3 to 4 months, it is difficult for infants to fall asleep by themselves. It is helpful for the parent to rock, walk, cuddle, or otherwise comfort the infant as he tries to fall asleep. After 4 months of age, the parent can help the baby learn to fall asleep at predictable times.
- There are wide variations of "normal" as to when babies sleep through the night. Some are able to do so by 6 to 7 weeks of age. Others may not until they are 3 or 4 months old.
- It does not help a baby sleep through the night to introduce solid foods too soon. A newborn's digestive system is immature and not ready to handle large protein molecules until approximately 4 months of age.

CRYING

- It is normal for a newborn to cry approximately 2 hours per day for the first 6 to 7 weeks of life.
- A "fussy period" during the day is to be expected.
- Crying is the way a baby communicates. First check the baby for physical causes of discomfort, such as a wet or dirty diaper or hunger. Then try all or some of the following suggestions to help quiet the baby.
  - Rock the baby.
  - Carry the baby and walk.
  - Take the baby for a stroll in the stroller.
  - Put the baby in a baby swing or a rocking cradle.
  - Gently pat or stroke the baby's back.
  - Swaddle the baby.
  - Take the baby for a ride in the car.
  - Turn on some white noise—washing machine, vacuum cleaner, air conditioner, radio not tuned to a station, etc.
- Never shake a baby for any reason. If you have tried everything and the baby continues to cry, put the baby down in a safe place and take a time-out. It won't hurt him to cry for a short time by himself. Also, you could ask someone else to take over for awhile.

SENSORY INPUT

- Babies' brains need stimulation to develop. Use the five senses to communicate with the baby.
- Visual stimulation can be as simple as making faces with your baby during periods of alertness. Mobiles are another means of visual enrichment.
- Talking, singing, and reading give the baby auditory stimulation.
- Holding and cuddling the baby and letting him touch different textures and shapes develops the sense of touch.
- Pay attention to your baby's cues. She will let you know when she has had enough stimulation and needs rest.

HEALTH MAINTENANCE

- Be sure to make an appointment with the pediatrician within the time frame given to you at discharge; usually at 2 weeks of age.
- Be sure to take the baby for follow-up screening and for immunizations at the appropriate times.
- Recognize signs of illness and follow up with the physician if these signs are present.
  - Fever
  - Vomiting
  - Unusually fussy
  - Diarrhea (frequent, watery stools)
  - Yellow or blue color to the skin
  - Breathing that appears stressed
  - Refuses to eat or has a poor suck
  - Appears listless.

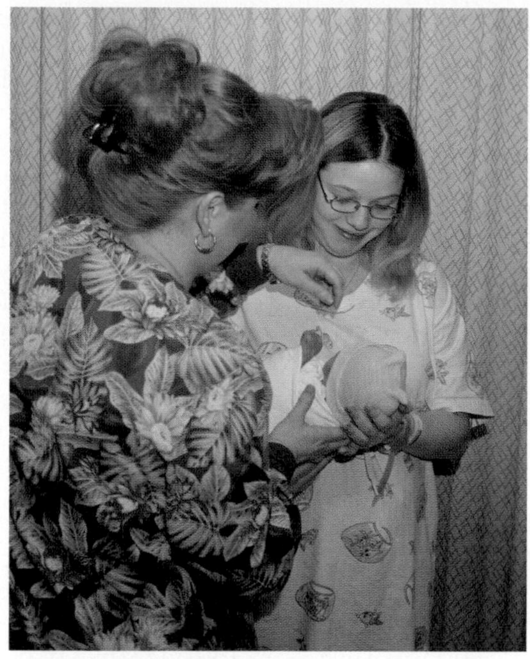

A

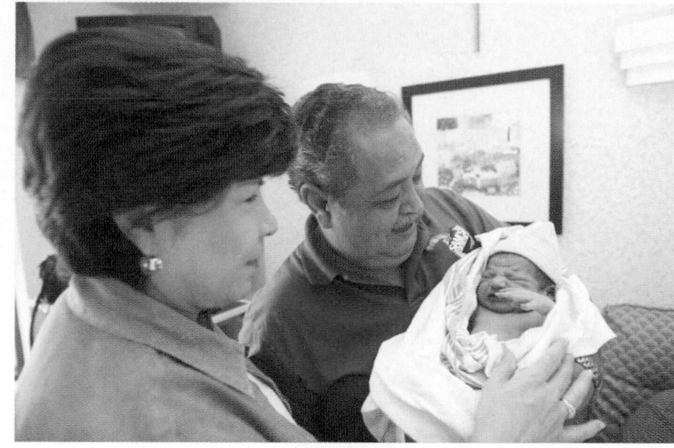

B

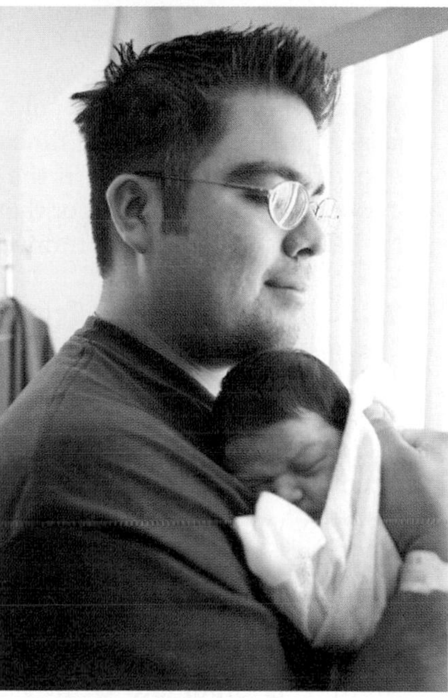

C

● ***Figure 15.8*** (**A**) The nurse teaches the new mother to support the newborn using the football hold. (**B**) The grandfather is using the familiar cradle hold. (**C**) The new father demonstrates the shoulder hold.

body with one hand because the body is tucked under the arm. This leaves one hand free for other tasks. Instruct the parents to use the football hold judiciously while walking because the head is largely unprotected with this hold. Cradling the baby is familiar to most parents, as is the shoulder hold, which is sometimes comforting for a colicky baby. Newborns should always be placed on their backs to sleep to reduce the risk for SIDS.

Teach the parents to swaddle the newborn. Swaddling gives the newborn a sense of security and is comforting. Demonstrate and then let the parents give a return demonstration. Place the blanket in such a way that the newborn is positioned diagonally on the blanket. Fold down the top corner of the blanket under the infant's head. Pull the left corner around the front of the infant and tuck it under his arm. Pull up the bottom corner and tuck it in the front. Pull the right corner around the front of the infant and tuck it under the left arm (Fig. 15-9).

Handwashing before and after handling the baby is the best way parents can protect their newborn from infection. They should also encourage visitors to wash their hands before touching the baby. Anyone with obvious illness should not visit until he or she is well again.

Clearing the Airway. Teach the parents how to use the bulb syringe. Depress the bulb first and then place it in the newborn's mouth, if excess secretions are noted. The nose is suctioned last. Clean the bulb with warm water and a mild soap. Sneezing is a normal response to particles in the

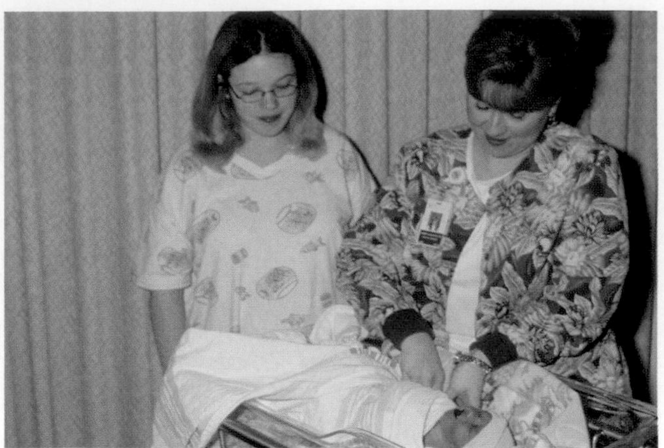

● ***Figure 15.9*** The nurse shows the new mother how to swaddle her newborn.

air and is not indicative of a cold. Yellow or green nasal drainage are signs of illness that should be reported to the physician. If the baby turns blue or stops breathing for longer than a few seconds, the parents should seek immediate emergency care (call 911).

Maintaining Adequate Temperature. Parents should be taught to protect their newborn from drafts and to adequately dress the infant. However, sometimes the temptation is to overdress the newborn. The best advice is to instruct the parents to dress the newborn in the amount and quality of clothes that would keep the parents comfortable in the environment. Check the baby's temperature if he seems ill. Temperatures of less than 97.7°F or greater than 100° F should be reported to the physician.

Monitoring Stool and Urine Patterns. It is normal for the newborn to have 6 to 10 wet diapers per day after the first day of life. Instruct the parents to report if the newborn does not void at all within a 12-hour period. Frequent, regular voiding indicates the newborn is getting enough milk.

Newborn stools initially are dark greenish-black and tarry. These stools are referred to as meconium. Transitional stools are lighter green or light green-yellow and are looser in character than is meconium. Most babies are having transitional stools by the time they are discharged home. In general, breast-fed babies have softer, less formed stools that have a sweetish odor to them. Bottle-fed babies tend to have more well-formed stools that are a little darker in color with a more unpleasant odor.

Signs of constipation are infrequent hard, dry stools. Babies normally turn red in the face and strain when passing stools. These signs do not indicate constipation. Diarrhea is defined as frequent stools with high water content. Because newborns dehydrate quickly, it is important for parents to notify the physician if the newborn has more than two episodes of diarrhea in one day.

Providing Skin Care. Teach new parents about normal, expected skin changes such as Mongolian spots and newborn rash (refer to Chapter 13 to review this material). A sponge bath should be given until the cord falls off, approximately 10 to 12 days after birth. Newborns need protection from chilling when they are bathed. It also is important for parents to monitor the water temperature to prevent scalding the newborn's tender skin. Daily tub baths are not necessary and may dry the skin. Some physicians want the parents to cleanse the cord site with alcohol several times daily.

Maintaining Safety. Newborns quickly learn to roll over and can move around on surfaces, even if unintentionally. For this reason, newborns and infants should never be left unattended on high surfaces, such as on dressing tables or beds. They also should not be left unattended around any amount of water to avoid the possibility of drowning. Plastic should not be used to cover infant mattresses or on any object to which the newborn has contact to protect from suffocation. Pillows are not needed and may be dangerous for the young infant.

Parents need to be taught to differentiate normal from abnormal newborn observations and behaviors. A yellow tint to the skin is indicative of jaundice and should be reported to the physician promptly. Untreated jaundice can lead to permanent brain damage. Listlessness and poor feeding behaviors are signs of illness that should be reported. Teach the parents normal behavior states of newborns and help them learn to read the special cues their baby gives regarding when and how much interaction he can tolerate (refer to Chapter 13).

Proper use of car seats is a critical skill for new parents to learn. Car seats save lives, and infants should never be transported in a car without one. Most states have laws regarding their use, and parents must be familiar with these laws. Newborns are safest in rear-facing seats placed in the middle of the back seat of the car. Parents should never place car seats in the front seat of cars equipped with air bags because death and injury have occurred when air bags deploy and infants are strapped into the front seat. If it is absolutely necessary to place the infant in a car seat in the front seat, there must be no air bag or the air bag must be professionally disabled. Parents should be thoroughly familiar with the operation of the car seat they choose.

EVALUATION: GOALS AND EXPECTED OUTCOMES

- **Goal:** The newborn will maintain an adequate level of comfort during the hospital stay.
  Expected Outcomes: The newborn shows signs of contentment, is not overly fussy, and does not show other signs of pain, particularly during and after painful procedures.
- **Goal:** The newborn remains free from signs and symptoms of preventable diseases.
  Expected Outcomes: The newborn is immunized against Hepatitis B, the parents describe when to take the newborn for repeat vaccinations for all childhood diseases, the newborn receives mandatory screening for metabolic and hearing disorders, and the parents explain what follow-up is necessary and what to do if the screens are abnormal.
- **Goal:** The parents will be able to adequately care for their newborn at home.
  Expected Outcomes: The parents demonstrate the skills needed to adequately care for their newborn; verbalize signs that should initiate a call to the physician when follow-up is needed, and how to find answers to questions that come up during the care of their newborn.

Test Yourself

- Name one advantage and one disadvantage of circumcision.
- What substance, in addition to the vaccination, is given to a newborn whose mother is positive for the hepatitis B surface antigen?
- List three ways parents can deal with newborn crying?

KEY POINTS

- The delivery room should be prepared for resuscitation of the newborn before birth. Resuscitation supplies should be checked and the warmer turned on in anticipation of the birth. If resuscitation is needed, Neonatal Resuscitation Program guidelines should be followed.
- The Apgar score is a way of determining how well the newborn is transitioning to life outside the womb. Five parameters (respiratory effort, heart rate, muscle tone, reflex irritability, and color) are all used to assign a score at 1 and 5 minutes of life. A healthy, vigorous newborn has a 5-minute score of 7 or greater.
- Steps should be taken to prevent the newborn from becoming overly cold or overly hot. A thermoneutral environment is ideal in which the temperature is maintained at a level so that heat is neither gained nor lost.
- Eye prophylaxis to prevent eye infection from gonorrhea should be instituted within the first hour after birth. Vitamin K is given IM to prevent bleeding problems.
- Identification bands are placed immediately in the delivery room before newborn and parents are separated.
- Hypoglycemia is a blood glucose level less than 40 mg/dL. Newborns can have no symptoms or may demonstrate multiple signs. The most common sign is shakiness or jitteriness. Hypoglycemia is best prevented and treated with early and regular feedings.
- Maintaining the newborn with his own crib and supplies, using excellent handwashing technique, and minimizing exposure to sick people are all measures nurses take to decrease the risk for cross-contamination and infection in the newborn.
- Nurses must be vigilantly on guard for suspicious activity in and around a nursery. The risk for abduction is a real threat. The nurse should teach the parents to ask to see identification before releasing their newborn to anyone.
- Newborns show behavioral and physiologic responses, such as crying, grimacing (or making other faces), and increased heart and respiratory rates, to painful procedures.
- Circumcision remains a controversial procedure. The AAP strongly recommends the use of analgesia and anesthesia for the procedure. If the parents choose not to circumcise, they must be taught proper hygiene for the uncircumcised penis.
- All newborns should receive a hepatitis B vaccination and screening for metabolic diseases such as phenylketonuria and congenital hypothyroidism that can lead to profound mental retardation and disability if left untreated.
- Parents need to learn how to hold and position their infant, how to clear the airway, maintain adequate body temperature, monitor stool and urine patterns, provide skin care, and maintain safety of their newborn.

REFERENCES AND SELECTED READINGS

Books and Journals

American Academy of Pediatrics. (2003). Campaign launched to avoid sudden death in child care settings. News release. Retrieved June 25, 2004, from http://www.aap.org/advocacy/archives/jansids.htm

American Academy of Pediatrics. (2002). Hearing: Newborn screening. Medical Library article. Retrieved August 29, 2002, from http://www.medem.com/MedLB/article_detaillb.cfm?article_ID = ZZZS5I9Y65D&sub_cat = 108

American Academy of Pediatrics NRP Steering Committee. (2000). *Neonatal Resuscitation Program: Textbook of Neonatal Resuscitation* (4th ed.). Elk Grave Village, IL: American Academy of Pediatrics.

American Academy of Pediatrics Policy Statement. (2000). Prevention and management of pain and stress in the neonate. *Pediatrics, 105*(2), 454–461. Retrieved August 29, 2002, from http://www.aap.org/policy/re9945.html

American Academy of Pediatrics Policy Statements. (1971, 1975, 1977, 1989). *Circumcision*. Found on the CIRP Circumcision Information and Resource Pages website. Retrieved August 29, 2002, from http://www.cirp.org/library/statements/aap/

Anand, K. J. S., & Hickey, P. R. (1987). Pain and its effects in the human neonate and fetus. *New England Journal of Medicine, 317*(21), 1321–1329. Retrieved August 29, 2002, from http://www.cirtl.org/pain.htm

Brooks, C. (1997). Neonatal hypoglycemia. *Neonatal Network, 16*(2), 15–21.

Burgess, A. W., & Lanning, K. V. (Eds.). (2003). *An analysis of infant abductions*. Developed from a study by the National Center for Missing and Exploited Children, the US Department of Justice, and the University of Pennsylvania's School of Nursing. 2nd ed. Retrieved January 20, 2004, from http://www.missingkids.com/en_US/publications/NC66.pdf

Cranmer, H., & Shannon, M. (2001). Pediatrics, hypoglycemia. D. Slapper, R. Konop, W. Wolfram, J. Halamka, & W. K. Mallon, (Eds.), *eMedicine*. Retrieved August 31, 2002, from http://www.emedicine.com/emerg/topic384.htm

Cunningham, F. G., Gant, N. F., Leveno, K. J., Gilstrap, L. C. III, Hauth, J. C., & Wenstrom, K. D. (2001). The newborn infant. *Williams obstetrics* (21st ed., pp. 385–402). New York: McGraw Hill Medical Publishing Division.

Evans, N. (1998). Hypoglycaemia. *Department of neonatal medicine protocol book, Royal Prince Alfred Hospital*. Retrieved August 30, 2002, from http://www.cs.nsw.gov.au/rpa/neonatal/html/newprot/hypogly.htm

Fletcher, M. A. (1999). Physical assessment and classification. In G. B. Avery, M. A. Fletcher, & M. G. MacDonald (Eds.), *Neonatology: Pathophysiology & management of the newborn* (5th ed., pp. 301–320). Philadelphia: Lippincott Williams & Wilkins.

Freij, B. J., & McCracken, G. H. (1999). Acute infections. In G. B. Avery, M. A. Fletcher, & M. G. MacDonald (Eds.), *Neonatology: Pathophysiology & management of the newborn* (5th ed., pp. 1189–1207). Philadelphia: Lippincott Williams & Wilkins.

Geyer, J., Ellsbury, D., Kleiber, C., Litwiller, D., Hinton, A., & Yankowitz, J. (2002). An evidence-based multidisciplinary protocol for neonatal circumcision pain management. *JOGNN, 31*(4), 403–410.

Kauffman, G. R., & Word, T. M. (1997). Neonatal hypoglycemia (medical negligence). *Trial, 33*(5), 42–46.

Kelly, J. M. (1999). General care. In G. B. Avery, M. A. Fletcher, & M. G. MacDonald (Eds.), *Neonatology: Pathophysiology & management of the newborn* (5th ed., pp. 333–343). Philadelphia: Lippincott Williams & Wilkins.

North American Nursing Diagnosis Association (NANDA). (2001). *NANDA nursing diagnoses: Definitions & classification 2001–2002*. Philadelphia: Author.

Owens, A. M. (2003). Researchers spend hours studying newborns' pain at being circumcised. *National Post*, Toronto, December 30, 2003. Retrieved January 20, 2004, from http://www.cirp.org/news/nationalpost12-30-03/

Richardson, H. (1997). Kangaroo care: Why does it work? *Midwifery Today, 44*(Winter):50–51. Retrieved August 28, 2002, from http://www.midwiferytoday.com/articles/kangaroocare.asp

Websites

Newborn Care

http://www.nlm.nih.gov/medlineplus/infantandnewborncare.html

Cord Care

http://www.rcp.gov.bc.ca/Guidelines/Newborn/Master.NB10.CordCare.February.pdf

Vitamin K

http://www.rcp.gov.bc.ca/Guidelines/Newborn/Master.NB12.VitK.pdf

WORKBOOK

NCLEX-STYLE REVIEW QUESTIONS

1. Baby Boy Alvarez is 5 minutes old. The nurse performs a quick assessment and determines that the newborn has a heart rate of 110 bpm, a weak cry, and acrocyanosis. His extremities are held in partial flexion, and he grimaces when a catheter is placed in his nose. What Apgar score does the nurse record?
   a. 5–The newborn is having extreme difficulty transitioning.
   b. 5–The newborn is having moderate difficulty transitioning.
   c. 6–The newborn is having moderate difficulty transitioning.
   d. 6–The newborn is vigorous and transitioning with minimal effort.
2. The delivery room nurse has just brought a 10-pound newborn to the nursery. You will be monitoring the newborn during the transition period. Which assessment parameter will *most* likely inhibit this newborn's transition?
   a. Apgar score
   b. Blood sugar
   c. Heart rate
   d. Temperature
3. The newborn has just been delivered. He is placed in skin-to-skin contact with his mother. A blanket covers all of his body except his head. His hair is still wet with amniotic fluid, etc. What is the most likely type of heat loss this baby may experience?
   a. Conductive
   b. Convective
   c. Evaporative
   d. Radiating
4. A woman dressed in hospital scrub attire without a name badge presents to the nursery and says that Mrs. Smith is ready for her baby. She offers to take the baby back to Mrs. Smith. What response by the nurse is best in this situation?
   a. "I don't know you. Are you trying to take a baby?"
   b. "Leave immediately! I'm calling security."
   c. "May I see your identification, please?"
   d. "You must be Mrs. Smith's sister. She said her sister is a nurse."

STUDY ACTIVITIES

1. Develop a poster that shows nurses ways to prevent transmitting infections in the nursery.
2. Develop a handout for nurses with helpful tips on preventing infant abductions. Use an Internet search to help you find material for the handout.
3. Make a discharge teaching handout for parents of a newborn.

CRITICAL THINKING: What Would You Do?

Apply your knowledge of the nurse's role in newborn care to the following situations.

1. A neighbor calls to tell you that his wife just delivered her newborn in the living room. The ambulance is on the way but is not yet there. You run to the house and find the baby loosely wrapped in a blanket. The neighbor says the baby was born approximately 2 minutes before you arrived.
   a. What actions do you take first and why?
   b. The newborn becomes jittery and irritable. What do you suspect may be the problem?
   c. What two interventions will need to be carried out as soon as the newborn and mother can be safely transported to a health care facility?
2. Mrs. Mathias just delivered a baby boy. He cries immediately and is pink. The newborn's cry sounds "wet" and "gurgly."
   a. What action should the nurse take first?
   b. If the respirations continue to sound wet, what step would the nurse take next?
3. Newborn Boy Hinojosa is crying and thrashing about after a circumcision.
   a. What is the likely cause of his crying?
   b. What should the nurse do in this situation?
4. A new mother calls the nursery from home. She and her newborn were discharged 2 days ago. She is worried about a small amount of yellow crust she notes at the circumcision site. She is also worried because the baby has been crying and fussy for the last hour.
   a. How would you advise the mother regarding the yellow crusting?
   b. What suggestions could you give her for the crying?

UNIT 6

Childbearing at Risk

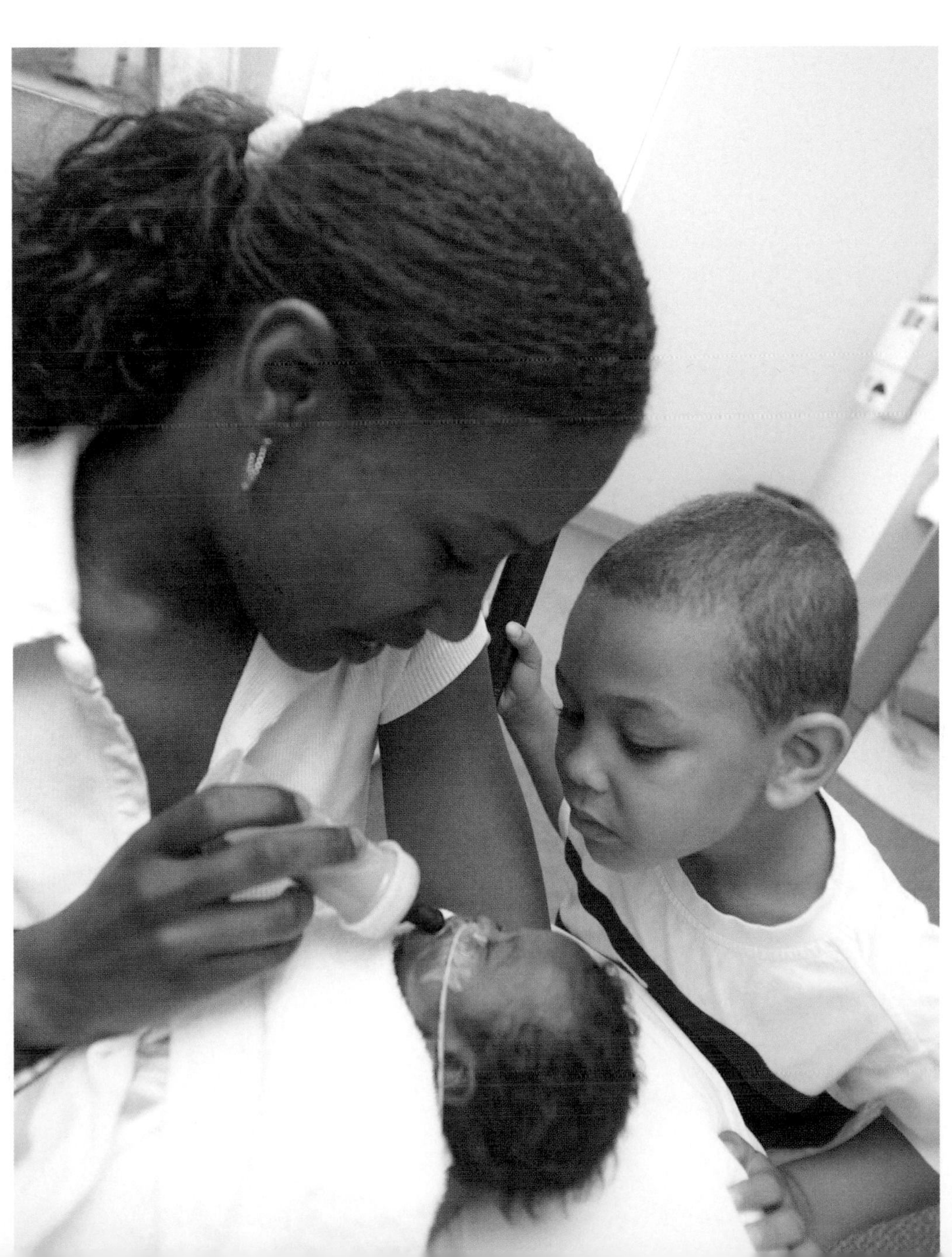

Pregnancy at Risk: Conditions That Complicate Pregnancy

16

STUDENT OBJECTIVES

On completion of this chapter, the student should be able to

1. List the advantages of tight glycemic control for the pregnant woman with diabetes.
2. Differentiate between the care of the pregnant woman with pregestational diabetes and one with gestational diabetes.
3. Describe typical nursing concerns for the pregnant woman with diabetes.
4. Explain the goals of treatment and nursing care for the pregnant woman with heart disease.
5. Differentiate between pregnancy concerns for the woman with iron-deficiency anemia and one with sickle cell anemia.
6. List treatment considerations for the pregnant woman with asthma.
7. Detail the risk to pregnancy from epilepsy.
8. Describe the impact on pregnancy from the TORCH infections.
9. Differentiate between common sexually transmitted infections according to cause, treatment, and impact on pregnancy.
10. Outline treatment for the pregnant woman with human immunodeficiency virus/acquired immunodeficiency syndrome (HIV/AIDS).
11. Describe nursing considerations for the pregnant woman with a sexually transmitted infection.
12. Outline components of a treatment plan for the pregnant woman who is the victim of intimate partner violence.
13. Delineate special concerns associated with adolescent pregnancy.
14. Describe the impact of delayed childbearing on pregnancy.

KEY TERMS

dermatome
diabetogenic effect of pregnancy
gestational diabetes
hyperglycemia
hyperinsulinemia
hypoglycemia
macrosomia
perinatologist
pregestational diabetes
status asthmaticus
status epilepticus
TORCH

In the very recent past, many women with chronic conditions were unable to successfully accomplish pregnancy and/or childbirth. Now that there are effective treatments available for many of these conditions, more women are entering pregnancy with chronic medical conditions. Consequently, the obstetric nurse is challenged to stay abreast of current research findings to intervene appropriately and to educate the woman carrying an at-risk pregnancy. The licensed vocational/practical nurse (LPN) assists the registered nurse (RN) to provide care for the pregnant woman at risk.

Highly specialized knowledge is needed to successfully manage the at-risk pregnancy. Maternal–fetal medicine is a branch of medical science that focuses on the perinatal period. A maternal–fetal medicine specialist is also referred to as a **perinatologist**. This physician specialist is an obstetrician who has received advanced training and specializes in the care of at-risk pregnancies. The perinatologist is competent in the diagnosis and treatment of the pregnant woman who presents with a pre-existing medical condition or who experiences a complication of pregnancy. The perinatologist sometimes provides consultations for the obstetrician who is managing the pregnancy. Alternatively, he or she may co-manage the woman's pregnancy with the obstetrician or be the primary care provider.

PREGNANCY COMPLICATED BY MEDICAL CONDITIONS

Chronic medical conditions and acute infections are risk factors for the pregnant woman. There are several ways in which pregnancy and medical conditions are interrelated. Pregnancy can affect the underlying medical disorder. The normal physiologic changes of pregnancy sometimes alleviate and at other times intensify the symptoms of illness. On the other hand, medical conditions can affect the progress and outcome of pregnancy. Frequently, the fetus is affected adversely by chronic medical conditions of the pregnant woman.

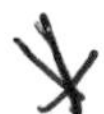

Diabetes Mellitus

Diabetes mellitus (DM) is a chronic disease in which glucose metabolism is impaired by lack of insulin in the body or by ineffective insulin utilization. DM, particularly if it is controlled poorly, can adversely affect pregnancy outcomes. Conversely, pregnancy affects glucose metabolism, which makes the disease challenging to manage. Approximately 4% of pregnancies are complicated by DM (Moore, 2002).

It is recommended that specialists be involved in the care of the pregnant woman with DM. Sometimes the obstetrician consults with an endocrinologist, who then manages the woman's DM throughout her pregnancy. At other times the obstetrician consults with the perinatologist or the perinatologist manages the woman with DM during her pregnancy. A team approach to the management of DM during pregnancy results in the best outcomes. It is recommended that the team be composed of the primary care physician, a registered nurse, a certified diabetic educator, a registered dietitian, and a social worker (Moore, 2002).

Classification of Diabetes Mellitus

There are two overall categories of DM: type 1 and type 2. These two diseases are very different in nature. They both affect glucose metabolism, but type 1 is characterized by a lack of insulin in the body, whereas type 2 is most often associated with insulin resistance. A woman who enters pregnancy with either type 1 or type 2 DM is said to have **pregestational diabetes**. According to the March of Dimes (2003), approximately 1 in 100 women of childbearing age has pregestational DM. Most women of childbearing age do not have full-blown type 2 DM. More often, a woman who is at risk for type 2 DM will develop **gestational diabetes** (GDM), a type of DM that is unique to pregnancy but in many respects mimics type 2 DM. The large majority (90%) of women whose pregnancies are complicated by DM have GDM (Moore, 2002).

Pregestational Diabetes Mellitus

Historically, the woman with pregestational type 1 DM had a higher incidence of spontaneous abortions (miscarriages). If the woman was able to carry the pregnancy to term, the fetus was at high risk for congenital anomalies and/or stillbirth. Fortunately, outcomes have been improved greatly with early monitoring and strict control of blood glucose levels. However, if DM is controlled poorly, particularly in the early weeks of pregnancy, the woman is two to four times more likely to experience a poor outcome, such as a child with a serious birth defect or stillbirth. Other pregnancy-related complications associated with pre-existing DM include pregnancy-induced hypertension, polyhydramnios (excess levels of amniotic fluid), preterm delivery, and shoulder dystocia (Cunningham et al., 2001c). The diabetic woman is three times as likely to experience a cesarean birth as a woman who does not have DM (Moore, 2002).

Some women who have had DM since childhood have damage to the blood vessels. Pregnancy has a tendency to speed up this damage. For example, if a woman has diabetic retinopathy (damage to the retina that can cause blindness), her vision may deteriorate during pregnancy. Fortunately, by approximately 6 months after delivery, vision returns to the prepregnant state. The most serious sequelae (consequences) of circulatory insufficiency occur in the kidneys, which can lead to renal damage and hypertension.

The placenta tends to be smaller, and maternal–fetal circulation is often decreased in longstanding DM, which may lead to chronic fetal hypoxemia and growth retardation, although, as with GDM (see discussion below), the fetus may be exceptionally large because of elevated maternal blood glucose levels. (Refer to Chapter 20 for a more detailed description of the newborn of the woman with diabetes.)

Gestational Diabetes Mellitus

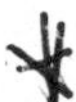

The woman who develops GDM is at increased risk for developing type 2 DM. In fact, more than half of these women will go on to develop type 2 DM within 20 years. It may be that the pancreas of the woman with GDM has sufficient resources to sustain normal blood sugars when she is not pregnant; however, the stress of pregnancy may be enough to bring on GDM. She then experiences sustained periods of hyperglycemia and hyperinsulinemia, which puts her and the unborn child at risk.

The underlying pathophysiology of GDM is insulin resistance. Normal pregnancy is marked by insulin resistance. Tissues become resistant to insulin to provide sufficient levels of glucose for the growing fetus. Although the exact cause of insulin resistance in pregnancy is not known, it is thought that the hormones estrogen, progesterone, and human placental lactogen (HPL) are at least partially responsible. As these pregnancy hormones rise, insulin resistance increases. The result in a normal pregnancy is threefold:

1. Blood glucose levels are lower than normal (mild hypoglycemia) when fasting.
2. Blood glucose levels are higher than normal (mild hyperglycemia) after meals.
3. Insulin levels are increased (**hyperinsulinemia**) after meals.

Together these changes are referred to as the **diabetogenic effect of pregnancy**. GDM develops when the woman cannot tolerate this normal pregnancy change. Risk factors for GDM are listed in Box 16-1.

The greatest risk for the fetus of the woman with GDM is excessive growth, resulting in macrosomia and birth trauma (shoulder dystocia). Insulin does not cross the placenta; however, blood sugar does. Large amounts of glucose cross the placenta when the woman's blood sugar levels are elevated. The fetus does not have insulin resistance, so her pancreas produces increased levels of insulin to handle the high sugar load. As with any disproportionate intake of sugar, the excess calories are stored in the fetus' body in the form of fat. The fetus is also at risk for delayed lung maturity and other complications seen in the newborn of the woman with DM (refer to Chapter 20). Research indicates that long-range complications for the infant include risk for obesity and type 2 DM.

BOX 16.1 Risk Factors for Gestational Diabetes Mellitus (GDM)

- History of a large-for-gestational age infant
- History of GDM
- Previous unexplained fetal demise
- Advanced maternal age (greater than 35 years)
- Family history of type 2 DM or GDM
- Obesity (greater than 200 pounds)
- Non-Caucasian ethnicity
- Fasting blood glucose of greater than 140 mg/dL
- Random blood glucose of greater than 200 mg/dL

Most women who develop GDM do not experience symptoms, although they may notice increased thirst, urinary frequency, hunger, or fatigue. Therefore, screening for GDM is a standard of obstetric care. Most obstetricians screen for GDM at approximately 24 to 28 weeks of pregnancy, although screening may be done as early as 20 weeks in states that have high rates (greater than 5%) of insulin resistance. If the woman has a history of GDM, she is usually screened at the first prenatal visit. The diagnosis of GDM is based on the results of the oral glucose tolerance test (OGTT). The OGTT is also referred to as a glucose challenge test. Box 16-2 outlines normal and diagnostic values of the OGTT.

Treatment

Prepregnancy Care

The woman who has type 1 DM is advised to consult with her physician before she becomes pregnant. Persistent maternal **hyperglycemia** (elevated blood glucose levels) is harmful to the growing fetus, particularly during the first 8 weeks of pregnancy, when organogenesis is occurring. Therefore, it is important for the woman to attain a state of euglycemia (normal blood glucose levels) in the months before becoming pregnant. It is also recommended that, several months before becoming pregnant, the woman with diabetes start taking a daily multivitamin supplement that contains at least 400

BOX 16.2 Diagnostic Values for the Oral Glucose Tolerance Test (OGTT)

Normal values are
- Fasting—less than 95 mg/dL
- 1 hour—less than 180 mg/dL
- 2 hours—less than 155 mg/dL
- 3 hours—less than 140 mg/dL

GDM is diagnosed if two or more values meet or exceed the levels listed above.

micrograms of folic acid. Adequate folic acid intake is the best way to prevent neural tube defects, for which the woman's fetus is particularly susceptible.

Monitoring Glycemic Control

It is important to track the pattern of glycemic control. Average blood sugar levels during the past 4 to 8 weeks are determined by measuring glycosylated hemoglobin (HbA_1C). HbA_1C is a blood test that determines the percentage of red blood cells (RBCs) that have glucose incorporated in the hemoglobin. Sustained periods of hyperglycemia result in higher HbA_1C levels. Because elevated glucose levels are the most damaging to the fetus during the 1st trimester, the goal is for the HbA_1C to be less than 7% for 2 to 3 months before pregnancy is achieved. At this level, the risk of congenital anomalies is equal to that of the general population (1% to 2%). As a comparison, when the HbA_1C is greater than 8.5%, the risk of fetal deformity increases to 22.4% (Moore, 2002). HbA_1C levels are monitored throughout the pregnancy.

Monitoring Renal Function

In addition to glucose assessments, the physician monitors renal function in the woman with long-standing (greater than 10 years) type 1 DM, or if vascular disease is present. Renal function is the best indicator of pregnancy success for the woman with DM (Moore, 2002). Plasma creatinine and blood urea nitrogen (BUN) along with a 24-hour urine for protein and creatinine clearance are measured in each trimester.

Maintaining Glycemic Control

The most important goal of treatment is for the woman to maintain tight glycemic (blood sugar) control before and throughout pregnancy. Because of the increased challenge of managing blood sugar during pregnancy, the woman must monitor her blood sugar many times during the day. Frequently she will need to check her glucose levels seven times per day: upon awakening, after breakfast, before and after lunch, before and after dinner, and before bedtime. The goal is to maintain fasting blood glucose levels of less than 90 mg/dL. Glucose levels should not exceed 120 mg/dL 2 hours after meals, and should generally measure 80 to 110 mg/dL between meals. There are three main facets to glycemic control for the woman with type 1 DM: insulin, diet, and exercise (Fig. 16-1). Glycemic control for the woman with GDM focuses heavily on diet therapy and exercise. Insulin therapy is used if these modalities fail to control the diabetes.

Insulin Therapy. Blood glucose levels vary with advancing gestation. In the first few months of pregnancy, the woman's insulin requirements fluctuate widely, and she is at risk for episodes of **hypoglycemia**, low blood glucose levels, particularly between meals. This phenomenon occurs because the rapidly growing embryo requires a constant supply of glucose, which may deplete maternal blood sugar levels. At the beginning of the 2nd trimester, insulin requirements stabilize, then begin to increase at approximately 24 weeks' gestation, continuing to increase until term. During labor, insulin needs are variable, and in the first 24 hours after delivery, insulin requirements fall dramatically. Because the pancreas of a woman with type 1 DM does not produce insulin, she must be on an insulin regimen. Twice-daily baseline doses of insulin may be ordered to be self-administered subcutaneously. Often a combination of regular and intermediate and/or long-acting insulin is ordered. The baseline doses are supplemented by regular insulin on a sliding scale basis, depending on glucose levels obtained throughout the day.

Insulin may be administered in low doses throughout the day with the use of an insulin pump. An insulin pump is a small device, approximately the size of a pager, that can be worn with a belt or placed in a pocket. A flexible tube placed in the subcutaneous tissue of the abdomen delivers the insulin. The pump has several advantages. Its action mimics that of a healthy pancreas. The woman gets a continuous basal flow of insulin, which helps keep her blood sugar stable throughout the day. She can give herself an insulin bolus by pushing a button before eating or if her glucose level is elevated above a predetermined level. Some women find the pumps more comfortable and less intrusive than self-administering insulin several times per day.

Insulin therapy is recommended for women with GDM when, despite diet and exercise, fasting blood sugar levels cannot be maintained lower than 95 mg/dL or 2 hour postprandial (after meals) sugars below 120 mg/dL. When insulin becomes necessary, the woman is usually hospitalized to titrate the dose and to provide education on self-administration.

Caution is in order! Although gestational diabetes (GDM) is similar to type 2 DM, oral hypoglycemic agents are not used because they are considered to be teratogenic (damaging to the fetus).

Diet Therapy. Another important part of diabetes management during pregnancy is diet therapy. In fact, the cornerstone of treatment for GDM is diet therapy, although insulin may be required, depending upon the severity of glucose intolerance. The goals of dietary intervention for any type of DM during pregnancy, in addition to supplying the nutritional needs of the woman and her fetus, are to maintain blood sugar levels in the normal range and to prevent

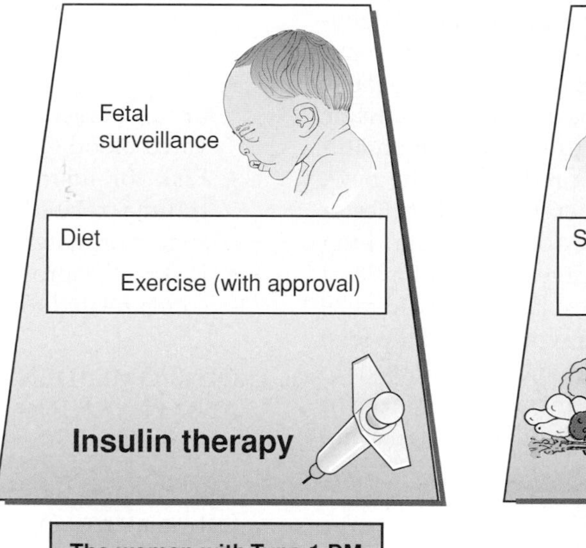

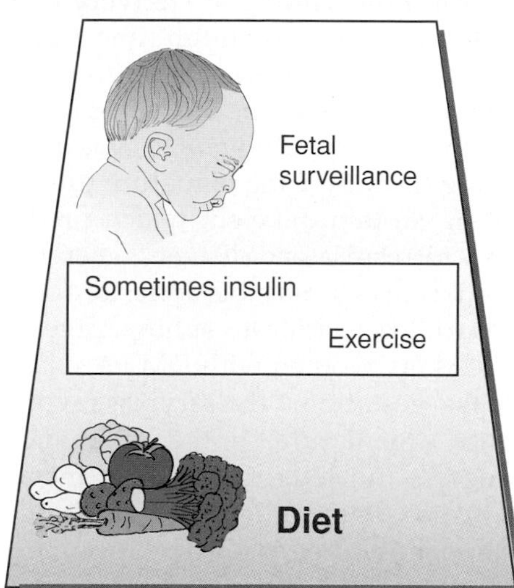

● ***Figure 16.1*** Treatment overview for diabetes in pregnancy. For women with pregestational type 1 DM, the foundation of glycemic management is insulin therapy along with dietary management, exercise, and fetal surveillance. For the woman who develops gestational diabetes (GDM), dietary modification is generally the foundation of treatment. Some women with GDM require insulin therapy, and others do not. Exercise and fetal surveillance are also important facets of care.

ketoacidosis. Consultation with a registered dietitian, preferably one who is also a certified diabetic educator, is recommended because diet requirements are individualized.

The objective is to eat so as to avoid surges and dips in blood sugar. The recommended diet includes a total caloric intake of 30 to 35 kcal/kg of ideal body weight per day. The nutrients are divided so that approximately 55% of dietary intake is composed of carbohydrates, 20% is protein, and 25% is fat (less than 10% should be saturated fat). Ideally the woman spreads her food intake over the day by eating three regular meals interspersed with three snacks.

Exercise. Exercise is another way to help control blood sugar for the woman with DM. However, the pregnant woman should always consult with her physician before exercising, particularly if her diabetes is poorly controlled or she has diabetes complications, such as vascular damage, hypertension, or renal insufficiency. It is generally recommended that exercises should put minimum stress on the trunk region to avoid fetal injury (Cunningham et al., 2001c). Exercise that involves the upper arm muscles, such as swimming, is ideal.

Fetal Surveillance

Fetal surveillance is critical for the woman with DM. An initial sonogram is done during the 1st trimester to determine gestational age and fetal viability. A more detailed, high-level sonogram is usually repeated at 18 to 20 weeks to look closely for structural defects in the fetus. Fetal anatomy is carefully assessed for abnormalities, and amniotic fluid volume is measured. Maternal serum alpha-fetoprotein levels are measured at 16 to 20 weeks to screen for neural tube defects. If HbA_1C levels were elevated in early pregnancy, a fetal echocardiogram is recommended in the 2nd trimester. Serial sonograms in the 3rd trimester (from approximately 26 weeks) are done every 4 to 6 weeks to measure fetal growth. The fetus of the woman with DM may grow to be unusually large, a condition known as **macrosomia**, which is diagnosed if the birth weight exceeds 4,500 grams (9.9 pounds) or the birth weight is greater than the 90th percentile for gestational age. Macrosomia occurs more commonly in women with gestational DM. Conversely, if the woman has longstanding DM or vascular disease, the fetus may be predisposed to intrauterine growth restriction (IUGR).

Third trimester fetal surveillance is vital to help detect signs of fetal stress that precede fetal death. Fetal activity counts are initiated daily at 28 weeks' gestation. At 28 to 34 weeks' gestation, twice-weekly nonstress testing (NST) is begun. A weekly biophysical profile (BPP) is generally recommended, and contraction stress tests (CSTs) are done if the NST is nonreactive or the BPP is nonreassuring. (Refer to Chapter 7 to review prenatal fetal testing.)

Determining Timing of Delivery
Determining the optimum time and method of delivery is a consideration in the care of the pregnant woman with DM. The challenge for the obstetrician is to schedule the delivery to avoid fetal death, while giving the fetus time to mature fully. Fetal lung maturation is often delayed, which predisposes the newborn to respiratory distress. Therefore, 3rd trimester amniocentesis may be done to document fetal lung maturity (a lecithin-to-sphingomyelin ratio of at least 2:1). Many women with DM have labor induced at 39 weeks' gestation if the cervix is favorable and the fetal lungs are mature. If the pregnancy is allowed to progress too long, there is an increased chance for delivery complications, such as shoulder dystocia and fetal demise.

● Nursing Process for the Pregnant Woman With DM

ASSESSMENT

The woman with type 1 DM usually has the disease diagnosed during childhood or adolescence. Therefore, she may be accustomed to monitoring her blood glucose levels and self-administering insulin. However, it is likely that she will need to increase the number of times she monitors daily. Have her do a return demonstration of self-glucose monitoring and recording of results. Be sure that she has a log and understands the importance of recording each blood sugar level.

Once GDM has been diagnosed, assess for understanding of therapeutic regimen management. Instruct the woman to bring her blood sugar log to every prenatal visit. Review the log with her and discuss blood sugar patterns noted. Assess her ability to self-manage her condition. Inquire regarding signs and symptoms of urinary tract infection and/or candidiasis. In the 3rd trimester, institute fetal surveillance as ordered by the physician.

During labor, frequent monitoring of blood glucose levels is required, sometimes as frequently as every hour. If the woman is unable to maintain normal glucose levels, an intravenous insulin drip may be initiated, with the insulin dose titrated to maintain glucose levels within a predetermined range. Chapter 20 covers care of the infant of the woman with diabetes.

SELECTED NURSING DIAGNOSES

- Ineffective Therapeutic Regimen Management
- Risk for Injury (maternal) related to unstable glucose levels: hypoglycemia or hyperglycemia and increased risk for obstetric complications
- Risk for Infection: vaginal candidiasis and/or urinary tract infection (UTI) related to elevated blood glucose levels
- Risk for Injury (fetal): fetal demise or birth trauma related to unstable maternal blood sugars or maternal hyperinsulinemia
- Risk for Disproportionate Growth: fetal macrosomia related to maternal hyperglycemia

OUTCOME IDENTIFICATION AND PLANNING

Appropriate goals may include that the woman will manage the therapeutic regimen successfully; maternal injury from hypoglycemia, hyperglycemia, and obstetric complications will be avoided; and the woman will remain free from infection. Fetal goals may include that the fetus will maintain health status, will be appropriate size for gestational age at birth, and will avoid birth trauma. Other goals and interventions are planned according to the individualized needs of the woman throughout pregnancy, birth, and the postpartum period.

IMPLEMENTATION

Monitoring Management of Therapeutic Regimen
With the assistance of the primary health care provider, information obtained regularly by self-monitoring or blood testing at home with a portable glucose monitor gives immediate feedback on effect of diet, activity, and medications on glucose levels. At every office visit carefully review the woman's blood sugar log. If she is having difficulty maintaining her blood glucose levels within the expected parameters, explore with her possible reasons.

Dietary recall for the past 3 days may be helpful for identifying patterns of food intake that interfere with blood sugar control. Refer the woman for a consult with a registered dietitian, if she is having difficulty following the prescribed dietary regimen. Review with the woman her exercise patterns to determine if improved blood sugar control might result from implementation of an exercise regimen

Carefully explore the woman's compliance with insulin administration. If she is having difficulty controlling her blood glucose levels, ask her to do a return demonstration by having her check her blood sugar levels. If possible, request that she do a return demonstration of insulin preparation and/or administration. Assist her to correct her technique, if necessary.

Frequent episodes of hypoglycemia may be caused by too much insulin or too little food. Explore her pattern of food intake in conjunction with insulin administration. Be certain she is eating three regular meals and three snacks daily. Food intake should follow insulin administration. A pattern of regular exercise may decrease insulin needs. Notify the physician of frequent episodes of hypoglycemia, particularly if the woman began a regular exercise program 3 to 4 weeks previously.

Preventing Maternal Injury

The woman with DM is at risk for unstable blood sugar levels and the associated risks. Take particular care to review the signs and symptoms of hypoglycemia (Box 16-3) with the woman and her family. The woman with pregestational DM is often aware of her hypoglycemic symptoms because she has been dealing with diabetes for some time. Explain that it is important to pay attention to the warning signals because she is more prone to hypoglycemia during pregnancy.

Pay close attention! One of the disadvantages of maintaining a euglycemic state is increased risk for hypoglycemia. Teach the woman the signs of hypoglycemia. Instruct her to keep a ready source of glucose (e.g., a candy bar or glass of orange juice) close by. Family members should know how to administer glucagon intramuscularly in the event of hypoglycemic coma.

Although any woman with DM is at risk for developing diabetic ketoacidosis (DKA), the woman with type 1 DM during pregnancy is at highest risk. She should know the signs of developing hyperglycemia and avoid triggers for DKA. Box 16-4 details these signs and triggers.

The woman with DM is at increased risk for pregnancy-induced hypertension (PIH). In the 3rd trimester the physician will likely recommend weekly blood pressure and urinary protein measurements. At every office visit carefully screen the woman for signs of PIH, such as headache, visual disturbances, epigastric pain, generalized edema, urinary protein, and elevated blood pressure. Inform the woman to immediately call the physician if she should experience any of the symptoms of PIH.

Monitoring for and Preventing Infection

The woman with diabetes is at increased risk for urinary tract infections (UTI) because of elevated blood sugar levels. Review with the woman the

BOX 16.3 Signs of Hypoglycemia

It is particularly important for the pregnant woman and her family to be familiar with the signs and symptoms of hypoglycemia because she is more vulnerable to the condition during pregnancy. Sometimes it helps to remember that the symptoms of hypoglycemia mimic those of the fight-or-flight response. The woman may experience any of the following symptoms.

- Anxiety
- Shakiness
- Confusion
- Headache
- Tingling sensations around the mouth
- Hunger
- Sudden behavior change
- Pale skin
- Cold, clammy skin
- Increased pulse
- Seizure
- Unresponsiveness

BOX 16.4 Diabetic Ketoacidosis (DKA) and Pregnancy

The onset of DKA is marked by the classic symptoms of hyperglycemia, which include

- Polydipsia (excessive thirst)
- Polyuria (increased frequency and amount of urine)
- Polyphagia (excessive hunger)

As DKA develops, the following symptoms appear

- Glucose >300 mg/dL
- Ketonuria
- Kussmaul respirations
- Acetone (like alcohol) breath
- Sleepiness
- Language slurring
- Decreased consciousness

Triggers for DKA include (but are not limited to) the following

- Too little insulin or too much food
- Infection
- Tocolytic therapy (to prevent preterm labor)
- Corticosteroid use
- Insulin pump failure

signs of a UTI, which include increased frequency, voiding small amounts, burning with urination, and cloudy urine. Teach her to drink 8 to 10 glasses of noncaffeinated beverages every day to help prevent UTI, and to wipe from front to back after using the restroom. Frequent handwashing (before and after meals and using the restroom) continues to be the best way to prevent infection. Remind the woman that if a UTI occurs, prompt treatment is essential because UTI can cause premature labor.

Candidiasis is another problem for which the woman with diabetes is prone. Signs of vaginal candidiasis include white, cheesy-type vaginal discharge, severe itching, and discomfort. The discharge does not have a foul odor but is highly irritating to tender vaginal tissue. Fluconazole (Diflucan) is an oral tablet that is sometimes prescribed for woman with vaginal candidiasis. However, normally the use of fluconazole during pregnancy is not recommended. Occasionally the benefits of treatment with this medication outweigh the possible risks to the fetus. The physician will discuss these risks with the woman. Most frequently the physician recommends treatment with over-the-counter vaginal creams and suppositories to control the symptoms of vaginal candidiasis during pregnancy. Verify that the woman understands treatment advice and that her questions have been adequately answered.

Monitoring Fetal Status

It is very important for the pregnant woman with DM to understand the risk of fetal demise, particularly if blood sugar levels are difficult to control and/or the woman requires insulin to manage her diabetes. The 3rd trimester is generally the time of greatest danger. Institute fetal surveillance per the physician's orders. It is always appropriate to teach the woman to monitor fetal activity and kick counts, starting at approximately 26 to 28 weeks' gestation. Perform twice-weekly NSTs in the physician office or as ordered. Give the fetal monitor tracing to the RN to assess and report results to the physician. Nonreactive NSTs usually are followed up with a CST and/or a BPP.

Estimating Fetal Weight

The fetus of the woman with DM is at risk for disproportionate growth resulting in fetal macrosomia (fetal weight greater than 4,000 grams). Assist the physician or RN to measure fundal height at each prenatal visit. Report findings that do not correlate with gestational age (refer to Chapter 7 to review fundal height assessment). Larger-than-expected size may be related to a large fetus or polyhydramnios.

Instruct the woman on the importance of serial sonograms to estimate the fetal weight. The macrosomic infant is much more likely to experience the delivery complication of shoulder dystocia (difficulty delivering fetal shoulders after delivery of the head), leading to birth trauma. Many physicians induce labor in the woman as soon as fetal lung maturity can be established in an attempt to prevent shoulder dystocia. Alternatively, the physician may elect to perform a cesarean delivery if macrosomia is suspected.

EVALUATION: GOALS AND EXPECTED OUTCOMES

- **Goal:** The woman will successfully manage the therapeutic regimen.
  Expected Outcomes:
  - Monitors and records blood sugar levels as ordered.
  - Adjusts her diet to recommendations by the physician and dietitian.
  - Exercises at least three times per week using recommended exercises.
  - Self-administers insulin, if ordered.
- **Goal:** Maternal injury from hypoglycemia and hyperglycemia will be avoided.
  Expected Outcomes:
  - Recognizes and treats hypoglycemia promptly.
  - Recognizes hyperglycemia and takes measures to prevent DKA.
- **Goal:** The woman will remain free from infection.
  Expected Outcomes:
  - Does not experience a UTI (or if she does, seeks prompt treatment).
  - Seeks prompt treatment for vaginal candidiasis.
- **Goal:** The fetus will maintain health status.
  Expected Outcomes:
  - Fetal activity counts are within normal limits.
  - NST is reactive.
  - BPP score is greater than 7.
  - CST is negative.
- **Goal:** The fetus will avoid birth trauma.
  Expected Outcomes:
  - Fetal weight is estimated to be appropriate for gestational age.
  - No birth injury results from shoulder dystocia.

Test Yourself

- What test is used to monitor long-term glucose control during pregnancy for the woman with diabetes?
- What term is used to describe the fetus whose weight exceeds 4,500 grams?
- What are the three cornerstones of therapy for the pregnant woman with diabetes?

Cardiovascular Disease

Heart disease is the third leading cause of death in women of childbearing age and complicates approximately 1% of all pregnancies (Cunningham et al., 2001a). In the past, most cases of heart disease during pregnancy were caused by rheumatic heart disease. Now, however, congenital heart disease is the underlying problem in at least 50% of pregnancies complicated by heart disease.

Significant cardiovascular changes occur in a normal pregnancy. Blood volume and cardiac output increase. Systemic vascular resistance drops. In a normal healthy woman, these cardiovascular changes are tolerated with minor notice. In the woman with heart or vessel disease, whose heart is already compromised, the increased demands of pregnancy can lead to cardiac failure. Heretofore undiagnosed heart disease can be unmasked or cardiac symptoms can worsen in the woman with pre-existing disease. The periods of greatest risk for the pregnant woman with cardiac disease are at the end of the 2nd trimester (when blood volume peaks), during labor, and in the early postpartum period secondary to fluid shifts.

The New York Heart Association's (NYHA) classification system (Table 16-1) is used to rate the severity of heart disease in the pregnant woman. Generally, women with Class I or II heart disease have a good prognosis for pregnancy. However, women with Class III or IV are at much higher risk for poor pregnancy outcomes and require more extensive monitoring and treatment throughout the pregnancy. In addition, the risk of maternal and fetal complications increases if the woman has any of the following conditions: cyanosis, erythrocytosis, stenotic lesions, or right-to-left shunt.

Clinical Manifestations and Diagnosis

Signs and symptoms (Box 16-5) vary depending on the underlying cause of heart disease. Tachycardia that lasts for more than several minutes accompanied by dizziness or light-headedness suggests a tachyarrhythmia and requires further investigation. The woman with an existing stenotic valve tends to have an increase in symptoms during pregnancy, whereas the woman with incompetent valves tends to experience fewer symptoms during pregnancy. Pregnancy is particularly dangerous for the woman with severe (greater than 80 mm Hg systolic) pulmonary hypertension.

The earliest warning sign of cardiac decompensation is persistent rales in the bases of the lungs. The woman will probably notice a nocturnal cough. Serious heart failure is marked by a sudden decrease in the ability to perform normal duties, exertional dyspnea, and attacks of coughing with a smothering feeling.

TABLE 16.1 NYHA's Clinical Classification of Heart Disease

Class	Amount of Compromise	Symptoms	Physical Limitations	Pregnancy Prognosis
I	Uncompromised	Asymptomatic	None	Good
II	Slightly compromised	• Asymptomatic at rest • Symptomatic with normal physical exertion	Slight	Good
III	Markedly compromised	Symptoms occur with minimal activity	Marked	Moderate; may need hemodynamic monitoring and special anesthetic management during labor
IV	Severely compromised	Symptoms occur at rest	Unable to perform any physical activity without discomfort	Poor, will need hemodynamic monitoring and special anesthetic, management during labor

BOX 16.5 Signs and Symptoms of Heart Disease

The woman may complain of
- Dyspnea
- Orthopnea
- Nocturnal cough
- Dizziness
- Fainting
- Chest pain

Physical examination may reveal
- Cyanosis
- Clubbing of the fingers
- Neck vein distention
- Tachycardia
- Heart murmurs
- Edema

Upon physical examination tachycardia, edema, and hemoptysis may be noted.

Treatment

A team approach is indicated to manage pregnancy complicated by heart disease. The obstetrician, cardiologist, perinatologist, and other specialists often collaborate in the care of the pregnant woman with heart disease. Treatment varies depending on the etiology of the heart condition; however, there are general principles for management. These principles involve activity levels, stress management, diet, and medication. No matter what the underlying cause of the condition, the main goal is prevention, early detection, and early treatment of cardiac decompensation.

Activity Levels

Activity is allowed as tolerated. The woman is cautioned to rest frequently and not allow herself to become overly fatigued. Because pregnancy greatly increases the workload of the heart, complete bed rest is sometimes necessary, particularly for the woman who is severely compromised (see Table 16-1).

Stress Management

Heart failure can be precipitated by any unusual stress that increases demands upon the cardiovascular system. Examples include infection, anemia, underlying medical disorders, and excessive emotional or physical stress. The physician carefully screens for any condition that might precipitate the stress response. Pneumococcal and influenza vaccines are recommended because infection is particularly harmful for the pregnant woman with heart disease. Antibiotic prophylaxis to prevent endocarditis is necessary before some high-risk procedures (e.g., some dental work and other invasive procedures) for the woman with moderate to severe heart disease.

Diet and Medications

The woman is advised to limit salt intake and weight gain during pregnancy. Most cardiac medications are continued during pregnancy, with the exception of warfarin (Coumadin) and angiotensin-converting enzyme (ACE) inhibitors. Warfarin crosses the placenta and increases the risk of congenital anomalies. An alternative is treatment with heparin. The large molecules of this anticoagulant do not cross the placental barrier. ACE inhibitors increase the risk of fetal mortality and can lead to intractable renal failure in the newborn.

Management During Labor and the Postpartum Period

Special precautions must be taken during labor. The supine position is contraindicated for any pregnant woman, but avoidance of supine hypotensive syndrome during labor for the woman with heart disease is imperative. Supine hypotensive syndrome can lead to decreased placental perfusion with resultant fetal compromise. The condition can also increase maternal cardiac output and quickly lead to maternal compromise.

Here's a helpful reminder. The signs of supine hypotensive syndrome include decreased blood pressure, dizziness, pallor, and clammy skin. It is imperative that you prevent this condition by positioning the woman in a semirecumbent position with a pillow or wedge under one hip. The pregnant woman with heart disease should never be flat on her back.

The stress and pain of labor greatly increases the demand on the heart, making pain relief a crucial part of labor management for the woman with heart disease. Epidural analgesia with narcotics and/or epidural anesthesia is the pain relief option of choice during labor. During the second stage of labor, vigorous pushing using Valsalva maneuver can lead to cardiac decompensation. Cesarean section is reserved for usual obstetric complications. Vaginal birth is preferred, if possible. It is no longer recommended that the woman with heart disease be given prophylactic antibiotics during labor and delivery, including cesarean delivery.

The woman remains at risk for heart failure in the postpartum period. She is monitored closely for signs of postpartum hemorrhage, anemia, infection, and thromboembolism. All of these complications greatly increase the risk of cardiac decompensation.

Nursing Care

The most important nursing action is to monitor for and teach the woman to recognize signs of cardiac decompensation. Listen to breath sounds at each office visit and during labor. Report rales in the bases of the lungs and complaints of nocturnal coughing. Elevated blood pressure and tachycardia are other warning signs that should be reported immediately. Increased respiration, shortness of breath and productive coughing may indicate the development of pulmonary edema or pulmonary emboli, either of which is life threatening.

It is especially important for the pregnant woman with heart disease to protect herself from infection. Instruct her to avoid crowds and anyone with signs of respiratory infection, even the common cold. Explain that cigarette smoking increases the risk of contracting an upper respiratory infection. Advise her of the importance of frequent handwashing. Administer pneumococcal and influenza vaccines, as ordered. Remind the woman of the importance of reporting her heart condition to all health care providers, including the dentist, so that prophylactic antibiotics can be administered, if necessary.

Inquire regarding illicit drug use and cigarette smoking in a nonjudgmental way. Explain that many illicit drugs and cigarette smoking adversely affect the heart and increase the risk for decompensation. Make clear that intravenous drug use increases the risk for infective endocarditis, a potentially lethal complication.

Assist the woman with tests for fetal well-being. Explain that serial ultrasound measurements allow the physician to monitor growth of the fetus. Instruct the woman to do fetal kick counts in the 2nd and 3rd trimesters. Decreased fetal movement should be reported immediately. Assist with amniocentesis, as indicated. Amniocentesis may be done to determine fetal lung maturity in anticipation of early delivery if the woman's cardiac status begins to deteriorate in the 3rd trimester.

Monitor the woman particularly closely during labor. Position her so that the gravid uterus does not compress the major blood vessels. Assess pain levels frequently. Administer intravenous analgesia as ordered. Assist with epidural anesthesia administration. Monitor vital signs as recommended for the at-risk pregnancy (see Chapter 10). Continue to observe for signs of cardiac decompensation in the postpartum period. Immediately report fever, increased bleeding, and any signs of decompensation.

Anemia

Anemia is a condition in which the blood is deficient in red blood cells (RBCs), hemoglobin, or in total volume. Anemia is not itself a disease. Rather, it is a symptom of an underlying disorder. There are three main causes of anemia: blood loss, hemolysis (increased RBC destruction), and decreased production of RBCs. There are multiple etiologies associated with each category. Iron-deficiency anemia is the most common anemia experienced during pregnancy. Other anemias that could complicate pregnancy include megaloblastic anemia from folate deficiency, pernicious anemia from vitamin B_{12} deficiency, sickle cell anemia, and thalassemia. This section focuses on iron-deficiency and sickle cell anemia.

Iron-Deficiency Anemia

Iron-deficiency anemia is characterized by reduced production of RBCs because the body does not have enough iron to manufacture the hemoglobin molecule. The RBCs that are produced are smaller in size (microcytic) and are pale in color (hypochromic). Because the pregnant woman has increased iron requirements, she is particularly vulnerable to iron-deficiency anemia.

Clinical Manifestations and Diagnosis

Common signs and symptoms of iron-deficiency anemia in the pregnant woman are tachycardia, tachypnea, dyspnea, pale skin, low blood pressure, heart murmur, headache, fatigue, weakness, and dizziness. Pica (ingestion of nonfood substances such as clay and laundry starch) and pagophagia (frequent chewing or sucking on ice) are both associated with iron-deficiency anemia.

Treatment

Treatment for iron-deficiency anemia is directed toward a diet rich in iron and folate in addition to iron and folate supplementation. Recent studies have shown that folate supplementation increases the effectiveness of iron therapy. Rarely does the pregnant woman with anemia require a blood transfusion.

Sickle Cell Anemia

Sickle cell anemia is a hemolytic anemia that is caused by an abnormal hemoglobin molecule called hemoglobin S (Hgb S). Individuals who have sickle cell anemia inherit two copies of the genetic mutation for Hgb S, one from the father and one from the mother. Some people are carriers of the trait because they inherit only one copy of the mutation. Individuals who are carriers are said to have sickle cell trait. In the United States, sickle cell anemia most commonly occurs in African-American individuals. Every year 1 in 400 African-American newborns is born with sickle cell anemia, and approximately 1 in 12 African-Americans has sickle cell trait (Mayfield, 1996).

Sickle cell anemia is a chronic condition characterized by acute exacerbations of the disease called "crises." Stress typically triggers a crisis, in which the abnormal hemoglobin causes RBCs to "sickle" when oxygen is released from the hemoglobin. The abnormal cells are sticky and clump together in such a way that they cannot flow easily through the capillaries. If enough of the cells clump, blood flow to the area is blocked, causing tissue ischemia and pain at the site of blockage. The reticuloendothelial system fights to rid the body of the abnormal hemoglobin by breaking down the sickled cells. Unfortunately, the bone marrow cannot produce enough RBCs to replace the damaged ones, so anemia results. The pregnant woman with sickle cell anemia is at higher risk for hypertension, particularly preeclampsia-eclampsia and preterm delivery. Newborns of the woman with sickle cell anemia are more likely to be small for gestational age.

Clinical Manifestations and Diagnosis

The woman with sickle cell trait rarely experiences symptoms, and when she does, the symptoms are generally mild. The woman with sickle cell anemia, however, is at risk for a sickle cell crisis at any time during the pregnancy. Dehydration and infection are two examples of conditions that predispose the woman to a crisis. Depending upon which area of the body is affected, the woman may experience recurrent bouts of pain in the joints, bones, chest, and abdomen. She also may experience nonspecific symptoms of anemia, such as fatigue, tachycardia, and dyspnea. Physical examination may reveal enlarged lymph nodes, enlarged spleen (splenomegaly), hematuria (bloody urine), or jaundice.

Treatment

Treatment between crises is directed at preventing a crisis, if possible. Maintaining adequate hydration, avoiding infection, getting adequate rest, and eating a balanced diet are all common sense strategies that decrease the risk of a crisis. Hydroxyurea (Hydrea), a medication that decreases the frequency and severity of crises, is not recommended during pregnancy because it is teratogenic in animals.

The initial prenatal visit requires additional laboratory work for the woman with sickle cell anemia to include hemoglobin electrophoresis, serum iron, total iron binding capacity, ferritin levels, liver function tests, electrolyte analysis, kidney function tests, urinalysis, and urine culture. Hepatitis B vaccine may be administered if the woman does not have hepatitis B. Asymptomatic bacteriuria is treated with antibiotics to prevent a full-blown urinary tract infection. The woman may be instructed to return for more frequent than normal prenatal visits. Prenatal visits are scheduled every 2 weeks in the 2nd trimester and every week throughout the 3rd trimester.

When the woman experiences a painful crisis, the physician orders a CBC, type and cross match, and sometimes arterial blood gas (ABG) measurements. Intravenous (IV) fluids are started to hydrate the patient and decrease blood viscosity. Narcotics are generally required to control the pain of an attack. Fetal monitoring is indicated, if the fetus is viable, and supplemental oxygen by face mask may be necessary. Antibiotics are given to treat infection, if it is present. Occasionally an exchange transfusion[1] may be indicated to reduce the amount of sickled RBCs in the circulation.

Nursing Care

At each visit do a 1- to 3-day diet recall to help identify patterns of food intake for the pregnant woman with any type of anemia. She may be embarrassed to give an accurate recall. In these instances, it may be helpful for a family member to assist with the dietary recall. Draw blood as ordered to monitor hemoglobin and hematocrit.

The woman with iron-deficiency anemia needs counseling regarding foods that are high in iron. These include animal protein, dried beans, fortified grains and cereals, dried fruits, and any food cooked in cast iron cookware. Instruct her that iron absorption will be enhanced if she includes foods high in vitamin C along with iron-rich foods. Absorption of her iron supplement will be enhanced if she drinks orange juice when she takes her supplement. Her diet should also contain adequate amounts of folate. Foods high in folic acid include fortified grains, dried beans, and leafy green vegetables.

Iron supplements predispose to constipation. The pregnant woman may be tempted to stop taking iron supplements because of constipation. Instruct her regarding the importance to her and her baby of continuing iron supplementation. All of the normal measures that help prevent constipation, such as maintaining adequate fluid intake, getting enough exercise, and establishing regular bowel habits are helpful for the pregnant woman taking iron supplements.

The woman with sickle cell anemia needs support and teaching throughout her pregnancy. Emphasize the importance of using common sense approaches to prevent crises. Instruct the woman to wash her hands frequently and to avoid highly crowded areas to decrease her risk of contracting an infection. Adequate fluid intake and rest are important for maintaining health in the pregnant woman with sickle cell anemia. Assist her to make and keep her prenatal appointments.

---

[1] For an exchange transfusion, a predetermined amount of blood is withdrawn from the patient (typically 500 cc) and 2 units of packed red blood cells are transfused.

Test Yourself

- What is the earliest sign of cardiac decompensation.
- Which are signs of supine hypotensive syndrome?
- Describe two conditions or situations that might trigger a crisis for the woman with sickle cell anemia.

Asthma

Asthma is a chronic, inflammatory disease of the airways characterized by acute exacerbations of reversible airway obstruction. As many as 4% of all pregnancies are complicated by asthma. This condition, also known as reactive airway disease (RAD), can be a severe threat to the health of the woman and her fetus, if the disease is not controlled properly. Pregnant women with poorly controlled asthma experience a higher incidence of preeclampsia-eclampsia, antepartum and postpartum hemorrhage, premature labor, respiratory failure, and death. Fetal complications include intrauterine growth restriction, fetal demise, and preterm birth. Perinatal outcomes are similar to those of the general population if the condition is well controlled throughout pregnancy.

Clinical Manifestations and Diagnosis

The course of the disease varies during pregnancy. Physical examination during remission may be completely normal. During an acute asthma episode the respiratory rate increases and the woman feels short of breath and anxious. An expiratory wheeze is characteristic. Other auscultation findings may include diffuse rhonchi, bronchovesicular sounds, or bronchial sounds throughout the lung fields. Retractions of the respiratory muscles may be noted. Complaint of nocturnal awakening is a classic symptom. Other symptoms frequently include a cough and chest tightness. Pulsus paradoxus, a pulse that weakens during inspiration, is often noted.

Treatment

The goals of antepartum asthma management are prevention of acute episodes, control of symptoms, maintenance of normal pulmonary function, and avoidance of emergency department visits and hospitalization.

The initial prenatal visit includes a thorough history of the course of the woman's asthma before pregnancy and in prior pregnancies, if applicable. The health care provider inquires as to the frequency of acute episodes, the severity of the disease, history of hospitalizations, and any known environmental stimuli that are asthma triggers for the woman. Medication history is carefully elicited. Baseline spirometry measurement is done to determine pulmonary function (Robinson & Norwitz, 2000). Other tests include allergen skin testing, pulse oximetry, ABG measurement, and chest x-ray (Miller & Greenberger, 1999).

Management of an Acute Exacerbation

Management of an acute attack often requires hospitalization for the pregnant woman. She may be treated on a 23-hour observation status, or her condition may necessitate a full admission. Oxygen is given by face mask to maintain the PO_2 above 60 mm Hg and the oxygen saturation greater than 95%. Fluids are given intravenously for hydration to loosen mucus in the airways. Epinephrine injected subcutaneously is often beneficial for relieving severe dyspnea. Frequent nebulizer treatments with a beta-agonist such as albuterol are done to bring the attack under control. Corticosteroids and/or theophylline may be started intravenously. Fetal well-being is generally assessed by external fetal monitoring methods after 20 weeks' gestation, although other measures of fetal well-being, such as ultrasound or biophysical profile, may also be ordered.

Status asthmaticus is a potentially fatal complication of an acute asthma attack. Severe asthma symptoms that do not respond after 30 to 60 minutes of treatment are diagnosed as status asthmaticus. This condition can lead to pneumothorax, pneumomediastinum, acute cor pulmonale, cardiac arrhythmias, and respiratory failure (Cunningham et al., 2001b). Status asthmaticus in the pregnant woman is treated aggressively, with early intubation and mechanical ventilation in the intensive care setting.

Labor and Birth Management

There are several important points to remember about managing the woman with asthma during labor. The woman may fear that asthma symptoms will be exacerbated by the stress of labor. This is not generally the case. In fact, symptoms tend to diminish during labor. Regularly scheduled asthma medications should continue to be administered throughout labor. Adequate hydration and analgesia minimize the risk of bronchospasm. Fentanyl is the narcotic of choice because it does not cause histamine release, which could lead to bronchospasm. Epidural analgesia is the ideal method of pain control for the laboring woman with asthma.

Vaginal delivery is attempted, if at all possible. If there are indications for a surgical delivery, epidural or spinal anesthesia is preferred over general anesthesia. If a general must be administered, atropine and glycopyrrolate (Robinul) may be ordered preoperatively to induce bronchodilation.

Nursing Care

Teaching is a major role when providing nursing care for the pregnant woman with asthma. Be sure that the woman does a return demonstration on the use of her inhaler. Do not assume that she knows how to use it. She should also do a return demonstration for use of the peak flow meter. Remind her of the importance of monitoring fetal activity and kick counts during the 2nd and 3rd trimesters. Family Teaching Tips: Managing Asthma During Pregnancy outlines the major points to make when educating the pregnant woman with asthma.

Epilepsy

Epilepsy is a group of neurologic disorders that involve a long-term tendency to have recurrent unprovoked seizures (Morrell, 2002). Approximately 1 in 200 pregnancies is complicated by epilepsy, making this disorder the most commonly encountered neurologic condition in pregnant women.

Clinical Manifestations

Several difficulties are encountered during pregnancy that relate to the condition of epilepsy. Drug metabolism is changed during pregnancy, making it more difficult to establish therapeutic antiepileptic drug (AED) levels. Thirty percent to 50% of women with epilepsy experience an increase in seizure frequency during pregnancy, whereas others experience a decrease or no change in seizure frequency. The major risk to the pregnancy during a seizure results from blunt trauma. Trauma can lead to miscarriage, premature rupture of membranes, and placental abruption.

The fetus of the woman with epilepsy is at almost two times greater risk of experiencing congenital malformations than is the fetus of a woman in the normal population. In the past it was thought that epilepsy itself increased the risk for birth defects. However, the latest research indicates that AEDs used to treat epilepsy are the major cause of fetal defects. Cleft lip and palate, cardiac defects, and neural tube defects comprise the majority of malformations noted in the fetus.

Treatment

Preconceptual care is highly recommended for the woman with epilepsy who wishes to become pregnant. A thorough history and physical examination establishes the diagnosis of epilepsy and the efficacy of the current treatment regimen in controlling seizures. If the woman has been seizure free for several years while receiving low-dose therapy, the physician may try to wean the woman from the AED. The woman with epilepsy should be followed by her obstetrician in consultation with a neurologist.

FAMILY TEACHING TIPS

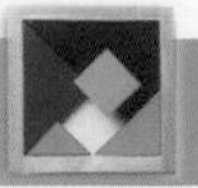

Managing Asthma During Pregnancy

- Do not stop taking your asthma medications. The risk to you and your baby is much higher from uncontrolled asthma than it is from taking your medications. Remember, you are "breathing for two."
- Check with your doctor before taking any over-the-counter medications. Some of these medications have been shown to cause harm to your developing baby.
- Protect yourself from asthma triggers.
  - Keep a symptom diary to identify your unique triggers.
  - Avoid cigarette smoke, exposure to animals, and dusty, damp environments.
  - Stay inside in air-conditioned surroundings during pollen seasons and when the pollution or mold index is high.
  - Wear a mask or scarf over your mouth on excessively cold days to help warm the air.
  - Protect yourself from colds and flu because respiratory infections can trigger acute asthma attacks.
    - Avoid crowds where viruses may be prevalent.
    - Wash your hands frequently.
    - Take the flu shot if you have moderate or severe asthma. The flu shot is based on a killed virus, so it is safe to use during pregnancy.
  - Avoid foods or chemicals that might have caused a reaction in the past, such as sulfites or MSG.
- Continue your allergy shots as long as you are not having reactions to the shots. If you are not currently taking allergy shots, it is usually not advised to begin doing so during pregnancy because of the risk of reactions.
- Monitor your peak expiratory flow rate (PEFR) regularly, as recommended by your doctor. If you have severe asthma, you will need to measure your PEFR at least twice daily. A decrease in the PEFR usually precedes an acute asthma attack hours to days before physical symptoms begin.
- Develop a crisis management plan in consultation with your physician. The plan should include how to recognize warning signs and what to do when early signs of worsening status occur. Go immediately to the nearest emergency department if any of the following occur after rescue drugs are taken.
  - Rapid improvement does not result.
  - Improvement is not sustained.
  - Condition worsens.
  - The episode is severe.
  - Fetal movement decreases.

At the very first sign of breathing difficulties use your peak flow meter to measure your PEFR. If it is low or has decreased from your last reading, call the doctor immediately. Other warning signs of an impending attack may include a headache, itchy throat, sneezing, coughing, or feeling tired.

High-dose (4 to 5 mg daily) folate supplementation is recommended in the months preceding and throughout pregnancy because AEDs increase the risk for neural tube defects. At 14 to 18 weeks' gestation, it is recommended that maternal serum alpha-fetoprotein levels be drawn and a high-resolution sonogram be performed to screen for neural tube defects. Beginning at 36 weeks, many physicians prescribe additional vitamin K supplementation because AED therapy can lead to vitamin K-deficient hemorrhage of the newborn.

Although there is an increased risk for cesarean delivery, epilepsy is not an indication for induction of labor or for cesarean delivery. Most women can expect a normal vaginal delivery. One percent to 2% of women experience seizures either during labor or after delivery. If the seizure is severe, a cesarean delivery may be indicated.

Status epilepticus is an emergency complication of epilepsy whereby seizure activity continues for 30 minutes or more after treatment is initiated or when three or more seizures occur without full recovery between seizures. Immediate measures are taken to protect the woman from injury while protecting the airway. Emergency intubation with mechanical ventilation is sometimes required. Blood work is drawn for glucose, electrolytes, CBC, AED levels, and blood and urine toxicology screens. An IV line is started to allow for IV administration of benzodiazepines, such as diazepam or lorazepam. Once seizures are under control, fosphenytoin is given via the IV route.

Nursing Care

Teach the woman the importance of carefully following her treatment regimen and of maintaining regular prenatal care. Emphasize the importance of eating a diet high in folic acid and of taking folic acid supplementation. Advise the woman to get plenty of rest and sleep and to exercise regularly. Assist her to schedule lab work at regular intervals. Provide support when prenatal testing is done to screen for fetal anomalies.

BOX 16.6 TORCH Infections

TORCH (an acronym for the infections)

Toxoplasmosis
Other: hepatitis B, syphilis, varicella and herpes zoster
Rubella
Cytomegalovirus (CMV)
Herpes simplex virus (HSV)

All are teratogenic. All cross the placenta. Fetal effect is determined by gestational age at exposure. TORCH syndrome is characterized by IUGR, microcephaly, hepatosplenomegaly, rash, thrombocytopenia, and CNS findings, such as ventricular calcifications and hydrocephaly.

Assessment

1. History: flu-like symptoms, fatigue, cat exposure, genital lesions, rash, exposure to sick children
2. Physical exam: lymphadenopathy, headache, malaise, jaundice, N/V, low-grade temperature, rash, ulcerated and painful lesions of the genitals
3. Psychosocial: fear, anxiety, apprehension

Diagnostics

1. Serologic tests
    - TORCH screen
    - CBC
    - HBsAg and HBeAg
    - Liver function tests
2. Cultures
    - CMV
    - HSV
3. Pap smear
4. Serial ultrasounds (monitor for IUGR and other defects throughout pregnancy)

Interventions

1. Instruct the woman regarding specifics of
    a. the infection
    b. transmission
    c. medication and medical management
2. Reinforce importance of handwashing
3. Encourage questions
4. Suggest a multidisciplinary conference with family members, if anxiety and fear levels are high
5. Encourage breast-feeding. These mothers may be afraid to breast-feed their babies.

Infectious Diseases

There are a number of infectious disease categories that present increased morbidity and mortality to the infant whose mother is victim of one or more of these infections. Some type of infective process is seen in approximately 15% of all pregnancies.

TORCH

TORCH (Box 16-6) is an acronym for a special group of infections that can be acquired during pregnancy and transmitted through the placenta to the fetus. The "T" stands for toxoplasmosis, the "O" for other infections (hepatitis B, syphilis, varicella and herpes zoster), the "R" is for rubella, the "C" is for cytomegalovirus (CMV), and the "H" stands for herpes simplex virus (HSV).

Each infection is teratogenic, and the effects are different, depending upon when during the pregnancy infection occurs. Fetal infection may lead to TORCH syndrome characterized by central nervous system (CNS) dysfunction. Mental retardation, microcephaly, hydrocephalus, CNS lesions, jaundice, hepatosplenomegaly, hearing deficits, and chorioretinitis are examples of sequelae for the newborn that is infected with one of the TORCH agents. Fetal infection may also lead to spontaneous abortion, intrauterine growth restriction (IUGR), stillbirth, and premature delivery. Prevention is the focus of interventions because many of the TORCH infections do not have effective treatment regimens.

A TORCH screen can be performed if the physician has reason to believe the woman might have one of the TORCH infections. Diagnosis is made by serial antibody titers. If the woman is seronegative (no antibodies in the blood) after two titers (taken 10 to 20 days apart), infection is ruled out. If the woman is seropositive (antibodies in the blood) for the first titer, but the titers do not rise by the second draw, she is considered to have a latent ("old") infection. This is important because it is very rare that a latent infection is passed to the fetus. However, if the woman's antibody titers have risen by the second draw, she is considered to be acutely infected.

Toxoplasmosis

Toxoplasmosis is an infection caused by the protozoan *Toxoplasma gondii*, also referred to as "*T. gondii*." It is transmitted via undercooked meat and through cat feces. Toxoplasmosis is a fairly common infection in humans and usually produces no symptoms. However, when the infection is transmitted from the woman through the placenta, a condition called congenital toxoplasmosis can occur. Approximately 400 to 4,000 cases of congenital toxoplasmosis occur per year in the United States (Jones, Lopez, & Wilson, 2003). The classic triad of symptoms for congenital toxoplasmosis is chorioretinitis, intracranial calcification, and hydrocephalus in the newborn.

Toxoplasmosis is difficult to diagnose because it rarely produces symptoms in the woman. This infection is particularly harmful to the fetus if it is contracted between 10 and 24 weeks of pregnancy. Treatment is with one or all of the following: spiramycin (Rovamycine, an investigational drug in the United States), pyrimethamine (Daraprim), and folinic acid. The newborn is also treated with antibiotics.

Infection can be prevented through several common sense approaches. Advise the pregnant woman to have someone else clean the cat litter box. If there is no one else to perform this duty, she should wear gloves and wash her hands thoroughly before and after cleaning the box. The box should be cleaned daily. She should wear gloves when working in the garden or when doing yard work. She should wash her hands thoroughly before and after handling raw meat, and she should eat only meats that have been completely cooked (i.e., no rare or medium rare meats). Any surface or item that is touched by raw meat should be thoroughly cleaned in hot, soapy water after contact. All fruits and vegetables need to be washed carefully before being served.

Other Infections: Hepatitis B, Syphilis, Varicella and Herpes Zoster

Hepatitis B. Hepatitis B virus (HBV) is transmitted sexually or through contact with blood or body fluids. It can also be transmitted to the fetus by contact with vaginal secretions and blood during delivery. In adults who become acutely infected, approximately 1% die of liver disease caused by the virus. Eighty-five percent to 90% completely recover and develop immunity to hepatitis B; 10% to 15% become chronic carriers and are at higher risk for developing cirrhosis and liver cancer.

Obstetricians screen their pregnant patients for hepatitis B surface antigen (HBsAg). A woman who has an acute HBV infection has elevated HBsAG titers. If the newborn is not treated, there is an increased risk that the infant will develop HBV infection. Approximately 25% of infants who become infected develop significant liver disease, and 50% develop chronic HBV infection.

As many as 90% of these neonatal infections can be prevented by neonatal immunoprophylaxis. If the mother is HBsAG positive, the neonate should receive hepatitis B immunoglobulin (HBIg) and the hepatitis B vaccine within 12 hours of birth. The immunoglobulin provides immediate protection, and the vaccine provides long-term protection from infection. Regardless of the woman's HBV status, all infants should be vaccinated against hepatitis B at birth, 1 to 2 months after birth, and again at 12 months of age.

Syphilis. Syphilis is a sexually transmitted infection (STI) with the bacterium (spirochete) *Treponema pallidum* (*T. pallidum*). The bacteria are transmitted via sexual contact or through broken skin. The main symptom of primary syphilis is a painless red pustule, which usually appears within 2 to 6 weeks after exposure. The pustule quickly erodes and develops a painless, bloodless ulcer called a chancre. Because it is painless, the newly infected person may not notice the chancre. The chancre, which sheds infectious fluid, usually appears on the body part that served as the portal of entry for the bacteria.

If the pregnant woman becomes infected with syphilis, the bacteria can cross the placenta, causing infection in the developing fetus. Spontaneous abortion occurs in 25% to 50% of women who develop acute syphilis early in the pregnancy. Preterm birth and fetal demise are other sequelae of active syphilis infection. If the woman carries the pregnancy to the age of viability, there is a 40% to 70% chance that the infant will be born infected with syphilis.

The infected infant may be born with birth defects, such as blindness, deafness, or other deformities.

Hutchinson's triad is characteristic and includes inflammation of the cornea, deafness, and notched teeth. Another characteristic of early congenital syphilis is snuffles, a nasal discharge that can be bloody. The newborn may have a vesicular or bullous rash that is contagious. On the other hand, the syphilis-infected infant may not immediately exhibit symptoms at birth. Symptoms can develop as long as weeks to months later. Swollen lymph glands, spleen and liver enlargement, jaundice, anemia, bone deformities, and vesicular rash may occur.

Screening for syphilis with the RPR or VDRL is one of the routine blood tests performed for every pregnant woman in the early part of pregnancy and repeated when she goes into labor. A positive screen requires further testing that is more specific to *T. pallidum*. Syphilis is curable, if properly treated. The treatment of choice for syphilis is benzathine penicillin B (Bicillin) administered intramuscularly as a single dose. Penicillin may be given during pregnancy and is safe to use while breast-feeding. Erythromycin is given to individuals who are sensitive to penicillin. Newborns with congenital syphilis are also treated with penicillin.

Varicella and Herpes Zoster. Varicella zoster is the virus that causes chickenpox. Herpes zoster is the recurrent form of the virus that lies dormant in the dorsal root ganglia of the spinal cord. Reactivation of herpes zoster results in shingles. Contact with shingles by persons who are nonimmune to chickenpox leads to the development of chickenpox in that individual. Varicella zoster and herpes zoster are members of the herpesvirus family.

Varicella zoster is transmitted by respiratory droplets and is highly contagious. The virus incubates for approximately 2 weeks and is contagious 2 days before onset of the skin lesions until the lesions crust over, generally 5 days after the initial onset. Herpes zoster (shingles) is characterized by a localized rash within a **dermatome**, an area on the body surface supplied by a particular sensory nerve. The rash is very painful. Occasionally pain precedes the rash. Anyone who has had chickenpox is at risk for developing shingles.

The incidence of varicella zoster during pregnancy is low, occurring in 1 to 5 of 10,000 pregnancies (Lie, 2003). Transmission of varicella zoster by the pregnant woman to her unborn child is very rare, occurring in 1 to 2 percent of cases (Van Earden & Bernstein, 2003). The highest risk (2%) occurs if the woman contracts varicella in the 2nd trimester, between 13 and 20 weeks' gestation. Transmission of herpes zoster is even more unlikely. However, the severity of fetal varicella syndrome, if it is contracted, gives cause to treat this infection during pregnancy with great care.

Fetal varicella syndrome is associated with low birth weight, scar-producing skin lesions, limb hypoplasia, and contractures. The syndrome can also result in damage to the ears, eyes, and CNS, leading to mental retardation, paralysis, and seizures. Prognosis for the neonate is poor. The newborn is at risk for neonatal varicella, a severe form of chickenpox with a 20% to 30% mortality rate, if the woman contracts varicella from 5 days before to 2 days after delivery. Another danger of varicella during pregnancy is the risk to the woman of developing varicella pneumonitis. This is a form of pneumonia that can be very severe, with a mortality rate as great as 40%. Even if the woman survives, the severity of the pneumonia could result in death of the fetus.

Any pregnant woman who reports a possible exposure to chickenpox or shingles should have a serologic test performed to detect varicella antibodies. Varicella zoster immune globulin (VZIG) may be given within 96 hours of exposure to help prevent the development of chickenpox. VZIG may also be given to the neonate (within 96 hours of exposure), if the woman develops chickenpox 5 days before, or within 48 hours after, delivery.

The best treatment is prevention. A woman of childbearing age who has not had chickenpox should be vaccinated. She should be instructed to avoid pregnancy for at least 1 month after vaccination. Pregnant women should not be vaccinated; however, susceptible individuals in the household of a pregnant woman who is susceptible to chickenpox should be vaccinated. This is the most effective way to prevent transmission to the pregnant woman. The nonimmune woman should receive one dose of varicella vaccine immediately after delivering her baby and a second dose at the 6-week postpartum visit.

Rubella

Rubella is a highly contagious disease caused by a virus. Rubella is usually a mild illness when it occurs in adults and children. Twenty percent to 50% of rubella infections are "silent," that is there are no symptoms. When symptoms occur, they are generally mild and include low-grade fever, rash, lymphadenopathy, general malaise, and conjunctivitis. Complications are rare.

The problem occurs when a woman contracts rubella while she is pregnant. Congenital rubella infection can result, which is anything but mild. Consequences of congenital rubella include spontaneous abortion, stillbirth, and congenital anomalies of varying severity. Hearing impairment is the single most common defect associated with congenital rubella infection. The greatest risk occurs if the woman develops rubella in the 1st trimester. Rubella contracted during the period of organogenesis (in the first 11 weeks of pregnancy) can result in multiple anomalies. Maternal rubella infection contracted after 20 weeks of pregnancy rarely results in birth defects. There is no cure for congenital rubella infection. Treatments are supportive and directed toward control of symptoms and complications.

The best treatment for congenital rubella infection is prevention. Ideally, all women of childbearing age would be tested for immunity to rubella before they become pregnant. Nonimmune women should be vaccinated before becoming pregnant and are advised to wait at least 28 days after vaccination to achieve pregnancy. Women are routinely tested for immunity to rubella in early pregnancy and again before delivery. The nonimmune woman is not vaccinated during pregnancy. She should be careful to avoid anyone with flu-like symptoms or rash during the pregnancy. Vaccination is administered in the early postpartum period before discharge from the hospital or birthing center. Breast-feeding is not a contraindication to receiving the rubella vaccine. Currently the Centers for Disease Control and Prevention (CDC, 2004) recommends that the combination measles, mumps, and rubella (MMR) vaccine be given to children at 12 to 15 months of age and a second dose at age 4 to 6 years before starting school. Routine vaccination of all children decreases spread of rubella and decreases the risk that a nonimmune pregnant woman will contract the infection.

Cytomegalovirus

Cytomegalovirus (CMV) is the silent menace. CMV is the most common cause of congenital viral infection, occurring in 0.2% to 2.2% percent of live births. A virus in the herpes family causes CMV. It is transmitted by contact with infected bodily fluids, such as saliva, blood, breast milk, urine, and semen. A common source of infection is young children.

Most individuals infected with CMV do not experience symptoms. If they do have symptoms, the symptoms mimic those of mononucleosis: sore throat, low-grade fever, swollen lymph glands, body aches, and fatigue. CMV is diagnosed by two or more antibody titers. If the antibody titers are rising, acute CMV infection is presumed.

A woman who contracts CMV for the first time while she is pregnant has a 30% to 40% risk of passing the infection to the fetus. The risk to the fetus from CMV infection is greatest during the first 20 weeks of pregnancy. Most affected newborns (approximately 90%) do not demonstrate symptoms at birth. However, as many as 15% of these infants develop one or more neurologic abnormalities, such as blindness, deafness, learning disabilities, and mental retardation. Signs that are more likely to be present at birth include hydrocephaly, microcephaly, IUGR, hepatosplenomegaly, jaundice, and rash. About 20% of newborns who have symptoms at birth will die. Ninety percent of the newborns who survive will develop serious neurologic deficits, such as mental retardation. The antiviral drug ganciclovir (Cytovene), which is used to treat adult AIDS patients with CMV-related eye infections, is currently being investigated for its efficacy in treating newborns with congenital CMV infection.

Because there is no cure for congenital CMV, prevention is strongly recommended. Pregnant women who have contact with small children should practice meticulous handwashing, particularly after contact with saliva and urine. Diapers, tissues, and other potentially infected items should be carefully disposed. Drinking glasses and eating utensils should not be shared. Pregnant health care workers should practice universal precautions. Although CMV is passed through breast milk, breast-feeding is not contraindicated because CMV infection contracted during birth or from breast-feeding rarely causes serious problems.

Herpes Simplex Virus

Herpes simplex virus (HSV) is a sexually transmitted infection caused by herpes simplex virus 1 (HSV-1) and herpes simplex virus 2 (HSV-2). The virus is spread by direct contact. In general, HSV-1 causes oral herpes, also known as cold sores, and HSV-2 causes genital herpes. However, both types can be transmitted to the mouth and/or genital region through kissing, oral-genital sex, and other sexual contact, and both types can cause serious illness in a newborn. Fortunately, neonatal herpes is rare, occurring in less than 0.1% of newborns.

Symptoms of genital herpes usually develop within 2 to 14 days after exposure to the virus. Without antiviral treatment, the lesions may last for as long as 20 days. The first attack is generally the most severe, although more than 75% of individuals with primary HSV infections have no symptoms. Painful lesions develop in the area that was exposed to the virus, usually the genital or anal regions. The lesions eventually completely heal and do not cause scarring. However, the virus lies dormant in the nervous system and can cause recurrent attacks. Flu-like symptoms, such as lymphadenopathy, headache, muscle aches, and low-grade fever, sometimes occur a day or two before an outbreak.

The majority of cases of neonatal herpes are contracted by contact with active virus in the birth canal, although a small percentage (5%) of fetuses are infected in utero. Most infants of women who have longstanding herpes do not develop neonatal herpes. This is thought to occur because maternal antibodies to herpes virus cross the placenta and protect the fetus. Preterm infants are more likely to contract herpes because antibodies do not begin to cross the placenta until approximately 28 weeks of gestation, so preterm infants do not have the same protection as full-term infants. The highest risk for neonatal herpes occurs in infants of women who develop herpes for the first time during the last trimester of pregnancy and who have active lesions in the birth canal at the time of delivery. In fact, the risk can be as high as 50%.

If the woman has a lesion at delivery, the safest alternative is cesarean delivery to prevent the baby from coming in contact with the virus in the birth canal. It is also recommended that no vaginal examinations be done, if there are active lesions. If there are no lesions present when the woman goes into labor, the American College of Obstetricians and Gynecologists recommends a vaginal delivery. It is recommended that internal monitoring with a fetal scalp electrode not be used during labor in women who have a history of genital herpes because the small break in the fetal scalp made by the electrode can serve as a portal of entry for the virus.

Sexually Transmitted Infections

A sexually transmitted infection (STI) is one that is transmitted primarily by sexual contact or through contact with blood or bodily fluids.[2] Many of the TORCH infections are STIs, including hepatitis B, syphilis, and herpes simplex. Other STIs of importance to the pregnant woman include trichomoniasis, gonorrhea, chlamydia, genital warts, and human immunodeficiency virus/acquired immunodeficiency syndrome (HIV/AIDS).

Many STIs are reportable diseases tracked by the CDC. Reportable infections include syphilis, chlamydia, gonorrhea, and AIDS. Some states require other STIs (in addition to those aforementioned) to be reported. One increasing concern is that many STIs increase the risk for the individual to contract HIV/AIDS. If symptoms of the infection include a break in the integrity of the skin or mucous membranes, these sites can provide a portal of entry for HIV.

Chlamydia

Chlamydia is the most prevalent reportable STI, occurring at a rate of 278.3 cases per 100,000 population in the year 2001. This represents a 10.4% increase over rates for the year 2000. Chlamydia is caused by infection with the bacterium *Chlamydia trachomatis* and is transmitted during oral, vaginal, and anal sex.

Approximately 75% of women who have chlamydia have no symptoms, which makes identification of the infection problematic. It also underscores that fact, that although this is the most prevalent STI, it is most likely grossly underreported. If the woman experiences symptoms, these may include vaginal discharge, abnormal vaginal bleeding, and abdominal or pelvic pain. Of several methods of diagnostic testing that are available, amplified DNA tests are the most sensitive. Acceptable specimens include urine and cervical secretions.

Fortunately, chlamydia is easily curable with antibiotics. Treatment is with one dose of azithromycin (Zithromax) or twice-daily dosing for 7 days with erythromycin. As with other STIs, the sexual partners of the individual also require treatment.

Untreated chlamydia increases the risk of contracting HIV/AIDS. The most frequent sequela of untreated chlamydia is pelvic inflammatory disease (PID), a serious infection of the reproductive tract that can lead to infertility and chronic pelvic pain. Inflammation of the fallopian tubes that occurs with PID often results in scarring, which increases the risk of ectopic pregnancy. A pregnant woman who contracts chlamydia is at increased risk for going into preterm labor. The fetus can come into contact with bacteria in the vagina during the birth process. If this happens, the newborn can develop pneumonia or conjunctivitis that can lead to blindness.

Gonorrhea

Gonorrhea is an STI caused by the bacterium *Neisseria gonorrhoeae* (*N. gonorrhoeae*). The years between 1975 and 1997 realized a 73.8% decline in cases of gonorrhea. In 1998, the rates increased by almost 8% and have remained steady through 2001 (CDC, 2001). Gonorrhea is second in prevalence only to chlamydia, with 361,705 cases reported for the year 2001. The highest percentage (approximately 75%) of cases occurs in adolescents and young adults (National Institute of Allergy and Infectious Diseases [NIAID], May 2002). The bacteria are transmitted during sexual contact. The primary site of infection for the woman is the cervix, although infection can occur anywhere along the genital tract, in the urethra and rectum, and in the oro- and nasopharynx (throat).

Initial symptoms, which usually develop within 2 to 10 days of exposure to the bacteria, are mild and may go unnoticed. The woman who contracts gonorrhea may have vaginal bleeding during sexual intercourse, pain and burning while urinating, and a yellow or bloody vaginal discharge. A discharge from the rectum, itching around the anus, and painful bowel movements with fresh blood on the feces are signs of rectal infection. Infrequently the infection is asymptomatic.

There are several methods used to diagnose gonorrhea. A culture taken from the cervix, rectum, or throat is the diagnostic method of choice because it positively identifies *N. gonorrhea*. However, a culture takes several days to grow, so results are not immediately available. Other tests are sometimes used that produce rapid, although less accurate, results. These tests include gram staining, oxidase testing, and acid

[2] Many references, including government resources, refer to STIs as sexually transmitted diseases (STDs). Because of the stigma associated with these diseases, this text uses sexually transmitted infection (STI).

production testing. A presumptive diagnosis of gonorrhea is made when the rapid tests yield positive results, so that treatment can begin before the culture results are available.

Treatment is usually with a combination of two antibiotics that treat both gonorrhea and chlamydia because these infections often occur together. Some antibiotics commonly prescribed to treat gonorrhea are not used during pregnancy. One problem that has arisen recently is strains of *N. gonorrhoeae* that are resistant to antibiotics. The CDC publishes guidelines for physicians to help prevent and treat antimicrobial resistance. Efforts are under way to develop a vaccine against gonorrhea.

Untreated gonorrhea can lead to PID, which can leave the woman infertile or susceptible to ectopic pregnancy because of scarring in the reproductive tract. The bacteria can also spread through the bloodstream and infect joints, heart valves, or the brain. Infection with gonorrhea greatly increases the risk of acquiring HIV infection.

Risk to pregnancy from gonococcal infection includes increased risk for abortion and preterm delivery. Risk to the fetus occurs if the fetal eyes become infected during birth, a condition known as ophthalmia neonatorum. Blindness can result from this infection; however, cases are rare because all newborns receive prophylactic treatment with ocular antibiotic ointment within the hour after birth.

Human Papillomavirus

Human papillomavirus (HPV) is spread by skin-to-skin contact, usually during sexual activity. This virus can cause condylomata acuminata (genital warts) and cervical cancer. An individual with asymptomatic HPV infection can unknowingly pass the virus on to sexual partners.

Condylomata acuminata develop in clusters on the vulva, within the vagina, on the cervix, or around the anus. The lesions may remain small, or they can develop into large clusters of warts that resemble cauliflower. An abnormal Papanicolaou (Pap) smear may be the first indication of HPV infection and should lead to further inspection for the virus. The diagnosis is made by visualization of the warts or by applying a solution of acetic acid to areas of suspected infection. Acetic acid causes infected areas to turn white. A biopsy of tissue can be taken and examined microscopically for evidence of infection.

Genital warts can disappear without treatment. The type of treatment chosen depends on many factors, including age of the patient; duration, location, extent, and type of warts; the patient's immune status; risk of scarring; and pregnancy status. Several medical treatments are available, most of which consist of topical applications. Many of these treatments involve the use of substances that are teratogenic and thus are contraindicated during pregnancy. Surgical removal of the warts through a variety of techniques, including blunt dissection, laser, and cryosurgery, is another treatment option.

Genital warts have a tendency to increase in size during pregnancy. This may result in heavy bleeding during vaginal delivery. The pregnant woman can pass HPV to her fetus during the birth process. In rare instances, neonatal HPV infection can result in life-threatening laryngeal papillomas. HPV infection can be transmitted to the infant but may not appear for as long as 3 years after birth.

Trichomoniasis

Trichomoniasis, or infection with Trichomonas, is an STI caused by one-celled protozoa. It can infect the urethra, vagina, cervix, and structures of the vulva. Trichomoniasis is transmitted during unprotected sexual contact with someone who has the infection. It is possible for the woman to transmit trichomoniasis to the fetus during vaginal delivery, although this is a rare occurrence.

Symptoms of trichomoniasis include large amounts of foamy, yellow-green vaginal discharge, vaginal itching, unusual vaginal odor, painful sex, and dysuria. As many as half of all women with trichomoniasis have no symptoms. The most common diagnostic test is called a "wet mount." The practitioner takes a swab of vaginal secretions and examines the sample under the microscope. Unique movements of the organism allow for accurate diagnosis in 40% to 60% of cases. A culture can also be done, which is more sensitive than a wet mount, but results are not available for several days.

Treatment is with metronidazole (Flagyl). Although metronidazole is available in vaginal suppository and cream formats, oral dosing is recommended by the CDC, even during pregnancy, because of its increased effectiveness in treating Trichomonas infection. Oral metronidazole is given as a 2-gram single dose or as a 500-mg, twice-daily dose for a period of 7 days. The cure rate is 90% to 95%. In rare cases in which symptoms persist despite adequate treatment, further treatment with high doses of metronidazole is recommended. There are a few documented cases of metronidazole-resistant strains of Trichomonas. Expected side effects of treatment with oral metronidazole are metallic taste and dark urine. Nausea and vomiting can occur with high doses or when alcohol is taken during treatment.

HIV/AIDS

In 1981, health care providers were first confronted with the STI acquired immunodeficiency syndrome (AIDS), which is caused by the human immunodeficiency virus (HIV). HIV attacks the protective cells of the immune system, leaving the body unprotected against pathogens that normally do not cause illness in humans. Individuals who die of AIDS usually succumb to these opportunistic infections.

Since 1981 there have been more than 816,000 cases of AIDS in the United States. Women are at a higher risk than men for heterosexual transmission of the virus because the vaginal rugae are perfect for harboring the virus over time. African-American and Latino women are becoming infected in greater proportion than nonminority women. Washington, DC; Texas; California; New York; New Jersey; and Florida have the highest AIDS rates among women.

HIV is most often transmitted during unprotected sexual activity with an infected partner. The virus can enter the body through the mucous membranes of the genitals, rectum, or mouth. People infected with HIV often do not look or feel sick and may transmit the virus to others before they know they are infected.

HIV can also be transmitted through contact with infected blood. The risk of contracting HIV infection through receiving a blood transmission is very small because of screening and treatment of donated blood. However, an individual can be exposed to HIV-infected blood by sharing needles for IV drug use, intramuscular injections of anabolic steroids, or tattooing.

A woman who has HIV during pregnancy is at risk for transmitting the infection to the fetus during pregnancy or childbirth and to the newborn while breast-feeding. This risk can be substantially decreased if the woman receives appropriate antiretroviral treatment during pregnancy and childbirth and if she refrains from breast-feeding.

Clinical Manifestations. There are several ways to stage HIV disease. This text describes three stages of HIV infection: early, intermediate, and advanced. These stages correspond to CD4-positive T-cell (CD4 cell) counts. In the early stage, CD4 counts remain above 500/mL of blood (normal). In the intermediate stage, the CD4 counts measure between 200/mL and 500/mL (below normal). The advanced stage, which is also known as AIDS, is characterized by CD4 counts below 200/mL. CD4 cells are specialized T-cells and key infection fighters of the immune system.

The early (initial) stage of infection may be characterized by flu-like symptoms, such as fever, headache, sore throat, aching joints, malaise, and lymphadenopathy, which last for several weeks. Conversely, approximately one-half of individuals do not experience symptoms at all during the early stage.

After the initial infection, the individual moves into the intermediate stage. This stage can be divided into two phases: latent and acute HIV disease. The latent stage is "silent" in that no symptoms occur. This phase lasts for an average of 8 to 10 years. Although the person has no symptoms, the virus is replicating rapidly and destroying CD4 cells. Unfortunately, unless the person is tested for HIV during the latent stage, he does not know that he is infected and may pass the virus on to others.

It is unknown why some HIV-positive individuals move rapidly into acute HIV disease in as little as 1 year, whereas others do not develop symptoms for 20 years or more. As stated previously, the average length of time before the onset of symptoms is 8 to 10 years. Once symptoms appear, the individual may seek treatment. Typical symptoms of acute HIV disease (Box 16-7) include swollen lymph nodes, feeling tired, weight loss, night sweats, fever, persistent oral or vaginal yeast infections, severe oral or genital herpes infections, shingles, skin rashes or scaly skin, and short-term memory loss. Women may develop severe PID that is not responsive to treatment.

The diagnosis of AIDS is made in the advanced stage of HIV infection. The CDC defines AIDS as an HIV-positive individual who has less than 200 CD4-positive T cells (CD4 cells) per milliliter of blood. It is at this stage that the person is immunosuppressed and becomes susceptible to opportunistic infections. Symptoms of opportunistic infections vary depending on the causative organism (bacteria, viruses, fungi, parasites, etc.). Symptoms may include extreme fatigue, dysphagia, coughing, dyspnea, nausea, vomiting, persistent diarrhea, severe weight loss, fever, confusion, ataxia,

BOX 16.7 Typical Symptoms of Acute HIV disease

Acute HIV disease describes the symptoms that appear during the latter part of the intermediate phase of HIV infection. CD4 cell counts remain above 200/mL of blood during this phase. Typical symptoms include:

- Persistent generalized lymphadenopathy
- Generalized malaise
- Weight loss
- Night sweats
- Fever
- Thrush (oral yeast infection)
- Candidiasis (vaginal yeast infection)
- Oral hairy leukoplakia (lesion characterized by white plaque on the lateral aspects of the tongue)
- Aphthous ulcers (painful, shallow ulcers of the oral mucosa)
- Herpes simplex virus (outbreaks are often severe)
- Shingles (herpes zoster)
- Anemia with associated pallor
- Thrombocytopenia
- Aseptic meningitis
- Peripheral neuropathies
- Short-term memory loss

seizures, blindness, and even coma. The individual is also susceptible to various rare cancers that are difficult to treat.

Diagnosis. A pregnant woman may become infected with HIV during pregnancy, or she may enter pregnancy with HIV. It is very important that the pregnant woman's HIV status is known. The CDC recommends that practitioners offer confidential HIV testing at the beginning of pregnancy and again during labor. The woman may refuse testing, but the practitioner is encouraged to counsel with the woman and explore reasons for refusal.

At present there are two methods to test for HIV infection: the enzyme-linked immunosorbent assay (ELISA) and the Western blot analysis. Both test for antibodies to the virus versus the virus itself. Antibodies to HIV usually develop within 6 to 12 weeks after exposure; however, it can take as long as 6 months for antibodies to appear. Researchers are trying to develop tests that can detect the HIV virus so that infection can be diagnosed much earlier and more reliably than is currently possible.

Unfortunately, all infants born to HIV-infected women have antibodies to HIV because the woman's antibodies cross the placenta. Therefore, an infant cannot be diagnosed with HIV infection using traditional testing methods until she is 18 months of age. Diagnosis in infants younger than 18 months of age requires viral culture on two separate specimens, both of which must be positive to make the diagnosis. This testing should be accomplished as soon as possible after birth so that therapy can be implemented quickly.

Treatment. The two main goals of treatment for the pregnant woman infected with HIV are to prevent progression of the disease in the woman and to prevent perinatal transmission of the virus to the fetus.[3] The best way to prevent perinatal transmission is to prevent HIV infection in the woman or to identify HIV infection before pregnancy or as early as possible during pregnancy. Therefore, early prenatal care for all women, regardless of risk, is imperative.

For the pregnant woman with HIV, therapy is composed of oral zidovudine (ZDV) prophylaxis, beginning as early as 14 weeks' gestation and continuing throughout pregnancy. Some studies have shown that adding a protease-inhibitor to the drug regimen may further reduce the risk of perinatal transmission of HIV. ZDV may be withheld in the 1st trimester of pregnancy to avoid possible teratogenic effects, although to date adverse fetal effects of ZDV administration in early pregnancy have not been demonstrated.

[3] Discussion of treatment for HIV for nonpregnant individuals is outside the scope of this textbook.

It is recommended that the HIV-positive woman be given the choice of cesarean delivery scheduled at 38 weeks' gestation to further reduce the risk of perinatal transmission. Several studies have shown that women who take antiretroviral medication during pregnancy and experience vaginal delivery have a 7% chance of transmitting the virus to their babies; whereas, women who take ZDV throughout pregnancy and have a cesarean delivery before the membranes rupture have as low as a 1% chance of perinatal transmission. If the woman elects for a vaginal delivery, IV ZDV is recommended to be given during labor and birth. Oral ZDV should be administered to the infant for the first 6 weeks of life. Breast-feeding is contraindicated. If these recommendations for prophylaxis are followed, the risk for perinatal transmission decreases from 25% to 35% for the untreated woman to as low as 2% for the treated woman.

If the woman is in an advanced stage of HIV disease during pregnancy, she should continue to receive treatment even in the 1st trimester. There have been no studies that show definite teratogenic properties of antiretroviral therapy. The risk to the woman and to her pregnancy from withholding treatment must be weighed against the potential risk to the fetus from drug therapy.

Nursing Care. Reassure the client that her confidentiality will be protected. Provide information concerning HIV infection and AIDS in an open, nonjudgmental manner. Explain the benefits of knowing HIV status early in pregnancy. Encourage the woman to be tested. Be certain that the woman knows how to protect herself from HIV infection by avoidance of high-risk behaviors.

If the woman is HIV positive, ensure that she understands the risk to her sexual partners and the importance of condom use. Counsel her regarding expected treatments. Explain the risks of perinatal transmission of HIV and the benefits of therapy. Explore her understanding of the treatment regimen.

● Nursing Process for the Pregnant Woman With an STI

Although different organisms cause STIs, avoiding high-risk behaviors can prevent them all. The nurse is in an excellent position to work with the pregnant woman who is diagnosed with an STI.

ASSESSMENT

Begin the assessment with a thorough history. Inquire regarding risk factors for STIs in a way that makes the woman feel safe to answer honestly. It is usually best to try to elicit the following information with open-ended questions, if possible. Is there a previous history of STI? Has she or her partner ever been treated for an STI? Has she had multiple sexual partners? Is she in a new sexual relationship? Does her partner always use a condom, or does she use the female condom for every sexual act including oral sex? Does she engage in anal sex with her partner? Does she or her sexual partner engage in IV drug use? Does she or her partner share needles for IV drug use?

The history should include questions regarding symptoms of STI. Does she have a vaginal discharge? If so, have her describe the discharge. Is sex painful? Does she bleed during or after sex? Has she noticed swollen lymph nodes? Has she been running low-grade fevers? Has she noticed any rashes or skin lesions? Has she experienced night sweats or lost weight without trying to do so?

Perform a physical assessment. Measure her weight. Compare her current weight to her previous or normal weight. Note any recent weight loss. Record her temperature and other vital signs. Some STIs cause a low-grade fever. Palpate the lymph nodes in the neck and groin regions. Report any swollen or nonmobile nodes. Inspect the oral mucosa and tongue for lesions. Inspect the skin thoroughly for rashes or lesions.

Take note of signs of emotional distress, anxiety, or low self-esteem. Does she practice good personal hygiene? Self-esteem issues can express themselves by self-neglect and poor grooming. Does she make appropriate eye contact? Inquire regarding her social support. Does she have friends? Does she live with anyone? Does she have a partner? Is he or she supportive of her? Notice nonverbal behaviors such as fidgeting, hand wringing, or inattention.

SELECTED NURSING DIAGNOSES

- Risk for Infection (STI) related to unsafe sexual practices, IV drug use, or needle sharing.
- Ineffective Protection related to altered immune status or broken skin barrier.
- Deficient Knowledge of STI and treatment regimen.
- Risk for Situational Low Self-Esteem related to the stigma associated with STIs.
- Anxiety related to pregnancy outcome and fetal safety.

OUTCOME IDENTIFICATION AND PLANNING

Goals for a pregnant woman with an STI include risk control, prevention of the spread of infection, adequate knowledge, maintaining positive self-esteem, anxiety control, and safe delivery of a healthy, infection-free infant. Goals and interventions are planned according to the individualized needs of the woman and her fetus throughout pregnancy, birth, and the postpartum period.

IMPLEMENTATION

Controlling Risks for STIs

Explain the risks of contact with infected bodily fluids and blood. Clarify that women are at higher risk than are men for contracting an STI during heterosexual intercourse. Make clear that the highest risk of STI transmission during sexual activity is engaging in anal intercourse without a condom. Emphasize the importance of using a latex condom for every act of sexual intercourse and a latex barrier for oral sex. Inform the woman to avoid sexual intercourse when there are open lesions or discharge on the genitals. Oral sex should also be avoided when lesions or discharge are present on the mouth or genitals.

Instruct the woman regarding proper handwashing techniques and the importance of frequent handwashing. If the woman is an IV drug user, assist her to find a needle exchange program, if one is available in the area. Help her devise a plan to avoid needle sharing. Assist her to enter a treatment program, if this is feasible and acceptable to the woman.

Maintaining Immune Status and Protection From Additional Infections

Teach the woman that infection with one STI puts her at higher risk for contracting another STI. This is particularly true for STIs that cause lesions or skin breakdown. Explain the importance of having all sexual partners treated for the infection. She should take her medication as directed.

Give instructions specific to the STI. If the woman is HIV positive, ensure that she understands the importance of diligently taking her antiretroviral medications daily. Explain that these medications control the viral load (amount of virus in the blood) and help maintain CD4 counts in the protective range.

Ensuring Knowledge of STI and Treatment Regimen

Teach the woman the specifics of the STI she is experiencing. Be sure that she can explain how the infection is transmitted, what the symptoms of infection are, how to avoid spreading the infection to her sexual partners, how to decrease the risk of transmitting the infection to her fetus, and what the treatment plan and goals are.

Verify understanding of the treatment regimen by asking the woman to describe the medications she is taking and when and how she is to take them. Have her explain the expected action of each medication, as well as expected side effects. Teach her to immediately report side effects she may find intolerable so that the physician can adjust her medications without jeopardizing her treatment. Explain the importance of completing the full course of treatment, even after symptoms subside, to prevent the development of resistant strains of the organism.

Enhancing Self-esteem

Maintain an open, accepting demeanor when interacting with the woman. Ensure she is in a comfortable, private place before interviewing her. Avoid asking potentially embarrassing questions in the presence of others.

Avoid negative criticisms and judgmental questions such as "Why didn't you?" or "You should have . . ." Encourage the woman to identify personal strengths. Convey confidence in the woman's ability to take care of her unborn child.

Reducing Anxiety

Use a calm, reassuring approach. Seek to understand the woman's perception of the risk to herself and to her fetus. Encourage the woman to verbalize her feelings. Use active listening. Ask for clarification when you do not understand.

Give factual information. Correct any misperceptions or misinformation the woman may have. Reassure the woman regarding the probable outcome of her pregnancy. Use up-to-date facts from reliable sources to avoid false reassurances. Help her understand the risks without causing unnecessary fear. For instance, you can explain that with treatment the risk of an HIV-positive woman transmitting HIV to her unborn child is less than 8%. Put another way, more than 90% of babies born to women with HIV disease who receive appropriate treatment will be born free of infection and will remain so.

EVALUATION: GOALS AND EXPECTED OUTCOMES

- **Goal:** The woman will control risks for STIs.
  Expected Outcomes:
  - Verbalizes ways she will reduce her risk for contracting or transmitting STIs.
  - Maintains a monogamous sexual relationship with one partner who is also monogamous or partner uses a latex condom for every act of sexual intercourse.
  - Avoids anal sex.
  - Avoids intravenous drug use or participates in a needle exchange program.
- **Goal:** The woman will not spread infection.
  Expected Outcomes:
  - Remains free of additional infections.
  - Maintains a plasma CD4 cell count above 200/mL (if HIV positive).
- **Goal:** The woman will have adequate knowledge of the STI and its treatment.
  Expected Outcomes:
  - Explains how the STI is transmitted.
  - Describes how to prevent transmission to sexual partners and decrease the risk of transmission to the fetus.
  - Explains her treatment regimen.
  - Verbalizes the goals of her treatment plan.
- **Goal:** The woman will maintain positive self-esteem.
  Expected Outcomes:
  - Demonstrates positive self-regard.
  - Makes positive statements about the self.
  - Maintains adequate personal hygiene.
  - Voices confidence in her ability to take care of her unborn child.
- **Goal:** The woman will have decreased anxiety.
  Expected Outcomes:
  - Expresses reasonable expectations regarding the outcome of the pregnancy.
  - Verbalizes decreased anxiety.

Test Yourself

- Which infection is best prevented by instructing the pregnant woman to avoid changing the cat litter box?
- Which sexually transmitted infection is most frequently diagnosed with a "wet mount?"
- What is the purpose of antiretroviral medications for the pregnant woman who is HIV positive?

PREGNANCY COMPLICATED BY INTIMATE PARTNER VIOLENCE

Intimate partner violence (IPV) is defined as abuse perpetrated by an individual against an intimate partner. The goal of the abusive behavior is to exert and maintain power and control over the partner. Abuse refers to any type of injury committed against a person, including physical, emotional, psychological, and

BOX 16.8 Examples of Abusive Acts

The terms "abuse" or "abused" are often misunderstood to refer only to egregious acts of violence that result in serious physical injury. Therefore, it is important for the health care professional to give specific examples of abuse when screening for intimate partner violence (IPV).

Physical Acts of Abuse

- Punching
- Hitting
- Kicking
- Slapping
- Shoving
- Biting
- Scratching
- Grabbing
- Choking
- Poking
- Shaking
- Hair pulling
- Burning

Emotional Acts of Abuse

- Threats of harm to self, the intimate partner, or others
- Refusing to interact with the intimate partner without explanation ("silent treatment")
- Name calling
- Put downs
- Derogatory comments
- Any act of control
    - Financial (controlling all the money)
    - Decision making (without consulting the partner)
    - Isolation from family or friends
    - Prohibiting access to transportation or telephone
- Threatening or completing acts of violence against pets or children
- Destroying property the intimate partner cares about
- Blaming the intimate partner for his or her violent outbursts

Sexual Acts of Abuse

- Forcing the partner to watch or perform any sexual act against the partner's will.

sexual maltreatment (Box 16-8). An intimate partner is any person who is now or who ever has been in an intimate relationship with the victim. This definition includes present and former spouses, boyfriends, girlfriends, and dating partners. IPV occurs in relationships without regard to sexual preference. In other words, IPV occurs between same sex partners, as well as between heterosexual partners. IPV crosses social, cultural, religious, and economic boundaries. Other terms used to describe IPV are domestic violence, spouse abuse, domestic abuse, and battering (CDC, 2003).

It is difficult to determine the extent of IPV, partly because it is unknown how many cases of IPV go unreported. Some of the difficulty is related to the varied definitions that are used to collect and report these data. The CDC is attempting to correct this problem through the use of standardized terminology and definitions. Although IPV can be directed against men, more women report being abused. Anywhere from 25% to 31% of American women have experienced physical or sexual assault at the hands of an intimate partner; whereas, only 7% of men report being victims of this type of abuse. Yearly, approximately 1.5 million women report criminal acts of violence from an intimate partner. Of these women, approximately 324,000 are pregnant at the time the violence occurs (CDC, 2003).

Pregnancy is a vulnerable time for a woman. IPV may begin or escalate during pregnancy, particularly if the pregnancy is unplanned (Gazmararian et al., 2000). According to the American College of Obstetricians and Gynecologists (ACOG) and the CDC (2004), 4% to 8% of all pregnant women experience abuse during the pregnancy. In a Maryland study of pregnancy-associated deaths, it was discovered that a pregnant, or recently pregnant, woman is more likely to die of homicide than any other cause, including cardiovascular causes, such as pregnancy-induced hypertension (Horon & Cheng, 2001).

The pregnant woman is at risk for certain complications associated with abuse. According to Cunningham et al. (2001b), a woman's risk of developing intrauterine infection or experiencing preterm labor is doubled if she is a victim of domestic violence. She is also at increased risk for abruptio placenta and delivering by cesarean section, and her infant is more likely to have a low birth weight (Anderson, 2002).

Clinical Manifestations and Diagnosis

Abuse may begin slowly and escalate with time, or abusive episodes may begin early in a relationship. There is a generally accepted model, the Cycle of Violence (Fig. 16-2), that explains the pathophysiology of IPV. Abusive episodes usually progress in three identifiable phases:

1. Tension building phase
2. Explosion phase
3. Absence of tension or the "honeymoon" phase

Although it is not always possible to identify IPV during interactions with the victim or abuser, there are warning signs. The perpetrator of IPV often exhibits an overly protective attitude toward the victim. The abuser may accompany the victim to all office visits and may answer questions for the victim. It is important to remember that he may seem pleasant and congenial. Conversely, he may make degrading remarks about the victim in front of health care providers or others.

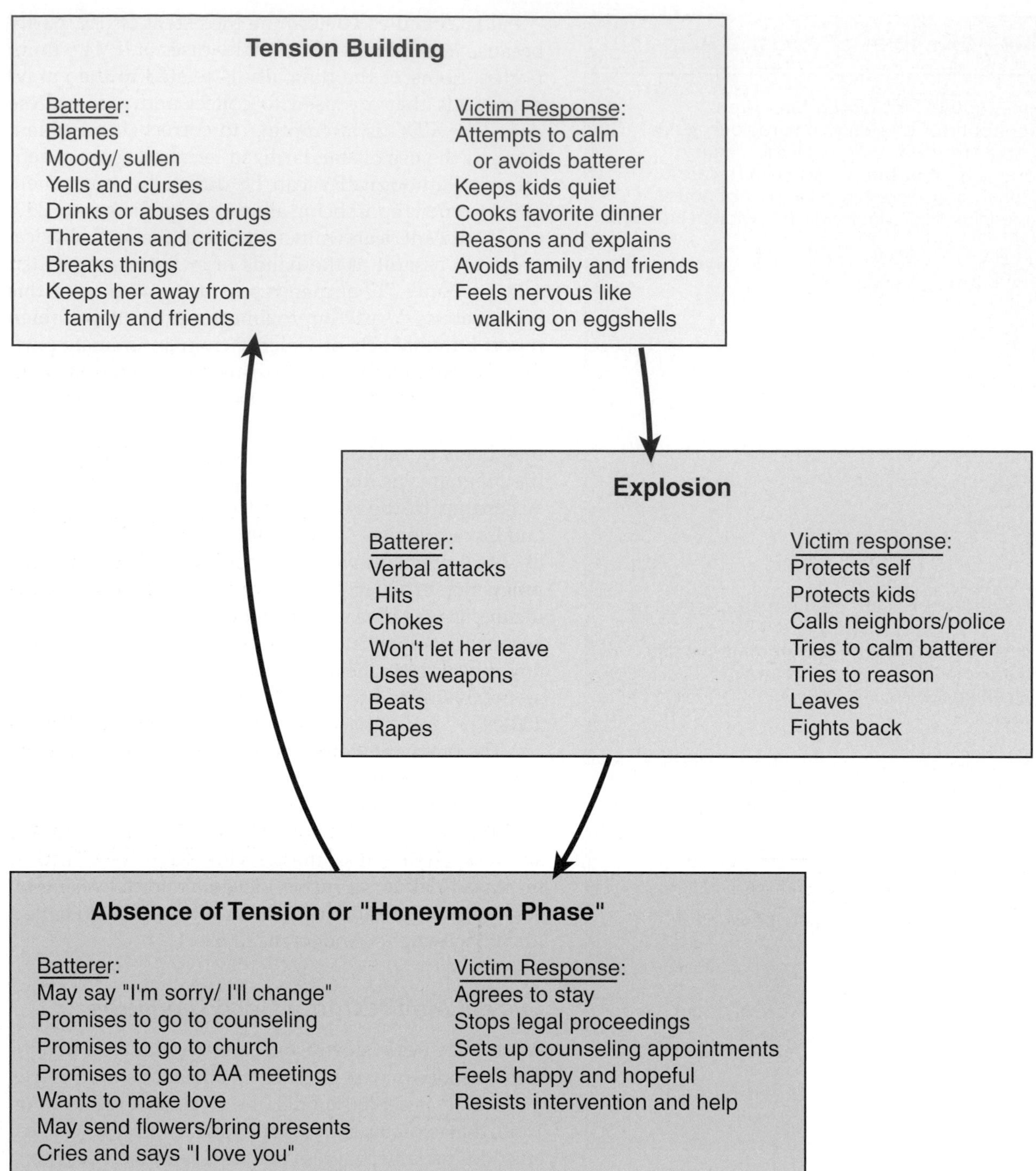
Tension Building
Batterer:
Blames
Moody/ sullen
Yells and curses
Drinks or abuses drugs
Threatens and criticizes
Breaks things
Keeps her away from family and friends
Victim Response:
Attempts to calm or avoids batterer
Keeps kids quiet
Cooks favorite dinner
Reasons and explains
Avoids family and friends
Feels nervous like walking on eggshells
Explosion
Batterer:
Verbal attacks
Hits
Chokes
Won't let her leave
Uses weapons
Beats
Rapes
Victim response:
Protects self
Protects kids
Calls neighbors/police
Tries to calm batterer
Tries to reason
Leaves
Fights back
Absence of Tension or "Honeymoon Phase"
Batterer:
May say "I'm sorry/ I'll change"
Promises to go to counseling
Promises to go to church
Promises to go to AA meetings
Wants to make love
May send flowers/bring presents
Cries and says "I love you"
Victim Response:
Agrees to stay
Stops legal proceedings
Sets up counseling appointments
Feels happy and hopeful
Resists intervention and help

● ***Figure 16.2*** The cycle of violence.

The victim may appear quiet and passive. She may avoid eye contact. She may have an unkempt appearance and may appear depressed. She may exhibit anxiety, nervousness, and suicidal tendencies. She may abuse alcohol or drugs in response to the abuse. Common medical complaints include headache or neck pain, chest pain, palpitations, numbness and tingling, pelvic pain, dyspareunia, and urinary tract infection (Wadman & Foral, 2003). Clues that should raise suspicion of abuse are listed in Box 16-9.

Treatment

Because every woman is at risk for IPV, routine screening of all women is the key to assisting those who are ready to report abuse and receive help. In particular,

BOX 16.9 Clues That May Indicate the Woman Is Being Abused

Any of the following signs should raise the suspicion of possible intimate partner violence (IPV). It is important to remember that a woman who is being abused may not show obvious signs of abuse.

- History of
  - Repeated assaults
  - Drug or alcohol abuse
  - Depression
  - Suicide attempts
- Injury* to the head, face, or neck
- Loose or broken teeth
- Injury to the breasts or abdomen
- Types of injury to include
  - Injury inflicted by a weapon
  - Cigarette and rope burns
  - Bite marks
  - Bruises and welts
- Pattern and distribution of injury to include
  - Areas normally covered by clothes
  - Occurring on both sides of the body (often on extremities)
  - Defensive posture injuries (such as to the hands or feet that occur when the victim tries to ward off the attacker)
- Injuries in various stages of healing
- Injuries that do not match the cause of trauma described by the woman or her partner

Signs unique to the pregnant woman may include

- Presents for late prenatal care or has no prenatal care
- Attends prenatal visits sporadically
- High gravidity and parity rates
- Poor weight gain during pregnancy
- History of
  - Spontaneous abortion(s)
  - STIs
  - Previous fetal death

* Injury can be evidenced by bruises, scrapes, scratches, or cuts, as well as burns, broken bones, etc.

Adapted from Anderson (2002), Wadman & Foral (2003), and others.

the prenatal period presents an excellent opportunity for screening for IPV. Prenatal visits offer opportunities for the health care provider to develop rapport and trust with the woman. The perinatal period is also a unique time of opportunity because the woman may be motivated to think about the future and the safety of her unborn child.

Although screening is a powerful tool, common barriers may get in the way (Williams, Dou, & Leal, 2003). The health care provider may feel the she does not have enough time to ask about IPV. Often providers feel uncomfortable addressing the issue. The provider may be afraid that he will embarrass or offend the woman. Many times screening is avoided because the provider feels helpless to do anything to change the situation. Because screening is a critical intervention for the victim of IPV, ACOG and the CDC recommend provider training to overcome these barriers.

Once IPV is identified, interventions are directed toward safety assessment and planning. Danger signals include statements from the woman that she or her children are in danger, that the violence has recently escalated, the partner has threatened to kill, or that there are lethal weapons (particularly guns) in the home. If the likelihood of danger exists, the health care provider assists the woman to develop a safety plan (Box 16-10).

Trained health care providers discuss options with the woman. Basically, the woman has three options:

- Stay with the abuser.
- Remove the abuser through arrest or with protective orders.
- Leave the relationship temporarily or permanently.

It is important for the provider to keep in mind that the woman is the only one who can truly determine which option is best for her.

Nursing Care

There are many reasons that it is difficult to discuss domestic violence with patients. Myths abound, such

BOX 16.10 Components of a Safety Plan

Whether or not the woman elects to stay in the abusive relationship, she should have a safety plan. The health care provider instructs her to

- Memorize the National Domestic Violence Hotline: 1-800-799-SAFE (7233) or 1-800-787-3224 (for hearing-impaired or deaf victims).
- Pack a bag in advance with cash, credit cards, and clothes for herself and children. The bag should remain at a trusted friend or family member's house.
- Have important personal documents readily accessible. These include
  - Birth certificates
  - Driver's license
  - Bank account information
  - Important telephone numbers
  - Insurance information and cards
  - Court documents or orders
  - Copies of utility bills
- Establish a code word with family and friends to indicate when violence is escalating and help is needed.
- Identify a safe place to go. This may be a women's shelter or other safe place. Each community has unique resources that should be identified for the woman.

as IPV happens in only certain socioeconomic or ethnic groups or the woman could just leave if she were not so weak or codependent. Often it is the nurse's own discomfort with the subject of abuse that keeps the silence. The nurse may feel powerless to do anything about the situation, and therefore does not bring up the subject. There may be a lack of knowledge about how to screen for abuse. Whatever the barrier, the nurse can learn to screen pregnant women for IPV.

Assist the RN to assess for abuse. Always screen the woman alone, away from children and the abuser (Cockey, 2003). Provide privacy. Ask simple, direct, open-ended questions in a nonjudgmental way to show the victim that you are a safe person when she is ready to disclose. Avoid questions that imply that the woman is responsible for the violence or that it is easy to walk away from a violent relationship. Questions to avoid include, "Why do you not just leave? What did you do to make your partner so angry? Why do you go back to your partner?" Remember, determining whether or not a woman should leave an abusive relationship is always only her decision to make.

Sometimes it is better to err on the side of caution! You may not be the best person to screen for IPV. If you haven't been trained, it is better to report your suspicions of abuse to an RN or other health care provider who has been trained to deal with victims of abuse. However, do not allow your discomfort with the subject to hinder you from learning how to screen for violence.

Always document the woman's responses to questioning about IPV. If the woman denies being in an abusive relationship, document her denial. It is important to quote the woman directly. Do not use terms such as "alleges" when you are documenting the woman's replies. This terminology may cast doubt on the veracity of the woman's answers if the medical record is ever used as evidence in a court of law.

If the woman discloses IPV, be careful to respond with supportive statements. One of the most important things you can communicate to the victim of abuse is the fact that the abuse is not her fault! You can say, "This is not your fault. No one deserves to be treated this way." Examples of other helpful statements include, "I'm sorry that you've been hurt. Do you want to talk about it? I am concerned for your safety. You have options. Help is available."

Document your assessment objectively. If there are physical indications of abuse, draw these on a body map, then use measurable terminology to describe each lesion or observation. Photographs can be invaluable aids in a courtroom. You must get the woman's written consent before photographing her, however.

Be knowledgeable about local resources that are available for the victim of IPV. Resources include office and hospital personnel with specialized training, IPV advocacy groups, women's shelters, hotlines, child protective services, and law enforcement resources. Many cities have city-wide plans to respond to IPV. Be familiar with your city's plan.

The compassionate nurse who develops the trust of the abused woman can help turn the tide of abuse. Recovery from IPV does not happen in only one or two interventions; rather, it is a consistent atmosphere of encouragement and esteem building that may assist the victim to become a survivor.

PREGNANCY COMPLICATED BY AGE-RELATED CONCERNS

The typical childbearing years envelop the ages of 15 through 44 years; however, females can, and sometimes do, become pregnant anywhere from ages 9 through 56 years of age. At either end of the age spectrum pregnancy carries higher risk for morbidity and mortality for the woman and her fetus. Although age-related concerns warrant special "at-risk" considerations, they are not in the pathophysiologic category, as are the medical conditions heretofore discussed. Instead, they are a natural part of the reproductive process requiring additional accommodations throughout the perinatal period.

Adolescent Pregnancy

Adolescent, or teen, pregnancy is defined as pregnancy occurring at 19 years of age or younger. The consequences of teenage pregnancy are well documented. According to the United States Department of Health and Human Services (2000), teenage mothers are "less likely to get or stay married, less likely to complete high school or college, and more likely to require public assistance and to live in poverty than their peers who are not mothers." There are also considerable consequences for the infants of adolescent mothers, particularly for those whose mothers are younger than 15 years. Infants of teen mothers are more likely to be below normal birth weight, experience higher neonatal mortality rate, and have a higher incidence of sudden infant death syndrome.

The good news is that the adolescent pregnancy rate has decreased steadily since 1990. Teen birth rates were at an all time low in 2001. The birth rate for teens younger than 15 years fell from 1.4 per 1,000 in 1991 to 0.8 per 1,000 in 2001. The 2001 rate for the youngest teens is the lowest it has been since 1966. The rate also fell for adolescents 15 through 19 years of age, from 38.6 in 1991 to 24.7 in 2001, which is a record low

(Hamilton, Sutton, & Ventura, 2003). The two foremost explanations for this decline are the number of female adolescents engaging in sexual intercourse has leveled off after increasing during the 1980s and condom use among sexually active teens has significantly increased (Anderson, Smiley, Flick, & Lewis, 2000).

Clinical Manifestations

Many pregnant teens seek late prenatal care, often in the 3rd trimester, or they return sporadically for prenatal visits. Sometimes they get no prenatal care. There are many factors that contribute to poor prenatal care and subsequent complications of pregnancy. Recent research points to the social situation of the adolescent as the root cause of increased pregnancy risk, rather than age itself. The pregnant teen is more likely than her older counterpart to be unmarried, have less education, be a member of an ethnic minority, and to live in poverty (Anderson et al., 2000).

The adolescent faces many barriers to receiving adequate prenatal care. The pregnant teen may be fearful of disclosing her pregnancy to her parents or caregivers, so she may attempt to hide the pregnancy by wearing loose clothing and avoiding prolonged interaction with adults. Or she may lack family support or transportation to regularly attend prenatal visits. Because body image is extremely important to the adolescent, she may use behaviors associated with eating disorders, such as purging or self-starvation, to avoid weight gain during the pregnancy. The pregnant adolescent may not get adequate nutrition secondary to poor food choices. There is increasing evidence that pregnant teens are at increased risk for domestic violence. This situation can also lead to sporadic attendance to prenatal visits. Whatever the reason for not receiving good prenatal care, the pregnant adolescent is at increased risk for complications, such as inadequate weight gain, anemia, and preeclampsia-eclampsia. All of these conditions can result in fetal complications, such as intrauterine growth restriction, low birth weight, and preterm birth.

Diagnosis of adolescent pregnancy is made with the same tests used for older women. However, the diagnosis can be easily missed if the practitioner does not keep in mind the prospect of pregnancy when performing a history and physical. Adolescents often deny the possibility of pregnancy (even to themselves), making diagnosis even more challenging. The adolescent should be screened for pregnancy if she reports irregular periods, nausea and vomiting, or fatigue.

Treatment

The best treatment for teenage pregnancy is prevention. Many physicians and advanced practice nurses are actively involved in programs designed to prevent adolescent pregnancy. Others are involved in research studies attempting to discover which methods work and which do not. Much of the literature on adolescent pregnancy concentrates on prevention.

The challenge of managing an adolescent pregnancy is considerable. Although obtaining information about the woman's physical and psychological response to pregnancy and social support available to her is notable for any pregnant woman's care, this part of the history is particularly valuable for the pregnant teen. If the adolescent does not have adequate social support, she is more likely to experience adverse outcomes. Other areas of the history to which the practitioner pays close attention include determining the teen's perception of options available to her, HIV and other STI risk factors, and school status. Because IPV is associated with adolescent pregnancy, it is particularly important for the practitioner to screen for domestic violence.

The informed practitioner does several things to assist the pregnant teen. Advocacy for the pregnant adolescent includes giving information in an open, nonjudgmental way and supporting the adolescent's choices. This approach requires that the practitioner treat the adolescent with dignity and respect by providing and protecting the right to privacy and confidentiality. Advocacy includes assisting the teen to freely make choices without coercion.

> **CULTURAL SNAPSHOT 16-1**
>
> Remember that each adolescent is an individual. Her beliefs and values are influenced by her culture. Plan interventions based on the unique needs of each teen.

One crucial part of management includes helping the teen to develop an adequate support network. Parents, teachers, friends, and the father of the baby are all potential resources for the pregnant adolescent. These individuals may benefit from guidance on ways they can effectively help.

Nursing Care

Caring for Developmental Needs

Keep in mind the developmental needs of the pregnant adolescent. Pregnancy does not change the developmental tasks, although it may complicate the issues. According to Erickson (Cramer, Flynn, & LaFave, 1997), developing an identity is an essential developmental task of the adolescent. It is important to help the pregnant teen to work on identity issues while she also begins to adopt the role of motherhood.

As with other teens, the pregnant adolescent's normal priorities include acceptance by her peer group and focusing on appearance. In addition, the adolescent, particularly the very young adolescent, is typically self-centered, a characteristic that can make it difficult for her to consider the needs of others. Take into account these priorities and characteristics as you plan your nursing care.

Caring for Physical Needs

Adequate nutrition is essential to the health of the pregnant teen. However, nutritional considerations may not have a high priority from the adolescent's viewpoint. Assist the teen to identify healthful foods that are appealing and easy to prepare. It may help to determine what foods the teen normally eats and then suggest more healthful alternatives. For instance, rather than forbidding desserts, help the teen to choose desserts that have nutritional value, such as fresh fruits or frozen yogurt. You might suggest that the teen try low-salt tortilla chips, baked potato chips, or whole grain crackers, rather than regular potato chips.

Cultural sensitivity is in order. Do not forget that food choices are influenced culturally. Be sure that you understand the teen's cultural context when you counsel her regarding prenatal nutrition.

Pregnant teens are at higher risk for delivering prematurely, particularly if they experience a repeat pregnancy during their teen years. One way to help decrease the risk of a repeat pregnancy is to counsel the teen regarding birth control methods. STIs are another potential problem. Encourage the use of barrier methods of birth control (particularly male use of latex condoms) that supply protection from STIs.

Caring for Emotional and Psychological Needs

The emotional and psychological needs of the adolescent are complex. When the emotional demands of pregnancy are added, the strain can be tremendous. It is frequently helpful to include significant support persons in the care planning. It is easier for them to provide meaningful support if they know how pregnancy might affect emotional functioning.

Be knowledgeable regarding community resources for the pregnant teen. If you or the primary practitioner refers the teen to another entity, follow up to make certain the adolescent receives the services for which she was referred. If not, try to determine the barriers that prevent her from following through with treatment. Assist her to work through the barriers to obtain needed services.

Remain nonjudgmental and open minded when dealing with pregnant teens. There are many factors working against the teen. Scolding and punishment are not helpful interventions. They tend to push the adolescent away and do little to resolve the real issues with which the teen must contend.

Pregnancy in Later Life

While adolescent birth rates have been steadily declining, births for women in their late 30s and early 40s have risen. In 1990, the birth rate for women 35 through 39 years of age was 31.7 per 1,000. The rate increased by 28% to 40.6 per 1,000 in 2001. For women ages 40 to 44 years, the birth rate increased by 47%, from 5.5 in 1990 to 8.1 per 1,000 in 2001. The rate for women aged 45 to 49 years has more than doubled from 0.2 in 1990 to 0.5 in 2001 (Hamilton et al., 2003).

There are risk factors that are associated with delayed childbearing. For women, fertility declines with age. Although assisted reproductive technology is much more effective than it was in the past, there is a higher incidence of multiple fetal pregnancies (i.e., twins, triplets) when these technologies are used to help a woman get pregnant. A woman older than 35 years is more likely to conceive a child with chromosomal abnormalities, such as Down's syndrome. She is also at higher risk for spontaneous abortion (miscarriage), pregnancy-induced hypertension, gestational diabetes, preterm delivery, and bleeding and placental abnormalities. She has almost twice the risk of a younger woman of having a fetal demise; she is more likely to have cesarean delivery; and she is more likely to deliver a low birth-weight baby. As ominous as these statistics sound, it is helpful to remember that the majority of pregnancies to women older than 35 years end with healthy babies and healthy moms.

Clinical Manifestations

In general the woman who waits to have her first baby until she is in her late 30s or early 40s has more education than her younger counterparts. Frequently she has chosen to postpone childbearing to pursue career choices. She is most likely to be married, to have financial resources, and to have planned the pregnancy. She is also more likely to have a chronic condition, such as diabetes or hypertension. It is of note that the older pregnant woman may be more likely to use alcohol during pregnancy, particularly if she is unmarried (CDC, 2002).

Some older women report more aches and pains during pregnancy, whereas others do not. If the older woman is physically fit, it is less likely that pregnancy will cause excessive tiredness and distress. The hormonal changes of pregnancy are often a cause of facial skin breakouts, even for the older woman.

Treatment

A preconceptual visit is recommended for any woman who wishes to become pregnant. For the older woman it is especially important that she have a complete physical before becoming pregnant, particularly if she has a chronic medical condition. Because it may be more difficult for the older woman to conceive, fertility experts recommend that she seek medical help if she is not pregnant within 6 months of trying.

Once pregnancy is achieved, genetic testing and counseling is offered to the woman older than 35 years. The miscarriage rate is higher as the woman ages, most likely because of chromosomal abnormalities of the conceptus. Trisomy 21 (Down's syndrome), trisomy 18 (Edward's syndrome), and trisomy 13 (Patau's syndrome) all occur with greater frequency as the woman ages. Therefore, chorionic villus sampling or early amniocentesis is offered.

Nursing Care

It is helpful to approach the older pregnant woman with an open mind. Be ready to answer questions and to suggest pregnancy and parenting resources. A woman that chooses to delay childbearing until she is past 35 years of age does not want to be constantly reminded that she is an "older" pregnant woman. Neither does she want to be reminded of the increased risks associated with late childbearing. If the woman complains of receiving "rude" remarks from strangers about her age, suggest that it is OK to ignore such remarks. If she has a good sense of humor, she may be able to make a joke out of the situation. For example, one woman who was asked if she had planned to have a child at her age replied that she was "certainly old enough to know better."

Suggest a good skin care routine to combat facial breakouts. The older pregnant woman may benefit from a trip to a spa for a facial. It will give her a chance to relax, and she can obtain advice from a skin expert. Caution her not to begin a vigorous exercise routine during pregnancy. If she enters pregnancy already physically fit, she may continue her exercise pattern as long as she does not experience a complication of pregnancy.

A PERSONAL GLIMPSE

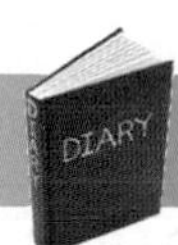

My husband and I married in our late 20s. We decided to wait until we were both in our 30s to have children because we had lots of school loans to pay off and wanted to be financially secure before raising a family. I got pregnant with my daughter when I was 33. It was a normal pregnancy; I felt great, and the baby and I were completely healthy throughout. When Libby was 3 years old, we decided to try and have another baby. I conceived easily and eagerly made my first doctor appointment to officially confirm the pregnancy. I assumed that this pregnancy would be as uncomplicated as my first. Imagine my surprise when I sat down with the nurse and she started grilling me about the potential for genetic problems and health problems in my baby because I was over 35 years old. She started talking about the need for me to have special blood tests and an amniocentesis. It was all rather overwhelming and scary. I was shocked. How could 3 years make such a difference in the way that my pregnancies would be managed?

Julia

LEARNING OPPORTUNITY: How can the nurse present information to the woman at risk without increasing her anxiety level? Does the risk level dramatically increase at the age of 35? Why or why not?

Test Yourself

- True or false: Intimate partner violence (IPV) occurs only in heterosexual relationships.
- List three components of a safety plan for a victim of IPV.
- Name two dysfunctional behaviors the pregnant adolescent might use to keep from gaining weight during pregnancy.

KEY POINTS

- Tight glycemic control for the pregnant woman with diabetes dramatically decreases the incidence of complications. Glucose levels over time are determined by measuring glycosylated hemoglobin (HbA1C).
- The pancreas of the woman with type 1 diabetes does not produce insulin, so it must be administered subcutaneously. Insulin can be self-injected or administered via an insulin pump. The cornerstone of therapy for gestational diabetes is diet therapy.
- Fetal surveillance is critical for the pregnant woman with diabetes. Fetal activity counts and nonstress testing is done to determine fetal well-being. Amniocentesis to determine fetal lung maturity may be done in the 3rd trimester to help determine the optimum time for delivery.
- Typical nursing concerns for the pregnant woman with DM include management of the therapeutic regimen, risk for maternal and fetal injury, risk for infection, and fetal macrosomia.

- The main goal of treatment for the pregnant woman with heart disease is prevention and early detection of cardiac decompensation. This goal is met by monitoring activity levels, managing stress, diet modification, and medication therapy.
- Iron-deficiency anemia requires iron supplementation and a diet high in iron-rich foods. Because iron supplements predispose to constipation, the nurse teaches the woman to maintain adequate hydration, exercise regularly, and get plenty of fiber in the diet.
- Preventing a crisis is the goal of treatment for the woman with sickle cell anemia. Interventions involve maintaining adequate hydration, avoiding infection, getting adequate rest, and eating a well-balanced diet.
- Teaching is an important part of asthma managment. The woman should be advised to continue taking her asthma medications during pregnancy. She should avoid over-the-counter medications and protect herself from asthma triggers and infection.
- Because antiepileptic drugs (AEDs) are a major cause of fetal defects, preconceptual care is recommended. High-dose folic acid supplements are given before and throughout pregnancy to help prevent neural tube defects, and vitamin K supplementation is often given during the last weeks of pregnancy to prevent neonatal hemorrhage.
- TORCH stands for toxoplasmosis, other (hepatitis B, syphilis, varicella, and herpes zoster), rubella, cytomegalovirus, and herpes simplex virus. These infections can lead to serious fetal anomalies and other complications. Prevention of infection is the best treatment strategy because many of the TORCH infections do not have effective treatment.
- Chlamydia is caused by sexual transmission of the bacterium *Chlamydia trachomatis*. It is frequently asymptomatic but easily treated with antibiotics.
- Gonorrhea is caused by the bacterium *Neisseria gonorrhoeae* and is treated with antibiotics. Gonorrhea increases the risk of PID, spontaneous abortion, and preterm delivery.
- Human papillomavirus (HPV) is a virus that causes genital warts. The warts have a tendency to increase in size during pregnancy and can lead to heavy bleeding during delivery. HPV can be transmitted to the fetus during birth.
- Trichomoniaisis is caused by a protozoan. It is treated with metronidazole (Flagyl) given orally.
- A pregnant woman with HIV/AIDS can pass the infection to her unborn child during pregnancy or childbirth or while breast-feeding. Disease progression and response to treatment are determined by measuring CD4 counts. Therapy during pregnancy is prophylactic administration of oral zidovudine (ZDV) throughout pregnancy. Breast-feeding is contraindicated.
- Nursing considerations for the pregnant woman with a sexually transmitted infection (STI) include risk for additional infection, ineffective protection, deficient knowledge, risk for low self-esteem, and anxiety. Education regarding STI prevention and treatment are important nursing functions.
- The Cycle of Violence describes the typical pathophysiology of IPV. Tension building is followed by the explosion phase, which leads to the honeymoon phase.
- Treatment of IPV includes the screening of all pregnant women. Once IPV is identified, interventions are directed toward safety assessment and planning. The victim should be assisted to develop a safety plan.
- A pregnant teen is at high risk for poor prenatal care. Body image is an important consideration that may lead to attempts to limit weight gain during pregnancy. She is also at risk for domestic violence, inadequate weight gain, anemia, and preeclampsia-eclampsia. Nutrition and social support are important areas of intervention for the pregnant adolescent.
- The woman who delays childbearing past 35 years of age is at increased risk for complications of pregnancy. However, she is frequently mature, has a career, is financially stable, and married. Most pregnancies to older women end successfully with a healthy mother and a healthy baby. Preconceptual care is ideal.

REFERENCES AND SELECTED READINGS

Books and Journals

American College of Obstetricians and Gynecologists (ACOG) & Centers for Disease Control (CDC). (2001). *Intimate partner violence during pregnancy: A guide for clinicians.* PowerPoint Training Slide Lecture. Released May 29, 2001. Retrieved September 14, 2003, from http://www.cdc.gov/reproductivehealth/violence/ipvdp.htm

American Diabetes Association. (2003). Gestational diabetes: Position statement. *Diabetes Care, 26*(Suppl 1), S103–S105.

Anderson, C. (2002). Battered and pregnant: A nursing challenge. *AWHONN Lifelines, 6*(2), 95–99.

Anderson, N. E., Smiley, D. V., Flick, L. H., & Lewis, C. Y. (2000). Missouri rural adolescent pregnancy project (MORAPP). *Public Health Nursing, 17*(5), 355–362.

Burnett, L. B., & Adler, J. (2001). Domestic violence. In S. A. Conrad, F. Talavera, R. C. Harwood, J. Halamka, & B. Brenner (Eds.), *eMedicine*. Last updated July 20, 2001. Retrieved September 14, 2003, from http://www.emedicine.com/emerg/topic153.htm

Burton, J., & Reyes, M. (2001). Breathe in breathe out: Controlling asthma during pregnancy. *AWHONN Lifelines, 5*(1), 24–30.

Caughey, A. B., & Sandberg, P. (2002). Seizure disorders in pregnancy. S. R. Trupin, F. Talavera, D. Chelmow, F. B. Gaupp, & L. P. Shulman (Eds.), *eMedicine*. Last updated June 28, 2002. Retrieved August 10, 2003, from http://www.emedicine.com/med/topic3433.htm

Centers for Disease Control and Prevention (CDC). (2000). National and state-specific pregnancy rates among adolescents—United States, 1995–1997. *MMWR, 49*(27). Retrieved September 20, 2003, from http://www.cdc.gov/ mmwr/preview/mmwrhtml/mm4927a1.htm

Centers for Disease Control and Prevention (CDC). (2001). *STD surveillance 2001*. Prepared by the Division of Sexually Transmitted Diseases of the National Center for HIV, STD and TB Prevention. Retrieved September 6, 2003, from http://www.cdc.gov/std/stats/TOC2001.htm

Centers for Disease Control and Prevention (CDC). (2002). Alcohol use among women of childbearing age—United States, 1991–1999. *MMWR, 51*(43), 273–276. Retrieved September 28, 2003, from http://www.cdc.gov/mmwr/preview/mmwrhtml/mm5113a2.htm

Centers for Disease Control and Prevention (CDC). (2003). *Intimate partner violence fact sheet*. Prepared by the Centers for Disease Control and Prevention and the National Center for Injury Preventions and Control. Last reviewed August 21, 2003. Retrieved September 13, 2003, from http://www.cdc.gov/ncipc/factsheets/ipvfacts.htm

Centers for Disease Control and Prevention (CDC). (2004). Recommended childhood and adolescent immunization schedule—United States, January—June 2004. Approved by the Advisory Committee on Immunization Practices, the American Academy of Pediatrics, and the American Academy of Family Physicians. Retrieved August 5, 2004, from http://www.cdc.gov/nip/recs/child-schedule.pdf

Cockey, C. D. (2003). Screening for violence in pregnancy: Nurses should ask about violence in private—but not all do. *AWHONN Lifelines, 7*(6), 495–497.

Cramer, C., Flynn, B., & LaFave, A. (1997). *Erick Erickson's 8 stages of psychosocial development summary chart*. Retrieved August 6, 2004, from http://web.cortland.edu/andersmd/ERIK/sum.HTML

Cunningham, F. G., Gant, N. F., Leveno, K. J., Gilstrap, L. C. III, Hauth, J. C., & Wenstrom, K. D. (2001a). Cardiovascular disease. In *Williams obstetrics* (21st ed., pp. 1181–1207). New York: McGraw-Hill Medical Publishing Division.

Cunningham, F. G., Gant, N. F., Leveno, K. J., Gilstrap, L. C. III, Hauth, J. C., & Wenstrom, K. D. (2001b). Critical care and trauma. In *Williams obstetrics* (21st ed., pp. 1159–1180). New York: McGraw-Hill Medical Publishing Division.

Cunningham, F. G., Gant, N. F., Leveno, K. J., Gilstrap, L. C. III, Hauth, J. C., & Wenstrom, K. D. (2001c). Diabetes. In *Williams obstetrics* (21st ed., pp. 1359–1381). New York: McGraw-Hill Medical Publishing Division.

Fischer, R. (2003). Genital herpes in pregnancy. In A. Witlin, F. Talavera, R. S. Legro, F. B. Gaupp, & L. P. Shulman (Eds.), *eMedicine*. Last updated March 20, 2003. Retrieved September 1, 2003, from http://www.emedicine.com/med/topic3554.htm

Gazmararian, J. A., Petersen, R., Spitz, A. M., Goodwin, M. M., Saltzman, L. E., & Marks, J. S. (2000). Violence and reproductive health: Current knowledge and future research directions [abstract]. *Maternal and Child Health Journal (special issue): Violence and Reproductive Health, 4*(2). Retrieved September 14, 2003, from http://www.cdc.gov/reproductivehealth/wh_viol_mchjv4n2.htm

Hamilton, B. E., Sutton, P. D., & Ventura, S. J. (2003). Revised birth and fertility rates for the 1990s and new rates for Hispanic populations, 2000 and 2001: United States. *National Vital Statistics Reports NVSS, 51*(12). Retrieved September 20, 2003, from http://www.cdc.gov/nchs/data/nvsr/nvsr51/nvsr51_12.pdf

Hicks, P. (2000). Gestational diabetes in primary care. *Medscape General Medicine, 2*(1). Retrieved August 3, 2003, from http://www.medscape.com/viewarticle/408910

Horon, I. L., & Cheng, D. (2001). Enhanced surveillance for pregnancy-associated mortality: Maryland, 1993–1998 [abstract]. *JAMA, 285*(11), 1455–1459. Retrieved September 14, 2003, from the JAMA&Archives website http://pubs.ama-assn.org/

Jones, J., Lopez, A., & Wilson, M. (2003). Congenital toxoplasmosis. *American Family Physician, 67*(10), 2131–2147. Retrieved August 31, 2003, from http://www.aafp.org/afp/20030515/2131.html

Kazzi, A. A., & Marachelian, A. (2001). Pregnancy, asthma. In A. J. Sayah, F. Talavera, M. Zwanger, J. Halamka, & S. H. Plantz (Eds.), *eMedicine*. Last updated June 6, 2001. Retrieved August 10, 2003, from http://www.emedicine.com/emerg/topic476.htm

Laino, C. (2003). Gestational diabetes raises risk of metabolic syndrome. In D. Flapan (Ed.), *Medscape Medical News*. Retrieved July 26, 2003, from http://www.medscape.com/viewarticle/457507

Lie, D. A. (2003). Varicella zoster in first trimester of pregnancy. *Medscape Primary Care, 5*(1). Posted March 21, 2003. Retrieved September 1, 2003, from http://www.medscape.com/viewarticle/450603

Liu, P., & Euerle, B. (2002). Syphilis. In D. R. Lucey, F. Talavera, J. L. Brusch, E. Mylonakis, & B. A. Cunha (Eds.), *eMedicine*. Last updated August 16, 2002. Retrieved September 1, 2003, from http://www.emedicine.com/med/topic2224.htm

March of Dimes. (Undated). Cytomegalovirus infection in pregnancy. *Quick reference: Infections and diseases*. Retrieved September 1, 2003, from http://www.marchofdimes.com/professionals/681_1195.asp

March of Dimes. (2003). *Diabetes in pregnancy*. Retrieved July 19, 2003, from http://www.marchofdimes.com/professionals/681_1197.asp

Mayfield, E. (1996). *New hope for people with sickle cell anemia*. U.S. Food and Drug Administration. (Last updated February 1999). Publication No. (FDA) 99-1251. Retrieved August 17, 2003, from http://www.fda.gov/fdac/features/496_sick.html

Metcalf-Wilson, K. (2002). Confidentiality, communication and compliance: The three 'C's' of female adolescent care. *AWHONN Lifelines, 6*(4), 344–348.

Miller, M. M., & Greenberger, P. A. (1999). Asthma and pregnancy: A review. *Medscape General Medicine, 1*(3). Retrieved August 3, 2003, from http://www.medscape.com/viewarticle/408736

Montgomery, K. S. (2003). Health promotion for pregnant adolescents. *AWHONN Lifelines, 7*(5), 432–444.

Moore, T. (2002). Diabetes mellitus and pregnancy. In R. K. Zurawin, F. Talavera, C. V. Smith, M. Cooper, & L. P. Shulman (Eds.), *eMedicine*. Last updated October 3, 2002. Retrieved July 17, 2003, from http://www.emedicine.com/med/topic3249.htm

Morrell, M. J. (2002). Epilepsy in women. *American Family Physician, 66*(8). Retrieved August 10, 2003, from http://www.aafp.org/afp/20021015/1489.html

National Institute of Allergy and Infectious Diseases (NIAID). (2002, May). *Gonorrhea*. Health matters fact sheet prepared by the NIAID. Retrieved September 6, 2003, http://www.niaid.nih.gov/factsheets/stdgon.htm

National Institute of Allergy and Infectious Diseases (NIAID). (2002, November). *Syphilis*. Health matters fact sheet prepared by the NIAID. Retrieved September 6, 2003, from http://www.niaid.nih.gov/factsheets/stdsyph.htm

National Institute of Allergy and Infectious Diseases (NIAID). (2003, June). *HIV infection and AIDS: An overview*. Fact sheet prepared by the Office of Communications and Public Liaison, National Institute of Allergy and Infectious Diseases, and National Institutes of Health, Bethesda, MD. Retrieved September 7, 2003, from http://www.niaid.nih.gov/factsheets/hivinf.htm

National Institutes of Health. (1993). *Report of the working group on asthma and pregnancy* (NIH Publication No. 93-3279). Retrieved August 9, 2003, from http://www.nhlbi.nih.gov/health/prof/lung/asthma/astpreg.txt

National Institutes of Health. (2002). Contraception and pregnancy. In *The management of sickle cell disease,* 4th ed. NIH publication No. 02-2117. Retrieved August 16, 2003, from http://www.nhlbi.nih.gov/health/prof/blood/sickle/sc_mngt.pdf

Ostlund, I., et al. (2003). Maternal and fetal outcomes if gestational impaired glucose tolerance is not treated. *Diabetes Care, 26*(7), 2107–2111.

Robinson, J. N., & Norwitz, E. R. (2000). Respiratory complications. In A. T. Evans & K. R. Niswander (Eds.), *Manual of obstetrics* (6th ed., pp. 82–89). Philadelphia: Lippincott, Williams & Wilkins.

Rochester, J. A., & Kirchner, J. T. (1997). Epilepsy in pregnancy. *American Family Physician, 56*(6). Retrieved August 10, 2003, from http://www.aafp.org/afp/971015ap/rochest.html

Rogers, M. F., Fowler, M. G., & Lindegren, M. L. (2001). Revised recommendations for HIV screening of pregnant women. *MMWR, 50*(RR19), 59–86. A CDC Report. Retrieved September 7, 2003, from http://www.cdc.gov/mmwr/preview/mmwrhtml/rr5019a2.htm

Schleiss, M. R. (2003). Cytomegalovirus infection. In D. Jaimovich, R. Konop, L. L. Barton, R. W. Tolan, & R. Steele (Eds.), *eMedicine*. Last updated April 1, 2003. Retrieved September 1, 2003, from http://www.emedicine.com/ped/topic544.htm

Silver, H. (2000). Cardiovascular complications. In A. T. Evans & K. R. Niswander (Eds.), *Manual of obstetrics* (6th ed., pp. 40–50). Philadelphia: Lippincott, Williams & Wilkins.

Smith, J. E., & Mattson, S. D. (2000). Domestic violence. In J. E. Smith & S. D. Mattson (Eds.), *Core curriculum for maternal–newborn nursing* (2nd ed.). Philadelphia: WB Saunders.

Spencer, D. (2002). Women's health and epilepsy. In A. S. Blum, F. Talavera, J. E. Cavazos, M. J. Baker, & N. Lorenzo (Eds.), *eMedicine*. Retrieved August 10, 2003, from http://www.emedicine.com/neuro/topic613.htm

United States Department of Health and Human Services. (2000). Family planning. *Tracking Healthy People 2010, Part B: Operational definitions*. Retrieved September 20, 2000, from http://www.healthypeople.gov/Document/html/tracking/od09.htm

Van Earden, P., & Bernstein, P. (2003). Varicella zoster infections in pregnancy. *Medscape Ob/Gyn and Women's Health, 8*(1). Posted June 10, 2003. Retrieved September 1, 2003, from http://www.medscape.com/viewarticle/455972

Wadman, M. C., & Foral, J. (2003). Domestic violence. In J. A. Salomone, F. Talavera, D. E. Houry, J. Adler, & J. S. Cohen (Eds.), *eMedicine*. Last updated March 18, 2003. Retrieved September 14, 2003, from http://www.emedicine.com/aaem/topic538.htm

Williams, G. B., Dou, M., & Leal, C. C. (2003). Violence against pregnant women. *AWHONN Lifelines, 7*(4), 348–354.

Winter, W. E., & Schatz, D. A. (2003). Current role of the oral glucose tolerance test. *Medscape Diabetes and Endocrinology, 5*(1). Retrieved July 26, 2003, from http://www.medscape.com/viewarticle/448038

Websites

Asthma and Pregnancy

http://allergy.mcg.edu/advice/preg.html

http://nationaljewish.org/medfacts/medfacts.html#AsthmaMedFacts

http://www.nhlbi.nih.gov/health/prof/lung/asthma/astpreg.txt

TORCH Infections and STIs

http://health.discovery.com/diseasesandcond/encyclopedia/1509.html

http://www.niaid.nih.gov/factsheets/stdsyph.htm

http://www.cdc.gov/nip/vaccine/varicella/faqs-clinic-vac-preg.htm

http://www.bcm.tmc.edu/pedi/infect/cmv/

Intimate Partner Violence

http://www.ndvh.org/

WORKBOOK

NCLEX-STYLE REVIEW QUESTIONS

1. A woman presents to the prenatal clinic for her 28-week prenatal visit. She has pregestational diabetes. Which type of diabetes does she *most* likely have?
   a. Type 1
   b. Type 2
   c. Undetermined
   d. Uncontrolled
2. A woman with Class III heart disease is in for a prenatal visit. If she is in early heart failure, which sign is *most* likely to be discovered during physical assessment?
   a. Audible wheezes
   b. Persistent rales in the bases of the lungs
   c. Elevated blood pressure
   d. Low blood pressure
3. A 30-year-old gravida 1 has sickle cell anemia. She is not currently in crisis. Which nursing intervention has the highest priority? Instructions on
   a. avoidance of infection
   b. constipation prevention
   c. control of pain
   d. iron-rich foods
4. A 25-year-old woman is in for her first prenatal visit at 28 weeks' gestation. Which assessment finding would most lead you to believe that she may be a victim of intimate partner violence?
   a. A calm demeanor
   b. Bilateral pedal edema
   c. A small bruise on her upper thigh
   d. Multiple bruises in varying stages of healing

STUDY ACTIVITIES

1. Use the following table to list and compare differences between gestational diabetes and type 1 diabetes during pregnancy.

	Gestational DM	Type I DM
Clinical presentation		
Treatment		
Nursing care		

2. Research the Internet to find at least five reliable websites that give patient education information regarding sickle cell anemia.
3. Investigate your community for resources to help adolescents during pregnancy and parenting. Share your findings with your clinical group.

CRITICAL THINKING: What Would You Do?

Apply your knowledge of medical conditions during pregnancy to the following situation.

1. Elizabeth, a 32-year-old gravida 2, has just received a diagnosis of gestational diabetes.
   a. What test was done to diagnose the condition? What were the results of the test?
   b. What risk factors for gestational diabetes may be present in Elizabeth's history?
   c. Explain the priorities of care for Elizabeth during her pregnancy.
2. Tanya is 29 years old and has asthma. She is pregnant with her first child.
   a. What will pregnancy likely do to Tanya's asthma severity?
   b. Outline a teaching plan for Tanya.
3. Rachel is pregnant with her third child. Her HIV test just came back positive. Rachel says she does not know how she contracted HIV. She thinks it could have been from a blood transfusion she received after her last delivery.
   a. What are the most common methods of HIV transmission? Name three risk factors for HIV.
   b. What are the priorities of care for Rachel?
   c. What medication will the physician likely prescribe for her?
   d. Rachel wants to know how best to protect her unborn child from the infection. How will you respond?
   e. Rachel asks if her other children should be tested. How do you respond? Why or why not?

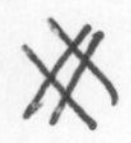

Pregnancy at Risk: Pregnancy-Related Complications

17

STUDENT OBJECTIVES

On completion of this chapter, the student should be able to

1. Choose appropriate nursing interventions for the woman with hyperemesis gravidarum.
2. Describe clinical manifestations of ectopic pregnancy.
3. Compare and contrast the six types of spontaneous abortion.
4. Discuss the treatment for incompetent cervix.
5. Provide patient teaching (e.g., pathology, treatment, and follow-up care) to a woman experiencing a hydatidiform mole.
6. Compare and contrast placenta previa and abruptio placenta according to characteristics of bleeding and other clinical manifestations.
7. Apply the nursing process to the care of a pregnant woman with a bleeding disorder.
8. Differentiate four categories of hypertensive disorders in pregnancy.
9. Discuss interventions that the nurse uses to care for the woman with preeclampsia-eclampsia.
10. Relate ways the management of a multiple gestation pregnancy is different from that of a singleton gestation.
11. Explain the threat to pregnancy posed by ABO and Rh incompatibilities.

KEY TERMS

abruptio placentae
cerclage
choriocarcinoma
eclampsia
ectopic pregnancy
gestational hypertension
hydatidiform mole
hyperemesis gravidarum
incompetent cervix
placenta previa
preeclampsia
proteinuria
salpingectomy
salpingitis
spontaneous abortion
vasospasm

In Chapter 16 the effect of pre-existing and acquired medical conditions on pregnancy was examined. This chapter focuses on conditions unique to pregnancy that place the woman and/or fetus at risk. Although an uneventful pregnancy is hoped for and often expected, complications can develop. Prenatal care is essential for early risk identification and early detection of developing complications.

The licensed practical or vocational nurse's (LPN's) role includes identification of risk factors for pregnancy-related complications through patient interview and data collection. Although the LPN does not independently provide care for a woman with a complicated pregnancy, he must be able to identify signs of complications and know what problems need prompt intervention. An understanding of the basic pathology and clinical manifestations of these conditions allows the nurse to intervene appropriately, to teach the patient about her condition and care, and to answer questions confidently.

The psychological and emotional impact a complication of pregnancy has on the woman and her family should not be forgotten or ignored. A complication that results in loss of the fetus can be devastating. The woman and her family will need support and guidance to help them cope with the loss. Sometimes the complication of pregnancy puts the woman's life in danger and difficult treatment choices must be made, such as the risk to the mother of continuing the pregnancy versus the risk to the fetus if he is delivered early. This chapter highlights information the nurse will need to provide basic physiologic and emotional care for the woman with a pregnancy at risk because of obstetric risk factors or complications.

HYPEREMESIS GRAVIDARUM

Hyperemesis gravidarum is a disorder of early pregnancy that is characterized by severe nausea and vomiting. Hyperemesis occurs in 0.5 to 10 cases per 1,000 pregnancies, with a higher incidence among white and younger women. The disorder most often appears between 8 and 12 weeks' gestation and usually resolves by week 16. The exact cause is unclear, although there is an association between hyperemesis and high levels of human chorionic gonadotropin (hCG) or estrogen. Some researchers have identified a connection between pyridoxine deficiency and hyperemesis. The risk of hyperemesis is increased with a multiple gestation (pregnancy with more than one fetus), molar pregnancy, or when there is a history of hyperemesis gravidarum. Stress and psychological factors can contribute to the condition.

Clinical Presentation

This disorder is distinguished from "morning sickness" because the nausea and vomiting are severe and result in dehydration, weight loss, and electrolyte imbalances, particularly hypokalemia. Acid-base imbalances may occur. Before a diagnosis of hyperemesis gravidarum is made, other causes of nausea and vomiting, such as hepatitis, hyperthyroidism, and disorders of the liver, gallbladder, and pancreas should be excluded. An ultrasound examination is helpful to rule out a molar pregnancy.

Clinical features of the disorder include symptoms of dehydration, such as poor skin turgor, postural hypotension, and elevated hematocrit. Although rare, esophageal tears or perforation can occur with unremitting vomiting. Prolonged starvation from severe or untreated hyperemesis can lead to thiamine deficiency and Wernicke's encephalopathy, a severe neurologic disorder marked by inflammation and hemorrhage in the brain.

Treatment

Emergency treatment is directed toward correcting fluid, electrolyte, and acid-base imbalances. Hospitalization becomes necessary when severe dehydration is present. Intravenous (IV) solutions that contain dextrose are frequently used to give the woman an energy source so that the body does not break down protein and fat for energy. Potassium is added to IV fluids because untreated hypokalemia can lead to cardiac disturbances. Other electrolytes or multivitamins may be added to the intravenous fluids as indicated to correct imbalances.

The woman is given nothing by mouth (NPO) for the first 24 hours or until the vomiting stops. Although vomiting sometimes ceases after rehydration, antiemetics are frequently required to control it. None of the antiemetics are approved by the United States Food and Drug Administration (FDA) for treatment of nausea and vomiting during pregnancy. Because many of these medications are in pregnancy Category C,[1] the physician must carefully weigh the benefit of using the drug against the possible harmful effects to the fetus.

When antiemetics are prescribed, they are usually more effective when ordered on a regular, around-the-clock schedule versus as-needed (PRN) dosing. Until vomiting is controlled, these medications are given by parenteral injection or via rectal suppository. Once the vomiting has subsided, antiemetics are given by mouth. Recent research has highlighted the benefits of several alternative therapies. In severe cases that do not respond to conventional treatment, additional measures may be taken. Steroid therapy is sometimes helpful, or the woman may require enteral feeding or parenteral nutrition.

---

[1]Pregnancy Drug Categories are described in Chapter 7 (Box 7-6).

CULTURAL SNAPSHOT

- Ginger is an herbal remedy commonly used to treat nausea. Some cultures consider ginger to be a "hot" herb that treats "cold" conditions. Although there is no information regarding possible adverse fetal effects during pregnancy, recent research demonstrates that ginger can reduce nausea significantly.
- Acupuncture/acupressure, specifically stimulation of the "P6 Neiguan point," located on the palmar aspect of the forearm above the wrist, has been shown to reduce nausea and vomiting by at least 50%. Some researchers recommend this traditional therapy as a first-line treatment before prescribing antiemetic medications.

Nutritional issues are addressed once the vomiting has stopped. A clear liquid diet is given and then advanced, as tolerated, to a bland diet. A dietitian is consulted to assist in determining caloric requirements. Pyridoxine supplementation may be ordered because deficiency of this B vitamin is associated with hyperemesis. Many physicians order thiamine supplements to prevent Wernicke's encephalopathy.

Nursing Care

Assess the woman for nausea and administer antiemetics, as ordered. It also is important to assess the amount and character of emesis. Record intake and output and weigh the woman daily. Assess for signs of dehydration, such as poor skin turgor and weight loss. Monitor laboratory values. An elevated hematocrit is associated with dehydration. Observe potassium levels, as ordered. Hypokalemia may result from severe vomiting, or hyperkalemia can occur with potassium supplementation. Monitor the fetal heart rate at least once per shift.

Did you know? A small amount of food taken at frequent intervals is easier to tolerate than one large meal, particularly for someone who is experiencing nausea.

After the vomiting has stopped, implement measures to promote intake. A relaxed, pleasant atmosphere is conducive to eating. The area for eating should be well ventilated and free of unpleasant odors. In addition, eating with others can promote intake. Every effort should be made to provide foods that the woman enjoys. Carbohydrates, such as breads, cereals, and grains, are sometimes easier to tolerate than other food types. Foods high in fat should be avoided because such foods may exacerbate nausea.

Provide mouth care before and after meals. This reduces unpleasant tastes in the mouth, thereby encouraging intake and retention of food. In addition, it is a good idea to restrict oral fluids at mealtime to avoid early satisfaction of hunger before sufficient nutrients are consumed.

Observe family dynamics. Because psychological factors can contribute to this disorder, a psychiatric or social worker consult might be indicated. Consult with the RN regarding this possibility. It may be therapeutic to allow the woman to ventilate her feelings regarding the pregnancy, her condition, and the hospitalization.

BLEEDING DISORDERS

Bleeding disorders can occur during early or late pregnancy. Bleeding disorders that occur during early pregnancy include ectopic pregnancy and spontaneous abortion. Although incompetent cervix is not technically a bleeding disorder, it is discussed in this section because it is a cause of early pregnancy loss. Molar pregnancy is most often found in early pregnancy but occasionally may not be diagnosed until midpregnancy. Placenta previa and abruptio placentae are bleeding disorders that become apparent during late pregnancy. These disorders can lead to hemorrhage during pregnancy and the birth process. The nurse must be alert to signs and symptoms of a bleeding disorder and must notify the physician if one is suspected. When the diagnosis is made promptly, hypovolemic shock from a bleeding episode may be avoided.

Ectopic Pregnancy

The term "ectopic" refers to an object that is located away from the expected site or position. An **ectopic pregnancy** is a pregnancy that occurs outside of the uterus. The fertilized ovum does not find its way to the uterus, so it implants in another location. In approximately 97.7% of all ectopic pregnancies, the pregnancy is found in a fallopian tube (Braun, 2003). This condition is referred to as a "tubal" pregnancy. Other sites, such as the abdomen, ovary, or cervix, can serve as implantation sites (Fig. 17-1), although this occurs rarely. The estimated incidence is 25 cases per 1,000 pregnancies, or 1 in 40 pregnancies (Braun, 2003). Ectopic pregnancy is the leading cause of pregnancy-related death in the first trimester.

Ectopic pregnancy occurs because some factor or condition prevents the fertilized egg from traveling down the fallopian tube, so it implants before it reaches the uterus. Adhesions, scarring, and narrowing of the tubal lumen may block the zygote's progress

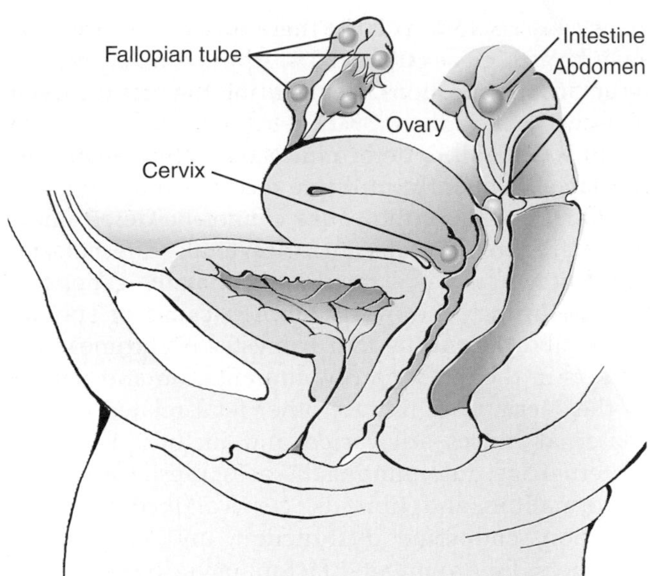

Figure 17.1 Possible implantation sites for an ectopic pregnancy.

to the uterus. Any condition or surgical procedure that can injure a fallopian tube increases the risk. Examples include **salpingitis**, infection of the fallopian tube, endometriosis, history of prior ectopic pregnancy, any type of tubal surgery, congenital malformation of the tube, or multiple elective abortions. Conditions that inhibit peristalsis of the tube can result in tubal pregnancy. Hormonal factors are thought to play a role because tubal pregnancy occurs more frequently in women who take fertility drugs or who use progesterone intrauterine contraceptive devices (IUDs).

Clinical Presentation

Symptoms usually appear 4 to 8 weeks after the last menstrual period (LMP), although the woman may not seek medical treatment until 8 to 12 weeks. The most commonly reported symptoms are pelvic pain and/or vaginal spotting. Other symptoms of early pregnancy, such as nausea and vomiting, also may be present.

Rarely, a woman may present with late signs, such as shoulder pain or hypovolemic shock. These signs are associated with tubal rupture, which occurs when the pregnancy expands beyond the tube's ability to stretch. The risk of tubal rupture increases with advancing gestation. Therefore, prompt diagnosis is critical to preventing rupture. If the tube ruptures, hemorrhage occurs into the abdominal cavity, which can lead to hypovolemic shock. Manifestations of shock include rapid, thready pulse; rising respiratory rate; shallow, irregular respirations; falling blood pressure; decreased or absent urine output; pale, cold, clammy skin; faintness; and thirst.

The diagnosis is not always immediately apparent because many women present with complaints of diffuse abdominal pain and minimal to no vaginal bleeding. Steps are taken to diagnose the disorder and to rule out other causes of abdominal pain. A serum or urine pregnancy test is done to detect the presence of hCG. Transvaginal ultrasound is used to locate the gestational sac and is often diagnostic. Culdocentesis (a procedure in which fluid is drawn from the cul-de-sac behind the vagina) may be done to identify the type of fluid located in the cul-de-sac. The presence of blood is associated with a ruptured tube. Laparoscopy may be required to confirm the diagnosis.

Treatment

Management depends on the condition of the woman. If she presents in shock with abdominal bleeding from a ruptured tube, she will be transported to surgery immediately for exploratory laparotomy, control of hemorrhage, and removal of the damaged tube. The ovaries and uterus are left intact. Volume expanders and blood transfusions may be used for massive hemorrhage.

In nonemergent diagnosed cases of tubal pregnancy, the physician must decide how best to remove the pregnancy. Laparoscopic surgery is the most common method of removing an ectopic pregnancy. If the woman desires to have children in the future, the physician makes every attempt to save the tube through the use of microsurgical techniques and minimally invasive surgery. When the tube cannot be saved or if the woman has finished childbearing, a **salpingectomy**, removal of the fallopian tube, is done.

A newer method of treating a small, unruptured ectopic pregnancy is the use of methotrexate, a drug that is also used in the treatment of cancer. The medication works by interfering with DNA synthesis, which disrupts cell multiplication. Because the cells of the zygote are rapidly multiplying, methotrexate targets the pregnancy for destruction. The medication is given intramuscularly. Sometimes a single dose is sufficient; at other times the physician may order multiple injections. The advantage to this approach is that surgery on the tube is avoided. Whatever treatment method is chosen, anti-D immunoglobulin (RhoGam) is given to the Rh-negative nonsensitized woman.

Think about this. Because surgery on a fallopian tube is a risk factor for ectopic pregnancy, treatment with the anticancer drug methotrexate can actually help prevent future ectopic pregnancies because surgery on the tube is avoided.

Nursing Care

Suspect ectopic pregnancy if the woman presents to the emergency department with abdominal pain and absence of menstrual periods for 1 to 2 months. Record vital signs and the amount and appearance of vaginal bleeding. Immediately report heavy bleeding or signs and symptoms of shock to the physician or registered nurse (RN).

If the physician decides surgery is necessary, assist the RN to prepare the patient. An IV line is started and laboratory testing done. At a minimum, a complete blood count (CBC) and blood type and cross-match are ordered. Check to see that written surgical consent is obtained and that the surgical preparatory checklist is completed.

Once the patient is in stable condition, emotional issues become the focus of nursing care. Be available for emotional support of the woman and her family. It is important to remember that the woman is grieving a loss, and each individual has her own way of expressing grief. Suggest outside sources of support, such as pastoral care or grief counseling.

Before discharge, instruct the woman regarding danger signs that should be reported, including fever, severe abdominal pain, or a vaginal discharge with bad odor. Explain that weekly follow-up care with her physician is necessary to measure hCG levels. Discuss contraceptive options and advise the woman that she should not attempt pregnancy until her hCG levels have returned to nonpregnant levels. If the woman desires more children, explain the possibility of another ectopic pregnancy and review the symptoms of ectopic pregnancy. Encourage her to seek grief counseling or attend a support group after discharge.

Early Pregnancy Loss

Early pregnancy loss is the most common complication of pregnancy and occurs in approximately 75% of women who are trying to conceive (Petrozza & O'Brien, 2002). A more specific term used to describe early pregnancy loss is **spontaneous abortion**, loss of a pregnancy before the age of viability (less than 20 weeks of gestation or fetal size of less than 500 grams). The common name for early pregnancy loss is *miscarriage*.

Here's a tip for you. It is best to use the term "miscarriage" when talking to patients about spontaneous abortion because the term "abortion" carries negative connotations for many people.

The rate of early pregnancy loss is difficult to determine because as many as 50% of losses occur before the woman realizes she is pregnant. The rate of recognized early pregnancy loss is 15% to 20%; therefore, the overall rate may be as high as 60% to 70%. Approximately 80% of spontaneous abortions occur during the first trimester (Puscheck & Pradhan, 2002).

It is difficult to determine the exact cause of miscarriage. Frequently, multiple factors contribute, and in many instances the cause cannot be determined. There are three overall categories: fetal, maternal, and environmental. Fetal factors are usually genetic in nature. In fact, the most common cause of spontaneous abortion in the first trimester is chromosomal defects in the fetus. Faulty implantation and defects in the sperm or ovum are other fetal-related causes. Maternal causes are varied and include advanced maternal age, autoimmune diseases, uterine anatomic abnormalities and fibroids, cervical incompetence, infection, endocrine dysfunction, and coagulation disorders. Environmental factors include poor nutrition; exposure to tobacco, chemicals, or radiation; and use of alcohol, street drugs, or certain prescription drugs.

Some authorities classify spontaneous abortion according to the timing of the loss. Early abortion occurs before 12 weeks and late abortion occurs between 12 and 20 weeks. Early abortion is most frequently caused by fetal factors, whereas maternal factors tend to cause late abortions.

Clinical Presentation

Typical symptoms of spontaneous abortion include cramping and spotting or frank bleeding, which can be severe. Blood clots or tissue may be expelled. Abdominal and suprapubic pain are common and may radiate to the lower back, buttocks, and perineum. Fever and chills are associated with sepsis.

There are several different types of spontaneous abortion: threatened, inevitable, incomplete, complete, and missed (Table 17-1). The definition of each type is related to whether or not the uterus is emptied, or for how long the products of conception are retained.

This is a good rule of thumb. Always consider any woman of childbearing age with vaginal bleeding to be pregnant until proven otherwise.

To make the diagnosis of spontaneous abortion the physician often orders laboratory and imaging studies. An hCG level is drawn to confirm that the woman is pregnant. A CBC can identify anemia associated with blood loss and can provide evidence of infection. Blood typing is important to determine if the woman is $Rh_o(D)$ negative. Blood cross-matching and coagulation studies may be ordered in cases of severe blood loss. Urinalysis is done to rule out a

TABLE 17.1 Comparison of Abortion Types

Abortion Type	Clinical Presentation	Treatment
Threatened abortion	Vaginal bleeding or spotting occurs. Cramping is often present, but the cervix does not dilate. The symptoms may resolve and the pregnancy may be maintained, or threatened abortion can progress to one of the other types.	Vaginal rest is indicated (e.g., no sexual intercourse or douches). Sometimes bed rest is prescribed. The woman is instructed to report bleeding heavier than a normal menstrual period, cramping, or fever. If tissue is passed, she is to save it for examination by the physician.
Inevitable abortion	Cramping and spotting or vaginal bleeding with cervical dilation. Amniotic fluid may leak.	Surgical removal of the pregnancy is the treatment of choice. The type of procedure performed depends largely on the gestational age. Pregnancies less than 14 weeks are usually evacuated by dilatation and curettage (D&C). (Refer to "Induced Abortion" in Chapter 4 for a discussion of specific techniques.)
Incomplete abortion	Some of the products of conception are expelled and others are retained. Usually, the fetus delivers and the placenta and membranes are retained.	Treatment is similar to that used for inevitable abortion.
Complete abortion	All of the products of conception (fetus, membranes, placenta) are expelled.	Usually no surgical procedures are recommended. The woman is dismissed home with instructions to monitor for complications such as heavy or increased bleeding or fever.
Missed abortion	The fetus dies, but remains in utero. Signs of pregnancy are present, but the fundus does not grow as expected in a normal pregnancy and may regress (get smaller). No fetal heart tones are present.	Ultrasound is used to confirm the diagnosis. If a dead fetus is carried for longer than 4 weeks, the risk of a hemorrhagic disorder is high; therefore, a coagulation profile is drawn. The uterus is then evacuated by D&C, or oxytocin or prostaglandin is used to induce labor, which results in passing of the products of conception.
Habitual (recurrent) abortion	The loss of three or more consecutive pregnancies before the fetus is viable.	Attempts are made to determine and treat the cause. For example, an incompetent cervix is often a cause of habitual abortion.

urinary tract infection. Transvaginal ultrasound is the diagnostic procedure of choice. The uterine cavity is visualized to determine if any products of conception are present and whether or not the embryo or fetus is alive.

Treatment

Treatment depends on which type of early pregnancy loss is occurring (see Table 17-1). Treatment for a threatened abortion is conservative because currently there is no specific therapy that can reliably prevent threatened abortion from progressing to spontaneous abortion. The physician develops a "wait-and-see" attitude. Usually she orders bed rest and pelvic rest, which includes no sexual intercourse, douches, or tampons. The woman is instructed to report heavy bleeding, cramping, or fever. Most other types of spontaneous abortion require some type of surgical intervention, unless all the products of conception are expelled (complete abortion). Vacuum aspiration or dilatation and curettage (D&C) are the most common methods used to clear the uterus of the products of conception (see Chapter 4 for discussion of the various procedures). Intravenous oxytocin (Pitocin) or oral Methergine may be ordered after uterine evacuation to help prevent bleeding. Ibuprofen may be ordered to control uterine cramping.

Nursing Care

Assess the woman's vital signs, amount and appearance of vaginal bleeding, and pain level. Count the number of perineal pads used or weigh perineal pads to assess the amount of bleeding. Document whether or not the pad is saturated and note if clots are present. Report a falling blood pressure and rising pulse, or other symptoms of shock, and an elevated temperature, which is associated with infection. If the pregnancy is greater than 10 to12 weeks, evaluate the fetal heart rate with a Doppler device. Save all expelled tissue for evaluation by the physician. Administer anti-D immunoglobulin (RhoGam) if the woman is Rh_0(D) negative.

After the pregnancy has been expelled, either spontaneously or through surgical intervention, continue to monitor vital signs and bleeding. Administer oxytocin or Methergine as ordered to control bleeding. Provide analgesics as ordered and comfort measures to treat pain. Usually the woman is dismissed home a few hours after vacuum aspiration or D&C, if she is in stable condition. Family Teaching Tips: Instructions for Self-Care After Spontaneous Abortion explains self-care at home.

This is important! If a woman is Rh_0(D) negative, she should receive Rh_0(D) immune globulin (RhoGAM) any time a pregnancy is terminated for any reason. The length or type of pregnancy does not change this need.

Grief reactions are to be expected. Allow the woman and her partner or support person privacy to discuss their feelings with each other. Offer parents the opportunity to view the fetus. It is important to acknowledge the loss and resist the temptation to reassure the woman that she "can always have more babies." The woman must work through her feelings and come to terms with the current loss before it is helpful or appropriate to focus on future pregnancies.

FAMILY TEACHING TIPS

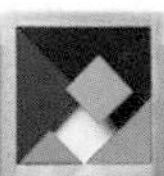

Instructions for Self-Care After Spontaneous Abortion

- Return for follow-up care if you experience any of the following danger symptoms.
  - Large amount of vaginal bleeding
  - Foul-smelling discharge
  - Severe pelvic pain
  - Temperature above 38°C (100.4°F)
- Do not use tampons or douche and refrain from sexual intercourse for approximately 2 weeks.
- Return for weekly physician visits to monitor hCG levels, if ordered. Avoid sexual intercourse or use contraception until hCG levels become negative.
- You will likely experience intermittent menstrual-like flow and cramps during the week after miscarriage. Ibuprofen is recommended to control painful cramping. Resume regular activities when you feel well.
- Grief counseling is beneficial.

A PERSONAL GLIMPSE

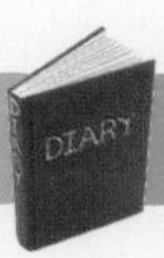

I was shocked when I found out I was pregnant with our fourth child. I was almost 40 years old and had a teenager and two school-age kids. At first, my husband and I were not eager to return to the days of sleepless nights and changing diapers. However, the idea of a sweet, new baby in our family grew on my husband and me, and our three kids were thrilled and excited. During the 10th week of my pregnancy, I started to have cramping and slight bleeding. I called my OB's office and the nurse said to come to the office immediately. I called my husband at work and asked him to come home and take me to the doctor. While I was waiting for him to arrive, the cramping grew stronger and the bleeding grew heavier. I started to cry because I knew I was losing my baby. After examining me, my doctor confirmed my fear; I had experienced a miscarriage. I was told that the miscarriage wasn't complete and that they would have to do a procedure to remove what remained in my uterus. No one really explained the procedure to us, and I felt so lonely lying on the table. After the procedure, the nurse gave me some medicine for pain and made sure I was comfortable; she told me that I could probably go home in a few hours. Before leaving the room, the nurse turned to my husband and me and said, "I know this has been difficult for you, but you and your husband are very fortunate to have three children at home." Although she may have meant no harm, this nurse made me feel guilty for grieving the loss of this unexpected, but wanted pregnancy.

Elisabeth

▶**LEARNING OPPORTUNITY:** In what ways can the nurse acknowledge that the loss of a pregnancy is a unique and deeply personal experience for the woman and her family?

Describe helpful things the nurse can say when a woman loses a pregnancy. Describe unhelpful responses.

The intensity and range of emotional responses of the woman experiencing a spontaneous abortion will vary greatly. The woman may feel overwhelmed by grief. She may feel guilty that she might have done something to cause the pregnancy loss. She may express anger with a divine power for allowing her to lose the baby. Accept and support the woman's emotions. The woman needs ongoing grief support after discharge; make sure the woman is referred for this service.

CULTURAL SNAPSHOT

Expressions of grief are influenced culturally. Some cultures discourage displays of emotion, whereas others encourage dramatic expression of grief. The degree of grief cannot be determined by the presence or absence of emotional expression.

Incompetent Cervix

When a woman has an **incompetent cervix**, painless cervical dilatation occurs with bulging of fetal membranes and parts through the external os. Usually loss of the pregnancy cannot be prevented. Therefore, although incompetent cervix is not technically a bleeding disorder, it often is a cause of habitual or recurrent abortion.

The exact cause of incompetent cervix is unknown, but there are factors that increase the risk. Any type of trauma to the cervix, such as surgical trauma (e.g., dilatation and curettage, conization or cauterization of the cervix) or exposure to diethylstilbestrol (DES) while in utero increases the likelihood that incompetent cervix will occur.

Treatment of incompetent cervix involves placing a purse-string type suture in the cervix to keep it from dilating. This procedure, known as **cerclage** is done between 14 and 26 weeks of gestation, generally after incompetent cervix has been diagnosed in a previous pregnancy. The suture is then removed when the pregnancy is at term or the woman goes into labor.

Test Yourself

- An elevation in what hormone is associated with hyperemesis gravidarum?
- List two conditions that increase the risk for ectopic pregnancy.
- Name two types of abortion in which the cervix dilates.

Hydatidiform Mole

A **hydatidiform mole**, also referred to as a molar pregnancy and gestational trophoblastic disease, is characterized by benign growth of placental tissue. There are two types of molar pregnancies: partial and complete. In both cases errors in chromosomal duplication occur during fertilization. The consequence is grapelike (hydatidiform) swelling of the chorionic villi and trophoblastic hyperplasia. Chromosomal abnormalities are present when there is a fetus; however, fetal tissue is found only in partial molar pregnancies. A molar pregnancy has some features of a malignancy in that the trophoblastic tissue proliferates (multiplies) out of control. In fact, 20% of women who experience a complete molar pregnancy develop **choriocarcinoma**, malignancy of the uterine lining, within 6 months to 1 year after molar pregnancy.

Fortunately, molar pregnancy occurs rarely. In Western countries, the rate is 1 per 1,000 to 1,500 pregnancies. The rate is uniform among ethnic groups living in the United States; however, in Asian countries the rate is much higher. Risk factors for a complete mole include extremes of age. Young women in their early teens and older women who are near the end of their reproductive lives are at highest risk. Women older than 40 years have a sevenfold increase in risk compared with younger women (Moore & Ware, 2002).

Clinical Presentation

Before the widespread use of ultrasound, molar pregnancy was most often diagnosed in the second trimester. Now the condition is diagnosed frequently in the first trimester before classic symptoms are evident. Thus, the most common presenting sign for both partial and complete moles is vaginal bleeding. Typically the woman presents between 8 and 16 weeks' gestation with complaints of painless (usually) brown to bright red vaginal bleeding. The bleeding may be intermittent or continuous and can be severe. An hCG level is obtained, the results of which is more often than not higher than expected for gestational age. Transvaginal ultrasound reveals the characteristic snowstorm pattern caused by grapelike vesicles that fill the uterus.

If a complete molar pregnancy continues into the second trimester undetected, other signs and symptoms appear. The woman often presents with complaints of dark to bright red vaginal bleeding and pelvic pain. Infrequently, she will report passage of grapelike vesicles. The physical examination may reveal a uterus that measures larger than expected for dates. Fetal heart tones are absent, and fetal parts cannot be detected. The snowstorm pattern is seen with abdominal ultrasound, and in 50% of the cases giant ovarian cysts are detected, which are the source of pelvic pain. Other less common findings include gestational hypertension (sometimes referred to as pregnancy-induced hypertension or PIH) before the 24th week (27%), hyperemesis gravidarum (26%), and hyperthyroidism (7%) (Kurowski & Yakoub, 2003).

Treatment

If the woman is hemorrhaging when she presents, the clinical team must move quickly to stabilize her condition. She requires IV volume expanders and blood transfusions. Clotting studies are ordered because coagulation disorders can develop as a complication of hemorrhage. Antihypertensives are administered if the blood pressure is elevated.

Once the woman is in stable condition, preparation for surgery begins. A chest x-ray is ordered to assess for vesicle emboli or lung metastasis. Blood samples are drawn to establish the baseline hCG level and to type and cross-match the blood, if this has not been previously accomplished.

Surgical treatment options include evacuation of the uterus by suction curettage, if the woman wishes to have children in the future. Abdominal hysterectomy is the treatment of choice when continued fertility is not desired. Labor induction techniques are not used because of the danger of hemorrhage. After the uterus is evacuated, RhoGAM is given to the woman who is Rh_o(D) negative.

Continued follow-up for 1 year is extremely important. The woman returns to the doctor's office every 1 to 2 weeks to have hCG levels drawn. This monitoring is done to detect the development of choriocarcinoma, which is highly treatable if caught early. The woman is instructed not to become pregnant during the year after a molar pregnancy and is usually placed on a regimen of oral contraceptives. Although the practice is controversial, some physicians recommend prophylactic chemotherapy because one in five women with a complete molar pregnancy will experience choriocarcinoma.

Nursing Care

The woman is at risk for several complications; therefore, it is important to watch her closely during the postpartum period. Vaginal bleeding and the condition of the uterine fundus must be monitored frequently. Observe vital signs and the woman's level of consciousness because shock can result from hemorrhage caused by uterine atony or accidental perforation of the uterus during surgery. Administer oxytocin as ordered to control uterine atony. Methergine or Hemabate are other medications that may be ordered to stimulate the uterine muscle to contract.

Disseminated intravascular coagulation (DIC), a bleeding disorder related to lack of clotting factors, is another possible complication. Molar tissue releases substances that break down clotting factors, increasing the woman's risk for DIC. Review clotting studies for abnormal values and monitor IV and injection sites for bleeding. Continual oozing from these sites should be reported immediately.

Trophoblastic embolus or pulmonary edema as a consequence of fluid overload is a possibly fatal condition; therefore, every nursing assessment should include a thorough evaluation of respiratory status and auscultation of the lung fields. Respiratory distress or crackles in the lungs must be reported to the RN or physician immediately. Continuous or intermittent pulse oximetry may be ordered. If oxygen saturation levels fall below 95%, supplemental oxygen is indicated.

In addition to nursing measures directed at preventing hemorrhage (see "Nursing Process for Caring of the Woman With a Bleeding Disorder") and detecting respiratory distress, emotional support is an important nursing function. The woman has to cope with a complication of pregnancy that can cause severe illness, but a baby will not result from her ordeal. Family Teaching Tips: Follow-up Care After Molar Pregnancy lists important aspects of patient education for a woman being discharged after treatment for a molar pregnancy.

Test Yourself

- What procedure is used to treat an incompetent cervix?
- How is hydatidiform mole diagnosed?
- Name three important discharge teaching points for the woman who has experienced a molar pregnancy.

FAMILY TEACHING TIPS

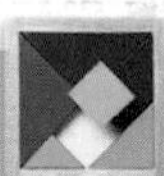

Follow-up Care After Molar Pregnancy

- Frequent physician visits will be necessary for 1 year after termination of a molar pregnancy to evaluate for the development of choriocarcinoma, a type of malignancy associated with molar pregnancy.
- Serum hCG levels are monitored at each visit to detect rising hCG levels, which may indicate the presence of choriocarcinoma.
- Avoid pregnancy for at least 1 year after treatment because hCG levels rise during pregnancy, making it difficult to differentiate between pregnancy and choriocarcinoma.
- Immediately report unexpected vaginal bleeding after evacuation of a molar pregnancy. Irregular vaginal bleeding is associated with choriocarcinoma.
- Report severe persistent headaches, cough, or bloody sputum. These are symptoms of metastasis, which requires immediate, aggressive treatment.

Placenta Previia

Placenta previa is a condition in which the placenta is implanted close to or covers the cervical os. Normally, the placenta implants in the upper uterine segment. In placenta previa, the placenta implants in the lower part of the uterus. As the pregnancy progresses, the part of the placenta that lies over the cervix bleeds because of rupture of blood vessels in the placenta.

The cause is not known. It may be that the site of normal implantation is scarred or damaged so that the embryo implants in a site that is more favorable for placental development. Conditions that increase the risk for placenta previa include history of elective abortions, multiparity, advanced maternal age (older than 35 years), previous cesarean birth or uterine incisions, maternal smoking, and prior placenta previa. The condition occurs approximately once for every 200 pregnancies (Queenan, 2000). The actual incidence of placenta previa at delivery is approximately one-tenth that diagnosed by ultrasound in the second trimester. However, this is true only for partial and marginal previas (see discussion in next paragraph). A complete placenta previa diagnosed in the second trimester rarely resolves to a normal implantation at delivery.

Placenta previa is classified according to the degree to which the placenta covers the cervix. Total placenta previa occurs when the placenta completely covers the cervix. If the placenta covers part of the cervix, the term partial placenta previa is used. Sometimes the placenta does not cover the cervix but is located on the border of the cervix. This condition is called marginal placenta previa. Figure 17-2 compares three classifications of placenta previa.

Clinical Presentation

Painless, bright red bleeding that begins with no warning is a strong indicator of placenta previa. Bleeding may be light to severe and usually stops spontaneously. However, bleeding will recur, and each subsequent episode usually produces heavier bleeding than the previous one. The first bleeding occurs on average between 27 and 32 weeks' gestation.

For any woman who presents with painless bleeding, a digital examination of the cervix should not be done until placenta previa has been excluded. This precaution is necessary because digital manipulation of placental tissue through the cervical os can cause uncontrollable bleeding. The diagnostic test of choice is transvaginal ultrasound because it is 100% predictive of placenta previa. Abdominal ultrasound is sometimes ordered. This method is 95% accurate in making the diagnosis.

Usually the first bleeding episode does not harm the fetus, unless it is unusually severe. The fetal heart rate should be within normal limits. Total placenta previa is associated with atypical fetal presentations, such as breech and transverse lie. It is thought that the abnormally located placenta prevents the fetus from assuming the expected head-down presentation. In severe bleeding episodes the fetus can become anemic, hypoxic, or develop hypovolemic shock because of loss of fetal blood and decreased oxygen transport across the placenta.

NEVER assist with a vaginal examination on a pregnant woman who is bleeding until the physician is sure that there is no placenta previa. During a vaginal examination, the fingers could penetrate the placenta, causing massive hemorrhage.

Treatment

If the initial bleeding episode does not stop or is massive, an immediate cesarean delivery is done to save the life of the woman and her fetus. If the initial bleeding episode stops and the fetus is still immature,

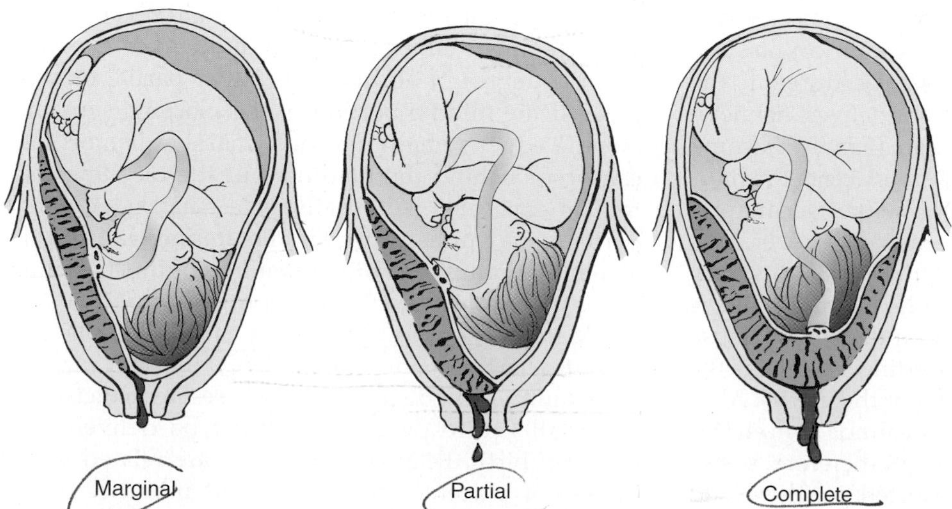

● ***Figure 17.2*** Three classifications of placenta previa.

hospitalization with bed rest is indicated. IV access is maintained, and at least two units of blood are placed on hold for immediate transfusion, if necessary.

If the woman is Rh_o(D) negative, a Kleihauer-Betke test is performed to determine if fetal blood cells are in the maternal circulation, which indicates fetal–maternal hemorrhage. This test helps to determine the appropriate dosage of anti-D immunoglobulin (RhoGam) to be given. Rh_oGam is injected for each bleeding episode to prevent isoimmunization, development of antibodies against Rho(D) positive blood in the pregnant woman. (See discussion later in this chapter.)

Serial nonstress tests (NSTs) are done to monitor fetal well-being. Continuous electronic fetal monitoring (EFM) is required during acute bleeding episodes. In some instances the woman is allowed to go home after the bleeding stops, but she must have someone with her at all times who can transport her immediately to the hospital if bleeding begins again.

A cesarean delivery is necessary in almost all cases of placenta previa. If the woman with a total previa were allowed to labor, massive hemorrhage could occur because placental blood vessels would break open and bleed as the cervix dilated. The physician often schedules the delivery as soon as it is reasonably certain that the fetal lungs are mature. The woman and fetus fare better when the delivery is accomplished in a planned fashion, as opposed to rushing to the operating room during an acute bleeding episode. Occasionally, a woman with a marginal placenta previa can deliver vaginally, as long as heavy bleeding does not occur during labor.

Nursing Care

The woman who has been diagnosed with placenta previa requires careful nursing observation. Maintain IV access at all times while the woman is hospitalized. Institute a perineal pad count so that bleeding can be quantified. Monitor the vital signs at regular intervals, and assess for signs of shock. Perform NSTs as ordered, and listen to the fetal heart rate at least every 4 hours. Instruct the woman to perform and record kick counts (see Chapter 7 for description of this procedure). If the woman is discharged home before she delivers her newborn, give her instructions for self-care (Family Teaching Tips: Home Care for the Woman With Placenta Previa).

Postpartum care of the woman with placenta previa is the same as for other women. However, it is important to observe her closely for signs and symptoms of infection and postpartum hemorrhage. She is at higher risk for both of these complications because of the proximity of the open, bleeding vessels at the former placenta site to the opening of the uterus. Also, the lower segment of the uterus cannot contract as effectively as can the upper segment; therefore, sometimes not enough pressure is exerted on the blood vessels to stop the bleeding.

FAMILY TEACHING TIPS

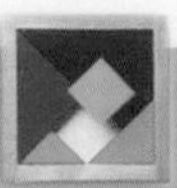

Home Care for the Woman With Placenta Previa

- Arrange for a dependable person with transportation to be available immediately to transport you to the hospital should a bleeding episode occur.
- Perform fetal kick counts at least daily. Decreased fetal activity is a sign of fetal stress. Kick counts are designed to measure fetal activity.
- Remain on bed rest (usually with bathroom privileges) while at home. Do no housework or lifting. Moderate-to-vigorous activity could bring about a bleeding episode.
- Vaginal rest is essential. Do not insert anything into the vagina (e.g., no sexual intercourse, no douching, no tampons). These activities could stimulate bleeding, and subsequent bleeding episodes tend to be more severe than the first.

Abruptio Placentae

Abruptio placentae, or placental abruption, is the premature separation of a normally implanted placenta. The incidence of abruptio placenta is 1% (Deering & Satin, 2002). Although the placenta is located in the normal place, it pulls away from the uterine wall before the end of labor. The cause of abruptio placentae is unknown; however, there are associated risk factors. Any condition that is characterized by elevated blood pressure puts the woman at risk for abruption. Preeclampsia and pre-existing chronic hypertension fall into this category. Maternal age greater than 35 years and multiparity increase the risk for placental abruption. Trauma (e.g., motor vehicle collisions or domestic violence), cigarette smoking, use of cocaine, and preterm premature rupture of the membranes are additional risk factors for abruption.

A placental abruption is classified in several ways. The bleeding is either concealed (hidden) or apparent, and the degree of abruption is either partial or complete. If the middle portion of the placenta separates but the edges remain attached, massive hemorrhage can occur behind the placenta but the bleeding may remain concealed. Alternatively, a small edge of the placenta may pull away from the uterine wall and the bleeding might be readily apparent. Figure 17-3 illustrates types of placental abruption.

Maternal complications of abruptio placenta include hemorrhagic shock, DIC, uterine rupture, renal failure, and death. If a classic cesarean incision is done, all future pregnancies must be delivered by cesarean birth. Fetal complications are related to the degree of placental separation and maturity of the fetus. Hypoxia, anemia, growth retardation, and even

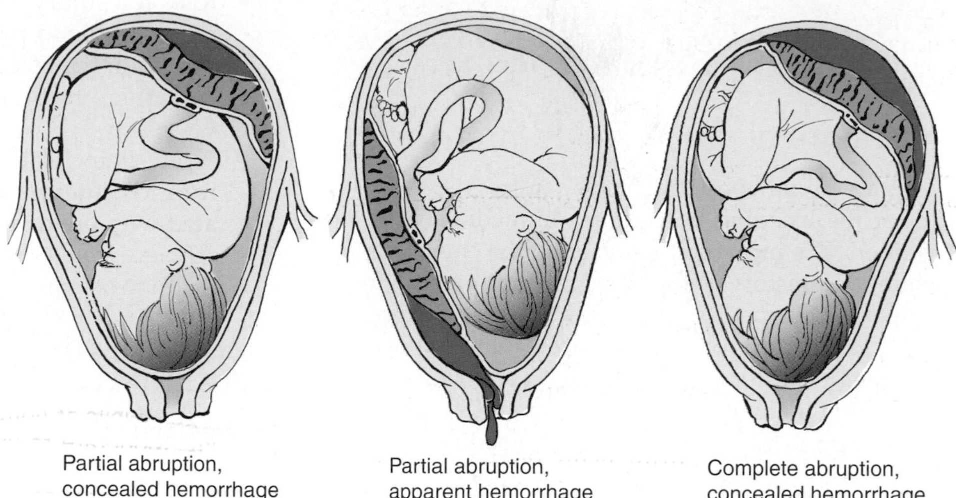

● ***Figure 17.3*** Types of placental abruption.

fetal death may occur. When preterm delivery is indicated, the neonate is at risk because of prematurity.

Clinical Presentation

The physician often makes the preliminary diagnosis based on signs and symptoms of the patient. The diagnosis is confirmed after delivery upon manual inspection of the placenta. The classic signs are pain, dark red vaginal bleeding, a tender abdomen that is rigid to palpation, and hypertonic labor. Pain has a sudden onset and is constant. Bleeding is apparent in most (approximately 80%) cases. The uterus may not relax well between contractions, the amniotic fluid often is bloody, and signs of maternal shock and fetal distress may be present. The fundal height may increase with severe intrauterine bleeding.

Ultrasound may assist with the diagnosis, but a negative sonogram does not rule out the possibility of abruption. As with other bleeding disorders, DIC is a potential complication of placental abruption. The physician carefully monitors fibrinogen levels and other clotting studies to detect the development of DIC.

Treatment

For cases in which there is severe bleeding, a large-bore IV is started and IV fluids are infused until cryoprecipitate, fresh frozen plasma, or whole blood is available for transfusion. Four units of packed red blood cells are cross-matched and are readily available from the laboratory. Oxygen is administered via face mask. The physician may perform an amniotomy to decrease intrauterine pressure. Immediate cesarean birth is done if the condition of either the woman or her fetus becomes unstable. After delivery of the fetus, if the physician is unable to control the bleeding, a hysterectomy may be done to save the woman's life.

Vaginal delivery is preferred to cesarean birth for small abruptions in which the woman and fetus remain hemodynamically stable or when the fetus has died. Contraindications for a vaginal birth include fetal distress, bleeding severe enough to threaten the life of the mother and fetus, or unsatisfactory progress of labor. The physician may rupture the membranes artificially to induce or augment labor, and oxytocin may be used. Although placental abruption is characterized by failure of the uterus to relax effectively, the benefits of vaginal delivery outweigh the risk of oxytocin induction in most cases (Cunningham et al., 2001b, pp. 629-630; Queenan, 2000, p. 301).

Maybe this will jog your memory on the exam! The classic way to tell the difference between placenta previa and abruptio placenta is that the bleeding with previa is bright red and *painless*, whereas the bleeding with an abruption is usually darker red (the blood may even be old) and *painful*. No pain = previa. Lots of pain = abruption.

Nursing Care

The woman with a suspected or diagnosed placental abruption requires careful monitoring. She is allowed nothing by mouth until her condition is stable. Assess for signs of shock. Watch for bleeding from the gums, nose, and venipuncture sites, which may indicate DIC. Insert a large-bore IV line and infuse IV fluid and blood products as ordered. Continuous EFM is necessary. The RN should evaluate the strip frequently. Immediately notify the RN if any signs of fetal distress become evident. Be prepared to quickly prepare the woman for an emergency cesarean birth if ordered.

After delivery, the woman requires close monitoring for postpartum hemorrhage because she is at risk for uterine atony. Continue to observe for signs of DIC. This complication may develop after delivery. Place the woman on strict monitoring of intake and output. Pay particular attention to the urinary output. Acute renal failure can occur.

● Nursing Process for the Woman With a Bleeding Disorder

ASSESSMENT

Take a thorough obstetric history, unless the severity of the bleeding necessitates immediate intervention. It is important to evaluate the chief complaint and history of the current condition and to note any risk factors for antepartum hemorrhage (e.g., grand multiparity, advanced maternal age, or previous history of a bleeding disorder).

During an acute bleeding episode it is critical to determine the characteristics of bleeding. How much is the woman bleeding? What is the color and consistency? Is pain present? If so, where and to what degree? In some conditions, bleeding can be hidden, such as a ruptured ectopic pregnancy and some placental abruptions. Ask yourself, "Is the fundal height increasing?" Take vital signs to determine if shock is present. Initial symptoms of shock include cool, clammy skin, restlessness, apprehension, and confusion. Late signs of shock include tachycardia and, when blood loss is severe, hypotension.

Obtain the fetal heart rate (FHR) and apply the EFM if the fetus is more than 20 weeks' gestation. It is important to assess and record the baseline FHR and to review the monitor strip for indications of fetal distress. Fetal tachycardia that progresses to bradycardia or decreased variability with late decelerations are ominous signs that must be reported to the charge RN or physician at once. Absence of the FHR is associated with fetal death or hydatidiform mole.

Palpate the uterus to determine if the resting tone is soft and to evaluate the characteristics of contractions, if present. Measure fundal height and compare it to previous measurements; concealed bleeding can cause increasing uterine distention.

Evaluate the woman's pain. Pelvic or shoulder pain in very early pregnancy is associated with ectopic pregnancy. Pain is generally not associated with placenta previa, unless the woman is also experiencing labor, in which case the pain will subside with each contraction. Cramping and abdominal pain may accompany spontaneous abortion and abruptio placentae.

SELECTED NURSING DIAGNOSES

- Ineffective Tissue Perfusion: placental related to hypovolemia from excessive blood loss
- Deficient Fluid Volume related to fluid volume loss from bleeding
- Risk for Injury (fetal) related to hypoxia and complications of prematurity
- Risk for Injury (maternal) related to fetal/maternal blood incompatibilities and complications of the bleeding disorder
- Risk for Infection related to open, bleeding vessels
- Acute Pain related to separation of placenta from the uterine wall or contractions associated with pregnancy loss
- Anxiety related to threat of harm and/or death to self and fetus

OUTCOME IDENTIFICATION AND PLANNING

Maintaining the safety of the pregnant woman and her fetus is the primary goal when planning care. Goals and interventions are planned according to the individual needs and situation of the woman. Appropriate goals may include that the woman's placental perfusion and fluid volume will be maintained; fetal injury from chronic or acute hypoxia will be avoided; maternal injury and Rh isoimmunization will be avoided; the woman will remain free of signs and symptoms of infection; she will express the ability to cope with her pain; and her anxiety will be reduced.

IMPLEMENTATION

Maintaining Placental Perfusion and Fluid Volume

The priority of care for any woman who is bleeding is to prevent and treat shock. For acute bleeding episodes, or when the potential for hemorrhage exists, start an IV line with a large-bore catheter per physician order. Infuse fluids, as ordered, to maintain blood volume. Collect blood specimens for type and cross-matching, and make certain that blood is available at all times for possible transfusion (2 to 4 units). If there is severe bleeding, administer blood and blood products as ordered.

It is important to monitor vital signs closely for signs of shock. Maintain strict intake and output monitoring with special attention to the urine output, which should remain above 30 milliliters (mL) per hour. In addition, maintain the woman in a lateral position to promote placental perfusion. Give oxygen by face mask if bleeding is heavy or if there are signs of fetal distress.

Sometimes the nurse will need to prepare the woman for surgery, either emergently to control the bleeding, or on a planned basis to prevent hemorrhage. In a planned situation, obtain informed consent, carry out preoperative orders, and complete the preoperative checklist. When the woman must be prepared for surgery emergently, move quickly and efficiently to get her ready.

If active bleeding is not occurring, but the potential for hemorrhage exists (e.g., placenta previa), assist the woman to remain on bed rest with bathroom privileges, as ordered. It is important to maintain an ongoing perineal pad count to monitor for increased bleeding. Evaluate fundal height for sudden size increase, a condition that may occur when there is concealed hemorrhage.

Avoiding Fetal Injury

When the pregnancy has reached the point of viability (usually considered 20 weeks and greater), the fetus should be monitored continuously during bleeding episodes until the woman is in stable condition. Watch the fetal monitoring tracing closely for signs of fetal distress, such as loss of variability, a gradually increasing or decreasing baseline, and late decelerations. If any of these signs are present, administer oxygen to the mother, reposition her to a side-lying position, and increase the rate of IV fluids. Notify the RN or physician immediately.

If the woman's condition has been stabilized and there are no signs of fetal distress, the woman may remain hospitalized for observation. Assist her to maintain bed rest, as ordered, and institute preterm labor precautions (refer to Chapter 18). Administer betamethasone as ordered to increase fetal lung maturity in the event delivery must occur before term.

Preventing Maternal Injury

Maternal injury can occur from complications, such as DIC, which are sometimes the sequelae of a bleeding disorder. Obtain specimens for laboratory studies as ordered. Typical blood work includes a complete blood count (CBC) to detect the presence of anemia and infection. Often coagulation studies are necessary because some disorders (such as abruptio placentae) are associated with a high risk of clotting dysfunction. Coagulation studies include platelet and fibrinogen levels, fibrin/fibrinogen degradation products, and prothrombin time/activated partial thromboplastin time.

In addition to close monitoring of laboratory results, observe for and report signs of DIC (e.g., bleeding from the nose, gums, and venipuncture sites). Watch for cough, dyspnea, fever, confusion and disorientation, symptoms that are also associated with DIC. Monitor the blood urea nitrogen and creatinine levels. Levels may be elevated secondary to renal failure. Assess the skin carefully for petechiae and purpura.

Injury can also result if bleeding causes fetal blood to come in contact with maternal blood. For this reason, blood typing is always done with any bleeding disorder of pregnancy. The woman who is Rh_0(D) negative may need a Kleihauer-Betke test to determine if any fetal blood has entered her circulation. This test can help the physician determine how much anti-D immunoglobulin (RhoGam) is needed. Every woman who is Rh_0(D) negative should receive anti-D immunoglobulin (RhoGam) if there is risk of fetal–maternal hemorrhage. All bleeding episodes and evacuation of the products of conception from the uterus increase this risk.

Preventing Infection

Take measures to prevent infection. It is important to use aseptic technique as indicated. In addition, teach the woman to wash her hands before and after eating, using the restroom, and performing perineal care. Monitor the temperature and white blood cell count. Report elevations in either parameter. Instruct the woman to report any vaginal discharge with a foul odor.

Managing Pain

Assess carefully regarding the woman's pain. It is important to ask the following questions regarding pain. Where is it? What is it like? When did it start? How often does it occur? What makes it worse? What makes it better? Intensity is best evaluated using a pain scale. Many nurses ask the woman to rate the pain on a scale of 0 to 10. Zero represents no pain at all and 10 represents the worst pain imaginable. If you use a pain scale, you can more effectively evaluate the success of your interventions.

Give the woman information about what is causing the pain (if you have that information) and how long she can expect it to last. Explain to her the medications the physician has ordered to help decrease her pain and tell her how frequently she can have them. For acute pain it is often better to schedule the pain medications, rather than waiting for the woman to ask for them. Explain that it is easier to treat pain before it becomes severe. Be sure that the room temperature, lighting, and noise level are at a comfortable level for the woman. It is also helpful to try to eliminate any factors that might be interfering with her ability to cope with the pain (e.g., if the woman is overly fatigued or bored, it will be more difficult for her to deal with the pain sensation). Consult with the RN regarding nonpharmacologic methods of pain relief, such as warm or cold applications, massage, or relaxation techniques. Be sure to inform the RN or the physician right away if measures to reduce pain are ineffective.

Reducing Anxiety

Care should be taken to attend to the woman's emotional needs. It can be frightening when there is active bleeding and health care providers are moving quickly to intervene. Use a calm and confident manner. It is a good idea to offer explanations for all procedures and treatments as they are being performed using language the woman and her family can understand. Promote expression of feelings and encourage the presence of supportive family members and friends, as appropriate. If the fetus dies because of complications of the bleeding disorder, or if the woman requires an unplanned, emergency hysterectomy, she will need additional support to deal with these losses. Request a social service consult if support is inadequate.

EVALUATION: GOALS AND EXPECTED OUTCOMES

- **Goal:** Placental perfusion and fluid volume are maintained
  Expected Outcomes: Skin and mucous membranes remain hydrated.
  - Hematocrit, serum electrolytes, and urine specific gravity remain within normal limits.
- **Goal:** Fetal injury is avoided.
  Expected Outcomes: Fetal monitor tracing shows presence of variability and reactivity without late decelerations.
- **Goal:** The woman remains injury free.
  Expected Outcomes: Coagulation studies remain within expected limits.
  - If DIC develops, the condition is caught early and treated immediately.
  - The woman who is Rh_o(D) negative does not become isoimmunized to Rh_o(D)-positive blood.
- **Goal:** The woman shows no signs of infection.
  Expected Outcomes: Vital signs remain within expected limits.
  - Fever is absent, and the white blood cell count remains within the normal range.
- **Goal:** The woman expresses the ability to cope with her pain.
  Expected Outcomes: She reports reduced pain (measured on a pain scale) after interventions.
  - She reports she is able to carry on with the activities of daily living and get enough sleep and rest despite the pain.
- **Goal:** The woman's anxiety is reduced.
  Expected Outcomes: Available social supports are used.
  - Effective coping strategies are used.
  - Decreased levels of anxiety are reported.

Test Yourself

- Name two characteristics that are different between abruptio placentae and placenta previa.
- Name three early symptoms of shock.
- Name one way to evaluate the extent of concealed hemorrhage.

HYPERTENSIVE DISORDERS IN PREGNANCY

Hypertension during pregnancy is the second leading cause of maternal morbidity and mortality in the United States, complicating 6% to 8% of all pregnancies (most of these are first-time pregnancies) and being responsible for almost 15% of maternal deaths. These disorders are not only dangerous for the pregnant woman, but also significantly increase the risk for the fetus (Lenfant, 2001). There are four basic categories of elevated blood pressure during pregnancy:

1. Gestational hypertension
2. Preeclampsia/eclampsia
3. Chronic hypertension
4. Preeclampsia superimposed on chronic hypertension

Gestational Hypertension

Gestational hypertension (formerly called pregnancy-induced hypertension or PIH) is the current term used to describe elevated blood pressure (greater than or equal to 140/90 mm Hg) that develops for the first time during pregnancy without the presence of protein in the urine. Gestational hypertension may resolve spontaneously after the baby is born, in which case the condition is referred to as transient hypertension. If the blood pressure remains elevated after delivery, the diagnosis becomes chronic hypertension. The concern is that gestational hypertension may develop into the more serious preeclampsia-eclampsia syndrome; therefore, urine checks for protein are done and blood pressure is monitored closely at each physician visit. If the blood pressure increases to a level that might endanger the woman or her fetus, the physician will prescribe antihypertensives.

Preeclampsia-Eclampsia

Preeclampsia is a serious condition of pregnancy in which the blood pressure rises to 140/90 mm Hg or higher accompanied by **proteinuria**, the presence of protein in the urine. Preeclampsia usually occurs after the 20th week of gestation and resolves when the pregnancy terminates. The syndrome may develop gradually, or it may appear suddenly without warning. The underlying cause of this disorder is unknown. It appears that exposure to trophoblastic tissue is the triggering factor, but it is not known what causes some pregnant women to develop sensitivity to the tissue while others do not. Risk factors for preeclampsia are listed in Box 17-1.

Medical researchers have been attempting to discover ways to prevent and predict preeclampsia-eclampsia

BOX 17.1	Risk Factors for Preeclampsia-Eclampsia

- Family history of preeclampsia-eclampsia
- African-American descent
- Nulliparity
- Pre-existing medical conditions such as
  - Chronic hypertension
  - Systemic lupus erythematosus
  - Renal disease
  - Diabetes
- Obstetric complications including
  - Multiple gestation
  - Hydatidiform mole (molar pregnancy)
  - Carrying a fetus that develops erythroblastosis fetalis
- Extremes of age
  - Younger than 20 years (increased risk probably due in large part to nulliparity)
  - Older than 35 years (increased risk most likely related to presence of chronic diseases)

because of the severe effects this condition can have on the woman and her fetus (Table 17-2). Various methods have been tried to prevent the condition, including high-protein, low-salt diets; low-dose aspirin therapy; and calcium supplementation. None of these therapies has been found to be effective in preventing preeclampsia.

Because there are no diagnostic tests available that can predict which woman will develop preeclampsia, early detection through regular prenatal care is the best alternative. Early prenatal care reduces morbidity and mortality associated with preeclampsia-eclampsia. However, a recent study indicates that there are differences in outcomes between ethnic groups.

Women who receive no prenatal care are more than seven times as likely to die of complications of preeclampsia and eclampsia as women who receive any prenatal care, according to a study in the April 2001 issue of *Obstetrics and Gynecology*. African-American women are 3.1 times more likely to die of preeclampsia or eclampsia than are white women. Although black and white women who received prenatal care had a lower risk of death, there is a far greater reduction for white women than for black women. This suggests that the quality of prenatal care may play a role, say researchers (ACOG News Release, 2001).

In a normal pregnancy a woman's blood pressure does not rise significantly above her baseline. In fact, during the second trimester the blood pressure decreases. However, in a pregnancy complicated by preeclampsia, the blood pressure rises. The elevated blood pressure occurs because the woman's blood vessels become more sensitive to substances that cause vasoconstriction, a condition that increases peripheral resistance and blood pressure. The rise in pressure is reinforced when the kidneys respond to decreased blood flow by releasing substances that raise the blood pressure.

The primary problem underlying the development of preeclampsia is generalized **vasospasm**, spasm of the arteries, which affects every organ in the body. Vasospasm causes generalized vasoconstriction, which leads to hypertension. The elevated blood pressure adversely affects the central nervous system and decreases blood flow to the kidneys, liver, and placenta. Vasospasm also leads to endothelial damage, which causes abnormal clotting. Tiny clots (microemboli) cause damage to internal organs, especially the liver and kidneys. Edema of the tissues, body organs, or both may result from this process (Fig. 17-4).

TABLE 17.2 Complications of Preeclampsia-Eclampsia That Can Cause Maternal and/or Fetal Injury or Death

Effects of Preeclampsia-Eclampsia	Potential Complications
Maternal Effects of Preeclampsia-Eclampsia	
Seizure activity	Bodily injury (especially the tongue), aspiration, placental abruption, or cerebral hemorrhage
Endothelial damage to pulmonary capillaries	Pulmonary edema
Severely elevated blood pressure and cerebral edema	Cerebral bleeding and complications associated with cerebral vascular accident (CVA or stroke). This complication is rare.
Edema and reduced blood flow to the liver	HELLP syndrome and/or rupture of the liver
Platelet aggregation and consumption of clotting factors	Thrombocytopenia and disseminated intravascular coagulopathy (DIC)
Fetal Effects of Preeclampsia-Eclampsia	
Reduced blood flow to the placenta	Intrauterine growth restriction (IUGR), oligohydramnios, and placental abruption
Preterm delivery to save mother or baby	Respiratory distress syndrome and other complications of prematurity

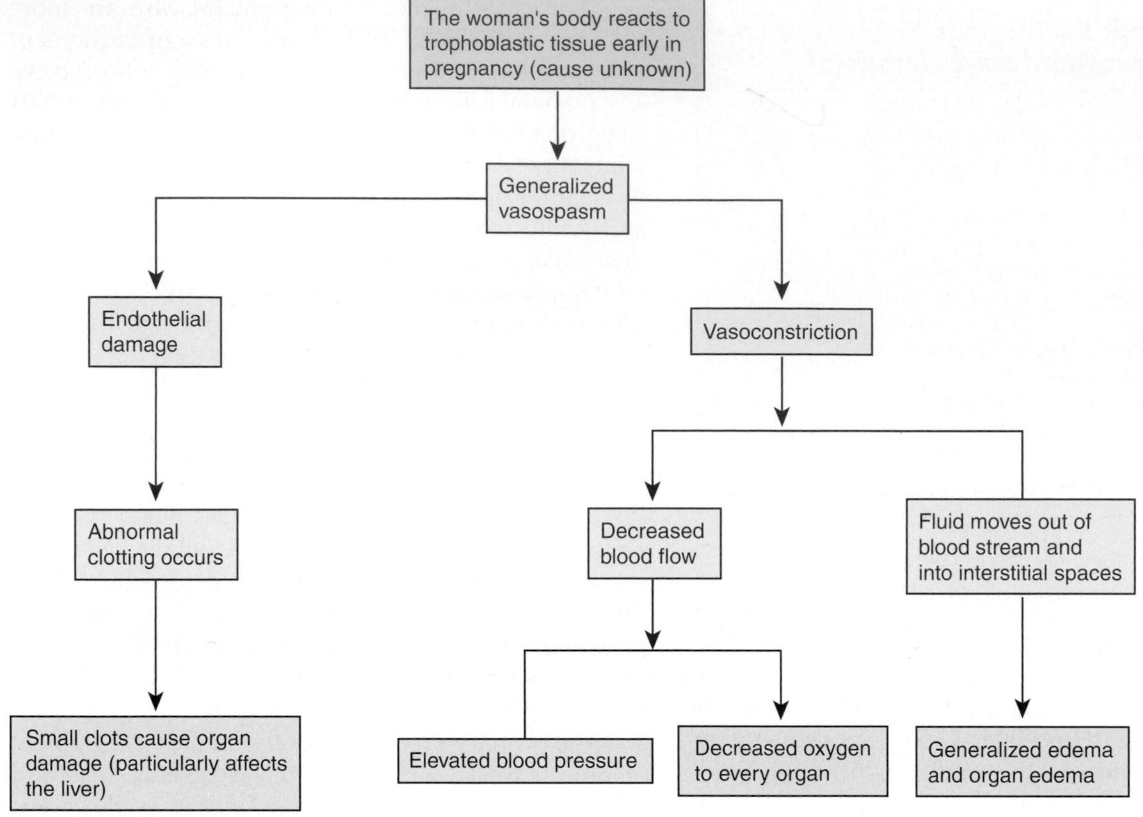

● ***Figure 17.4*** Pathophysiology of preeclampsia. Every body organ is affected.

Clinical Presentation

Preeclampsia is diagnosed when blood pressures of greater than 140 mm Hg systolic or 90 mm Hg diastolic develop after the 20th week of gestation. The hypertension must be documented on at least two different occasions and be accompanied by proteinuria (measured initially by dipstick of a clean-catch or catheterized urine specimen followed by a 24-hour urine collection). The presence of edema or weight gain is no longer considered a criterion for diagnosis of this disorder because edema occurs commonly in pregnancy and is not specific to preeclampsia. However, edema is significant if it is nondependent or if it involves the face and hands.

Depending on symptoms, preeclampsia is categorized as mild or severe (Table 17-3). Symptoms of mild preeclampsia are limited to slightly elevated blood pressure and limited protein in the urine. Severe preeclampsia is manifested by blood pressure above 160/110 mm Hg, greater than 2+ of protein in the urine, and symptoms related to edema of body organs and decreased blood flow to tissues. The central nervous system (CNS), especially the brain, is sensitive to small changes in fluid volume. Nervous system irritability occurs, resulting in hyperactive deep tendon reflexes and clonus (Fig. 17-5). A severe headache may indicate the presence of cerebral edema. If the retina of the eye becomes edematous, the woman will report blurred or double vision and spots before her eyes. Visual changes and a severe headache indicate that a seizure is likely to occur. Liver involvement results in elevation of liver enzymes. Severe edema of the liver causes nausea and pain in the epigastric region. In addition, a low platelet count may result in prolonged bleeding time, and pulmonary edema may occur when the disease process affects the lungs.

If the woman with severe preeclampsia experiences a convulsion or a coma, she has progressed from preeclampsia to **eclampsia**, the presence of seizure activity or coma in a woman with preeclampsia. Seizures are typically generalized tonic-clonic in nature and only rarely progress to status epilepticus. Potential complications of eclamptic seizure activity include cerebral hemorrhage, stroke,

Be careful! Don't let the term "mild" (when applied to preeclampsia) fool you. Mild preeclampsia can progress rapidly to severe preeclampsia or full-blown eclampsia with seizures. This is a serious disorder. Any woman with signs of preeclampsia should be monitored closely.

TABLE 17.3 Comparison of Mild and Severe Preeclampsia and Eclampsia

	Mild Preeclampsia	Severe Preeclampsia	Eclampsia
Blood pressure	140/90 mm Hg or higher; diastolic pressure remains below 100 mm Hg	160/110 mm Hg or higher	Same as for severe preeclampsia
Proteinuria	Trace to 1+ in a random specimen; 300 mg or greater in 24-hour specimen	Persistent 2+ or more; 500 mg or greater in 24-hour specimen	Same as for severe preeclampsia
Serum creatinine	Normal	Elevated	Elevated
Platelet count	Normal	Low (thrombocytopenia)	Same as for severe preeclampsia; may develop HELLP syndrome
Liver enzymes	Normal to minimally elevated	Markedly elevated	Same as for severe preeclampsia
Headache, visual disturbances, epigastric (abdominal) pain	Absent	Present	Present; epigastric pain is an important warning of an impending seizure
Fetal growth	Normal (not restricted)	May be restricted, unless there is a sudden onset near term and the baby is delivered promptly	Same as for severe preeclampsia
Edema	Trace to 1+ pedal, if present	May or may not be present; edema of the face or hands is significant	May or may not be present
Pulmonary edema	Absent	May be present	May be present
Seizure activity or coma	Absent	Absent	Present

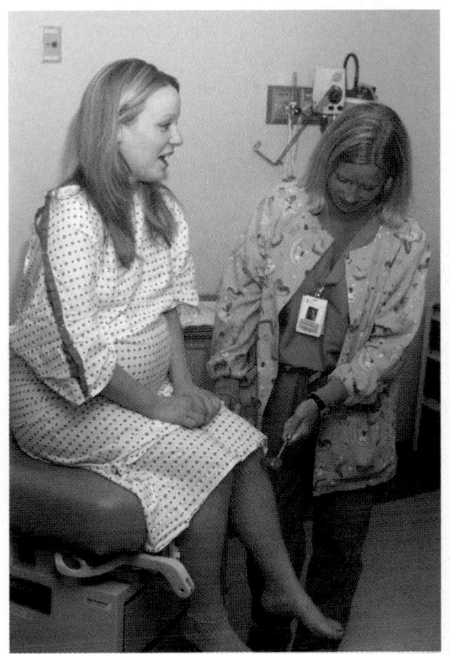

A

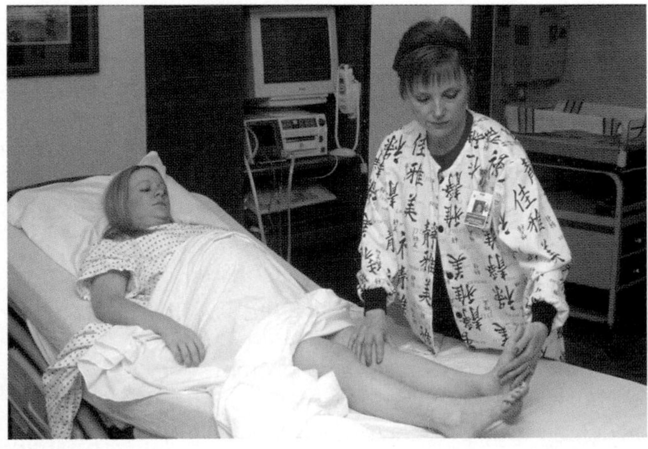

B

● ***Figure 17.5*** (**A**) Patellar reflexes are best checked with the woman in a sitting position and the legs hanging freely. Absent reflexes are graded as "0," hypoactive reflexes are "1+," normal reflexes are "2+," brisk reflexes are "3+" and "4+." (**B**) The nurse checks for clonus by dorsiflexing the foot, then quickly letting go. Normally the foot rebounds smoothly against the nurse's hand. If clonus is present, the foot jerks rapidly. Clonus is recorded in "beats." One beat means the foot made one jerky movement against the hand, and so on.

hepatic rupture, abruptio placentae, fetal compromise, and death of the woman or fetus. The woman with preeclampsia remains at risk for seizure activity throughout pregnancy, labor, and in the first few days of the postpartum period. In fact, the signs of preeclampsia-eclampsia may occur suddenly in the postpartum period even if they were not noticeable before delivery.

HELLP syndrome is a severe form of preeclampsia-eclampsia. HELLP is an acronym for *h*emolysis, *e*levated *l*iver enzymes, and *l*ow *p*latelets, which are the laboratory findings in a woman with this complication of preeclampsia-eclampsia. The presence of HELLP syndrome or eclampsia greatly increases the mortality associated with preeclampsia.

Treatment

The primary goals of therapy are to deliver a healthy baby and restore the woman to a healthy state. To accomplish these goals the physician must consider several issues.

The most important decision regarding management of preeclampsia involves the timing of delivery because the only cure for preeclampsia is to end the pregnancy. If the fetus is at term (>37 weeks), the physician will usually induce labor because a vaginal birth is preferred to a cesarean delivery. If the fetus is preterm, management depends upon the severity of the disease and determination of fetal lung maturity. The benefits and risks of conservative management (bed rest and observation) are weighed against the benefits and risks of a preterm delivery. If the woman's condition deteriorates rapidly or the intrauterine environment becomes hostile, the physician delivers the baby promptly to save the life of the woman, the baby, or both.

Conservative management may be chosen for the woman with mild preeclampsia. If she is compliant with the treatment plan and understands the danger signals, she may receive care at home. Otherwise, hospitalization is required. Activity restriction is implemented, which usually involves bed rest on the left side with bathroom privileges. The woman should stay in a minimally stimulating environment; therefore, visitors are usually restricted to one or two support persons. The blood pressure is monitored at least every 4 hours and the weight is measured daily. Urine protein is determined via a 24-hour urine collection, or a protein dipstick is used to check each voiding. Deep tendon reflexes are assessed, and the presence of clonus is determined at lease once per shift. The woman is asked to report signs of worsening condition, such as headache, visual disturbances, or epigastric pain.

If conservative management is attempted to allow a preterm fetus to mature, close observation of the fetus is indicated. Fetal kick counts are done after every meal, and NSTs are done at least twice weekly. A biophysical profile (see Chapter 7) and serial sonograms may be done to monitor fetal status and growth. In addition, amniocentesis may be done to determine lung maturity using the lecithin/sphingomyelin (L/S) ratio. A ratio of 2:1 is indicative of lung maturity. If imminent delivery seems necessary and the baby is preterm, glucocorticoids (usually betamethasone) may be administered to the woman in an attempt to hasten maturity of the fetal lungs.

Preventing maternal seizures is another important goal of therapy. If severe preeclampsia ensues, bed rest in a darkened, quiet room is implemented and visitors are restricted. The most effective medication to prevent and treat eclamptic seizures is magnesium sulfate, which is usually administered via the IV route (Box 17-2). This medication is reserved for the woman with severe disease. The drug works by directly relaxing skeletal muscles and raising the seizure threshold. IV $MgSO_4$ is the drug of choice to treat eclamptic seizures, although other anticonvulsants such as phenytoin (Dilantin) or diazepam (Valium) are sometimes ordered.

BOX 17.2 Pharmacology Focus: Magnesium Sulfate

Method of Action:
Prevents seizures by relaxing muscles and through direct action on the central nervous system (CNS).

Usual Dosage and Administration
IV route: Loading dose of 4 to 6 grams diluted in 100 mL fluid infused over 15 to 20 minutes, followed by maintenance dose of 2 grams per hour
Antidote: Calcium gluconate 1gram IV push over 2 minutes

Nursing Interventions
1. Carefully prepare and administer magnesium sulfate exactly as ordered.
2. Use a pump to regulate flow when administering via IV route.
3. Monitor vital signs per agency protocol every 15 to 30 minutes.
4. Perform hourly assessments of the following parameters
   a. Urinary output and protein levels
   b. Deep tendon reflexes
   c. Edema
5. Request serum magnesium levels every 4 to 6 hours, as ordered.
6. Discontinue magnesium sulfate and notify the physician if deep tendon reflexes are absent, respirations are less than 14 per minute, or urinary output is less than 30 mL/hour.
7. Therapeutic levels of magnesium sulfate are between 4 and 7 mEq/L. Patellar reflexes disappear at 10 mEq/L; respiratory arrest occurs at 12 mEq/L.

Note: The RN administers this medication. However, the LPN may assist with monitoring of the patient who is receiving IV magnesium.

Administration of magnesium sulfate requires careful management. If the medication is given intravenously, an IV pump must be used to control the rate of the infusion. Fluid overload could lead to pulmonary edema, a complication for which the woman with preeclampsia is at risk.

Magnesium sulfate is eliminated via the kidneys, and preeclampsia can cause kidney damage. Therefore, close attention must be given to urinary output, which is measured hourly. An hourly output of less than 30 mL must be reported because a low urinary output can lead to high serum levels of magnesium. The therapeutic level of magnesium sulfate is 4 to 8 mg/dL. This level is effective to in preventing seizures without causing toxicity. Magnesium toxicity begins when serum magnesium levels approach 9 mg/dL. First the reflexes disappear, then as the levels increase, respiratory depression and cardiac arrest can occur. For this reason, the reflexes and respiratory rate of the woman receiving magnesium sulfate are monitored at frequent intervals. Serum magnesium levels are drawn at prescribed intervals. Calcium gluconate is the antidote to magnesium sulfate. The RN gives this medication by IV push to treat magnesium overdose.

Because magnesium sulfate causes muscular relaxation, uterine contractions are inhibited. If delivery is indicated, the woman usually requires oxytocin induction of labor. She is at risk for postpartum hemorrhage because the uterine muscle may be unable to contract effectively. Careful monitoring for this complication is indicated after delivery.

The treatment of hypertension is controversial. Antihypertensives are only given to treat severely elevated blood pressure (greater than 160/105 mm Hg) because a rapid drop in the blood pressure can lead to decreased placental perfusion, resulting in fetal distress. Hydralazine (Apresoline) is the drug of choice for severely elevated blood pressure. Nifedipine (Procardia) is another antihypertensive that might be administered.

Nursing Care

Care of the woman with preeclampsia or eclampsia is challenging. The woman and fetus require frequent monitoring for symptoms of worsening condition. The experienced RN is responsible for assessment and care of the woman with preeclampsia, although the practical nurse may assist.

In the hospital, monitor blood pressure at least every 4 hours for mild preeclampsia and more frequently for severe disease (Nursing Procedure 17-1). In addition, it is important to auscultate the lungs every 2 hours. Adventitious sounds may indicate developing pulmonary edema. Weigh the woman daily on the same scale at the same time of day while she is wearing

Nursing Procedure 17.1 Measuring Blood Pressure in Preeclampsia

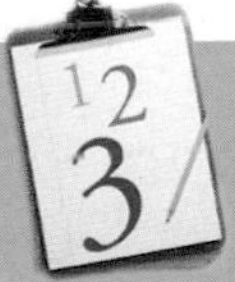

EQUIPMENT

Blood pressure cuff appropriate to the size of the woman*
Sphygmomanometer
Stethoscope

PROCEDURE

1. Wash hands.
2. Assist the woman to the same position for each reading; preferably she should be sitting.
3. Apply the blood pressure cuff to the arm in the usual fashion and support the arm.
4. Auscultate carefully. Note the systolic pressure; use phase 1 Korotkoff (the reading where the first clear, rhythmic sound becomes audible).
5. Diastolic pressure is noted at phase 5 Korotkoff (the number at which the sound completely disappears).
6. If the pressure is greater than 140/90 mm Hg, reposition the woman to her left side, wait 5 minutes and repeat the reading.
7. If the pressure continues to be elevated, determine if the woman is experiencing headache, blurred vision, or epigastric pain.
8. Reposition the woman comfortably on her left side, supported by pillows.
9. Replace equipment appropriately and wash hands.
10. Report immediately to the RN blood pressures greater than 140/90 mm Hg and/or abnormal symptoms.
11. Record the blood pressure per agency protocol. If the pressure was taken twice, record each reading, noting the time of each and maternal position.

Note: Most facilities use automated blood pressure equipment such as a Dinamap blood pressure device. These devices can be set to automatically take and record the blood pressure at preset intervals. There is also a manual override feature. Many fetal monitoring systems include automated blood pressure monitoring capabilities. With these systems the blood pressures are automatically taken and recorded on the fetal monitor strip.

* Care should be taken to choose a cuff that fits the woman correctly. If a small cuff is used to measure the blood pressure for a large woman, the reading may be elevated falsely. Conversely, if a large cuff is used on a small woman, the reading may be lowered falsely.

the same amount of clothing. Report any sudden increase in weight.

Teach the woman to report headache, visual changes, and epigastric pain, which are warning signs of an impending seizure. It is important to keep the environment quiet and nonstimulating because bright lights and loud noises could precipitate a seizure. Institution of seizure precautions is a must. Seizure precautions include padding the side rails and keeping suction equipment, an oral airway, supplemental oxygen, and medications readily available for use at the bedside. If a seizure does occur, follow proper procedure (Nursing Procedure 17-2).

The woman should remain on bed rest in the left lateral position, although some women with mild preeclampsia are allowed bathroom privileges. Maintain strict monitoring of intake and output. IV fluids may be ordered. It is important to control the infusion carefully with an IV pump to maintain adequate hydration without causing overload. Report urinary output of less than 30 mL/hour.

Adequate nutrition is important to promote fetal growth and maternal well-being. There is no special diet for preeclampsia, but careful attention is needed so that nutrients are consumed in adequate amounts (see Chapter 7). Salt does not need to be restricted below normal levels, but care should be taken to avoid excessive intake. See Nursing Care Plan 17-1.

The nurse also cares for the psychosocial needs of the woman hospitalized for preeclampsia. Boredom may be an issue because of prolonged bed rest. Encourage the woman to read, keep a journal, or do crafts. The woman may be anxious about the well-being of her fetus or because she had to leave older children at home. Keep the woman informed of the results of NSTs and other tests of fetal well-being. Reassure her that she can monitor fetal well-being by doing kick counts regularly. Allow her to ventilate her feelings of fear or frustration. Short daily visits by older children or telephone calls may also help alleviate anxiety.

Postpartum care of the woman varies depending on whether magnesium sulfate was used during the intrapartum period. If it was, the woman receives care in the labor and delivery unit or a high-risk antepartum unit for the first 24 to 48 hours after delivery. During that time magnesium sulfate administration is continued, and close monitoring of respirations, deep tendon reflexes, clonus, and urinary output is continued as before delivery. Close observation for postpartum hemorrhage is indicated.

If the medication was not used, the woman may be transferred to a postpartum unit. In addition to normal

Nursing Procedure 17.2
What to Do in the Event of an Eclamptic Seizure

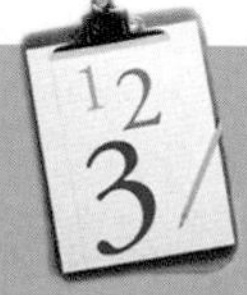

EQUIPMENT

Suction equipment
Equipment to deliver oxygen
Magnesium sulfate
IV access materials
Fetal monitor

PROCEDURE

When the seizure begins:

1. If you are in the room when a seizure begins, summon help with the call bell and note the time the seizure began.
2. Gently attempt to place the woman on her side, if possible. Do not force her to this position if injury will result.
3. Provide oxygen by face mask.

During the seizure:

4. The RN will prepare and administer IV magnesium sulfate loading dose per orders or standing protocol to stop the seizure.
5. If IV access is not in place, establish access as soon as it is safe to do so.
6. Suction PRN, if it is safe to do so, because aspiration is a real threat. Do not force the suction catheter into the mouth, particularly if you are using a hard plastic suction tip.
7. Watch for signs of spontaneous birth of the baby. Sometimes a seizure will precipitate birth.
8. Note the characteristics of the seizure so that you may accurately record a description after the emergency is over.

After the seizure:

9. Continue to suction PRN.
10. Continue administering oxygen to prevent/treat maternal–fetal hypoxia.
11. Begin continuous monitoring of the fetal heart rate, if a continuous monitor is not already in place.
12. Notify the physician of the seizure, if another nurse has not already completed this task.
13. Document the following parameters.
    a. Time the seizure began
    b. Characteristics of the seizure: tonic-clonic activity, fecal or urinary incontinence, cyanosis, etc.
    c. All nursing actions completed and medications administered
    d. Response of the woman to interventions
    e. Evaluation of the electronic fetal monitor tracing

NURSING CARE PLAN 17-1

The Woman With Preeclampsia

CASE SCENARIO

Hilda Rodriguez is a 35-year-old Gravida 1, Para 0 at 33 weeks' gestation. She was admitted to the hospital with the diagnosis of mild preeclampsia. Admitting vital signs are BP 150/98 mm Hg, T 98.7°F, P 70 bpm, R 20/min. She denies contractions, headache, blurred vision, or epigastric pain. Her deep tendon reflexes are 2+ (normal), and she does not have clonus (also a normal finding). Proteinuria of 1+ is found in a random voided specimen. Fetal heart rate is in the 150s, and a nonstress test at the physician's office today was reactive.

NURSING DIAGNOSIS

Ineffective Tissue Perfusion (maternal vital organs, peripheral tissues and placenta) related to constriction of blood vessels (vasospasms).

GOAL

Maintenance of adequate arterial blood supply to major organs, peripheral tissues, and placenta.

EXPECTED OUTCOMES

- The woman remains alert, awake, and responsive
- Blood pressure remains 140/90 mm/Hg or lower
- Urinary output is at least 30 mL/hour
- Extremities remain warm to touch
- Peripheral edema +1 or less
- No facial edema or ascites
- Weight remains stable without sudden increases

NURSING INTERVENTIONS	*RATIONALE*
Maintain bed rest in side-lying position, as ordered (strict or with bathroom privileges).	Bed rest in a side-lying position improves blood flow to the kidneys and other vital organs.
Monitor neurologic status (level of responsiveness) as per facility protocol.	Lowered levels of consciousness may indicate the presence of cerebral edema.
Monitor vital signs q 4 hours or more frequently as ordered; report blood pressure >140/90 mm Hg or as ordered.	A highly elevated blood pressure can interfere with blood flow to major body organs and extremities.
Perform strict intake and output measurements.	Vasospasms associated with preeclampsia can lead to hypovolemia, a condition that decreases blood flow to vital organs.
Monitor urinary output q 4 hours or as ordered; report outputs totaling less than 30 mL/hour, or 120 mL per 4-hour time period.	Reduced urinary output can indicate decreased blood flow to the kidneys, which should be treated promptly to prevent kidney damage.
Measure daily weights. a. Use the same scale at the same time each day with the same amount of clothing. b. Report sudden weight gain. c. Monitor for edema.	Sudden weight gain and edema indicates that fluid is being retained. Although the woman has more overall body water, the fluid is trapped in tissues so that less fluid is in the blood, a condition that leads to decreased perfusion.

NURSING DIAGNOSIS:

Risk for Injury (maternal) related to cerebral irritability and possible progression of preeclampsia to eclampsia.

GOAL

Freedom from injury related to seizure activity.

EXPECTED OUTCOMES

The woman will

- Not experience injury from seizure activity
- Maintain a clear airway

(nursing care plan continues on page 422)

NURSING CARE PLAN 17-1 continued

The Woman With Preeclampsia

NURSING INTERVENTIONS	*RATIONALE*
Monitor vital signs as ordered; assess for increasing blood pressure.	Increasing blood pressure indicates a worsening of status. The woman is then at risk for seizure activity.
Institute seizure precautions a. Side rails up and padded b. Airway, suction, and oxygen equipment set up at bedside. c. Quiet, minimally stimulating environment (low lights, sound, etc.)	A noisy, stimulating environment increases the risk for a seizure. If the woman does have a seizure, padded side rails, airway, suction equipment and oxygen will all be needed to prevent serious injury from the seizure (e.g., aspiration)
Monitor for signs of impending seizure. d. Headache e. Blurred vision f. Epigastric pain g. Hyperactive reflexes: 4+ h. Presence of clonus	All listed signs are indicators that seizure activity will likely occur unless there is intervention.
Assist the RN to administer magnesium sulfate, as ordered.	Magnesium sulfate is a muscle relaxant and a central nervous system depressant that can prevent eclamptic seizures.

NURSING DIAGNOSIS

Risk for Injury (fetal) related to chronic hypoxia secondary to ineffective tissue perfusion of the placenta and episodes of acute hypoxia during maternal seizure activity.

GOAL

Maintenance of adequate fetal oxygenation.

EXPECTED OUTCOMES

The fetus will

- Maintain a heart rate between 120 and 160 bpm
- Remain active with normal kick counts
- Demonstrate well-being with reactive nonstress tests
- No injury occurs and fetus remains reactive if a maternal seizure occurs.

NURSING INTERVENTIONS	*RATIONALE*
Maintain in side-lying position, or with a wedge under one hip.	A side-lying position increases perfusion to the placenta.
Monitor fetal heart tones and reactivity, as ordered.	Monitoring is done to determine fetal status.
Instruct the client to monitor fetal kick counts after each meal. (Chapter 7 outlines the procedure for performing fetal kick counts.)	If the fetus is moving as often as expected, there is reassurance the fetus is doing well. A decrease in fetal movement is an ominous sign.
Assist the RN to perform nonstress tests (NST), as ordered.	Serial NSTs will be ordered to closely monitor fetal status. A nonreactive NST indicates the fetus may be in distress.

postpartum care, closely observe the blood pressure and monitor for other signs of worsening preeclampsia because a seizure can occur as long as several days after delivery. Observe the woman closely because she is at increased risk for postpartum hemorrhage. Monitor the platelet count, as ordered, and watch for development of complications, such as bleeding from the mouth, gums, nose, or injection sites. If the neonate is in the neonatal intensive care unit (NICU), assist the woman to visit as soon as she is able. If she cannot visit, provide pictures of the infant and provide a daily update on the baby's condition.

Chronic Hypertension and Preeclampsia Superimposed on Chronic Hypertension

Chronic hypertension is high blood pressure that is present and diagnosed before the woman becomes pregnant. When a woman with preexisting hypertension becomes pregnant, the pregnancy is already at risk. Sustained high blood pressure can be damaging to blood vessels and eventually can decrease placental perfusion, leading to fetal growth restriction. In addition, the woman with chronic hypertension is at a much higher risk of developing superimposed preeclampsia. Box 17-3 lists the complications associated with chronic hypertension in the pregnant woman.

Clinical Presentation

Chronic hypertension is said to exist if the blood pressure has been elevated consistently above 140/90 mm/Hg when the woman is not pregnant. If hypertension develops before the 20th week of gestation, the diagnosis is suspected but is not confirmed until after pregnancy. If the elevation continues after the end of the pregnancy, the diagnosis of chronic hypertension is made. Some women with preexisting hypertension may begin the pregnancy with mild disease, but then experience severe disease after the 24th week.

The diagnosis of superimposed preeclampsia is made when a woman who has chronic hypertension experiences proteinuria. The presence of preeclampsia superimposed on chronic hypertension is a particularly lethal one. In these cases, the preeclampsia tends to develop earlier in the pregnancy and runs a more severe course. The risk of placental abruption and incidence of fetal growth restriction is increased significantly.

Treatment and Nursing Care

Ideally, the woman with chronic hypertension meets with the physician before becoming pregnant to modify her treatment regimen. If she is taking a hypertensive medication that may be teratogenic, the physician changes her medication to one that is recommended for use during pregnancy. The physician often recommends a sodium-restricted diet, explains work and exercise limitations, and recommends weight loss, if the woman is overweight. Once pregnancy is achieved, prenatal visits are done more frequently, usually every 2 weeks during the first half of pregnancy, and weekly thereafter. Fetal surveillance is intensified with serial ultrasound tests, frequent NSTs, and biophysical profiles.

Mild, uncomplicated cases of chronic hypertension tend to fare well without significant increases in perinatal mortality. In fact, pharmacologic therapy may not be needed in women with mild disease. However, in cases of severe hypertension (i.e., if the diastolic blood pressure exceeds 110 mm/Hg) antihypertensive therapy is almost always indicated.

Certain antihypertensive agents are typically used to control the blood pressure. Methyldopa (Aldomet), beta blockers, and calcium channel blockers may be prescribed. The benefit of treatment with one of these agents generally outweighs the risk of fetal effects when hypertension is severe. Angiotensin-converting enzyme (ACE) inhibitors and angiotensin II receptor antagonists/blockers are contraindicated, and thiazide diuretics are not recommended for use during pregnancy because of adverse fetal effects.

BOX 17.3 Complications Associated With Chronic Hypertension in Pregnancy

Medical Complications
- Ventricular hypertrophy
- Cardiac decompensation
- Cerebrovascular accident (CVA)
- Chronic renal damage

Complications of Pregnancy
- Superimposed preeclampsia
- Placental abruption
- Fetal growth restriction

Source: Cunningham, F. G., et al. (2001b). Hypertensive disorders in pregnancy. In *Williams Obstetrics* (21st ed., pg. 571). New York: McGraw-Hill.

Test Yourself

- List four categories of high blood pressure during pregnancy.
- What is the underlying process that causes most of the problems associated with preeclampsia?
- HELLP is an acronym for __________.

MULTIPLE GESTATION

A multiple gestation refers to a pregnancy in which the woman is carrying more than one fetus.[2] Twins are the most common manifestation of multiple gestation. In the general population twins (two fetuses) occur once in 83 deliveries, triplets (three fetuses) occur once in 6,900 deliveries, and quadruplets (four fetuses) occur once in 575,000 pregnancies (Elliot, 2003). Most pregnancies resulting in more than two fetuses are the result of fertility treatments. The incidence of twins is also increased with fertility techniques.

Twins can be identical (monozygotic), resulting from one ovum fertilized by one sperm, or fraternal (dizygotic), the result of two ova fertilized by two sperm (see Chapter 5 for review). A woman has an

[2]Singleton gestation is the term used when the woman is carrying one fetus.

increased chance of conceiving dizygotic twins if she has one or more of the following risk factors: older maternal age, multiparity, or family history of dizygotic twins. Monozygotic twins may have one or two placentas and one or two amniotic sacs. The best situation occurs when monozygotic twins each have their own placenta and amniotic sac.

When twins share a placenta, a serious condition called twin-to-twin transfusion syndrome (TTTS) can occur. In this situation, one twin receives more blood from the placenta than his sibling. This twin is called the recipient. The recipient twin gets too much blood, which can overload the cardiovascular system and result in polycythemia and heart failure. The other twin, called the donor twin, does not get enough blood from the placenta. This twin can become severely anemic and experience intrauterine growth restriction.

A multifetal pregnancy is considered to be at risk. The woman with multifetal pregnancy is at increased risk for hyperemesis gravidarum, pyelonephritis, preterm labor, placenta previa, and pregnancy-induced hypertension. The fetuses are at risk to be conjoined, to experience growth restriction, or to be born prematurely. During labor there is a higher risk for umbilical cord prolapse. During the postpartum period the woman is at risk for postpartum hemorrhage.

There also is increased fetal demand for nutrients in a multifetal pregnancy. This situation can easily lead to maternal anemia. Insufficient iron leads to iron-deficiency anemia, whereas insufficient folic acid may result in megaloblastic anemia.

Clinical Presentation

The woman carrying multiple fetuses usually presents with a uterus that is large for dates. She is more likely than a woman carrying one fetus to experience anemia, fatigue, severe nausea and vomiting, and hyperemesis gravidarum. The practitioner will perform an ultrasound examination to date the pregnancy and to rule out polyhydramnios, fibroid tumors, and molar pregnancy.

Treatment

Management of a multifetal pregnancy often includes consultation with a perinatologist. There is increased emphasis on the woman's diet, multivitamin and iron supplements, and rest. Obstetric ultrasounds are done every 4 to 6 weeks after diagnosis to assess fetal growth and presentation, and placental location. After 24 weeks' gestation, the woman is asked to schedule prenatal visits every 2 weeks, which include a cervical evaluation at every visit. Weekly NSTs are scheduled after 32 weeks.

The practitioner must choose (or recommend) a mode of delivery. In general, a cesarean delivery is indicated if twin A (the first twin) is not in a vertex presentation. If twin A is vertex, the practitioner may opt to try a vaginal delivery. Success for this method is increased if both twins are vertex. If twin B (the second twin) is breech, the practitioner may schedule a cesarean delivery, or attempt a vaginal delivery but only if twin B is not larger than twin A. If a vaginal delivery is attempted, the practitioner may perform podalic version to turn twin B after twin A is delivered. Or the practitioner may attempt a breech delivery for twin B. If twin B experiences fetal distress, or the practitioner experiences difficulty delivering twin B vaginally, a cesarean delivery may be performed for twin B.

Nursing Care

Assist the physician to perform assessments to detect complications throughout the pregnancy. Instruct the woman regarding symptoms of preterm labor (Chapter 18). Teach the woman to perform fetal movement counts daily after 32' weeks gestation. Encourage the woman to get adequate rest and a well-balanced diet.

BLOOD INCOMPATIBILITIES

There are several situations that can cause problems for the fetus related to blood incompatibilities between the woman's blood and the fetus' blood. Normally the two bloodstreams never meet. But occasionally some type of trauma occurs that allows intermingling of the two bloodstreams. This situation is more likely to occur during invasive procedures such as amniocentesis or active labor, after spontaneous abortion, or when the placenta separates at birth. Two types of blood incompatibilities are discussed: Rh incompatibility and ABO incompatibility.

Rh Incompatibility

The Rh_o(D) factor is an antigen (protein) that is found on the surface of blood cells. When this factor is present on the blood cells, the individual is Rh positive, and when the factor is lacking, the person is Rh negative. If a woman who is Rh negative is exposed to Rh-positive blood, such as through an incorrectly cross-matched blood transfusion, her immune system produces antibodies to fight the Rh_o(D) antigen. Once her body has produced antibodies to the Rh_o(D) factor, she is sensitized to Rh-positive blood, a condition referred to as *isoimmunization*.

The problem arises when a woman who is Rh negative carries a fetus with Rh-positive blood. If the pregnant woman has been sensitized, the antibodies to the Rh_o(D) factor readily cross the placenta and attack the fetus' blood cells. The fetus develops hemolytic anemia and often requires exchange transfusions in utero or shortly after birth. In years past, a woman who was Rh negative often became sensitized while carrying her first child. Sensitization most often occurred during childbirth, when fetal blood can leak into the woman's bloodstream during delivery. Thereafter, with each subsequent pregnancy, the fetus with Rh-positive blood would develop hemolytic anemia, with the disease becoming increasingly severe with each pregnancy. Now sensitization rarely occurs because the Rh-negative woman is given Anti-D immunoglobulin (RhoGam) within 72 hours of delivering an Rh-positive baby.

Clinical Presentation

The goal is to identify the woman at risk for Rh incompatibility and to prevent sensitization from occurring. The routine blood and Rh typing that are done during the first prenatal visit serve this function. Antibody screening is done to determine if the woman is sensitized. A positive antibody screen indicates that sensitization has occurred. In this instance the woman will have no symptoms at all; however, the fetus may be severely affected. The physician often performs amniocentesis or cordocentesis to diagnose and assess hemolytic disease in the fetus. If sensitization has not occurred (i.e., the antibody screen is negative), the woman will be instructed that she needs RhoGam after any invasive procedure, trauma of any kind (e.g., motor vehicle collision or physical trauma), and delivery, whether it be by abortion, miscarriage, removal of ectopic pregnancy, or vaginal or cesarean birth.

Treatment

RhoGam is a product derived from blood that prevents the Rh-negative woman from developing antibodies to the Rh_0(D) factor. It is critical for a woman who is Rh-negative to receive RhoGam after childbirth, miscarriage or abortion, ectopic pregnancy, or any invasive procedure, such as amniocentesis or chorionic villus sampling. It is during these times that fetal blood is most likely to come into contact with maternal blood. Most physicians also administer a prophylactic minidose of RhoGam at 28 weeks of pregnancy.

CULTURAL SNAPSHOT

Some religions ban the use of blood products. Inform the woman that Anti-D immunoglobulin (RhoGam) is derived from blood and obtain her consent before administering the treatment. If a woman refuses RhoGam, alert the RN or physician immediately. The woman must be fully informed of the risks and consequences of refusing the treatment.

If the woman is sensitized, she is not a candidate for RhoGam, and the fetus requires close observation. As the pregnancy progresses, fetal well-being is assessed with amniocentesis, cordocentesis, biophysical profiles, NSTs, or contraction stress tests. If hemolytic disease is severe, the fetus may require exchange transfusions, or the physician may opt to deliver the fetus prematurely (refer to Chapter 20 for discussion of hemolytic disease of the newborn).

It is important to note that Rh incompatibility does not occur if the woman is Rh positive. It doesn't matter what the fetus' Rh factor is, if the woman is Rh positive, she is not a candidate for RhoGam. An Rh-negative woman who delivers an Rh-negative child is also not a candidate for RhoGam. Because the gene for Rh-negative blood is autosomal recessive, if the woman's partner is Rh negative and she is Rh negative, the fetus will be Rh negative, and RhoGam will be unnecessary. RhoGam is never to be administered to the newborn.

Think of it this way. A problem with Rh incompatibility can only exist if the woman is Rh negative. So first determine the blood type of the woman. If she is Rh positive, then there isn't a problem. If she is Rh negative, a problem exists only if the fetus is Rh positive.

Nursing Care

The nurse's responsibility in cases of Rh incompatibility is to always check the woman's blood type on laboratory reports and the prenatal record. If there is a discrepancy, notify the physician. Before discharging a woman after any invasive procedure, abdominal trauma, abortion, ectopic pregnancy, or childbirth, check her blood type. If she is Rh negative, it is important to follow up to see if she is a candidate for RhoGam. If she is a candidate, obtain orders and administer the RhoGam. Instruct the woman regarding the purpose and importance of RhoGam to subsequent pregnancies. Make certain that she understands under what circumstances she is to receive RhoGam.

ABO Incompatibility

ABO incompatibility is another cause of hemolytic disease of the newborn. The problem most frequently arises when the woman's blood type is O and the fetus' blood type is A, B, or AB. Type O blood has naturally occurring antibodies against types A, B, and AB. However, these antibodies are large and generally do not cross the placenta. Occasionally during pregnancy fetal blood may leak into the maternal circulation, causing the woman's immune system to produce antibodies to fetal blood. These antibodies are smaller than the naturally occurring antibodies and readily cross the placenta, where they work to destroy fetal blood. Fortunately, this type of blood incompatibility usually results in a much less severe form of hemolytic disease than does Rh incompatibility. The neonate rarely requires exchange transfusions, although she will likely require treatment for jaundice.

Test Yourself

- List three complications for which a multiple gestation is at risk.
- Name two situations that place the fetus at increased risk for blood incompatibilities.
- What product is administered to an Rh-negative woman after she has delivered an Rh-positive fetus?

KEY POINTS

- Nursing care of hyperemesis gravidarum focuses on assisting the woman to regain fluid balance and to obtain nutrition needed for healthy fetal development.
- Signs and symptoms of ectopic pregnancy include missed menstrual period, nausea and vomiting, abdominal pain, shoulder pain, and vaginal spotting or bleeding. If the tube ruptures, the woman will experience hemorrhage into the abdominal cavity and hypovolemic shock.
- Spontaneous abortion is loss of a pregnancy before the fetus is able to survive outside the uterus on his own (before viability). Abortions are classified according to whether or not the uterus is emptied, or for how long the products of conception are retained. The six types of spontaneous abortion are threatened, inevitable, incomplete, complete, missed, and habitual (recurrent).
- Cerclage is the surgical procedure used to treat incompetent cervix. A suture is used to close the cervix so that the pregnancy can be carried to term.
- The nurse provides patient education regarding follow-up care to the woman who experiences molar pregnancy, including the importance of frequent physician visits, monitoring of serum hCG levels, avoiding pregnancy for at least 1 year, and reporting any symptoms of metastasis (e.g., severe persistent headache, cough or bloody sputum, or unexpected vaginal bleeding).
- Placenta previa causes painless, bright red bleeding during pregnancy because the placenta is implanted abnormally, either close to or covering the cervix. Abruptio placentae is associated with dark red, painful bleeding caused by separation of the placenta from the wall of the uterus at any time before the end of labor.
- The nursing process is used to develop the plan of care for a woman with a bleeding disorder. The focus of the care plan is maintaining placental perfusion and fluid volume, avoiding fetal injury (dealing with hypoxia), preventing maternal injury (dealing with isoimmunization), preventing infection, and reducing anxiety and pain.
- Hypertensive disorders are classified according to when in relation to the pregnancy the high blood pressure is first diagnosed, the presence or absence of proteinuria, and whether or not the condition resolves spontaneously after delivery. The four categories of hypertension are gestational hypertension, preeclampsia/eclampsia, chronic hypertension, and preeclampsia superimposed on chronic hypertension.
- Priority nursing interventions for the woman with preeclampsia-eclampsia include maintaining bed rest in a side-lying position; monitoring neurologic status, blood pressure, urinary output, and daily weights; instituting seizure precautions; observing for signs of an impending seizure (headache, blurred vision, epigastric pain, hyperactive reflexes, presence of clonus); assisting the RN to administer magnesium sulfate; and monitoring the fetus (fetal kick counts, fetal heart rate, NSTs).
- A multiple gestation, also known as multifetal pregnancy, is at risk. The woman is more likely to experience hyperemesis gravidarum, pyelonephritis, preterm labor, placenta previa, preeclampsia-eclampsia, and postpartum hemorrhage. Close observation of the pregnancy with special attention to diet and fetal well-being is recommended. Frequently, a perinatologist manages the pregnancy. The mode of delivery is dependent on several factors, the most important of which is the presentation of each twin.
- Rh and ABO incompatibilities can cause hemolytic disease of the fetus/newborn. Prevention of Rh incompatibilities through the use of RhoGam for the Rh-negative woman is the goal of therapy. If sensitization (isoimmunization) has occurred, the focus of assessment and care becomes the fetus, who may require exchange transfusions.

REFERENCES AND SELECTED READINGS

Books and Journals

ACOG News Release. (2001). Pregnancy-related mortality from preeclampsia and eclampsia. Retrieved February 15, 2003, from http://www.acog.com/from_home/publications/press_releases/nr03-31-01-4.cfm

Braun, R. D. (2003). Surgical management of ectopic pregnancy. *eMedicine*. J. J. Kavanagh, F. Talavera, G. F.

Whitman-Elia, F. B. Gaupp, & L. P. Shulman (Eds.). Retrieved January 28, 2003, from http://www.emedicine.com/med/topic3316.htm

Chamberlain, G., & Steer, P. (Eds.). (1999). Obstetric emergencies. *British Medical Journal, 318*, 1342.

Chudacoff, R. (2000). *Hyperemesis gravidarum*. The American Surrogacy Center, Inc. Retrieved January 17, 2003, from http://www.surrogacy.com/medres/article/hyperem.html

Cunningham, F. G., Gant, N. F., Leveno, K. J., Gilstrap, L. C. III, Hauth, J. C., & Wenstrom, K. D. (2001a). Gastrointestinal disorders. In *Williams obstetrics* (21st ed., pp. 1275–1276). New York: McGraw Hill Medical Publishing Division.

Cunningham, F. G., Gant, N. F., Leveno, K. J., Gilstrap, L. C. III, Hauth, J. C., & Wenstrom, K. D. (2001b). Section VII. Common complications of pregnancy. In *Williams obstetrics* (21st ed., pp. 565–810). New York: McGraw Hill Medical Publishing Division.

Deering, S. H., & Satin, A. (2002). Abruptio placentae. *eMedicine*. B. A. Meyer, F. Talavera, A. V. Sison, F. B. Gaupp, & L. P. Shulman (Eds.). Retrieved February 9, 2003, from http://www.emedicine.com/med/topic6.htm

Edelman, A., & Logan, J. R. (2001). Pregnancy, hyperemesis gravidarum. *eMedicine*. A. J. Saya, F. Talavera, M. Zwanger, J. Halamks, & R. O'Conner (Eds.). Retrieved January 17, 2003, from http://www.emedicine.com/emerg/topic479.htm

Elliot, J. P. (2003). *Multiple gestation*. Condition summary from Best Doctors website. Retrieved November 15, 2003, from http://www.bestdoctors.com/en/conditions/g/gestation/gestation_100200.htm

Ernst, E., & Pittle, M. H. (2000). Efficacy of ginger for nausea and vomiting: A systematic review of randomized clinical trials. *British Journal of Anaesthesia, 84*(3), 367–371. Abstract retrieved January 19, 2003, from http://www.jr2.ox.ac.uk/bandolier/booth/alternat/AT128.html

Gaufberg, S. V. (2001). Threatened abortion. *eMedicine*. R. Alson, F. Talavera, M. Zwanger, J. Halamka, & J. Adler (Eds.). Retrieved February 8, 2003, from http://www.emedicine.com/emerg/topic11.htm

Kurowski, K., & Yakoub, N. (2003). Staying alert for gestational trophoblastic disease: Implications for primary care clinicians. *Women's Health in Primary Care, 6*(1), 39–47.

Lenfant, C. (2001). Management of hypertension in pregnancy. *Journal of Clinical Hypertension, 3*(2), 71–72. Retrieved August 10, 2001, from Medscape database. http://www.medscape.com

Magee, L. A. (1998). The safety and effectiveness of antiemetic therapy for NVP. Presented at the 1st International Conference on Nausea and Vomiting of Pregnancy. Retrieved January 19, 2003, from http://www.nvpvolumes.org/index.htm

Mattson, S., & Smith, J. E. (Eds.). (2000). *Core curriculum for maternal–newborn nursing. AWHONN publication* (2nd ed.). Philadelphia: WB Saunders Company.

Moore, L. E., & Ware, D. (2002). Hydatidiform mole. *eMedicine*. J. G. Pritzker, F. Talavera, A. D. Barnes, F. B. Gaupp, & L. P. Shulman (Eds.). Retrieved January 17, 2003, from http://www.emedicine.com/med/topic1047.htm

National High Blood Pressure Education Program Working Group Report on High Blood Pressure in Pregnancy. (2001). Working Group Report on high blood pressure in pregnancy. *Journal of Clinical Hypertension, 3*(2), 75–88. Retrieved August 10, 2001, from http://www.medscape.com/LeJacq/JCH/2001/v03.n02/jch0302.02/pnt-jch0302.02.html

Nettina, S. M. (2001). Complications of the childbearing experience. In *The Lippincott manual of nursing practice* (7th ed., pp. 1179–1219). Philadelphia: Lippincott Williams & Wilkins.

Petrozza, J. C., & O'Brien, B. (2002). Early pregnancy loss. *eMedicine*. B. D. Cowan, F. Talavera, C. V. Smit, F. B. Gaupp, & L. P. Shulman (Eds.). Retrieved February 8, 2003, from http://www.emedicine.com/med/ topic3241.htm

Puscheck, E., & Pradhan, A. (2002). Complete abortion. *eMedicine*. S. R. Trupin, F. Talavera, R. S. Legro, F. B. Gaupp, & L. P. Shulman (Eds.). Retrieved February 8, 2003, from http://www.emedicine.com/med/ topic3310.htm

Queenan, R. A. (2000). Third trimester bleeding. In A. T. Evans & K. R. Niswander (Eds.), *Manual of obstetrics* (6th ed., pp. 298–305). Philadelphia: Lippincott Williams & Wilkins.

Saju, J., & Lyons, D. L. (2002). Placenta previa. *eMedicine*. R. Levine, F. Talavera, R. S. Legro, F. B. Gaupp, & L. P. Shulman (Eds.). Retrieved February 9, 2003, from http://www.emedicine.com/med/topic3271.htm

Sepilian, V., & Wood, E. (2002). Ectopic pregnancy. *eMedicine*. R. K. Zurawin, F. Talavera, A. D. Barnes, F. B. Gaupp, & L. P. Shulman (Eds.). Retrieved February 8, 2003, from http://www.emedicine.com/med/ topic3212.htm

Williams, M. C. (2000). Hepatic, biliary, and gastrointestinal complications. In A. T. Evans & K. R. Niswander (Eds.), *Manual of obstetrics* (6th ed., pp. 90–126). Philadelphia: Lippincott Williams & Wilkins.

Yoon, Y., & Ko, P. (2001). Placenta previa. *eMedicine*. J. J. Sachter, F. Talavera, M. Zwanger, J. Halamka, & S. H. Plantz (Eds.). Retrieved February 9, 2003, from http://www.emedicine.com/emerg/topic427.htm

Websites

Hyperemesis Gravidarum

http://www.am-i-pregnant.com/hg.shtml

Early Pregnancy Loss

http://www.miscarriageassociation.org.uk/
http://www.babycenter.com/refcap/252.html

Cervical Incompetence

http://www.dyspareunia.org/html/cervical_cerclage.htm

Ectopic and Molar Pregnancy

http://www.modimes.org/professionals/681_1189.asp

Bleeding During Pregnancy

http://www.perinatalmed.com/articles/vaginalbleeding.html
http://www.smartmoms.org/health-safety/health1.html

Preeclampsia

http://www.preeclampsia.org/index.asp

Rh Incompatibility and RhoGam

http://folsomobgyn.com/rh_testing_and_rhogam.htm

Package Insert for RhoGam

http://www.babycenter.com/rhogam/info.pdf

WORKBOOK

NCLEX-STYLE REVIEW QUESTIONS

1. A 28-year-old gravida 4 para 0 is seen at the prenatal clinic for complaints of lower abdominal cramping and spotting at 12 weeks' gestation. The nurse midwife performs a pelvic examination and finds that the cervix is closed. What does the nurse suspect is the cause of the cramps and spotting?
   a. Ectopic pregnancy
   b. Habitual abortion
   c. Incompetent cervix
   d. Threatened abortion
2. A 32-year-old gravida 1 para 0 at 36 weeks' gestation is brought to the obstetric department reporting abdominal pain. Her blood pressure is 164/90 mm Hg, her pulse is 100 beats per minute, and her respirations are 24 per minute. She is restless and slightly diaphoretic with a small amount of dark red vaginal bleeding. What assessment should the nurse make next?
   a. Check deep tendon reflexes.
   b. Measure fundal height.
   c. Palpate the fundus and check fetal heart rate.
   d. Obtain a voided urine specimen and determine blood type.
3. Which assessment finding best correlates with a diagnosis of hydatidiform mole?
   a. Bright red painless vaginal bleeding
   b. Brisk deep tendon reflexes and shoulder pain
   c. Dark red, "clumpy" vaginal discharge
   d. Painful uterine contractions and nausea
4. Which instruction is appropriate to give to a woman with hyperemesis gravidarum?
   a. Eat mainly high-fat foods to supply sufficient calories.
   b. Limit fluids with meals to increase retention of food.
   c. Do all your own cooking so you will build up a tolerance for food odors.
   d. Take your antinausea medicine after meals to help control the nausea.

STUDY ACTIVITIES

1. Fill in the table to indicate how ectopic pregnancy, threatened abortion, inevitable abortion, and incompetent cervix are alike and how they are different according to the signs and symptoms listed.

	Pain	Bleeding	Nauses and Vomiting	Cervical Dilation
Ectopic pregnancy				
Threatened abortion				
Inevitable abortion				
Incompetent cervix				

2. Go to the following Internet site: http://www-medlib.med.utah.edu/WebPath/webpath.html
   a. Click on "Systemic Pathology."
   b. Click on "Female Genital Tract Pathology."
   c. Choose images of the ectopic pregnancy (number 51 in the "Fallopian Tube" section), and of a molar pregnancy (numbers 84 to 86 in the "Placenta" section).
3. Think of an experience you, a relative, or a friend has had that involved a miscarriage. Be ready to share your story with your clinical group. Discuss interventions the nurse can use to help the parents to cope after a miscarriage.

CRITICAL THINKING: What Would You Do?

Apply your knowledge of hypertensive disorders of pregnancy to the following situation.

1. Maria, a 38-year-old primigravida, presents to the doctor's office for a scheduled prenatal visit at 28 weeks' gestation. During the assessment, Maria comments that she must be eating more than she thought because she gained 5 pounds during the course of 2 days. Her blood pressure is 150/92 mm Hg while sitting.
   a. What should the nurse ask next? Why?
   b. What additional assessments should be done?

c. Based on these data, what management plan is the physician likely to implement?

2. Maria is admitted to the hospital to rule out preeclampsia. The doctor's orders include bed rest with bathroom privileges, regular diet, private room, limit visitors, 24-hour urine specimen for protein and creatinine clearance, complete blood count, blood urea nitrogen and creatinine levels, liver profile, and coagulation studies.
   a. How should the nurse prepare the room for Maria? What supplies are needed? Why?
   b. If Maria has preeclampsia, what results does the nurse anticipate to see on the laboratory report for each test?
   c. Why did the doctor write an order for a private room and to limit visitors?
3. Maria receives a diagnosis of mild preeclampsia. She is to remain in the hospital on bed rest.
   a. What fetal assessment tests should be done? How frequently?
   b. What special instructions and recurring assessments should be included on the care plan?
   c. Maria asks the nurse, "Since my condition is mild, why can't I just go home? I could stay in bed there and I'd be so much more comfortable." How should the nurse reply?
4. The nurse is doing the a.m. assessment. Maria says, "I woke up with a terrible headache, and I can't seem to wake up enough to see well this morning. Everything looks blurry." Maria's blood pressure is 164/110 mm Hg.
   a. How is Maria's condition classified now?
   b. What other assessments should the nurse make? What should be done next after the assessment is completed?
   c. How does the nurse expect the treatment plan will change?

Labor at Risk

18

STUDENT OBJECTIVES

On completion of this chapter, the student should be able to

1. Choose appropriate nursing interventions for the client with labor dystocia.
2. Compare and contrast PROM with preterm PROM.
3. Describe clinical manifestations of preterm labor.
4. Discuss treatment options for preterm labor.
5. Apply the nursing process to the care of a woman in preterm labor.
6. Develop a patient teaching plan for the woman with a post-term pregnancy.
7. Describe nursing interventions for the woman experiencing fetal demise.
8. Compare and contrast obstetric emergencies according to clinical manifestations, treatment, and nursing care.

KEY TERMS

chorioamnionitis
labor dystocia
pelvic rest
precipitous labor
tocolytic

There are situations that sometimes arise that put the laboring woman and her fetus at risk. It is for this reason that many women prefer to deliver in a hospital setting. However, a well-trained practitioner who monitors the laboring woman closely can often catch signs of developing complications so that intervention can prevent harm no matter what the treatment setting. The following discussion describes complications that might be encountered during labor. Although the licensed practical nurse/licensed vocational nurse (LPN/LVN) may not be directly responsible for the laboring woman, it is helpful to know the signs of labor complications to be able to summon help when needed.

DYSFUNCTIONAL LABOR (DYSTOCIA)

Labor dystocia is an abnormal progression of labor. Dystocia occurs as a result of a malfunction in one or more of the "four Ps" of labor that were discussed in Chapter 8: passageway, passenger, powers, or psyche. The pelvis may be small or contracted because of disease or injury. The fetus may be malpositioned, excessively large (macrosomic), or have an anomaly, such as hydrocephalus or omphalocele, which may not allow him to fit through the birth canal. Uterine contractions may be of insufficient quality or quantity. The woman may be unable to push effectively during the second stage of labor because of exhaustion. The woman may "fight" the contractions because of fear or pain. Frequently it is a combination of factors that results in dysfunctional labor.

Complications

Difficult labor is associated with increased maternal and fetal morbidity and mortality. The risk for infection is increased when labor is prolonged, particularly in association with ruptured membranes. Bacteria can ascend the birth canal, resulting in fetal or maternal bacteremia and sepsis. Neonatal pneumonia can result from the fetus aspirating infected amniotic fluid. Uterine rupture can result from obstructed labor. This complication can be lethal for the woman and her fetus. Labor dystocia is the most common reason cited for performing a primary cesarean delivery, which carries increased risk for mother and baby.

Some complications of labor dystocia relate only to the woman. Fistula formation is more common in prolonged labor because the presenting part exerts pressure for prolonged periods on maternal soft tissue, a situation that can result in tissue necrosis and subsequent fistula development. Pelvic floor injury is more common for the woman who experiences a difficult labor or delivery.

TABLE 18.1 Expected Labor Progress

	Primipara	Multipara
Expected length of the latent phase of labor	<20 hours	<14 hours
Expected rate of dilation during active labor	At least 1.2 centimeters per hour	At least 1.5 centimeters per hour
Expected rate of fetal descent during active labor	At least 1 centimeter per hour	At least 2 centimeters per hour

Clinical Manifestations and Diagnosis

Before abnormal labor can be diagnosed, the clinician must be aware of what constitutes normal labor. Table 18-1 compares expected rates of labor progress for the primipara and multipara. For additional review of normal labor, refer to Chapters 8 and 10.

Labor dystocia can occur in any stage of labor, although it is diagnosed most commonly once the woman is in active labor or when she reaches the second stage of labor. Dystocia is characterized by disorders of protraction and arrest. A protraction disorder occurs when there is abnormally slow progression of labor. An arrest disorder refers to total lack of progress. A primipara in active labor receives a diagnosis of protraction of dilation if cervical dilation progresses at less than 1.2 centimeters/hour. She has a diagnosis of protraction of descent if the fetal head descends at less than 1 centimeter/hour. If a multipara in active labor experiences less than 1.5 centimeters/hour cervical dilation or fetal descent of less than 2 centimeters/hour, she is diagnosed with protraction disorder. Arrest disorders occur when there is no change in cervical dilation or fetal descent for a period of 2 hours provided adequate labor has been established.

Causes of Labor Dysfunction

Labor dysfunction can occur as a result of problems with the uterus or problems with the fetus.

Uterine Dysfunction

There are two types of uterine dysfunction: hypotonic and hypertonic. The most common is hypotonic dysfunction. This labor pattern is manifested by uterine contractions that may or may not be regular, but the quantity or strength is insufficient to dilate the cervix.

Hypertonic dysfunction presents in two ways. The most common is frequent ineffective contractions. Some clinicians refer to this syndrome as uterine "irritability." The underlying problem with this disorder is that the uterine muscle cells do not contract in a coordinated fashion. The end result is an elevated resting uterine tone with small, short, but frequent contractions.

The other type of hypertonic dysfunction manifests as increased frequency and intensity of uterine contractions. This type of hypertonic dysfunction often results in **precipitous labor**—labor that lasts less than 3 hours from the start of uterine contractions to birth. The complication that most frequently results from a precipitous labor is maternal soft tissue damage, such as lacerations of the cervix, vaginal wall, and perineum; and bruising or other trauma to the infant from rapid descent through the birth canal.

Be careful! Don't confuse precipitous labor with precipitous delivery, although precipitous labor may result in a precipitous birth. Precipitous labor is an abnormally fast labor (lasting less than 3 hours); whereas, a precipitous delivery refers to a delivery that is unattended by the physician or nurse midwife. A precipitous delivery may be totally unattended or it may be nurse controlled. This type of delivery may occur outside or inside of the health care facility.

Cephalopelvic Disproportion (CPD)

Labor arrest is sometimes referred to as "failure to progress." If hypotonic labor is ruled out as the cause of failure to progress, the practitioner may suspect CPD. In this situation the diameters of the fetal head are too large to pass through the birth canal. CPD can be due to a condition that causes an enlarged fetal head, such as fetal macrosomia or hydrocephalus. CPD can also result from a small maternal pelvis. In the past, maternal rickets frequently was the cause of a contracted pelvis. Improved nutrition has decreased the incidence of rickets, so today most cases of CPD are due to other causes. Nongynecoid pelvic types, such as android, anthropoid, or platypelloid, may result in CPD.

Fetal Malposition

Fetal malposition can cause prolonged labor. When the back of the fetal head is positioned toward the posterior portion of the maternal pelvis, the position is referred to as occiput posterior (see Chapter 8 for a review of fetal positions). A labor complicated by occiput posterior position is usually prolonged and characterized by maternal perception of increased intensity of back discomfort. The lay term for this type of labor is "back labor." Face presentation is another cause of prolonged labor. When the fetal face presents, the largest diameters of the fetal head are presented to the maternal pelvis, and labor is generally prolonged. Breech presentation, transverse lie, and compound presentations may also cause labor dystocia. Any of these fetal positions may result in the need for cesarean delivery, although vaginal delivery may be possible.

Treatment

Treatment depends on the cause of labor dystocia. However, because the cause is not always known, clinicians usually give what is called a "trial of labor." If uterine hypofunction is the cause of inadequate progress, augmentation of labor with artificial rupture of membranes or intravenous (IV) oxytocin infusion or both is usually the treatment of choice. Augmentation is carried out using the same process as that for labor induction. (See Chapter 11 for discussion of labor induction.) Oxytocin augmentation is the treatment of choice for uterine irritability in the absence of placental abruption. In this situation, oxytocin assists the uterus to contract more effectively so that the pattern spaces out, but individual contractions are stronger and more effective.

Hypertonic labor may result from an increased sensitivity of uterine muscle to oxytocin induction or augmentation. Treatment for this iatrogenic cause of hypertonic labor is to decrease or shut off the oxytocin infusion. If the hypertonic pattern causes the fetal heart rate to drop precipitously, the practitioner may order administration of a **tocolytic**, a substance that relaxes the uterine muscle, to slow the labor.

If the cause of labor dystocia is fetal malposition, the practitioner may attempt to manipulate the fetus to a more favorable position. For occiput posterior position, the fetus may rotate unaided to an anterior position, although the labor is generally prolonged because the fetus must rotate 180 degrees, as compared with 90 degrees if the fetal head begins descent in a transverse position. If the woman completes the first stage of labor and the fetal head has not rotated, the practitioner may use the vacuum extractor or forceps to attempt to rotate the head to an anterior position. This requires that the fetal head be at +2 station, or lower. It is possible for the fetus to deliver from an occiput posterior position. In this situation, the fetus is born face up.

There are three basic options for a breech presentation. The practitioner may use a version procedure (see Chapter 11) in an attempt to turn the fetus to a cephalic presentation. Frequently this procedure is effective; however, sometimes the fetus turns back to a breech presentation before labor ensues. Some practitioners will allow the woman to labor with the fetus in a breech presentation and attempt a vaginal delivery, although this practice has become less common because of successful version techniques and malpractice concerns. A cesarean delivery is the third option for delivering a breech presentation.

This is a good review tip. When you prepare a table in anticipation of a vaginal breech delivery, be sure to include a set of piper forceps. Piper forceps are often used to deliver the head after the rest of the body has delivered in a breech presentation.

For a transverse lie (shoulder presentation), there are two options. Either the practitioner will use external version to try to turn the fetus to a cephalic presentation, or she will deliver by cesarean. If the fetus remains in a transverse lie, he cannot deliver vaginally.

Nursing Care

Carefully assess fetal lie, presentation, and position when the woman presents to the labor and delivery area. During the active phase, assess the contraction pattern every 30 minutes. Check for uterine contractions of adequate frequency and intensity. Assess fetal response to uterine contractions. Perform a thorough pain assessment every hour to include a pain scale to rate intensity. Ask the woman to describe her pain. Inquire regarding the presence of intense back pain.

Plot cervical changes and fetal descent on a labor graph. Observe for slow progression or arrest of labor. Identify slow progression if a primipara in active labor dilates more slowly than 1.2 centimeters/hour or the fetal head descends at less than 1 centimeter/hour; or if a multipara in active labor dilates more slowly than 1.5 centimeters/hour or the fetal head descends at less than 1.5 centimeters/hour over a period of several hours. Identify arrest of dilation if no cervical change occurs during a period of 2 hours, and arrest of descent if no descent occurs during a 2-hour period.

If a disorder of dilation or descent is noted, the physician must be notified. However, there are several assessments that must first be made. Check to see if the woman has a full bladder. Remember that a full bladder can interfere with the progress of labor. Next, determine if the contraction pattern is adequate. Contractions should occur every 2 to 3 minutes apart, last 60 to 90 seconds, and be of moderate to strong intensity during the active phase of labor.

If the bladder is empty and the contraction pattern is adequate, try to determine if the fetus is in an occiput posterior position. Inquire regarding the character of the woman's pain. Suspect occiput posterior position if the woman complains of severe lower back pain. Remember, counterpressure applied to the lower back with a fisted hand sometimes helps the woman to cope with the "back labor" that is characteristic of occiput posterior positioning.

Determine if the woman might benefit from pain relief measures. Intravenous sedation or epidural anesthesia might be helpful. If the woman is "fighting" the contractions, pain control might help her relax and allow the cervix to dilate.

Call a full report of your labor assessments to the physician. Carefully note any orders for sedation, anesthesia, or oxytocin augmentation. After carrying out the ordered interventions, continue to evaluate for adequate labor progress. Notify the physician if interventions do not result in progression of labor or if signs of fetal distress occur.

Test Yourself

- Name four complications that are associated with labor dystocia.
- What is the usual medical treatment for uterine hypofunction?
- List three nursing assessments that must be made before notifying the physician of a disorder of dilation or descent?

PREMATURE RUPTURE OF MEMBRANES

Premature rupture of membranes (PROM) refers to spontaneous rupture of the amniotic sac before the onset of labor. PROM occurs in approximately 10% of pregnancies at term (Wilkes & Galan, 2002b). This condition is to be differentiated from preterm labor, which is the onset of labor before the end of 37 weeks' gestation, and preterm PROM, which refers to rupture of the amniotic sac before the onset of labor in a woman who is less than 37 weeks' gestation. Complications associated with PROM include abruptio placentae, umbilical cord compression or prolapse, and infection.

Preterm PROM is the leading known cause of preterm delivery and occurs in approximately 2% of all pregnancies. Risk factors for preterm PROM include cigarette smoking, previous preterm delivery, vaginal bleeding, low socioeconomic conditions, sexually transmitted infections, and unknown causes. The farther along in the pregnancy that PROM occurs, the better the chance for a healthy outcome. Most women with preterm PROM deliver within 1 week after the amniotic sac ruptures. PROM before the age of viability rarely results in a good outcome.

Clinical Manifestations and Diagnosis

The woman with PROM usually presents to the delivery suite with reports of a large gush or continuous, uncontrollable leaking of fluid from the vagina. She may report vaginal discharge or bleeding and pelvic pressure. However, she does not present with regular uterine contractions because she is not in labor.

Sometimes the diagnosis is obvious when large amounts of amniotic fluid are visible. A definitive diagnosis of PROM is made by speculum examination. The practitioner looks for pooling of amniotic fluid and then tests the fluid with Nitrazine paper, which turns blue in the presence of amniotic fluid. If the Nitrazine test is equivocal (uncertain), the practitioner may elect to perform a fern test. For this test, the practitioner collects a specimen of fluid from the vagina on a sterile cotton swab and then smears the specimen on a slide. When the specimen is viewed under the microscope, a ferning pattern indicates that amniotic fluid is present.

Treatment

The major problem for the woman with PROM at term is the increased risk for infection, specifically **chorioamnionitis**, bacterial or viral infection of the amniotic fluid and membranes. With each hour that passes after PROM that delivery has not occurred, the risk for infection increases. Fortunately, most women go into spontaneous labor within 24 hours of PROM. However, many practitioners prefer to induce labor with oxytocin rather than wait for nature to take its course. Both treatment options, expectant management (wait and see) and induction of labor, should be carried out in the hospital. Research has shown that the neonate born to the woman who stays at home with PROM and waits for labor to ensue before presenting to the hospital or birthing clinic for care has a much higher risk of being admitted to the neonatal intensive care unit (NICU) with neonatal sepsis (Wilkes & Galan, 2002b).

Management of preterm PROM is more complicated. If there are signs of infection, such as elevated maternal temperature; maternal tachycardia; cloudy, foul-smelling amniotic fluid; and uterine tenderness, cultures are obtained, antibiotics started, and delivery facilitated, regardless of gestational age. However, if there is no infection, expectant management may be chosen. The goal is to allow the fetus time to mature and achieve delivery before the woman or her fetus becomes infected.

The usual practice is to administer 7 days of antibiotic therapy. The practitioner often orders a course of IV antibiotics (usually ampicillin and erythromycin) for 48 hours, followed by oral antibiotics for 5 days. Antibiotic therapy for longer than 7 days is not recommended because of the risk that resistant strains of bacteria might emerge.

The woman may be put on strict bed rest or bed rest with bathroom privileges. **Pelvic rest**, a situation in which nothing is placed in the vagina (including tampons and the practitioner's fingers to perform a cervical examination), is instituted because the risk for infection increases whenever the cervix is manipulated. The practitioner may elect to perform periodic sterile speculum examinations to check for cervical changes. A digital examination is not necessary unless signs of labor, such as pelvic pressure, cramping, regular contractions, or bloody show, are present.

Fetal surveillance is performed at least daily. Generally, the woman is instructed to perform kick counts after every meal. Daily nonstress tests (NSTs) may also be ordered. If the woman is less than 32 weeks' gestation, intramuscular injections of a corticosteroid (e.g., Betamethasone and Dexamethasone) are given to hasten fetal lung maturity. Some practitioners administer a tocolytic to prolong the pregnancy long enough for the steroid injections to work. Tocolytics are not administered in the presence of infection.

Nursing Care

Assess the woman who presents with reports of PROM. Ask the woman to describe the sequence of events that occurred in association with the rupture of the amniotic sac. Check for visible signs of PROM—pooling of fluid and positive Nitrazine or fern test.

Here's a tip for you. Always give a thorough report! The length of time the membranes were ruptured before delivery is an important part of the report to the pediatrician and to the nurse assuming care of the infant. This information will alert them to monitor the newborn closely for signs of sepsis in the event of prolonged rupture of membranes.

Once the diagnosis has been established, follow the practitioner's orders for management of PROM. If the woman is at term, expect continuous fetal heart rate monitoring. Watch for the sudden onset of deep variable decelerations, which may indicate umbilical cord prolapse. Take the temperature at least every 2 hours. Promptly report temperature elevation, prolonged maternal or fetal tachycardia, and cloudy or foul-smelling amniotic fluid. Watch for the natural onset of labor, or administer oxytocin induction, if ordered.

PRETERM LABOR

Preterm labor is labor that occurs after 19 weeks' and before the end of 37 weeks' gestation. Preterm labor often leads to preterm birth, which accounts for 70% of neonatal morbidity and mortality. Despite years of research, the incidence of preterm birth has actually increased from approximately 8% to 9% in the 1980s to 11.9% in 2001 (Bernhardt & Dorman, 2004). The current rate is much higher than the Healthy People 2010 goal of 7.6% (Church-Balin & Damus, 2003). It is widely accepted that the development of effective treatments for preterm labor would greatly reduce the health care burden of sick neonates.

Often the cause of preterm labor is not readily apparent. In fact, there is no associated risk factor in one-half of woman presenting with preterm labor (Moos, 2004). The top three risk factors associated with preterm labor are current multiple gestation pregnancy (twins, triplets, or more), history of previous preterm birth, and uterine or cervical abnormalities. Although history of previous preterm labor is one of the better predictors, this association is not helpful for predicting preterm labor for the primigravida. Other risk factors are listed in Box 18-1.

Clinical Manifestations and Diagnosis

It is not always easy to diagnose preterm labor. The presence of painful uterine contractions does not by itself indicate that the woman is in preterm labor because pain is a subjective phenomenon that can be affected by many variables. The definitive diagnosis is made when uterine contractions result in cervical change. The earlier the diagnosis is made, the greater the likelihood that treatment will be effective. If the diagnosis is made after the woman has progressed to greater than 3 centimeters, it is unlikely that preterm birth will be avoided.

The woman in preterm labor often presents with signs that include uterine contractions, which may be painless; pelvic pressure; menstrual-like cramps; vaginal pain; and low, dull backache accompanied by vaginal discharge and bleeding. The membranes may or may not be ruptured. The most frequent examinations used to diagnose preterm labor include assessment of contraction frequency, fetal fibronectin test (Box 18-2), and measurement of cervical length. No change in cervical length in the presence of a negative fetal fibronectin test indicates that the woman has less than 10% chance of delivering prematurely.

BOX 18.1 Risk Factors for Preterm Labor and Birth

Obstetric and Gynecologic Risk Factors
- Multiple gestation (twins, triplets)
- History of preterm birth
- Uterine or cervical abnormalities
  - Fibroid tumors
  - Bicornuate uterus
  - Incompetent cervix
- Preterm premature rupture of membranes
- Placenta previa
- Retained intrauterine device
- Short time period (less than 6 to 9 months) between pregnancies

Demographic and Lifestyle Risk Factors
- Extremes of maternal age (<17 years of age or >35 years of age)
- Member of an ethnic minority
- Low socioeconomic status
- Late or no prenatal care
- Smoking
- Alcohol use
- Illicit drug use
- Intimate partner violence
- Lack of social support
- High levels of stress
- Long working hours with long periods of standing

Medical Risk Factors
- Infection
  - Chorioamnionitis
  - Bacterial vaginosis
  - Bacteriuria
  - Acute pyelonephritis
  - Sexually transmitted infections
- High blood pressure
- Diabetes
- Clotting disorders
- Entering the pregnancy underweight
- Obesity

Fetal-Related Risk Factors
- Fetal demise
- Intrauterine growth restriction (IUGR)
- Congenital anomalies

Treatment

Standard obstetric care includes evaluation of risk factors for preterm delivery as early as the first office visit. If risk factors are identified, the cervix is examined for evidence of injury. A workup is done to detect asymptomatic bacteriuria, sexually transmitted infections, and bacterial vaginosis. These infections are treated, if present. At 20 and 26 weeks' gestation a transvaginal ultrasound may be done to measure the length of the cervix. A cervical length of less than 2.5 centimeters is considered abnormal. Education is given regarding the

BOX 18.2 Fetal Fibronectin Test

Fetal fibronectin is a protein that serves as an adhesive between the amniotic sac and the uterine lining. This protein is normally found in cervical secretions up to approximately 22 weeks' gestation, after which it is normally absent. The test is performed during a speculum examination of the cervix. A cotton swab is used to collect a sample of cervical secretions, which is sent to a laboratory for analysis. It takes anywhere from 6 to 36 hours to get the results of the test.

The presence of fetal fibronectin in cervical secretions (a positive test) in association with signs of preterm labor may indicate that the adhesive is coming apart too early and that preterm birth is imminent. The absence of fetal fibronectin (a negative test) is a more reliable indicator than is a positive test. A negative test indicates that the woman will not likely deliver for at least 2 weeks.

signs and symptoms of preterm labor. Weekly telephone contact with a nurse and regular prenatal visits are encouraged.

Once active preterm labor is diagnosed, the practitioner must determine how best to treat it. Often bed rest and hydration with either oral or IV fluids is enough to stop uterine irritability and prolong the pregnancy. The decision must be made as to whether or not tocolytics (Table 18-2) should be used. A fetus less than 23 weeks' gestation has almost no chance of surviving outside of the womb, so tocolytics generally are not used below this gestational age. Likewise, tocolytics are not often prescribed after 34 weeks' gestation because neonatal morbidity and mortality are very low at this point in the pregnancy. Tocolytics are administered most frequently between 24 and 33 weeks' gestation. Although the medication may not prevent preterm birth, it often allows the practitioner to buy enough time to allow corticosteroid injections to help mature the fetal lungs or to allow transfer to a facility with a higher level of neonatal intensive care.

TABLE 18.2 Tocolytic Agents

Medication	Route of Administration	Maternal Side Effects	Fetal/Neonatal Side Effects
Magnesium sulfate	IV	*At therapeutic levels*: Pulmonary edema *At toxic levels*: Respiratory depression, tetany, paralysis, profound hypotension, cardiac arrest	*At therapeutic levels*: Nonreactive nonstress test; decreased to no fetal breathing movements
Ritodrine (Yutopar)	IV	Hypokalemia, hyperglycemia, tachycardia, hypotension, palpitations, anxiety, shortness of breath, headache, nausea or vomiting, pulmonary edema, cardiac ischemia, cardiac insufficiency, maternal death	Tachycardia, elevated serum glucose
Terbutaline (Bricanyl)	Subcutaneously	Same as ritodrine	Same as ritodrine
Indomethacin	*Loading dose*: Rectal suppository *Maintenance dose*: Orally	Renal failure, hepatitis, gastrointestinal bleeding	Premature closure of the ductus arteriosus, oligohydramnios, neonatal necrotizing enterocolitis, intraventricular hemorrhage
Nifedipine (Procardia)	Sublingually	Transient hypotension	Unknown

● Nursing Process for the Woman With Preterm Labor

ASSESSMENT

Collect a thorough history, including previous preterm births, multiple gestation pregnancies, infections, cigarette smoking, and other risk factors for preterm labor (see Box 18-1). Inquire if the woman is experiencing symptoms of preterm labor, such as uterine contractions; uncontrollable leaking of fluid from the vagina; backache; menstrual-like cramps; or vaginal pain, discharge, or bleeding.

The physical assessment includes Nitrazine testing. If the Nitrazine test results are uncertain, prepare to assist the RN or practitioner to perform a speculum exam to check for pooling of fluid and to obtain a fern test. Place the woman on the fetal monitor. Observe for uterine irritability or contractions. Palpate the uterus carefully. A hard, board-like uterine rigidity and pain that does not relent may indicate placental abruption.

Assess the woman's emotional response. The threat of preterm labor may cause apprehension, fear, and anxiety. The woman and her partner may be concerned for the well-being of the fetus. Once the diagnosis is established, the woman may be concerned about the side effects of tocolytic therapy.

SELECTED NURSING DIAGNOSES

- Risk for Imbalanced Fluid Volume related to dehydration, infusion of high volumes of IV fluid, and/or side effects of tocolytic therapy
- Risk for Injury related to side effects of tocolytic therapy
- Acute Pain related to labor contractions
- Anxiety related to threat of harm to or death of self and fetus

PLANNING AND GOALS

Maintaining the safety of the pregnant woman and her fetus is the primary goal when planning care. Appropriate goals may include that the woman will maintain a balanced fluid volume with clear lung fields; she will not experience injury from tocolytic therapy; she will report a tolerable pain level; and she will report a reduction in anxiety. Additional goals and interventions are planned according to the individual needs and situation of the woman.

IMPLEMENTATION

Maintaining a Balanced Fluid Volume

Monitoring fluid status is an important nursing function for the woman in preterm labor. Sometimes hydration with IV fluids is all that is needed to stop the premature contractions. Monitor the IV site and the rate of infusion. Administer a fluid bolus of 500 to 1,000 mL as ordered and then reduce to the ordered maintenance rate.

Monitor vital signs. A normal blood pressure in conjunction with a rising pulse upon moving from a recumbent to a sitting or standing position is associated with low fluid volume. Hypotension is associated with severe dehydration. Monitor urinary output. Record urine characteristics. Concentrated urine with a high specific gravity may indicate dehydration.

Watch for signs of fluid overload. Normally a healthy pregnant woman can withstand high fluid volumes; however, if she is receiving tocolytics, watch closely for signs of developing pulmonary edema, such as dyspnea, tachycardia, productive cough, and adventitious breath sounds.

Preventing Injury

If the woman is receiving magnesium sulfate therapy to stop preterm labor, assess her at least once per hour. Report dyspnea, tachycardia, productive cough, or adventitious breath sounds to the RN or primary care provider. Monitor respiratory rate. Report bradypnea or periods of apnea. Check the deep tendon reflexes at least hourly. Report decreased or absent reflexes immediately. Refer to Chapter 17 for other nursing actions necessary for magnesium infusion.

If the woman is receiving a $Beta_2$-adrenergic receptor agonist, such as ritodrine or terbutaline, monitor serum potassium and glucose levels, as ordered. Report low potassium or elevated glucose to the RN or primary care provider. Monitor for and report any significant changes in the vital signs, in particular tachycardia or hypotension. The primary care provider usually leaves orders detailing the pulse and blood pressure levels that should be reported. Assess for shortness of breath, anxiety, and palpitations. Immediately report any complaints of chest pain. Monitor for signs of pulmonary edema.

Managing Pain

Assess the woman's pain using a pain scale at the frequency ordered by the RN. Ask the woman at what level the pain is tolerable. Be sure to assess and record location, characteristics, and intensity. Administer pain medication as ordered by the primary care provider. Keep in mind that a sudden increase in pain intensity or pain that does not relent may be the sign of a developing complication. Report any changes in the character or intensity of pain.

Reducing Anxiety
Encourage the woman and her partner to verbalize their fears and concerns. Answer questions honestly and to the best of your ability. If you do not know the answer, say so, and explain that you will find the answer as soon as possible. Make certain that the woman and her partner know the treatment plan. Explain procedures before performing them. Allow the woman to ventilate regarding her feelings. Explore with the RN coping strategies that the woman is using. Assist the woman to use positive coping strategies whenever possible. If she is alone without a support system, ask for a social services or pastoral care consult.

EVALUATION: GOALS AND EXPECTED OUTCOMES

- **Goal:** Fluid volume balance is maintained.
  Expected Outcomes:
  - Skin and mucous membranes remain hydrated.
  - Lung fields remain clear to auscultation.
  - Hematocrit, serum electrolytes, and urine specific gravity remain within normal limits.
- **Goal:** The woman remains injury free.
  Expected Outcomes:
  - The woman reports onset of respiratory distress immediately, such as
    - Dyspnea.
    - Productive cough.
  - The woman reports cardiac signs immediately, such as
    - Chest pain.
    - Heart palpitations.
    - Racing pulse
- **Goal:** The woman expresses the ability to cope with her pain.
  Expected Outcomes:
  - Reports reduced pain (measured on a pain scale) after interventions.
  - Reports she is able to get sufficient sleep and rest despite the pain.
- **Goal:** The woman verbalizes that she is coping with her anxiety.
  Expected Outcomes:
  - Available social supports are used.
  - Effective coping strategies are used.
  - Decreased levels of anxiety are reported.

Test Yourself

- What is the difference between PROM and preterm PROM?
- Describe four nursing interventions appropriate for the woman with PROM.
- Name three treatment options for the woman in preterm labor.

POST-TERM PREGNANCY AND LABOR

A post-term pregnancy is one that lasts longer than 2 weeks after the due date (i.e., 42 weeks). The incidence of post-term pregnancy is 3% to 12% (Wilkes & Galan, 2002a). Some pregnancies are erroneously diagnosed as post-term because of miscalculation of gestational age. Certainty of pregnancy dating is diminished when the woman seeks late prenatal care and is unsure of her last menstrual period. This is true because early sonograms are the most accurate at determining gestational age.

A post-term pregnancy is at risk for increased perinatal mortality, particularly during labor. The post-term pregnancy is more likely to be complicated by oligohydramnios and meconium staining of the amniotic fluid. Oligohydramnios increases the incidence of cord compression, with subsequent development of fetal distress during labor. Thick meconium-stained fluid increases the risk for meconium aspiration syndrome (discussed in Chapter 20). The risk for birth of an unusually large infant increases as the gestation advances. The woman in labor with a large infant is at higher risk for shoulder dystocia. A post-term pregnancy that is also complicated by intrauterine fetal growth restriction (IUGR) is particularly at risk for perinatal mortality. The theory that a post-term pregnancy is at risk for decreased placental functioning has not been verified by clinical studies (Cunningham et al., 2001a).

Clinical Manifestations and Diagnosis

The woman presents with an intrauterine pregnancy that has been determined to be at or past 42 completed weeks. Usually the primary care provider will attempt to use several methods to determine fetal age, such as when the fetal heart rate could first be heard by Doppler and by fetoscope, early ultrasound measurements, and recorded fundal height measurements. Amniotic fluid volume may be decreased, as measured by ultrasound. Fetal macrosomia may be suspected.

When an amniotomy is done, meconium staining frequently is noted.

Treatment

There are two basic treatment plans for the woman who is carrying a post-term pregnancy. One is called expectant management. This treatment protocol involves frequent testing for fetal well-being (Searing, 2001). The woman is instructed to report decreased fetal movement immediately. NSTs are performed at least twice weekly. Ultrasound to measure amniotic fluid volume and biophysical profiles (BPPs) are frequently performed. The second strategy for managing a post-term pregnancy is induction of labor at 42 weeks' gestation. (Chapter 11 discusses labor induction.) Clinical research has shown that similar outcomes occur using either strategy.

Nursing Care

Teach the woman who is post-term to monitor fetal movements daily. (Refer to Chapter 7 for description of fetal kick counts.) Explain the importance of reporting decreased fetal movement to her primary care provider immediately. She may be anxious regarding the well-being of her fetus. Provide realistic reassurances. Be certain that the primary care provider has answered all her questions and concerns adequately. If you identify a knowledge deficit, instruct her appropriately or refer her to the RN or primary care provider for clarification.

During labor, observe the fetal monitor strip closely for signs of fetal distress. Report these immediately to the RN in charge. Carefully note and record the color and amount of amniotic fluid that is released when the water bag breaks. No fluid is worrisome because it may indicate oligohydramnios with thick meconium staining. If you assisted with the amniotomy, be sure to inform the RN of this finding.

INTRAUTERINE FETAL DEATH

Fetal death is defined as death of the fetus in utero (lack of cardiac activity) at 20 weeks' or greater gestation or a weight of 500 grams or more. This definition distinguishes fetal death from early pregnancy loss, such as occurs with spontaneous abortion.

Causes of fetal death can be categorized into four general types: fetal, placental, maternal, and unknown. Approximately 25% to 40% of fetal deaths can be attributed to fetal causes, 25% to 35% placental causes, 25% to 35% unknown causes, and 5% to 10% maternal causes (Cunningham et al., 2001c). Examples of fetal causes include genetic or congenital abnormalities and infection. The most common cause of fetal demise is placental abruption. This is usually categorized under placental causes; however, preeclampsia and other disorders can increase the risk for placental abruption. Cord accidents (such as prolapse or true knot), premature rupture of the membranes, and twin-to-twin transfusion syndrome are other placental causes. Maternal causes include advanced maternal age; medical disorders, such as diabetes mellitus and hypertension; and pregnancy-related complications, such as preeclampsia-eclampsia, Rh disease, uterine rupture, and infection.

Clinical Manifestations and Diagnosis

It is when the woman no longer detects fetal movement that she often presents for treatment. Inability to find the fetal heart rate leads the primary care provider to suspect fetal death. Confirmation of death is made by sonogram. The fetal heart is visualized. Lack of cardiac activity is diagnostic.

Treatment

In the past, the woman was advised to wait until labor spontaneously ensued; however, the longer a woman carries a dead fetus, the greater her risk for developing disseminated intravascular coagulopathy (DIC). Currently the recommendation is to induce labor within the next few days.

Induction is carried out as described in Chapter 11 for fetal demise at or near term. When the gestational age is less than 28 weeks, the cervix is rarely favorable for induction. In these cases, the woman may be induced with prostaglandin E_2 vaginal suppositories or oral or intravaginal misoprostol.

Nursing Care

Physical care of the woman is carried out as for other women having labor induced. Careful attention to the history is warranted because the woman with a uterine scar from previous surgery is at risk for rupture. For the woman at term, the tocodynamometer is used to monitor uterine contractions during labor. Postpartum care is the same as for other women.

Emotional care of the woman is more complex. She may experience shock, denial, anger, and depression. Remember that grief responses vary from individual to individual. Allow the woman and her family space to comfort one another, but do not avoid her. Offer to call a pastor or other spiritual leader she may desire. Be sure to determine if the woman wishes any religious sacraments or rituals to be done. Most institutions provide postpartum care in a unit or room away from the nursery.

Don't forget the golden rule!
A woman who has just received a diagnosis of fetal demise is experiencing a terrific loss. Be available to her without intruding. Answer her questions honestly. Encourage her to hold and name her baby, if she is able.

Be sure that mementos are collected. Take pictures as dictated by institutional policy. Pictures are usually taken even if the woman refuses them. The pictures are kept on file for a year or more. The woman is told that she can change her mind and come get the pictures at any time. Collect a lock of hair, footprints, and other reminders of the baby. Refer to Chapter 19 for further discussion of how to care for the grieving woman.

Test Yourself

- Name five complications for which the post-term pregnancy is at risk.
- What condition is the woman at greater risk of developing if a fetal demise is not delivered within a few days of fetal death?
- Describe at least three ways the nurse can provide support for the woman with a fetal demise?

EMERGENCIES ASSOCIATED WITH LABOR AND BIRTH

Amniotic Fluid Embolism

Amniotic fluid embolism is a rare obstetric emergency that frequently results in death or severe neurologic impairment of the woman and her fetus. Recently a new name has been proposed for the disorder: anaphylactoid syndrome of pregnancy. The proposed new name resulted from research that indicates that amniotic fluid embolism more resembles anaphylaxis and septic shock than it does pulmonary embolism.

Amniotic fluid embolism occurs in 1 in 20,000 to 1 in 80,000 pregnancies. Maternal mortality ranges from 26% to 61%; however, very few (approximately 15%) survive without neurologic damage (De Jong & Fausett, 2003). Amniotic fluid embolism is often divided into two major phases: respiratory distress, followed by hemodynamic instability, which includes pulmonary edema and hemorrhage. The woman may become comatose, and if she survives, may remain in a vegetative state.

Clinical Manifestations and Diagnosis

In most cases, symptoms of amniotic fluid embolism occur suddenly during or immediately after labor. The woman usually develops symptoms of acute respiratory distress, cyanosis, and hypotension. If she is in labor, the fetus typically demonstrates signs of fetal distress, with bradycardia occurring in most cases.

Diagnosis is made based on the clinical symptoms and laboratory studies. Arterial blood gases (ABGs) demonstrate acidosis and hypoxemia. Bleeding times are usually prolonged. Evidence of pulmonary edema may be seen on a chest x-ray (Moore & Ware, 2002).

Treatment

Because amniotic fluid embolism is still poorly understood, varied clinical approaches have been tried in an effort to increase survival rates. Unfortunately, there is currently no curative therapy; therefore, treatment is aimed at supporting vital functions. An immediate response to the woman's initial complaint of respiratory distress is necessary to increase the woman's chances of survival. The woman often progresses quickly to full cardiopulmonary arrest and requires advanced cardiac life support, including mechanical intubation and ventilation. Delivery of the infant by cesarean within 5 minutes after the start of cardiopulmonary resuscitation (CPR) is recommended (Curran, 2003). Typically, disseminated intravascular coagulopathy is treated with massive fluid resuscitation and blood product replacement therapy. Once the woman is in stable condition, she requires care in an adult intensive care unit (ICU).

Nursing Care

Respond promptly and summon for immediate assistance if a laboring or postpartum woman reports dyspnea. Administer oxygen via face mask. Measure the vital signs, particularly the blood pressure and pulse. Hypotension, tachycardia, and other signs of shock are usually evident. Initiate CPR, if needed, and be prepared to assist with a cesarean delivery at the bedside, if needed. Be prepared to assist the RN during fluid resuscitation and blood product administration. Anticipate transfer to the ICU as soon as the woman is stable enough to transfer.

Shoulder Dystocia

Shoulder dystocia is an obstetric emergency that is dreaded by all obstetric practitioners. The fetal head delivers, but the shoulders become stuck in the bony pelvis, preventing delivery of the body. Unless the condition is remedied within a few minutes, the fetus can suffer permanent brain damage because his chest cannot expand, and he cannot take his first breath. Although macrosomia (fetal weight greater than 4,000 grams) and

A PERSONAL GLIMPSE

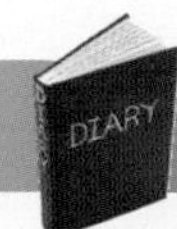

My wife, Sally, had just delivered our daughter. We had waited to have a child until we were in our 30s, and then it had taken us 2 years to get pregnant. I was so awed by the whole birth experience. I was taking pictures of my daughter when I heard Sally say to the nurse, "I can't breathe!" I looked over and saw that she was very pale, almost gray. In the blink of an eye she stopped breathing and one of the nurses started helping her breathe. The other nurse took the baby and me to the nursery. The nursery nurse was very kind. She let me stay with the baby as long as I wanted; however, I couldn't concentrate on the baby because I was so worried about my wife. I went to the waiting room and I was pacing up and down. After what seemed like an eternity the doctor came to talk to me. He said that he thought Sally had an embolism. He told me that she had a breathing tube and was connected to a machine that was helping her breathe. The nurse came out and took me to the ICU. I felt so frightened by all the tubes and machines that were connected to my wife. I felt very helpless. I also felt guilty for putting my wife through this. I didn't know if I could forgive myself if she didn't make it. Slowly, over the next week Sally started to get better. I have never felt more thankful in my life than on the day I was able to take Sally home. She was very weak, but she was alive. It was such a joy to see her finally able to hold our little Jessica.

Bill

LEARNING OPPORTUNITY: What could the nurses in this situation have done to help the husband cope with his wife's severe illness? What interventions could the nurse use to help promote attachment between the newborn and the woman when the woman who has been critically ill begins to get better?

maternal diabetes are the two risk factors known to be associated with shoulder dystocia, many cases occur in fetuses of normal weight. Therefore, this complication should be anticipated at every delivery.

Shoulder dystocia puts the woman and the fetus at risk. Even if correct maneuvers are used, injury can still result. The woman is at increased risk for uterine rupture and/or bladder rupture. The fetus is at increased risk for brachial plexus injuries and fractures of the humerus and clavicle (Rose, 1998).

Clinical Manifestations and Diagnosis

The "turtle sign" is the classic sign that alerts the practitioner to the probability of shoulder dystocia. The fetal head delivers, but then retracts similar to a turtle. The practitioner tries gentle downward pressure on the fetal head in an attempt to deliver the anterior shoulder, but is unable to do so using normal maneuvers.

Treatment

There are several maneuvers the practitioner can attempt to relieve shoulder dystocia. Two of them require the direct assistance of the nurse (Fig. 18-1).

- McRoberts maneuver (see Fig. 18-1*A*) is often tried first and is frequently successful. Two nurses are needed to assist with this maneuver. With the woman in lithotomy position, each nurse holds one leg and sharply flexes the leg toward the woman's shoulders. This opens the pelvis to its widest diameters and allows the anterior shoulder to deliver in almost half of the cases.
- In addition to McRoberts maneuver, one nurse can use a fist to apply suprapubic pressure (see Fig. 18-1*B*). This will sometimes dislodge the impacted shoulder.

The birth attendant can try other maneuvers, such as placing a hand in the vagina and attempting to push one of the shoulders in a clockwise or counterclockwise motion. The birth attendant may intentionally fracture a clavicle in an attempt to dislodge the fetus. In some cases the birth attendant has placed the head back in the birth canal and done an emergency cesarean delivery. This maneuver, called Zavanelli maneuver, has been successful, but is associated with increased risk of trauma.

Nursing Care

Assist the birth attendant with maneuvers, as described above. Be prepared to go for a stat cesarean delivery if the body cannot be delivered. If maneuvers are successful and a vaginal delivery is accomplished, perform a careful assessment of the newborn. Check for crepitus in the area of the clavicle, which might indicate the bone is broken. Check for spontaneous movements of both arms. Sometimes the newborn will move only one arm, which may indicate Erb's palsy. This injury is characterized by (usually temporary) nerve damage and inability to move the arm. When edema subsides, full function normally returns, although injury can persist.

This is important! Don't EVER apply pressure to the fundus (fundal pressure). This action has been linked to increased incidence of birth trauma. The shoulder can actually become more impacted, and the woman has an increased chance of uterine or bladder rupture when this maneuver is used in instances of shoulder dystocia.

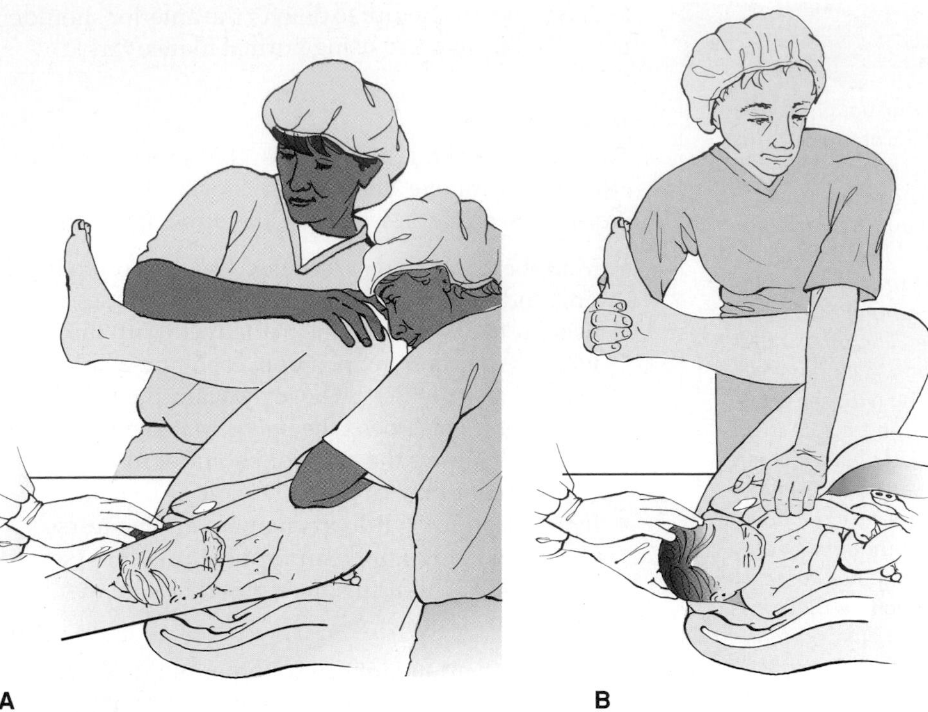

● ***Figure 18.1*** Techniques to relieve shoulder dystocia. (**A**) McRoberts maneuver. Two nurses (or the nurse and the woman's coach) each take one of the woman's legs and sharply flex them onto the woman's abdomen. This position maximally opens the pelvis, which sometimes dislodges the impacted shoulder. (**B**) Suprapubic pressure. The nurse puts pressure just above the pubic bone. Sometimes this maneuver in conjunction with McRoberts maneuver is successful in dislodging the impacted shoulder.

Umbilical Cord Prolapse

Umbilical cord prolapse occurs when the umbilical cord slips down in front of the presenting part. It occurs rarely in vertex presentations. Factors that increase the risk include fetal malpresentation, multiple gestation, intrauterine fetal growth restriction, prematurity, and rupture of the membranes with the fetus at a high station (Curran, 2003).

Clinical Manifestations and Diagnosis

Prolapse of the umbilical cord can occur at any time. Infrequently the condition may be detected before the membranes rupture. The woman may report feeling "something coming out" when the membranes rupture. Sometimes she presents with a cord prolapse. The cord may be visible at the introitus, or it may be palpable in the vaginal vault. An occult prolapse results in cord compression, but the cord is not easily palpable. Frequently a prolapse is detected immediately after spontaneous or artificial rupture of the membranes. The fetal heart rate usually drops precipitously. Vaginal examination typically confirms the diagnosis.

Treatment

When the cord is compressed against the bony pelvis, it can compromise fetal circulation and result in fetal death unless interventions are carried out quickly. The examiner who discovers the condition should push upward on the presenting part with the fingers to move the fetus away from the cord. Immediate cesarean delivery should be accomplished to save the fetus' life.

Nursing Care

Always check fetal heart tones after spontaneous or artificial rupture of the membranes. If the fetal heart rate drops, perform a vaginal examination (or call the RN to do one), and palpate for the umbilical cord. If the woman presents with a visible prolapse, quickly place her in bed and gently palpate the cord for pulsations to verify fetal viability. Then use your fingers to press upward on the presenting part. Continue to hold the presenting part off of the cord until the infant is delivered by cesarean delivery. (You will be transported with the woman to the operating room. The sterile drapes will be placed over you.) If you discover the condition and are unable to call for help, place the patient in knee–chest position, call for help, and then continue to intervene as previously described (Curran, 2003). If another nurse is holding the presenting part off of the cord, move quickly to prepare the woman for emergency cesarean delivery.

Uterine Rupture

Uterine rupture occurs when the uterus tears open, leaving the fetus and other uterine contents exposed to the peritoneal cavity. Rarely is this a spontaneous occurrence. It is usually associated with a uterine scar

TABLE 18.3 Placental Abnormalities

Condition	Description	Risk Factors	Maternal and Fetal Implications
Placenta accreta	Abnormal adherence of the placenta to the uterine wall. Variations of penetration occur, including • Placenta increta—the placenta invades the uterine muscle. • Placenta percreta—the placenta penetrates through the uterine muscle, sometimes invading the bladder and other pelvic structures.	History of previous uterine surgery; such as • Cesarean delivery (risk increases with each subsequent C section) • Myomectomy • Dilation and curettage • Induced abortion Other risk factors include • Age older than 35 • Placenta previa	*Maternal implications*: Interferes with normal placental separation in the 3rd stage of labor, resulting in hemorrhage, which may require hysterectomy to control. May also cause uterine rupture during pregnancy or labor. *Fetal implications*: Fetal death may occur if the condition results in uterine rupture.
Velamentous insertion of the umbilical cord	The umbilical cord is attached to the side (versus the center) of the placenta, and the fetal vessels separate in the membranes before reaching the placenta. Vasa previa is a variation in which the fetal vessels are in the part of the membrane that is in front of the presenting part.	Low-lying placenta, antepartum hemorrhage, in vitro fertilization (IVF) pregnancy	*Fetal implications*: Exsanguination (the fetus may bleed out) resulting in fetal death may occur when the membranes rupture.
Succenturiate placenta	An "accessory" placenta that develops at a distance from the main placenta. Vasa previa can occur in this situation when the fetal vessels traverse the membranes between the two placentas.	Same as for velamentous placenta	*Maternal implications*: May result in hemorrhage when the accessory placenta is retained. Hemorrhage may require blood transfusions and/or hysterectomy to control. *Fetal implications*: The same as for vasa previa.
Nuchal cord	The umbilical cord is wrapped once (or more) around the fetus' neck.	This condition occurs frequently in normal pregnancies with no identifiable risk factors.	*Fetal implications*: Moderate-to-deep variable decelerations may occur during labor. Rarely, a tight nuchal cord can lead to fetal death.
True knot	A true knot occurs when the umbilical cord is tied in a knot.	This condition can occur in an active fetus with a long cord.	*Fetal implications*: A true knot sometimes results in fetal death.

from previous uterine surgery. Often the scar results from a prior cesarean delivery; however, any surgery that requires an incision into the uterus can place the woman at risk for uterine rupture. Traumatic rupture can occur in connection with blunt trauma, such as occurs in an automobile collision or intimate partner violence. Incidence of uterine rupture is 0.1% to 1.5% when the previous incision type was a low cervical transverse incision, and 4% to 9% when the incision type is classical or T-shaped (Curran, 2003).

Clinical Manifestations and Diagnosis

Abrupt change in the fetal heart rate pattern is often the most significant sign associated with uterine rupture (Dauphinee, 2004). Another sign is pain in the abdomen, shoulder, or back that is not masked by epidural anesthesia. Sometimes the woman will begin to report intense pain when the epidural has been giving relief until that point. Falling blood pressure and rising pulse may be associated with hypovolemia caused by occult bleeding. A vaginal examination may demonstrate a higher fetal station than was present previously. There may or may not be changes in the contraction pattern.

Treatment

As soon as uterine rupture is recognized, the treatment is immediate cesarean delivery. This action is necessary to save the woman's life and, it is hoped, that of the fetus, as well, although uterine rupture is associated with a high incidence of fetal death. This is true because the fetus can withstand only approximately 20 minutes in utero after uterine rupture. This time period can be even shorter if the cord prolapses through the tear in the uterine wall and becomes compressed.

Nursing Care

Recognizing the signs of uterine rupture is critical for the obstetric nurse because the complication requires quick recognition and action to avoid fetal and maternal death. In cases of trial-of-labor-after-cesarean (TOLAC), the RN should monitor the woman during labor, particularly if oxytocin is used to induce or augment the labor. If signs of rupture occur, the woman is immediately prepared for cesarean delivery, and other interventions are instituted to treat hypovolemic shock.

Placental and Umbilical Cord Abnormalities

Although technically abnormalities of the placenta and umbilical cord are not obstetric emergencies, they can lead to emergency situations and can have dire outcomes for the woman and her fetus. Selected conditions that can result in maternal and fetal complications are listed in Table 18-3.

Test Yourself

- Describe three clinical manifestations of amniotic fluid embolism.
- Describe two maneuvers for which the nurse can assist when shoulder dystocia complicates delivery.
- Define vasa previa.

KEY POINTS

- Nursing interventions for labor dystocia include carefully assessing the fetal lie, presentation, and position and the woman's labor pattern throughout labor. Compare the woman's progress with expected norms and notify the practitioner when progress deviates from the expected. Assist the woman to keep her bladder empty, frequently assess adequacy of the contraction pattern, and administer pain relief interventions.
- PROM is spontaneous rupture of the amniotic sac before the onset of labor in a full-term fetus; preterm PROM is PROM in a pregnancy that is less than 37 weeks' gestation. In both cases, the woman presents to the delivery suite with uncontrollable leaking of fluid from the vagina. The woman's temperature must be monitored frequently to detect early signs of infection.
- Clinical manifestations of preterm labor include uterine contractions, with or without pain; pelvic pressure; cramping; backache; and vaginal discharge and bleeding.
- Bed rest and hydration with oral or IV fluids often is the first way the practitioner attempts to stop symptoms of preterm labor. Urinalysis and other lab work are also done to detect infection. If the membranes are not ruptured, the practitioner may prescribe tocolytics and injectable steroids to stop the labor long enough to allow the fetal lungs to mature.
- Nursing interventions for the woman in preterm labor include maintaining a balanced fluid volume, preventing injury, managing the woman's pain, and reducing anxiety.
- Patient teaching for the woman carrying a post-term pregnancy includes discussing the plan of care, whether it be expectant management or labor induction. Expectant management involves frequent fetal kick counts and NSTs to monitor fetal well-being. Instruct the woman to report decreased fetal movement immediately.
- During labor induction of a woman with fetal demise, monitor the contraction pattern to avoid uterine rupture. Monitor the woman for signs of DIC. Provide emotional care for the woman and her family.
- Amniotic fluid embolism occurs suddenly during labor or in the immediate postpartum period. The woman becomes acutely dyspneic, apprehensive, hypotensive, and cyanotic. Treatment is supportive, and the woman requires care in the ICU.
- Shoulder dystocia occurs when the fetal head is born but the shoulders fail to deliver. McRoberts maneuver and suprapubic pressure are two interventions that require the active involvement of the

nurse. Carefully observe the newborn for signs of birth injury.

- Umbilical cord prolapse occurs when the umbilical cord slips down in front of the presenting part. Unless pressure is immediately relieved, the fetus will die or will experience permanent brain damage from lack of oxygen. An immediate cesarean delivery is required.
- History of a previous uterine scar increases the risk of uterine rupture during labor. Ominous fetal heart rate patterns on the fetal monitor are usually the most significant sign of rupture. Prompt cesarean delivery is necessary to save the fetus and the woman.

REFERENCES AND SELECTED READINGS

Books and Journals

Bernhardt, J., & Dorman, K. (2004). Pre-term birth risk assessment tools: Exploring fetal fibronectin and cervical length for validating risk. *AWHONN Lifelines, 8*(1), 38–44.

Church-Balin, C., & Damus, K. (2003). Commentary: Preventing prematurity. *AWHONN Lifelines, 7*(2), 97–101.

Crowley, P. (2003). Antenatal corticosteroids—current thinking. *BJOG: An International Journal of Obstetrics and Gynaecology, 110*(Suppl 20), 77–78. Retrieved December 2, 2003, from http://www.womenshealth-elsevier.com/doc/journals/pdf/bjog%20sup%2015.pdf

Cunningham, F. G., Gant, N. F., Leveno, K. J., Gilstrap L. C. III, Hauth, J. C., & Wenstrom, K. D. (2001a). Postterm pregnancy. In *Williams obstetrics* (21st ed., pp. 729–742). New York: McGraw-Hill Medical Publishing Division.

Cunningham, F. G., Gant, N. F., Leveno, K. J., Gilstrap, L. C. III, Hauth, J. C., & Wenstrom, K. D. (2001b). Preterm birth. In *Williams obstetrics* (21st ed., pp. 689–727). New York: McGraw-Hill Medical Publishing Division.

Cunningham, F. G., Gant, N. F., Leveno, K. J., Gilstrap, L. C. III, Hauth, J. C., & Wenstrom, K. D. (2001c). Section V: Abnormal labor. In *Williams obstetrics* (21st ed., pp. 423–482). New York: McGraw-Hill Medical Publishing Division.

Curran, C. A. (2003). Intrapartum emergencies. *JOGNN, 32*(6), 802–813.

Dauphinee, J. D. (2004). VBAC: Safety for the patient and the nurse. *JOGNN, 33*(1), 105–115.

Davis, D. (2003). Amniotic fluid embolism: Exploring this rare but typically fatal condition. *AWHONN Lifelines, 7*(2), 126–131.

De Jong, M. J., & Fausett, M. B. (2003). Anaphylactoid syndrome of pregnancy: A devastating complication requiring intensive care. *Critical Care Nurse, 23*(6), 42–48.

Divon, M. Y., Haglund, B., Nisell, H., Otterblad, P. O., & Westgren, M. (1998). Fetal and neonatal mortality in the postterm pregnancy: The impact of gestational age and fetal growth restriction. *American Journal of Obstetrics and Gynecology, 178*(4), 726–731.

Fisk, N. M., & Chan, J. (2003). The case for tocolysis in threatened preterm labour. *BJOG: An International Journal of Obstetrics and Gynaecology, 110*(Suppl 20), 98–102. Retrieved December 2, 2003, from http://www.womenshealth elsevier.com/doc/journals/pdf/bjog%20sup%2020.pdf

Freda, M. C. (2003). Nursing's contribution to the literature on preterm labor and birth. *JOGNN, 32*(5), 659–667.

Glimore, D. A., Wakim, J., Secrest, J., & Rawson, R. (2003). Anaphylactoid syndrome of pregnancy: A review of the literature with latest management and outcome data. *AANA Journal, 71*(2), 120–126.

Lindsey, J. L. (2002). Evaluation of fetal death. *eMedicine*. Witlin, A., Talavera, F., Smith, C. V., Gaupp, F. B., & Shulman, L. P. (Eds.). Retrieved January 11, 2004, from http://www.emedicine.com/med/topic3235.htm

Moore, L. E., & Ware, D. (2002). Amniotic fluid embolism. *eMedicine*. Kavanagh, J. J., Talavera, F., Barnes, A. D., Gaupp, F. B., & Shulman, L. P. (Eds.). Retrieved April 30, 2004, from http://www.emedicine.com/med/topic122.htm

Moore, M. L. (2003). Preterm labor and birth: What have we learned in the past two decades? *JOGNN, 32*(5), 638–649.

Moos, M. (2004). Understanding prematurity. *AWHONN Lifelines, 8*(1), 32–37.

Newton, E. R. (2002). Preterm labor. *eMedicine*. Trupin, S. R., Talavera, F., Legro, R. S., Gaupp, F. B., & Shulman, L. P. (Eds.). Retrieved November 30, 2003, from http://www.emedicine.com/med/topic3245.htm

Oyelese, K. O., Schwarzler, P., Coates, S., Sanusi, F. A., Hamid, R., & Campbell, S. (1998). A strategy for reducing the mortality rate from vasa previa using transvaginal sonography with color doppler. *Ultrasound Obstetrics and Gynecology, 12*(6), 434–438.

Rose, V. L. (1998). ACOG releases practice pattern on shoulder dystocia. *American Family Physician, 57*(10), 2546–2547.

Saju, J., & Lyon, D. (2003). Diagnosis of abnormal labor. *eMedicine*. Zurawin, R. K., Talavera, F., Legro, R. S., Gaupp, F. B., & Shulman, L. P. (Eds.). Retrieved November 3, 2003, from http://www.emedicine.com/med/topic3488.htm

Searing, K. A. (2001). Induction versus post-date pregnancies: Exploring the controversy and who's really at risk. *AWHONN Lifelines, 5*(2), 44–48.

Walling, A. D. (1999). Risk of hemorrhage and scarring in placenta accreta. *American Family Physician, 60*(2), 636.

Weismiller, D. G. (1999). Preterm labor. *American Family Physician*, 59, 593–604. Retrieved December 2, 2003, from http://www.aafp.org/afp/990201ap/593.html

Wilkes, P. T., & Galan, H. (2002a). Postdate pregnancy. *eMedicine*. Cowan, B. D., Talavera, F., Legro, R. S., Gaupp, F. B., & Shulman, L. P. (Eds.). Retrieved January 11, 2004, from http://www.emedicine.com/med/topic3248.htm

Wilkes, P. T., & Galan, H. (2002b). Premature rupture of membranes. *eMedicine*. Trupin, S. R., Talavera, F., Whitman-Elia, G. F., Gaupp, F. B., & Shulman, L. P. (Eds.). Retrieved November 23, 2003, from http://www.emedicine.com/med/topic3246.htm

Websites.

http://www.moonlily.com/obc/complications.html

Post-term Pregnancy

http://www.aafp.org/afp/080196/960801c.html

Shoulder Dystocia

http://pregnancy.about.com/cs/laborbirth/a/aa081801a.htm

http://www.obgyn.net/pb/pb.asp?page=/pb/articles/dystocia-casereport

WORKBOOK

NCLEX-STYLE REVIEW QUESTIONS

1. A 35-year-old Gravida 1 delivered after 24 hours of labor. Her membranes ruptured 4 hours after she started labor. Two hours before she delivered, she spiked a temperature of 101°F. For which of the following complications is her newborn most at risk?
   a. ABO incompatibility
   b. Fistula formation
   c. Pelvic floor injury
   d. Pneumonia
2. A 26-year-old primigravida is attempting natural childbirth. Her doula has been supporting her through the past 16 hours of labor. The laboring woman is now 6 centimeters dilated. She continues to report severe pain in her back with each contraction. She finds it comforting when her doula uses the ball of her hand to put counterpressure on her lower back. What do you think is the likely cause of the woman's back pain?
   a. Breech presentation
   b. Fetal macrosomia
   c. Occiput posterior position
   d. Nongynecoid pelvis
3. A 31-year-old Gravida 3 Para 1 calls the clinic. She is at 29 weeks' gestation. She says that she has been having uterine contractions every 10 minutes for the past 2 hours. She also feels "heaviness" in her vaginal area. Her first baby was born prematurely at 28 weeks' gestation. What advice by the nurse is best for this woman?
   a. "Come into the hospital immediately. These signs strongly indicate that you may be in premature labor."
   b. "Drink two large glasses of water. Lie down on your left side. If the contractions don't stop in an hour, come in to the hospital."
   c. "Monitor your contractions for 1 more hour. If they increase in frequency, or get stronger, come in right away."
   d. "It is not likely that you will deliver a second baby prematurely. Don't panic. If you continue to have contractions, come in to be checked."
4. You are assisting in a delivery that is complicated by shoulder dystocia. Which nursing action is indicated?
   a. Give fundal pressure.
   b. Start rescue breathing.
   c. Assist the RN to flex the woman's thighs.
   d. Watch the fetal monitor for signs of fetal distress.

STUDY ACTIVITIES

1. Use the table provided to compare fetal and maternal causes of labor arrest.

Fetal Causes of Labor Arrest	Maternal Causes of Labor Arrest

2. Interview your local March of Dimes representative to see what is being done in your community to learn more about and prevent preterm labor. Share your findings with your clinical group.
3. Develop a teaching plan for a woman with a post-term pregnancy that is being managed expectantly.

CRITICAL THINKING: What Would You Do?

Apply your knowledge of labor at risk to the following situations.

1. Julia, a Gravida 2 Para 0, just found out that her fetus is in a breech position at 36 weeks' gestation. Julia is afraid that she will have to have a cesarean delivery. What options does Julia have in this situation?
2. Julia's pregnancy proceeds to 39 weeks' gestation. She presents to labor and delivery because her "water bag broke." After the midwife confirms that the membranes have ruptured, she explains to Julia that the plan is for Julia and her husband to wait in the hospital until labor begins. Julia wants to know why she and her husband can't just go home to wait for contractions to begin.

a. How do you reply to Julia?

b. What nursing interventions will you plan for Julia during the wait before labor begins?

c. How would your care be different if Julia were at 30 weeks' gestation with ruptured membranes versus 39 weeks?

3. Kimberly has been receiving the tocolytic terbutaline for the past 12 hours. You are taking Kimberly's vital signs at the beginning of your shift. You notice that Kimberly's pulse is 130 and her blood pressure is 88/50 mm Hg. When you ask her how she is feeling, she replies, "I feel out of breath, and I have a feeling of pressure in my chest." What should you do?

Postpartum Woman at Risk

19

STUDENT OBJECTIVES

On completion of this chapter, the student should be able to

1. Identify major conditions that place a woman at risk during the postpartal period.
2. Differentiate between early and late postpartum hemorrhage
3. Describe appropriate nursing interventions for the woman with postpartum hemorrhage, regardless of the cause.
4. Compare and contrast four types of infection that may occur in the postpartum period.
5. Identify factors that place a postpartum woman at risk for a thromboembolic disorder.
6. Describe three different psychiatric problems that can complicate the postpartum period.
7. Discuss the nurse's role when caring for a postpartal woman who is grieving.
8. Identify behaviors that would suggest malattachment.

KEY TERMS

cystitis
endometritis
exudate
hematoma
hypovolemic shock
malattachment
mastitis
pyelonephritis
uterine atony
uterine subinvolution

Often considered the "fourth trimester of pregnancy," the postpartum period encompasses the first 6 weeks after childbirth. After delivery, the woman begins to experience physiologic and psychological changes that return her body to the prepregnancy state. These changes usually occur without difficulty. However, factors such as blood loss, trauma during delivery, infection, or fatigue can place the postpartum woman at risk. The nurse plays a key role in identifying the woman at risk for complications to ensure early detection and prompt intervention. Most often, the nurse is the person who identifies the problem and alerts the primary medical provider of the pressing need for intervention. Nursing interventions for the postpartum woman at risk focus on treating the complication, thereby minimizing the effects on the woman's return to her prepregnant state; promoting adaptation to her role as mother of a new infant; and supporting and enhancing maternal–infant bonding.

This chapter addresses major complications associated with the postpartum period, including hemorrhage, infection, thromboembolic disorders, and psychiatric disorders. The priority aspects of nursing care are emphasized for each complication. In addition, the chapter describes special postpartum situations, such as postpartal grieving and malattachment. The nurse's role in each situation is presented.

POSTPARTUM HEMORRHAGE

Postpartum hemorrhage is one of the leading causes of maternal deaths, accounting for approximately 30% of all pregnancy-related deaths (Roman & Rebarber, 2003). It can occur early, within the first 24 hours after delivery, or late, anytime after the first 24 hours through the 6-week postpartum period. The woman is most vulnerable to hemorrhage during the first 24 hours after delivery, with the greatest risk occurring in the first hour after delivery.

Traditionally, postpartum hemorrhage has been defined as any blood loss in an amount greater than 500 mL after a vaginal delivery or greater than 1,000 mL after a cesarean birth. However, because blood loss estimates during delivery are often inaccurate, the American College of Obstetricians and Gynecologists (ACOG) has defined postpartum hemorrhage as a decrease in the hematocrit of 10% or greater after delivery when compared with that before delivery (AGOG, 1998; Roman & Rebarber, 2003).

The causes of postpartum hemorrhage can be grouped into four major categories: **uterine atony**, inability of the uterus to contract effectively; lacerations to the uterus, cervix, vagina, or perineum; retained placenta; and disruption in maternal clotting abilities. It is important to monitor all postpartum women for excessive bleeding because two-thirds of the women who experience postpartum hemorrhage have no risk factors. However, certain factors are known to increase the risk for postpartum hemorrhage (Box 19-1). Early detection and prompt intervention are necessary to control the hemorrhage. Otherwise the woman can progress to shock, renal failure, and ultimately death from the loss of blood.

Early Postpartum Hemorrhage

Early postpartum hemorrhage refers to blood loss (greater than 500 mL) within the first 24 hours after delivery. Early postpartum hemorrhage results from one of the three following conditions:

- Uterine atony
- Lacerations
- Hematoma

BOX 19.1 Risk Factors for Postpartum Hemorrhage

Each risk factor is listed by cause.

Uterine Atony
- Multiparity
- Intrauterine infection
- Previous uterine surgery
- Prolonged or difficult labor
- History of postpartum hemorrhage
- Placenta previa or abruptio placentae
- Use of oxytocin for labor stimulation or augmentation
- Use of agents during labor that relax the uterus (tocolytics), such as
  - magnesium sulfate
  - terbutaline
  - certain anesthetics
  - nitroglycerin
- Overdistention of the uterus, such as occurs with
  - multiple gestation
  - polyhydramnios
  - fetal macrosomia

Lacerations and Hematomas
- Episiotomy
- Macrosomia
- Precipitous labor
- Traumatic delivery
- Use of forceps or vacuum extraction for delivery

Retained Placenta
- Abruptio placentae
- Placenta accreta
- Prolonged third stage of labor

Disruption in Maternal Clotting Abilities
- Fetal demise
- Thrombocytopenia
- Pregnancy-induced hypertension

Most cases of early postpartum hemorrhage result from uterine atony. With this condition, the uterus does not contract as it should. Thus, the muscles of the uterus remain relaxed and exert no compression on the open uterine blood vessels. As a result, the vessels continue to bleed. This blood loss can be extensive and rapid. Lacerations can occur as small tears or cuts in the perineal tissue, vaginal sidewall or cervix. A **hematoma** is a clot of blood that collects within tissues and leads to concealed blood loss.

Regardless of the cause, the woman is at risk for developing hypovolemia, a system-wide decrease in blood volume from too much blood loss. If the blood loss continues, the woman may develop **hypovolemic shock**, which is characterized by a weak, thready, rapid pulse; drop in blood pressure; cool, clammy skin; and changes in level of consciousness. These findings may occur abruptly and be dramatic if the blood loss is large and occurs quickly. However, with bleeding of a more gradual onset, these signs and symptoms may be extremely subtle because of the woman's ability to compensate for the blood loss over time. With continued bleeding, the woman's body eventually is overwhelmed and no longer able to compensate for the loss. At that point she exhibits the typical signs and symptoms of shock.

The woman who experiences postpartum hemorrhage is also at risk for developing anemia from the blood loss. Other complications connected with postpartum hemorrhage include complications associated with blood transfusions, further bleeding that may occur if clotting factors are used up or if disseminated intravascular coagulation (DIC) develops, need for emergency surgical intervention to include hysterectomy with loss of childbearing capability, and multiple organ failure.

Clinical Manifestations

Clinical manifestations of early postpartum hemorrhage differ according the cause of the hemorrhage.

Hemorrhage Caused by Uterine Atony. If the underlying cause of hemorrhage is uterine atony, the woman's fundus usually will be difficult to palpate. When the fundus is identified on palpation, it is soft (boggy), relaxed, and located above the level of the umbilicus. The woman's bladder may be distended, further interfering with uterine contraction. A full bladder may cause the uterus to be pushed to one side, rather than being at the midline. Vaginal bleeding (lochia) typically is moderate to heavy, possibly with numerous large clots.

Hemorrhage Caused by Lacerations. When lacerations are the cause of bleeding, the fundus is firm on palpation. However, the bleeding continues in a steady trickle. Characteristically, the bleeding is bright red in color, in contrast to the dark red color of lochia.

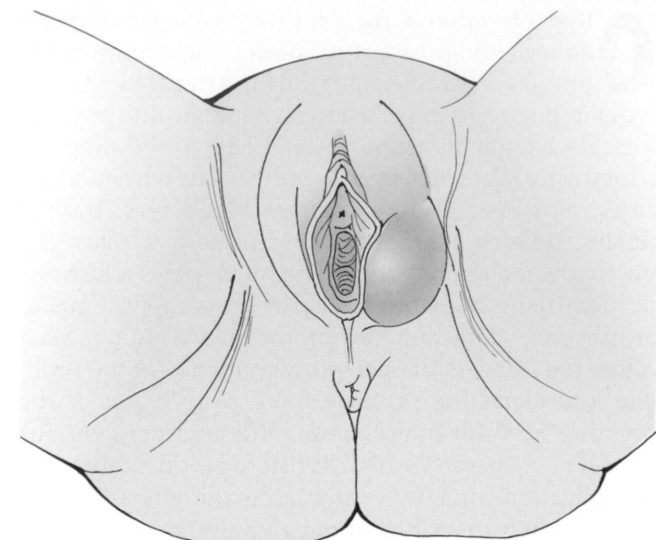

● ***Figure 19.1*** Perineal hematoma. Notice the localized area of swelling. A perineal hematoma usually results from trauma to the area that breaks a blood vessel, causing bleeding into the tissue. The main symptom is severe perineal pain unrelieved by normal measures, and a soft, palpable mass.

Hemorrhage Caused by Hematoma. Unlike uterine atony and lacerations, the bleeding associated with hematoma formation may not be apparent (Fig. 19-1). A blood vessel ruptures and leaks into the surrounding tissue. This causes pressure, pain, swelling (edema), and dark red or purple discoloration, most commonly on one side of the perineum. Initially, the area may feel soft. However, as leakage into the tissues continues, the area becomes firm to the touch. In addition, the area is tender on palpation.

A hematoma also can form deep in the pelvis. This is a much more difficult problem to identify. The primary symptom is deep pain unrelieved by comfort measures or medication and accompanied by vital sign instability. Regardless of where the hematoma occurs, the woman's lochia usually is within expected parameters. However, if the hematoma is large, she may experience a significant loss of blood into the tissues, leading to signs and symptoms of hypovolemic shock.

Diagnosis

Diagnosis is made on clinical signs and changes in laboratory values. Because of blood loss, the woman's hemoglobin and hematocrit levels will be decreased from her prelabor (baseline) levels, approximately 1 to 1.5 g/dL and 2% to 4%, respectively. In addition, if the woman has an underlying coagulation defect, clotting times will be increased and platelet and prothrombin levels will be decreased.

Treatment

The goal of treatment for postpartal hemorrhage is to correct the underlying cause while attempting to control the hemorrhage and reduce its effects on the woman. If the woman is exhibiting signs and symptoms of hypovolemic shock, emergency measures are instituted to support vital functions. These include rapid IV fluid replacement, blood transfusions, oxygen administration, and frequent close monitoring of all vital functions. Insertion of an indwelling urinary catheter may be necessary to monitor the woman's urine output hourly.

Treatment for Uterine Atony. If uterine atony is present, fundal massage (refer to Nursing Procedure 12-1 in Chapter 12) is initiated first. Massage attempts to help the uterus to contract, thereby compressing the blood vessels and ultimately decreasing the bleeding. Once the uterus is contracted, firm gentle pressure is applied to the uterus to help express any clots that may have collected in the uterus. The woman's bladder must be empty when fundal massage is initiated. Otherwise the uterus will not remain contracted once the massage stops.

Don't do it! Never, never, never, attempt uterine massage without first placing one hand over the symphysis pubis. Doing so could cause the uterus to turn inside out (inversion). Once this occurs, massive hemorrhage ensues and can quickly lead to death.

Drug therapy may be necessary if fundal massage fails to maintain the uterus in a contracted state. Oxytocic agents, such as oxytocin (Pitocin), ergonovine (Ergotrate), methylergonovine (Methergine), carboprost (Hemabate), and misoprostol (Cytotec) may be administered parenterally. If drug therapy is ineffective, the primary care provider may need to intervene. Bimanual compression of the uterus is frequently the first method attempted. Exploration of the uterine cavity may be the next option when other treatment measures fail. Uterine packing may be done to control hemorrhage. Another option is uterine artery embolization or ligation to control bleeding. When postpartum hemorrhage due to uterine atony continues despite all efforts to control it, a hysterectomy may be done, usually only as a last resort.

Treatment for Lacerations and Hematomas. Postpartal hemorrhage caused by lacerations is treated by surgical repair of the lacerations. Small hematomas usually require no additional treatment other than application of ice and analgesics to control pain. In most instances, small hematomas absorb spontaneously, usually during a period of 4 to 6 weeks. Surgical incision, with drainage and evacuation of clots and ligation of the bleeding vessel may be required if the hematoma is large.

● Nursing Process for the Woman With Early Postpartum Hemorrhage

The nurse plays an important role in monitoring the woman's status, assisting with measures to control bleeding, providing support to the woman and her family, and educating the woman about her condition. Maintaining the woman's safety is paramount.

ASSESSMENT

As with any patient, thorough, frequent assessment is necessary to allow for early detection and prompt intervention should hemorrhage occur. Be aware of the woman's history, labor progress, and risk factors for postpartum hemorrhage. Note the use of any analgesia or anesthesia during labor and delivery or the use of oxytocin for labor induction or augmentation. This information helps to identify potential factors that would place the woman at risk for hemorrhage.

Ask the woman about the onset of the bleeding, if appropriate. For example, "Did the bleeding seem to increase suddenly or have you noticed a constant trickling?" Ask about any associated symptoms, such as "Do you have any pain or pressure?" These types of questions help to provide information about the possible cause of the hemorrhage. Ask the woman how frequently she is changing her perineal pads, how saturated they appear, and when she changed the pad last. The bleeding of a woman who has changed her perineal pads twice in the last hour with each pad containing approximately a half-dollar sized amount of lochia is far different from that of a woman who has changed her perineal pads twice in the last hour because they were saturated. Additional evaluation of the second woman is necessary. In this case, the primary health care provider also needs to be notified.

Assess the fundus for consistency, shape, and location. Remember that the uterus should be firm, in the midline, and decrease 1 centimeter each postpartum day. Inability to locate the fundus suggests that it is not firm and contracting. Displacement to one side suggests that the woman has a distended bladder.

Observe lochia for color, amount, odor, and character, including evidence of any clots. When evaluating the lochia, turn the woman to her side and look under the buttocks for any pooling of blood that may occur while she is in bed. Note amount and characteristics of the bleeding. Dark red is the normal color of lochia in the first few postpartum days. A bright red color is associated with fresh bleeding, such as that from a laceration. Note whether or not bleeding decreases with fundal massage.

Here's an objective way to determine the quantity of blood loss!

Remember that 1 gram of weight is approximately equal to 1 milliliter (mL) of fluid. First weigh a dry, clean perineal pad. Next, weigh the used pad and then subtract the dry pad weight from this amount. The result will be the amount of blood lost. For example, a dry perineal pad weighs 5 grams. A used perineal pad weighs 34 grams. 34 − 5 = 29 grams, which is equivalent to 29 mL of blood loss.

Determine when the woman last urinated. Remember that a full bladder can impede uterine contraction, predisposing her to hemorrhage. Inspect the woman's perineal area closely for evidence of lacerations or hematomas. Do not mistake an episiotomy for a laceration. Typically an episiotomy is approximately 1 to 2 inches in length and has clean, regular sutured edges, whereas a laceration varies in length, and its edges appear irregular and somewhat jagged. Evaluate pain and other associated symptoms. Severe pain and pressure that are unrelieved by ordinary pain control measures may indicate the presence of a hematoma.

Assess the woman's vital signs to obtain a baseline and then monitor vital signs as ordered, noting any changes suggesting hypovolemic shock. Also note the color and temperature of the woman's skin and her level of consciousness. Recall that cool, clammy skin and decreasing level of consciousness may indicate hypovolemic shock. Table 19-1 highlights assessment findings for the major causes of postpartum hemorrhage.

CULTURAL SNAPSHOT

For people of color (e.g., African American, Hispanic, and Asian), assess skin "color" (pale, red, cyanotic, jaundiced) by looking at the mucous membranes of the mouth, tongue, and gums. The unpainted nail bed also gives a clear, nonpigmented view of color.

SELECTED NURSING DIAGNOSES

- Deficient Fluid Volume related to excessive blood loss
- Risk for Injury related to hemorrhage and possible development of hypovolemic shock
- Ineffective Tissue Perfusion related to decreased circulating blood volume subsequent to postpartum hemorrhage and development of hypovolemic shock

OUTCOME IDENTIFICATION AND PLANNING

Appropriate goals for the woman experiencing postpartum hemorrhage include the following: the woman will demonstrate signs and symptoms of restored fluid balance; she will remain free of any injury; and she will exhibit signs of adequate tissue perfusion.

IMPLEMENTATION

Nursing care for the woman experiencing postpartum hemorrhage focuses on stopping the bleeding, restoring fluid balance, preventing injury, and promoting adequate tissue perfusion. As with any postpartal complication, be sure to provide emotional support to the woman and her family, explaining all events and procedures to minimize anxiety and fear. Keep the family informed of the situation, explaining laboratory tests, procedures, and signs of improvement. Allow the partner and family to discuss feelings, which may be very intense. Frustration, anger, blame, disbelief, and sorrow often are expressed. Listen, be patient, be present, and acknowledge that this is a difficult time.

Controlling and Restoring Fluid Balance

Key to restoring fluid balance is stopping the bleeding. First, try fundal massage to stop the bleeding (see Nursing Procedure 12-1 in Chapter 12). Administer oxytocics, as ordered. If an IV line with oxytocin is present, increase the rate of flow to a fast drip. Prepare the woman for surgical intervention if less drastic measures do not control bleeding. If the woman is scheduled for surgery, withhold all food and fluids, unless allowed by the physician. Be sure to explain all treatments and procedures to the woman and her family to help reduce anxiety. If the woman continues to hemorrhage, expect her to be transferred to the intensive care unit for closer, more frequent monitoring.

When a woman experiences postpartum hemorrhage, fluid is lost. If she is allowed oral intake, encourage her to increase her oral fluid intake. If

TABLE 19.1 Assessing the Source of Postpartum Hemorrhage

	Uterine Atony	Subinvolution of the Uterus	Lacerations	Retained Placental Fragments	Hematoma
Occurrence	Early	Late	Early	Early or late	Early
Condition/ placement of uterus	Fundus will be boggy and high. If the bladder is full, the fundus will also be displaced to one side.	Fundus may be firm when palpated but boggy a short time later.	Normal	Fundus will be slightly boggy when assessed but often becomes firm when massaged.	Normal
Characteristics of lochia	Moderate to heavy lochia (i.e., when a perineal pad fills up with blood in less than 1 hour)	Initially, lochia flow is normal. Then the lochia will increase over what is expected and/or will revert to an earlier type of flow (e.g., the lochia will become rubra after it has changed to serosa, etc.).	Bleeding is heavy, bright red, and continues in a steady trickle or flow.	Intermittent clots will characterize bleeding.	Normal
Characteristics of pain	May be absent.	May be absent or there may be constant cramping. Backache may be present.	May be constant.	May be characterized by intermittent or heavier than normal cramping.	Pressure and severe pain at the site (perineal hematoma). Deep pain unrelieved by comfort measures or medication (deep pelvic hematoma)
Other signs and symptoms	Tachycardia, hypotension, and other signs of hypovolemic shock if blood loss is severe.	Dizziness, light-headedness, and fatigue when changing positions or doing simple self-care tasks. Fever and other signs of infection may be present.	Bruising may be apparent.	Portions of maternal surface of placenta are missing.	Swelling (edema) and dark red or purple discoloration (perineal hematoma). Accompanied by instability of blood pressure, pulse, and hemoglobin and hematocrit (deep pelvic hematoma).

the woman is not able to drink oral fluids, or if fluid loss is significant, expect to administer fluids intravenously. Typically, isotonic IV solutions, such as normal saline or lactated Ringer's solution, are ordered for replacement. Assist with IV catheter insertion if the woman does not have one already inserted, and administer fluids as ordered. Use care in administering fluids to avoid circulatory overload from too rapid or too great an infusion.

Continue to monitor the woman's fundus and lochia frequently for changes indicating continuation or resolution of the hemorrhage. If uterine atony is causing the bleeding and the woman received IV oxytocin, fundal assessment is crucial. Although oxytocin helps to contract the uterus, and this effect is immediate, the drug has a short duration of action, placing the woman at risk for hemorrhage secondary to a recurrence of atony once the IV rate of administration is slowed or stopped.

Inspect the perineum closely for evidence and amount of bleeding. Monitor pad count and weigh pads to determine the amount of blood lost. Be sure to turn the woman on her side and inspect the area under the buttocks because blood can pool, presenting a misleading picture. Assist as necessary with fundal massage to keep the uterus in a contracted state. Be aware that the uterus may relax quickly when massage stops, placing the woman at risk for continued hemorrhage.

Monitor the woman's intake and output closely, possibly every hour if necessary, to determine the effectiveness of therapy and progression or resolution of the fluid imbalance. Urine output should be at least 30 mL/hour, indicating adequate renal function. Encourage the woman to void frequently to prevent bladder distention from interfering with uterine contraction, increasing the risk for continued hemorrhage. If the woman has difficulty voiding, try measures such as running warm water over the perineum, placing the woman's hand in a basin or sink of warm water, or having the woman hear running water at the sink. If all else fails and the woman is unable to void, anticipate the need for insertion of an indwelling urinary catheter.

Expect to assist with obtaining blood specimens for laboratory testing, such as complete blood count, electrolyte levels, coagulation studies, and type and cross-matching for blood. If ordered, administer blood component therapy to aid in replacing fluid and blood loss.

Continue to monitor the woman's vital signs frequently for changes. Be alert for a rising pulse rate, changing pulse characteristics to rapid and thready, or decreasing blood pressure, which may indicate hypovolemic shock.

Preventing Injury

A postpartum woman who is hemorrhaging is at risk for injury. Reduction in blood supply to the brain can lead to changes in the woman's level of consciousness, placing her at risk for injury from confusion, disorientation, and falls. Therefore, safety measures are necessary to ensure that the woman remains free from injury.

Keep the call light close by and urge the woman to remain in bed. Check on her frequently, and encourage a family member to stay with her, if necessary. If the woman is allowed to ambulate to the bathroom, have her sit at the side of the bed for a short time before arising to prevent orthostatic hypotension. Then assist her to ambulate and stay nearby in the event that she complains of lightheadedness or dizziness.

Continue to monitor the woman's vital signs for changes. If she reports dizziness or lightheadedness when getting up, obtain her blood pressure while lying, sitting, and standing, noting any change of 10 mm Hg or more. Should the woman's blood pressure drop with position changes, notify the primary care provider.

Promoting Adequate Tissue Perfusion

A decrease in circulating blood volume secondary to hemorrhage affects tissue perfusion because oxygen, carried by the blood, is not transported to the required areas in adequate amounts. Therefore, oxygen must be provided. Expect to administer oxygen therapy via nasal cannula as ordered. Depending on the woman's need, oxygen may be administered via mask. Institute continuous pulse oximetry to evaluate oxygen saturation levels. Notify the physician if the oxygen saturation falls below 95%.

Arterial blood gas (ABG) studies may be performed to evaluate the woman's acid-base balance and provide a more definitive evaluation of the woman's current status. Be prepared to adjust the oxygen flow rate based on the ABG findings.

Continue to assess the woman's skin color and temperature for changes. Cold, clammy skin may indicate that constriction of the peripheral vessels is occurring, suggesting that the woman is developing hypovolemic shock or that the woman's condition is worsening. Also check nail beds for color and capillary refill. Keep in mind that a capillary refill greater than 3 seconds suggests impaired blood flow.

Monitor the woman's level of consciousness for changes. A woman who is alert and oriented is exhibiting adequate cerebral perfusion. However, confusion, disorientation, or deteriorating levels of consciousness suggest diminished blood flow and inadequate cerebral perfusion.

When adequately perfused, the kidneys function to produce urine. Adequate renal function is evidenced by a urine output of at least 30 mL/hour. Therefore, monitor the woman's urine output for changes. Report any urine output less than this amount immediately.

EVALUATION: GOALS AND EXPECTED OUTCOMES

- **Goal:** The woman will demonstrate evidence of fluid balance.
- Expected Outcomes:
  - Intake and output are within acceptable parameters.
  - Output is at least 30 mL/hour.
  - Vital signs are within normal limits.
  - Lochia is moderate in amount, without clots.
  - Laboratory test results, including hemoglobin and hematocrit levels, have returned to acceptable levels.
- **Goal:** The woman will remain free of injury.
- Expected Outcomes:
  - Vital signs are maintained within acceptable parameters.
  - The woman demonstrates no signs and symptoms of hypovolemic shock.
  - The uterus remains in a contracted state.
  - The woman is alert and oriented.
  - The woman remains free of falls.
- **Goal:** The woman will exhibit signs of adequate tissue perfusion.
- Expected Outcomes:
  - The woman is alert and oriented to person, place, and time.
  - The woman's skin is pink, warm, and dry with quick capillary refill.
  - Vital signs are within acceptable parameters.
  - Oxygen saturation remains above 95%.
  - Urine output is at least 30 mL/hour.

Late Postpartum Hemorrhage

Late postpartum hemorrhage refers to blood loss (more than 500 mL) occurring after the first 24 hours after delivery, and at any time throughout the 6-week postpartum period. Most cases of late postpartum hemorrhage result from retained placental fragments or **uterine subinvolution**, a condition in which the uterus returns to its prepregnancy shape and size at a rate that is slower than expected (usually the result of retained placental fragments or an infection). The woman who has had uterine surgery, including a previous cesarean birth or an abortion, is at high risk for retained placental fragments along the surgical scar.

Clinical Manifestations

As with early postpartum hemorrhage, the woman with late postpartal hemorrhage notices an increase in bleeding. This increase usually occurs abruptly several days after discharge. Along with an abrupt onset of bleeding, the woman exhibits a uterus that is not contracted firmly. On palpation, the uterus is not descending at the usual rate of 1 centimeter or fingerbreadth per postpartum day. Lochia is heavier than that which would be expected. The woman may report episodes of intermittent, irregular, or excessive vaginal bleeding. In addition, the woman may report backache, fatigue, and general malaise. She may also report pelvic pain or heaviness. Her temperature may be elevated slightly and lochia may be foul smelling if an infection is present.

Diagnosis

Similar to the findings of early postpartum hemorrhage, the woman's hemoglobin and hematocrit levels will be decreased. If retained placental fragments are the cause, the woman's serum human chorionic gonadotropin levels will be elevated. Ultrasound may reveal evidence of placental fragments. An elevated white blood cell count may be noted with an infection. However, this result may not be conclusive because a postpartal woman's white blood cell count typically is elevated in the early postpartum period.

Treatment

Treatment of late postpartum hemorrhage focuses on correcting the underlying cause of the hemorrhage. Drug therapy, similar to that used for uterine atony, may be administered to aid in contracting the uterus. Often, uterine contraction aids in removing any fragments from the uterus. If necessary, surgery, specifically dilation and curettage (D&C) may be done to remove the fragments from the myometrium. Usually, this procedure is performed only when other treatment measures have been ineffective because it can traumatize the uterus further, leading to additional bleeding. Antibiotic therapy is indicated if an infection is present.

Nursing Care

Most cases of late postpartum hemorrhage occur after the woman has been discharged from the health care or birthing facility. Therefore, patient education before discharge about expected changes and danger signs and symptoms is crucial. Instruct the woman to call her primary care provider if she experiences any signs of infection, such as fever greater than 100.4°F, chills, or foul-smelling lochia. She should also report lochia that increases (versus decreasing) in amount, or reversal of the pattern of lochia (i.e., moves from serosa back to rubra).

Test Yourself

- What is the definition of postpartum hemorrhage?
- Name the most common cause of early postpartum hemorrhage.
- Name three nursing actions that should be used for the woman who is experiencing postpartum hemorrhage secondary to uterine atony.

POSTPARTUM INFECTION

Postpartum infection, also called puerperal infection, refers to any infection that occurs after delivery. Most commonly, the infection involves the reproductive tract, but it also can involve other areas, such as the breast, wound, or urinary tract. Current research suggests that postpartum infections occur in approximately 1% to 8% of all postpartum women, with the maternal mortality rate attributable to postpartum infection ranging from 4% to 8% (Kennedy, 2003).

A postpartum infection is suspected when the woman develops a fever of 100.4°F (38°C) or greater on two consecutive occasions at least 6 hours apart during the first 10 days postpartum, but not including the first 24 hours (Simpson & Creehan, 2001). Various organisms are associated with postpartum infections, including but not limited to staphylococcus, streptococcus, *Escherichia coli*, and Chlamydia.

Specific risk factors are associated with the development of a postpartum infection, primarily involving the reproductive tract. Antepartum risk factors include: history of infection; history of chronic conditions, such as diabetes, anemia, or poor nutrition; infections of the genital tract; smoking; and obesity. Intrapartal risk factors include:

- Cesarean birth
- Urinary catheterization
- Episiotomy or lacerations
- Frequent vaginal examinations
- Retained placenta or one requiring manual removal
- Prolonged rupture of membranes (usually more than 24 hours)
- Chorioamnionitis (infection/inflammation of the fetal membranes)
- Traumatic birth, including the use of instruments such as forceps or vacuum extractor
- Use of invasive procedures, such as internal fetal monitoring, fetal scalp sampling, and amnioinfusion

Use of poor aseptic technique and inadequate handwashing are also risk factors. In addition, a woman who experiences postpartum hemorrhage has a greater risk for postpartal infection because of her weakened state and reduced ability to fight off the infection.

Although postpartal infection usually is localized, it can progress and spread to nearby structures such as the peritoneum, causing peritonitis, or to the blood, causing septicemia and posing a significant risk to the woman's well-being. Most postpartal infections occur once the woman is discharged from the health care facility. Therefore, patient teaching about possible signs and symptoms is crucial to ensure early detection and prompt intervention.

Endometritis

Endometritis refers to an infection of the uterine lining. It is the most common postpartal infection, occurring in as many as 3% of women who delivered vaginally and as many as 15% of women who had a cesarean birth (Franzblau & Witt, 2002). Bacteria, often normal vaginal flora, gain entrance to the uterus during birth or the immediate postpartum period.

Typically, endometritis is considered a polymicrobial infection. This means that anaerobic and aerobic organisms enter the uterus from the lower reproductive tract. Common causative organisms include group A streptococci (usually associated with endometritis occurring on day 1 or 2 postpartum); *E. coli* (usually associated with endometritis occurring on day 3 or 4 postpartum); *Klebsiella pneumoniae*; proteus; *Chlamydia trachomatis* (usually associated with endometritis occurring after day 7 postpartum); and Bacteroides species (usually associated with endometritis with cesarean birth).

Endometritis is a serious complication because the infection can spread to nearby organs, such as the fallopian tubes (causing salpingitis), ovaries (causing oophoritis), connective tissues and ligaments (causing parametritis), and the peritoneum (causing peritonitis).

Clinical Manifestations

The woman with endometritis typically looks ill and commonly develops a fever of 100.4°F (38°C) or higher (more commonly 101°F [38.4°C], possibly as high as 104°F [40°C]) on the 3rd to 4th postpartum day. The rise in temperature at this specific time is the most significant finding. The woman exhibits tachycardia, typically a rise in pulse rate of 10 beats per minute for each rise in temperature of 1 degree. In addition, the woman may report chills, anorexia, and general malaise. She also may report abdominal cramping and pain, including strong afterpains. Fundal assessment reveals uterine subinvolution and tenderness. Lochia commonly is increased in amount, dark, purulent, and foul smelling. However, if the woman's temperature is high, her lochia may be scant or absent.

Diagnosis

A complete blood count reveals an elevated white blood cell (WBC) count with increased eosinophiles or polymorphonuclear leukocytes. Urine culture, which may be done to rule out possible urinary tract infection, is negative. Vaginal cultures confirm the diagnosis and reveal the offending organisms. Blood cultures are positive in approximately 10% to 30% of the cases (Simmons & Bammel, 2001). Pelvic ultrasound may reveal an abscess or possible retained placental fragments that have become infected.

Pay close attention! Remember that the WBC count of a postpartal woman is elevated normally, ranging as high as 20,000 to 30,000/mm^3. So use caution when interpreting this laboratory result as an indicator for infection. Do suspect infection if the woman's WBC count is near the upper range of 30,000/mm^3 or higher, or if it has increased significantly above her immediate postpartum count.

Treatment

The mainstay of treatment is antibiotic therapy. Typically the woman is admitted to the health care facility for IV therapy. Until culture and sensitivity reports are available, the woman is started on broad-spectrum antibiotic therapy. Commonly used agents include combination therapy with clindamycin (Cleocin) and gentamicin. Ampicillin may be added to the treatment regimen if there is no response to the initial therapy. Cefoxitin (Mefoxin) or moxalactam are alternative agents that may be used. Oral antibiotic therapy is initiated once the woman has been afebrile for approximately 48 hours.

In addition to antibiotics, the primary care provider may prescribe oxytocic agents to aid in uterine involution and promote uterine drainage. Analgesics may be necessary if the woman is experiencing strong afterpains or abdominal discomfort. Hydration with IV and oral fluids and adequate nutrition also are important treatment measures.

Nursing Care

The woman with endometritis is visibly ill. Therefore, nursing care focuses on administering drug therapy to combat the infection, promoting physical and emotional comfort, alleviating anxiety, and teaching the woman about measures used to treat the infection and to prevent a recurrence, including proper perineal care and handwashing.

Managing Antibiotic Therapy. Administer prescribed broad-spectrum antibiotics intravenously and assess the woman for changes indicating an improvement. Monitor the woman's vital signs every 2 to 4 hours, or more often if indicated. Expect to see a reduction in temperature and a return of the pulse rate to preinfection levels as the infection resolves. Monitor for a decrease in abdominal pain and tenderness and a change in the woman's lochia to normal color (based on the postpartum day) and amount. Palpate the fundus to evaluate for uterine contraction. Expect to administer oxytocic agents as ordered to promote uterine involution. As with the administration of any medication, check with the primary care provider or lactation consultant to determine whether the woman can continue to breastfeed. In most cases the woman will be able to continue breast-feeding. If breast-feeding is contraindicated, encourage the woman to pump her breasts to maintain the milk supply.

Keep in mind that many antibiotics can be nephrotoxic (damaging to the kidneys). Encourage an increase in fluid intake, intravenously and orally, preferably to 3,000 mL/day, and monitor the woman's intake and output. Report any decrease in urine output to less than 30 mL/hour.

In conjunction with antibiotic therapy, position the woman in the semi-Fowler's position to promote uterine drainage and prevent extension of the infection. If possible and allowed by the physician, encourage the woman to ambulate to promote drainage. Be alert for signs and symptoms of peritonitis, such as pronounced abdominal pain, and distention, a rigid, boardlike abdomen and absent bowel sounds. Also assess the woman for tachycardia, tachypnea, hypotension, changes in sensorium, and decreased urine output. These suggest septic shock, a serious, possibly fatal complication.

Encourage frequent changing of perineal pads to remove infected drainage, reminding the woman to remove the pad using a front-to-back motion to avoid contaminating the perineal area. Reinforce the need to wash her hands after each change. Offer perineal care every 2 hours or as necessary. Be sure to wear gloves when handling the woman's soiled perineal pads to prevent infection transmission.

Providing Comfort Measures. The woman needs comfort care during this time. Provide cool washcloths and frequent linen changes, especially if the woman is febrile and diaphoretic. If the woman reports chills, add extra blankets to keep her warm; however, be careful that she doesn't become overheated. Keep the room calm and quiet to ensure the woman rests.

Expect to administer analgesics for reports of abdominal pain. Encourage the woman to change positions frequently while maintaining the semi-Fowler's position. The woman probably will be fatigued because of the stress of the infection. Allow for frequent rest periods so that she does not overtax herself. In addition, assist with personal hygiene measures, including perineal care.

Alleviating Anxiety. The woman who develops endometritis typically has been discharged from the health care facility. She may become anxious and upset when readmission is necessary because now she will be separated from her newborn. Allow her to verbalize her feelings. Provide support and guidance as necessary. Enlist the aid of the woman's spouse or significant other and family to help in alleviating her anxiety.

If breast-feeding is allowed, encourage the woman to pump her breasts for feedings. Alternatively, the primary care provider may allow the baby to be brought in for feedings. If not, encourage the family to bring in pictures of the baby for the woman to keep in her room.

Providing Patient Teaching. Patient teaching is a major focus of nursing care. One key area of teaching is medication therapy, especially if the woman is to continue the therapy at home. Other areas to address include proper handwashing techniques; perineal care; expected changes in lochia; signs and symptoms of a recurrent infection; danger signs to notify the physician. Family Teaching Tips: Endometritis outlines the major discharge teaching points.

FAMILY TEACHING TIPS

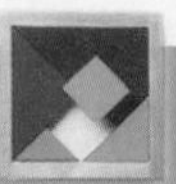

Endometritis

- Be sure to complete all of your antibiotics, even though you are feeling better.
- Call your care provider if you have any of the following symptoms of recurrent infection:
  - Temperature greater than 100.4°F (38°C)
  - Chills
  - Abdominal pain that does not go away with pain medication
  - Vaginal discharge that smells bad (like rotten meat)
- You should do the following things to prevent additional infection:
  - Wash your hands thoroughly before and after eating, using the restroom, or touching your vaginal area.
  - Wipe from front to back after using the restroom.
  - Remove soiled sanitary pads from front to back. Fold the pad so that the discharge is contained in the middle section of the pad, and then wrap it in toilet paper, or preferably a plastic bag. Dispose in the trash.
  - Wash hands before applying a new pad. Apply the pad from front to back. Do not touch the middle section of the pad. This part should remain very clean because it will be touching your vaginal area.
- You will heal faster and be less likely to get sick again if you do the following things:
  - Get at least 8 hours of sleep every night.
  - Rest frequently. Take a nap when the baby is napping.
  - Eat a nutritious diet.
  - Gradually increase your activity as you are able to tolerate it.
  - Drink plenty (1 to 2 liters) of fluids each day.
- Be sure to attend your scheduled follow-up visits with your primary care provider.

Wound Infection

Postpartal wound infections typically involve infections of the perineum that develop at the site of an episiotomy or laceration. Wound infection also can occur at the site of the abdominal incision after a cesarean birth. Perineal wound infections, although rare, commonly develop on the 3rd or 4th postpartum day. Factors increasing the risk of perineal wound infections include infected lochia, fecal contamination of the wound, and inadequate hygiene measures. In most cases, the infectious organism is normal vaginal flora.

Post-cesarean delivery incisional infections usually develop about the 4th postpartum day, often after the woman has developed endometritis. Although these infections most commonly are caused by contamination with vaginal flora, *Staphylococcus aureus* from the skin or another outside source has been identified as a cause in some cases.

Risk Factors

Risk factors for the development of a postpartum wound infection include:

- History of a chronic medical disorder, such as diabetes or hypertension
- Anemia or malnutrition
- Obesity
- Chorioamnionitis
- Immunosuppression, including treatment with corticosteroids
- Development of a hematoma
- Prolonged labor, rupture of membranes, or operative time
- Hemorrhage (Franzblau & Witt, 2002; Simpson & Creehan, 2001).

Clinical Manifestations

The woman with a perineal wound infection most likely will report pain out of proportion to what is expected. Inspection of the perineum reveals redness of the area and edema of the surrounding tissue. Separation of the wound edges may be noted. Often there is a foul-smelling, possibly purulent, vaginal drainage. The area will be tender on palpation. Fever and general malaise also may be present.

The woman experiencing an incisional infection after a cesarean birth often develops endometritis before the onset of the incisional infection. In this case, the woman continues to be febrile, even with antibiotic treatment. Inspection of the abdominal wound reveals erythema and induration (area of hardened tissue). In addition, the wound edges may be separated (Fig. 19-2). **Exudate** (drainage; fluid accumulation) may or may not be present, and the drainage may or may not be purulent. A small area of fluid collection may be noted near the incision. When opened, the area may ooze serosanguinous or purulent fluid (Franzblau & Witt, 2002). The area of the wound typically is warm and tender on palpation, and the woman reports pain.

Diagnosis

A complete blood count (CBC) with differential may reveal an elevation in WBC count. A culture of the area reveals the causative organism and guides treatment. Ultrasound may be used to determine if an abscess is present (Singhal & Zammit, 2002).

Additional laboratory studies may include serum protein, albumin, pre-albumin, and transferrin. These are done to assess nutritional status, which affects wound healing. Coagulation studies and a metabolic profile may be ordered (Stillman, 2002).

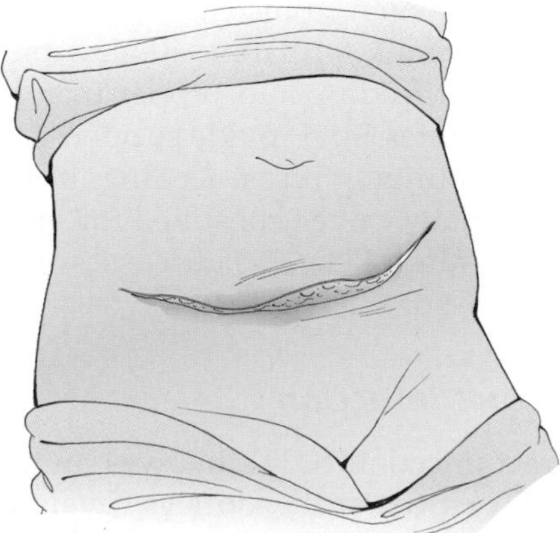

● ***Figure 19.2*** Postcesarean wound infection. A wound infection usually has an area of induration (raised and firm to palpation) surrounded by erythema. The wound may or may not be separated, as is shown in the illustration.

Treatment

Antibiotic therapy is indicated for treatment of the infection. For the woman with a perineal infection, therapy is supportive to include analgesics, local anesthetic sprays, warm compresses, and sitz baths. If an abscess develops, surgical incision and drainage are performed.

For the woman with an incisional infection, wound care, involving opening the wound for drainage (possibly requiring a trip to the operating room), irrigation, debridement, and possibly packing may be necessary. The goal is to clean the wound and promote granulation.

Nursing Care

For the woman with a perineal infection, provide warm compresses to the wound site and sitz baths to provide comfort. These measures also aid the healing process by increasing circulation to the area. Typically these are ordered for 20 minutes several times a day. When assisting with the application of warm compresses, be sure to adhere to standard precautions and perform handwashing.

Keeping the perineal area clean also is important. Encourage the woman to change her perineal pads and to perform perineal care frequently. Urge her to use a front-to-back motion when removing perineal pads and when cleaning the perineum after voiding and moving her bowels. Also remind her to wash her hands after performing any perineal care and using the bathroom. Although always important, thorough handwashing is absolutely essential when the woman is being cared for at home. Handwashing is critical to prevent transmitting the infection to the newborn.

For the woman with an incisional infection, wound care may be ordered. This may include dressing changes, irrigations, debridement, or possibly wound packing. Always use aseptic technique when performing wound care. With each dressing change or procedure, inspect the wound for signs and symptoms indicating resolution of the infection and evidence of healing. If necessary, record measurements of the wound to aid in evaluating progress. If wound care will need to be continued after discharge or if wound care is being provided in the home, teach the woman or another family member how to perform the care. She should also be able to detect signs and symptoms of increasing infection and know the signs that indicate the wound is healing. Have the person perform a return demonstration of any procedure.

Mastitis

Mastitis refers to an infection of the mammary gland (breast). This infection is most common in women who are breast-feeding for the first time. Typically, only one breast is affected. Although the infection can occur at any time when the woman is breast-feeding, it is most common during the 2nd and 3rd weeks after delivery.

Mastitis occurs when organisms are transferred from the woman's hands, staff's hands, or newborn's mouth to the breast and enter the breast tissue through a small, often microscopic, crack, fissure, or injured area on the nipple or breast tissue. Certain risk factors have been identified as contributing to the development of mastitis. These include

- Inadequate or incomplete breast emptying during feeding or lack of frequent feeding leading to milk stasis
- Engorgement
- Clogged milk ducts
- Cracked or bleeding nipples (Simpson & Creehan, 2001)

If left untreated, mastitis can progress to an abscess, which may require surgical drainage.

Clinical Manifestations

The woman with mastitis usually develops the infection after discharge, when she is at home. Common complaints include general flu-like symptoms that occur suddenly; such as fever, malaise, and possibly chills. In addition, the woman often reports tenderness, pain, and heaviness in her breast. Inspection reveals erythema and edema in an area on one breast but not the other (Fig. 19-3). The area is hard, warm, and tender on palpation. Purulent drainage may or may not be noted.

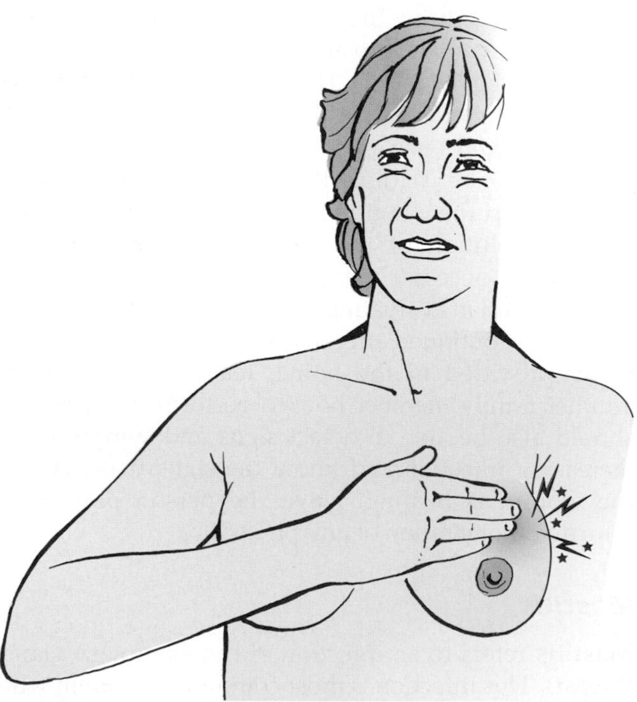

● ***Figure 19.3*** Mastitis. The woman with mastitis usually has a reddened, painful area on one breast that is warm to palpation.

Diagnosis

No specific tests are used to confirm the diagnosis of mastitis. Typically, the diagnosis is made based on the woman's signs and symptoms. A sample of breast milk may be sent for analysis, but the results fail to yield accurate and reliable data (Franzblau & Witt, 2002).

Treatment

Supportive care in conjunction with antibiotic therapy is used to treat mastitis. Penicillinase-resistant agents such as dicloxacillin (Dynapen) are the drugs of choice. Therapy usually is continued for 10 days. Analgesics may be prescribed for comfort.

Nursing Care

Nursing care focuses on resolving the infection and preventing further milk stasis. Preventing milk stasis is important for relieving the discomfort and preventing extension of the infection with possible abscess formation. Encourage the woman to breast-feed (unless contraindicated) every 1½ to 2 hours. Frequent feeding enhances complete emptying of the breast. If the woman is unable to breast-feed, for example because the affected breast is too sore or antibiotic therapy contraindicates breast-feeding, encourage the woman to manually express breast milk or use a breast pump to empty her breasts.

If the woman is breast-feeding, recommend the use of warm compresses or a warm shower before feeding to promote the let-down reflex and stimulate the flow of milk. Warm compresses also are soothing and increase blood flow to the area to stimulate healing. Suggest that the woman begin breast-feeding on the affected breast first, if possible. Doing so promotes the milk ejection reflex in the affected breast, thereby making complete emptying more efficient. Massaging the affected area over the breast during feeding also helps to ensure complete emptying.

As with any woman who is breast-feeding, encourage the woman to increase her fluid intake to ensure adequate milk formation. Review proper techniques for breast-feeding and proper infant positioning (refer to Chapter 14). Provide support and encouragement for continuing breast-feeding. If necessary, a lactation consultant can be consulted for specific assistance. Nursing Care Plan 19-1 discusses the care of a woman with mastitis.

Urinary Tract Infection

Urinary tract infection (UTI) involves an infection of the bladder (**cystitis**) or the kidneys (**pyelonephritis**). Anatomically, a woman's urethra is shorter than a man's urethra, thereby increasing the woman's risk for UTI. In addition, trauma during birth and inadequate bladder emptying may lead to urinary stasis

A PERSONAL GLIMPSE

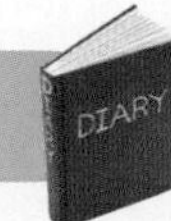

Breast-feeding my daughter was a challenge from the very beginning. She didn't want to latch on, she arched her back and cried, and she fussed at the breast. It took us several months to finally get a good pattern down. When she was about 6 months old, she and I were visiting my grandmother at the beach. One morning I woke up and felt awful. I had a hard, red spot on my breast and I felt hot and cold and exhausted. I took my temperature and it was 103°F. The only option I had was to go the emergency room. I knew it had to be mastitis, and the emergency room doctor verified this. All I wanted was the prescription for antibiotics so that I could get back to my daughter. While writing the prescription, the doctor said to me, "You know you should really stop breast-feeding." I must have looked at him rather strangely because he said, "The infection and the antibiotics aren't good for the baby." I did not want to stop nursing my daughter after all we had been through. As soon as I got home I called a friend who is a nurse. I told her what antibiotic I was taking, and she assured me that it was perfectly fine for me to continue breast-feeding my daughter. In fact, she told me that I should breast-feed frequently to help unclog the blocked milk duct in my breast. I was very relieved.

Jill

LEARNING OPPORTUNITY: Why is it important for breast-feeding to continue while the woman is being treated for mastitis? What can the nurse do to help a woman with mastitis continue breast-feeding?

intrapartally and postpartally, increasing the woman's risk for developing a UTI. Moreover, frequent vaginal examinations during delivery, urinary catheterizations, and delivery involving instrumentation further compound the risk.

Clinical Manifestations

The signs and symptoms exhibited by a woman with cystitis differ from those of a woman with pyelonephritis. Typically, those associated with pyelonephritis are more dramatic and severe. The woman with cystitis characteristically reports burning and pain on urination. She reports urgency and frequency and voids only small amounts at a time. The woman usually has a low-grade fever and possibly suprapubic pain.

In addition to burning, pain, urgency, and frequency, the woman with pyelonephritis presents with a high, spiking fever that rises and falls abruptly. Often she has shaking chills and reports nausea and vomiting. Flank pain and tenderness are common. In addition, tenderness at the costovertebral angle (the area on the back just above the waistline) is noted on palpation.

Diagnosis

A urinalysis and clean catch urine for culture and sensitivity are done to determine evidence of an infection. The urinalysis typically reveals white blood cells, protein, blood, and presence of bacteria. The clean catch urine specimen, considered diagnostic for UTI, reveals greater than 10^5 colony-forming units. In addition, a complete blood count may reveal an elevated white blood cell count.

Treatment

Antibiotic therapy is the treatment of choice based on the urine culture and sensitivity results. For the woman with cystitis, antibiotics are administered orally. For the woman with pyelonephritis, antibiotic therapy is ordered intravenously. Typically therapy begins with a broad-spectrum antibiotic and is later adjusted based on the urine culture and sensitivity reports.

In addition to antibiotic therapy, antipyretics and analgesics, such as acetaminophen (Tylenol); antispasmodics; urinary analgesics; such as phenazopyridine hydrochloride (Pyridium); and antiemetics may be ordered. Hydration and good perineal hygiene also are important.

Nursing Care

Nursing care focuses on promoting comfort, ensuring adequate hydration, and providing patient teaching. The woman with cystitis typically does not require admission to a health care facility for treatment. However, the woman with pyelonephritis usually is admitted for IV hydration and antibiotic therapy.

Providing Comfort. Providing comfort measures is important. The woman with a UTI typically has pain and burning on urination, which can make voiding difficult. In addition, this discomfort can prevent the woman from emptying her bladder completely, resulting in urinary stasis. Urinary stasis provides a good medium for organism growth, further compounding her risk for infection, and possibly increasing her risk for extension of the infection, for

Pay attention! If the woman is experiencing pain and burning on urination, she may be hesitant to drink the necessary amount of fluid, fearing that increasing fluid intake will increase the number of times she will need to void and thus increase her pain. Explain that a high urinary output often decreases the pain associated with UTI.

NURSING CARE PLAN 19.1

The Woman With Mastitis

CASE SCENARIO:
Jessica Thompson is a 22-year-old gravida 1 para 1, who delivered her baby vaginally 2 weeks ago. She is breast-feeding. She has just been readmitted to the postpartum ward of the hospital with a diagnosis of mastitis in the right breast. Her admitting vital signs are BP 128/70, T 101.2°F, P 106 bpm, R 22/minute. She says that she feels like she has the flu. She is very tired all the time, and her body aches all over. Assessment of her breast-feeding techniques indicates that the baby feeds better from the left breast, so Jessica usually starts with the left breast. Since her right breast began hurting 2 days ago, she has avoided using that breast to feed the baby because she says, "It just hurts too much." She also reports that sometimes the baby uses a pacifier between feedings. Jessica says that she isn't sure that she should keep breast-feeding because she is afraid that "the infection might hurt my baby." The physician has ordered clindamycin (Cleocin) 900 mg IV every 8 hours; acetaminophen (Tylenol) 1,000 mg PO every 4 to 6 hours PRN temperature greater than 100.4°F; ibuprofen (Motrin) 800 mg PO every 8 hours PRN pain.

NURSING DIAGNOSIS:
Hyperthermia related to inflammation secondary to infectious process as evidenced by T 101.2°F.

GOAL: Regulation of temperature.

EXPECTED OUTCOMES:
- Temperature will decrease to less than 100.4°F.
- Pulse rate will decrease to less than 100 bpm.
- Muscle aches will resolve.

NURSING INTERVENTIONS	*RATIONALE*
Monitor vital signs, including temperature every 4 hours until it has been less than 100.4°F for at least 24 hours.	Monitoring the vital signs will allow tracking of temperature spikes and overall response to therapy.
Monitor WBC, as ordered.	White blood cell count will begin decreasing as the infection resolves.
Administer the antipyretic, acetaminophen, as ordered.	Antipyretics control body temperature.
Administer antibiotic, clindamycin, as ordered.	Antibiotics will treat the infection that is causing the fever.
Place a pitcher of ice water at the bedside and refill it frequently, as needed. Offer juices, popsicles, and other liquids every 1 to 2 hours.	Temperature elevation can result in fluid loss. Also, adequate hydration is needed so that the body can effectively fight infection.

NURSING DIAGNOSIS
Ineffective Breast-feeding Pattern related to incomplete emptying of the right breast and pacifier use.

GOAL: Maintenance of effective breast-feeding.

EXPECTED OUTCOMES:
- Initiates breast-feeding on demand at least every 1.5 to 2 hours.
- Infant exhibits proper latch during breast-feeding.
- Empties both breasts regularly.

NURSING INTERVENTIONS	*RATIONALE*
Encourage Jessica to continue breast-feeding.	Breast-feeding with mastitis is safe for the baby. In fact, stopping breast-feeding does not help the woman recover and may cause her condition to get worse.
Request a consult with a lactation specialist.	A lactation specialist can evaluate the woman for subtle factors that may be interfering with the breast-feeding process and can help the baby to latch on well.

NURSING CARE PLAN 19.1 continued

The Woman With Mastitis

NURSING INTERVENTIONS	*RATIONALE*
Assist Jessica to breast-feed every 1.5 to 2 hours until symptoms begin to resolve.	Regular emptying of the breasts improves milk flow and decreases stasis, which can lead to blocked milk ducts and further infection.
Instruct Jessica to start on the right breast first, if she is able. If not, it may help to assist her to use a breast pump on the right breast while she is feeding on the left breast.	It is important that Jessica completely empty the affected breast at every feeding to increase milk flow and circulation to the area.
Instruct Jessica to gently massage the affected area (the lump that is warm and tender) as the breast is emptied (i.e., during breast-feeding or pumping).	Gentle massage is indicated to help unclog the clogged duct that is causing the problem.
Encourage rooming in with the infant, as long as someone can stay at the bedside with Jessica.	Rooming in allows for breast-feeding on demand, which is ideal. A competent adult must remain at the bedside to take responsibility for the baby, because the baby is not a patient. It is not appropriate for the patient to have responsibility for the infant until she is well enough to go home.
If the baby must go home at any time, assist Jessica to pump her breasts every 2 hours. The milk can be refrigerated for later consumption by the baby.	Pumping the breasts stimulates milk production, increased blood flow, and increased milk flow, all of which help decrease the symptoms of mastitis.
Discourage pacifier use.	Sucking on a pacifier or artificial nipple can decrease the amount that the infant suckles, thereby increasing the risk for milk stasis.

NURSING DIAGNOSIS
Acute Pain related to mastitis (particularly associated with breast-feeding).

GOAL: Tolerable pain levels

EXPECTED OUTCOMES:
- Verbalizes adequate relief from pain after interventions.
- Empties affected breast without undue pain.

NURSING INTERVENTIONS	*RATIONALE*
Administer ibuprofen, as ordered. In the first 24 to 48 hours, administer the medication around the clock versus PRN.	Ibuprofen usually provides excellent pain relief for the pain associated with mastitis. It also has anti-inflammatory properties, which further help reduce pain. Around-the-clock dosing prevents acute pain from becoming severe. Once pain becomes severe, it is more difficult to treat.
Assist Jessica to apply warm compresses or a heating pad to the affected breast. Alternatively, or additionally, encourage her to take warm showers.	Warmth helps to decrease pain and increases blood flow to the area, which increases milk flow.

NURSING DIAGNOSIS
Fatigue related to infectious process.

GOAL: Ability to perform self- and baby-care functions.

EXPECTED OUTCOMES:
- Verbalizes feeling rested.
- Reports increased energy levels.
- Performs self- and baby-care without complaints of fatigue.

(nursing care plan continues on page 464)

NURSING CARE PLAN 19.1 continued

The Woman With Mastitis

NURSING INTERVENTIONS	*RATIONALE*
Encourage frequent rest periods.	Promotes healing.
Encourage adequate nutrition.	Promotes healing and provides energy source.
Encourage wakefulness during the early evening hours. Discourage late afternoon naps.	Promotes sleep during the night, which provides the most restful sleep.
Encourage the use of bedtime rituals, preferably ones she uses at home.	Promotes sleep.
Limit visitors, as appropriate.	Reduces stimuli and allows for rest.
Reduce light and noise stimuli at bedtime.	Promotes sleep.
Encourage significant other to care for the baby (other than feedings) during the night.	Promotes periods of uninterrupted sleep.
Group nursing interventions and care activities.	Avoids unnecessary interruptions and promotes rest.

NURSING DIAGNOSIS
Deficient Knowledge: Self-care after discharge

GOAL: Demonstrates ability to care for self at home.

EXPECTED OUTCOMES:
- Washes hands before and after using the restroom, eating, touching the breasts.
- Answers questions accurately regarding self-care.
- Breast-feeds infant every 2 to 3 hours without prompting.

NURSING INTERVENTIONS	*RATIONALE*
Teach importance of handwashing. Encourage frequent handwashing at appropriate times.	Helps prevent the spread and recurrence of infection.
Encourage Jessica to continue breast-feeding as instructed (refer to breast-feeding guidelines above).	Proper breast-feeding techniques decrease the likelihood that mastitis will recur.
Instruct regarding early warning signs, which include • Breast engorgement • Nipple soreness or cracking • A painful lump in one breast, which is a sign of a plugged duct	If the woman initiates intervention at the first warning sign, she may be able to prevent a recurrence of mastitis.
If she has any of the warning symptoms, she should do the following • Rest in bed, if possible. • Breast-feed frequently from the affected breast. • Put a warm compress on the affected breast. • Gently massage lumpy areas while the infant is feeding. • Call her physician if she develops fever 100.4°F or above or if she does not get better within 24 hours.	These measures encourage the flow of milk; help prevent milk stasis; and prevent early mastitis from becoming more severe.

example, from the bladder to the kidneys. Therefore, assist the woman with comfort measures, such as running warm water over the perineum or using a sitz bath when voiding. In addition, administer analgesics such as acetaminophen (Tylenol) as ordered. A urinary analgesic (e.g., phenazopyridine hydrochloride [Pyridium]) is comforting, if ordered.

Promoting Adequate Hydration. Adequate hydration is necessary to dilute the bacterial concentration in the urine and aid in clearing the organisms from the urinary tract. Encourage the woman to drink at least 3,000 mL of fluid a day. Suggest she drink one glass per hour to ensure adequate intake and to keep a record of her intake.

Advise the woman to drink fluids that make the urine acidic, deterring organism growth. Fluids such as cranberry, plum, prune, or apricot juices are examples. Tell the woman to avoid carbonated beverages because they increase the alkalinity of urine, which promotes organism growth. If the woman has pyelonephritis, expect to administer fluids intravenously in addition to oral fluid to ensure adequate hydration.

Providing Patient Teaching. Patient teaching is essential for ensuring compliance with therapy and preventing a recurrence of cystitis or pyelonephritis. Instruct the woman to complete the full drug regimen, which can range from 5 to 10 days. Although the woman with pyelonephritis will receive antibiotic therapy intravenously, she probably will be switched to an oral form that will be continued after discharge (depending on her length of stay in the health care facility). If the woman is breast-feeding, provide instruction concerning the safety of her continuing to breast-feed based on the particular antibiotic she is taking. Other important patient teaching topics include hydration measures; comfort measures; perineal care; and preventive measures, including signs and symptoms of a recurrence.

Test Yourself

- List five risk factors for postpartum infection.
- Name five signs and symptoms of endometritis.
- Describe four clinical manifestations of postpartum wound infection.

THROMBOEMBOLIC DISORDERS

Thromboembolic disorders in the postpartum period typically involve three types:

- Superficial thrombophlebitis
- Deep vein thrombophlebitis
- Pulmonary embolism

Of these three, pulmonary embolism is the most serious and possibly fatal.

Risk Factors

The postpartal woman is at risk for thromboembolic disorders for three reasons: (1) Clotting factors that increased during pregnancy are still elevated, promoting blood clotting; (2) During pregnancy and birth, the fetal head exerted pressure on the veins of the lower extremity, causing them to dilate; and (3) The woman has spent a relative amount of time during labor and delivery being inactive or with her extremities placed in stirrups, leading to venous pooling and stasis. In addition, some women may have other factors that further increase their risk for thromboembolic disorders. These may include

- Varicose veins
- Past history of thrombophlebitis
- Obesity
- Smoking
- Age greater than 35 years
- History of three or more pregnancies
- Prolonged labor
- Use of forceps or cesarean birth

Superficial and Deep Vein Thrombophlebitis

Thrombophlebitis refers to an inflammation of the lining of the vein with the formation of clots. It can be categorized as superficial or deep vein. Superficial thrombophlebitis typically involves the saphenous veins of the lower extremities, usually affecting the calf area. Deep vein thrombophlebitis (DVT) usually affects the deeper veins of the calf, thigh, or pelvis. These deep veins carry the majority of venous return from the legs to the heart, making it a more serious condition than superficial thrombophlebitis.

Clinical Manifestations

In most cases, signs and symptoms of superficial thrombophlebitis develop within the first 3 postpartum days. The woman with deep vein thrombophlebitis may develop signs and symptoms during pregnancy or at any time during the postpartum period.

Typically the postpartum woman with superficial thrombophlebitis exhibits a tender, painful area along a vein in the calf, most commonly a varicose vein. On inspection the area is reddened and the vein is enlarged and highly visible. The area is warm and cordlike to the touch (Schreiber, 2002). The affected extremity may be swollen, and the woman may report pain when walking.

The woman with deep vein thrombophlebitis may have no symptoms. If the woman does exhibit signs, these typically include increased calf pain and tenderness. The leg is swollen visibly and, when circumference of the thigh and calf is measured, is larger than the other leg. Pedal edema also may be present. The area is warm, tender, and red. Homans' sign (pain on dorsiflexion of the foot) may be positive. Historically, a positive Homans' sign was indicative of deep vein thrombophlebitis. However, this is no longer considered a reliable sign because the pain may be attributable to muscle strain or contusion. In addition, the woman may exhibit indications of an arterial spasm, causing a decrease in circulation to the affected area. As a result, the leg may appear visibly pale or white, and pedal pulses may be diminished. Other signs and symptoms include chills, low-grade fever (usually not greater than 101°F [38.3°C]), malaise, stiffness of the affected leg, and pain on ambulation (Schreiber, 2002).

Diagnosis

Confirmation of superficial thrombophlebitis is based on the woman's signs and symptoms. For the woman with deep vein thrombophlebitis, the physician may order several diagnostic tests, such as Doppler ultrasonography or venography with a contrast medium, which reveals altered blood flow confirming the inflammation and blood clots.

Treatment

The primary goals of medical therapy are to prevent further thrombus formation and to prevent pulmonary embolism, a potentially fatal complication. Treatment for superficial thrombophlebitis includes analgesics, elevation of the affected extremity, bed rest, and local application of heat. Anticoagulant therapy such as Heparin or low-molecular-weight-heparin (enoxaparin [Lovenox]) may be ordered and is usually administered subcutaneously. Heparin is administered with caution in the postpartum period and usually is not given in the immediate postpartum period because of bleeding concerns. As the woman's condition improves, ambulation is encouraged.

For the woman with deep vein thrombophlebitis, treatment is similar to that for superficial thrombophlebitis, including analgesics, heat, bed rest, application of compression stockings, and elevation of the leg. In addition, anticoagulant therapy typically is ordered. Heparin is usually given intravenously by continuous infusion pump; enoxaparin (Lovenox) is given subcutaneously. After several days of heparin or enoxaparin therapy, the woman is started on oral anticoagulant therapy with warfarin (Coumadin). Heparin therapy is decreased gradually as the warfarin therapy reaches therapeutic levels. Oral anticoagulant therapy is continued for approximately 6 weeks.

Nursing Care

Nursing care for the woman with superficial thrombophlebitis and deep vein thrombophlebitis includes instituting bed rest; applying compression stockings, as ordered; and elevating the affected extremity to promote venous return. Inspect the lower extremities for changes in color, temperature, and size. Palpate pedal pulses and measure the circumference of each lower extremity and compare the results bilaterally to determine the degree of edema. Assist the woman to remove the compression stockings for an hour every 8 to 12 hours.

Apply warm compresses as ordered. When applying the compresses, ensure that they are at the proper temperature to avoid burning the woman. Because of altered blood flow, the woman's ability to sense temperature extremes may be diminished, placing her at risk for a burn injury. Also be sure that the weight of the compresses does not rest on the leg, causing a further compromise in blood flow. In addition, check the woman's bed linens and change them as necessary because the linens may become damp or wet from the moist heat applications. If possible, use a waterproof pad to protect the linens. Warm moist compresses can cool quickly. Provide the woman with extra blankets if necessary to prevent chilling. Also use chemical heat packs or a pad such as an Aquathermia pad to help keep the compresses warm.

For the woman with deep vein thrombophlebitis, it is important to monitor the woman's vital signs closely for slight elevations in temperature, possibly to 101°F (38.3°C), and report this finding to the physician. Because the woman with deep vein thrombophlebitis has an increased risk for developing a pulmonary embolism, be alert for and immediately report any sudden onset of breathing difficulties.

Consistency equals accuracy!

Use this guideline to measure swelling. Compare one extremity on the woman to the other when deciding if swelling is abnormal. Use an indelible pen to mark a line on the back of the leg at the largest part of the extremity to be measured. This line can be as small as 1 inch. At the same level, mark the other extremity. Use a paper tape to measure and record the circumference of both extremities. Compare these results to see if there is a difference. If you make this recording every 4 hours, it will be easy to see if the swelling is increasing or decreasing. The mark allows all nurses to measure at the same point.

Expect to administer anticoagulant therapy as ordered. When administering heparin, always have the antidote, protamine sulfate, readily available should the woman experience bleeding. Place the woman on bleeding precautions, which includes monitoring for evidence of bleeding, applying 5 to 10 minutes of pressure to injection or venipuncture sites, and avoiding unnecessary injections. Be sure to urge the woman to report any increase in vaginal bleeding, saturation of perineal pads or evidence of bruising, oozing at IV sites, or gingival bleeding.

The woman typically is discharged on oral anticoagulant therapy. Therefore, teach the woman about the drug and signs and symptoms to report immediately (Family Teaching Tips: Anticoagulant Therapy).

Pulmonary Embolism

Pulmonary embolism refers to a clot (thrombus) that breaks free from the vessel wall and travels to the heart and through the pulmonary circulation, where it becomes lodged and interrupts the blood flow to the

FAMILY TEACHING TIPS

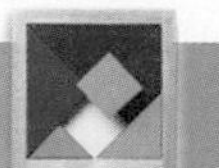

Anticoagulant Therapy

While you are on anticoagulant therapy, you are at risk for bleeding. Look for the following signs of bleeding:

- Bruising
- Bleeding gums
- Nosebleed
- Oozing from scratches and scrapes
- Blood in the urine
- Black or tarry stools
- Increased vaginal bleeding
- Notify the primary care provider of any change in level of consciousness, decreased ability to follow commands, or decreased sensation or ability to move extremities. These signs may indicate the presence of a cerebral bleed. This is an emergency that requires immediate intervention.

The following precautions will help prevent excessive bleeding:

- Use a soft toothbrush.
- Avoid use of razor blades (use an electric razor to shave).
- Avoid aspirin-containing products.
- Check with the primary care provider before taking any over-the-counter (OTC) medications.
- Notify your dentist and any other health care provider that you are on anticoagulant therapy.
- Apply pressure for 5 to 10 minutes after any injections or after blood is drawn or if you accidentally cut or scrape yourself.

Heparin and warfarin (Coumadin) are both considered safe for use in breast-feeding mothers (Anderson, 2002; Zimmerman, undated).

lungs. Thrombus formation occurs most commonly in the pelvic vein in postpartum women. If a large area of blood flow is compromised, cardiovascular collapse ultimately occurs, which can be fatal.

Pulmonary embolism is a complication that can result from deep vein thrombophlebitis. It also may result from superficial thrombophlebitis, but this is rare. Pulmonary embolism is the leading cause of maternal mortality.

Clinical Manifestations

The postpartum woman who develops a pulmonary embolism typically exhibits a sudden onset of dyspnea, pleuritic chest pain, and an impending sense of severe apprehension or doom. If the woman experiences any of these, report them immediately. In addition, the woman may be tachypneic, tachycardic, and hypotensive. She may have a cough with bloody sputum (hemoptysis) and report abdominal pain. Cyanosis and changes in level of consciousness also may occur.

Diagnosis

Arterial blood gases reveal a decrease in the partial pressure of oxygen and partial pressure of carbon dioxide. Ventilation/perfusion scan demonstrates a mismatching between lung tissue perfusion and ventilation, that is, a decrease in or absence of perfusion in lung areas that are being normally ventilated. Pulmonary angiography will reveal a defect in filling or an abrupt cessation of blood flow at the location of the embolus. A chest radiograph may show atelectasis, infiltrates, or pleural effusions, all of which suggest a pulmonary embolism.

Treatment

Development of a pulmonary embolism is considered a life-threatening emergency requiring immediate treatment. Administration of oxygen therapy via face mask and medication administration to treat the woman's symptoms are used. For example, if the woman is hypotensive, dopamine may be used to raise the woman's blood pressure. Heparin therapy is administered to prevent further clot formation. Thrombolytic agents may be administered to dissolve the existing clot.

Continuous monitoring via pulmonary artery catheterization and continuous electrocardiogram monitoring often are necessary. Because of the woman's critical status, she most likely will be transferred to the intensive care unit.

Nursing Care

Immediate action by the nurse is crucial for the woman who develops a pulmonary embolism. After assessing signs and symptoms of a pulmonary embolism, notify the physician at once and immediately raise the head of the bed to at least 45 degrees to facilitate breathing. Begin oxygen therapy at 8 to 10 liters per minute via face mask. Be prepared to assist with obtaining specimens for arterial blood gas analysis and prepare the woman for diagnostic testing. Monitor the woman's vital signs closely. Provide emotional support and explain all procedures and treatments to the woman, who is most likely apprehensive about what is happening. Prepare the woman for transfer to the intensive care unit.

Test Yourself

- What three factors put the postpartum woman at risk for thrombus formation?
- Name four nursing interventions appropriate for the woman with DVT.
- What symptoms are associated with pulmonary embolism?

POSTPARTUM PSYCHIATRIC DISORDERS

Three separate psychiatric conditions have been identified as occurring during the postpartum period. These include: postpartum blues (also known as "baby blues" or "maternity blues"); postpartum depression; and postpartum psychosis. Of these three conditions, postpartum blues is the most common and least serious. Research reveals that at least 50% of all postpartum women experience this transitory phase of sadness and crying. (See Chapter 12 for more discussion of this condition.)

Postpartum depression and postpartum psychosis are considered mood disorders involving one's view of life. Depression affects the woman's ability to function; however, her perception of reality remains intact. Conversely, the woman with postpartum psychosis experiences a severe distortion in her view of reality, often accompanied by hallucinations and delusions.

The exact cause of these disorders is unknown. Researchers believe that multiple factors are responsible for their development. These factors may include:

- Stress arising from the pregnancy and responsibilities associated with child rearing
- Sudden decrease in endorphins with labor and abrupt changes in hormonal levels (estrogen and progesterone) after delivery
- Low serum levels of free tryptophan (which are associated with the psychiatric diagnosis of major depression)
- Possible thyroid gland dysfunction

Regardless of the cause, the nurse plays a key role in teaching the woman about the signs and symptoms of each disorder and in early detection so that prompt treatment can be initiated.

Postpartum Depression

Postpartum depression is described as a mood disorder that involves a pervasive and sustained emotion in which the woman demonstrates a lack of interest or pleasure in usual activities. This disorder is believed to affect as many as 15% of new mothers. Some research provides evidence that this rate is even higher, possibly as high as 25% in women with multiple births and in those who deliver preterm newborns. In addition, as many as 50% of women with postpartum depression may go undiagnosed because of the stigma associated with mental illness (Beck, 2003).

Duration of the disorder is variable. Symptoms may begin at any time after delivery. Although the disorder may resolve within 3 to 6 months, research has revealed that approximately 25% of women will continue to experience depression after 1 year (Franzblau & Witt, 2002). Certain factors have been identified as possibly increasing a woman's risk for postpartum depression. These factors are highlighted in Box 19-2.

BOX 19.2 Risk Factors for Postpartum Depression

The following factors increase a woman's risk for developing postpartum depression:

- Episodes of depression or anxiety during the pregnancy at any trimester
- Stressful life events, such as loss of employment, change in family situation, serious illness, or loss of family member
- Problems in relationship with partner or spouse
- Inadequate or lack of social support from family, friends, or partner
- Anger at the pregnancy or an undesired pregnancy
- Personal history of depression before pregnancy or family history of psychological problems
- History of sexual abuse or intimate partner abuse

Clinical Manifestations

The woman with postpartum depression commonly demonstrates strong feelings of sadness and irritability. She is frequently tearful. She may have a lack of interest in her surroundings and have trouble motivating herself to do normal activities. She may show disinterest in others and a lack of enjoyment with life. Often intense feelings of inadequacy, inability to cope, ambivalence, guilt, and unworthiness are noted.

In conjunction with these signs and symptoms, the woman may report problems sleeping, loss of libido, decreased appetite, inability to concentrate, overwhelming fatigue, feelings of insecurity and loss of control, and obsessive thinking. In addition, the woman may contemplate harming herself (suicide) or the infant.

Diagnosis

Diagnosis is made on the basis of signs and symptoms, which must be present on most days for at least 2 weeks for the diagnosis to apply. The primary care provider usually screens the woman for hypothyroidism because this condition can cause symptoms of depression.

Treatment

Treatment for the woman with postpartum depression is usually accomplished on an outpatient basis, although severe cases may require hospitalization in a psychiatric facility. A trained mental health professional guides the treatment plan, which includes the woman's family. Antidepressant therapy may be prescribed. Agents such as selective serotonin reuptake inhibitors (SSRIs), including paroxetine (Paxil), fluoxetine (Prozac), and sertraline (Zoloft), are first-line drugs in the treatment of postpartum depression. Research demonstrates that these agents are safe for use in women who are breast-feeding. Electroconvulsive treatment (ECT), which has been shown to be effective for women with major depression, may be used for the woman with postpartum depression.

Nursing Care

Early detection and treatment are critical because the disorder can be totally disruptive of the woman's life and frequently interferes with interpersonal relationships. Therefore, all postpartum women and their families need information regarding the warning signs and symptoms. This teaching should be done as a part of routine postpartum discharge instructions. In fact, some states have mandated that every pregnant woman be given written information about postpartum depression along with a list of local resources as a part of prenatal care and again before discharge from the hospital after giving birth.

It is normal for the postpartum woman to be reluctant to verbalize any feelings of sadness or lack of enthusiasm about motherhood or child caring and rearing because of fear of rejection or feelings of guilt. Thus, the nurse plays a key role in dispelling the myth that happiness automatically occurs after the birth of a child.

Instruct the woman and her family that postpartum depression can occur at any time after delivery Therefore, the family needs to keep a listening ear to the woman's concerns. Instruct the family to be especially alert for complaints about problems sleeping, lack of energy or interest in daily activities, or fatigue out of proportion to the woman's status. It is especially important the woman understand that she should seek help immediately if she has thoughts of harming herself or her baby.

Once postpartum depression has been diagnosed, acknowledge any feelings that the woman expresses. Avoid statements that provide false reassurance or that discount the woman's feelings, such as, "Don't worry, you'll feel better soon," or "Your baby is so cute. You shouldn't feel so sad!" Assist the woman in obtaining support as necessary. Contact with others in a support group can help to alleviate feelings of isolation.

A PERSONAL GLIMPSE

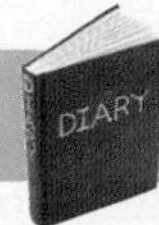

When I gave birth to our oldest daughter, my husband and I were living away from our families and friends. I remember bringing our daughter home from the hospital and feeling completely overwhelmed and anxious. Our daughter was fussy and didn't nurse well. I had no mother, sister, or girlfriend nearby to talk with or get advice from. My husband was calm and very supportive, but he worked full-time shift work. I remember feeling so lonely and depressed. I kept thinking that these feelings would go away after a few weeks. But they didn't. I wasn't eating or sleeping well, and I know I was miserable to be around. I felt completely inadequate as a mother. Finally, after 8 weeks of this my husband suggested we go see the doctor. Reluctantly, I made an appointment. When we first got to the doctor's office, the nurse sat down with us to ask us questions. When she asked why we were there, I started crying but managed to explain what I had been feeling since the birth of our daughter. She handed me some tissues and put her hand on my arm. She assured me that she and the doctor would work with me to help me feel better and return to my normal emotional state.

I am so glad that my husband suggested I get help. The doctor gave me a prescription for Paxil, and the nurse gave me all sorts of great suggestions, like joining a new mom support group and making sure that I got daily exercise. In just a few weeks, I felt so much better and now have much more confidence in my ability to be a mother to our daughter.

Lynne

LEARNING OPPORTUNITY: What clues did this woman give that indicate she was suffering from postpartum depression versus the "baby blues?" What specific actions can the nurse take to quickly recognize and provide support for the woman who has postpartum depression?

Postpartum Psychosis

Postpartum psychosis refers to a condition that usually occurs within the first 2 to 3 weeks after delivery, possibly as early as the 1st or 2nd day. With this disorder, the woman exhibits severe distortions of reality. This condition occurs in approximately 1 to 2 women for every 1,000 births (Beck, 2003; Simpson & Creehan, 2001). It is considered an emergency situation requiring immediate treatment. With treatment, postpartum psychosis generally spans 2 to 3 months.

Clinical Manifestations

Typically the woman with postpartum psychosis exhibits manifestations similar to those for any woman experiencing psychosis. Symptoms often associated with schizophrenia, bipolar disorder, or major depression may be noted. The woman with postpartum psychosis may demonstrate the following:

- Delusions that may cause her to believe that the infant is dead or defective

- Hallucinations, which may involve voices telling the woman to kill herself or her child
- Severe agitation, restlessness, or irritability
- Hyperactivity, euphoria, or little concern for self or infant (manic phase of bipolar disorder)
- Depression including preoccupation with guilt, feelings of worthlessness and isolation, extreme overconcern for the infant's health, and sleep disturbances
- Poor judgment and confusion

Because of the woman's misperception of reality, suicide and infanticide are possible.

Treatment

Postpartum psychosis is a psychiatric emergency requiring immediate treatment. Typically the woman requires hospitalization with treatment focusing on her specific symptoms. Medications such as antipsychotic agents and antidepressants are used. In addition, suicide precautions may be necessary. The woman's family should be involved in the treatment plan.

Nursing Care

The care of the woman with postpartum psychosis requires specialized psychiatric training beyond the scope of practice for the obstetric nurse. However, all nurses need to be aware of the signs and symptoms of postpartum psychosis so that early detection and prompt intervention can occur.

SPECIAL POSTPARTUM SITUATIONS

In addition to complications that can occur in the postpartum period, two other situations may require nursing intervention. These include grief and malattachment.

Grief in the Postpartal Period

Typically, the postpartum period is thought of as a happy time of celebrating the birth of a newborn. However, not all pregnancies conclude in a happy family taking home a healthy newborn. These situations may include the woman who is placing her newborn for adoption; the family faced with a newborn with congenital anomalies; and the family whose newborn (fetus) dies.

Grief is a universal process that is experienced uniquely by each individual. Grief is a natural response to a loss; whether the loss is the result of a choice, such as occurs with adoption; or when the situation is completely out of the individual's control, such as occurs when the newborn has a congenital anomaly or dies. Shock and disbelief are most frequently the first feelings experienced. The feeling of numbness or unreality may last hours, days, or weeks. Anger, even to the point of rage, bargaining, and depression are natural stages of the grieving process. It is normal for individuals to pass in and out of the stages several times as they work through their feelings. When the individual reaches the acceptance stage, healing has usually occurred.

Frequently men and women differ in their responses to grief. These differences can cause a rift between the woman and her spouse unless the couple receives intervention to help them work through the differences. Sometimes the woman will respond to feelings of sadness and guilt with tearfulness and isolation. The man may respond to these same feelings by throwing himself into his work. The woman may misperceive that her spouse "doesn't care" or isn't grieving. Counseling is frequently beneficial.

The Woman Placing the Newborn for Adoption

Giving the newborn up for adoption is a complicated and difficult choice facing some women. The woman often enters into a very somber period of grief and detachment. Each case is unique and must be handled as the circumstances develop. Sometimes she is emotional and needs to discuss the dreams and hopes that she is releasing with this decision. Sometimes circumstances are beyond her control, leading her to this decision. In all cases, the woman requires support, personal care, and comfort through the early postpartum period.

The woman who is placing her newborn for adoption requires nonjudgmental support. It is critical for you to be aware of your own attitudes about the situation to avoid the temptation to influence the outcome toward your beliefs. Be very aware that your role is to be an advocate for the woman, which involves keeping her informed of her rights and options and supporting her in whatever decision that she makes. It is also important for you to recognize that each state has laws that govern the rights of each party in the adoption process. Be knowledgeable of your institution's policies regarding handling of the adoption process.

The Family Whose Newborn Has Congenital Anomalies

Helping parents adjust to a newborn with congenital anomalies is a challenge for the postpartum nurse. Involving a newborn specialist very early in this situation is important because many anomalies can be corrected with early interventions and neonatal surgery. Despite early positive interventions, the family still experiences a measure of loss and grief for the normal newborn, the perfect son or daughter.

For the family with a newborn who has a congenital anomaly, encourage frequent interaction. Point out positive features of the newborn. Role model healthy behaviors by talking and playing with the baby as you would with any newborn. Give the parents information about the disorder or point them in the direction of resources that can assist them as they make treatment decisions, etc. When the family goes home, they may benefit by participation in a parent support group.

The Family Whose Newborn (Fetus) Has Died

Death often forces individuals to face core issues and personal values; it leaves emotions raw while people struggle for meaning. When a newborn or fetus dies, the parents are often totally unprepared to deal with their new reality. They frequently voice questions to which there are no good answers. Each person and family will respond to the situation in their own way.

Coping with death of the fetus or newborn can be stressful for the nurse, as well as the family. You may feel inadequate to help and be tempted to withdraw from the situation. In planning care for the family whose newborn or fetus has died, it is important to recognize your feelings so that you don't let your feelings interfere with your ability to care for the woman and her family. It may be helpful to talk through your feelings with a friend or co-worker. Do not let personal beliefs and values overshadow the family's beliefs and values. Allow the family to experience their own grief process; provide assistance and support to the family in ways that are meaningful and helpful to them.

Several measures can help provide meaning to the family during this difficult time. Grief is not a process of forgetting sad occasions. Rather, it is a process of remembering good things about the person who died. The baby who died is a part of a family and has a place with them. The family can name their newborn, even if it was stillborn. Memory items such as footprints and hand prints, a name record, blessing, and souvenir birth record identify this baby as a member of a particular family. Parents have identified photos of the newborn as a precious memory. Keep in mind that the photos must be comforting photos, that is, ones with the baby clothed, washed, and positioned comfortably. Allow the family or mother to assist with clothes, bathing, animal toys, or blankets. The more the family is involved, the more memories they will have when they recall this difficult time. Each family is unique in their beliefs regarding death and burial. For some, this will be a very quiet process; for others it will be emotional and surrounded by many friends and family. Follow the cues set by the family.

Malattachment in the Postpartal Period

The relationship of attachment begins when a women first finds out that she is pregnant. Through the prenatal visits, the information about the well-being of her baby reinforces this attachment. As she hears the heart beat, sees the baby's movements on ultrasound, and feels the movement inside her uterus, the woman begins to perceive this something inside her body as a "someone" other than herself. Preparations of the nursery and choosing names continue this bonding process.

Many things influence the degree of attachment. A stable relationship, good prenatal course, and positive anticipation of a healthy infant help a woman to begin an internal relationship with her baby before he or she is born. This enduring emotional bond between the baby and a primary caregiver is called attachment. Difficulties during the pregnancy, immaturity of the woman, or an unreliable support system puts the family at risk for **malattachment** or emotional distancing in the maternal–infant relationship. Pregnancies after a miscarriage or infant death often give rise to fears that interfere with normal attachment. Pregnancy complications or difficult relationships with the father of the baby can also adversely affect attachment. In addition, alcohol and drug abuse can contribute to malattachment and infant neglect.

Key signs of malattachment include lack of eye contact, lack of verbal stimulation, and a lack of response to the newborn's cries or cues. Other direct observations that show evidence of malattachment are listed in Table 19-2. If you observe any of these signs, report them to the RN. Lack of bonding between the mother and her newborn can be very serious if the woman is allowed to go home without proper support. Therefore, interventions include involving the whole family in the bonding and care of the infant. Discharge planning includes a predischarge consult with a clinical psychologist or clinical social worker to assess

CULTURAL SNAPSHOT

In the United States, fathers take a more active role in the direct care of their newborns shortly after birth. Families from different cultures may incorporate other relatives in newborn care. Be careful not to misinterpret lack of the father's involvement as malattachment. Family cultural beliefs may prescribe that only female members, such as the woman's sisters, mother, or mother-in-law, are allowed to handle the baby until the child is older. In some cultures, the woman is expected to remain secluded at home for approximately 4 to 6 weeks after delivery. Ask the family directly about who will be attending to the needs of the woman and infant once they go home.

TABLE 19.2 Comparing Attachment and Malattachment

Attachment	Malattachment
Uses endearments and pet names	Speaks of the newborn as an object; "it"
Speaks softly and uses "baby talk"	Makes no eye contact with the newborn
Calls newborn by name, often	Does not use the newborn's name
Becomes involved in routine care of diapering, bathing, and feeding	Shows disinterest in daily care and feeding of the newborn
Holds newborn close to body or in direct face-to-face contact	Places newborn in crib or lays newborn on lap facing away from mother
Responds to crying, smiling, feeding, and elimination with positive reinforcement	Ignores crying and newborn cue behaviors; reacts negatively to elimination needs
Easily calms upset newborn	Does not perceive newborn's needs; newborn is frustrated and nervous

support systems available for the mother. A referral for home care may be appropriate.

Test Yourself

- What signs indicate that the woman may be experiencing postpartum depression versus the "baby blues?"
- Name five stages of grief that individuals normally experience when faced with a loss.
- List three things the nurse can do to help a family cope with the birth of a newborn with a congenital anomaly.

KEY POINTS

- Hemorrhage, infection, thromboembolic disorders, and psychiatric disorders are conditions that put the postpartum woman at risk.
- Early postpartum hemorrhage occurs in the first 24 hours after birth and is most frequently caused by uterine atony. Late postpartum hemorrhage can occur anytime after the first 24 hours. Frequent causes are infection, subinvolution, and retained placental fragments.
- Nursing interventions for the woman with postpartum hemorrhage are focused on identifying the cause and stopping the bleeding. Establishing an IV line and frequent monitoring of vital signs and urinary output are critical actions. To determine the cause, assess the condition of the uterine fundus and characteristics of the lochia, and observe for shock and pain out of proportion with the observed blood loss, which may indicate concealed bleeding.
- Endometritis, infection of the uterine lining, is the most common postpartal infection. IV antibiotics are necessary for serious infections.
- Wound infection can involve the episiotomy or laceration or cesarean incision. Risk factors include chronic medical conditions, obesity, and any factor that decreases a woman's resistance. Antibiotic therapy and drainage of the wound may be required.
- Mastitis is a localized infection of breast tissue that is caused by milk stasis in a milk duct and infection with organisms that enter the breast through a crack or fissure in the nipple. Treatment involves antibiotics, emptying the breasts (preferably by breast-feeding), and warm compresses.
- Urinary tract infection (UTI) is the fourth type of infection that can complicate the postpartum period. Symptoms include frequency, urgency, and burning upon urination. Pyelonephritis is a more serious infection than cystitis because it involves the kidneys. Pyelonephritis is accompanied by high, intermittent fever with flank tenderness. Antibiotics are the therapy of choice.
- All postpartum women are at risk for thromboembolic disorders because of increased clotting factors that remain elevated after birth, exertion of the fetal head on the veins of the lower extremities during pregnancy, and the length of time in labor and delivery of being inactive or placed in stirrups, which can lead to stasis and pooling of blood in the extremities.
- The three psychiatric disorders that can affect the woman in the postpartum period include the postpartum blues, postpartum depression, and postpartum psychosis. Postpartum blues is temporary and self-limited tearfulness and blue mood. Depression is diagnosed if symptoms are interfering with the woman's ability to function in daily life for a period of 2 weeks or more. Psychosis occurs when the woman's perception of reality is distorted. Depression and psychosis require treatment by a mental health professional.
- The nurse's role is to support the woman who is grieving. Listen and be accepting of her feelings. Encourage the use of a support group and counseling for the couple. If the newborn dies, help

the family make memories by encouraging them to hold the baby and say goodbye, by taking pictures, and by giving them a memento box with clothes the baby wore or blankets, etc.

- Malattachment may be occurring if the woman does not interact with or hold her baby. If she turns away or doesn't talk to the baby or call him by name, she may be having problems with attachment. Notify the RN if you notice any of these symptoms.

REFERENCES AND SELECTED READINGS

Books and Journals

American College of Obstetricians and Gynecologists (ACOG). (1998). *Postpartum hemorrhage*. ACOG Technical Bulletin, 243. Washington, DC. Author.

Anderson, P. O. (2002). *Safety of commonly used drugs in nursing mothers*. UCSD Medical Center Department of Pharmacy. Retrieved April 25, 2004, from http://health.ucsd.edu/pharmacy/resources/breastfeeding.htm

Beck, C. T. (2003). Recognizing and screening for postpartum depression in mothers of NICU infants. *Advances in Neonatal Care, 3*(1), 37–46. Retrieved April 25, 2004, from http://www.medscape.com/viewarticle/450938

Chandran, L. (2003). Endometritis. In E. Alderman, R. Konop, W. Wolfram, P. D. Petry, & M. Strafford (Eds.), *eMedicine*. Retrieved April 23, 2004, from http://www.emedicine.com/ped/topic678.htm

Cheng, D. (2003). *Postpartum depression*. Focus on Women's Health Article: U.S. Department of Health and Human Services, Office on Women's Health. Retrieved April 24, 2004, from http://www.4woman.gov/HealthPro/healtharticle/

Cheng, D., & D'Agnati, D. D. (2002). *About postpartum depression*. State of Maryland, Department of Health and Mental Hygiene. Retrieved September 27, 2002, from http://mdpublichealth.org/womenshealth/pdf/postpartum_booklet.pdf

Cockey, C. D. (2003). Low-dose warfarin prevents clot recurrence. *AWHONN Lifelines, 7*(2), 106–108.

Cunningham, F. G., Gant, N. F., Leveno, K. J., Gilstrap, L. C. III, Hauth, J. C., & Wenstrom, K. D. (2001). *Williams obstetrics* (21st ed.). New York: McGraw-Hill Medical Publishing Division.

Depression After Delivery, Inc. (2001). *Postpartum psychosis*. Retrieved September 27, 2002, from http://www.depressionafterdelivery.com

Franzblau, N., & Witt, K. (2002). Normal and abnormal puerperium. In R. Levine, F. Talavera, G. F. Whitman-Elia, G. B. Gaupp, & L. P. Shulman (Eds.), *eMedicine*. Retrieved April 23, 2004, from http://emedicine.com/med/topic3240.htm

Hanna, B., Jarman, H., Savage, S., & Layton, K. (2004). The early detection of postpartum depression: Midwives and nurses trial a checklist. *JOGNN, 33*(2), 191–197.

Kennedy, E. (2003). Pregnancy, postpartum infections. In A. J. Sayah, F. Talavera, M. Zwanger, J. Halamka, & R. O'Connor (Eds.), *eMedicine*. Retrieved April 23, 2004, from http://www.emedicine.com/emerg/topic482.htm

Mandeville, L. K., & Troiano, N. H. (Eds.). (1999). *High-risk and critical care intrapartum nursing*. AWHONN publication (2nd ed.). Philadelphia: Lippincott Williams & Wilkins.

Maternal & Neonatal Health. (Undated). Preventing postpartum hemorrhage: Active management of the third stage of labor. *Maternal & Neonatal Health: Best Practices*. Retrieved September 1, 2002, from http://www.mnh.jhpiego.org/best/pphactmng.pdf

Mattson, S., & Smith, J. E. (Eds.). (2000). *Core curriculum for maternal–newborn nursing*. AWHONN publication (2nd ed.). Philadelphia: WB Saunders.

Roman, A. S., & Rebarber, A. (2003). Seven ways to control postpartum hemorrhage. *Contemporary OB/GYN, 48*(3), 34–53. Retrieved April 23, 2004, from http://www.medscape.com/viewarticle/451545

Schreiber, D. (2002). Deep vein thrombosis and thrombophlebitis. In F. Counselman, F. Talavera, G. Setnik, J. Halamka, & B. Brenner (Eds.), *eMedicine*. Retrieved April 24, 2004, from http://www.emedicine.com/emerg/topic122.htm

Simmons, G. T., & Bammel, B. (2001). Endometritis. In A. C. Sciscione, F. Talavera, A. V. Sison, F. B. Gaupp, & L. P. Shulman (Eds.), *eMedicine*. Retrieved April 23, 2004, from http://www.emedicine.com/med/topic676.htm

Simpson, K. R., & Creehan, P. A. (2001). *AWHONN Association of Women's Health, Obstetric and Neonatal Nurses: Perinatal Nursing*. Philadelphia: Lippincott Williams & Wilkins.

Singhal, H., & Zammit, C. (2002). Wound infection. In B. J. Daley, F. Talavera, A. L. Friedman, M. E. Zevitz, & J. Geibel (Eds.), *eMedicine*. Retrieved April 24, 2004, from http://www.emedicine.com/med/topic2422.htm

Stillman, R. M. (2002). Wound care. In B. J. Daley, F. Talavera, A. L. Friedman, M. E. Zevitz, & J. Geibel (Eds.), *eMedicine*. Retrieved April 24, 2004, from http://www.emedicine.com/med/topic2754.htm

Wainscott, M. P. (2003). Pregnancy, postpartum hemorrhage. In A. J. Sayah, F. Talavera, M. Zwanger, J. Halamka, & S. H. Plantz (Eds.), *eMedicine*. Retrieved April 23, 2004, from http://www.emedicine.com/emerg/topic481.htm

Yokoe, D. S., Christiansen, C. L., Johnson, R., Sands, K. E., Livingston, J., Shtatland, E. S., & Platt, R. (2001). Epidemiology of and surveillance for postpartum infections. *Emerging Infectious Diseases, 7*, 837–841. Retrieved April 23, 2004, from www.cdc.gov/ncidod/eid/vol7no5/pdf/yokoe.pdf

Zimmerman, D. (undated). *Medical care of the breastfeeding mother*. Retrieved April 24, 2004, from http://www.terem.com/abstracts40.htm

Websites

Postpartum Hemorrhage

http://www.babycenter.com/refcap/baby/physrecovery/1152328.html

http://pregnancy.about.com/cs/postpartumrecover/a/pph.htm

Postpartum Depression

http://www.nimh.nih.gov/publicat/depwomenknows.cfm

http://www.4woman.gov/faq/postpartum.pdf

WORKBOOK

NCLEX-STYLE REVIEW QUESTIONS

1. A woman is in for her postpartum checkup. She has a fever of 101°F and reports abdominal pain and a "bad smell" to her lochia. What diagnosis do you suspect?
   a. Mastitis
   b. Endometritis
   c. Subinvolution
   d. Episiotomy infection
2. The nurse enters the room of a woman who delivered 12 hours ago. The woman is leaning forward in bed and is obviously having difficulty breathing. The area around her mouth is blue. What should the nurse do first?
   a. Administer oxygen by nasal cannula.
   b. Obtain arterial blood for blood gas analysis.
   c. Raise the head of the bed.
   d. Tell the woman that she doesn't need to worry.
3. A woman delivered a healthy baby girl 2 days ago. Which observation by the nurse indicates the need for additional assessment and follow-up? The woman
   a. actively participates in the care of her baby.
   b. comments that her baby has red hair like her grandmother.
   c. reports that she will be happy to get home because she doesn't like hospital food.
   d. tells a friend, referring to her baby, "it just cries all the time."
4. When caring for a postpartum woman who exhibits a large amount of bleeding, which areas would the nurse need to assess before the woman ambulates?
   a. Attachment, lochia color, complete blood cell count
   b. Blood pressure, pulse, complaints of dizziness
   c. Degree of responsiveness, respiratory rate, fundus location
   d. Height, level of orientation, support systems

STUDY ACTIVITIES

1. Use the following table to compare superficial and deep vein thrombophlebitis.

	Superficial Thrombophlebitis	Deep Vein Thrombophlebitis
Clinical manifestations		
Diagnosis		
Treatment		
Nursing care		

2. Research the resources in your community for postpartum depression. How many of these are available at no charge to the woman? How can the woman find out about these resources? Share your findings with your clinical group.
3. Develop a teaching plan for young teenage mothers to help them decrease their chances for developing a postpartum infection.

CRITICAL THINKING: What Would You Do?

Apply your knowledge of postpartum complications to the following situation.

1. Josie is an outgoing 15-year-old girl who delivered a baby girl 24 hours ago. You walk in because you hear the newborn crying. Josie is talking to a friend on the telephone about the football game next week. When you check on the baby in the crib beside Josie's bed, the baby is jittery and red in the face.
   a. What is your impression of this situation? What ongoing assessments will you do to evaluate this situation?
   b. What do you need to do for the baby? Which individuals do you need to involve in the discharge planning process?
2. You just received Tiffany from the labor and delivery (L&D) unit after a normal delivery of a little girl. Her fundus is slightly firm, above the umbilicus, and positioned to the right. Her sanitary pad is full, but the L&D nurse reported that she received perineal care just before transport.

a. What is the likely source of the heavy lochia? What nursing interventions should be done?

b. If the fundus remains firm and in the midline, but a steady flow of lochia is noted despite fundal massage, what do you suspect is causing the problem? What nursing interventions should be done in this instance?

3. A woman who had a cesarean birth 3 days ago asks you to look at her incision, which is red and warm to touch with a small amount of yellow drainage along the edges.

a. What conclusions do you reach as a result of your assessment? What additional assessments should be made? What interventions are appropriate in this situation?

b. What if the woman reported hardness in an area of one of her breasts? How would you assess her breasts? What instructions would you give her?

The Newborn at Risk: Gestational and Acquired Disorders

20

STUDENT OBJECTIVES

On completion of this chapter, the student will be able to

1. Explain the various components of the gestational age assessment.
2. Classify the high-risk newborn by birth weight and gestational age while anticipating related problems.
3. Differentiate symmetric and asymmetric growth retardation in SGA infants.
4. Compare and contrast the characteristics of premature, full-term, and post-term newborns.
5. List possible contributing factors for preterm birth.
6. Identify five complications associated with preterm newborns.
7. List the characteristics of a post-term newborn.
8. Identify the major acquired disorders associated with newborns.
9. Describe the signs and symptoms commonly assessed in newborns with an acquired disorder, such as meconium aspiration syndrome.
10. Discuss the care needed for a newborn of a chemically dependent mother and one with a congenitally acquired infection.

KEY TERMS

apnea
appropriate for gestational age (AGA)
asphyxia
aspiration
Erb palsy
erythroblastosis fetalis
gestational age
hemolysis
hydramnios
hyperbilirubinemia
hypoglycemia
intrauterine growth restriction (IUGR)
intraventricular hemorrhage
kernicterus
large for gestational age (LGA)
lecithin
low birth weight (LBW)
macroglossia
macrosomia
meconium aspiration
necrotizing enterocolitis (NEC)
polycythemia
post-term
preterm
respiratory distress syndrome (RDS)
retinopathy of prematurity (ROP)
ruddy
small for gestational age (SGA)
surfactant
term
very low birth weight (VLBW)

The majority of newborns are born around 40 weeks' gestation weighing from 5.5 to 10 lb (2.5 to 4.6 kg) and measuring 18 inches to 23 inches (45 to 55 cm) in length. However, variations in **gestational age** (the length of time between fertilization of the egg and birth of the infant) and variations in birth weight occur. These variations increase the newborn's risk for perinatal problems. In addition, newborns also may develop problems at birth or soon after birth. These problems may be the result of conditions present in the woman during pregnancy or at the time of delivery, events occurring or factors present with delivery, or possibly the result of an unknown cause. Regardless, these acquired disorders also place the newborn at risk for serious health problems.

VARIATIONS IN SIZE AND GESTATIONAL AGE

Newborns may be classified based on their size or gestational age. When using size, the newborn's weight, length, and head circumference are considered. Size classifications include:

- **small for gestational age (SGA),** which is a newborn whose weight, length, and/or head circumference falls below the 10th percentile for gestational age;
- **appropriate for gestational age (AGA),** which is a newborn whose weight, length, and/or head circumference falls between the 10th and 90th percentiles for gestational age; and
- **large for gestational age (LGA),** which is an infant whose weight, length, and/or head circumference is above the 90th percentile for gestational age.

Two other classifications, based on weight, may be used to classify newborns by size. **Low birth-weight (LBW)** newborns are those who weigh less than 2,500 g. **Very low–birth-weight (VLBW)** newborns weigh less than 1,500 g.

Newborn classification based on gestational age includes:

- **preterm,** or premature, a newborn born at 37 weeks' gestation or less; commonly called premature
- **post-term,** or postmature, a newborn born at 42 weeks' or more gestation
- **term,** a newborn who is born between the beginning of week 38 and the end of week 41 of gestation.

A gestational age assessment is key to determining a newborn's classification.

GESTATIONAL AGE ASSESSMENT

Assessment of gestational age is a critical evaluation. The registered nurse (RN) is ultimately responsible for performing the gestational age assessment. However, the licensed vocational/practical nurse (LPN) should be familiar with the instruments used and be able to differentiate characteristics of the full-term newborn from those of the premature or post-term newborn. Although prenatal estimates, particularly the sonogram, are fairly accurate in determining gestational age, the most precise way to assess gestational age is through direct evaluation of the newborn. Several tools are available to assist the nurse in determining gestational age. The Newborn Maturity Rating and Classification developed by Ballard (Fig. 20-1) is a common gestational age assessment tool used in newborn nurseries. This tool is used as a basis for the discussion below.

Gestational age assessment typically involves the evaluation of two main categories of maturity: physical and neuromuscular maturity. Physical maturity can be assessed immediately after birth. Generally, the physical characteristics remain fairly constant and do not change rapidly with time. However, neuromuscular maturity, as evidenced by neuromuscular characteristics, can be influenced by several factors, such as medications given to the mother during labor and the time that has elapsed since birth. Therefore, it is best to do a gestational age assessment within the first few hours after birth. If the newborn is premature or postmature, it is important to have that information early on because his needs will differ from those of the term newborn.

Physical Maturity

Six categories are rated to determine physical maturity. These include:

1. Skin
2. Lanugo
3. Plantar creases
4. Breast buds
5. Ears
6. Genitals

Each category is rated on a scale of 0 to 5, with 5 being the highest or most completed development. Table 20-1 summarizes the gestational assessment findings in a term, premature, and postmature newborn.

Neuromuscular Maturity

Like physical maturity, six categories are rated. These categories are:

	0	1	2	3	4	5
SKIN	gelatinous red, transparent	smooth pink, visible veins	superficial peeling &/or rash, few veins	cracking pale area, rare veins	parchment, deep cracking, no vessels	leathery, cracked, wrinkled
LANUGO	none	abundant	thinning	bald areas	mostly bald	
PLANTAR CREASES	no crease	faint red marks	anterior transverse crease only	creases ant. 2/3	creases cover entire sole	
BREAST	barely percept.	flat areola, no bud	stippled areola, 1–2 mm bud	raised areola, 3–4 mm bud	full areola, 5–10 mm bud	
EAR	pinna flat, stays folded	sl. curved pinna, soft with slow recoil	well-curv. pinna, soft but ready recoil	formed & firm with instant recoil	thick cartilage, ear stiff	
GENITALS Male	scrotum empty, no rugae		testes descending, few rugae	testes down, good rugae	testes pendulous, deep rugae	
GENITALS Female	prominent clitoris & labia minora		majora & minora equally prominent	majora large, minora small	clitoris & minora completely covered	

A

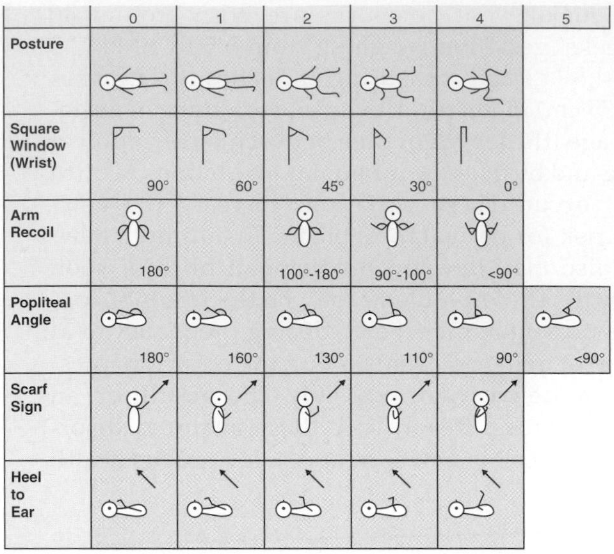

	0	1	2	3	4	5
Posture						
Square Window (Wrist)	90°	60°	45°	30°	0°	
Arm Recoil	180°		100°-180°	90°-100°	<90°	
Popliteal Angle	180°	160°	130°	110°	90°	<90°
Scarf Sign						
Heel to Ear						

B

Score	Wks
5	26
10	28
15	30
20	32
25	34
30	36
35	38
40	40
45	42
50	44

C

● ***Figure 20.1*** Ballard's assessment of gestational age criteria. (**A**) Physical maturity assessment criteria. (**B**) Neuromuscular maturity assessment criteria. *Posture*: With infant supine and quiet, score as follows: arms and legs extended = 0; slight or moderate flexion of hips and knees = 2; legs flexed and abducted, arms slightly flexed = 3; full flexion of arms and legs = 4. *Square Window*: Flex hand at the wrist. Exert pressure sufficient to get as much flexion as possible. The angle between hypothenar eminence and anterior aspect of forearm is measured and scored. Do not rotate wrist. *Arm Recoil*: With infant supine, fully flex forearm for 5 sec, then fully extend by pulling the hands and release. Score as follows: remain extended or random movements = 0; incomplete or partial flexion = 2; brisk return to full flexion = 4. *Popliteal Angle*: With infant supine and pelvis flat on examining surface, flex leg on thigh and fully flex thigh with one hand. With the other hand, extend leg and score the angle attained according to the chart. *Scarf Sign*: With infant supine, draw infant's hand across the neck and as far across the opposite shoulder as possible. Assistance to elbow is permissible by lifting it across the body. Score according to location of the elbow: elbow reaches opposite anterior axillary line = 0; elbow between opposite anterior axillary line and midline of the thorax = 1; elbow at midline of thorax = 2; elbow does not reach midline of thorax = 3; elbow at proximal axillary line = 4. *Heel to Ear*: With infant supine, hold infant's foot with one hand and move it as near to the head as possible without forcing it. Keep pelvis flat on examining surface. (**C**) Scoring for a Ballard assessment scale. The point total from assessment is compared to the left column. The matching number in the right column reveals the infant's age in gestation weeks. (From: Ballard, J. L. [1991]. New Ballard score expanded to include extremely premature infants. *Journal of Pediatrics, 119,* 417–423.)

1. Posture
2. Square window (measurement of wrist angle with flexion toward forearm until resistance is met)
3. Arm recoil (extension and release of arm after arm is completely flexed and held in position for approximately 5 seconds)
4. Popliteal angle (measurement of knee angle on flexion of thigh with extension of lower leg until resistance is met)
5. Scarf sign (arm pulled gently in front of and across top portion of body until resistance is met)
6. Heel to ear (movement of foot to near the head as possible)

Each category is rated on a scale of 0 to 5. See Table 20-1 for a summary of the findings associated with term, premature, and postmature newborns.

THE SMALL-FOR-GESTATIONAL-AGE NEWBORN

Small for gestational age (SGA) is a term used to describe a baby who is born smaller than the average size in weight for the number of weeks' gestation at the time of delivery. The criterion is that the SGA newborn's weight falls below the 10th percentile of that

TABLE 20.1 Comparing Gestational Age Assessment Findings

Assessment Parameter	Term Newborn	Preterm Newborn	Post-term Newborn
Physical Maturity			
Skin	Cracking of the skin and few visible veins	Very thin with little subcutaneous fat and easily visible veins	Leathery, cracked, and wrinkled
Lanugo	Thinning of lanugo with balding areas	Abundance of fine downy hair up to 34 weeks	Almost absent lanugo with many balding areas
Plantar creases	Creases covering at least the anterior 2/3 of foot	Smooth feet with few creases	Creases covering entire foot
Breast buds	Raised areola with 3- to 4-mm breast bud	Flat areola with little to no breast bud	Full areola with 5- to 10-mm breast bud
Ear	Cartilage present within pinna with ability for natural recoil when folded	Little cartilage, allowing shape to be maintained when folded	Cartilage thick; pinna stiff
Genitals	Male with pendulous scrotum covered with rugae; testicles descended	Male with smooth scrotum and undescended testicles	Male with pendulous scrotum with deep rugae
	Female with large labia major covering minora	Female with prominent clitoris; labia minora not covered by majora	Female with clitoris and labia minora completely covered by labia majora
Neuromuscular Maturity			
Posture	Flexed position with good muscle tone	Hypotonic with extension of the extremities	Full flexion of arms and legs
Square window	Flexible wrists with a small angle, usually ranging from 0 to 30 degrees	Angle greater than 45 degrees	Similar to that for term newborn
Arm recoil	Quick recoil with angle at elbow less than 90 degrees	Slowed recoil time with angle greater than 90 degrees	Similar to that for term newborn
Popliteal angle	Resistance to extension with knee angle 90 degrees or less	Decreased resistance to extension with large angle at knee	Similar to that for term newborn
Scarf sign	Increased resistance to movement with elbow unable to reach midline	Increased flexibility with elbow extending past midline	Similar to that for term newborn
Heel to ear	Moderate resistance to movement	Little to no resistance to movement	Similar to that for term newborn

which is expected. Gestationally, the newborn may be preterm, term, or post-term. It is preferred that the SGA baby is identified before birth, typically using the ultrasound method, allowing the health care team to determine anticipated treatment.

The SGA newborn usually appears physically and neurologically mature but is smaller in size than other infants of the same gestational age. These infants are often weak, unable to tolerate large feedings, and experience difficulty staying warm.

Although some SGA babies are small because their parents are small (genetics), most are small because of circumstances that occurred during the pregnancy, causing limited fetal growth. This condition is known as **intrauterine growth restriction (IUGR)**. It occurs when the fetus does not receive adequate amounts of oxygen and nutrients necessary for the proper growth and development of organs and tissues. IUGR can begin at any time during the pregnancy.

Contributing Factors

IUGR, the most common underlying condition leading to SGA newborns, results from interference in the supply of nutrients to the fetus. Lack of adequate maternal nutrition may be a contributing factor. As a result, the mother is unable to meet the increased nutritional demands of pregnancy. Thus, the fetus does not receive the necessary nutrients for growth. Another factor may involve an abnormality in the placenta or its function. The placenta may have become damaged, such as when the placenta separates prematurely, or a decrease in blood flow to the placenta reduces its ability to transport nutrients. Maternal conditions that interfere with adequate blood flow to the placenta, such as pregnancy-induced hypertension or uncontrolled diabetes, contribute to placental malfunction. In some situations, placental functioning may be normal, but the fetus is unable to use the nutrients being supplied, such as when the fetus develops an intrauterine infection.

If a mother smokes during pregnancy, the newborn's birth weight can be reduced by 200 grams. Maternal tobacco use is the most common preventable cause of IUGR.

Common factors leading to a restriction in growth rate associated with SGA newborns include:

- Chromosomal abnormalities
- Congenital defects
- Congenital infections
- Multiple gestations in which each fetus competes for supplied nutrients in the blood
- Maternal history of long-term problems, such as chronic kidney disease, high blood pressure, severe malnutrition or anemia, intrauterine infection, substance abuse, and cigarette smoking
- Fetal nutritional deficiencies
- Maternal complications during pregnancy, such as gestational diabetes, placental abruption or placenta previa, preeclampsia, or pregnancy-induced hypertension (PIH)

Characteristics of the SGA Newborn

Typically, SGA newborns experiencing IUGR are classified as symmetrically growth restricted or asymmetrically growth restricted, based on appearance.

Symmetrically Growth-Restricted Newborns

The symmetrically growth-restricted newborn accounts for 90% of IUGR newborns. These newborns have not grown at the expected rate for gestational age on standard growth charts. Generally, all three growth measurements (weight, length, and head circumference), when plotted on a standard growth chart, fall below the 10th percentile. Because there is prolonged limited growth in the size of organs affecting body growth, both head and body parts are in proportion but are below normal size for gestational age.

The newborn may appear active on inspection and demonstrate more developed neurologic responses because of a more advanced age in comparison to size. However, the newborn typically appears wasted with poor skin turgor. Sutures in the skull may be separated widely, and the abdomen may be sunken.

If the fetus experienced hypoxia early on in gestation and this hypoxia continued throughout the pregnancy, the newborn is at an increased risk for central nervous system (CNS) abnormalities and developmental delays.

Asymmetrically Growth-Restricted Newborns

The asymmetrically growth-restricted newborn has not grown at the expected rate for gestational age based on standard growth charts. When the three growth measurements (weight, length, and head circumference) are plotted on a standard growth chart, one of the measurements falls below the 10th percentile. Accounting for 10% of IUGR, these newborns typically are those with normal measurements for head circumference and length but demonstrate a comparatively low birth weight.

Asymmetrically growth-restricted newborns typically appear thin and pale with loose dry skin. They have a wasted, wide-eyed look, with a head that is disproportionately large when compared with body size. The umbilical cord appears thin and dull looking, compared with the shiny, plump cord of an AGA or LGA newborn.

Typically, these newborns demonstrate more developed organ systems, resulting in fewer neurologic complications and an improved survival rate when compared with newborns with symmetrical growth restriction. However, the newborn still may encounter many other risks and complications.

Potential Complications

Harsh conditions in utero can lead to a decrease in the amount of oxygen available to the fetus (hypoxia), causing the fetus to experience chronic fetal distress. Unable to meet the demands of normal labor and birth because of intrauterine fetal distress, the fetus will gasp in utero or with the first breaths at delivery, resulting in **aspiration** (when the baby breaths fluid into the lungs) of amniotic fluid or fluid containing the first stool called meconium.

The growth-restricted fetus is at increased risk for cesarean delivery because of fetal distress. Birth by cesarean predisposes the newborn to a respiratory distress condition called transient tachypnea of the newborn (TTN), which is caused by retained fetal lung fluid.

Because of the high demand for metabolic fuel and loss of brown fat used to survive in utero, coupled with the large ratio of body surface area to weight, the SGA newborn may experience thermoregulation problems (difficulty maintaining body temperature). As a result, the newborn may develop hypothermia. In addition, the newborn typically experiences **hypoglycemia** (low blood sugar) because of a high metabolic rate in response to heat loss and low glycogen stores. Hypoglycemia is the most common complication.

In response to chronic hypoxia in utero, red blood cell production increases, leading to **polycythemia** (excess number of red blood cells). Polycythemia also is caused by endocrine, metabolic, or chromosomal disorders of the SGA newborn and can occur with placental transfusion at the time of delivery.

Nursing Care

The care provider or RN is responsible for assessing gestational age and identifying potential complications. The LPN aids in carrying out the measures as identified in the plan of care for the SGA newborn at risk. Expect to perform routine newborn care with a focus on breathing and blood glucose patterns, thermoregulation, and parental interaction.

Review the maternal history and note any factors that might contribute to SGA. Estimate gestational age to determine SGA status and establish if IUGR is symmetric or asymmetric. Be alert for potential complications and risk factors of the newborn related to respiratory distress, hypothermia, hypoglycemia, polycythemia, and altered parental interaction with the newborn. Conduct and document routine nursing care with special emphasis on the following:

- Monitor respiratory status, including respiratory rate and pattern and observe for signs and symptoms of respiratory distress, such as cyanosis, nasal flaring, and expiratory grunting
- Provide measures to maintain skin temperature between 36.5°C and 37.0°C (97.7°F to 98.6°F)
- Monitor blood glucose levels to maintain levels >40 mg/dL
- Monitor results of other blood studies, such as hematocrit (<65%), hemoglobin (<22 g/dL), and bilirubin (<12 mg/dL)
- Observe feeding tolerance, including amounts taken and any difficulties or problems encountered, such as inability to suck at breast, fatigue, excessive spitting up, or diarrhea
- Monitor intake and output and daily weights
- Observe for jaundice
- Encourage parents to visit frequently and care for their infant

THE LARGE-FOR-GESTATIONAL AGE NEWBORN

A large-for-gestational age (LGA) newborn is one who is larger than the average baby. More precisely, an LGA newborn is one whose weight when plotted on a standard growth chart is above the 90th percentile. Typically the newborn weighs more than 4,000 grams. Generally, the newborn's overall body size is proportional, but both head and weight fall in the upper limits of intrauterine growth charts. Most LGA infants are genetically or nutritionally adequate. However, their size is misleading because development often is immature because of gestational age.

Some newborns are categorized as LGA incorrectly due to miscalculation of the date of conception. Therefore a thorough assessment of gestational age is essential to identify potential problems and requirements of these newborns.

Contributing Factors

In the majority of cases, the underlying cause of the large size of the LGA newborn is unknown. However, certain factors have been identified. Genetic factors may contribute to the development of large size in the newborn. For example, parents who are large have an increased tendency for a LGA newborn. Male newborns also are typically larger than female newborns. In addition, multiparous women have two to three times the number of LGA newborns than do primiparous women. The belief is that with each succeeding pregnancy, the fetus grows larger.

Congenital disorders also have been implicated. Beckwith's syndrome, a rare genetic disorder is associated with excessive intrauterine growth, causing hormonally induced excessive weight gain and **macroglossia** (abnormally large tongue), which can cause feeding difficulties. Transposition of the great vessels, a congenital heart disease, also is associated with LGA newborns. Other factors include umbilical abnormalities, such as omphalocele, hypoglycemia, and hyperinsulinemia of the newborn.

Maternal diabetes is the most widely known contributing factor. LGA newborns are frequently born to diabetic women with poor glucose control. Continued high blood glucose levels in the women lead to an increase in insulin production in the fetus. Increased insulin levels act as a fetal growth hormone, causing **macrosomia**, an unusually large newborn with a birth weight of greater than 4,500 grams (9 lbs 14 oz). After birth, the pancreas of the LGA newborn continues to produce high levels of insulin. However, the newborn is no longer exposed to the elevated glucose levels of the mother; therefore, the newborn's blood sugar falls leading to hypoglycemia.

Characteristics of the LGA Newborn

A newborn who is LGA typically demonstrates less motor skills ability and difficulty in regulating behavioral states (more difficult to arouse and maintain a quiet alert state). Commonly, a LGA newborn exhibits immaturity with reflex testing and possibly signs and symptoms of birth trauma, such as bruising or a broken clavicle. In addition, the newborn's skull may show evidence of molding, cephalohematoma, or caput succedaneum.

Potential Complications

Most commonly, LGA newborns develop complications associated with the increase in body size. This increased size is a leading cause of breech position and shoulder dystocia, which results in an increased incidence of birth injuries and trauma from a difficult extraction. Subsequent problems include fractured skull or clavicles; cervical or brachial plexus injury from peripheral nerve damage; and **Erb palsy** (a facial paralysis resulting from injury to the cervical nerves).

Trauma to the central nervous system can occur during birth. As a result, perfusion to the fetus is decreased. Oxygen and carbon dioxide exchange is diminished, ultimately resulting in **asphyxia** (severe hypoxia). CNS trauma also can interfere with the newborn's ability to maintain thermoregulation.

Frequently the LGA infant's head size diameter is disproportionately larger than the mother's pelvic outlet, creating cephalopelvic disproportion (CPD). As a result, cesarean delivery may be necessary. Subsequently, the LGA newborn is at risk for additional complications, such as those associated with effects of anesthesia. Other complications may include respiratory distress syndrome and transient tachypnea of the newborn.

Nursing Care

Identifying the newborn at risk for LGA is important for anticipating the plan of care. Carefully review the maternal history for any risk factors that would contribute to an LGA newborn. Note any prenatal ultrasound reports, such as fetal skull size measurement. Estimate gestational age to determine LGA status. Conduct and document routine nursing care with a special emphasis on the following:

- Monitor vital signs frequently, especially respiratory status for changes indicating respiratory distress
- Observe for signs and symptoms of hypoglycemia, including monitoring results of blood glucose levels
- Note any signs of birth trauma or injury
- Help parents verbalize feelings about any bruising or trauma they notice, including their fears of causing their newborn more pain
- Encourage parent–newborn bonding by providing interaction and support, such as showing how to arouse a sleepy newborn, console a fussy newborn, and offer feedings

Test Yourself

- What two major areas are evaluated with a gestational age assessment?
- What is the underlying factor commonly associated with most SGA newborns?
- LGA newborns are at an increased risk for what complications associated with their size?

THE PRETERM NEWBORN

At one time, prematurity was defined only on the basis of birth weight: any live infant weighing 2,500 g (5 lb 8 oz) or less at birth. Time proved this definition inadequate because some term infants weigh less than 2,500 g, and some premature infants weigh more than 2,500 g. The American Academy of Pediatrics advocates the use of the term "preterm": (premature) infant to mean any infant of less than 37 weeks' gestation.

Determining the gestational age of the preterm newborn is crucial. The Dubowitz scoring system was devised as an assessment tool based on external and neurologic development. Variations of the system are currently in use in many hospitals (see discussion of gestational age assessment and Figure 20-1 earlier in this chapter). The newborn is evaluated by the criteria on the chart, and the gestational age of the infant is calculated from the score. This assessment usually is performed within the first 24 hours of life and at least by the time the newborn is 42 hours old.

The preterm infant's untimely departure from the uterus may mean that various organs and systems are not sufficiently mature to adjust to extrauterine life. Often, small community hospitals or birthing centers are not equipped to care adequately for the preterm infant. When preterm delivery is expected, the woman often is taken to a facility with a neonatal intensive care unit (NICU) before delivery. However, if delivery occurs before the woman can be transported, transportation of the newborn may be necessary. Teams of specially trained personnel may come from the NICU to transport the neonate by ambulance, van, or helicopter. The newborn is transported in a self-contained, battery-powered unit that provides warmth and oxygen. Intravenous (IV) fluids, monitors, and other emergency equipment also may be used during the transport of the newborn.

Contributing Factors

The underlying cause of preterm birth, in most cases, is unknown. Despite development of medication to control preterm uterine activity, controlling preterm labor to prevent preterm delivery remains a problem.

Most often, preterm births result from a combination of factors, such as poor health habits and diet, inadequate living conditions, and overwork of the pregnant woman. Other contributing factors include low income, frequent pregnancies occurring in close succession, and maternal age extremes (younger than 20 years and older than 40 years).

One of the most common factors contributing to preterm delivery is premature rupture of membranes (PROM). This may be due to various underlying conditions, such as acute or chronic maternal infection or disease.

Multiple births are often preterm because of **hydramnios** (excessive amniotic fluid), a larger than average intrauterine mass, and/or early cervical dilation. Other factors related to the birth of preterm newborns involve the need for earlier delivery to ensure maternal or fetal well-being. These include eclampsia from pregnancy-induced hypertension, placenta previa, and abruptio placenta.

Preterm births also may result from emotional or physical trauma to the woman, such as when the woman requires nonobstetric-related surgery; habitual abortion or habitual premature birth; fetal infection, such as syphilis; and fetal malformations.

Characteristics of the Preterm Newborn

Compared with the term infant, the preterm infant is tiny, scrawny, and red. The extremities are thin, with little muscle or subcutaneous fat. The head and abdomen are disproportionately large, and the skin is thin, relatively translucent, and usually wrinkled. Veins of the abdomen and scalp are more visible. Lanugo is plentiful over the extremities, back, and shoulders. The ears have soft, minimal cartilage and thus are extremely pliable. The soft bones of the skull tend to flatten on the sides, and the ribs yield with each labored breath. Testes are undescended in the male; the labia and clitoris are prominent in the female. The soles of the feet and the palms of the hands have few creases (Fig. 20-2). Many of the typical newborn reflexes are weak or absent.

Complications of the Preterm Newborn

The preterm newborn's physiologic immaturity causes many difficulties involving virtually all body systems, the most critical of which is respiratory. Typically, respirations are shallow, rapid, and irregular, with periods of apnea (temporary interruption of the breathing impulse). Respirations may become so labored that the chest wall, perhaps even the sternum, is retracted.

Pediatricians and nursery staff should be alerted to the impending birth of a preterm infant so that equipment for resuscitation and emergency care is ready. If the birth occurs in a facility without a NICU, plans should be made to transport the newborn immediately after birth.

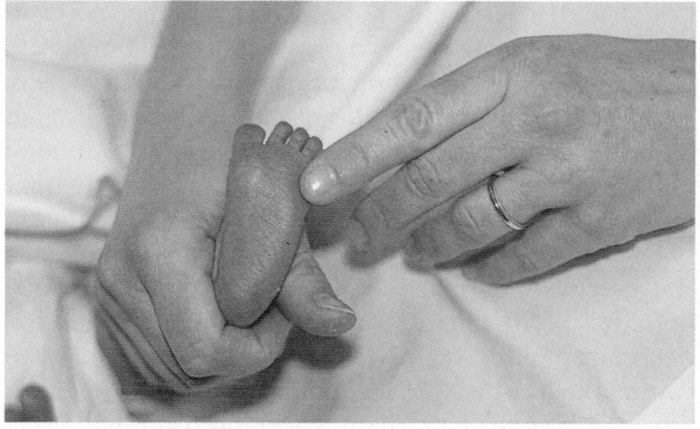
A

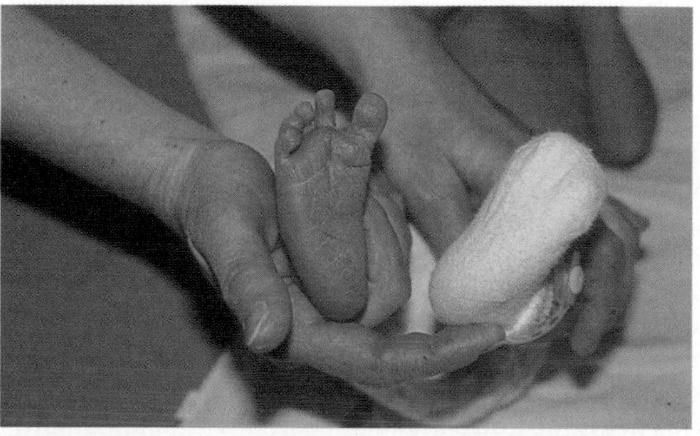
B

● ***Figure 20.2*** Sole creases in a preterm newborn (**A**) and a term newborn (**B**).

Respiratory Distress Syndrome

Respiratory distress syndrome (RDS), also known as hyaline membrane disease, occurs in about 50,000 of the 250,000 premature infants born in the United States each year. It occurs because the lungs are too immature to function properly. Normally, the lungs remain partially expanded after each breath because of a substance called **surfactant**, a biochemical compound that reduces surface tension inside the air sacs. The premature infant's lungs are deficient in surfactant and thus collapse after each breath, greatly reducing the infant's vital supply of oxygen. This damages the lung cells, and these damaged cells combine with other substances present in the lungs to form a fibrous substance called hyaline membrane. This membrane lines the alveoli and blocks gas exchange in the alveoli.

The preterm newborn with RDS may exhibit problems breathing immediately or a few hours after birth. Typically, respirations will be increased, usually greater than 60 breaths per minute. Nasal flaring and retractions may be noted. Mucous membranes may appear cyanotic. As respiratory distress progresses, the newborn exhibits see-saw like respirations in which the chest wall retracts and the abdomen protrudes on inspiration and then the sternum rises on expiration. Breathing becomes noticeably labored, the respiratory rate continues to increase, and expiratory grunting occurs. Breath sounds usually are diminished, and the newborn may develop periods of apnea.

If premature delivery is expected, an attempt may be made to prevent RDS. Through amniocentesis, the amount of **lecithin**, the major component of surfactant, may be measured to determine lung maturity. If insufficient lecithin is present 24 to 48 hours before delivery, the mother may be given a glucocorticosteroid drug (betamethasone) that crosses the placenta and causes the infant's lungs to produce surfactant. The infant begins to produce surfactant about 72 hours after birth; therefore, the critical time comes within these first several days. Infants who survive the first 4 days have a much improved chance of recovery unless other problems are overwhelming.

After birth, surfactant replacement therapy with synthetic or naturally occurring surfactant, obtained from animal sources or extracted from human amniotic fluid, has proved successful in the treatment of RDS. Surfactant is administered as an inhalant through a catheter inserted into an endotracheal tube, at or soon after birth. The therapy may be used as preventive treatment ("rescue") to avoid the development of RDS in the newborn at risk. Newborns with RDS usually receive additional oxygen through continuous positive airway pressure, using intubation or a plastic hood. This helps the lungs to remain partially expanded until they begin producing surfactant, usually within the first 5 days of life. The preterm newborn who develops RDS requires supportive care that focuses on measures to promote adequate oxygenation.

Intraventricular Hemorrhage

Intraventricular hemorrhage (IVH) is a complication of preterm birth that occurs more often in the newborn of less than 32 weeks' gestation. In addition to early gestational age, other factors commonly associated with IVH include birth asphyxia, low birth weight, respiratory distress, and hypotension. Ultrasonography, computed tomography, and magnetic resonance imaging can be used to determine if bleeding has occurred.

Signs of possible IVH include hypotonia, apnea, bradycardia, a full (or bulging) fontanelle, cyanosis, and increased head circumference. Neurologic signs such as twitching, convulsions, and stupor are also possible warning signs. However, mild bleeding can occur without these symptoms.

Preventing IVH focuses on avoiding situations that increase or cause fluctuations in the cerebral blood pressure. Appropriate measures include keeping the head and body in alignment when moving and turning the newborn (avoiding twisting the head at the neck), reducing procedures that cause crying (as a result of pain), and minimizing endotracheal suctioning. Any unnecessary disturbances of the newborn are to be avoided. In addition, analgesics may be administered to relieve or reduce discomfort and lessen the danger of increased intracranial blood pressure.

Cold Stress

All newborns are subject to heat loss, and maintaining thermoregulation is crucial. For the preterm newborn, thermoregulation is a major problem. The preterm newborn has a large body surface area when compared to the body weight, allowing for greater heat loss through evaporation, radiation, conduction, and convection. In addition, the preterm newborn has little subcutaneous fat to act as insulation. This in conjunction with the preterm newborn's immature muscular development interfering with the newborn's ability to keep his body flexed and to actively move about to generate heat. Moreover, the preterm newborn cannot shiver or sweat, mechanisms useful for generating and dissipating heat, respectively. Immaturity of the central nervous system and the lack of integrated reflex control of peripheral blood vessels (to cause vasodilation or vasoconstriction) also affect the preterm newborn's ability to maintain body temperature. Therefore, cold stress is a greater threat to the preterm newborn than it is to the term newborn. Cold stress may result in hypoxia, metabolic acidosis, and hypoglycemia. To prevent heat loss and to control other aspects of the premature infant's environment, an isolette or a radiant warmer is used (Fig. 20-3). The isolette has a clear Plexiglas top that allows a full view of the newborn from all aspects. The isolette

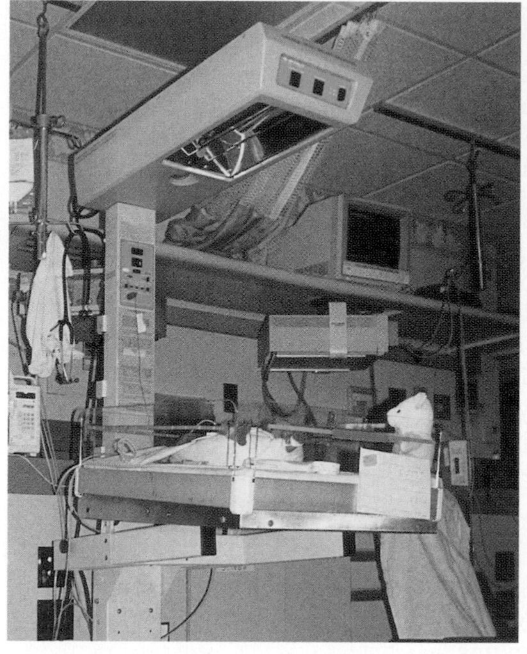

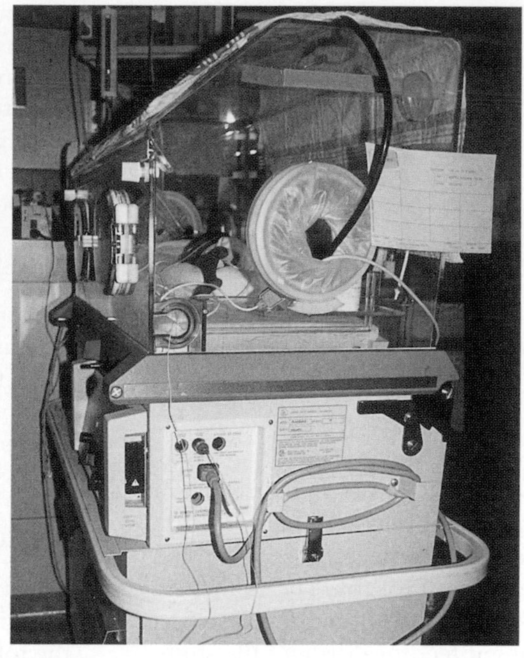

A B

● ***Figure 20.3*** Maintenance of thermoregulation. (**A**) Newborn under a radiant warmer. (**B**) Newborn in an isolette.

maintains ideal temperature, humidity, and oxygen concentrations and isolates the infant from infection. Portholes at the side allow access to the newborn with minimal temperature and oxygen loss. A heat-sensing probe attached to the newborn's skin controls the temperature of the isolette or the radiant warmer. Oxygen typically is administered. If oxygen is administered through an oxygen hood, it must be warmed and moisturized before it is administered.

Retinopathy of Prematurity

Retinopathy of prematurity (ROP) refers to a complication commonly associated with the preterm newborn. It results from the growth of abnormal immature retinal blood vessels. Preterm birth may be a factor contributing to this growth. In addition, the use of high concentrations of oxygen has been identified as a major cause. The immature blood vessels constrict when high levels of oxygen are given, depriving the retinal tissues of adequate nutrition. In addition, in some newborns capillaries increase, leading to scarring and eventually retinal detachment. These events lead to varying degrees of blindness.

Remember that usually the younger the preterm infant, the higher the probability of ROP.

ROP was once thought to be irreversible, but laser therapy and cryosurgery have been effective in reducing the degree of blindness. Laser treatment has proved more effective and less damaging to surrounding eye tissues than cryosurgery. Prevention of this complication is key by monitoring the preterm newborn's blood oxygen level and keeping it within normal limits. Levels greater than 100 mm Hg greatly increase the risk of ROP.

Necrotizing Enterocolitis

Necrotizing enterocolitis (NEC) is an acute inflammatory disease of the intestine. Although it may occur in full-term neonates, it most often occurs in small preterm newborns. The cause is not clearly defined. Precipitating factors are hypoxia, causing poor tissue perfusion to the bowel; bacterial invasion of the bowel; and feedings of formula, which provide material on which bacterial enzymes can work. Clinical manifestations include distention of the abdomen, return of more than 2 mL of undigested formula when the gastric contents are aspirated before a feeding, and occult blood in the stool. The newborn feeds poorly and may experience vomiting and periods of apnea. This disorder usually occurs within the first 10 days of life. Diagnosis is confirmed by abdominal radiographs. The infant with necrotizing enterocolitis is gravely ill and must be cared for in the NICU.

Initially, oral feedings are discontinued and nasogastric suction, IV fluids, and antibiotics are given. There is a danger that a necrotic area will rupture, causing peritonitis. A temporary colostomy may be needed to relieve the obstruction, and surgical removal of the necrotic bowel may be necessary.

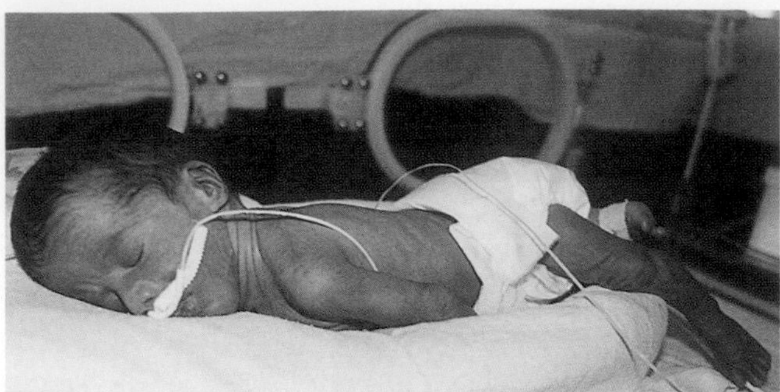

● ***Figure 20.4*** Typical resting posture of preterm newborn. Note the lax position and immature muscular development.

Other Complications

The preterm newborn desperately needs nourishment but has a digestive system that may be unprepared to receive and digest food. The stomach is small, with a capacity that may be less than 1 to 2 oz. The sphincters at either end of the stomach are immature, causing regurgitation or vomiting if feedings distend the stomach. The immature liver cannot manage all the bilirubin produced by **hemolysis** (destruction of red blood cells with the release of hemoglobin), making the infant prone to jaundice and high blood bilirubin levels **(hyperbilirubinemia)** that may result in brain damage.

The preterm infant does not receive enough antibodies from the mother and cannot produce them. This characteristic makes the infant particularly vulnerable to infection.

Muscle weakness in the premature infant contributes to nutritional and respiratory problems and to a posture distinct from that of the term infant (Fig. 20-4). The infant may not be able to change positions and is prone to fatigue and exhaustion, even from eating and breathing. Skilled, gentle intensive care is needed for the newborn to survive and develop. The parents also need supportive, intensive care.

Test Yourself

- When is a newborn classified as preterm?
- What is observed on the hands and feet of a preterm newborn?
- Which complication associated with preterm newborns is due to a surfactant deficiency?

● Nursing Process for the Preterm Newborn

The physical condition of a preterm newborn demands the skilled assessment and planning of nursing care, emphasizing maintenance of adequate oxygenation, continuous electronic cardiac and respiratory monitoring, frequent manual monitoring of vital signs, thermoregulation, infection control, hydration, provision of adequate nutrition and sensory stimulation for the newborn, and emotional support for the parents.

ASSESSMENT

Although assessment of the preterm newborn is similar to that for any newborn, the initial assessment focuses on the status of the respiratory, circulatory, and neurologic systems to determine the immediate needs of the infant. Box 20-1 highlights the assessment findings of a preterm newborn.

SELECTED NURSING DIAGNOSES

Based on the initial assessment, some of the nursing diagnoses that may be appropriate include the following:

- Ineffective Breathing Pattern related to an immature respiratory system

A PERSONAL GLIMPSE

My son was born 8.5 weeks before his expected due date. I was unable to hold him until 12 hours after his birth. I was discharged from the hospital with a Polaroid snapshot of him and the phone number of the hospital's neonatal intensive care unit.

For 2 weeks I visited him, learning new medical terms and gaining an understanding of all the obstacles he would have to overcome before being released. These days were an emotional roller coaster filled with feelings of joy over being blessed with a son; enormous concern over his condition; and a great deal of guilt. The thing I wanted most in the world was to take him home, healthy and without the IVs, equipment, monitors, and the hard hospital chairs. When I left him each day, I was leaving a part of myself, and I felt as though I would not be whole until he was home with me.

Looking back, I so appreciated that the staff was optimistic when informing me of things, but not overly so. Unmet expectations can be devastating! There is not a moment that I am not thankful for my son and his health and not a night that I don't sleep better after I have checked on him sleeping in bed.

Kerry

LEARNING OPPORTUNITY: Give specific examples of what the nurse could do to support this mother and help decrease her fears and anxieties.

BOX 20.1 Assessment Findings of a Preterm Newborn

- Skin: Usually thin, translucent to gelatinous with vessels easily seen, becoming loose and wrinkled after a few days. Generalized edema and ecchymosis (typically from birth trauma to presenting parts) are normally seen, along with a small amount of vernix caseosa and subcutaneous fat (for insulation to maintain heat) and inadequate stores of brown fat. Lanugo is characteristically present on sides of face, extremities, and back with thin and fine hair on head and eyebrows and soft and thin nails.
- Color: Ranging from pink or dark red (**ruddy**) to acrocyanosis, a bluish discoloration of the palms of the hands and soles of the feet. (This condition is considered normal immediately after birth but should not persist longer than 48 hours.) Generalized cyanosis is possible because of the preterm newborn's ill state; jaundice may be seen by day 2 to day 8.
- Behavior/activity level: Incapable of moving smoothly from one state or level of alertness to another to control his environmental input. The preterm newborn maintains a hypersensitive/hyperalertness; may have a feeble or even absent cry and show an exaggerated response to unpleasant stimuli. Typically, the preterm newborn shows less spontaneous activity than a term newborn; will become lethargic with onset of illness; agitation may be revealed by vital signs such as an increased heart rate and blood pressure, an increase or decrease in respiratory rate, or decreased oxygen saturation levels.
- Muscle tone: Characteristically weak, leaving a flaccid and open resting position and allowing for increased heat loss of body temperature, as well as an increased inability to control his behavioral state.
- Breasts: Engorgement rarely seen. Nipples and areola are usually not easily noted.
- Head: Large in proportion to body size; bones of the skull are soft, with overriding sutures and small fontanels, leaving a narrow, flattened appearance to head and face.
- Eyes: Small and sometimes fused; eyelids may become edematous after treatment.
- Ears: Soft, flat, and small with little cartilage, allowing for the pinna to bend and fold, leading to potential injury to ear.
- Nose: Small with visible milia; breathing predominately through nose; nasal flaring indicative of respiratory distress.
- Chest: Weak musculoskeletal structure; lung auscultation typically wet and noisy; heart beat rapid and difficult to hear over lung sounds. Apnea common.
- Abdomen: Full and soft with a weak muscle tone, allowing for visible bowel loops and marked abdominal distention.
- Genitalia: In female, labia minora and clitoris prominent because the labia majora are underdeveloped; in male, small scrotum and, frequently, undescended testes.

- Ineffective Thermoregulation related to immaturity and transition to extrauterine life
- Risk for Infection related to an immature immune system and environmental factors
- Risk for Imbalanced Nutrition, Less Than Body Requirements related to an inability to suck
- Risk for Impaired Skin Integrity related to urinary excretion of bilirubin and exposure to phototherapy light
- Activity Intolerance related to poor oxygenation and weakness
- Risk for Disorganized Infant Behavior related to prematurity and excess environmental stimuli
- Parental Anxiety related to a seriously ill newborn with an unpredictable prognosis
- Risk for Impaired Parenting related to separation from the newborn and difficulty accepting loss of ideal newborn
- Interrupted Family Processes related to the effect of prolonged hospitalization on the family

OUTCOME IDENTIFICATION AND PLANNING

The major goals for the preterm newborn include improving respiratory function, maintaining body temperature, preventing infection, maintaining adequate nutrition, preserving skin integrity, conserving energy, and promoting sensory stimulation. Goals for the family include reducing anxiety and improving parenting skills and family functioning. The premature newborn is cared for by highly skilled nurses in an NICU. Nursing care is planned and implemented to address each of the goals identified.

IMPLEMENTATION

Improving Respiratory Function

Not all preterm newborns need extra oxygen, but many do. Isolettes are made with oxygen inlets and humidifiers for raising the oxygen concentration inside from 20% to 21% (room air) to a higher percentage. In addition, a clear plastic hood placed over the infant's head supplies humidified oxygen at the concentration desired. Oxygen saturation of the blood may be monitored by pulse oximetry, or the oxygen and carbon dioxide levels may be measured by transcutaneous monitoring. Both of these methods help establish the desirable oxygen concentration in the newborn. In the absence of pathologic lung changes, it is safer to keep the oxygen concentration lower than 40%, unless hypoxia is documented.

Observing the preterm newborn's respirations is obviously of utmost importance. Also monitor the pulse rate and note skin color, muscle tone, alertness, and activity.

Measure the rate of respiration and identify retractions to help determine proper oxygen concentrations. Ensure that oxygen support or ventilator settings and placement of an endotracheal (ET) tube, if ordered, is as prescribed to ensure adequacy of ventilation and respiration assistance. Repositioning the newborn every 2 hours helps to reduce the risk for pneumonia and atelectasis. Frequent suctioning may be necessary to prevent airway obstruction, hypoxia, and asphyxiation. If not contraindicated, elevate the head of the bed as needed to maintain a patent airway.

Observe for changes in respiratory effort, rate, depth, breath sounds, and regularity of respirations. Note any expiratory grunting or chest retractions (substernal, suprasternal, intercostal, subcostal), including severity, and nasal flaring to determine the newborn's ability to maintain respirations.

One of the most hazardous characteristics of the preterm newborn is the tendency to stop breathing periodically (**apnea**). The hypoxia caused by this apnea and general respiratory difficulty may lead to mental retardation or other neurologic problems.

Electronic apnea alarms are used routinely. Electrodes are placed across the infant's chest with leads to the apnea monitor, providing a continuous reading of the respiratory rate. Visual and audio alarms may be set to alert the nurse when the rate goes too high or too low or if the infant waits too long to take a breath.

It is a nursing responsibility to place, check, and replace the leads on the newborn. Each day, remove electrodes and reapply them in a slightly different location to protect the infant's sensitive skin from being damaged by the electrode paste and adhesive. Cleanse the skin carefully between applications of the electrodes. Many false alarms are the result of leads that have come loose. Some of these false alarms may be prevented by using a small amount of electrode paste and being careful to keep the paste inside the circle of adhesive on the electrode.

Respiratory assistance may be used to handle apnea. Usually, gentle stimulation, such as wiggling a foot, is enough to remind the newborn to breathe. However, sometimes respirations need to be assisted by a bag and mask. Every nursery nurse should know how to "bag" an infant. The principles of this form of assisted respiration are similar to those of mouth-to-mouth rescue breathing:

1. Slightly extend the neck to open the airway.
2. Cover the infant's mouth and nose with the mask. Maintain a tight seal between the mask and the infant's face.
3. Quickly but gently squeeze the small bag filled with oxygen or air. The quantity of air needed is relatively small, and the pressure is gentle to prevent damage to the immature lungs.

Promote rest times between procedures because organized care helps to conserve the newborn's energy and reduce oxygen consumption. Supportive medications may be ordered to stimulate the central respiratory chemoreceptors, relax bronchial smooth muscle, and stimulate the CNS to increase respiratory skeletal activity.

Maintaining Body Temperature

The preterm newborn's body temperature must be monitored closely and continuously. Monitors that record temperature, pulse, respirations, and blood pressure; transcutaneous oxygen and carbon dioxide monitors; and pulse oximeters (monitors used to measure oxygen saturation) are all routinely used in the NICU. However, close observation by a nurse who is regularly assigned to the same newborn remains an essential part of the infant's care. Observe the monitoring and life-support equipment, making sure it is functioning properly, and systematically assess the infant. Time assessment and other procedures so that the infant is disturbed as little as possible to conserve energy. In addition, be sure to expose as little of the newborn's skin as possible during procedures to minimize heat loss.

Observe for signs of cold stress, such as low temperature, body cold to touch, pallor, and lethargy. The preterm newborn has weak muscle tone and activity. Therefore, leaving the newborn in an extended posture decreases heat conservation. Be aware of and avoid heat loss via the following mechanisms:

- Evaporation, such as through wet skin during bathing
- Conduction, such as when lying on a cold surface such as a scale for weighing
- Radiation, such as when the newborn is exposed to but not in contact with surfaces, for example, isolette walls near a window

- Convection, such as when the newborn is exposed to drafts

Most isolettes have a control system for temperature regulation. Attach a temperature-sensitive electrode to the infant's abdomen and connect it to the isolette thermostat. The unit may then be set to turn the heater on and off according to the infant's skin temperature. Open units with overhead radiant warmers allow maximum access to the infant when sophisticated equipment or frequent manipulation for treatment and assessment is necessary. The temperature remains more constant than in the closed unit, which is constantly having the door or portholes opened and the atmosphere breached.

The preterm newborn must not be overheated because this causes increased consumption of oxygen and calories, possibly jeopardizing the newborn's status. Use clothing, a head covering (such as a stockinette cap), and blankets when removing the newborn from the warm environment of the isolette or radiant warmer for feeding or cuddling. It is still standard practice to take and record axillary temperatures when the infant is being warmed by either of these methods.

Although monitoring equipment provides a continual reading of the heart rate, take apical pulses periodically, listening to the heart through the chest using a stethoscope for 1 full minute so as not to miss an irregularity in rhythm. Observations should include rate, rhythm, and strength. The pulse rate is normally rapid (120 to 140 beats per minute [bpm]) and unstable. Premature newborns are subject to dangerous periods of bradycardia (as low as 60 to 80 bpm) and tachycardia (as high as 160 to 200 bpm). The nurse's observations of the pulse rate, rhythm, and strength are essential to determining how the infant is tolerating treatments, activity, feedings, and the temperature and oxygen concentration of the isolette.

Preventing Infection

Infection control is an urgent concern in the care of the preterm newborn. The preterm infant cannot resist bacterial invasions, so the caregivers must provide an atmosphere that protects him or her from such attacks. The primary means of preventing infection is handwashing. All persons who come in contact with the newborn must practice good handwashing immediately before touching the newborn and when moving from one newborn to another. Handwashing is the most important aspect of infection control.

Other important aspects of good housekeeping include regular cleaning or changing of humidifier water, IV tubing, and suction, respiratory, and monitoring equipment. The NICU is separate from the normal newborn nursery and usually has its own staff. This separation helps eliminate sources of infection. Personnel in this area usually wear scrub suits or gowns. Personnel from other departments (radiology, respiratory therapy, or laboratory) put a cover gown over their uniforms while working with these newborns.

Observe the newborn frequently for signs and symptoms of infection including:

- Temperature instability (decrease or increase)
- Glucose instability and metabolic acidosis
- Poor sucking
- Vomiting
- Diarrhea
- Abdominal distention
- Apnea
- Respiratory distress and cyanosis
- Hepatosplenomegaly
- Jaundice
- Skin mottling
- Lethargy
- Hypotonia
- Seizures

Close observation allows for successful intervention if infection occurs. Obtain diagnostic laboratory work as ordered and report results that indicate the source and treatment of infection. Routine laboratory tests used to diagnose and treat infections include blood cultures, cerebral spinal fluid analysis, urine tests, tracheal aspirate culture, and superficial cultures. Expect antibiotics to be ordered to treat suspected or confirmed bacterial infections.

Maintaining Adequate Nutrition

When born, a preterm newborn may be too weak to suck or may not yet have developed adequate sucking and swallowing reflexes. Commonly, the preterm newborn has poorly coordinated suck, swallow, and gag reflexes, leading to possible aspiration; a limited stomach capacity, contributing to distention and inadequate intake; poor muscle tone of the cardiac sphincter, leading to regurgitation and secondary apnea and bradycardia; and finally, muscle weakness, which leads to exhaustion. In addition, preterm newborns do not tolerate carbohydrates and fats well.

For several hours or even 1 day, the preterm newborn may be able to manage without fluids, but soon IV fluids will be necessary. In many instances, an IV "life line" is established immediately after delivery. Fluids are infused through a catheter passed into the umbilical vein in the stub of the umbilical cord if it is still fresh. Intravenous fluids may be given through other veins, particularly the peripheral veins of the hands or feet. Extremely small amounts of fluid are needed, perhaps as little as 5 to 10 mL/hour or even less. They may be measured accurately and administered at a steady rate by using an infusion pump. Keep accurate, complete records of IV fluids and frequently observe for infiltration or overhydration.

Measure and record all urinary output by weighing the diapers before and after they are used. Urine volume is normally 35 to 40 mL/kg per 24 hours during the first few days, increasing to 50 to 100 mL. Also observe and record the number of urinations, the color of the urine, and edema. Edema changes the loose, wrinkled skin to tight, shiny skin.

At first, some preterm newborns receive all their fluid, electrolyte, vitamin, and calorie needs by the IV route; others can start with a nipple and bottle. Special nipples and smaller bottles may be used to prevent too much formula from flowing into the newborn's mouth.

Premature newborns are likely to have problems with aspiration because the gag reflex does not develop until about the 32nd to 34th week of gestation. As a result, gavage feedings may be necessary. The frequency and quantity of gavage feedings are individualized. Usually, feedings are given every 2 hours. Extending the feeding time too long may tire the infant (Fig. 20-5).

Typically a feeding should be completed in less than 30 minutes. If the stomach is not empty by the next feeding, allow more time between feedings or give smaller feedings. Usually, the quantity given is just as much as the infant can tolerate and is increased milliliter by milliliter as quickly as tolerated. Commonly amounts as small as 5 to 10 mL per feeding are given. Special preterm newborn nursers are available. These nursers are calibrated in 1-mL markings.

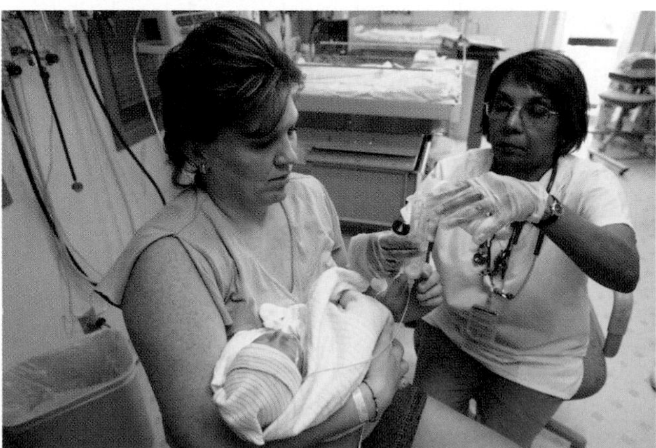

● ***Figure 20.5*** The nurse helps the caregiver administer a gavage feeding to her premature infant.

The feeding is too large if the newborn's stomach becomes so distended that it causes respiratory difficulty, vomiting, or regurgitation and if there is formula left in the stomach by the next feeding.

Breast milk, the preferred source of nutrition for the preterm newborn, is thought to be higher in protein, sodium, chloride, and immunoglobulin A than is the breast milk of mothers of term infants. Mothers can pump their breast milk and freeze it to use for bottle or gavage feedings until the preterm newborn is strong enough to breastfeed. The use of her own milk to nourish her newborn is a tremendous boost to the emotional satisfaction of the mother.

The most common premature infant formula has 13 calories/oz (often called half-strength formula). A formula with 20 calories/oz (the usual strength for newborns) also may be used. If the formula is too rich (too high in carbohydrates and fats), vomiting and diarrhea may occur. If the infant does not gain weight after the initial postnatal weight loss, the formula may be too low in calories.

When a preterm newborn who is being gavage fed begins to suck vigorously on the fingers, hands, pacifier, or gavage tubing and demonstrates evidence of a gag reflex, nipple feeding should be tried. The infant who can take the same quantity of formula by nipple that was tolerated by gavage feeding without becoming too tired is ready. Alternating gavage and nipple feedings may be necessary in some cases to assist the preterm newborn in making the transition. The nipple for a preterm newborn usually is made of softer rubber than the regular nipple. It is also smaller, but no shorter, than the regular nipple.

Burp preterm newborns often during and after feedings. Sometimes simply changing the infant's position is enough assistance; at other times, it may help to gently rub or pat the infant's back. Throughout feedings, be careful to prevent aspiration. Hold the infant for the feeding, keeping oxygen available as needed. After a feeding, the best position for the preterm newborn is probably on his or her right side, with the head of the mattress slightly elevated.

Other feeding methods can be used if neither gavage nor nipple feeding is tolerated and if IV fluids are inadequate. Some preterm newborns do better if fed with a rubber-tipped medicine dropper. Others may require gastrostomy feedings. The preterm newborn who is not receiving nipple feedings should be given nonnutritive sucking opportunities, such as a pacifier.

Weigh the preterm newborn daily. These daily weights give an indication of overall health and indicate whether enough calories are being consumed. The physicians and parents probably will want to know the infant's current weight each day. Weigh the newborn with the same clothing, using the same scale at the same time each day to help ensure accurate, comparable data.

Preserving Skin Integrity

Assess skin integrity frequently but at least every shift for changes in color, turgor, texture, vascularity, and signs of irritation or infection. Pay special attention to areas in which equipment is attached or inserted. Frequent skin assessment allows for early detection and prompt intervention. A preterm newborn's skin is extremely fragile and can be injured easily. Reposition the preterm newborn every 2 to 4 hours and PRN as necessary. Handle the preterm newborn gently when repositioning. If the preterm newborn is placed on the back, make sure that aspiration does not occur. Preterm infants have a knack for wriggling into corners and cracks from which they cannot extract themselves, so close observation is necessary.

Changing the diaper as soon as possible after soiling will maintain clean and dry skin. Keep the skin clean and dry but avoid excessive bathing, which furthers dries the skin. Pad pressure prone areas by using sheep skin blankets, waterbeds, pillows, or egg crate mattresses to help prevent additional skin breakdown to these areas. In addition monitor intake and output and avoid dehydration and over hydration.

Apply creams and ointments and medication as prescribed for relief of itching, infections, and to prevent breakdown. Be sure to record the use of any special equipment or procedures.

Promoting Energy Conservation and Sensory Stimulation

The preterm newborn uses the most energy to breathe and pump blood. Plan the newborn's day to avoid exhaustion from constant handling and movement. In addition, help conserve the preterm newborn's energy by eliminating regular bathing and giving only "face and fanny" care as needed. Preterm newborns usually are dressed in only a diaper, if anything, to conserve energy, provide more freedom of movement, and allow a better opportunity to observe the infant. However, do not be misled into ignoring or avoiding the newborn or discouraging the contact essential to establishing a normal relationship.

The environment of the NICU, with its lights, noises, frequent handling, and invasive procedures can be overwhelming to the preterm newborn's immature central nervous system. Overstimulation can be as much of a problem as lack of stimulation. Therefore, assist with measures to balance the amount of stimulation the newborn receives. Speak gently and softly and minimize the amount of handling. If the preterm newborn is in an isolette, avoid tapping on the sides and opening and closing the portholes too frequently to reduce the amount of noise in the newborn's environment.

Older preterm infants have a special need for sensory stimulation. Mobiles hung over the isolette and toys placed in or on the infant unit may provide visual stimulation. A radio with the volume turned low, a music box, or a wind-up toy in the isolette may provide auditory stimulation. An excellent form of auditory stimulation comes from the voices of the infant's family, physicians, and nurses talking and singing. Being bathed, held, cuddled, and fondled provides needed tactile stimulation. Contact is essential to the infant and the family. Some NICUs have "foster grandparents" who regularly visit long-term NICU infants and provide them with sensory stimulation, cuddling, loving, crooning, and talking. These programs have proven beneficial to both the infants and the volunteer grandparents.

Reducing Parental Anxiety

Birth of a preterm newborn creates a crisis for the family caregivers. Often their long-awaited baby is whisked away from them, sometimes to a distant neonatal center, and hooked up to a maze of machines. Parents feel anxiety, guilt, fear, depression, and perhaps anger. They cannot share the early, sensitive attachment period. It may take weeks to establish touch and eye contact, ordinarily achieved in 10 minutes with a term infant. Parents often leave the hospital empty-handed, without the perfect, healthy infant of their dreams. How can they learn to know and love the strange, scrawny creature that now lives in that plastic box? These feelings are normal, but studies have shown that if these feelings are not expressed and resolved, they can damage the long-term relationship of parents and child, even resulting in child neglect or abuse.

The mother's condition also must be considered. If the infant was delivered by cesarean birth, or if the labor was difficult or prolonged, she may feel abandoned or too weak to become involved with the baby.

Nurses who work with high-risk infants can do much to help families cope with the crisis of prematurity and early separation. To ease some of the apprehension of the family caregivers, transport teams prepare the newborn for transportation, then take the newborn in the transport incubator into the mother's room so that the parents may see (and touch, if possible) the newborn before the child is whisked away. In many cases, instant photos provide the family some concrete reminder of the newborn until they can visit in person.

Explain what is happening to the newborn in the NICU and periodically report on his or her condition (by phone if the NICU is not in the same hospital) to reassure the family that the child is receiving excellent care and that they are being kept informed. Listen to the family and encourage them to express their feelings and support one another. As soon as possible, the family should see, touch, and help care for the newborn. Most NICUs do not restrict visiting hours for parents or support persons, and they encourage families to visit often, whenever it is convenient for them. Many hospitals offer 24-hour phone privileges to families so that they are never out of touch with their newborn's caregivers.

Improving Parenting Skills and Family Functioning

Before the mother is discharged from the hospital, plans are made for both parents and other support persons to visit the preterm newborn and to participate in the care. They need to feel that the newborn belongs to them, not to the hospital. To help foster this feeling and strengthen the attachment, work closely with families to help them progress toward successful parenthood. Siblings should be included in the visits to see the preterm newborn (Fig. 20-6). The monitors, warmers, ventilators, and other equipment may be frightening to siblings and family caregivers. Make the family feel welcome and comfortable when they visit. A primary nurse assigned to care for the infant gives the family a constant person to contact, increasing their feelings of confidence in the care the newborn is receiving.

Support groups of families who have experienced the crisis that a preterm newborn causes are of great value to the families. Members of these support groups can visit the families in the hospital and at home, helping the parents and other family members to deal with their feelings and solve the problems that may arise when the infant is ready to come home or if the infant does not survive.

As the time for discharge of the infant nears, the family is understandably apprehensive. The NICU nurses must teach the parents and support persons the skills they need to care for the infant. This knowledge gives them confidence that they can take care of the infant. Some hospitals allow caregivers to stay overnight before the infant's discharge so that they can participate in around-the-clock care. The knowledge that they can telephone the physician and nurse at any time after discharge to have questions answered is reassuring.

Before discharge, most preterm newborns will have successfully made the transition from isolette to open crib, thriving without artificial support systems. In addition to feeding, bathing, and general care of the infant, many families of premature newborns need to learn infant cardiopulmonary resuscitation and the use of an apnea monitor before the infant is discharged (Fig. 20-7). Some preterm infants are being sent home with oxygen, gastrostomy feeding tubes, and many other kinds of sophisticated equipment. This helps place the infant in the home much earlier, but it requires intensive training and support of the family members who care for the infant.

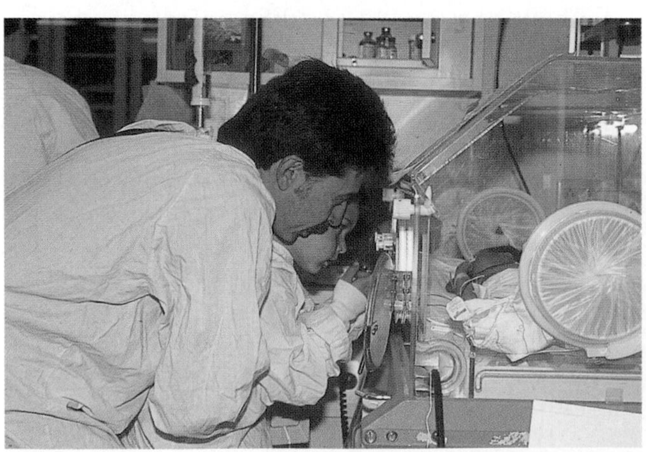

● ***Figure 20.6*** Encouraging sibling interaction with the preterm newborn.

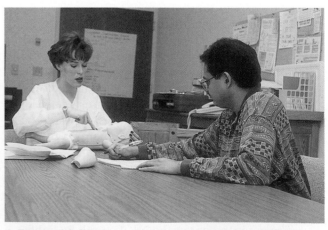

● ***Figure 20.7*** Teaching a parent how to perform CPR before discharge.

After the baby goes home, a nurse, usually a community health nurse, visits the family to check on the health of the mother and the baby. The nurse provides additional support and teaching about the infant's care, if necessary, and answers any questions the family might have.

EVALUATION: GOALS AND EXPECTED OUTCOMES

Evaluation of the preterm newborn is an ongoing process that demands continual readjustment of the nursing diagnoses, planning, and implementation. Goals and expected outcomes include:

- **Goal:** The preterm newborn's respiratory function will improve.
  Expected Outcomes: Respiratory rate remains less than 60 bpm; no grunting or retractions evidenced; breath sounds clear; oxygen saturation level greater than 95%; symmetrical chest expansion; no episodes of apnea.
- **Goal:** The preterm newborn's temperature will remain stable.
  Expected Outcome: Temperature is maintained at 97.7°F to 98.6°F (36.5°C to 37.0°C).
- **Goal:** The infant will remain free of infection.
  Expected Outcome: Signs of infection are not noted, as evidenced by vital signs within normal limits; breath sounds clear; and skin intact.
- **Goal:** The preterm newborn's nutritional status will remain adequate.
  Expected Outcomes: The infant ingests increased amounts of oral nutrition and gains weight daily; skin turgor improves.
- **Goal:** The preterm newborn will remain free of skin breakdown.
  Expected Outcome: The newborn's skin is intact and free of redness, rashes, and irritation.
- **Goal:** The preterm newborn will show improved tolerance to activity.
  Expected Outcomes: Vital signs remain stable and skin color remains pink during activity; supplemental oxygen is required in decreasing amounts until no longer necessary.
- **Goal:** The preterm newborn demonstrates appropriate behavior in response to stimulation.
  Expected Outcome: The newborn responds appropriately to stimuli cues.
- **Goal:** The parents demonstrate a reduction in anxiety level.
  Expected Outcome: Parents and family caregivers express feelings and anxieties concerning the newborn's condition, visit and establish a relationship; demonstrate interaction with the newborn, holding and helping to provide care.
- **Goal:** Parents demonstrate appropriate parenting skills.
  Expected Outcomes: Parents and family caregivers learn how to care for the newborn in the hospital and at home; parents hold, cuddle, talk to, and feed the preterm newborn; family caregivers demonstrate knowledge of appropriate infant care.
- **Goal:** The family adapts to the crisis and begins functioning at an appropriate level.
  Expected Outcome: Family has an adequate support system and uses it; contacts a support group for families of high-risk infants.

THE POST-TERM NEWBORN

When pregnancy lasts longer than 42 weeks, the infant is considered to be post-term (postmature), regardless of birth weight.

Contributing Factors

About 12% of all infants are post-term. The causes of delayed birth are unknown. However, some predisposing factors include first pregnancies between the ages of 15 and 19 years, the woman older than 35 years with multiple pregnancies, and certain fetal anomalies, such as anencephaly.

Characteristics of the Post-term Newborn

Some post-term newborns have an appearance similar to term infants, but others look like infants 1 to 3 weeks old. Little lanugo or vernix remains, scalp hair is abundant, and fingernails are long. The skin is dry, cracked, wrinkled, peeling, and whiter than that of the normal newborn. These infants have little subcutaneous fat and appear long and thin. This lack of subcutaneous fat may lead to cold stress. These infants are threatened by failing placental function and are at risk for intrauterine hypoxia during labor and delivery. Thus, it is customary for the physician or nurse–midwife to induce labor or perform a cesarean delivery when the baby is markedly overdue. Many physicians believe that pregnancy should be terminated by the end of 42 weeks.

Potential Complications

Often, the post-term infant has expelled meconium in utero. At birth, the meconium may be aspirated into the lungs, obstructing the respiratory passages and irritating the lungs. This may lead to pneumonia. Whenever meconium-stained amniotic fluid is detected in any delivery, oral and nasopharyngeal suctioning often is performed as soon as the head is born. After delivery, gastric lavage also may be performed to remove any meconium swallowed and to prevent aspiration of vomitus.

In the last weeks of gestation, the infant relies on glycogen for nutrition. This depletes the liver glycogen stores and may result in hypoglycemia. Another complication of the post-term infant may be polycythemia in response to intrauterine hypoxia. Polycythemia puts the infant at risk for cerebral ischemia, hypoglycemia, thrombus formation, and respiratory distress as a result of hyperviscosity of the blood.

Nursing Care

Special care can be taken when knowledge of a post-term newborn is evident. Early in the pregnancy, typically before 20 weeks, ultrasound examinations are performed to help establish more accurate dating by measurements taken of the fetus. Later in the pregnancy (after 42 weeks), ultrasound is used to evaluate fetal development, weight, the amount of amniotic fluid, and the placenta for signs of aging. This information allows the physician to make an informed decision regarding the safest form of delivery.

To reduce the chances of meconium aspiration, upon delivery of the post-term newborn's head and just before the baby takes his first breath, the physician or clinical nurse will suction the infant's mouth and nose and also check for respiratory problems related to meconium aspiration.

Typically, postmature newborns are ravenous eaters at birth. With this in mind, if the newborn is free from respiratory distress, the practical nurse can offer feedings at 1 or 2 hours of age, being observant for potential aspiration and possible asphyxia. Serial blood glucose levels will be monitored because the post-term newborn is at risk for hypoglycemia because of the increased use of glucose stores. Intravenous glucose infusions may be ordered to stabilize the newborn's glucose level.

Provide a thermoregulated environment, such as a radiant heat warmer or isolette, and use measures to minimize heat loss, such as reducing drafts and drying the skin thoroughly after bathing. With an increased production in red blood cells in response to hypoxia, venous and arterial hematocrit levels may be drawn to evaluate for polycythemia. If polycythemia is suspected, a partial exchange transfusion may be done to prevent hyperviscosity.

Anticipate that the stressed post-term newborn will not tolerate the labor and delivery process too well. Therefore, expect to observe and monitor the newborn's cardiopulmonary status closely. Administer supplemental oxygen therapy as ordered for respiratory distress.

Post-term newborns can appear very different from what parents had expected to see. Help facilitate a positive parent–newborn bond by explaining the newborn's condition and reasons for treatments and procedures. Encourage them to express their feelings and to participate in their newborn's care, if possible, to alleviate their stresses and fears about the newborn's condition.

Test Yourself

- What should be provided to a preterm newborn who is not receiving nipple feedings?
- What are three potential complications associated with post-term newborns?

ACQUIRED DISORDERS

RESPIRATORY DISORDERS

A newborn is at risk for developing respiratory disorders after birth as the newborn adapts to the extrauterine environment. The risk for these disorders increases when the newborn experiences a gestational age variation.

Transient Tachypnea of the Newborn

Transient tachypnea of the newborn (TTN) involves the development of mild respiratory distress in a newborn. It typically occurs after birth, with the greatest degree of distress occurring approximately 36 hours after birth. TTN commonly disappears spontaneously around the 3rd day.

TTN results from a delay in absorption of fetal lung fluid after birth. Before birth, the fetus receives nutrients, including oxygen, via the placenta. Thus, the fetus does not breathe, and the lungs are filled with fluid. As the fetus passes through the birth canal during delivery, some of the fluid is expelled as the thoracic area is compressed. After birth, the newborn breathes and fills the lungs with air, thus expelling additional lung fluid. Any fluid that remains is later expelled by coughing or absorbed into the bloodstream.

Contributing Factors

TTN is commonly seen in newborns born by cesarean delivery. Here, the newborn does not experience the compression of the thoracic cavity that occurs with passage through the birth canal. Newborns who are preterm or SGA or whose mothers smoked during pregnancy or have diabetes also are at risk for TTN.

Clinical Manifestations

A newborn who develops TTN typically exhibits mild respiratory distress, with a respiratory rate greater than 60 breaths per minute. Mild retractions, nasal flaring, and some expiratory grunting may be noted. However, cyanosis usually does not occur. Often the newborn has difficulty feeding because he or she is breathing at such a rapid rate and is unable to suck and breathe at the same time.

Diagnosis and Treatment

Arterial blood gases may reveal hypoxemia and decreased carbon dioxide levels. A chest x-ray usually indicates some fluid in the central portion of the lungs with adequate aeration. Treatment depends on the newborn's gestational age, overall status, history, and extent of respiratory distress. Unless an infection is suspected, medication therapy usually is not given. IV fluids and gavage feedings may be used to meet the newborn's fluid and nutritional requirements. Oral feedings typically are difficult because of the newborn's increased respiratory rate. Supplemental oxygen often is ordered, and oxygen saturation levels are monitored via pulse oximetry.

Nursing Care

Caring for the newborn with TTN requires close observation and monitoring and providing supportive care. Monitor the newborn's vital signs and oxygen saturation levels closely, being alert for changes that would indicate that the newborn is becoming fatigued from the rapid breathing. Administer IV fluids and supplemental oxygen as ordered. Assist the parents in understanding what their newborn is experiencing to help allay any fears or anxieties that they may have.

Meconium Aspiration Syndrome

Meconium aspiration syndrome (MAS) refers to a condition in which the fetus or newborn develops respiratory distress after inhaling meconium mixed with amniotic fluid. Meconium is a thick, pasty, greenish-black substance that is present in the fetal bowel as early as 10 weeks' gestation. **Meconium aspiration** occurs when the fetus inhales meconium along with amniotic fluid. Meconium staining of amniotic fluid usually occurs as a reflex response that allows the rectal sphincter to relax. Subsequently, meconium is released into the amniotic fluid. The fetus may aspirate meconium while in utero or with his or her first breath after birth. The meconium can block the airway partially or completely and can irritate the newborn's airway, causing respiratory distress.

Contributing Factors

Typically, meconium aspiration syndrome is associated with fetal distress during labor. Most commonly, the fetus experiences hypoxia, causing peristalsis to increase and the anal sphincter to relax. The fetus then gasps or inhales the meconium-stained amniotic fluid.

Additional factors that contribute to the development of MAS include a maternal history of diabetes or hypertension, difficult delivery, advanced gestational age, and poor intrauterine growth.

Clinical Manifestations

MAS is suspected whenever amniotic fluid is stained green to greenish black. Other manifestations include:

- Difficulty initiating respirations after birth
- Low Apgar score
- Tachypnea or apnea
- Retractions
- Hypothermia
- Hypoglycemia
- Cyanosis

Diagnosis and Treatment

Typically, diagnosis is confirmed with a chest x-ray that shows patches or streaks of meconium in the lungs. Air trapping or hyperinflation also may be seen. Treatment begins with suctioning the newborn during delivery, before the shoulders are delivered. Tracheal and bronchial suctioning may be indicated to remove any meconium plugs that may be lower in the respiratory tract. Oxygen therapy and assisted ventilation may be necessary to support the newborn's respiratory status. In some case, extracorporeal membrane oxygenation (ECMO) may be used to support the newborn's need for oxygen. Antibiotic therapy may be ordered to prevent the possible development of pneumonia. The physician may order chest physiotherapy with clapping and vibration to help in removing any remaining meconium from the lungs.

Nursing Care

Newborns with MAS are extremely ill and often require care in the NICU. Nursing care focuses on observing the neonate's respiratory status closely and ensuring adequate oxygenation. Measures to maintain thermoregulation are key to reducing the body's metabolic demands for oxygen. Be prepared to administer respiratory support and medication therapy as ordered.

Sudden Infant Death Syndrome

Sudden infant death syndrome (SIDS) has caused much grief and anxiety among families for centuries. One of the leading causes of infant mortality worldwide, SIDS claims an estimated 2,500 lives annually in the United States alone. Although there has been a dramatic drop in the incidence of deaths during the past 20 years, SIDS is still the leading cause of death in infants between 7 and 365 days of age (Carroll & Laughlin, 1999).

Commonly called "crib death," SIDS is the sudden and unexpected death of an apparently healthy infant in whom the postmortem examination fails to reveal an adequate cause. The term SIDS is not a diagnosis but rather a description of the syndrome.

Varying theories have been suggested about the cause of SIDS. Over the years, much research has been done, but no single cause has been identified.

Contributing Factors

Infants who die of SIDS are usually 2 to 4 months old, although some deaths have occurred during the 1st and 2nd week of life. Few infants older than 6 months of age die of SIDS. It is a greater threat to low birthweight infants than to term infants. It occurs more often in winter and affects more male infants than female infants, as well as more infants from minority and lower socioeconomic groups. Infants born to mothers younger than 20 years of age, infants who are not first born, and infants whose mothers smoked during pregnancy also have been found to be at greater risk. Research has revealed that a greater number of infants with SIDS have been sleeping in a prone (face down) position than in a supine (lying on the back with the face up) position. As a result of these studies, the American Academy of Pediatrics recommends that infants must not be placed in a prone position to sleep until they are 6 months old.

Clinical Manifestations

SIDS is rapid and silent and occurs at any time of the day. The history reveals that no cry has been heard, and there is no evidence of a struggle. People who have been sleeping nearby claim to have heard nothing unusual before the death was discovered. It is not uncommon for the infant to have been recently examined by a physician and found to be in excellent health. The autopsy often reveals a mild respiratory disorder but nothing considered serious enough to have caused the death.

A closely related syndrome is apparent life-threatening event (ALTE). This is an episode in which the infant is found in distress but when quickly stimulated, recovers with no lasting problems. These were formerly called "near-miss SIDS." These infants are placed on home apnea monitors (Fig. 20-8). The apnea monitor is set to sound an alarm if the infant has not taken a breath within a given number of seconds. Family caregivers are taught infant cardiopulmonary resuscitation (CPR) so that they can respond quickly if the alarm sounds. Infants who have had an episode of

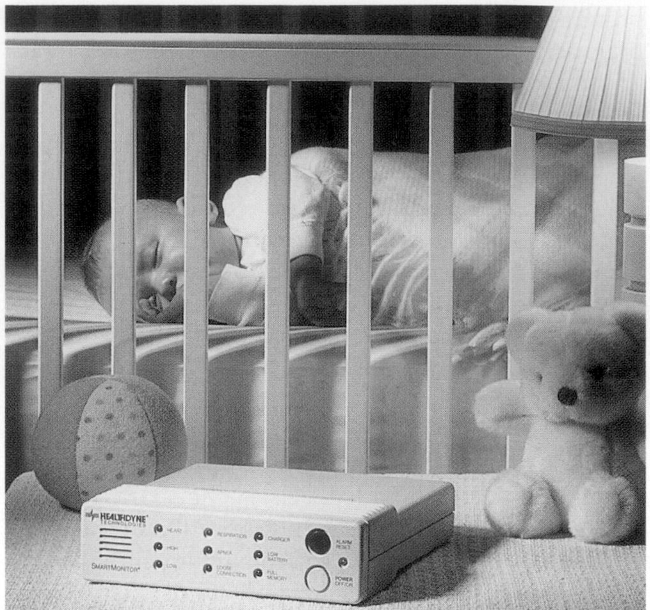

● ***Figure 20.8*** An apnea monitor for home monitoring.

ALTE are at risk for additional episodes and may be at risk for SIDS. Infants are usually kept on home apnea monitoring until they are 1 year old. This is a stressful time for the family because someone who is trained in infant CPR must be with the infant at all times.

Nursing Care

The effects of SIDS on caregivers and families are devastating. Grief is coupled with guilt, even though SIDS cannot be prevented or predicted. Disbelief, hostility, and anger are common reactions. An autopsy must be done and the results promptly made known to the family. Even though the family caregivers are told that they are not to blame, it is difficult for most not to keep searching for evidence of some possible neglect on their part. Prolonged depression usually follows the initial shock and anguish over the infant's death.

The immediate response of the emergency department staff should be to allow the family to express their grief, encouraging them to say good-by to their infant and providing a quiet, private place for them to do so. Compassionate care of the family caregivers includes helping to find someone to accompany them home or to meet them there. Referrals should be made to the local chapter of the National SIDS Foundation immediately. Sudden Infant Death Alliance is another resource for help. In some states, specially trained community health nurses who are knowledgeable about SIDS are available. These nurses are prepared to help families and can provide written materials, as well as information, guidance, and support in the family's home. They maintain contact with the family as long as necessary and provide support in a subsequent pregnancy.

One concern of the caregivers is how to tell other children in the family what has happened and how to help them deal with their grief and anger. Many books and booklets are available.

Caregivers are particularly concerned about subsequent infants. Recent studies have indicated that the risk for these infants is no greater than that for the general population. Many care providers, however, continue to recommend monitoring these infants for the first few months of life to help reduce the family's stress. Monitoring is usually maintained until the new infant is past the age of the SIDS infant's death.

HEMOLYTIC DISEASE OF THE NEWBORN

Hemolytic disease of the newborn is another name for **erythroblastosis fetalis**, a condition in which the infant's red blood cells are broken down (hemolyzed) and destroyed, producing severe anemia and hyperbilirubinemia. This rapid destruction of red blood cells may produce heart failure, brain damage, and death.

Before the mid-1960s, hemolytic disease was largely the result of Rh incompatibility between the blood of the mother and the blood of the fetus. The introduction of immune globulin, or RhoGAM, in the mid-1960s has markedly reduced the incidence of this disorder. Hemolytic disease occurring today is principally the result of ABO incompatibility and is generally much less severe than the Rh-induced disorder.

Rh Incompatibility

Rh factor, a protein substance (antigen), is found on the surface of red blood cells. The antigen is named "Rh" because it was first identified in the blood of rhesus monkeys. Persons who have the factor are Rh_o(D) positive; those lacking the factor are Rh_o(D) negative. A person's blood type is inherited and follows the rules of hereditary dominance and recession. Rh_o(D) positive trait is dominant. Therefore, if both members of a couple are Rh_o(D) negative, the couple's children will also be Rh_o(D) negative, and there will be no hemolytic disorder. However, if the woman is Rh_o(D) negative and the man is Rh_o(D) positive, the child may inherit Rh_o(D) positive blood and the disorder may occur.

If the man is homozygous positive for the trait, then both of his genes carry the Rh_o(D) positive (dominant) trait. In this case, if the woman is Rh_o(D) negative, then all of the couple's children will be Rh_o(D) positive and are vulnerable to hemolytic disease. However, if the man is heterozygous positive for the trait, then one of his genes carries the antigen and the other does not. In this case, if the woman is Rh_o(D) negative, then there is a 50-50 probability that the child will be Rh_o(D) positive and therefore vulnerable to hemolytic disease.

The Rh_o(D) positive fetus is only vulnerable to hemolytic disease if his mother is Rh_o(D) negative and has been sensitized to Rh_o(D) positive blood. The woman may only become sensitized (develop antibodies) against the Rh_o(D) antigen if she is exposed to the antigen. This situation may occur if the Rh_o(D) negative woman receives a transfusion with Rh_o(D) positive blood or it may occur during abortion or miscarriage, amniocentesis or other traumatic procedure, placental abruption, or during birth when the placenta separates and fetal blood cells escape into the woman's circulation. Because sensitization normally occurs only during birth, the first-born child is not usually affected by hemolytic disease.

With the next pregnancy, the maternal antibodies enter the fetal circulation and begin to hemolyze the baby's red blood cells. Rapid destruction of red blood cells causes excretion of bilirubin into the amniotic fluid. The fetus makes a valiant attempt to replace the red blood cells being destroyed by sending out large amounts of immature red blood cells (erythroblasts) into the bloodstream (thus the name erythroblastosis fetalis). As the process of rapid destruction of red blood cells continues, anemia develops. If the anemia is severe enough, heart failure and death of the fetus in utero may result.

ABO Incompatibility

The major blood groups are A, B, AB, and O, and each has antigens that may be incompatible with those of another group. The most common incompatibility in the newborn occurs between an infant with type O blood and a mother with type A or B blood. The reactions are usually less severe than in Rh incompatibility.

Prevention

The dramatic reduction in the incidence of erythroblastosis fetalis is due largely to the introduction of RhoGAM. It is effective only in mothers who do not have Rh antibodies, and it must be administered by injection within 72 hours after delivery of an Rh-positive infant or after abortion. Most obstetricians also give the mother an injection of RhoGAM in the 28th week of pregnancy to prevent any sensitization occurring during the pregnancy. RhoGAM essentially neutralizes any Rh_o(D) positive cells that may have escaped into the mother's system, preventing isoimmunization. As mentioned, RhoGAM also must be given to the Rh_o(D) negative mother after an abortion. It is never given to an infant or to a father. The use of RhoGAM on all patients who are candidates for it offers the hope of eliminating hemolytic disease caused by Rh incompatibility. The criteria for giving RhoGAM are:

- The woman must be Rh_0(D) negative.
- The woman must not be sensitized.
- The infant must be Rh_0(D) positive.
- The direct Coombs' test (a test for antibodies performed on cord blood at delivery) must be weakly reactive or negative.

All expectant women should have their blood tested for blood group and Rh type at the initial prenatal visit. If the woman is found to be Rh_0(D) negative, she should then be followed closely throughout her pregnancy. The woman should have blood titers performed periodically as a screening method to detect the presence of antibodies. This allows the physician to evaluate the health of the fetus and plan for the infant's delivery and care.

No preventative measures exist for ABO incompatibility.

Diagnosis

When titers show the presence of antibodies, the physician tries to determine to what degree the fetus is affected. Because there is no direct way to sample fetal blood to determine the degree of anemia, indirect means must be used.

Diagnosis may be made through the use of amniocentesis. Through a needle inserted into the amniotic sac, 10 to 15 mL of amniotic fluid is removed. The fluid is sent to the laboratory for spectrophotometric analysis, which shows the amount of bile pigments (bilirubin) in the amniotic fluid. Thus, it can be determined if the fetus is mildly, moderately, or severely affected.

If analysis of the amniotic fluid shows that the fetus is severely affected, the obstetrician will either perform an intrauterine transfusion of Rh_0(D) negative blood or, if the fetus is beyond 32 weeks' gestation, induce labor or perform a cesarean delivery. After delivery, the baby is turned over to a pediatrician or neonatologist, who will arrange for exchange transfusions.

Clinical Manifestations

Infants with known incompatibility (either Rh or ABO) to the mother's blood are examined carefully at birth for pallor, edema, jaundice, and an enlarged spleen and liver. If prenatal care was inadequate or absent, a severely affected infant may be stillborn or have hydrops fetalis, a condition marked by extensive edema, marked anemia and jaundice, and enlargement of the liver and spleen. These babies are in critical condition and need exchange transfusions at the earliest possible moment. If untreated, severely affected infants are at risk for severe brain damage or **kernicterus** from excess bilirubin levels. Death occurs in about 75% of infants with kernicterus; those who survive may be mentally retarded or develop spastic paralysis or nerve deafness. Exchange transfusions are given at once to infants who have signs of neurologic damage when first seen, although there is no proof that the damage is reversible. Fortunately, our current ability to detect and treat hemolytic disease has reduced the number of infants who become permanently damaged to just a few.

Treatment and Nursing Care

A severely affected newborn usually is transfused without waiting for laboratory confirmation. All other suspected infants have a sample of cord blood sent to the laboratory for a Coombs' test for the presence of damaging antibodies, Rh and ABO typing, hemoglobin and red blood cell levels, and measurement of plasma bilirubin. A positive direct Coombs' test indicates the presence of antibodies on the surface of the infant's red blood cells. A negative direct Coombs' test indicates that there are no antibodies on the infant's red blood cells.

A positive Coombs' test indicates the presence of the disease but not the degree of severity. If bilirubin and hemoglobin levels are within normal limits, the infant is watched carefully and frequent laboratory blood tests are performed. Bilirubin levels may be measured noninvasively with transcutaneous bilirubinometry or by a heel stick, results of which may be interpreted by the nursery nurse with specialized equipment. Exchange transfusions are performed at the discretion of the physician. The infant is cared for in the NICU.

Any infant admitted to the newborn nursery should be examined for jaundice during the first 36 hours or more. Early development of jaundice (within the first 24 to 48 hours) is a probable indication of hemolytic disease.

Phototherapy

Phototherapy refers to the use of special lights to help reduce bilirubin levels. These specially designed fluorescent lights help to prevent bilirubin levels from reaching the danger point of 20 mg/dL, beyond which kernicterus is a threat.

The criteria for treatment with phototherapy vary with the infant's size and age. The lights are placed above and outside the isolette (Fig. 20-9). The infant is nude (except for possibly a diaper under the perineal area to collect urine and feces), with the eyes shielded from the ultraviolet light. The eye patches may promote infection if they are not clean and changed frequently, or they may cause eye damage if they are not applied so that they stay in place. The light may cause the infant to have skin rashes; "sunburn" or tanning;

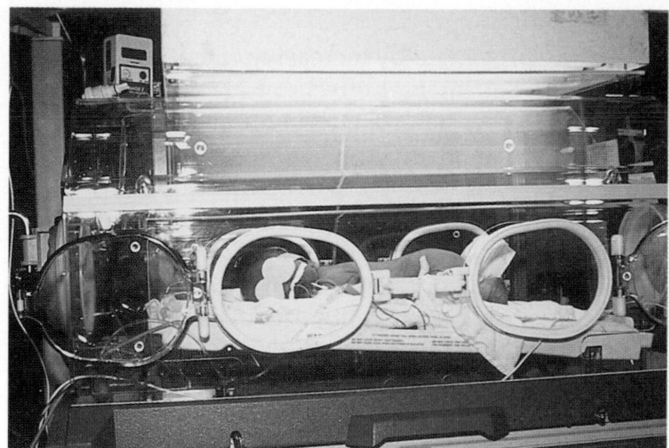

● ***Figure 20.9*** A newborn receiving phototherapy.

loose, greenish stools; hyperthermia; an increased metabolic rate; increased evaporative loss of water; and priapism (a perpetual abnormal erection of the penis). Infants undergoing phototherapy need as much as 25% more fluids to prevent dehydration. Monitor the serum bilirubin levels routinely when the infant is receiving phototherapy.

A fiberoptic blanket consisting of a pad attached to a halogen light source with illuminating plastic fibers also can be used. The blanket is covered with a disposable protective cover and can be wrapped about the infant to disperse therapeutic light. These blankets can be used at home, cutting hospitalization costs for the infant with hyperbilirubinemia and reducing the separation time for the infant and family. The neonate's eyes do not need to be covered when the fiberoptic blanket is used. The light can stay on all the time, and the neonate is available for care as needed.

Infants whose bilirubin has been restored to normal levels may be discharged to routine home care like any well newborn. The nurse should be sensitive to the parents' feelings of guilt and anxiety. They may feel that they caused the condition and need to ventilate their feelings. They must never be made to feel that they are responsible for the condition.

NEWBORN OF A DIABETIC MOTHER

The severity of the mother's diabetes has a direct relation to the risk for the infant. The diabetic woman who can closely control her blood glucose level before conception and throughout pregnancy, particularly in the early months, can avoid having an infant with the congenital anomalies commonly associated with diabetes. Infants of mothers with poorly controlled type 2 or gestational diabetes have a distinctive appearance. They are large for gestational age, plump and full-faced, and coated with vernix caseosa. Both the placenta and the umbilical cord are oversized. In contrast, infants of mothers with poorly controlled, long-term, or severe type 1 diabetes actually may suffer from intrauterine growth retardation.

Newborns of diabetic mothers often are at risk for hypoglycemia in the first few hours after birth (Box 20-2). The woman's high blood glucose levels increase the blood glucose level of the fetus before birth and cause the fetal pancreas to secrete increased amounts of insulin. This process leads to the increased intrauterine growth of the fetus. After birth, however, the high levels of glucose are suddenly cut off when the umbilical cord is cut, but the newborn's pancreas cannot readjust quickly enough and it continues to produce insulin. Thus, hypoglycemia (or hyperinsulinism) occurs. This condition may be fatal if not detected quickly and treated with oral or IV glucose to raise the level of the infant's blood glucose. Hypoglycemia, if untreated, may cause severe, irreversible damage to the central nervous system.

The usual range of blood glucose levels for newborns is 45 to 90 mg/dL. If the newborn's blood glucose level is 40 mg/dL or lower, the infant is treated with IV fluids, early feedings, and IV or oral glucose. The newborn's blood glucose level is checked by heel stick on a frequent schedule for the first 24 hours of life.

These infants are subject to many other hazards, including congenital anomalies, hypocalcemia, hyperbilirubinemia, and respiratory distress syndrome. Newborns of diabetic mothers require especially careful observation.

BOX 20.2 Signs and Symptoms of Hypoglycemia in the Newborn

Central Nervous System Signs
- Jitteriness
- Tremors
- Twitching
- Limpness
- Lethargy
- Weak or high-pitched cry
- Apathy
- Seizures
- Coma

Other Signs
- Cyanosis
- Apnea
- Irregular, rapid respirations
- Poor feeding
- Sweating

Test Yourself

- What respiratory disorder is associated with a delay in the absorption of fetal lung fluid after birth?
- When meconium aspiration is suspected, how does the amniotic fluid appear?
- What medication has dramatically reduced the incidence of erythroblastosis fetalis?

NEWBORN OF A CHEMICALLY DEPENDENT MOTHER

Alcohol and illicit drug use by the mother during pregnancy can lead to many problems in the newborn. Newborns of mothers who use alcohol are at risk for fetal alcohol syndrome (FAS). Typically, newborns of chemically dependent mothers are SGA and experience withdrawal symptoms.

Unfortunately, identifying the pregnant woman who abuses alcohol or drugs may be difficult. Many of these women have no prenatal care or only infrequent care. They may not keep appointments because of apathy or simply because they are not awake during the day. As a result, many of these infants have suffered prenatal insults that result in intrauterine growth retardation, congenital abnormalities, and premature birth.

Fetal Alcohol Syndrome

Alcohol is one of the many teratogenic substances that cross the placenta to the fetus. Fetal alcohol syndrome (FAS) is often apparent in newborns of mothers with chronic alcoholism and sometimes appears in newborns whose mothers are low to moderate consumers of alcohol. No amount of alcohol is believed to be safe, and women should stop drinking at least 3 months before they plan to become pregnant. The ability of the mother's liver to detoxify the alcohol is apparently of greater importance than the actual amount consumed.

Clinical Manifestations

FAS is characterized by low birth weight, smaller height and head circumference, short palpebral fissures (eyelid folds), reduced ocular growth, and a flattened nasal bridge. These newborns are prone to respiratory difficulties, hypoglycemia, hypocalcemia, and hyperbilirubinemia. Their growth continues to be slow, and their mental development is retarded, despite expert care and nutrition.

Nursing Care

FAS can be prevented by increasing the public's awareness of the detrimental effects of alcohol use during pregnancy. Other helpful interventions include screening women of reproductive age for alcohol problems and encouraging women to obtain adequate prenatal care and use appropriate resources for decreasing alcohol use.

Nursing care for the newborn with FAS is supportive and focuses on preventing complications such as seizures. Sedatives or anticonvulsants may be ordered to prevent stimulation that may lead to seizure activity. Providing adequate nutrition is key to supporting weight gain. The newborn's sucking reflex may be weak, and he or she may be too irritable to feed. Monitor the newborn's daily weights and intake and output. Encourage the parents to feed the newborn. This measure also helps to promote bonding.

Newborn With Withdrawal Symptoms

Newborns of mothers addicted to cocaine, heroin, methadone, or other drugs are born addicted, and many of these infants suffer withdrawal symptoms during the early neonatal period. However, the time of onset varies widely. For example, newborns experiencing withdrawal from opiates typically experience withdrawal symptoms within 24 to 48 hours after birth. However, it may take up to 10 days before the newborn exhibits any symptoms. For the newborn withdrawing from heroin, some may develop symptoms within 72 hours after birth, whereas others may not experience symptoms for as long as 2 weeks.

Clinical Manifestations

Withdrawal symptoms commonly include tremors, restlessness, hyperactivity, disorganized or hyperactive reflexes, increased muscle tone, sneezing, tachypnea, vomiting, diarrhea, disturbed sleep patterns, and a shrill high-pitched cry (Fig. 20-10). Ineffective sucking and swallowing reflexes create feeding problems, and regurgitation and vomiting occur often after feeding.

Nursing Care

Care of the newborn experiencing drug withdrawal focuses on providing physical and emotional support. Medications, such as chlorpromazine, clonidine, diazepam, methadone, morphine, paregoric, or phenobarbital, may be ordered to aid in withdrawal and prevent complications such as seizures.

Because of neuromuscular irritability, many of these newborns respond favorably to movement and close body contact with their caregivers. Therefore, some nurseries place the newborns in special carriers that hold them close to the nurse's chest while the nurse moves about the nursery. Swaddling the infant

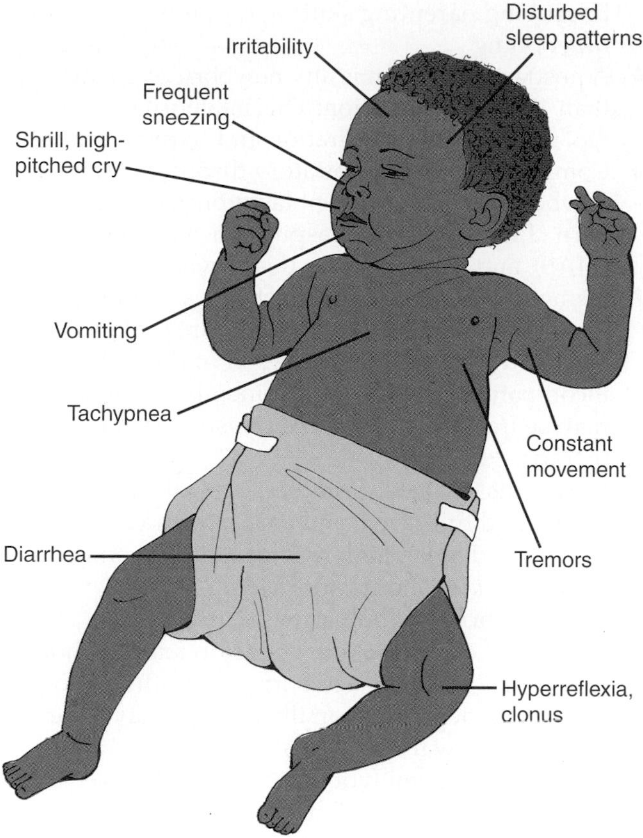

● ***Figure 20.10*** Manifestations of a newborn with withdrawal.

(wrapping securely in a small blanket) with arms across the chest also is recommended as a method of quieting the agitated newborn. Keep the newborn's environment dimly lit to minimize stimulation. Maintain the newborn's airway and monitor the newborn's respiratory status closely for changes. Provide small frequent feedings, keeping the newborn's head elevated to promote effective sucking and reduce the risk of aspiration. Vomiting and diarrhea may lead to fluid and electrolyte imbalances. Monitor intake and output closely and give supplemental fluids as ordered. Use a nonjudgmental approach when interacting with the newborn and his or her mother.

NEWBORN WITH A CONGENITALLY ACQUIRED INFECTION

Newborns are at increased risk for infections because their immune systems are immature and they cannot localize infections. High-risk newborns are even more susceptible than normal newborns. Infections may be acquired prenatally from the mother (through the placenta), during the intrapartum period (during labor and delivery) from maternal vaginal infection or inhalation of contaminated amniotic fluid, and after birth from cross-contamination with other infants, health care personnel, or contaminated equipment.

Infections in the newborn can be caused by a variety of organisms. The major cause is group B beta-hemolytic streptococcal infection. The newborn can acquire this infection from the mother because this organism is naturally found in the female reproductive tract. Another means of transmission is from one newborn to another if good handwashing is not used.

The rubella virus may be transmitted to the fetus if the mother becomes infected during the 1st trimester of pregnancy. The newborn is at risk for numerous congenital anomalies, such as cataracts, heart disease, deafness, microcephaly, and motor and cognitive impairments.

Infection with *Chlamydia trachomatis* or *Neisseria gonorrhoeae* may lead to ophthalmia neonatorum, a very serious form of conjunctivitis. The organisms may be transmitted to the newborn during vaginal birth. The routine administration of erythromycin ointment to the eyes of a newborn after birth aids in preventing this infection.

A mother infected with hepatitis B can transmit the virus to the newborn via contact with infected blood at the time of delivery. To prevent the complications associated with infection, newborns of mothers who are positive for the virus are given hepatitis B immune globulin within 12 hours after birth.

Infection with herpes virus type 2 can occur in newborns in one of two ways. The virus may be transmitted via the placenta to the fetus when the mother has an active infection during pregnancy. However, the most common method of transmission is via contact with the vaginal secretions of a mother who has active herpes lesions in the vaginal area at the time of delivery.

Human immunodeficiency virus (HIV) may be transmitted to the fetus across the placenta, from the mother's body fluids during birth, or through breast milk. If the mother is known to be positive for HIV, she should not breast-feed her newborn. The infant's test results are positive for HIV antibodies for as long as 15 months because he or she has passively acquired antibodies from the mother. Only 20% to 40% of infants born to known HIV-infected mothers are infected themselves (Ahuwalia, Merritt, Beck, & Rogers, 2001). To help prevent transmission to the fetus, antiretroviral therapy is ordered for HIV-positive women during the 2nd and 3rd trimesters of pregnancy and during labor and delivery. The newborns also may receive therapy during the first 6 weeks of life.

The newborn often does not have any specific signs of illness. The clue that alerts the nurse to a possible problem may be signs such as cyanosis, pallor, thermal instability (difficulty keeping temperature within normal range), convulsions, lethargy, apnea, jaundice, or just "not looking right." Diagnosis is made through blood, urine, and cerebrospinal fluid cultures and other laboratory and radiographic tests necessary to isolate the specific organism. Treatment consists of intensive antibiotic therapy, IV fluids, respiratory therapy, and other supportive measures.

The newborn of an HIV-positive mother may not show any signs of infection at birth and appears much the same as any other newborn. Signs of HIV infection usually are not seen in infants younger than 4 to 6 months of age. By 1 year of age, about half of those who are infected have symptoms, and by 2 years of age, most HIV-infected infants have symptoms. The prognosis is poor for infants who have symptoms before 1 year of age and those who develop *Pneumocystis carinii* pneumonia. Bacterial infections, such as pneumonia, meningitis, and bacteremia, are common in infected newborns. These infants also commonly have thrush, mouth sores, and severe diaper rash. Gloves must be worn by personnel when they are performing the first bath on every newborn. Gloves also must be worn by the nurse when performing any procedure in which the nurse could be exposed to blood or body fluids that may contain blood.

KEY POINTS

- Newborns are classified by size as small for gestational age (SGA), appropriate for gestational age (AGA), and large for gestational age (LGA).
- Newborns are classified by gestational age as preterm, post-term, or term.
- A gestational age assessment usually evaluates two major categories of maturity: physical maturity and neuromuscular maturity.
- Intrauterine growth restriction (IUGR) is the most common underlying condition leading to SGA newborns; the underlying cause for LGA newborns is not known.
- A preterm newborn is any newborn of less than 37 weeks' gestation. This newborn typically is tiny, scrawny, and red with little muscle or subcutaneous fat. The skin appears translucent and thin.
- Common complications associated with preterm newborns include respiratory distress syndrome, intraventricular hemorrhage, cold stress, retinopathy of prematurity, and necrotizing enterocolitis.
- Care of the preterm newborn focuses on improving respiratory function, maintaining body temperature, preventing infection, maintaining adequate nutrition, preserving skin integrity, promoting energy conservation and sensory stimulation, reducing parental anxiety, and improving parenting skills and family functioning.
- A postterm newborn is any newborn of greater than 42 weeks' gestation. This newborn is at high risk for meconium aspiration and hypoglycemia.
- Common acquired respiratory disorders of the newborn include transient tachypnea of the newborn (TTN), meconium aspiration syndrome (MAS), and sudden infant death syndrome (SIDS).
- Hemolytic disease of the newborn, a condition in which the infant's red blood cells are broken down and destroyed, may be the result of Rh or ABO incompatibility. Hyperbilirubinemia occurs and may be treated by exchange transfusions or phototherapy.
- Newborns of diabetic mothers typically are LGA, plump and full-faced, and coated with vernix caseosa and are at high risk for hypoglycemia during the first few hours after birth.
- The newborn of a mother who is chemically dependent on alcohol may develop fetal alcohol syndrome (FAS); the newborn of a mother who is chemically dependent on illicit drugs may experience withdrawal symptoms.
- Group B beta hemolytic streptococcus is the major cause of infection in the newborn. Other causes include rubella virus; *Chlamydia trachomatis* or *Neisseria gonorrhoeae* (leading to ophthalmia neonatorum); hepatitis B; herpes virus type 2; and human immunodeficiency virus (HIV).

REFERENCES AND SELECTED READINGS

Books and Journals

Ahuwalia, I. B., Merritt, R., Beck, L. F., & Rogers, M. (2001). Multiple lifestyle and psychosocial risks and delivery of small for gestational age infants. *Obstetrics and Gynecology, 97*(5 Pt 1):649–656. PMID: 11339910 [PubMed - indexed for MEDLINE]

Ballard, J. L. Khoury, J. C., Wedig, K., Wang, L., Eilers-Walsman, B. L., & Lipp, R. (1991). New Ballard score expanded to include extremely premature infants. *Journal of Pediatrics, 119*(3), 417–423.

Carroll, J. L., & Laughlin, G. M. (1999). Sudden infant death syndrome. In *Oski's pediatrics: Principles and practices* (3rd ed.). Philadelphia: Lippincott Williams & Wilkins.

Farrell, M. (2003). Gestational diabetes. *The American Journal of Maternal/Child Nursing, 28*(5), 301–305.

Hockenberry, M. J., Wilson, D., Winkelstein, M. L., & Kline, N. E. (2003). *Wong's nursing care of infants and children* (7th ed.). St. Louis: Mosby.

Johnson, T. (2003). Hypoglycemia and the full-term newborn: How well does birth weight for gestational age predict risk? *Journal of Obstetric, Gynecologic, and Neonatal Nursing (JOGNN), 32*(1), 48–57.

Pillitteri, A. (2003). *Maternal and child health nursing* (4th ed.). Philadelphia: Lippincott Williams & Wilkins.

Thomas, K. (2003). Infant weight and gestational age effects on thermoneutrality in the home environment. *Journal of Obstetric, Gynecologic, & Neonatal Nursing (JOGNN), 32*(6), 745–752.

White, R. C., et al. (2004). Developmental patterns of physiological response to a multisensory intervention in extremely premature and high-risk infants. *Journal of Obstetric, Gynecologic, & Neonatal Nursing (JOGNN), 33*(2), 266–275.

Web Addresses

Fetal Alcohol Syndrome

http://www.niaaa.nih.gov/publications/brochure.htm

Prematurity

http://kidshealth.org/parent/system/ill/nicu_diagnoses.html

http://www.marchofdimes.com/prematurity

http://premature-infant.com/index.cfm

WORKBOOK

NCLEX-STYLE REVIEW QUESTIONS

1. The nurse is assisting in a newborn assessment of gestational age using the Newborn Maturity Rating and Classification (Ballard) scoring system. Of the following characteristics, which would be noted in a newborn with the oldest gestational age? The newborn has
   a. abundant lanugo, flat areola, and pinna flat.
   b. anterior transverse plantar crease, ear recoil, and few scrotal rugae.
   c. transparent skin, no lanugo, and prominent clitoris.
   d. bald areas, plantar creases cover sole, and 3- to 4-mm breast bud.
2. A newborn is considered large for gestational age (LGA) when the newborn is larger than the average baby. Which of the following is *most* likely to be a contributing factor in a newborn that is LGA? The mother of the newborn has
   a. no other children.
   b. gained little weight during pregnancy.
   c. a diagnosis of diabetes.
   d. a history of smoking during pregnancy.
3. The nurse is caring for a preterm newborn. When developing a plan of care for the preterm newborn, which of the following nursing interventions would be the *most* important intervention to include?
   a. Repositioning at least every 2 hours
   b. Monitoring body temperature
   c. Promoting rest periods between procedures
   d. Recording urinary output
4. The nurse is caring for the newborn of a mother who abused cocaine during her pregnancy. Which of the following characteristics would the nurse likely see in this newborn? The newborn
   a. weighs above average when born.
   b. sleeps for long periods of time.
   c. cries when touched.
   d. has facial deformities.
5. The preterm newborn has specific characteristics, which differ from those of the term newborn. Identify characteristics that may be seen in the preterm newborn.
   Select all that apply:
   a. Extremities are thin, with little muscle or subcutaneous fat.
   b. Skin is thickened and without wrinkles.
   c. Head and abdomen are disproportionately large.
   d. Veins of the abdomen and scalp are visible.
   e. Lanugo is not evident on the back and shoulders.
   f. Ears have soft, minimal cartilage and are pliable.

STUDY ACTIVITIES

1. Research your community to find sources of help for families who have lost children to sudden infant death syndrome (SIDS). What support groups and organizations are available that you might recommend to families who have lost a child because of SIDS? Discuss with your peers what you found and make a list of resources to share.
2. Go to the following Internet site: http://kidshealth.org.
   Click on "Enter Parents." Type "premature" in the search box.
   Click on "A Primer on Preemies."
   a. What are the two basic needs of a premature infant discussed on this site?
   b. What are the common health problems often seen in premature infants?
   c. What suggestions does this site offer to families of children who have a premature infant?

CRITICAL THINKING: What Would You Do?

1. Andrea, the mother of Andrew, a newborn, has just been told that her son's bilirubin level is elevated and he is going to be given phototherapy. Andrea appears concerned and anxious and looks as if she is about to cry.
   a. What is the first thing you would do and say to Andrea?
   b. What would you explain to Andrea regarding the purpose of the phototherapy for Andrew?

c. What will you teach this mother in regards to what she might expect while Andrew is under the light?

2. You are teaching a nutrition class to a group of pregnant women. One of the women says that she heard it was not a problem to drink a little alcohol while she was pregnant. Another member of the group says she has heard about something called fetal alcohol syndrome.

   a. What will you teach this group regarding the use of alcohol during pregnancy?

   b. What is fetal alcohol syndrome?

   c. What are the characteristics of infants with fetal alcohol syndrome?

   d. What are the possible long-term complications of fetal alcohol syndrome?

The Newborn at Risk: Congenital Disorders

21

STUDENT OBJECTIVES

On completion of this chapter, the student should be able to

1. Differentiate between cleft lip and cleft palate.
2. Identify the early signs that indicate the presence of an esophageal fistula.
3. Name the greatest preoperative danger for newborns with tracheoesophageal atresia.
4. List and describe the five types of hernias that newborns may have.
5. Differentiate the three types of spina bifida that may occur.
6. Name the type of spina bifida that is most difficult to treat and state why.
7. Describe the two types of hydrocephalus that may occur.
8. State the most obvious symptoms of hydrocephalus.
9. Describe two types of shunting performed for hydrocephalus.
10. List five common types of congenital heart defects and trace the blood flow of each defect.
11. State the two most common skeletal deformities in the newborn.

KEY TERMS

atresia
bilateral
brachycephaly
chordee
congestive heart failure (CHF)
cyanotic heart disease
ductus arteriosus
ductus venosus
foramen ovale
galactosemia
hernia
hip dysplasia

STUDENT OBJECTIVES

12. List three signs and symptoms of congenital dislocation of the hip.
13. Describe the treatment for congenital dislocation of the hip.
14. Identify the test to detect phenylketonuria in the newborn.
15. Describe the treatment for phenylketonuria.
16. Name the tests performed on newborns to detect congenital hypothyroidism.
17. State the one serious outcome that is common to untreated phenylketonuria, congenital hypothyroidism, and galactosemia.
18. Discuss the reason Down syndrome is also called trisomy 21.
19. List 10 signs and symptoms of Down syndrome.

KEY TERMS

hypothermia
imperforate anus
overriding aorta
phenylketonuria
pulmonary stenosis
right ventricular hypertrophy
spina bifida
supernumerary
talipes equinovarus
unilateral
ventricular septal defect
ventriculoatrial shunting
ventriculoperitoneal shunting

Malformations that occur during the prenatal period and are present at birth are termed *congenital anomalies*. Many times these can be corrected during the first months or years of life. Some congenital conditions are termed inborn errors of metabolism, which are hereditary disorders that affect metabolism. Other congenital defects are caused by chromosomal abnormalities. These types of congenital malformations and disorders are discussed within this chapter. Gestational and acquired disorders of the newborn are present at birth and are caused by prenatal and perinatal damage due to maternal infection, substance use, maternal disorders or disease, birth trauma, or abnormalities specific to pregnancy. These disorders are discussed in Chapter 20.

The birth of a newborn with a congenital defect (anomaly) is a crisis for parents and caregivers. Depending on the defect, immediate or early surgery may be necessary. Early, continuous, skilled observation and highly skilled nursing care are required. Rehabilitation of the newborn and education of the family caregivers in the newborn's care are essential. The emotional needs of the newborn and the family must be integrated into the plans for nursing care. Many of these newborns have a brighter future today as a result of increased diagnostic and medical knowledge and advances in surgical techniques.

Family caregivers experience a grief response whether the newborn's defect is a result of abnormal intrauterine development or a chromosomal abnormality. They mourn the loss of the perfect child of their dreams, question why it happened, and may wonder how they will show the newborn to family and friends without shame or embarrassment. This grief may interfere with the process of parent–newborn attachment. Parents need to understand that their response is normal and that they are entitled to honest answers to their questions about the newborn's condition. Other children in the family should be informed gently but honestly about the newborn and should be allowed to visit the newborn when accompanied by adult family members. Sufficient time and attention must be devoted to the older siblings to avoid jealousy toward the newborn.

CONGENITAL MALFORMATIONS

Congenital anomalies or malformations may be caused by genetic or environmental factors. Approximately 2% to 3% of all infants born have a major malformation (Holmes, 1999). These anomalies include defects of the gastrointestinal, central nervous, cardiovascular, skeletal, and genitourinary systems. Defects such as cleft lip and severe neural tube defects are apparent at birth, but others may be discovered only after a complete physical examination. Congenital anomalies account for a large percentage of the health problems seen in newborns and children.

Gastrointestinal System Defects

Most gastrointestinal system anomalies are apparent at birth or shortly thereafter. The anomalies are often the result of embryonic growth interrupted at a crucial stage. Many of these anomalies interfere with the normal nutrition and digestion essential to the newborn's normal growth and development. Many anomalies require immediate surgical intervention.

Cleft Lip and Cleft Palate

The birth of a newborn with a facial deformity may change the atmosphere of the delivery from one of joyous anticipation to one of awkward tension. Parents and family are naturally eager to see and hold their newborn and must be prepared for the shock of seeing the facial disfigurement of a cleft lip. Their emotional reaction to such an obvious malformation is usually much stronger than to a "hidden" defect, such as congenital heart defect. They need encouragement and support, as well as considerable instruction about the newborn's feeding and care.

The most common facial malformations, cleft lip and cleft palate, occur either alone or in combination. Cleft lip occurs in about one in 1,000 live births and is more common in males. Cleft palate occurs in one newborn in 2,500, more often in females. Their cause is not entirely clear; they appear to be influenced genetically but sometimes occur in isolated instances with no genetic history. Although a cleft lip and a cleft palate often appear together, either defect may appear alone. In embryonic development, the palate closes later than the lip, and the failure to close occurs for different reasons.

The cleft lip and palate defects result from failure of the maxillary and premaxillary processes to fuse during the 5th to 8th week of intrauterine life. The cleft may be a simple notch in the vermilion line, or it may extend up into the floor of the nose (Fig. 21-1). It may be either **unilateral** (one side of the lip) or **bilateral** (both sides). Cleft palate occurs with a cleft lip about 50% of the time, most often with bilateral cleft lip. The child born with a cleft palate, but with an intact lip, does not have the external disfigurement that may be so distressing to the new parent. However, the problems are more serious. Cleft palate, which develops sometime between the 7th and 12th weeks of gestation, is often accompanied by nasal deformity and dental disorders, such as deformed, missing, or **supernumerary** (excessive in number) teeth.

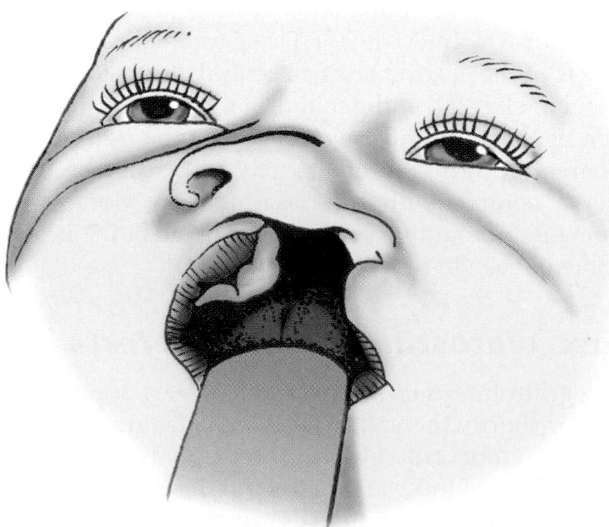

● ***Figure 21.1*** A cleft lip may extend up into the floor of the nose.

In an 8-week-old embryo, there is still no roof to the mouth; the tissues that are to become the palate are two shelves running from the front to the back of the mouth and projecting vertically downward on either side of the tongue. The shelves move from a vertical position to a horizontal position; their free edges meet and fuse in midline. Later, bone forms within this tissue to form the hard palate.

Normally the palate is intact by the 10th week of fetal life. Exactly what happens to prevent this closure is not known for sure. The incidence of cleft palates is higher in the close relatives of people with the defect than it is in the general population, and some evidence indicates that environmental and hereditary factors play a part in this defect.

Clinical Presentation

The physical appearance of the newborn confirms the diagnosis of cleft lip. Diagnosis of cleft palate is made at birth with the close inspection of the newborn's palate. To be certain that a cleft palate is not missed, the examiner must insert a gloved finger into the newborn's mouth to feel the palate to determine that it is intact. If a cleft is found, consultation is set up with a clinic specializing in cleft palate repair.

Treatment

Surgery, usually performed by a plastic surgeon, is a major part of the treatment of a newborn with a cleft lip, palate, or both (Fig. 21-2). Total care involves many other specialists, including pediatricians, nurses, orthodontists, prosthodontists, otolaryngologists, speech therapists, and occasionally psychiatrists. Long-term, intensive, multidisciplinary care is needed for newborns with major defects.

Plastic surgeons' opinions differ as to the best time for repair of the cleft lip. Some surgeons favor early repair, before the newborn is discharged from the hospital. They believe early repair can alleviate some of the family's feelings of rejection of the newborn. Other surgeons prefer to wait until the newborn is 1 or 2 months old, weighs about 10 lb, and is gaining weight steadily. Newborns who are not born in large medical centers with specialists on the staff are discharged from the birth hospital and referred to a center or physician specializing in cleft lip and palate repair.

If early surgery is contemplated, the newborn should be healthy and of average or above-average weight. The newborn must be observed constantly because a newborn has a higher likelihood of aspiration than does an older infant. These newborns must

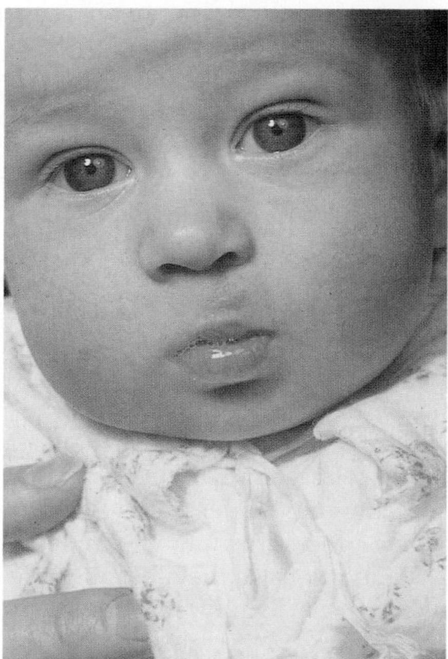

● ***Figure 21.2*** Infant with a surgical repair of a cleft lip.

be cared for by competent plastic surgeons and experienced nurses.

The goal in repairing the cleft palate is to give the child a union of the cleft parts to allow intelligible and pleasant speech and to avoid injury to the maxillary development. The timing of cleft palate repair is individualized according to the size, placement, and degree of deformity. The surgery may need to be done in stages over a period of several years to achieve the best results. The optimal time for surgical repair of the cleft palate is considered to be between 6 months and 5 years of age. Because the child cannot make certain sounds when starting to talk, undesirable speech habits are formed that are difficult to correct. If surgery must be delayed beyond the 3rd year, a dental speech appliance may help the child develop intelligible speech.

● Nursing Process in Caring for the Newborn With Cleft Lip and Cleft Palate

ASSESSMENT

One primary concern in the nursing care of the newborn with a cleft lip with or without a cleft palate is the emotional care of the newborn's family. In interviewing the family and collecting data, the nurse must include exploration of the family's acceptance of the newborn. Practice active listening with reflective responses, accept the family's emotional responses, and demonstrate complete acceptance of the newborn.

The family caregivers who return to the hospital with their infant for the beginning repair of a cleft palate have already faced the challenges of feeding their infant. Conduct a thorough interview with the caregiver that includes a question about the methods they found to be most effective in feeding the infant.

Physical examination of the infant includes temperature, apical pulse, and respirations. Listen to breath sounds to detect any pulmonary congestion. Observe skin turgor and color, noting any deviations from normal. In addition, observe the infant's neurologic status, noting alertness and responsiveness. Document a complete description of the cleft.

SELECTED NURSING DIAGNOSIS

Nursing diagnoses for the newborn before surgery may include:

- Imbalanced Nutrition: Less than Body Requirements related to inability to suck secondary to cleft lip
- Compromised Family Coping related to visible physical defect
- Anxiety of family caregivers related to the child's condition and surgical outcome
- Deficient Knowledge of family caregivers related to care of child before surgery and the surgical procedure

Nursing diagnoses applicable to the newborn after the surgical repairs are:

- Risk for Aspiration related to a reduced level of consciousness after surgery
- Ineffective Breathing Pattern related to anatomic changes
- Risk for Deficient Fluid Volume related to NPO status after surgery
- Imbalanced Nutrition: Less than Body Requirements related to difficulty in feeding after surgery
- Acute Pain related to surgical procedure
- Risk of Injury to the operative site related to newborn's desire to suck thumb or fingers and anatomic changes
- Risk for Infection related to surgical incision
- Risk for Delayed Growth and Development related to hospitalizations and surgery
- Deficient Knowledge of family caregivers related to long-term aspects of cleft palate

OUTCOME IDENTIFICATION AND PLANNING: PREOPERATIVE CARE

Goal setting and planning must be modified to adapt to the surgical plans. If the newborn is to be discharged from the birth hospital to have surgery a month or two later, the nurse may focus on preparing the family to care for the newborn at home and helping them cope with their emotions. The major goals include maintaining adequate nutrition, increasing family coping, reducing the parents' anxiety and guilt regarding the newborn's physical defect, and preparing parents for the future repair of the cleft lip and palate.

IMPLEMENTATION

Maintaining Adequate Nutrition. The newborn's nutritional condition is important to the planning of surgery because the newborn must be in good condition before surgery can be scheduled. However, feeding the newborn with a cleft lip or palate before repair is a challenge. The procedure may be time consuming and tedious because the newborn's ability to suck is inadequate. Breastfeeding may be successful because the breast tissue may mold to close the gap. If the newborn cannot breast-feed, the mother's breast milk may be expressed and used instead of formula until after the surgical repair heals. Various nipples may be tried to find the method that works best. A soft nipple with a crosscut made to promote easy flow of milk or formula may work well. A large nipple with holes that allow the milk to drip freely makes sucking easier. If the cleft lip is unilateral, the nipple should be aimed at the unaffected side. The infant should be kept in a upright position during feeding.

If the infant does not have a cleft lip or if the lip has had an early repair, sucking may be learned more easily, even though the suction generated is not as good as in the infant with an intact palate. Lamb's nipples (extra-long nipples) and special cleft palate nipples molded to fit into the open palate area to close the gap have been used with success.

One of the simplest and most effective methods may be the use of an eyedropper or an Asepto syringe with a short piece of rubber tubing on the tip (Breck feeder) (Fig. 21-3). The dropper or syringe is used carefully to drip formula into the newborn's mouth at a rate slow enough to allow the newborn to swallow. As the newborn learns to eat, much coughing, sputtering, and choking may occur. The nurse or family caregiver feeding the newborn must be alert for signs of aspiration.

Whatever feeding method is used, the experience may be frustrating for both the feeder and the newborn. Have family caregivers practice the feeding techniques under supervision. During the teaching process, give them ample opportunity to ask questions so they feel able to care for the newborn (see Family Teaching Tips: Cleft Lip/Cleft Palate).

Promoting Family Coping. Encourage family members to verbalize their feelings regarding the defect and their disappointment. Convey to the family that their feelings are acceptable and normal. While caring for the newborn, demonstrate behavior that clearly displays acceptance of the newborn. Serve as a model for the family caregivers' attitudes toward the child.

Reducing Family Anxiety. Give the family caregivers information about cleft repairs. Pamphlets are available that present photographs of before and after corrections that will answer some of their questions. Encourage them to ask questions and reassure them that any question is valid.

Providing Family Teaching. By the time the infant is actually admitted for the repair, the family will have received a great amount of information, but all families need additional support

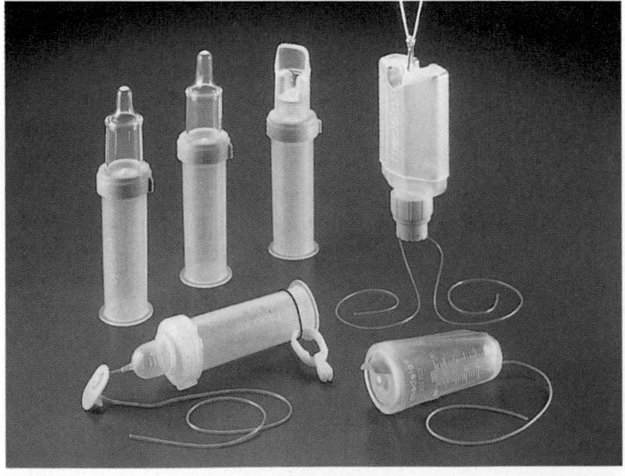

A

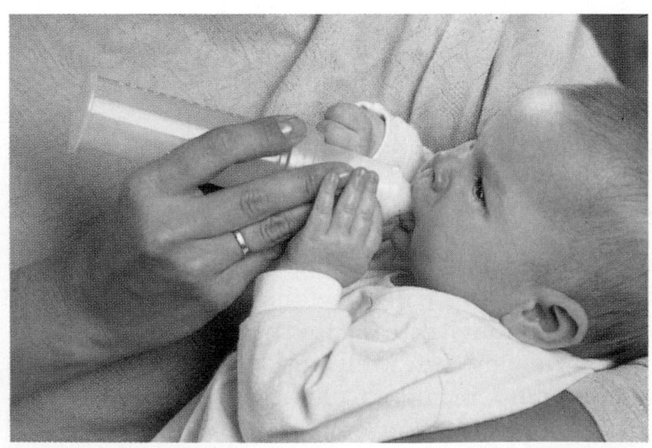

B

● ***Figure 21.3*** Specialty feeding devices used for the newborn with a cleft lip or palate include (**A**) special nipples and devices and (**B**) a special feeder.

FAMILY TEACHING TIPS

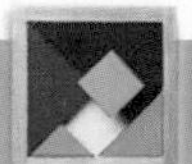

Cleft Lip/Cleft Palate

- Sucking is important to speech development.
- Holding the baby upright while feeding helps avoid choking.
- Burp the baby frequently because a large amount of air is swallowed during feeding.
- Don't tire the baby. Limit feeding times to 20 to 30 minutes maximum. If necessary, feed the baby more often.
- Feed strained foods slowly from the side of the spoon in small amounts.
- Don't be alarmed if food seeps through the cleft and out the nose.
- Have baby's ears checked any time he or she has a cold or upper respiratory infection.
- Talk normally to baby (no "baby talk"). Talk often; repeat baby's babbling and cooing. This helps in speech development.
- Try to understand early talking without trying to correct baby.
- Good mouth care is very important.
- Early dental care is essential to observe teething and prevent caries.

throughout the procedure. Explain the usual routine of preoperative, intraoperative, and postoperative care. Written information is helpful, but be certain the parents understand the information. Simple things are important; show families where they may wait during surgery, inform them how long the surgery should last, tell them about the postanesthesia care unit procedure, and let them know where the surgeon will expect to find them to report on the surgery.

OUTCOME IDENTIFICATION AND PLANNING: POSTOPERATIVE CARE

Major goals for the postoperative care of the infant who is hospitalized for surgical repair of cleft lip or palate include preventing aspiration, improving respiration, maintaining adequate fluid volume and nutritional requirements, relieving pain, preventing injury and infection to the surgical site, promoting normal growth and development, and increasing the family caregivers' knowledge about the child's long-term care.

IMPLEMENTATION

Preventing Aspiration. To facilitate drainage of mucus and secretions, position the infant on the side, never on the abdomen, after a cleft lip repair. The infant may be placed on the side after a cleft palate repair. Watch the infant closely in the immediate postoperative period. Do not put anything in the infant's mouth to clear mucus because of the danger of damaging the surgical site, particularly with a palate repair.

Changing Breathing Pattern. Immediately after a palate repair, the infant must change from a mouth-breathing pattern to nasal breathing. This change may frustrate the infant, but the infant positioned to ease breathing and given encouragement should be able to adjust quickly.

Monitoring Fluid Volume. In the immediate postoperative period, the infant needs parenteral fluids. Follow all the usual precautions: check placement, discoloration of the site, swelling, and flow rate every 2 hours. Document intake and output accurately. Parenteral fluids are continued until the infant can take oral fluids without vomiting.

Maintaining Adequate Nutrition. As soon as the infant is no longer nauseated (vomiting should be avoided if possible), the surgeon usually permits clear liquids. After the cleft lip repair, no tension should be placed on the suture line, to prevent the sutures from pulling apart and leaving a scar. A specialized feeder may need to be used because bottle- or breast-feeding may increase the tension on the suture line.

For an infant who has had a palate repair, no nipples, spoons, or straws are permitted; only a drinking glass or a cup is recommended. A favorite cup from home may be reassuring to the older infant. Offer clear liquids such as flavored gelatin water, apple juice, and synthetic fruit-flavored drinks. Red juices should not be given because they may conceal bleeding. Infants do not usually like broth. The diet is increased to full liquid, and the infant is usually discharged on a soft diet. When permitted, foods such as cooked infant cereals, ice cream, and flavored gelatin are often favorites. The surgeon determines the progression of the diet. Nothing hard or sharp should be placed in the infant's mouth. After each feeding, clear water is used to rinse the mouth and suture line.

Relieving Pain. Observe the infant for signs of pain or discomfort from the surgery. Administer

CULTURAL SNAPSHOT

In some cultures genetic defects are blamed on the mother—something she did or ate; stress or trauma that occurred during pregnancy; viewing a child with a defect caused her child to have the same defect. The mother may have feelings of guilt or fears of being an unacceptable mother and needs to be supported by the nurse.

ordered analgesics as needed. Relieving pain not only comforts the infant, but may also prevent crying, which is important because of the danger of disrupting the suture line. Make every effort to prevent the infant with a lip repair from crying to prevent excessive tension on the suture line.

Preventing Postoperative Injury. Continuous, skilled observation is essential. Swollen mouth tissues cause excessive secretion of mucus that is handled poorly by a small infant. For the first few postoperative hours, never leave the infant alone because aspiration of mucus occurs quickly and easily. Because nothing is permitted in the infant's mouth, particularly the thumb or finger, elbow restraints are necessary. The thumb, although comforting, may quickly undo the repair or cause undesirable scarring along the suture line. The infant's ultimate happiness and well-being must take precedence over immediate satisfaction. Accustoming the infant to elbow restraints gradually before admission is helpful.

Elbow restraints must be applied properly and checked frequently (see Figure 30-1). Place the restraints firmly around the arm and pinned to the infant's shirt or gown to prevent them from sliding down below the elbow. The infant's arms can move freely but cannot bend at the elbows to reach the face. Apply the restraint snugly but do not allow the circulation to be hindered. The older infant may need to be placed in a jacket restraint. The use of restraints must be documented.

Some nurses find this approach helpful. For the infant in restraints, playing "Peek-a-Boo" and other infant games will help to comfort and entertain the baby; however "Patty Cake" does not work well with an infant in elbow restraints.

Remove restraints at least every 2 hours, but remove them only one at a time and control the released arm so that the thumb or fingers do not pop into the mouth. Comfort the infant and explore various means of comforting. Talk to the infant continuously while providing care. Inspect and massage the skin, apply lotion, and perform range-of-motion exercises. Replace restraints when they become soiled.

Preventing Infection. Gentle mouth care with tepid water or clear liquid may be recommended to follow feeding. This care helps clean the suture area of any food or liquids to promote a cleaner incision for optimal healing.

Care of Lip Suture Line. The lip suture line is left uncovered after surgery and must be kept clean and dry to prevent infection and subsequent scarring. A wire bow called a Logan bar or a butterfly closure is applied across the upper lip and attached to the cheeks with adhesive tape to prevent tension on the sutures caused by crying or other facial movement (Fig. 21-4). Carefully clean the sutures after feeding and as often as necessary to prevent collection of dried formula or serum. Frequent cleaning is essential as long as the sutures are in place. Clean the sutures gently with sterile cotton swabs and saline or the solution of the surgeon's choice. Application of an ointment such as bacitracin may also be ordered. Care of the suture line is extremely important because it has a direct effect on the cosmetic appearance of the repair. Teach the family how to care for the suture line because the infant will probably be discharged before the sutures are removed (7 to 10 days after surgery). The infant probably will be allowed to suck on a soft nipple at this time.

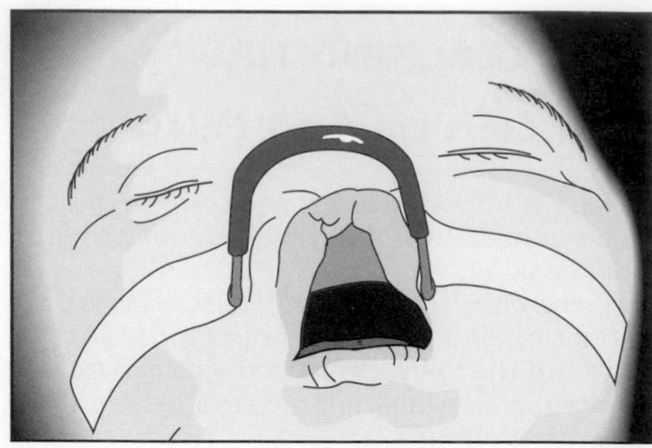

● ***Figure 21.4*** Logan bar for easing strain on sutures.

Aseptic technique is important while caring for the infant undergoing lip or palate repair. Good handwashing technique is essential. Instruct the family caregivers about the importance of preventing anyone with an upper respiratory infection from visiting the infant. Observe for signs of otitis media that may occur from drainage into the eustachian tube.

Promoting Sensory Stimulation. The infant needs stimulating, safe toys in the crib. The nurse and family caregivers must use every opportunity to provide sensory stimulation. Talking to the infant, cuddling and holding him or her, and responding to cries are important interventions. Provide freedom from restraints within the limitations of safety as much as possible. One caregiver should be assigned to provide stability and consistency of care. Family caregivers and health care personnel must encourage the older child to use speech and help enhance the child's self-esteem. A baby experiences emotional frustration because of restraints, so satisfaction must be provided in other ways. Rocking, cuddling, and other soothing techniques are an important part of nursing care. Family members and other caregivers are the best people to supply this loving care.

Providing Family Teaching. After effective surgery and skilled, careful nursing care, the appearance of the baby's face should be improved greatly. The scar fades in time. Family caregivers need to know that the baby will probably need a slight adjustment of the vermilion line in later childhood, but they can expect a repair that is barely, if at all, noticeable (see Fig. 21-2).

Cleft lip and cleft palate centers have teams of specialists who can provide the services that these children and their families need through infancy, preschool, and the school years. Explain to the caregivers the services offered by the pediatrician, plastic surgeon, orthodontist, speech therapist, nutritionist, and public or home health nurse. These professionals can give explanations and counseling about the child's diet, speech training, immunizations, and general health. Encourage family caregivers to ask them any questions they may have. Be alert for any evidence that the caregivers need additional information and arrange appropriate meetings.

Dental care for the deciduous teeth is even more important than usual. The incidence of dental caries is high in children with a cleft palate, but preservation of the deciduous teeth is important for the best results in speech and appearance.

EVALUATION: GOALS AND EXPECTED OUTCOMES

Preoperative

- **Goal:** The newborn will show appropriate weight gain.
  Expected Outcomes: The newborn's weight increases at a predetermined goal of 1 oz or more per day.
- **Goal:** The family will demonstrate acceptance of the newborn.
  Expected Outcomes: Family caregivers verbalize their feelings about the newborn and cuddle and talk to the newborn.
- **Goal:** The family caregiver's anxiety will be reduced.
  Expected Outcomes: Family caregivers ask appropriate questions about surgery, openly discuss their concerns, and voice reasonable expectations.
- **Goal:** The family will learn how to care for the newborn and will have an understanding of surgical procedures.
  Expected Outcomes: Family caregivers ask appropriate questions, demonstrate how to feed the newborn before surgery, and describe the surgical procedures.

Postoperative

- **Goal:** The infant's respiratory tract will remain clear, the infant will breathe easily, and the respiratory rate will be within normal limits.
  Expected Outcomes: The infant has clear lung sounds with no aspiration, and the respiratory rate stays within normal range.
- **Goal:** The infant will adjust his or her breathing pattern.
  Expected Outcomes: The infant breathes nasally with little stress and maintains normal respirations.
- **Goal:** The infant will show signs of adequate hydration during NPO period.
  Expected Outcomes: The newborn's skin turgor is good, mucous membranes are moist, and urine output is adequate; there is no evidence of parenteral fluid infiltration.
- **Goal:** The infant will have adequate caloric intake and retain and tolerate oral nutrition.
  Expected Outcomes: The infant gains 0.75 to 1 oz (22 to 30 g) per day if younger than 6 months of age or 0.5 to 0.75 oz (13 to 22 g) per day if older than 6 months and does not experience nausea or vomiting.
- **Goal:** The infant's pain and discomfort will be minimized.
  Expected Outcomes: The infant rests quietly, does not cry, and is not fretful.
- **Goal:** The surgical site will remain free of injury.
  Expected Outcomes: The surgical site is intact; the infant puts nothing into the mouth such as straws, sharp objects, thumb, or fingers.
- **Goal:** The infant's incision site will remain free of signs and symptoms of infection.
  Expected Outcomes: The incisional site is clean with no redness or drainage. The infant's temperature is within normal limits. The caregivers and family members practice good handwashing and aseptic technique.
- **Goal:** The infant will show evidence of normal growth and development.
  Expected Outcomes: The infant is content most of the time and responds appropriately to the caregiver and family. The infant engages in age- and development-appropriate activities within the limits of restraints.
- **Goal:** The family will learn how to care for the infant's long-term needs.
  Expected Outcomes: The family caregivers ask appropriate questions, respond appropriately to staff queries, and describe services available for the child's long-term care.

Esophageal Atresia

Atresia is the absence of a normal body opening or the abnormal closure of a body passage. Esophageal atresia with or without fistula into the trachea is a serious congenital anomaly and is among the most common anomalies causing respiratory distress. This condition occurs in about 1 in 2,500 live births. Several types of esophageal atresia occur; in more than 90% of affected newborns, the upper, or proximal, end of the esophagus ends in a blind pouch and the lower, or distal, segment from the stomach is connected to the trachea by a fistulous tract (Fig. 21-5).

Clinical Presentation

Any mucus or fluid that a newborn swallows enters the blind pouch of the esophagus. This pouch soon fills and overflows, usually resulting in aspiration into the trachea. Few other conditions depend so greatly on careful

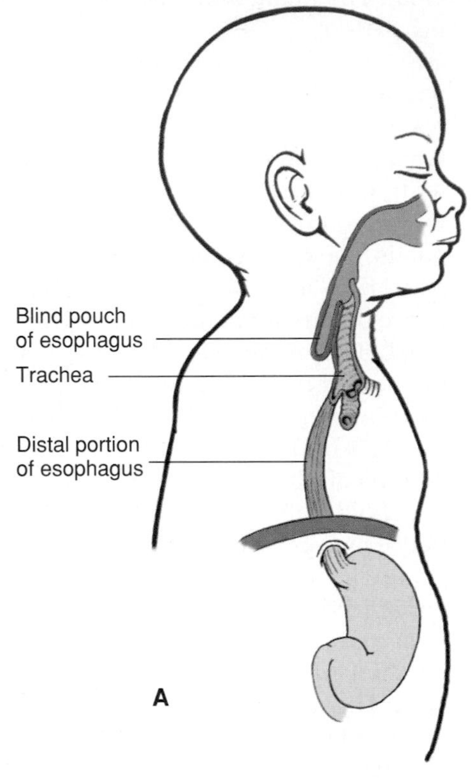

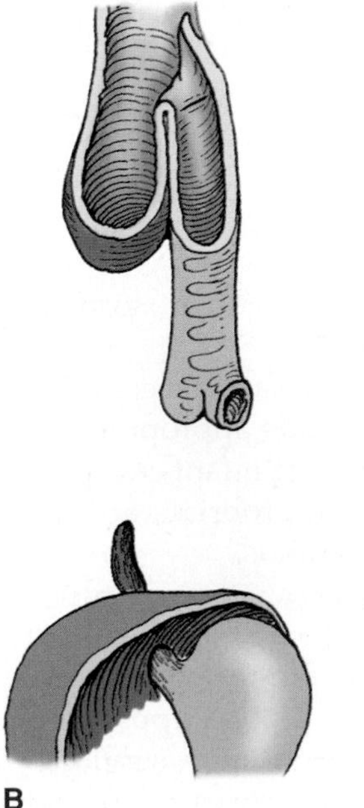

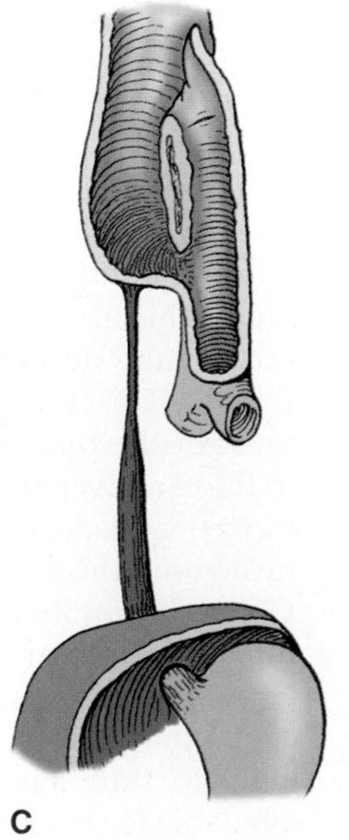

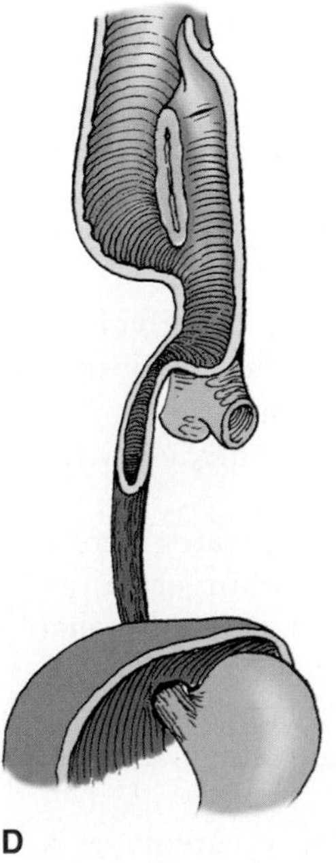

● ***Figure 21.5*** (**A**) The most common form of esophageal atresia. (**B**) Both segments of the esophagus are blind pouches. (**C**) Esophagus is continuous but with narrowed segment. (**D**) Upper segment of esophagus opens into trachea.

nursing observation for early diagnosis and, therefore, improved chances of survival. The newborn with this disorder has frothing and excessive drooling and periods of respiratory distress with choking and cyanosis. Many newborns have difficulty with mucus, but the nurse should be alert to the possibility of an anomaly and report such difficulties immediately. No feeding should be given until the newborn has been examined.

If early signs are overlooked and feeding is attempted, the newborn chokes, coughs, and regurgitates as the food enters the blind pouch. The newborn becomes deeply cyanotic and appears to be in severe respiratory distress. During this process, some of the formula may be aspirated, resulting in pneumonitis and increasing the risk of surgery. This newborn's life may depend on the careful observations of the nurse. If there is a fistula of the distal portion of the esophagus into the trachea, the gastric contents may reflux into the lungs and cause a chemical pneumonitis.

Treatment and Nursing Care

Surgical intervention is necessary to correct the defect. Timing of the surgery depends on the surgeon's preference, the anomaly, and the newborn's condition. Aspiration of mucus must be prevented, and continuous, gentle suction may be used. The newborn needs intravenous fluids to maintain optimal hydration. The first stage of surgery may involve a gastrostomy and a method of draining the proximal esophageal pouch. A chest tube is inserted to drain chest fluids. An end-to-end anastomosis is sometimes possible. If the repair is complex, surgery may need to be done in stages.

Often these defects occur in premature newborns, so additional factors may complicate the surgical repair and prognosis (Fig. 21-6). If there are no other major problems, the long-term outcome should be good. Regular follow-up is necessary to observe for and dilate esophageal strictures that may be caused by scar tissue.

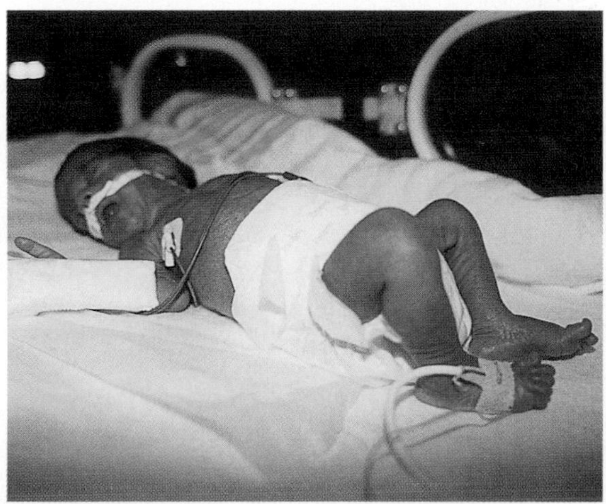

● ***Figure 21.6*** Repair of tracheal esophageal atresia in premature newborns may be complicated by other factors.

Imperforate Anus

Early in intrauterine life, the membrane between the rectum and the anus should be absorbed, and a clear passage from the rectum to the anus should exist. If the membrane remains and blocks the union between the rectum and the anus, an **imperforate anus** results. In a newborn with imperforate anus, the rectal pouch ends blindly at a distance above the anus; there is no anal orifice. A fistula may exist between the rectum and the vagina in females or between the rectum and the urinary tract in males.

Clinical Presentation

In some newborns, only a dimple indicates the site of the anus (Fig. 21-7A). When the initial rectal temperature is attempted, it is apparent that there is no anal opening. However, a shallow opening may occur in the anus, with the rectum ending in a blind pouch some distance higher (Fig. 21-7B). Thus, being able to pass a thermometer into the rectum does not guarantee that the rectoanal canal is normal. More reliable presumptive evidence is obtained by watching carefully for the first meconium stool. If the newborn does not pass a stool within the first 24 hours, the physician should be notified. Abdominal distention also occurs. Definitive diagnosis is made by radiographic studies.

Treatment

If the rectal pouch is separated from the anus by only a thin membrane, the surgeon may repair the defect from below. For a high defect, abdominoperineal resection is indicated. In these newborns, a colostomy is performed, and extensive abdominoperineal resection is delayed until 3 to 5 months of age or later.

Nursing Care

When the newborn goes home with a colostomy, the family must learn how to give colostomy care. Teach caregivers to keep the area around the colostomy clean with soap and water and to diaper the baby in the usual way. A protective ointment is useful to protect the skin around the colostomy.

Hernias

A **hernia** is the abnormal protrusion of a part of an organ through a weak spot or other abnormal opening in a body wall. Complications occur depending on the amount of circulatory impairment involved and how much the herniated organ impairs the functioning of another organ. Most hernias can be repaired surgically.

Diaphragmatic Hernia

In a congenital hernia of the diaphragm, some of the abdominal organs are displaced into the left chest

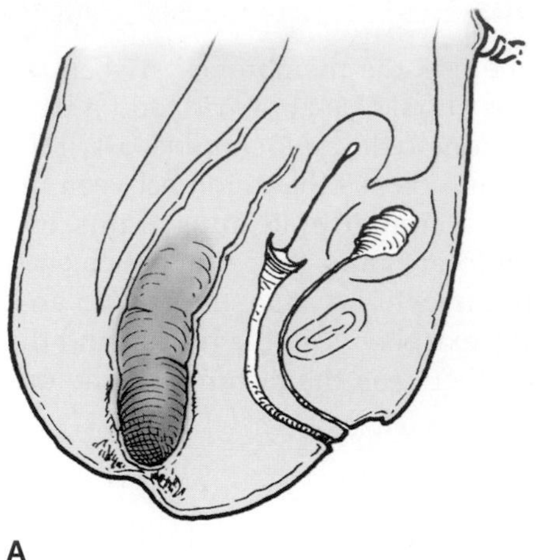

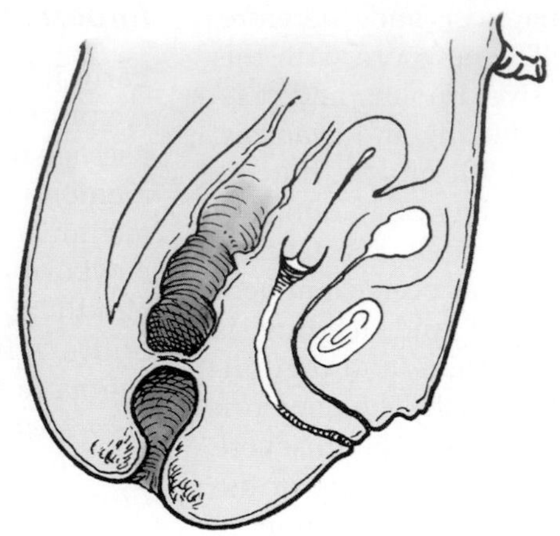

● ***Figure 21.7*** Imperforate anus (anal atresia). (**A**) Membrane between anus and rectum. (**B**) Rectum ending in a blind pouch at a distance above the perineum.

through an opening in the diaphragm. The heart is pushed toward the right, and the left lung is compressed. Rapid, labored respirations and cyanosis are present on the first day of life, and breathing becomes increasingly difficult. Surgery is essential and may be performed as an emergency procedure. During surgery, the abdominal viscera are withdrawn from the chest and the diaphragmatic defect is closed.

This defect may be minimal and repaired easily or so extensive that pulmonary tissue has failed to develop normally. The outcome of surgical repair depends on the degree of pulmonary development. The prognosis in severe cases is guarded.

Hiatal Hernia

More common in adults than in newborns, hiatal hernia is caused when the cardiac portion of the stomach slides through the normal esophageal hiatus into the area above the diaphragm. This action causes reflux of gastric contents into the esophagus and subsequent regurgitation. If upright posture and modified feeding techniques do not correct the problem, surgery is necessary to repair the defect.

Omphalocele

Omphalocele is a relatively rare congenital anomaly. Some of the abdominal contents protrude through into the root of the umbilical cord and form a sac lying on the abdomen. This sac may be small, with only a loop of bowel, or large and containing much of the intestine and the liver (Fig. 21-8). The sac is covered with peritoneal membrane instead of skin. These defects may be detected during prenatal ultrasonography so that prompt repair may be anticipated. At birth, the defect should be covered immediately with gauze moistened in sterile saline, which then may be covered with plastic wrap to prevent heat loss. Surgical replacement of the organs into the abdomen may be difficult with a large omphalocele because there may not be enough space in the abdominal cavity. Other congenital defects often are present.

With large omphaloceles, surgery may be postponed and the surgeon will suture skin over the defect, creating a large hernia. As the child grows, the abdomen may enlarge enough to allow replacement.

Umbilical Hernia

Normally the ring that encircled the fetal end of the umbilical cord closes gradually and spontaneously after birth. When this closure is incomplete, portions of omentum and intestine protrude through the opening. More common in preterm and African-American newborns, umbilical hernia is largely a cosmetic problem (Fig. 21-9). Although upsetting to

Did you know? Some people believe that taping a coin on an umbilical hernia will help reduce the hernia. This can actually result in a serious problem for the newborn and should not be done.

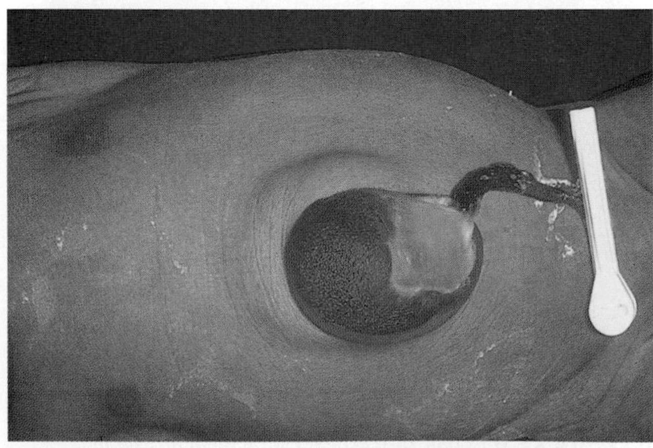

● ***Figure 21.8*** Large omphalocele with liver and intestine.

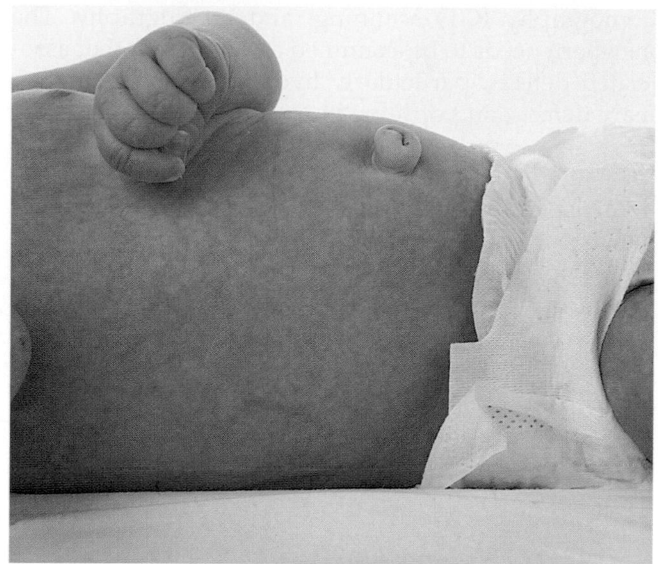

● ***Figure 21.9*** Small umbilical hernia in newborn.

parents, umbilical hernia is associated with little or no morbidity. In rare instances, the bowel may strangulate in the sac and require immediate surgery. Almost all these hernias close spontaneously by the age of 3 years; hernias that do not close should be corrected surgically before the child enters school.

Inguinal Hernia

Primarily common in males, inguinal hernias occur when the small sac of peritoneum surrounding the testes fails to close off after the testes descend from the abdominal sac into the scrotum. This failure allows the intestine to slip into the inguinal canal, with resultant swelling. If the intestine becomes trapped (incarcerated) and the circulation to the trapped intestine is impaired (strangulated), surgery is necessary to prevent intestinal obstruction and gangrene of the bowel. As a preventive measure, inguinal hernias normally are repaired as soon as they are diagnosed.

Test Yourself

- What are two major concerns for the newborn with a cleft lip or cleft palate?
- What is a potential complication for the newborn who has esophageal atresia?
- How are hernias most often treated?

Central Nervous System Defects

Central nervous system defects include disorders caused by an imbalance of cerebrospinal fluid (as in hydrocephalus) and a range of disorders resulting from malformations of the neural tube during embryonic development (often called "neural tube defects"). These defects vary from mild to severely disabling.

Spina Bifida

Caused by a defect in the neural arch generally in the lumbosacral region, **spina bifida** is a failure of the posterior laminae of the vertebrae to close; this leaves an opening through which the spinal meninges and spinal cord may protrude (Fig. 21-10).

Clinical Presentation

Signs and Symptoms. A bony defect that occurs without soft-tissue involvement is called *spina bifida occulta*. In most instances, it is asymptomatic and presents no problems. A dimple in the skin or a tuft of hair over the site may cause one to suspect its presence, or it may be overlooked entirely.

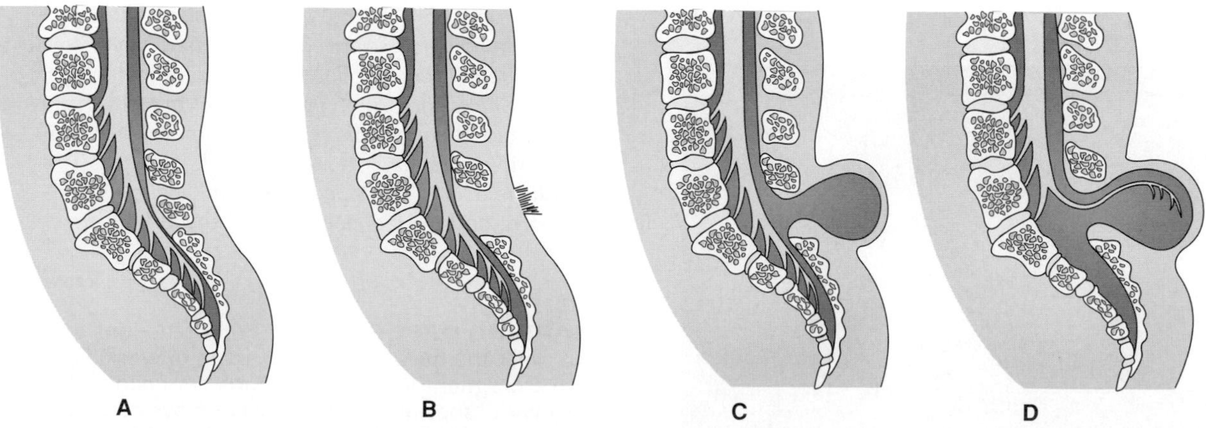

● ***Figure 21.10*** Degrees of spinal cord anomalies. (**A**) The normal spinal closure. (**B**) Occulta defect. (**C**) Meningocele defect. (**D**) Myelomeningocele defect clearly shows the spinal cord involvement.

When part of the spinal meninges protrudes through the bony defect and forms a cystic sac, the condition is termed *spina bifida with meningocele.* No nerve roots are involved, so no paralysis or sensory loss below the lesion appears. However, the sac may rupture or perforate, introducing infection into the spinal fluid and causing meningitis. For this reason, as well as for cosmetic purposes, surgical removal of the sac with closure of the skin is indicated.

In *spina bifida with myelomeningocele,* there is a protrusion of the spinal cord and the meninges, with nerve roots embedded in the wall of the cyst (Fig. 21-11). The effects of this defect vary in severity from sensory loss or partial paralysis below the lesion to complete flaccid paralysis of all muscles below the lesion. Complete paralysis involves the lower trunk and legs, as well as bowel and bladder sphincters.

Making a clear-cut differentiation in diagnosis between a meningocele and a myelomeningocele on the basis of symptoms alone is not always possible. Myelomeningocele may also be termed *meningomyelocele;* the associated "spina bifida" is always implied but not necessarily named. *Spina bifida cystica* is the term used to designate either of these protrusions.

Laboratory and Diagnostic Test Results. Elevated maternal alpha-fetoprotein (AFP) levels followed by ultrasonographic examination of the fetus may show an incomplete neural tube. An elevated AFP level in the maternal serum or amniotic fluid indicates the probability of central nervous system abnormalities. Additional examination may confirm this and allow the pregnant woman the opportunity to consider terminating the pregnancy. The best time to perform these tests is between 13 and 15 weeks' gestation, when peak levels are reached. Most obstetricians perform AFP testing.

Diagnosis of the newborn with spina bifida is made from clinical observation and examination. Additional evaluation of the defect may include magnetic resonance imaging (MRI), ultrasonography, computed tomography (CT) scanning, and myelography. The newborn needs to be examined carefully for other associated defects, particularly hydrocephalus, genitourinary defects, and orthopedic anomalies.

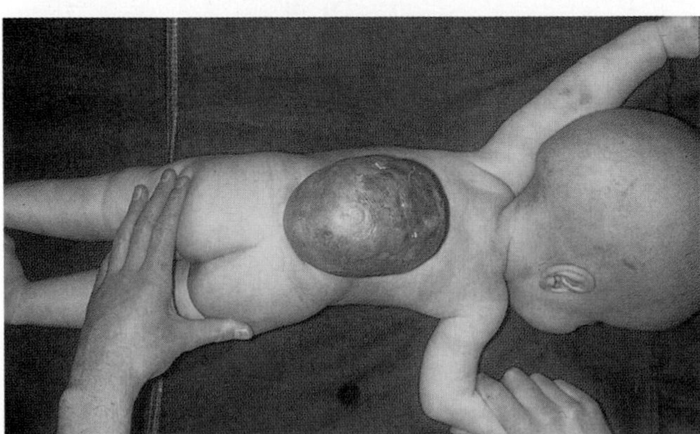

● ***Figure 21.11*** A newborn with a myelomeningocele and hydrocephalus.

Treatment

Many specialists are involved in the treatment of these newborns, especially in the case of myelomeningocele. These specialists may include neurologists, neurosurgeons, orthopedic specialists, pediatricians, urologists, and physical therapists. After a thorough evaluation of the newborn, a plan of surgical repair and treatment is developed.

Highly skilled nursing care is necessary in all aspects of the newborn's care. The child requires years

A PERSONAL GLIMPSE

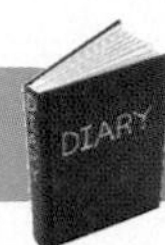

A child with "special needs." I never thought I would have to understand just what that really means. Courtney was our second child. A perfect pregnancy. Absolutely no problems. I didn't drink, never smoked, so I planned on a perfectly healthy baby. Until the AFP test. I will never forget that test now. I was 4 months pregnant and went in for the routine test. A few days later the results were in. A neurotube defect. . . . what in the world was that?

I have been asked many times if I was glad I knew before I had Courtney that she would have problems. I've thought a lot about it and even though it made the last several months of the pregnancy a little (well, maybe more than a little) worrisome, yes, I'm very glad we knew. Courtney was born C-section at a regional medical center that is about 60 miles from home. She was in surgery just a few hours after she was born.

Words like spina bifida, hydrocephalus, v. p. shunt, catheterizations, glasses, walkers, braces, kidney infections, all became everyday words at our home. We have learned a lot in the last 5 years. Courtney has frequent doctor visits to all her specialists. She is the only 5-year-old concerned if her urine is cloudy and making sure her mom gives her medication on time.

A little over 5 years ago a "special" child was born, and we feel very blessed she was given to us!!

Rhonda

LEARNING OPPORTUNITY: What reactions do you think the nurse might anticipate in working with a pregnant woman who finds her child will be born with "special needs?" In what ways could the nurse encourage this mother to share with other parents in similar situations?

of ongoing follow-up and therapy. Surgery is required to close the open defect but may not be performed immediately, depending on the surgeon's decision. Waiting several days does not seem to cause additional problems, and this period gives the family an opportunity to adjust to the initial shock and become involved in making the necessary decisions.

● Nursing Process in Caring for the Newborn With Myelomeningocele

ASSESSMENT

A routine newborn examination is conducted with emphasis on neurologic impairment. When collecting data during the examination, observe the movement and response to stimuli of the lower extremities. Carefully measure the head circumference and examine the fontanelles. Thoroughly document the observations made. When the newborn is handled, take great care to prevent injury to the sac.

The family needs support and understanding during the newborn's initial care and for the many years of care during the child's life. Determine the family's knowledge and understanding of the defect, as well as their attitude concerning the birth of a newborn with such serious problems.

SELECTED NURSING DIAGNOSES

- Risk for Infection related to vulnerability of the myelomeningocele sac
- Risk for Impaired Skin Integrity related to exposure to urine and feces
- Risk for Injury related to neuromuscular impairment
- Compromised Family Coping related to the perceived loss of the perfect newborn
- Deficient Knowledge of the family caregivers related to the complexities of caring for a newborn with serious neurologic and musculoskeletal defects

OUTCOME IDENTIFICATION AND PLANNING: PREOPERATIVE CARE

The preoperative goals for care of the newborn with myelomeningocele include preventing infection, maintaining skin integrity, preventing trauma related to disuse, increasing family coping skills, education about the condition, and support.

IMPLEMENTATION

Preventing Infection Monitor the newborn's vital signs, neurologic signs, and behavior frequently to observe for any deviations from normal that may indicate an infection. Prophylactic antibiotics may be ordered. Carry out routine aseptic technique with conscientious handwashing, gloving, and gowning as appropriate. Until surgery is performed, the sac must be covered with a sterile dressing moistened in a warm sterile solution (often sterile saline). Change this dressing every 2 hours; do not allow it to dry to avoid damage to the covering of the sac. The dressings may be covered with a plastic protective covering. Maintain the newborn in a prone position so that no pressure is placed on the sac. After surgery, continue this positioning until the surgical site is well healed.

Diapering is not advisable with a low defect, but the sac must be protected from contamination with fecal material. Placing a protective barrier between the anus and the sac may prevent this contamination. If the anal sphincter muscles are involved, the newborn may have continual loose stools, which adds to the challenge of keeping the sac free from infection.

Promoting Skin Integrity. The nursing interventions discussed in the previous section on infection also are necessary to promote skin integrity around the area of the defect and the diaper area. As mentioned, leakage of stool and urine may be continual. This leakage causes skin irritation and breakdown if the newborn is not kept clean and the diaper area is not free of stool and urine. Scrupulous perineal care is necessary.

Preventing Contractures of Lower Extremities. Newborns with spina bifida often have **talipes equinovarus** (clubfoot) and congenital **hip dysplasia** (dislocation of the hips), both of which are discussed later in this chapter. If there is loss of motion in the lower limbs because of the defect, conduct range-of-motion exercises to prevent contractures. Position the newborn so that the hips are abducted and the feet are in a neutral position. Massage the knees and other bony prominences with lotion regularly, then pad them, and protect them from irritation. When handling the newborn, avoid putting pressure on the sac.

Promoting Family Coping. The family of a newborn with such a major anomaly is in a state of shock on first learning of the problems. Be especially sensitive to their needs and emotions. Encourage family members to express their feelings and emotions as openly as possible. Recognize that some families express emotions much more freely than others do, and adjust your responses to the family with this in mind. Provide privacy as needed for the family to mourn together over their loss, but do not avoid the family because this only exaggerates their feelings of loss and depression. If possible, encourage the family members to cuddle or touch the newborn using proper precautions for the safety of the defect. With the permission of the physician, the newborn may be held in a chest-to-chest position to provide closer contact.

Providing Family Teaching. Give family members information about the defect and encourage them to discuss their concerns and ask questions. Provide information about the newborn's present state, the proposed surgery, and follow-up care. Remember that anxiety may block understanding and processing knowledge, so information may need to be repeated. Information should be provided in small segments to facilitate comprehension.

After surgery, the family needs to be prepared to care for the newborn at home. Teach the family to hold the newborn's head, neck, and chest slightly raised in one hand during feeding. Also teach them that stroking the newborn's cheek helps stimulate sucking. Showing the family how to care for the newborn, allowing them to participate in the care, and guiding them in performing return demonstrations are all methods to use in family teaching.

For long-term care and support, refer the family to the Spina Bifida Association of America (*http://www.sbaa.org*). Give them materials concerning spina bifida. These children need long-term care involving many aspects of medicine and surgery, as well as education and vocational training. Although children with spina bifida have many long-term problems, their intelligence is not affected; many of these children grow into productive young adults who may live independently (Fig. 21-12).

EVALUATION: GOALS AND EXPECTED OUTCOMES

- **Goal:** The newborn will be free from signs and symptoms of infection.
  Expected Outcomes: The newborn's vital signs and neurologic signs are within normal limits; the newborn shows no signs of irritability or lethargy.
- **Goal:** The newborn will have no evidence of skin breakdown.
  Expected Outcomes: The newborn's skin will remain clean, dry, and intact and will have no areas of reddening or signs of irritation.
- **Goal:** The newborn remains free from injury.
  Expected Outcomes: The newborn's lower limbs show no evidence of contractures.

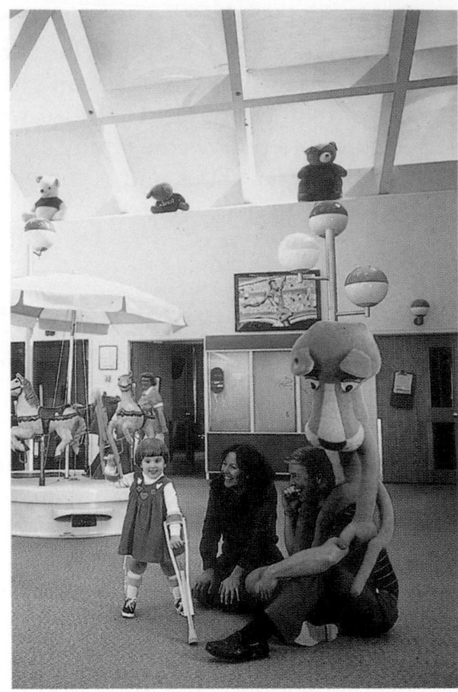

● ***Figure 21.12*** Learning to use new braces and a crutch, this girl underwent successful surgery for repair of a myelomeningocele during infancy.

- **Goal:** The family caregivers will show positive signs of beginning coping.
  Expected Outcomes: The family members verbalize their anxieties and needs and hold, cuddle, and soothe the newborn as appropriate.
- **Goal:** The family caregivers will learn to care for the newborn.
  Expected Outcomes: The family demonstrates competence in performing care for the newborn, verbalizes understanding of the signs and symptoms that should be reported, and has information about support agencies.

Hydrocephalus

Hydrocephalus is a condition characterized by an excess of cerebrospinal fluid (CSF) within the ventricular and subarachnoid spaces of the cranial cavity. Normally a delicate balance exists between the rate of formation and absorption of CSF: the entire volume is absorbed and replaced every 12 to 24 hours. In hydrocephalus, this balance is disturbed.

Cerebrospinal fluid is formed mainly in the lateral ventricles by the choroid plexus and is absorbed into the venous system through the arachnoid villi. Cerebrospinal fluid circulates within the ventricles and the subarachnoid space. It is a colorless fluid consisting of water with traces of protein, glucose, and lymphocytes.

In the *noncommunicating* type of congenital hydrocephalus, an obstruction occurs in the free circulation

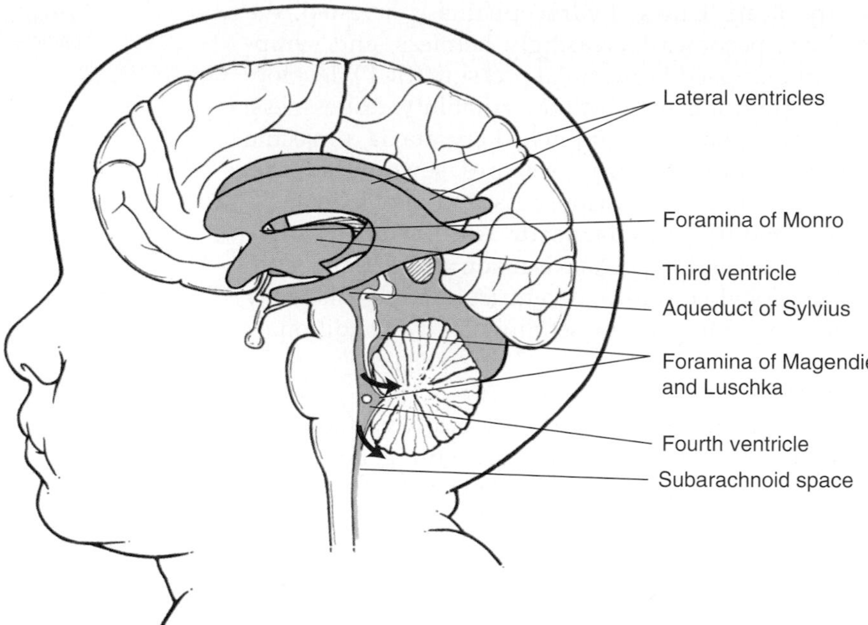

● ***Figure 21.13*** Ventricles of the brain and channels for the normal flow of cerebrospinal fluid.

of CSF. This blockage causes increased pressure on the brain or spinal cord. The site of obstruction may be at the foramen of Monro, the aqueduct of Sylvius, the foramen of Luschka, or the foramen of Magendie (Fig. 21-13). In the *communicating* type of hydrocephalus, no obstruction of the free flow of CSF exists between the ventricles and the spinal theca; rather the condition is caused by defective absorption of CSF, thus causing increased pressure on the brain or spinal cord. Congenital hydrocephalus is most often the obstructive or noncommunicating type.

Hydrocephalus may be recognized at birth, or it may not be evident until after a few weeks or months of life. The condition may not be congenital but instead may occur during later infancy or during childhood as the result of a neoplasm, a head injury, or an infection such as meningitis.

When hydrocephalus occurs early in life before the skull sutures close, the soft, pliable bones separate to allow head expansion. This condition is manifested by a rapid increase in head circumference. The fact that the soft bones can yield to pressure in this manner may partially explain why many of these newborns fail to show the usual symptoms of brain pressure and may exhibit little or no damage in mental function until later in life. Other newborns show severe brain damage, which often has occurred before birth.

Clinical Presentation

Signs and Symptoms. An excessively large head at birth is suggestive of hydrocephalus. Rapid head growth with widening cranial sutures is also strongly suggestive and may be the first manifestation of this condition. An apparently large head in itself is not necessarily significant. Normally every newborn's head is measured at birth, and the rate of growth is checked at subsequent examinations. If a newborn's head appears to be abnormally large at birth or appears to be enlarging, it should be measured frequently.

As the head enlarges, the suture lines separate and the spaces may be felt through the scalp. The anterior fontanelle becomes tense and bulging, the skull enlarges in all diameters, and the scalp becomes shiny and its veins dilate (Fig. 21-14). If pressure continues to increase without intervention, the eyes appear to be pushed downward slightly with the sclera visible above the iris—the so-called "setting sun" sign.

If the condition progresses without adequate drainage of excessive fluid, the head becomes increasingly heavy, the neck muscles fail to develop sufficiently, and the newborn has difficulty raising or turn-

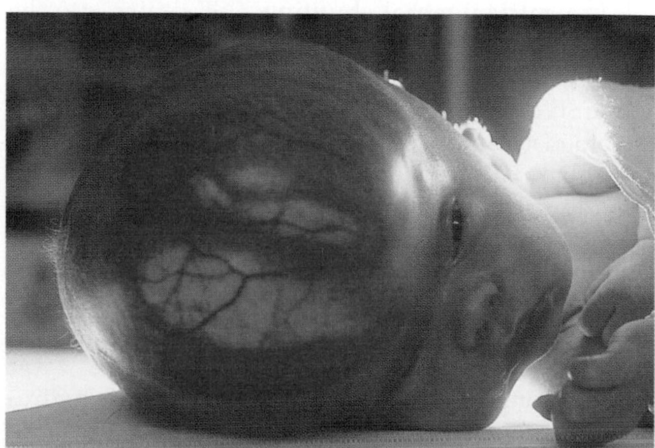

● ***Figure 21.14*** A newborn with hydrocephalus. Note the pull on the eyes giving the "setting sun" appearance.

ing the head. Unless hydrocephalus is arrested, the newborn becomes increasingly helpless, and symptoms of increased intracranial pressure (IICP) develop. These symptoms may include irritability, restlessness, personality change, high-pitched cry, ataxia, projectile vomiting, failure to thrive, seizures, severe headache, changes in level of consciousness, and papilledema.

Laboratory and Diagnostic Test Results. Positive diagnosis of hydrocephalus is made with CT and MRI. Echoencephalography and ventriculography also may be performed for further definition of the condition.

Treatment

Surgical intervention is the only effective means of relieving brain pressure and preventing additional damage to the brain tissue. If minimal brain damage has occurred, the child may be able to function within a normal mental range. Motor function is usually retarded. In some instances, surgical intervention may remove the cause of the obstruction, such as a neoplasm, a cyst, or a hematoma, but most children require placement of a shunting device that bypasses the point of obstruction, draining the excess CSF into a body cavity. This procedure arrests excessive head growth and prevents additional brain damage.

Many shunt procedures use a silicone rubber catheter that is radiopaque so that its position may be checked by radiographic examination. The silicone rubber catheter reduces the problem of tissue reaction. A valve or regulator is an essential part of each catheter that prevents excessive build-up of fluid or too-rapid decompression of the ventricle. The most common procedure, particularly for newborns and small children, is **ventriculoperitoneal shunting** (VP shunt). In this procedure, the CSF is drained from a lateral ventricle in the brain; the CSF runs through the subcutaneous catheter and empties into the peritoneal cavity. This procedure allows the insertion of some excess tubing to accommodate growth. As the child grows, the catheter needs to be revised and lengthened (Fig. 21-15).

In **ventriculoatrial shunting,** CSF drains into the right atrium of the heart. This procedure cannot be used in children with pathologic changes in the heart. The CSF drained from the ventricle is absorbed into the bloodstream.

Other pathways of drainage have been used with varying degrees of success. All types of shunts may have problems with kinking, blocking, moving, or shifting of tubing. The danger of infection in the tubing is a constant concern. Children with shunts must be observed constantly for signs of malfunction or infection.

The long-term outcome for a child with hydrocephalus depends on several factors. If untreated, the outcome is very poor, often leading to death. With shunting, the outcome depends on the initial cause of the increased fluid, the treatment of the cause, the brain damage sustained before shunting, complications with the shunting system, and continued long-term follow-up. Some of these children can lead relatively normal lives if they have follow-up and revisions as they grow.

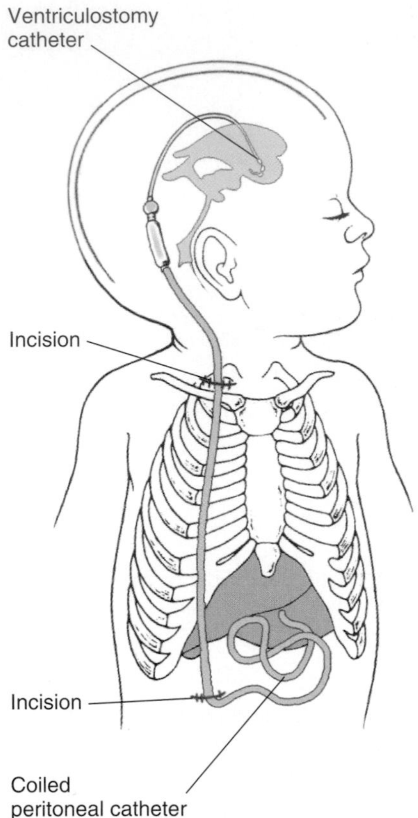

● ***Figure 21.15*** Ventriculoperitoneal shunt.

● Nursing Process in Caring for the Postoperative Newborn With Hydrocephalus

ASSESSMENT

Obtaining accurate vital and neurologic signs is necessary before and after surgery. Measurement of the newborn's head is essential. If the fontanelles are not closed, carefully observe them for any signs of bulging. Observe, report, and document all signs of IICP. If the child has returned for revision of an existing shunt, obtain a complete history before surgery from the family caregiver to provide a baseline of the child's behavior.

Determine the level of knowledge family members have about the condition. For the family of the newborn or young newborn, the diagnosis will probably come as an emotional shock.

Conduct the interview and examination of the newborn with sensitivity and understanding.

SELECTED NURSING DIAGNOSES

- Risk for Injury related to increased ICP
- Risk for Impaired Skin Integrity related to pressure from physical immobility
- Risk for Infection related to the presence of a shunt
- Risk for Delayed Growth and Development related to impaired ability to achieve developmental tasks
- Anxiety related to the family caregiver's fear of the surgical outcome
- Deficient Knowledge related to the family's understanding of the child's condition and home care

OUTCOME IDENTIFICATION AND PLANNING

The goals for the postoperative care of the newborn with shunt placement for hydrocephalus include preventing injury, maintaining skin integrity, preventing infection, maintaining growth and development, and reducing family anxiety. Family goals include increasing knowledge about the condition and providing loving, supportive care to the newborn.

IMPLEMENTATION

Preventing Injury. At least every 2 to 4 hours, monitor the newborn's level of consciousness. Check the pupils for equality and reaction, monitor the neurologic status, and observe for a shrill cry, lethargy, or irritability. Measure and record the head circumference daily. Carry out appropriate procedures to care for the shunt as directed. To prevent a rapid decrease in ICP, keep the newborn flat. Observe for signs of seizure, and initiate seizure precautions. Keep suction and oxygen equipment convenient at the bedside.

Promoting Skin Integrity. After a shunting procedure, keep the newborn's head turned away from the operative site until the physician allows a change in position. If the newborn's head is enlarged, prevent pressure sores from forming on the side where the child rests. Reposition the newborn at least every 2 hours as permitted. Inspect the dressings over the shunt site immediately after the surgery, every hour for the first 3 to 4 hours, and then at least every 4 hours.

Preventing Infection. Infection is the primary threat after surgery. Closely observe for and promptly report any signs of infection, which include redness, heat, or swelling along the surgical site, fever, and signs of lethargy. Perform wound care thoroughly as ordered. Administer antibiotics as prescribed.

Promoting Growth and Development. Every newborn has the need to be picked up and held, cuddled, and comforted. An uncomfortable or painful experience increases the need for emotional support. A newborn perceives such support principally through physical contact made in a soothing, loving manner.

This is important! Always support the head of a newborn with hydrocephalus when picking up, moving, or positioning. Using egg-crate pads, lamb's wool, or a special mattress can prevent pressure and breakdown of the scalp.

The newborn needs social interaction and needs to be talked to, played with, and given the opportunity for activity. Provide toys appropriate for his or her physical and mental capacity. If the child has difficulty moving about the crib, place toys within easy reach and vision: a cradle gym, for example, may be tied close enough for the newborn to maneuver its parts.

Unless the newborn's nervous system is so impaired that all activity increases irritability, the newborn needs stimulation just as any child does. If repositioning from side-to-side means turning the newborn away from the sight of activity, the crib may be turned around so that vision is not obstructed.

A newborn who is given the contact and support that all newborns require develops a pleasing personality because he or she is nourished by emotional stimulation. Use the time spent on physical care as a time for social interaction. Talking, laughing, and playing with the newborn are important aspects of the newborn's care. Make frequent contacts, and do not limit them to the times when physical care is being performed.

Reducing Family Anxiety. Explain to the family the condition and the anatomy of the surgical procedure in terms they can understand. Discuss the overall prognosis for the child. Encourage family members to express their anxieties and ask questions. Giving accurate, nontechnical answers is extremely helpful. Give the family information about support groups such as the National Hydrocephalus Foundation (*www.nhfonline.org*) and encourage them to contact the groups.

Providing Family Teaching. Demonstrate care of the shunt to the family caregivers and have them perform a return demonstration. Provide them with a list of signs and symptoms that should be reported. Review these with the family members and make sure they understand them. Discuss appropriate growth and developmental expectations for the child, and stress realistic goals.

EVALUATION: GOALS AND EXPECTED OUTCOMES

- **Goal:** The newborn will be free from injury related to complications of excessive cerebrospinal fluid.
  Expected Outcomes: The newborn has no signs of IICP, such as lethargy, irritability, and seizure activity, and has a stable level of consciousness.
- **Goal:** The newborn's skin will remain intact.
  Expected Outcomes: The newborn's skin shows no evidence of pressure sores, redness, or other signs of skin breakdown.
- **Goal:** The newborn will remain free of infection.
  Expected Outcomes: The newborn shows no signs of infection; vital signs are stable; and there is no redness, drainage, or swelling at the surgical site.
- **Goal:** The newborn will have age-appropriate growth and development.
  Expected Outcomes: The newborn's social and developmental needs are met. The newborn interacts and plays appropriately with toys and surroundings.
- **Goal:** The family caregiver's anxiety will be reduced.
  Expected Outcomes: The family expresses fears and concerns and interacts appropriately with the newborn.
- **Goal:** The family will learn care of the child.
  Expected Outcomes: The family participates in the care of the newborn, asks appropriate questions, and lists signs and symptoms to report.

Cardiovascular System Defects: Congenital Heart Disease

Cardiovascular system defects range from mild to severe. They may be detected immediately at birth or may not be detected for several months. When a newborn is suspected of having a heart abnormality, the family is understandably upset. The heart is *the* vital organ; a person can live without a number of other organs and appendages, but life itself depends on the heart. The family caregivers will have many questions: the nurse may answer some; the physician must answer others. Many answers will not be available until after various evaluation procedures have been conducted.

Technological advances have progressed rapidly in this field, making earlier detection and successful repair much more likely. However, heart defects are still the leading cause of death from congenital anomalies in the first year of life. A brief discussion of the development and function of the embryonic heart is useful to understanding the malformations that occur.

Development of the Heart

The heart begins beating early in the 3rd to 8th week of intrauterine life. When first formed, the heart is a simple tube receiving blood from the placenta and pumping it out into its developing body. During this period, the heart rapidly develops into its normal, but complex, four-chambered structure.

Adjustments in circulation must be made at birth. During fetal life the lungs are inactive, requiring only a small amount of blood to nourish their tissues. Blood is circulated through the umbilical arteries to the placenta, where waste products and carbon dioxide are exchanged for oxygen and nutrients. The blood is then returned to the fetus through the umbilical vein.

At birth, the umbilical cord is cut, and the newborn's own independent circulatory system is established. Certain circulatory bypasses, such as the **ductus arteriosus,** the **foramen ovale,** and the **ductus venosus,** are no longer necessary. They close during the first several weeks after birth. In addition, the pressure in the heart, which has been higher on the right side during fetal life, now changes so that the left side of the heart has the higher pressure (Fig. 21-16).

During this period of complex development, any error in formation may cause serious circulatory difficulty. The incidence of cardiovascular malformations is about 8 in 1,000 live births. Some abnormalities are slight and allow the person to lead a normal life without correction. Others cause little apparent difficulty but need correction to improve the chance for a longer life and for optimal health. Some severe anomalies are incompatible with life for more than a short time; others may be helped but not cured by surgery.

Common Types of Congenital Heart Defects

Traditionally, congenital heart defects have been described as cyanotic or acyanotic conditions. **Cyanotic heart disease** implies an oxygen saturation of the peripheral arterial blood of 85% or less. This condition occurs when a heart defect allows any appreciable amount of oxygen-poor blood in the right side of the heart to mix with the oxygenated blood in the left side of the heart. Defects that permit right-to-left shunting may occur at the atrial, ventricular, or aortic level.

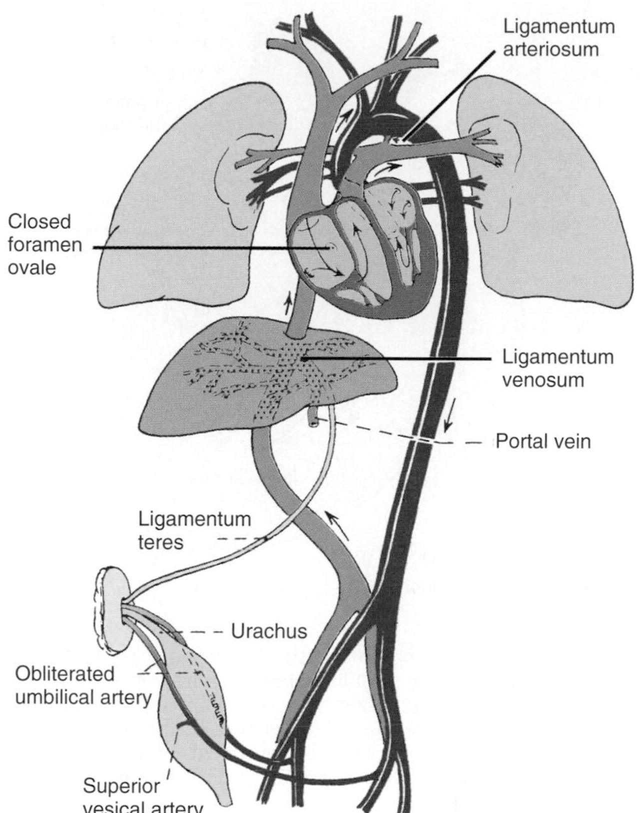

● ***Figure 21.16*** Normal blood circulation. Highlighted ligaments indicate pathways that should close at or soon after birth. *Arrows* indicate normal flow of blood.

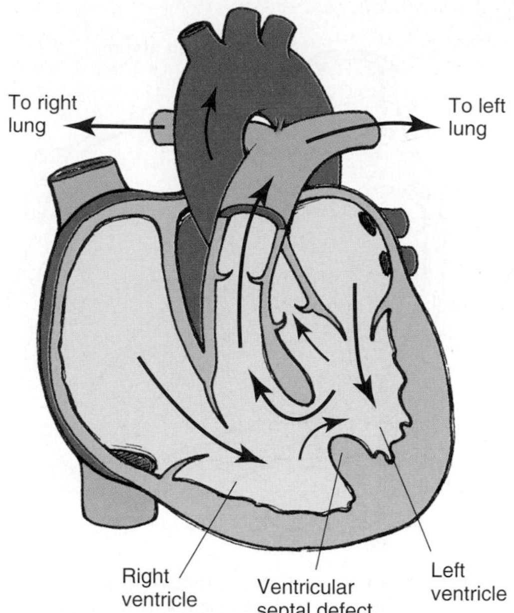

● ***Figure 21.17*** A ventricular septal defect is an abnormal opening between the right and left ventricle. Ventricular septal defects vary in size and may occur in the membranous or muscular portion of the ventricular septum. Owing to higher pressure in the left ventricle, a shunting of blood from the left to the right ventricle occurs during systole. If pulmonary vascular resistance produces pulmonary hypertension, the shunt of blood is then reversed from the right to the left ventricle, with cyanosis resulting.

However, because defects are often complex and occur in various combinations, this is an inadequate means of classification. A more clear-cut classification system is based on blood flow characteristics. These are:

1. Increased pulmonary blood flow (e.g., ventricular septal, atrial septal, and patent ductus arteriosus)
2. Obstruction of blood flow out of the heart (e.g., coarctation of the aorta)
3. Decreased pulmonary blood flow (e.g., tetralogy of Fallot)
4. Mixed blood flow, where saturated and desaturated blood mix in the heart, aorta, and pulmonary vessels (e.g., transposition of the great arteries)

Because defects often occur in combination, they give rise to complex situations. Most nurses may never see many of the complex defects and most of the rare, isolated defects. The conditions discussed here are common enough that the pediatric nurse needs to be familiar with their diagnosis and treatment.

Ventricular Septal Defect

Ventricular septal defect is the most common intracardiac defect. It consists of an abnormal opening in the septum between the two ventricles, which allows blood to pass directly from the left to the right ventricle. No unoxygenated blood leaks into the left ventricle, so cyanosis does not occur (Fig. 21-17).

Small, isolated defects are usually asymptomatic and often are discovered during a routine physical examination. A characteristic loud, harsh murmur associated with a systolic thrill occasionally is heard on examination. A history of frequent respiratory infections may occur during infancy, but growth and development are unaffected. The child leads a normal life.

Corrective surgery may be postponed until the age of 18 months to 2 years, when the surgical risk is less than that for newborns. However, surgical techniques have improved to the degree that the repair may be made in the first year of life with high rates of success. The child is observed closely and may be prescribed a regimen of prophylactic antibiotics to prevent frequent respiratory infections. If pulmonary involvement becomes a problem, the repair is done without further delay. Repairs in children who are at high risk are done by the use of cardiac catheterization procedures.

Atrial Septal Defects

In general, left-to-right shunting occurs in all true atrial septal defects. However, the atrial septum of many healthy people houses a patent **foramen ovale** that normally causes no problems because its valve is

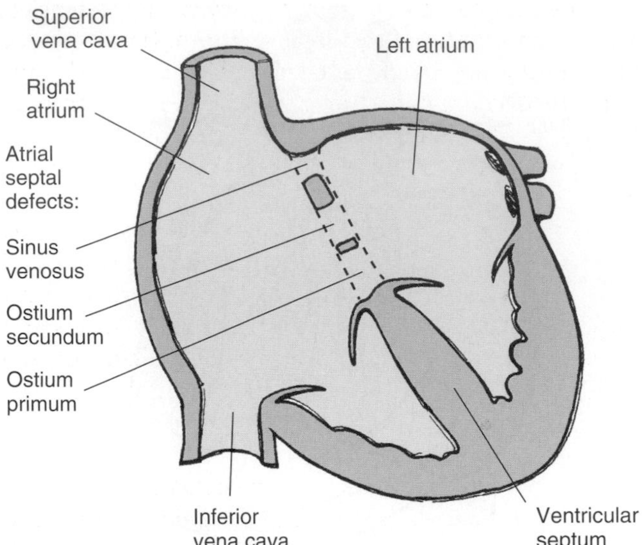

● ***Figure 21.18*** An atrial septal defect is an abnormal opening between the right and left atria. Basically, three types of abnormalities result from incorrect development of the atrial septum. An incompetent foramen ovale is the most common defect. The ostium secundum defect results from abnormal development of the septum secundum and causes an opening in the middle of the septum. Improper development of the septum primum produces an opening at the lower end of the septum known as an ostium primum defect, frequently involving the atrioventricular valves. In general, left-to-right shunting of blood occurs in all atrial septal defects.

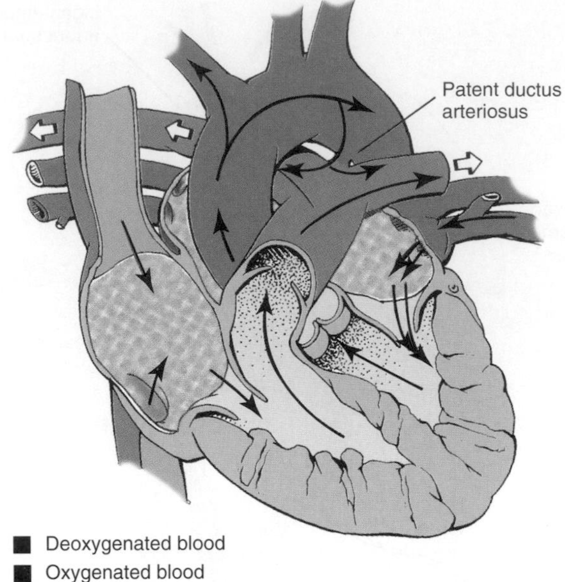

● ***Figure 21.19*** The patent ductus arteriosus is a vascular connection that, during fetal life, short-circuits the pulmonary vascular bed and directs blood from the pulmonary artery to the aorta. Functional closure of the ductus normally occurs soon after birth. If the ductus remains patent after birth, the higher pressure in the aorta reverses the direction of blood flow in the ductus.

anatomically structured to withstand left chamber pressure, rendering it functionally closed (Fig. 21-18).

True atrial septal defects are common heart anomalies and may occur as isolated defects or in combination with other heart anomalies. Atrial septal defects are amenable to surgery with a low surgical mortality risk. Since the advent of the heart–lung bypass machine, this repair may be performed in a dry field, replacing the older "blind" technique. The opening is closed with sutures or a Dacron patch.

Patent Ductus Arteriosus

The **ductus arteriosus** is a vascular channel between the left main pulmonary artery and the descending aorta. In fetal life it allows blood to bypass the nonfunctioning lungs and go directly into the systemic circuit. After birth the duct normally closes, eventually becoming obliterated and forming the ligamentum arteriosum. However, if the ductus arteriosus remains patent, blood continues to be shunted from the aorta into the pulmonary artery. This situation results in a flooding of the lungs and an overloading of the left heart chambers (Fig. 21-19).

Normally the ductus arteriosus is nonpatent after the 1st or 2nd week of life and should be obliterated by the 4th month. Why it fails to close is unknown. Patent ductus arteriosus is common in newborns who exhibit the rubella syndrome, but most newborns with this anomaly have no history of exposure to rubella during fetal life. It is also common in preterm newborns weighing less than 1,200 g and in newborns with Down's syndrome.

Symptoms of patent ductus arteriosus are often absent during childhood. Growth and development may be retarded in some children with an easy fatigability and dyspnea on exertion. The diagnosis may be based on a characteristic machinery-like murmur over the pulmonary area, a wide pulse pressure, and a bounding pulse. Cardiac catheterization is diagnostic but is not required in the presence of classic clinical features.

Indomethacin (Indocin), a prostaglandin inhibitor, may be administered with some success to premature newborns to promote closure of the ductus arteriosus. If this fails to close the ductus, surgery is indicated in all diagnosed cases, even if they are asymptomatic. Some persons live a normal life span without correction, but the risks involved far outweigh the surgical ones. Surgical correction consists of closure of the defect by ligation or by division of the ductus. Division is the method of choice if the child's condition permits because the ductus occasionally reopens after ligation. The optimal age for surgery is before the age of 2 years, with earlier surgery for severely affected newborns. Prognosis is excellent after a successful repair.

Coarctation of the Aorta

This congenital cardiovascular anomaly consists of a constriction or narrowing of the aortic arch or the descending aorta usually adjacent to the ligamentum arteriosum (Fig. 21-20).

Most children with this condition have no symptoms until later childhood or young adulthood. A few newborns have severe symptoms in their first year of life; they show dyspnea, tachycardia, and cyanosis, which are all signs of developing congestive heart failure.

In older children, the condition is diagnosed easily based on hypertension in the upper extremities and hypotension in the lower extremities. The radial pulse is readily palpable, but the femoral pulses are weak or even impalpable. Blood pressure is normal or elevated in the arms and is low or undetectable in the legs. A high-pitched systolic murmur is usually present and heard over the base of the heart and over the interscapular area of the back. The diagnosis may be confirmed by aortography.

Obstruction to blood flow caused by the constricted portion of the aorta does not cause early difficulty in an average child because the blood bypasses the obstruction by way of collateral circulation. The bypass is chiefly from the branches of the subclavian and carotid arteries that arise from the arch of the aorta. Eventually the enlarged collateral arteries erode the rib margins, and the rib notching may be visualized by radiographic examination.

Uncorrected coarctation may cause hypertension and cardiac failure later in life. The optimal age for elective surgery is before the age of 2 years. Early surgery may be necessary for a gravely ill newborn who presents with severe congestive heart failure. In early infancy, the mortality rate depends on the presence of other congenital heart problems.

Surgery consists of resection of the coarcted area with an end-to-end anastomosis of the proximal and distal ends of the aorta. Occasionally a long defect may necessitate an end-to-end graft using tubes of Dacron or similar material. Prognosis is excellent for the restoration of normal function after surgery.

Tetralogy of Fallot

This is a fairly common congenital heart defect involving 50% to 70% of all cyanotic congenital heart diseases. It consists of a grouping of heart defects (tetralogy denotes four abnormal conditions): (1) **pulmonary stenosis,** (2) **ventricular septal defect,** (3) **overriding aorta,** and (4) **right ventricular hypertrophy.** The pulmonary stenosis is usually seen as a narrowing of the upper portion of the right ventricle and may include stenosis of the valve cusps. Pulmonary stenosis results, in turn, in right ventricular hypertrophy. The aorta appears to straddle the ventricular septum, overriding the ventricular septal defect. This defect allows a shunt of unsaturated blood from the right ventricle into the aorta or into the left ventricle (Fig. 21-21).

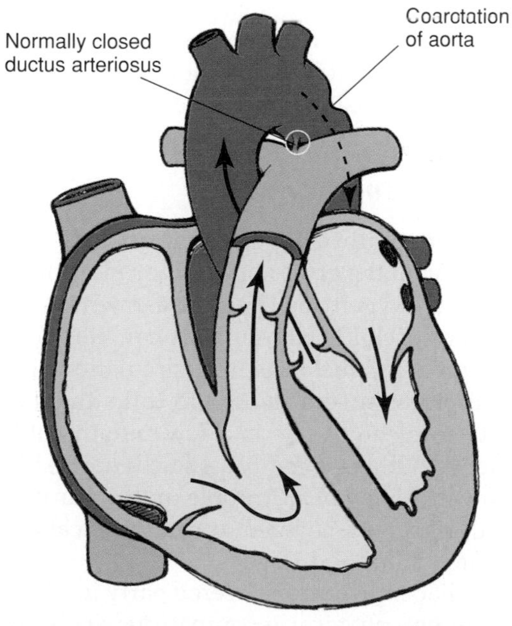

Normally closed ductus arteriosus

Coarctation of aorta

● ***Figure 21.20*** Coarctation of the aorta is characterized by a narrowed aortic lumen. It exists as a preductal or postductal obstruction, depending on the position of the obstruction in relation to the ductus arteriosus. Coarctations exist with great variation in anatomic features. The lesion produces an obstruction to the flow of blood through the aorta, causing an increased left ventricular pressure and workload.

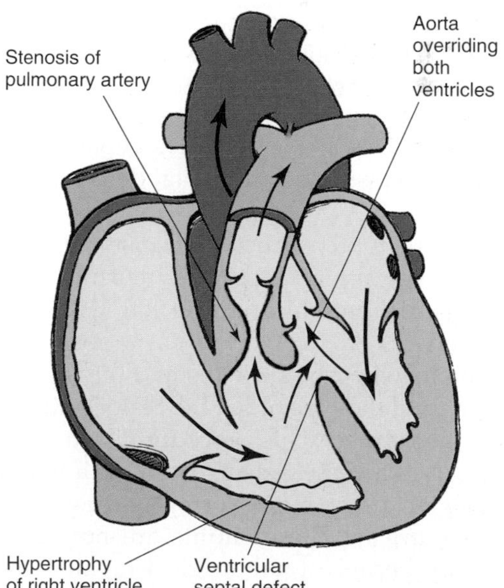

● ***Figure 21.21*** Tetralogy of Fallot is characterized by the combination of four defects: (1) pulmonary stenosis, (2) ventricular septal defect, (3) overriding aorta, and (4) hypertrophy of the right ventricle. It is the most common defect causing cyanosis in patients surviving beyond 2 years of age. The severity of symptoms depends on the degree of pulmonary stenosis, the size of the ventricular septal defect, and the degree to which the aorta overrides the septal defect.

The child with tetralogy of Fallot may be precyanotic in early infancy, with the cyanotic phase starting at 4 to 6 months of age. However, some severely affected newborns may show cyanosis earlier. As long as the ductus arteriosus remains open, enough blood apparently passes through the lungs to prevent cyanosis.

The infant presents with feeding difficulties and poor weight gain, resulting in retarded growth and development. Dyspnea and easy fatigability become evident. Exercise tolerance depends in part on the severity of the disease; some children become fatigued after little exertion. In the past, on experiencing fatigue, breathlessness, and increased cyanosis, the child was described as assuming a squatting posture for relief. Squatting apparently increased the systemic oxygen saturation. However, squatting rarely is seen today because these newborns' defects usually are repaired by the time they are 2 years old.

Attacks of paroxysmal dyspnea are common during infancy and early childhood. An anoxic spell is heralded by sudden restlessness, gasping respiration, and increased cyanosis that lead to a loss of consciousness and, possibly, convulsions. These attacks, called "tet spells," last from a few minutes to several hours and appear to be unpredictable, although stress does seem to trigger some episodes.

The history and clinical manifestations are usually sufficient to make a diagnosis. However, cardiac catheterization, electrocardiography, chest radiography, and laboratory tests to determine polycythemia and arterial oxygen saturation may be performed for additional definition.

The preferred repair of these defects is total surgical correction. This procedure requires the use of a cardiopulmonary bypass machine. The heart is opened, and extensive resection is done. The repair relieves the pulmonary stenosis, and the septal defect is closed by use of a patch.

Successful total correction transforms a grossly abnormal heart into a functionally normal one. However, most of these children are left without a pulmonary valve.

In infants who cannot withstand the total surgical correction until they are older, the Blalock-Taussig procedure is performed. This procedure is an end-to-end anastomosis of a vessel arising from the aorta, usually the subclavian artery, to the corresponding right or left pulmonary artery. These shunts are now seen only occasionally because total surgical repair is meeting with much greater success and lower mortality rates.

Transposition of the Great Arteries

This severe defect was at one time almost always fatal. Advancements in diagnosis and treatment have increased the success rate in treatment of this disorder. In transposition of the great arteries, the aorta arises from the right ventricle instead of the left, and the pulmonary artery arises from the left ventricle instead of the right. These newborns are usually cyanotic from birth.

Test Yourself

- What is the difference between spina bifida with meningocele and spina bifida with myelomeningocele?
- What does the newborn have an excess of in the condition of hydrocephalus? How is hydrocephalus treated?
- List the five common types of congenital heart defects.
- In children with heart conditions what is the most common manifestation or symptom?

Risk Factors

Maternal alcoholism, maternal irradiation, ingestion of certain drugs during pregnancy, maternal diabetes, and advanced maternal age (older than 40 years) increase the incidence of heart defects in newborns. Rubella in the expectant mother during the first trimester can also cause cardiac malformations. Maternal malnutrition and heredity may be contributing factors. Recent studies have shown that the offspring of mothers who had congenital heart anomalies have a much higher risk of having congenital heart anomalies. If one child in the family has a congenital heart abnormality, later siblings have a very high risk for such a defect.

Clinical Presentation

The newborn with a severe abnormality, such as a transposition of the great vessels, is cyanotic from birth and requires oxygen and special treatment. A less seriously affected child, whose heart can compensate to some degree for the impaired circulation, may not have symptoms severe enough to call attention to the difficulty until he or she is a few months older and more active. Others may live a fairly normal life and not be aware of any heart trouble until a murmur or an enlarged heart is discovered during physical examination in later childhood.

A cardiac murmur discovered early in life necessitates frequent physical examinations. This murmur may be a functional, "innocent" murmur that may disappear as the child grows older, or it may be the chief manifestation of an abnormal heart or an abnormal circulatory system. The most common parental concern is that of feeding difficulties. Newborns with cardiac anomalies severe enough to cause circulatory difficulties have a history of being poor eaters, tiring easily from the effort to suck, and failing to grow or thrive normally. These manifestations of **congestive heart failure** (CHF) may appear during the first year of life in newborns with conditions such as large ventricular septal defects, coarctation of the aorta, and other defects that place an increased workload on the ventricles. See Chapter 36 for a full discussion of CHF.

Treatment and Nursing Care

Advances in medical technology have enabled heart repairs to be performed in newborns as young as less than 1 day old. Miniaturization of instruments, earlier diagnosis through the use of improved diagnostic techniques, pediatric intensive care facilities staffed with highly skilled nurse specialists, and more sophisticated monitoring techniques have all contributed to these advances.

Most physicians now think it is important to operate as early as possible to repair defective hearts. Inadequate circulation may prevent adequate growth and development and cause permanent, irreparable physical, mental, and emotional damage. If the child is receives a diagnosis early and correction or repair is possible, CHF may be avoided.

In cases where the child has CHF, it is important that the CHF be treated. The primary goals in the treatment of CHF are to reduce the workload of the heart and to improve the cardiac functioning, thus increasing oxygenation of the tissues. This is done by removing excess sodium and fluids, slowing the heart rate, and decreasing the demands on the heart. See Chapter 36 for a complete discussion of CHF and its treatment.

Care at Home Before Surgery

A child with congenital heart disease may show easy fatigability and retarded growth. If the child has a cyanotic type of heart disease with clubbing of the fingers or toes, periods of cyanosis and reduced exercise tolerance are evident. This young child may assume a squatting position, which reduces the return flow to the heart, thus temporarily reducing the workload of the heart.

Such a child should be allowed to lead as normal a life as possible. Families are naturally apprehensive and find it difficult not to overprotect the child. They often increase the child's anxiety and cause fear in the child about participating in normal activities. Children are rather sensible about finding their own limitations and usually limit their activities to their capacity if they are not made unduly apprehensive.

Some families can adjust well and provide guidance and security for the sick child. Others may become confused and frightened and show hostility, disinterest, or neglect; these families need guidance and counseling. The nurse has a great responsibility to support the family. The nurse's primary goal is to reduce anxiety in the child and family. This goal may be accomplished through open communication and ongoing contact.

Routine visits to a clinic or a physician's office become a way of life, and the child may come to feel different from other people. Physicians and nurses have a responsibility both to the family caregivers and the child to give clear explanations of the defect, using readily understandable terms and diagrams, pictures, or models. A child who knows what is happening can accept a great deal and can continue with the business of living.

Cardiac Catheterization

Cardiac catheterization may be performed before heart surgery to obtain more accurate information about the child's condition. The child or newborn is sedated or anesthetized for this process, and a radiopaque catheter is inserted through a vein into the right atrium. In the newborn or young child, the femoral vein often is used. Close observation of the child after the procedure is essential. Carefully monitor the site used and check the extremity for pulses, edema, skin temperature and color, and any other signs of poor circulation or infection. A pressure dressing is used over the catheterization site and left in place until the day after the procedure. The dressing should be snug and intact and monitored closely for any signs of bleeding from the site. The child is kept flat in bed with the extremity straight for as long as 6 hours after the procedure. Vital signs are monitored closely.

Preoperative Preparation

When a child enters the hospital for cardiac surgery, it is seldom a first admission; generally, it has been preceded by cardiac catheterization or perhaps other hospitalizations. The child may be admitted a few days before surgery to allow time for adequate preparation. With the current emphasis on cost containment, however, many preoperative procedures are done on an outpatient basis. Preoperative teaching should be intensive for the family and the child at an age appropriate level. They should understand that blood might be obtained for typing and crossmatching and for other determinations as ordered. Additional x-ray studies may be done.

The equipment to be used after surgery should be described with drawings and pictures. If possible, the family caregivers and the child should be taken to a cardiac recovery room and shown chest tubes and an oxygen tent. They should meet the nursing personnel and see the general appearance of the unit. Of course, nurses should use good judgment about the timing and the extent of such preparation; nothing is gained by arousing additional anxiety with premature or excessively graphic descriptions. A young child may become familiar with the surgical clothing worn by personnel and with the oxygen tent and can perhaps listen to a heartbeat. The child should be taught how to cough and should practice coughing. He or she should understand that coughing is important after surgery and must be done regularly, even though it may hurt.

Cardiac Surgery

Open-heart surgery using the heart–lung machine has made extensive heart correction possible for many children who otherwise would have been disabled throughout their limited lives. Machines have been refined for use with newborns and small children. Heart transplants may be performed when no other treatment is possible.

Hypothermia—reducing the body temperature to 68°F to 78.8°F (20°C to 26°C)—is a useful technique that helps to make early surgery possible. A reduced body temperature increases the time that the circulation may be stopped without causing brain damage. The blood temperature is reduced by the use of cooling agents in the heart–lung machine. This also provides a dry, bloodless, motionless field for the surgeon.

Postoperative Care

At the end of surgery, the child is taken to the pediatric intensive care unit for skillful nursing by specially trained personnel for as long as necessary. Children who have had closed-chest surgery need the same careful nursing as those who have had open-heart surgery.

By the time the child returns to the regular pediatric unit, chest drainage tubes usually have been removed and the child has started taking oral fluids and is ready to sit up in bed or in a chair. The child probably feels weak and helpless after such an experience and needs encouragement and reassurance. However, with recovery a child is usually ready for activity. Family caregivers usually need to reorient themselves and to accept their child's new status. This attitude is not easy to acquire after what seemed like a long period of anxious watching. The surgeon and the surgical staff evaluate the results of the surgery and make any necessary recommendations regarding resumption of the child's activities. Plans should be made for follow-up and supervision, as well as counseling and guidance.

Skeletal System Defects

Skeletal system defects in the newborn may be noted and treatment begun soon after birth. Some skeletal system defects may not be evident until later in the child's life. Congenital talipes equinovarus (clubfoot) is usually evident at birth. Another common skeletal system defect is congenital hip dysplasia (dislocation of the hip). Children with these conditions and their parents often face long periods of exhausting, costly treatment; therefore, they need continuing support, encouragement, and education.

Congenital Talipes Equinovarus

Congenital clubfoot is a deformity in which the entire foot is inverted, the heel is drawn up, and the forefoot is adducted. The Latin *talus,* meaning ankle, and *pes,* meaning foot, make up the word *talipes,* which is used in connection with many foot deformities. Equinus, or plantar flexion, and varus, or inversion, denotes the kind of foot deformity present in this condition. The equinovarus foot has a club-like appearance, thus the term "clubfoot" (Fig. 21-22A).

Congenital talipes equinovarus is the most common congenital foot deformity, occurring in about 7 in 1,000 births. It appears as a single anomaly or in connection with other defects, such as myelomeningocele. It may be

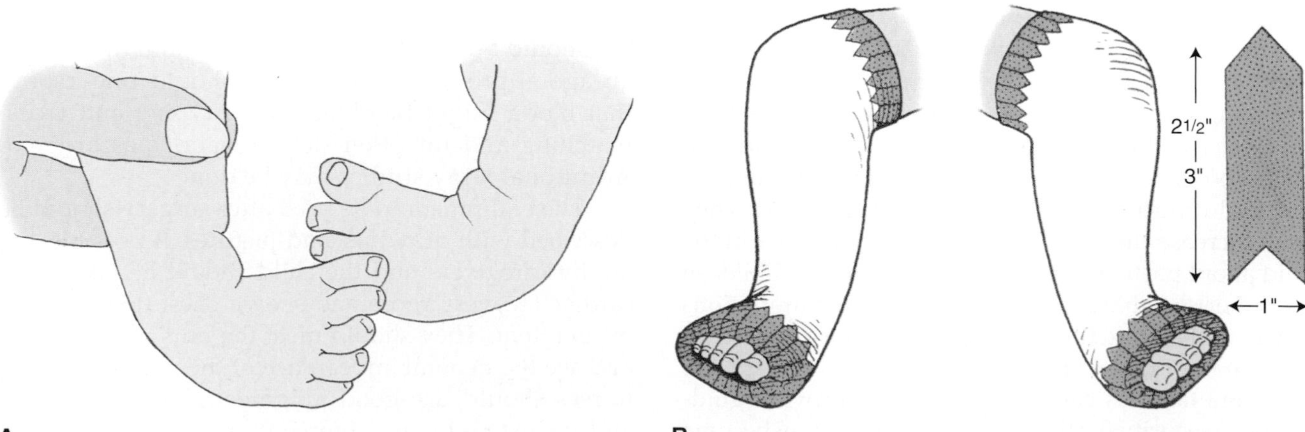

● ***Figure 21.22*** (**A**) Bilateral clubfoot. (**B**) Casting for clubfoot in typical overcorrected position showing petalling of cast.

bilateral (both feet) or unilateral (one foot). The cause is unclear, although a hereditary factor is observed occasionally. A hypothesis that has received some acceptance proposes an arrested embryonic growth of the foot during the first trimester of pregnancy.

Clinical Presentation

Talipes equinovarus is detected easily in a newborn but must be differentiated from a persisting "position of comfort" assumed in utero. The positional deformity may be corrected easily by the use of passive exercise, but the true clubfoot deformity is fixed. The positional deformity should be explained to the parents at once to prevent anxiety.

Treatment

Nonsurgical Treatment. If treatment is started during the neonatal period, correction usually may be accomplished by manipulation and bandaging or by application of a cast. The cast often is applied while the newborn is still in the neonatal nursery. While the cast is applied, the foot is first moved gently into as nearly normal a position as possible. Force should not be used. If the family caregiver can be present to help hold the newborn while the cast is applied, the caregiver will have the opportunity to understand what is being done. The very young newborn gets satisfaction from sucking, so a pacifier helps prevent squirming while the cast is applied.

The cast is applied over the foot and ankle (and usually to midthigh) to hold the knee in right-angle flexion (Fig. 21-22*B*). Casts are changed frequently to provide gradual, atraumatic correction—every few days for the first several weeks, then every week or two. Treatment is continued usually for a matter of months until radiograph and clinical observation confirm complete correction.

Any cast applied to a child's body should have some type of waterproof material protecting the skin from the cast's sharp plaster edges. One method is to apply strips of adhesive vertically around the edges of the cast in a manner called "petaling" (Fig. 21-22*B*). To petal a cast, strips of adhesive are cut 2 inches or 3 inches long and 1 inch wide. One end is notched, and the other end is cut pointed to aid in smooth application. Family caregivers must be taught cast care.

After correction with a cast, a Denis Browne splint with shoes attached may be used to maintain the correction for another 6 months or longer (Fig. 21-23). After overcorrection has been attained, the child should wear a special clubfoot shoe, which is a laced shoe whose turning out makes it appear that the shoe is being worn on the wrong foot. The Denis Browne splint still may be worn at night, and the caregivers should carry out passive exercises of the foot. The older infant may resist wearing the splint, so family caregivers must be taught the importance of gentle, but firm, insistence that the splint be worn.

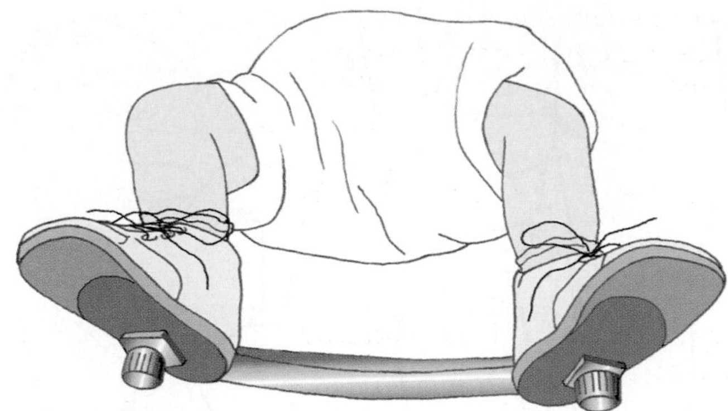

● ***Figure 21.23*** A Denis Browne splint with shoes attached is used to correct clubfoot.

Surgical Treatment. Children who do not respond to nonsurgical measures, especially older children, need surgical correction. This approach involves several procedures, depending on the age of the child and the degree of the deformity. It may involve lengthening the Achilles tendon and operating on the bony structure for the child older than 10 years. Prolonged observation after correction by either means should be carried out, at least until adolescence; any recurrence is treated promptly.

Congenital Hip Dysplasia

Congenital hip dysplasia results from defective development of the acetabulum with or without dislocation. The malformed acetabulum permits dislocation, with the head of the femur becoming displaced upward and backward. The condition is difficult to recognize during early infancy. When there is a family history of the defect, increased observation of the young newborn is indicated. The condition is often bilateral and about seven times more common in girls than in boys.

Clinical Presentation

Early recognition and treatment before an infant starts to stand or walk are extremely important for successful correction. The first examination should be part of the newborn examination. Experienced examiners may detect an audible click when examining the newborn using the Barlow's sign and Ortolani's maneuver (see Chapter 13, Nursing Procedure 13-2). These tests, used together on one hip at a time, show a tendency for dislocation of the hip in adduction and abduction and should be conducted only by an experienced practitioner. The tests are effective only for the 1st month, after this time the clicks disappear. Signs that are useful after this include:

- Asymmetry of the gluteal skin folds (higher on the affected side) (Fig. 21-24*A*).

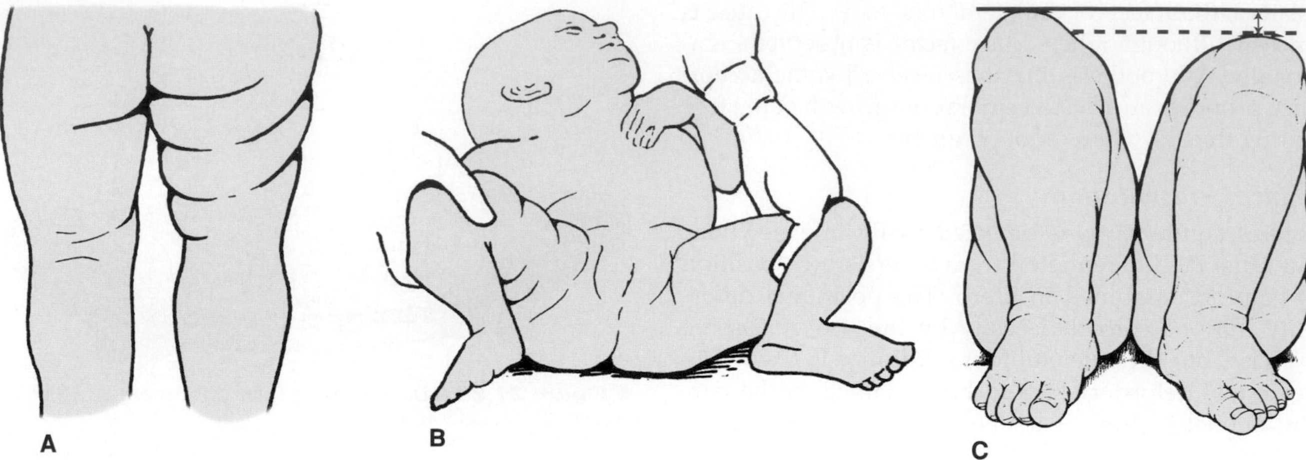

● *Figure 21.24* Congenital hip dislocation. (**A**) Asymmetry of the gluteal folds of the thighs. (**B**) Limited abduction of the affected hip. (**C**) Apparent shortening of the femur.

- Limited abduction of the affected hip (Fig. 21-24*B*). This is tested by placing the infant in a dorsal recumbent position with the knees flexed, then abducting both knees passively until they reach the examination table without resistance. If dislocation is present, the affected side cannot be abducted more than 45 degrees.
- Apparent shortening of the femur (Fig. 21-24*C*).

After the child has started walking, later signs include lordosis, swayback, protruding abdomen, shortened extremity, duck-waddle gait, and a positive Trendelenburg sign. To elicit this sign, the child stands on the affected leg and raises the normal leg. The pelvis tilts down, rather than up toward the unaffected side. X-ray studies usually are made to confirm the diagnosis in the older newborn. Uncorrected dislocation causes limping, easy fatigue, hip and low back discomfort, and postural deformities.

Treatment

Correction may be started in the newborn period by placing two or three diapers on the infant to hold the legs abducted, in a frog-like position. Cloth diapers work best for this purpose. Another treatment option, when the dislocation is discovered during the first few months, consists of manipulation of the femur into position and the application of a brace. The most common type of brace used is the Pavlik harness (Fig. 21-25). The primary care provider assesses the infant weekly while the infant is in the harness and adjusts the harness to align the femur gradually. Sometimes no additional treatment is needed.

If treatment is delayed until after the child has started to walk or if earlier treatment is ineffective, open reduction followed by application of a spica cast usually is needed. A spica or "hip spica cast," as it is often called, covers the lower part of the body, from the waist down and either one or both legs, usually leaving the feet open. The cast maintains the legs in a frog-like position, with the hips abducted. There may be a bar placed between the legs to help support the cast. After the cast is removed, a metal or plastic brace is applied to keep the legs in wide abduction.

● Nursing Process in Caring for the Infant in an Orthopedic Device or Cast

ASSESSMENT

Although the actual hospitalization of the infant is relatively short (if no other abnormalities

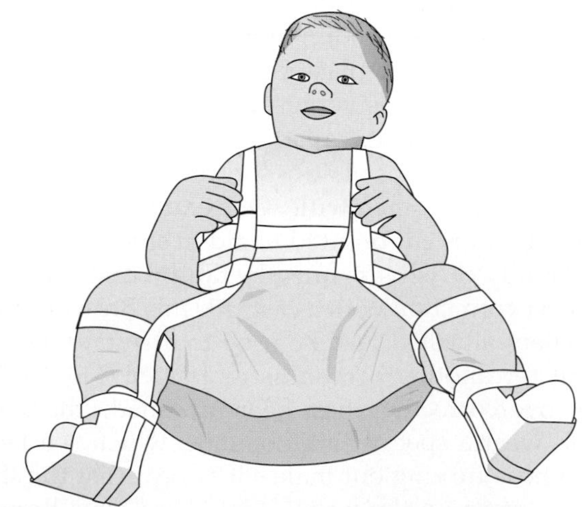

● *Figure 21.25* Proper positioning of an infant in a Pavlik harness. The harness is composed of shoulder straps, stirrups, and a chest strap. It is placed on both legs, even if only one hip is dislocated.

require hospitalization), the nurse must teach the family about cast care or care of the infant in an orthopedic device such as a Pavlik harness. Determine the family caregiver's ability to understand and cooperate in the infant's care. Emotional support of the family is important.

The observation of the infant varies depending on the orthopedic device or cast used. Immediately after the application of a cast, observe for signs that the cast is drying evenly. Check the toes for circulation and movement. Check the skin at the edges of the cast for signs of pressure or irritation. If an open reduction has been performed, observe the child for signs of shock and bleeding in the immediate postoperative period.

SELECTED NURSING DIAGNOSES

- Acute Pain related to discomfort of orthopedic device or cast
- Risk for Impaired Skin Integrity related to pressure of the cast on the skin surface
- Risk for Delayed Growth and Development related to restricted mobility secondary to orthopedic device or cast
- Deficient Knowledge of family caregivers related to home care of the infant in the orthopedic device or cast

OUTCOME IDENTIFICATION AND PLANNING

Goals include relieving pain and discomfort, maintaining skin integrity, promoting growth and development, and increasing family knowledge about the infant's home care. Goals for the family focus on the desire for correction of the defect with minimal disruption to the infant's growth and development and care of the infant at home.

IMPLEMENTATION

Providing Comfort Measures. The infant may be irritable and fussy because of the restricted movement caused by the device or cast. Useful methods of soothing the infant include nonnutritive sucking, stroking, cuddling, and talking. If irritability seems excessive, check the infant for signs of irritation from the device or cast. The infant in a cast may be held after the cast is completely dry. Do not remove the harness unless specific permission for bathing is granted by the provider. Teach the family caregivers how to reapply the harness correctly. The infant in a Pavlik harness is not as difficult to handle as the infant in a cast.

Promoting Skin Integrity. For the first 24 to 48 hours after application of a cast, place the infant on a firm mattress and support position changes with firm pillows. When handling the cast, use the palms of the hands to avoid excessive pressure on the cast. Carefully inspect the skin around the cast edges for signs of irritation, redness, or edema. Petal the edges of the cast around the waist and toes and protect the cast with plastic covering around the perineal area. Take great care to protect the diaper area from becoming soiled and moist. If the covering becomes soiled, remove it, wash and dry thoroughly, then reapply or replace it. With the Pavlik harness, monitor the skin under the straps frequently and massage it gently to promote circulation. To relieve pressure under the shoulder straps, place extra padding in the area.

Avoid using powders and lotions because caking of the powder or lotion can cause areas of irritation. Daily sponge baths are important and must include close attention to the skin under the straps of the device or around the edge of the cast.

Observe the infant in a cast carefully for any restriction of breathing caused by tightness over the abdomen and lower chest area. Vomiting after a feeding may be an indication that the cast is too tight over the stomach. In either case, the cast may have to be removed and reapplied.

Prevent the older infant or child from pushing any small particles of food or toys down into the cast. Diapering can be a challenge for the infant in a cast. Disposable diapers are usually the most effective way to provide good protection of the cast and prevent leakage.

Providing Sensory Stimulation Because the infant will be in the device or cast for an extended period when much growth and development occur, provide him or her with stimulation of a tactile nature. Provide mobiles, musical toys, and stuffed toys. Do not permit the infant to cry for long periods. Keep feeding times relaxed. Hold the infant if possible and encourage interaction. Provide a pacifier if the infant desires it. Encourage activities that use the infant's free hands. The older infant may enjoy

CULTURAL SNAPSHOT

Cradleboards are devices used as baby carriers and to provide security for newborns in some cultures. Using a cradleboard can sometimes aggravate hip dysplasia. The nurse can encourage the caregivers to use thick diapers, sometimes more than one, to help in keeping the hips in a slightly abducted position when the child is carried on a cradleboard. Cloth diapers work better than disposable diapers for this purpose.

looking at picture books and interacting with siblings. Diversionary activities should include transporting the infant to other areas in the home or in the car. Strollers and car seats may be adapted to allow safe transportation.

Here's an idea. For older infants or toddlers in a hip spica cast, a wagon may provide a convenient and fun way to explore the environment, encourage stimulation, and promote independence.

Providing Family Teaching. Determine the family caregiver's knowledge and design a thorough teaching plan because the infant will be cared for at home for most of the time. Use complete explanations, written guidelines, demonstrations, and return demonstrations. Provide the family with a resource person who may be called when a question arises and encourage them to feel free to call that person. Make definite plans for return visits to have the device or cast checked. The caregiver needs to understand the importance of keeping these appointments. Provide a public or home health nurse referral when appropriate (see Nursing Care Plan 21-1: The Infant With an Orthopedic Cast).

EVALUATION: GOALS AND EXPECTED OUTCOMES

- **Goal:** The infant will show signs of being comfortable.
  Expected Outcomes: The infant is alert and content with no long periods of fussiness. The infant interacts with caregivers with cooing, smiling, and eye contact.
- **Goal:** The infant's skin will remain intact.
  Expected Outcomes: The infant's skin around the edges of the cast shows no signs of redness or irritation. The diaper area is clean, dry and intact, and protected from soiling.
- **Goal:** The infant will attain appropriate developmental milestones.
  Expected Outcomes: The infant responds positively to audio, visual, and diversionary activities. The infant shows age-appropriate development.
- **Goal:** The family caregivers will learn home care of the infant.
  Expected Outcomes: The family demonstrates care of the infant in the orthopedic device or cast, asks pertinent questions, and identifies a resource person to call.

Test Yourself

- How is congenital clubfoot treated?
- What three signs are seen in the infant with a congenital hip dysplasia?
- List five nursing interventions used to promote skin integrity for an infant in a cast.

Genitourinary Tract Defects

Most congenital anomalies of the genitourinary tract are not life threatening but may present social problems with lifelong implications for the child and family. Thus, early recognition and supportive, understanding care are essential.

Hypospadias and Epispadias

Hypospadias is a congenital condition in which the urethra terminates on the ventral (underside) surface of the penis, instead of at the tip. A cordlike anomaly (a **chordee**) extends from the scrotum to the penis, pulling the penis downward in an arc. Urination is not affected, but the boy cannot void while standing in the normal male fashion. Surgical repair is desirable between the ages of 6 and 18 months, before body image and castration anxiety become problems. Microscopic surgery makes early repair possible. Surgical repair is often accomplished in one stage and is often done as outpatient surgery. These newborns should not be circumcised because the foreskin is used in the repair. Severe hypospadias may require additional surgical procedures.

In epispadias, the opening is on the dorsal (top) surface of the penis. This condition often occurs with exstrophy of the bladder. Surgical repair is indicated.

Exstrophy of the Bladder

This urinary tract malformation occurs in 1 in 30,000 live births in the United States and is usually accompanied by other anomalies, such as epispadias, cleft scrotum, cryptorchidism (undescended testes), a shortened penis, and cleft clitoris. It also is associated with malformed pelvic musculature, resulting in a prolapsed rectum and inguinal hernias. Children with this defect have a widely split symphysis pubis and posterolaterally rotated hip sockets, causing a waddling gait.

In this condition, the anterior surface of the urinary bladder lies open on the lower abdomen (Fig. 21-26). The exposed mucosa is red and sensitive to touch and allows direct passage of urine to the outside. This condition makes the area vulnerable to infection and trauma.

NURSING CARE PLAN 21-1

The Infant With an Orthopedic Cast

Six-month-old Melissa Davis has right congenital hip dysplasia. After a trial with a Pavlik harness, she has been placed in a hip spica cast. The cast has just been applied. This is a new experience for her and her caregiver.

NURSING DIAGNOSIS
Acute Pain related to discomfort of hip spica cast

GOAL: The infant will show signs of being comfortable.

OUTCOME CRITERIA

- The infant is alert and contended.
- The infant has no long periods of fussiness.
- The infant interacts with caregivers by cooing, smiling, and eye contact.

NURSING INTERVENTIONS	*RATIONALE*
Check edges of cast for smoothness; petal edges of cast.	Rough edges can cause irritation and discomfort.
Soothe by stroking, cuddling, and talking to infant.	These comfort measures help the infant feel safe, secure, and loved and provide distraction from discomfort and restriction of cast.
Provide infant with a pacifier.	Nonnutritive sucking is a means of self-comfort.

NURSING DIAGNOSIS
Risk for Impaired Skin Integrity related to pressure of the cast on the skin surface

GOAL: The infant's skin will remain intact.

OUTCOME CRITERIA

- The infant's skin around the cast shows no signs of redness or irritation.
- The infant's skin in the diaper area is clean, dry, and intact with no signs of perineal redness of irritation.

NURSING INTERVENTIONS	*RATIONALE*
Place infant on firm mattress for 24 to 48 hours until cast is dry.	The cast is still pliable until dry. Undue pressure on any point must be avoided.
Use palms when handling damp cast.	Using palms instead of fingers prevents excessive pressure in any one area.
Petal all edges of cast.	Petalling provides a smooth edge along cast to avoid irritation.
Inspect skin around the cast edges for redness and irritation during each shift.	Early signs of irritation indicate areas that may need added protection.
Protect perineal area of cast with waterproof covering.	Urine and feces can easily cause irritation, skin breakdown, or a softened and malodorous cast.
Remove, wash, and thoroughly dry perineal covering if wet or soiled.	A clean, dry perineal cast protective covering decreases the problem of breakdown.

NURSING DIAGNOSIS
Risk for Delayed Growth and Development related to restricted mobility secondary to hip spica cast

GOAL: The infant will attain appropriate developmental milestones.

OUTCOME CRITERIA

- The infant responds positively to audio, visual, and diversional activities.
- The infant smiles, coos, and squeals in response to family caregivers.
- The infant shows age appropriate development.

(nursing care plan continues on page 536)

NURSING CARE PLAN 21-1 continued

The Infant With an Orthopedic Cast

NURSING INTERVENTIONS	*RATIONALE*
Provide mobiles, musical toys, stuffed toys, and toys infant can manipulate.	Visual, tactile, and auditory stimulation are important for infant development.
Encourage caregiver to interact with infant during feeding.	Interacting (babbling, cooing) with others in her or his environment encourages development.
Plan activities that include changes of environment such as moving to the playroom in the hospital or to a different room in the home.	Environmental variety provides increased visual, auditory, and tactile stimulation.

NURSING DIAGNOSIS

Deficient Knowledge of family caregivers related to the home care of the infant in a cast

GOAL: The family caregivers will learn home care of the infant.

OUTCOME CRITERIA

- The family caregivers demonstrate care of the infant in the hip spica cast.
- The family caregivers ask pertinent questions.
- The family caregiver identifies a resource person to call.

NURSING INTERVENTIONS	*RATIONALE*
Determine the family caregivers' knowledge level and design a teaching plan.	An effective teaching plan is tailored to begin with the knowledge base of the family.
Choose teaching methods most suited to family caregivers' recognized needs and learning style.	The family's ability to read, understand, and follow directions and their cognitive abilities affect the results.
Before discharge, schedule follow-up appointment for return visit to have the cast checked.	Scheduling the follow-up appointment emphasizes to family caregivers the importance of close follow-up.

Surgical closure of the bladder is preferred within the first 48 hours of life. Final surgical correction is completed before the child goes to school. If bladder repair is not done early in the child's life, the family caregivers must be taught how to care for this condition and how to deal with their feelings toward this less-than-perfect child. Their emotional reaction may be further complicated if the malformation is so severe that the sex of the child may be determined only by a chromosome test (see the following section on ambiguous genitalia).

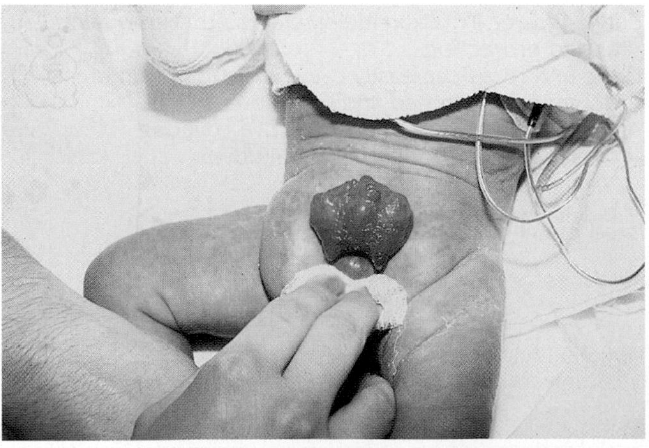

A

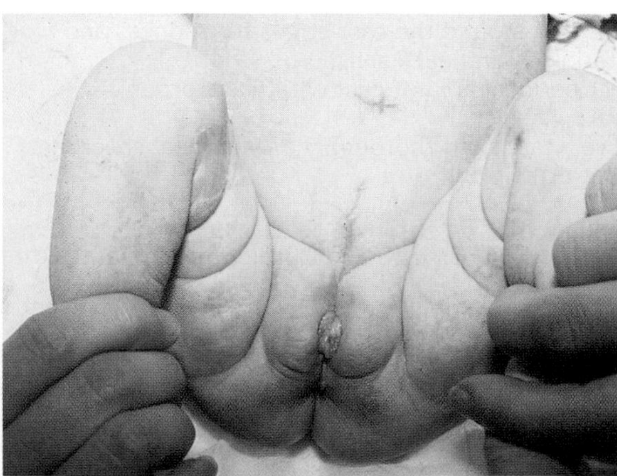

B

● ***Figure 21.26*** Exstrophy of the bladder. (**A**) Prior to surgery, note the bright-red color of the bladder. (**B**) Following surgical repair.

Nursing care of the newborn with exstrophy of the bladder should be directed toward preventing infection, preventing skin irritation around the seeping mucosa, meeting the newborn's need for touch and cuddling, and educating and supporting the family during this crisis.

Ambiguous Genitalia

If a child's external sex organs did not follow a normal development in utero, at birth it may not be possible to determine by observation if the child is a male or female. The external sexual organs are either incompletely or abnormally formed. This condition is called ambiguous genitalia. Although rare, the birth of a newborn with ambiguous genitalia presents a highly charged emotional climate and has possible long-range social implications. Regardless of the cause, it is important to establish the genetic sex and the sex of rearing as early as possible, so that surgical correction of anomalies may occur before the child begins to function in a sex-related social role. Authorities believe that the newborn's anatomic structure, rather than the genetic sex, should determine the sex of rearing. It is possible to construct a functional vagina surgically and to administer hormones to offer an anatomically incomplete female a somewhat normal life. Currently it is impossible to offer comparable surgical reconstruction to males with an inadequate penis. Parents may feel guilt, anxiety, and confusion about their child's condition and need empathic understanding and support to help them cope with this emergency.

INBORN ERRORS OF METABOLISM

Disorders referred to as inborn errors of metabolism are hereditary disorders that affect metabolism. Inborn errors of metabolism include phenylketonuria, galactosemia, congenital hypothyroidism, maple syrup urine disease, and homocystinuria. Nursing care for the newborn involves prompt diagnosis and initiation of treatment. Family teaching might include dietary guidelines, information about the disorder, and genetic counseling. The family also needs support and information to prepare for the long-term care of a chronically ill child (see Chapter 32).

Phenylketonuria

Phenylketonuria (PKU) is a recessive hereditary defect of metabolism that, if untreated, causes severe mental retardation in most but not all affected children. It is uncommon, appearing in about 1 in 10,000 births. Children with this condition lack the enzyme that normally changes the essential amino acid phenylalanine into tyrosine.

As soon as the newborn with this defect begins to take milk (either breast or cow's milk), phenylalanine is absorbed in the normal manner. However, because the affected newborn cannot metabolize this amino acid, phenylalanine builds up in the blood serum to as much as 20 times the normal level. This build-up occurs so quickly that increased levels of phenylalanine appear in the blood after only 1 or 2 days of ingestion of milk. Phenylpyruvic acid appears in the urine of these newborns between the 2nd and the 6th week of life.

Most untreated children with this condition develop severe and progressive mental deficiency. The high levels of phenylalanine in the bloodstream and tissues cause permanent damage to brain tissues. The newborn appears normal at birth but begins to show signs of mental arrest within a few weeks. Therefore, this disorder must be diagnosed as early as possible, and the child must be placed immediately on a low-phenylalanine formula.

Clinical Presentation

Signs and Symptoms. Untreated newborns may experience frequent vomiting and have aggressive and hyperactive traits. Severe, progressive retardation is characteristic. Convulsions may occur, and eczema is common, particularly in the perineal area. There is a characteristic musty smell to the urine.

Laboratory and Diagnostic Test Results. Most states require newborns to undergo a blood test to detect the phenylalanine level. This screening procedure, the Guthrie inhibition assay test, uses blood from a simple heel prick. The test is most reliable after the newborn has ingested some form of protein. The accepted practice is to perform the test on the second or third day of life. If the newborn leaves the hospital before this time, the newborn is brought back to have the test performed. The test may be repeated in the third week of life if the first test was done before the newborn was 24 hours old. Health practitioners caring for newborns not born in a hospital are responsible for screening these newborns. When screening indicates an increased level of phenylalanine, additional testing is done to make a firm diagnosis.

Treatment and Nursing Care

Dietary treatment is required. A formula low in phenylalanine should be started as soon as the condition is detected; Lofenalac and Phenyl-free are low-phenylalanine formulas. Best results are obtained if the special formula is started before the newborn is 3 weeks of age. A low-phenylalanine diet is a very restricted one; foods to be omitted are breads, meat, fish, dairy products, nuts, and legumes. A nutritionist should supervise the diet carefully. The child remains on the diet at least into early adulthood, and it may even be recommended indefinitely. If a woman who has PKU decides to have a child and is not following a diet low in phenylalanine, she should return to following the dietary treatment for at least 3 months before becoming pregnant. The diet is continued through the pregnancy to help in preventing the child from being born with a mental impairment. Routine blood testing is done to maintain the serum phenylalanine level at 2 to 8 mg/dL.

Maintaining the newborn on the restricted diet is relatively simple compared with the problems that arise as the child grows and becomes more independent. As the child ventures into the world beyond home, more and more dietary temptations are available, and dietary compliance is difficult. The family and child need support and counseling throughout the child's developmental years. The length of time that the restrictions are necessary remains unclear. Although difficult, it seems best to follow the diet into adolescence.

Galactosemia

Galactosemia is a recessive hereditary metabolic disorder in which the enzyme necessary to convert galactose into glucose is missing. The newborns generally appear normal at birth but experience difficulties after ingesting milk (breast, cow's, or goat's) because one of the component monosaccharides of milk lactose is galactose.

Clinical Presentation

Early feeding difficulties with vomiting and diarrhea severe enough to produce dehydration and weight loss and jaundice are primary manifestations. Unless milk is withheld early, other difficulties include cataracts, liver and spleen damage, and mental retardation, with a high mortality rate early in life. A screening test (Beutler test) can be used to test for the disorder.

Treatment and Nursing Care

Galactose must be omitted from the diet, which in the young newborn means a substitution for milk. Nutramigen and Pregestimil are formulas that provide galactose-free nutrition for the newborn. The diet must continue to be free of lactose when the child moves on to table foods, but the diet allows more variety than does the phenylalanine-free diet.

Congenital Hypothyroidism

At one time referred to by the now unacceptable term "cretinism," congenital hypothyroidism is associated with either the congenital absence of a thyroid gland or the inability of the thyroid gland to secrete thyroid hormone. The incidence is about 1 in 5,000 births or about twice as common as PKU.

Clinical Presentation

Signs and Symptoms. The newborn appears normal at birth, but clinical signs and symptoms begin to be noticeable at about 6 weeks of life. The facial features are typical and include depressed nasal bridge, large tongue, and puffy eyes. The neck is short and thick (Fig. 21-27). The voice (cry) is hoarse, the skin is dry and cold, and the newborn has slow bone development. Two common features are chronic constipation and abdomen enlargement caused by poor muscle tone. The newborn is a poor feeder and often characterized as a "good" baby by the parent or caretaker because he or she cries very little and sleeps for long periods.

Laboratory and Diagnostic Test Results. Most states require a routine test for triiodothyronine (T_3) and thyroxine (T_4) levels to determine thyroid function in all newborns before discharge for early diagnosis of congenital hypothyroidism. This test is done as part of the heel-stick screening, which includes the Guthrie screening test for PKU.

Treatment and Nursing Care

The thyroid hormone must be replaced as soon as the diagnosis is made. Levothyroxine sodium, a synthetic thyroid replacement, is the drug most commonly used. Blood levels of T_3 and T_4 are monitored to prevent overdosage. Unless therapy is started in early infancy, mental retardation and slow growth occur. The later that therapy is started, the more severe the mental retardation. Therapy must be continued for life.

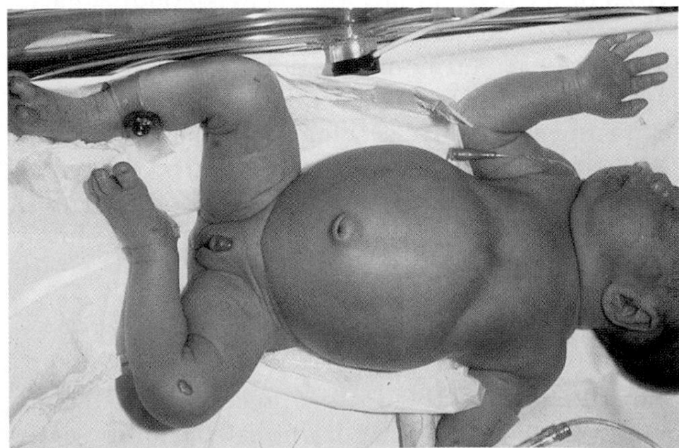

● ***Figure 21.27*** A newborn with congenital hypothyroidism; note the short, thick neck and enlarged abdomen.

Test Yourself

- Why is it desirable for genitourinary tract defects such as hypospadias to be corrected by the time the child is 18 months old?
- What is a serious outcome that can occur if phenylketonuria, congenital hypothyroidism, and galactosemia are not treated?

Maple Syrup Urine Disease

Maple syrup urine disease (MSUD) is an inborn error of metabolism of the branched chain amino acids. It is autosomal recessive in inheritance. It is rapidly progressive and often fatal.

Clinical Presentation

The onset of MSUD occurs very early in infancy. In the 1st week of life, these newborns often have feeding problems and neurologic signs such as seizures, spasticity, and opisthotonos. The urine has a distinctive odor of maple syrup. Diagnosis is made through a blood test for the amino acids leucine, isoleucine, and valine. This is easily done at the same time the heel stick for PKU is performed.

Treatment and Nursing Care

Treatment of MSUD is dietary and must be initiated within 12 days of birth to be successful. The special formula is low in the branched chain amino acids. The special diet must be continued indefinitely.

CHROMOSOMAL ABNORMALITIES

Chromosomal abnormalities are often evident at birth and frequently cause physical and cognitive challenges for the child throughout life. There are various forms of chromosomal abnormalities, including nondisjunction, deletion, translocation, mosaicism, and isochromosome abnormalities.

The most common abnormalities are nondisjunction abnormalities, which occur when the chromosomal division is uneven. Normally during cell division of the cells of reproduction, the 46 chromosomes divide in half, with 23 chromosomes in each new cell. Nondisjunction abnormalities occur when a new cell has an extra chromosome (e.g., 24) or not enough chromosomes (e.g., 22). When this defective chromosome joins with a normal reproductive cell having 23 chromosomes, an abnormality occurs. Down syndrome, the most common chromosomal abnormality, most often is a result of chromosomal nondisjunction with an extra chromosome on chromosome 21. Two other common chromosomal abnormalities that may be seen include the Turner and Klinefelter syndromes, which are nondisjunction abnormalities occurring on the sex chromosomes.

Down Syndrome

Down syndrome is the most common chromosomal anomaly, occurring in about 1 in 700 to 800 births. Langdon Down first described the condition in 1866, but its cause was a mystery for many years. In 1932, it was suggested that a chromosomal anomaly might be the cause, but the anomaly was not demonstrated until 1959.

Down syndrome has been observed in nearly all countries and races. The old term "mongolism" is inappropriate and no longer used. Most people with Down syndrome have trisomy 21 (Fig. 21-28); a few have partial dislocation of chromosomes 15 and 21. A woman older than 35 years of age is at a greater risk of bearing a child with Down syndrome than is a younger woman, but children with Down syndrome are born to women of all ages. Older women and increasing numbers of younger women are choosing to undergo screening at 15 weeks' gestation for low maternal serum alpha-fetoprotein levels and high chorionic gonadotropin levels, which indicates the possibility of Down syndrome in the fetus. Amniocentesis and chorionic villus sampling are more accurate and will confirm the blood test results. These screening tests give women the option of aborting the fetus or continuing with the pregnancy and preparing themselves for the birth of a disabled child.

Clinical Presentation

All forms of the condition show a variety of abnormal characteristics. Mental status is usually within the moderate to severe range of retardation, with most children being moderately retarded. The most common anomalies include:

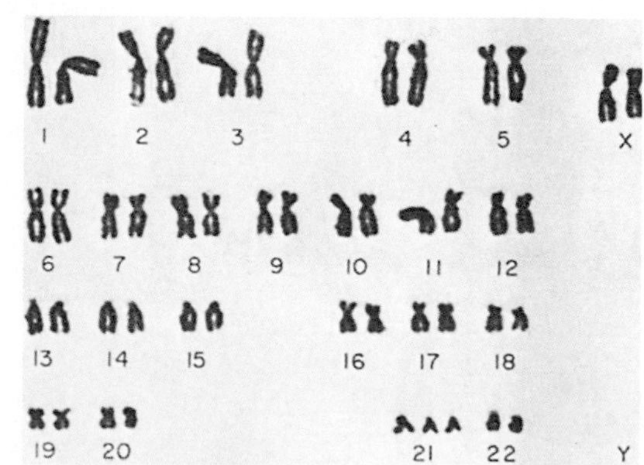

● *Figure 21.28* Karotype showing trisomy 21. Note three chromosomes in the 21 position.

- **Brachycephaly** (shortness of head)
- Retarded body growth
- Upward and outward slanted eyes (almond-shaped) with an epicanthic fold at the inner angle
- Short, flattened bridge of the nose
- Thick, fissured tongue
- Dry, cracked, fissured skin that may be mottled
- Dry and coarse hair
- Short hands with an incurved fifth finger
- A single horizontal palm crease (simian line)
- Wide space between the first and second toes
- Lax muscle tone (often referred to as "double jointed" by others)
- Heart and eye anomalies
- Greater susceptibility to leukemia than that of the general population

Not all these physical signs are present in all people with Down syndrome. Some may have only one or two characteristics; others may show nearly all the characteristics (Fig. 21-29).

Treatment and Nursing Care

The physical characteristics of the child with Down syndrome determine the medical and nursing management. Lax muscles, congenital heart defects, and dry skin contribute to a large variety of problems. The child's relaxed muscle tone may contribute to respiratory complications as a result of decreased respiratory expansion. The relaxed skeletal muscles contribute to late motor development. Gastric motility is also decreased, leading to problems with constipation. Congenital heart defects and vision or hearing problems add to the complexities of the child's care.

In infancy, the child's large tongue and poor muscle tone may contribute to difficulty breast-feeding or ingesting formula and can cause great problems when the time comes to introduce solid foods. The family caregivers need support during these trying times. As the child gets older, concern about excessive weight gain becomes a primary consideration.

The family caregivers of the child with Down syndrome need strong support and guidance from the time the child is born. Early intervention programs have yielded some encouraging results, but depending on the level of cognitive impairment, the family may have to decide if they can care for the child at home or if other living arrangements need to be considered for the child. A cognitively impaired child who is undisciplined or improperly supervised may threaten the safety of others in the home and the neighborhood. Caring for the child may demand so much sacrifice from other family members that the family structure may be significantly affected. However, with consistent care, patience, and guidelines, families of children with Down syndrome often find joy and pleasure in the gentle and loving nature of the child.

Turner Syndrome

The newborn with Turner syndrome has one less X chromosome than normal. Characteristics of Turner syndrome include short stature, low set ears, a broad-based neck that appears webbed and short, a low-set

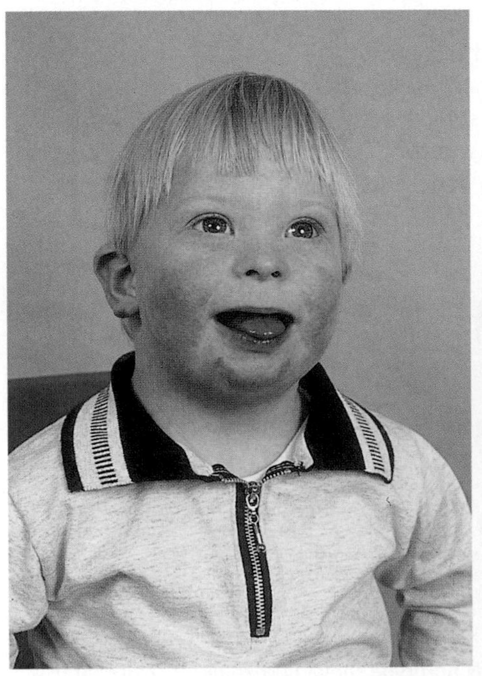

A

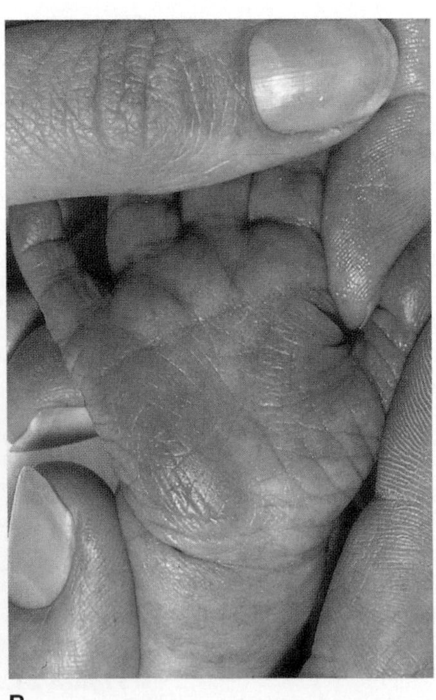

B

● ***Figure 21.29*** Typical features of a child with Down syndrome: (**A**) facial features; (**B**) horizontal palm crease (simian line).

hairline at the nap of the neck, broad chest, an increased angle of the arms, and edema of the hands and feet. These children frequently have congenital heart defects as well. Females are most often affected by Turner syndrome and, with the exception of pubic hair, do not develop secondary sex characteristics.

Children with Turner syndrome have normal intelligence but may have visual-spatial concerns, learning disabilities, problems with social interaction, and may lack physical coordination. Growth hormones are given to increase the height, as well as the hormonal levels, but females with Turner syndrome rarely can become pregnant.

Klinefelter Syndrome

The presence of an extra X chromosome causes Klinefelter syndrome. The syndrome is most commonly seen in males. Characteristics are not often evident until puberty, when the child does not develop secondary sex characteristics. The testes are usually small and do not produce mature sperm. Increased breast size and a risk of developing breast cancer are frequently seen.

Boys with Klinefelter syndrome often have normal intelligence but frequently have behavior problems, show signs of immaturity and insecurity, and have difficulty with memory and processing. Hormone replacements of testosterone may be started in the early teens to promote normal adult development.

KEY POINTS

- A failure of the maxillary and premaxillary processes to fuse during fetal development can cause a cleft lip on one or both sides of the lip or a cleft palate, in which the tissue in the roof of the mouth does not fuse properly.
- Early signs that a newborn may have an esophageal fistula include frothing and excessive drooling and periods of respiratory distress with choking and cyanosis.
- The greatest preoperative danger for the newborn with tracheoesophageal atresia is the possibility of aspiration and pneumonitis, as well as respiratory distress.
- Diaphragmatic hernias occur when abdominal organs are displaced into the left chest through an opening in the diaphragm. If the cardiac portion of the stomach slides into the area above the diaphragm, a hiatal hernia is caused. A rare occurrence, the omphalocele is seen when the abdominal contents protrude through the umbilical cord and form a sac lying on the abdomen. If the end of the umbilical cord does not close completely and a portion of the intestine protrudes through the opening, an umbilical hernia is formed. Inguinal hernias occur mostly in males when a part of the intestine slips into the inguinal canal.
- Spina bifida is caused when the spinal vertebrae fail to close and an opening is left where the spinal cord or meninges may protrude. Spina bifida occulta is seen when soft tissue is not involved and only a dimple in the skin may be seen. Spina bifida with meningocele occurs when the spinal meninges protrude through and forms a sac, and spina bifida with myelomeningocele occurs when both the spinal cord and meninges protrude. The later condition is the most difficult to treat because of the concern of complete paralysis below the lesion.
- If an obstruction in the circulation of cerebral spinal fluid (CSF) occurs, the condition is called "noncommunicating hydrocephalus." With communicating hydrocephalus, there is defective absorption of CSF. The most obvious symptom of hydrocephalus is the rapid increase in head circumference. Ventriculoperitoneal shunting (VP shunt) drains CSF from the brain into the peritoneal cavity. With ventriculoatrial shunting, the CSF is drained into the heart.
- Ventricular septal defects allow the blood to pass from the left to the right ventricle; in the atrial septal defect the blood flows from the left to the right atria. With a patent ductus arteriosus, blood is shunted from the aorta into the pulmonary artery. When coarctation of the aorta occurs there is a narrowing of the aortic arch and an obstruction of blood flow.
- Tetralogy of Fallot is a group of heart defects including pulmonary stenosis, ventricular septal defect, overriding aorta, and right ventricular hypertrophy. The child with Tetralogy of Fallot has cyanosis and low oxygen saturation. The severe and usually fatal defect, transposition of the great arteries, causes cyanosis and occurs because the aorta arises from the right ventricle, instead of the left, and the pulmonary artery arises from the left ventricle, instead of the right.
- Clubfoot, talipes equinovarus, and congenital hip dysplasia are the most common skeletal deformities in the newborn. Signs and symptoms of congenital dislocation of the hip include asymmetry of the gluteal skin folds, limited abduction of the affected hip and shortening of the femur. To treat hip dislocation, the femur is manipulated and a brace applied. A hip spica cast may be used after an open reduction, if necessary.
- Phenylketonuria is detected by doing a blood test called the Guthrie inhibition assay test to detect phenylalanine levels. Dietary treatment using a formula and diet low in phenylalanine is started and continued as the child gets older.

- Congenital hypothyroidism is detected by performing tests for triiodothyronine (T_3) and thyroxine (T_4) levels to determine thyroid function.
- If phenylketonuria, congenital hypothyroidism, and galactosemia are not treated, the newborn often has severe mental retardation.
- Down syndrome is sometimes called trisomy 21 because of the three-chromosome pattern seen on the 21st pair of chromosomes. Signs and symptoms seen in children with Down syndrome include brachycephaly (shortness of head); slowed growth; slanted (almond shaped) eyes; short, flattened nose; thick tongue; dry, cracked, fissured skin; dry and coarse hair; short hands with an incurved fifth finger; single horizontal palm crease (simian line); wide space between the first and second toes; lax muscle tone; heart and eye anomalies; and a greater susceptibility to leukemia.

REFERENCES AND SELECTED READINGS

Books and Journals

Finesilver, C. (2002). Down syndrome. *RN*, 65(11), 43–49.

Fishman, M. A. (1999). Developmental defects. In *Oski's pediatrics: Principles and practice* (3rd ed.). Philadelphia: Lippincott Williams & Wilkins.

Goldberg, M. J. (2001). Early detection of developmental hip dysplasia. *Pediatrics in Review, 22*(4), 131–134.

Gorlin, R. J. (1999). Craniofacial defects. In *Oski's pediatrics: Principles and practice* (3rd ed.). Philadelphia: Lippincott Williams & Wilkins.

Holmes, L. B. (1999). Congenital malformations. In *Oski's pediatrics: Principles and practice* (3rd ed.). Philadelphia: Lippincott Williams & Wilkins.

Lewanda, A. F., & Jabs, E. W. (1999). Dysmorphology: Genetic syndromes and associations. In *Oski's pediatrics: Principles and practice* (3rd ed.). Philadelphia: Lippincott Williams & Wilkins.

McDaniel, N. L. (2001). Heart ventricular and atrial septal defects. *Pediatrics in Review, 22*(8), 265.

North American Nursing Diagnosis Association (NANDA). (2001). *NANDA nursing diagnoses: Definitions and classification 2001–2002*. Philadelphia: Author.

Oxley, J. (2001). Are arm splints required following cleft lip/palate repair? *Pediatric Nursing, 13*(1) 27–30.

Pillitteri, A. (2003). *Maternal and child health nursing* (4th ed.). Philadelphia: Lippincott Williams & Wilkins.

Purnell, L., & Paulanda, B. (2003). *Transcultural health care: A culturally competent approach* (2nd ed.). Philadelphia: FA Davis.

Robinson, D., & Drumm, L. (2001). Maple syrup disease: A standard of nursing care. *Pediatric Nursing, 27*(3), 255.

Sommerlad, B. C. (2002). The management of cleft lip and palate. *Current Pediatrics, 12*(1), 36–42.

Springhouse nurse's drug guide (3rd ed.). (2000). Springhouse, PA: Springhouse Corporation.

Sparks, S., & Taylor, C. (2001). *Nursing diagnosis reference manual* (5th ed.). Springhouse, PA: Springhouse Corporation.

Suddaby, E. C. (2001). Contemporary thinking for congenital heart disease. *Pediatric Nursing*, 27(3), 233.

Wedge, J. H., et al. (2001). Congenital clubfoot. *Current Pediatrics*, 11(5), 332–340.

Wong, D. L., & Hockenberry-Eaton, M. (2001). *Wong's essentials of pediatric nursing* (6th ed.). St. Louis: Mosby.

Wong, D. L., Perry, S., & Hockenberry, M. (2002). *Maternal child nursing care* (2nd ed.). St. Louis: Mosby.

Websites

Spina Bifida

http://www.sbaa.org

Cleft Lip and Cleft Palate

http://www.cleft.org

WORKBOOK

NCLEX-STYLE REVIEW QUESTIONS

1. The nurse is doing an admission examination on a newborn with a diagnosis of hydrocephalus. If the following data were collected, which might indicate a common symptom of this diagnosis?
   a. Sac protruding on the lower back
   b. Respiratory rate of 30 breaths a minute
   c. Gluteal folds higher on one side than the other
   d. Head circumference of 18 inches
2. When collecting data during an admission interview and examination on a newborn, the nurse finds the newborn has cyanosis, dyspnea, tachycardia, and feeding difficulties. These symptoms might indicate the newborn has which of the following conditions?
   a. Spina bifida
   b. Tetralogy of Fallot
   c. Congenital rubella
   c. Hip dysplasia
3. In caring for a newborn who has had a cleft lip/cleft palate repair, the *highest* priority for the nurse is to
   a. document the time period the restraints are on and off.
   b. observe the incision for redness or drainage.
   c. teach the caregivers about dental care and hygiene.
   d. provide sensory stimulation and age-appropriate toys.
4. In planning care for an infant who had a spica cast applied to treat a congenital hip dysplasia, which of the following nursing interventions would be included in this newborn's plan of care?
   a. Inspect skin for redness and irritation.
   b. Change bedding and clothing every 4 hours.
   c. Weigh every morning and evening using same scale.
   d. Monitor temperature and pulse every 2 hours.
5. The nurse is caring for a newborn who has a myelomeningocele and has not yet had surgery to repair the defect. Which of the following measures will be used to prevent the site from becoming infected? (Select all that apply.)
   a. Give antibiotics as a prophylactic measure.
   b. Cover the sac with a saline soaked sterile dressing.
   c. Maintain the newborn in a supine position.
   d. Place a plastic protective covering over the dressing.
   e. Change the dressing every 8 hours.

STUDY ACTIVITIES

1. Using the table below, list the common types of congenital heart defects. Include the description of the defect (chambers and parts of the heart involved), the blood flow characteristics, symptoms, and treatment.

Detect	Description of Defect	Blood Flow Characteristics	Symptoms	Treatment

2. Make a list of the maternal risk factors that may cause congenital heart defects. For each of these risk factors, state what could be done to decrease the occurrence of these risks.
3. Develop a teaching project by creating a mobile or gathering a collection of appropriate toys and activities that could be used for sensory stimulation with a newborn who is in an orthopedic cast. Present your project to your classmates and explain why and how these items would be appropriate to use for developmental stimulation.
4. Go to the following Internet site: http://www.pediheart.org
   a. Click on "Parent's Place."
   b. Click on "Prepare for Surgery."
   c. Read the section "Preparing Your Child for Surgery."
   d. Read the section "Helpful Parent Tips."

5. List eight tips to share with parents whose child is having heart surgery.
6. List three books that parents could use with the child who is having heart surgery.

CRITICAL THINKING: What Would You Do?

1. Diane's baby was born with a bilateral cleft lip and cleft palate. When you bring the baby to her for feeding, she breaks down and sobs uncontrollably.
   a. Describe what your immediate response would be.
   b. What feelings and emotions do you think Diane is experiencing?
   c. Write out an example of a therapeutic response you could make?
2. Cody was born with hydrocephalus and has been admitted to the pediatric unit to have a ventriculoperitoneal (VP) shunt placed. You walk into Cody's room after the pediatrician has discussed the procedure with Cody's parents. They seem anxious and begin asking you questions. How will you answer the following questions?
   a. What is hydrocephalus and what caused Cody to have the disorder?
   b. Why does Cody need to have a shunt and how does it work?
   c. What long-term problems will Cody have because of the disorder?
3. *Dosage calculation:* The nurse is preparing the preoperative medication of Demerol (meperidine) for an infant who is having a surgical procedure to correct a congenital heart defect. The infant weighs 9.9 pounds (9 pounds, 14.4 ounces). The usual dosage range of this medication is 1 to 2.2 mg per kg. Answer the following:
   a. How many kilograms does the infant weigh?
   b. What is the low dose of Demerol (in milligrams) that this infant could be given?
   c. What is the high dose of Demerol (in milligrams) that this infant could be given?

Glossary

abruptio placentae, or placental abruption the premature separation of a normally implanted placenta.
abstinence (as related to birth control); refraining from vaginal sexual intercourse.
abuse misuse, excessive use, rough or bad treatment; used to refer to misuse of alcohol or drugs (substance abuse) and mistreatment of family members (domestic abuse).
accelerations spontaneous elevations of the fetal heart rate (FHR).
actual nursing diagnoses diagnoses that identify existing health problems.
alcohol abuse drinking sufficient alcoholic beverages to induce intoxication.
alcoholism chronic alcohol abuse.
amenorrhea absence of menstruation.
amniocentesis a diagnostic procedure whereby a needle is inserted into the amniotic sac and a small amount of fluid is withdrawn and used for biochemical, chromosomal, and genetic studies.
amnioinfusion infusion of normal saline into the uterus.
amnion a thick fibrous lining, made up of several layers, that helps to protect the fetus and forms the inner part of the sac in which the fetus grows.
amniotic fluid the specialized fluid that fills the amniotic cavity and serves to protect the fetus.
amniotomy artificial rupture of membranes (AROM).
analgesia the use of medication to reduce the sensation of pain.
android pelvis the typical male pelvis; in the woman, the heart shape of the android pelvis is not favorable to a vaginal delivery.
anesthesia the use of medication to partially or totally block all sensation to an area of the body.
anthropoid pelvis woman's pelvis that is elongated in its dimensions and is sometimes referred to as apelike.
anticipatory grief preparatory grieving that often helps caregivers mourn the loss of their fetus or newborn when death actually comes.
appropriate for gestational age (AGA) a newborn whose weight, length, and/or head circumference falls between the 10th and 90th percentiles for gestational age
areola darkened area around the nipple.
artificial nutrition infant formula.
asphyxia suffocation caused by interference with the oxygen supply of the blood.
aspiration breathing fluid into the lungs.
attachment the enduring emotional bond that develops between the parent and infant.
ballottement a probable sign of pregnancy that occurs when the examiner pushes up on the uterine wall during a pelvic examination, then feels the fetus bounce back against the examiner's fingers.
biophysical profile (BPP) a method that uses a combination of factors to determine fetal well-being.
Bishop score one commonly used scoring method to determine cervical readiness that evaluates five factors: cervical consistency, position, dilation, effacement, and fetal station.
blastocyst the structure that forms about 5 days after fertilization when the dividing cell mass develops a hollow, fluid-filled core.
blended family both partners in a marriage bring children from a previous marriage into the household: his, hers, and theirs.
boggy uterus a uterus that feels soft and spongy, rather than firm and well contracted.
bonding development of a close emotional tie between the newborn and the parent or parents.
bottle mouth (nursing bottle) caries condition caused by the erosion of enamel on the infant's deciduous teeth from sugar in formula or sweetened juice that coats the teeth for long periods. This condition also can occur in infants who sleep with their mothers and nurse intermittently throughout the night.
bradycardia decreased pulse rate
Braxton Hicks contractions the painless, intermittent, "practice" contractions of pregnancy.
breakthrough pain pain that occurs when the basal dose of analgesia does not control the pain adequately.

brown fat a specialized form of heat-producing tissue found only in fetuses and newborns.

capitation a method that managed care plans use to reduce costs by paying a fixed amount per person to the health care provider to provide services for enrollees.

caput succedaneum edematous swelling of the soft tissues of the scalp caused by prolonged pressure of the occiput against the cervix during labor and delivery. The edema disappears within a few days.

cardinal movements the turns and movements made during the journey of the fetus; referred to as the mechanisms of delivery.

case management a systematic process to ensure that a client's health and service needs are met.

cavernous hemangiomas congenital malformations that are subcutaneous collections of blood vessels with bluish overlying skin. Although these lesions are benign tumors, they may become so extensive as to interfere with the functions of the body part on which they appear.

cerclage procedure that involves placing a purse string type suture in the cervix to keep it from dilating.

cesarean birth the delivery of a fetus through abdominal and uterine incisions: laparotomy and hysterotomy, respectively. Cesarean comes from the Latin word "caedere," meaning "to cut."

Chadwick's sign the bluish-purplish color of the cervix, vagina, and perineum during pregnancy.

chloasma or mask of pregnancy; brown blotchy areas on the forehead, cheeks, and nose of the pregnant woman.

chorioamnionitis bacterial or viral infection of the amniotic fluid and membranes.

choriocarcinoma malignancy of the uterine lining.

chorion a second layer of thick fibrous tissue that surrounds the amnion.

chorionic villi finger-like projections that extend out from the chorion giving it a rough appearance.

chorionic villus sampling (CVS) a newer procedure that can provide chromosomal studies of fetal cells similar to that of amniocentesis.

chromosomes thread-like structures that occur in pairs and carry genetic information.

circumcision surgical removal of all or part of the foreskin (prepuce) of the penis.

classification ability to group objects by rank, grade, or class.

cleavage the process of mitotic division performed by the zygote.

client advocacy speaking or acting on behalf of others to help them gain greater independence and to make the health care delivery system more responsive and relevant to their needs.

climacteric the interlude surrounding menopause in which changes take place.

co-dependent parent parent who supports, directly or indirectly, the other parent's addictive behavior.

cohabitation family a living situation in which a man and woman live together but are not legally married.

coitus interruptus or withdrawal; requires the man to pull the penis out of the vagina before ejaculation to avoid depositing sperm in or near the vagina.

colostomy a surgical procedure in which a part of the colon is brought through the abdominal wall to create an outlet for elimination of fecal material.

colostrum thin, yellowish, milky fluid secreted by the mother's breasts during pregnancy or just after delivery (before the secretion of milk).

communal family alternative family in which members share responsibility for homemaking and child rearing. All children are the collective responsibility of adult members.

community-based nursing a type of nursing practice focused on wellness and a holistic approach to caring for the child in a community setting.

compartment syndrome a serious neurovascular concern that occurs when increasing pressure within the muscle compartment causes decreased circulation.

cordocentesis or **percutaneous umbilical blood sampling (PUBS)**, a procedure similar to amniocentesis, except that fetal blood is withdrawn, rather than amniotic fluid.

corpus luteum a yellow body that forms after ovulation from the remnants of the follicle which is caused by elevated luteinizing hormone (LH) levels.

couplet care postpartum care in which the mother and newborn remain together and receive care from one nurse.

couvade syndrome phenomenon in which some fathers actually experience some of the physical symptoms of pregnancy, such as nausea and vomiting, along with their partner.

cradle cap accumulation of oil and dirt that often forms on an infant's scalp; seborrheic dermatitis.

craniotabes softening of the occipital bones caused by a reduction of mineralization of the skull.

cretinism a congenital condition marked by stunted growth and mental retardation.

critical pathways standard plans of care used to organize and monitor the care provided.

croup general term that typically includes symptoms of a barking cough, hoarseness, and inspiratory stridor.

cultural competency the capacity of the nurse to work with people by integrating their cultural needs into their nursing care.

cystitis infection of the bladder.

decidua the endometrium that has changed to support a pregnancy.
dependence compulsive need to use a substance for its satisfying or pleasurable effects.
dependent nursing actions nursing actions that the nurse performs as a result of a physician's orders, such as administering analgesics for pain.
dermatome an area on the body surface supplied by a particular sensory nerve.
diabetogenic effect of pregnancy condition that occurs when blood glucose levels are lower than normal (mild hypoglycemia) when fasting, blood glucose levels are higher than normal (mild hyperglycemia) after meals, and insulin levels are increased (hyperinsulinemia) after meals.
diagonal conjugate area that extends from the symphysis pubis to the sacral promontory, which is measured to provide an estimate of the size of the obstetric conjugate.
diastasis recti abdominis separation of the rectus abdominis muscle that supports the abdomen.
dizygotic fraternal twins that develop from separate egg and sperm fertilizations.
doula Greek for servant; birth assistants who are trained to provide the highest quality emotional, physical, and educational support to women and their families during childbirth and the postpartum period.
ductus arteriosus prenatal blood vessel between the pulmonary artery and the aorta that closes functionally within the first 3 or 4 days of life.
ductus venosus prenatal blood vessel between the umbilical vein and the inferior vena cava; does not achieve complete closure until the end of the 2nd month of life.
dysfunctional family family that cannot resolve routine stresses in a positive, socially acceptable manner.
dyspareunia painful intercourse.
early deceleration the dip in the fetal heart rate (FHR) tracing that occurs in conjunction with and mirrors a uterine contraction.
eclampsia condition in which the woman with severe preeclampsia experiences a convulsion or a coma.
ectopic pregnancy a pregnancy that occurs outside of the uterus.
effacement shortening of the cervix during labor.
effleurage a form of touch that involves light circular fingertip movements on the abdomen; a technique a woman can use in early labor.
elective abortion an abortion performed at the woman's request that does not involve preservation of health.
elective induction induction of labor in which the physician and woman decide to end the pregnancy in the absence of a medical reason to do so.
embryo the developing conceptus.
en face position establishment of eye contact in the same plane between the caregiver and infant; extremely important to parent–infant bonding; also called mutual gazing.
endometriosis a painful reproductive and immunologic disorder in which tissue implants resembling endometrium grow outside of the uterus.
endometritis an infection of the uterine lining.
endometrium the vascular mucosal inner layer of walls of the corpus and fundus that changes under hormonal influence every month in preparation for possible pregnancy.
engagement occurs when the presenting part of the fetus has settled into the true pelvis at the level of the ischial spines.
engorgement occurs when the milk comes in and the woman's body responds with increasing the blood supply to the breast tissues.
epididymis an intricate network of coiled ducts on the posterior portion of each testis that is approximately 6 meters (20 feet) in length.
episiotomy a surgical incision made into the perineum to enlarge the vaginal opening just before the baby is born.
epispadias condition in which the opening of the urinary meatus is located abnormally on the dorsal (upper) surface of the glans penis.
Epstein's pearls small white cysts found on the midline portion of the hard palate of some newborns.
Erb's palsy a facial paralysis resulting from injury to the cervical nerves.
erythema toxicum fine rash of the newborn that may appear over the trunk, back, abdomen, and buttocks. It appears about 24 hours after birth and disappears in several days.
erythroblastosis fetalis a condition in which the infant's red blood cells are broken down (hemolyzed) and destroyed, producing severe anemia and hyperbilirubinemia.
esotropia eye deviation toward the other eye.
estimated date of confinement (EDC) the estimated date that the baby will be born.
estimated date of delivery (EDD) the estimated date that the baby will be born.
extended family consists of one or more nuclear families plus other relatives; often crosses generations to include grandparents, aunts, uncles, and cousins. The needs of individual members are subordinate to the needs of the group, and the children are considered an economic asset.
exudate drainage; fluid accumulation.
false pelvis the flared upper portion of the bony pelvis.

fertilization process by which the male's sperm unites with the female's ovum.

fetal alcohol syndrome (FAS) syndrome seen in an infant born to a woman who abused alcohol during pregnancy, including shorter stature, lower birth weight, possible microcephaly, facial deformities, hearing disorders, poor coordination, minor joint and limb abnormalities, heart defects, delayed development, and mental retardation.

fetal attitude the relationship of the fetal parts to one another.

fetal fibronectin a protein found in fetal membranes and amniotic fluid.

fetal lie the long axis of the fetus in relation to the long axis of the pregnant woman.

fetal mortality rate perinatal mortality rate calculated by dividing the number of deaths that occur in utero at 20 or more weeks of gestation by the number of live births plus fetal deaths.

fetal presentation the foremost part of the fetus that enters the pelvic inlet.

fetus term for the organism after it has reached the 8th week of life and acquires a human likeness.

fontanel "soft spot" covered by a tough membrane at the junctures of the six bones of a newborn's skull. At birth, two fontanels can be detected—the anterior fontanel at the junction of the frontal and parietal bones and the posterior fontanel at the junction of the parietal and occipital bones. They are ossified (filled in by bone) during the normal growth process.

foramen ovale opening between the left and right atria of the fetal heart that closes with the first breath.

forceps metal instruments with curved, blunted blades (somewhat like large hollowed-out spoons) that are placed around the head of the fetus by the birth attendant to facilitate delivery.

forceps marks noticeable marks on the infant's face that may occur if delivery was assisted with forceps; usually disappear within a day or two.

foremilk breast milk that is very watery and thin and may have a bluish tint. This is what the infant receives first during the breast-feeding session.

gametes sex cells.

gametogenesis the formation and development of gametes or germ cells by the process of meiosis.

gavage feeding nourishment provided directly through a tube passed into the stomach.

genes units threaded along chromosomes that carry genetic instructions from one generation to another. Like chromosomes, genes also occur in pairs. There are thousands of genes in the chromosomes of each cell nucleus.

genetic counseling study of the family history and tissue analysis of both partners to determine chromosome patterns for couples concerned about transmitting a specific disease to their unborn children.

gestational age the length of time between fertilization of the egg and birth of the infant.

gestational diabetes (GDM) a type of diabetes mellitus (DM) that is unique to pregnancy but in many respects mimics type 2 DM.

gestational hypertension (formerly called pregnancy-induced hypertension or PIH) the current term used to describe elevated blood pressure (greater than or equal to 140/90 mm Hg) that develops for the first time during pregnancy without the presence of protein in the urine.

gestational surrogate or surrogate mother; a woman who donates the use of her uterus, or she may also donate her ovum and agree to be inseminated with the male partner's sperm.

glycosuria glucose in the urine.

Goodell's sign softening of the cervix during pregnancy.

grand multiparity five or more pregnancies.

gravida the number of pregnancies the woman has had (regardless of the outcome).

growth result of cell division and marked by an increase in size and weight; physical increase in body size and appearance caused by increasing numbers of new cells.

gynecoid pelvis categorized as a typical female pelvis (although only about half of all women have this type of pelvis); the rounded shape of the gynecoid inlet allows the fetus room to negotiate the dimensions of the bony passageway.

Harlequin sign or Harlequin coloring characterized by a clown-suit–like appearance of the newborn. The newborn's skin is dark red on one side of the body while the other side of the body is pale. The dark red color is caused by constriction of blood vessels, and the pallor is caused by dilation of blood vessels.

health maintenance organizations (HMOs) professional groups of physicians, laboratory service personnel, nurse practitioners, nurses, and consultants who care for the family's health on a continuing basis and are geared to health care and disease prevention. The family pays a set fee for total care; that fee covers any necessary hospitalization. The emphasis is on health and prevention.

Hegar's sign softening of the uterine isthmus during pregnancy.

hematoma a clot of blood that collects within tissues and leads to concealed blood loss.

heterosexual relationship intimate relationship between two people of the opposite sex.

hind milk breast milk that is thicker and whiter. It contains a higher quantity of fat than foremilk and therefore has a higher caloric content than foremilk.

hip dysplasia see congenital hip dysplasia.

homosexual relationship intimate relationship between two people of the same sex.

homozygous term used to describe a particular trait of an individual when any two members of a pair of genes carry the same genetic instructions for that trait.

hydatidiform mole, also referred to as a molar pregnancy and gestational trophoblastic disease; a condition characterized by benign growth of placental tissue.

hydramnios excessive amniotic fluid.

hyperbilirubinemia high blood bilirubin levels.

hyperemesis gravidarum a disorder of early pregnancy that is characterized by severe nausea and vomiting.

hyperglycemia elevated blood glucose levels.

hyperinsulinemia increased insulin levels.

hypoglycemia low blood sugar levels.

hypospadias condition that occurs when the opening to the urethra is on the ventral (under) surface of the glans.

hypovolemic shock condition characterized by a weak, thready, rapid pulse; drop in blood pressure; cool, clammy skin; and changes in level of consciousness.

immunologic properties properties from the woman that help protect the newborn from infections and strengthen the newborn's immune system.

imperforate anus congenital disorder in which the rectal pouch ends blindly above the anus and there is no anal orifice.

incompetent cervix painless cervical dilation that occurs with bulging of fetal membranes and parts through the external os.

independent nursing actions nursing actions that may be performed based on the nurse's own clinical judgment.

induced abortion the purposeful interruption of pregnancy before 20 weeks' gestation.

infant mortality rate the number of deaths during the first 12 months of life, which includes neonatal mortality.

infertility the inability to conceive after a year or more of regular and unprotected intercourse, or the inability to carry a pregnancy to term.

insulin reaction excessively low blood sugar caused by insulin overload; results in too-rapid metabolism of the body's glucose; insulin shock; hypoglycemia.

interdependent nursing actions nursing actions that the nurse must work with other health team members to accomplish, such as meal planning with a dietary therapist and teaching breathing exercises with a respiratory therapist.

intermittent infusion device a type of device that is used for administering medications by the intravenous route and can be left in place and used at intervals.

intrauterine growth restriction (IUGR) condition in which babies are small because of circumstances that occurred during the pregnancy, causing limited fetal growth.

intraventricular hemorrhage (IVH) bleeding within a ventricle of the heart or brain.

involution the shrinking or returning to normal size of the uterus, cervix, and vagina.

isoimmunization development of antibodies against Rh_o(D) positive blood in the pregnant woman.

jacket restraint used to secure the child from climbing out of bed or a chair or to keep the child in a horizontal position; must be the correct size for the child.

jaundice a yellow staining of the skin that occurs when a large amount of unconjugated bilirubin is present (serum levels of 4 to 6 mg/dL and greater)

kangaroo care a way to maintain the newborn's temperature and promote early bonding; the nurse dries the newborn quickly, places a diaper or blanket over the genital area and a cap on the head, then places the newborn in skin-to-skin contact with the mother or father and covers them both with blankets.

kernicterus neurologic complication of unconjugated hyperbilirubinemia in the infant.

labor dystocia an abnormal progression of labor.

lactation consultant a nurse or layperson who has received special training to assist and support the breast-feeding woman.

laminaria cervical dilators.

lanugo fine, downy hair that covers the skin of the fetus.

large for gestational age (LGA) an infant whose weight, length, and/or head circumference is above the 90th percentile for gestational age.

late decelerations decelerations that are offset from the labor contraction. Late decelerations begin late in the contraction and recover after the contraction has ended.

lecithin major component of surfactant.

libido sexual drive.

linea nigra a darkened line that develops on the skin in the middle of the abdomen of pregnant women.

lochia vaginal discharge after birth.

long-term variability (LTV) the wider fluctuations that make the electronic fetal monitoring (EFM) tracing look wavy over time.

low birth weight (LBW) newborns that weigh less than 2,500 g.
macroglossia abnormally large tongue.
macrosomia condition that is diagnosed if the birth weight exceeds 4,500 grams (9.9 pounds) or the birth weight is greater than the 90th percentile for gestational age.
malattachment emotional distancing in the maternal–infant relationship.
mastitis infection of the breast tissue.
maternal mortality rate the number of maternal deaths per 100,000 live births caused by a pregnancy-related complication that occurs during pregnancy or during the 42 days after pregnancy.
meconium first stools of the newborn; amniotic fluid together with a sticky, greenish-black substance composed of bile, mucus, cellular waste, intestinal secretions, fat, hair, and other materials swallowed during fetal life.
meconium aspiration occurs when the fetus inhales some meconium along with amniotic fluid.
menarche beginning of menstruation.
menorrhagia heavy or prolonged uterine bleeding.
metrorrhagia menstrual bleeding that is normal in amount but occurs at irregular intervals between menstrual periods.
microcephaly a very small cranium.
milia pearly white cysts usually seen over the bridge of the nose, chin, and cheeks of a newborn. They are usually retention cysts of sebaceous glands or hair follicles and disappear within a few weeks without treatment.
mittelschmerz pain experienced midcycle in the menstrual cycle at the time of ovulation.
molding elongation of the fetal skull to accommodate the birth canal.
mongolian spots areas of bluish-black pigmentation resembling bruises; most often seen over the sacral or gluteal regions of infants of African, Mediterranean, Native American, or Asian descent; usually fade within 1 or 2 years.
monozygotic identical twins that are derived from one zygote; one egg and one sperm divide into two zygotes shortly after fertilization.
mons pubis or mons; a rounded fatty pad located atop the symphysis pubis.
Montgomery's tubercles sebaceous glands on the areolas that produce secretions that lubricate the nipple. Montgomery's tubercles become more prominent during pregnancy.
morbidity the number of persons afflicted with the same disease condition per a certain number of population.
Moro reflex abduction of the arms and legs and flexion of the elbows in response to a sudden loud noise, jarring, or abrupt change in equilibrium: fingers flare, except the forefinger and thumb, which are clenched to form a C shape. Occurs in the normal newborn to the end of the 4th or 5th month.
mortality rate statistics recorded as the ratio of deaths in a given category to the number of individuals in that category of the population.
morula the solid cell cluster that forms about 3 days after fertilization, when the total cell count has reached 32.
mottling a red and white lacy pattern sometimes seen on the skin of newborns who have fair complexions.
multigravida a woman who has had more than one pregnancy.
mutation fundamental change that takes place in the structure of a gene; results in the transmission of a trait different from that normally carried by that particular gene.
mutual gazing see *en face position.*
myometrium the muscular middle layer of the walls of the corpus and fundus that is responsible for the contractions of labor.
nadir the lowest point of the deceleration of the fetal heart rate (FHR).
Nagele's rule a formula used to determine the pregnancy due date by adding 7 days to the date of the first day of the last menstrual period (LMP), then subtracting 3 months.
necrotizing enterocolitis an acute inflammatory disease of the intestine.
neonatal adjective used to describe the time period from birth through the first 28 days or 1 month of life.
neonatal abstinence syndrome (NAS) symptoms seen in the newborn of the woman who has abused substances during pregnancy; withdrawal symptoms.
neonatal mortality rate the number of infant deaths during the first 28 days of life for every 1,000 live births.
neonate term used to describe a newborn in the first 28 days of life.
nuclear family family structure that consists of only the father, the mother, and the children living in one household.
nulligravida a woman who has never been pregnant.
nursing process proven form of problem solving based on the scientific method. The nursing process consists of five components: assessment, nursing diagnosis, planning, implementation, and evaluation.
nutrition history information regarding the client's eating habits and preferences.
objective data in the nursing assessment, the data gained by the nurse's direct observation.
obstetric conjugate the smallest diameter of the inlet through which the fetus must pass.

open-glottis pushing method of expelling the fetus that is characterized by pushing with contractions using an open glottis so that air is released during the pushing effort.

opioids medications with opium-like properties (also known as narcotic analgesics); the most frequently administered medications to provide analgesia during labor.

opisthotonos arching of the back so that the head and the heels are bent backward and the body is forward.

ophthalmia neonatorum a severe eye infection contracted in the birth canal of a woman with gonorrhea or Chlamydia.

orchiopexy surgical procedure used to bring an undescended testis down into the scrotum and anchor it there.

outcomes goals that are specific, stated in measurable terms, and have a time frame for accomplishment.

ovulation releasing the mature ovum into the abdominal cavity, which occurs on day 14 of a 28-day cycle.

palmar grasp reflex phenomenon that results when pressure is placed on the palm of the hand near the base of the digits causing flexion or curling of the fingers.

parity or para, communicates the outcome of previous pregnancies in the obstetric history.

pelvic rest a situation in which nothing is placed in the vagina, including tampons and the practitioner's fingers, to perform a cervical examination.

percutaneous umbilical blood sampling (PUBS) or cordocentesis a procedure similar to amniocentesis, except that fetal blood is withdrawn, rather than amniotic fluid.

perimenopause the time before menopause when vasomotor symptoms (hot flashes, night sweats) and irregular menses begin.

perimetrium the tough outer layer of the walls of the corpus and fundus, which is made of connective tissues and supports the uterus.

perinatal the period surrounding birth, from conception throughout pregnancy and birth.

perinatal mortality rate the number of fetal/neonatal deaths that occur from 28 weeks of gestation through the first 7 days of life.

perinatologist a maternal–fetal medicine specialist.

periodic changes variations in the fetal heart rate (FHR) pattern that occur in conjunction with uterine contractions.

personal history data collected about a client's personal habits, such as hygiene, sleeping, and elimination patterns, as well as activities, exercise, special interests, and favorite objects (toys).

phenylketonuria (PKU) recessive hereditary defect of metabolism that results in a congenital disease caused by a defect in the enzyme that normally changes the essential amino acid, phenylalanine, into tyrosine. If untreated, PKU results in severe mental retardation.

phimosis adherence of the foreskin to the glans penis.

physiologic jaundice icterus neonatorum; jaundice that occurs in a large number of newborns but has no medical significance; result of the breakdown of fetal red blood cells.

pica compulsive eating of nonfood substances.

placenta previa a condition in which the placenta is implanted close to, or covers, the cervical os.

plantar grasp reflex phenomenon that results when pressure is placed on the sole of the foot at the base of the toes; causes the toes to curl downward.

platypelloid pelvis pelvis that is flat in its dimensions with a very narrow anterior-posterior diameter and a wide transverse diameter; this shape makes it extremely difficult for the fetus to pass through the bony pelvis.

polyuria dramatic increase in urinary output, often with enuresis.

postcoital test evaluates the interaction of the man's sperm with the woman's cervical mucus.

postpartum blues, sometimes called the "baby blues," a temporary depression that usually begins on the 3rd day after delivery and lasts for 2 or 3 days, in which the woman may be tearful, have difficulty sleeping and eating, and feel generally let down.

postterm or postmature, a newborn born at 42 weeks' or more gestation.

precipitous labor labor that lasts less than 3 hours from the start of uterine contractions to birth.

preeclampsia a serious condition of pregnancy in which the blood pressure rises to 140/90 mm Hg or higher accompanied by proteinuria, the presence of protein in the urine.

pregestational diabetes condition in which a woman enters pregnancy with either type 1 or type 2 diabetes mellitus.

premenstrual syndrome (PMS) symptoms in the period before menstruation, including edema (resulting in weight gain), headache, increased anxiety, mild depression, or mood swings; premenstrual tension.

prepuce or foreskin; a layer of tissue that covers the glans of the penis.

preterm, or premature, a newborn born at 37 weeks' gestation or less; commonly called premature.

priapism prolonged, abnormal erection of the penis.

primary nursing system whereby one nurse plans the total care for a child and directs the efforts of nurses on the other shifts.

primary prevention limiting the spread of illness or disease by teaching, especially regarding safety, diet, rest, and exercise.

prospective payment system predetermined rates to be paid to the health care provider to care for patients with certain classifications of diseases.
proteinuria the presence of protein in the urine.
pseudomenses (pseudomenstruation) false menstruation; a slight red-tinged vaginal discharge in female infants resulting from a decline in the hormonal level after birth compared with the higher concentration in the maternal hormone environment before birth.
puberty period during which secondary sexual characteristics begin to develop and reproductive maturity is attained.
puerperal fever an illness marked by high fever caused by infection of the reproductive tract after the birth of a child.
puerperium the postpartum period.
pulse oximeter photoelectric device used to measure oxygen saturation in an artery; can be attached to a newborn's finger, toe, or heel.
pyelonephritis infection of the kidneys.
pyrosis heartburn caused by acid reflux through the relaxed lower esophageal sphincter (LES).
recessive gene gene carrying different information for a trait within a pair that is not expressed (e.g., blue eyes versus brown eyes). A recessive gene is detectable only when present on both chromosomes.
regurgitation spitting up of small quantities of milk; occurs rather easily in the young infant.
respiratory distress syndrome (RDS) see *hyaline membrane disease*.
retinopathy of prematurity (ROP) a complication commonly associated with the preterm newborn that results from the growth of abnormal immature retinal blood vessels.
risk nursing diagnoses category of diagnoses that identifies health problems to which the patient is especially vulnerable.
ritual a routine; in labor, a repeated series of actions that the woman uses as an individualized way of dealing with the discomfort of labor.
rooting reflex infant's response of turning the head when the cheek is stroked toward the stroked side.
rumination voluntary regurgitation.
salpingectomy removal of the fallopian tube.
salpingitis infection of the fallopian tube.
scurvy a disease that results from severe vitamin C deficiency and is characterized by spongy gums, loosened teeth, and bleeding into the skin and mucous membrane.
seborrhea a scalp condition characterized by yellow, crusty patches; also called cradle cap.
sebum oily secretion of the sebaceous glands.
secondary prevention limiting the impact or reoccurrence of disease by focusing on early diagnosis and treatment.
seminiferous tubules tiny coils of tissue in the lobes of the testis in which spermatogenesis occurs.
sexual abuse sexual contact between a child and someone in a caregiving position, such as a parent, baby-sitter, or teacher.
sexual assault sexual contact made by someone who is not functioning in the role of the child's caregiver.
short-term variability (STV) the moment-to-moment changes in fetal heart rate (FHR) that result in roughness of the electronic fetal monitor (EFM) tracing.
simian crease a single straight palmar crease; an abnormal finding that is associated with Down syndrome.
single-parent family household headed by one adult of either sex. There may be one or more children in the family.
small for gestational age (SGA) a newborn whose weight, length, and/or head circumference falls below the 10th percentile for gestational age.
smegma the cheeselike secretion of the sebaceous glands found under the foreskin.
spermatogenesis production of sperm.
spina bifida failure of the posterior lamina of the vertebrae to close; leaves an opening through which the spinal meninges and spinal cord may protrude.
spinnbarkeit an elastic quality of cervical mucus that allows it to be stretched 5 centimeters or more between the thumb and forefinger.
spontaneous abortion loss of a pregnancy before the age of viability (less than 20 weeks of gestation or fetal size of less than 500 grams). The common name for early pregnancy loss is miscarriage.
startle reflex follows any loud noise; similar to the Moro reflex, but the hands remain clenched. This reflex is never lost.
station the relationship of the presenting part of a fetus to the ischial spines.
status asthmaticus a potentially fatal complication of an acute asthma attack involving severe asthma symptoms that do not respond after 30 to 60 minutes of treatment.
status epilepticus an emergency complication of epilepsy whereby seizure activity continues for 30 minutes or more after treatment is initiated or when three or more seizures occur without full recovery between seizures.
step reflex also called the dance reflex; tendency of infants to make stepping movements when held upright.
stepfamily consists of custodial parent, children, and a new spouse.
striae stretch marks.

subjective data in the nursing assessment, data spoken by the child or family.

substance abuse the misuse of an addictive substance, such as alcohol or drugs, that changes the user's mental state.

sucking reflex infant's response of strong, vigorous sucking when a nipple, finger, or tongue blade is put in his or her mouth.

supernumerary excessive in number (e.g., more than the usual number of teeth).

supine hypotensive syndrome condition that occurs during late pregnancy in which the gravid uterus can compress the woman's vena cava and aorta, causing the blood pressure to fall when the woman is in the supine position.

surfactant a substance found in the lungs of mature fetuses that keeps the alveoli from collapsing after they first expand.

suture narrow band of connective tissue that divides the six nonunited bones of a newborn's skull.

symmetry a balance in shape, size, and position from one side of the body to the other; a mirror image.

tachypnea rapid respirations.

talipes equinovarus clubfoot with plantar flexion.

teratogens from the Greek *terato,* meaning monster, and *genesis,* meaning birth; an agent or influence that causes a defect or disruption in the prenatal growth process. The effect of a teratogen depends on when it enters the fetal system and the stage of differentiation of the organs or organ systems at that time. Generally the fetus is most vulnerable to teratogens during the 1st trimester.

term a newborn who is born between the beginning of week 38 and the end of week 41 of gestation.

tertiary prevention a focus on rehabilitation and teaching to prevent additional injury or illness.

therapeutic abortion a pregnancy termination performed for reasons related to maternal or fetal health or disease.

thermoneutral environment an environment in which heat is neither lost nor gained.

thermoregulation regulation of temperature.

thrush A fungal infection (caused by *Candida albicans*) in the oral cavity.

tocolytic a substance that relaxes the uterine muscle.

tolerance in substance abuse, ability of body tissues to endure and adapt to continued or increased use of a substance.

tonic neck reflex also called the fencing reflex; seen when the infant lies on the back with the head turned to one side, the arm and leg on that side extended, and the opposite arm flexed as if in a fencing position.

TORCH an acronym for a special group of infections that can be acquired during pregnancy and transmitted through the placenta to the fetus. The "T" stands for toxoplasmosis, the "O" for other infections (Hepatitis B, syphilis, varicella and herpes zoster), the "R" is for rubella, the "C" is for cytomegalovirus (CMV), and the "H" stands for herpes simplex virus (HSV).

total parenteral nutrition (TPN) the administration of dextrose, lipids, amino acids, electrolytes, vitamins, minerals, and trace elements into the circulatory system to meet the nutritional needs of the child whose needs cannot be met through the gastrointestinal tract.

true pelvis the portion of the pelvis below the linea terminalis.

tympanic membrane sensor device used to determine the temperature of the tympanic membrane by rapidly sensing infrared radiation from the membrane. The tympanic thermometer offers the advantage of recording the temperature rapidly with little disturbance to the newborn.

urge-to-push method method of expelling the fetus in which the woman bears down only when she feels the urge to do so using any technique that feels right for her.

urostomy a surgical opening created to help with the elimination of urine.

uterine atony inability of the uterus to contract effectively.

uterine subinvolution a condition in which the uterus returns to its prepregnancy shape and size at a rate that is slower than expected (usually the result of retained placental fragments or an infection).

uteroplacental insufficiency diminished or deficient blood flow to the uterus and placenta.

utilization review a systematic evaluation of services delivered by a health care provider to determine appropriateness and quality of care, as well as medical necessity of the services provided.

vaginitis inflammation of the vagina.

variability fluctuations in fetal heart rate (FHR).

variable deceleration a change in the FHR that may occur at any point during a contraction and has a jagged, erratic shape on the electronic fetal monitor (EFM) tracing.

vas deferens the muscular tube in which sperm begin their journey out of the man's body.

vascular nevus commonly known as a strawberry mark; a slightly raised, bright-red collection of hypertrophied skin capillaries that does not blanch completely on pressure.

vasectomy male sterilization.

vasospasm spasm of the arteries.

ventricular septal defect abnormal opening in the septum of the heart between the ventricles; allows blood to pass directly from the left to the right side of the heart; the most common intracardiac defect.

ventriculoatrial shunting plastic tubing implanted into the cerebral ventricle passing under the skin to the cardiac atrium; provides drainage for excessive cerebrospinal fluid.

ventriculoperitoneal shunting plastic tubing implanted into the cerebral ventricle passing under the skin to the peritoneal cavity, providing drainage for excessive cerebrospinal fluid. Excessive tubing can be inserted to accommodate the child's growth.

vernix caseosa greasy, cheeselike substance that protects the skin during fetal life; consists of sebum and desquamated epithelial cells.

version a process of manipulating the position of the fetus while in utero.

very low birth weight (VLBW) newborns weighing less than 1,500 g.

vestibule the area within the boundaries of the labia minora, which includes the urethral meatus, vaginal opening, and Bartholin glands.

viable able to live outside of the uterus (fetus).

vigorous pushing method of expelling the fetus in which the woman is told to take a deep breath, hold the breath, and push while counting to 10. She is encouraged to complete three "good" pushes in this manner with each contraction.

vulva the external genitalia of the female reproductive system.

wellness nursing diagnoses diagnoses that identify the potential of an individual, family, or community to move to a higher level of wellness.

Wharton's jelly a clear gelatinous substance that gives support to the cord and helps prevent compression of the cord, which could impair blood flow to the fetus.

withdrawal symptoms in substance abuse, physical and psychological symptoms that occur when the drug is no longer being used.

zygote or conceptus, results when an ovum and a spermatozoon unite. The zygote has the full complement of 46 chromosomes, arranged in 23 pairs.

English–Spanish Glossary

Helpful Explanatory Phrases

Both the tu (informal for younger people) and the usted (more formal for people, not known, older than one) forms are offered. In each case the informal is stated first.

Hello. My name is _______.	*Hola. Me llamo _________.*
I am your nurse.	*Soy tu enfermera.*
I don't understand much Spanish. When I ask you questions, please answer with one or two words.	*No entiendo mucho español. Por favor contesta con una o dos palabras.* *Por favor conteste con una o dos palabras.*
Please speak more slowly.	*Habla más despacio, por favor.* *Hable más despacio, por favor.*
I'm sorry, but I don't understand.	*Lo siento, pero no entiendo.*

Admission Questions

What is your name, including your last name?	*¿Cómo te llamas? Incluye tu apellido.* *¿Cómo se llama? Incluya su apellido.*
How many times have you been pregnant?	*¿Cuántas veces has estado embarazada?* *¿Cuántas veces ha estado embarazada?*
When did your contractions begin?	*¿Cuándo empezaron los dolores?*
Did your water bag break?	*¿Se te rompió la bolsa?* *¿Se le rompió la bolsa?*
Is the baby moving normally?	*¿Está moviéndose normalmente el bebé?*
Have you had any problems with this pregnancy?	*¿Has tenido problemas con este embarazo?* *¿Ha tenido problemas con este embarazo?*
Do you have any chronic illnesses, such as asthma, diabetes, tuberculosis, heart disease?	*¿Tienes alguna enfermedad crónica, como asma, diabetes, tuberculosis, enfermedades del corazón?* *¿Tiene alguna enfermedad crónica, como asma, diabetes, tuberculosis, enfermedades del corazón?*
Are you taking any medications?	*¿Estás tomando alguna medicina?* *¿Está tomando usted alguna medicina?*
How much alcohol do you drink?	*¿Tomas bebidas alcohólicas? ¿Cuánto tomas?* *¿Toma bebidas alcohólicas? ¿Cuánto toma?*
How many cigarettes do you smoke per day?	*¿Fumas cigarillos? ¿Cuántos fumas por día?* *¿Fuma cigarillos? ¿Cuántos fuma por día?*
What plans do you have for pain management?	*¿Qué planes tienes para manejar los dolores?* *¿Qué planes tiene para manejar los dolores?*
Do you want an epidural?	*¿Quieres una inyección epidural?* *¿Quiere una inyección epidural?*
Do you plan to breast-feed?	*¿Piensas dar pecho? ¿Piensas amamantar?* *¿Piensa dar pecho? ¿Piensa amamantar?*
Do you want the baby circumcised?	*¿Deseas circuncisión para el bebé?* *¿Desea circuncisión para el bebé?*

Admission Procedures	
Please put on this gown.	*Por favor, ponte esta bata.* *Por favor, póngase esta bata.*
Wipe with these, then urinate in this cup.	*Límpiate con éstas. Luego orina en este vaso.* *Límpiese con éstas. Luego orine en este vaso.*
Press this button when you need the nurse.	*Empuja este botón cuando necesitas a la enfermera.* *Empuje este botón cuando necesite a la enfermera.*
This is a fetal monitor.	*Esta máquina es para checar al bebé.*
This part monitors the contractions.	*Esta parte es para checar los dolores.*
This part monitors the baby's heartbeat.	*Este es para checar el latido del corazón del bebé.*
Intrapartum Procedures	
I am going to check your labor progress.	*Voy a checar como esta progresando el parto.*
Put your heels together and let your legs relax outward to each side.	*Pon juntos los talones y deja relajar las piernas hacia fuera para cada lado.* *Ponga juntos los talones y deje relajar las piernas hacia fuera para cada lado.*
Take a deep breath in, exhale, and then breathe with me.	*Respira profundo, exhala, y luego respira conmigo.* *Respire profundo, exhale, y luego respire conmigo.*
Please turn to your left (right) side.	*Por favor, voltéate a tu lado izquierdo (derecho).* *Por favor, voltéese a su lado izquierdo (derecho).*
I am going to insert a catheter into your vein.	*Voy a meterte una aguja a la vena.* *Voy a meterle una aguja a la vena.*
I am going to put a catheter into your bladder to drain the urine, and then I will remove the catheter.	*Voy a meterte(le) un catéter (un tubo) en la vejiga para vaciarla (sacar la orina), y después voy a quitar el catéter.*
Don't push. Blow out, like this.	*No empujes. Sopla, así.* *No empuje. Sople, así.*
Push!	*¡Empuja!* *¡Empuje!*
It's a boy (girl)!	*¡Es varón!* *¡Es mujer!*
Congratulations!	*¡Felicidades!*
Cesarean Delivery	
You need a cesarean section.	*Usted necesita una sección cesariana*
I am going to shave your abdomen and your upper thighs.	*Voy a rasurar el abdomen (estomago) y los muslos.*
I am going to put a catheter into your bladder. The urine will drain into the bag. The nurses will take the catheter out 24 hours after your surgery.	*Voy a insertarte(le) un catéter en la vejiga. La orina va a drenarse en la bolsa. Las enfermeras te(le) sacaran el catéter unas veinticuatro horas después de tu(su) cirugía.*
Hold the pillow over your incision, and then cough.	*Pon (ponga) la almohada sobre la incisión (cortada) y luego tose (tosa).*
What kind of pain do you have? Is it your incision? Is it cramping? Is it gas pains?	*¿Qué clase de dolor tienes (tiene)?* *¿Es tu (su) incisión (cortada)?* *¿Son calambres (espasmos)?* *¿Son dolores de gas?*
Are you having any nausea?	*¿Tienes (tiene) nausea?*
Have you vomited?	*¿Has (Ha) vomitado?*
Are you passing gas?	*¿Estás (Está) pasando gas?*
Have you had a bowel movement?	*¿Has (Ha) defecado?* *¿Has (Ha) hecho del baño?*

Answers to Workbook Questions

CHAPTER 1

NCLEX-Style Review Questions

1. d
   Rationale. Treatment advances for preterm infants have done the most to improve neonatal mortality statistics. Control of puerperal fever has helped improve maternal morbidity and mortality. Use of anesthesia during labor has led to the most births occurring in hospitals. Enforcement of strict rules in hospitals is generally not a helpful technique. If you had trouble with this question, review the section on Maternal–Infant Health Status.
2. b
   Rationale. The nursing process is a form of problem solving. Although using the nursing process may help contain costs, this is not a primary benefit. Oral communication and health teaching are two tools used in carrying out the nursing process, but these methods do not describe the entire process. If you had trouble answering this question, review the introductory material on the nursing process.
3. a
   Rationale. Data collection and physical assessment are all part of assessment. Planning includes goal setting and planning appropriate interventions. Implementation is the step in which the plan is carried out. Evaluation is the step in which the nurse determines whether or not goals and outcomes were achieved and whether or not the problem has been solved or the care plan needs to be revised. If you answered this question incorrectly, review the section on the steps of the nursing process.
4. c
   Rationale. Nursing care is carried out in the implementation step of the nursing process. Assessment includes data collection and establishing rapport with the patient. Planning includes goal setting and planning appropriate interventions. Evaluation is the step in which the nurse determines whether or not goals and outcomes were achieved and whether or not the problem has been solved, or the care plan needs to be revised. If you answered this question incorrectly, review the section on the steps of the nursing process.

Critical Thinking: What Would You Do?

1. *Suggested answers:*
   a. Explain the CHIP program to the woman. She may not realize that there is a state-sponsored insurance program that charges her for her child's insurance on a sliding scale basis (based on family income). Although her child may not qualify for Medicaid, she will likely be able to purchase affordable insurance for the child's health care needs.
   b. Yes. She does have options. See answer above.
2. *Suggested answers:*
   Newborns are more secure and as a result usually happier and recover more quickly when they are in the presence of the individuals in their lives with whom they have developed a sense of trust; in most cases these individuals are the child's caregivers. The presence of the caregivers also gives the nurse an opportunity to provide teaching that will benefit the child after discharge. Caregivers can give the child support in a threatening or uncomfortable situation.

CHAPTER 2

NCLEX-Style Review Questions

1. b
   Rationale. In a stepfamily a parent brings children from a previous relationship into a relationship with a new partner. If both partners in this new relationship bring children to this relationship, the family is known as a blended family. This often occurs with the increasing rate of divorce.
2. d
   Rationale. Although the nurse may use the Internet and previous knowledge she obtained when caring for a Korean client, the nurse should use a variety of sources to learn about the culture. The most

important factor is to involve the woman and her family in planning care. This action will best promote integration of cultural aspects into the plan of care.

3. a

Rationale. Primary prevention activities focus on promoting wellness to prevent problems from arising. Counseling a woman to stop smoking before she becomes pregnant is an excellent way to protect her unborn baby from the adverse effects of smoking. Screening activities are examples of secondary prevention. Assisting the parents of a premature baby to learn to work with an apnea monitor is an example of tertiary prevention. Sharing information about birth settings with a pregnant woman gives the woman information upon which she can base her decision, but it is not an example of primary prevention.

4. c

Rationale. Although some of the other statements may be true, it is best to explore with the woman her reasons for wanting a home birth. As an advocate for the woman, the nurse should give her the facts about each setting so that the woman can make an informed decision.

5. d

Rationale. When doing teaching in a community-based setting, the nurse must know the needs of the audience to best be able to convey the information to the particular group of individuals. The nurse can then use appropriate teaching strategies and resources to teach the group.

Critical Thinking: What Would You Do?

1. *Suggested answers:*

In teaching this family, it would be important to include information regarding phototherapy treatment for the infant, including purpose of treatment; safety factors involved with the treatment; procedure for carrying out the treatment; and follow-up appointments and care for the infant. You should also provide information about the illness of the 6-year-old child, including reviewing what has been done for this child to this point; recommendations for having the child seen by a care provider if she has not been seen; clarification of information and treatments this child's care provider has given the family if a provider has seen the child; follow-up needed for this child; preventive measures to reduce possibilities of further infection; and teaching regarding smoking in the home, including exploration with the parents about their understanding of the effects of smoking on their children and themselves, teaching regarding the effects of smoking on their children and themselves, and recommending community resources and support regarding smoking cessation.

2. *Suggested answers:*

a. In teaching any group of individuals it is important for the nurse to know the age, educational level, ethnic and gender mix, language barriers, and previous teaching the group has had regarding the subject.

b. In presenting the lesson to these adolescents, the nurse would review growth and development principles of the teen and plan the lesson to be at the appropriate level of understanding, as well as to include activities to enhance learning at their level of development. Keeping in mind that an open-minded nonjudgmental attitude when presenting the lesson would also be important.

CHAPTER 3

NCLEX-Style Review Questions

1. d

Rationale. The seminal vesicles contribute alkaline fluid and fructose to semen. The fructose is a simple sugar that provides energy for sperm movement. Bartholin glands provide lubrication to the vestibule in the female. Bulbourethral glands provide lubrication to the male urethra and add to the volume of semen. The epididymis is a coiled structure on top of each testis in which sperm mature. If this question was difficult for you, review the section on semen formation.

2. b

Rationale. The vagina has an acidic pH, an environment that is hostile to sperm. Therefore, semen has an alkaline pH, which protects sperm from the acid of the vagina. Testosterone is a testicular hormone that influences sperm development and maturation. The seminiferous tubules are the site within the testes in which male gametes are formed. If you had difficulty with this question, review the section on semen formation.

3. d

Rationale. The urinary meatus is found below the clitoris and is one of the structures of the vestibule. It is located above the vaginal opening (between the clitoris and vaginal opening). The true perineum is the structure found between the vestibule and anus.

4. d

Rationale. The isthmus is called the lower uterine segment during pregnancy. This is the thinnest area of the uterus, making it the most vulnerable site for uterine rupture.

5. c
   Rationale. Estrogen stimulates regeneration and growth of the endometrial lining by stimulating blood vessel development. This is the hormone that most influences the proliferative phase of the endometrial cycle. FSH and LH are both anterior pituitary hormones that govern the hormone production of the ovaries. Progesterone is an ovarian hormone that most influences the secretory phase of the endometrial cycle.

Critical Thinking: What Would You Do?

1. *Suggested answers:*
   a. Because Doug wears tight jeans and works in a hot environment, his sperm count might be decreased. The formation and maturation of sperm require a temperature that is a little lower than body temperature. Tight clothing keeps the testes close to the body and increases the temperature.
   b. It would be helpful for Doug to find some looser clothing to wear during the hot days when he is working outside. His tight jeans could be saved for other occasions and for when the weather is cool.
2. *Suggested answers:*
   a. It would be helpful to know if Nancy is taking antibiotics for any reason. It would also be helpful to know if she uses tampons, deodorant-style sanitary napkins, or any type of highly perfumed substances near the vulva.
   b. The practice of douching and using products with deodorant on the external genitalia can change the pH of the vagina. Normally the pH is acidic, but if it becomes more alkaline, the protective function is lost. Nancy would be well advised to discuss the use of these products with her physician. Together they can come up with a plan to meet her hygiene objectives without compromising her reproductive health.

CHAPTER 4

NCLEX-Style Review Questions

1. d
   Rationale. Female health screening recommends that the woman should have her first Pap smear 3 years after first intercourse or age 21 years, whichever comes first.
2. d
   Rationale. The nurse would document that the woman reports menorrhagia, which refers to heavy or prolonged menstrual bleeding. Dysmenorrhea refers to difficult or painful menses. Metrorrhagia is irregular bleeding. Amenorrhea is absence of menses.
3. d
   Rationale. Although medications can be helpful, other measures, including stress reduction and regular exercise, may have the most overall effect. Prostaglandins, not infection, cause the symptoms of PMS, so antibiotics are not appropriate therapy for this disorder. Diuretics may be used to treat the bloating associated with PMS but are not necessarily the most helpful overall medications.
4. a
   Rationale. Cloudy urine may indicate a bladder infection. This condition would need immediate evaluation and treatment by a physician to prevent complications. If she forgot to do Kegel exercises, the appropriate reply would be to go ahead and do them now. Urine escaping during coughing is a symptom associated with a cystocele but does not require immediate intervention. Pessaries should be removed periodically and washed. If the woman forgets to reapply it, then she should reinsert it when she remembers.

Critical Thinking: What Would You Do?

1. *Suggested answers:*
   a. Amanda can expect a detailed history and thorough physical examination to include a pelvic examination and Pap smear.
   b. Amanda is experiencing primary infertility. She and her husband have been trying for 2 years without success. One year of unprotected intercourse is enough to qualify for the diagnosis of infertility. It is primary infertility because Amanda has never before been pregnant.
   c. It may be helpful to point out to Amanda that many women wait until their late 30s to begin having children. This is a normal phenomenon of our culture. It may also help to explain that guilt feelings are a very normal response to initial infertility. Explain that the physician will work with Amanda and her husband to try to determine what the problem is and to do everything possible to help her have a child.
2. *Suggested answers:*
   a. A semen analysis requires that her husband obtain a sperm sample, usually by masturbation. If this is unacceptable to either of them, they may use a special condom to collect the sample during intercourse. It is important that all of the ejaculate be collected and placed into the sterile specimen cup provided for that purpose. The specimen must be delivered to the lab within 30 minutes of collection. The postcoital test

involves determination of ovulation by using FAM techniques. Just before ovulation the couple should have intercourse without using lubricants. Amanda must go to the clinic 8 to 12 hours after intercourse; at the clinic, a sample of her cervical mucus will be collected for testing.
b. ICSI is an advanced reproductive therapy used to treat infertile couples in whom the man has a low sperm count. A sperm sample is obtained through masturbation or testicular biopsy. One sperm is paralyzed by stroking the distal portion of its tail. An ovum is harvested from the woman, then the sperm is injected into the ovum, and the fertilized cell is placed into the woman's uterus.

3. *Suggested answers:*
   a. Hot flashes are caused by low estrogen levels and periodic surges of luteinizing hormone, but the physiology is not completely understood.
   b. The physician may recommend low dose HRT; although this is a controversial therapy. Other options include treatment with a progestin, certain antihypertensives, anticonvulsants, and antidepressants.
   c. Cindy should be careful to get adequate weight-bearing exercise. She may also increase her comfort by lowering the temperature in her house, wearing comfortable lightweight clothing in layers, and avoiding spicy foods, alcohol, and caffeine. She should continue taking calcium and vitamin D supplements. Vaginal estrogen creams and lotions can be used to treat vaginal dryness and decrease sexual discomfort. She should continue having mammograms annually.

CHAPTER 5

NCLEX-Style Review Questions

1. c
   Rationale. A teratogen will have the most damage upon the developing embryo. During the pre-embryonic stage a teratogen will have an all-or-nothing effect. A teratogen can affect the developing fetus, but the effect will not be as damaging as a teratogen ingested during the embryonic stage. During the embryonic stage there is tissue differentiation and development of all the organ systems.
2. c
   Rationale. The embryonic stage begins at the end of the 2nd week after fertilization and is complete at the end of the 8th week after fertilization. Before this time frame is the pre-embryonic stage, and after this time frame is the fetal stage.
3. d
   Rationale. The chorionic villi project into the intervillous spaces, where they are surrounded by maternal blood that enters the spaces from the endometrial arteries. Nutrients from the maternal blood are transferred into the chorionic villi to be taken to the fetus, and waste products from the fetus are transferred into the maternal blood to be removed by the woman's body. They are anchoring villi that help to adhere the placenta to the decidua basalis, but their primary function is to exchange wastes for nutrients.
4. b
   Rationale. The foramen ovale is a fetal shunt. The foramen primum and the septum secundum are cardiac structures but are not involved in fetal circulation. The ductus deferens is another name for the vas deferens located in the male. The two other fetal shunts are the ductus venosus and ductus arteriosus.
5. a
   Rationale. Identical twins are also known as monozygotic and share the same chromosomal material. Fraternal twins are classified as dizygotic. Trizygotic refers to three zygotes.

Critical Thinking: What Would You Do?

1. *Suggested answers:*
   a. Rebecca is approximately 8 weeks' gestation. The fetus is approximately 1 inch long. All of the organs are formed. The heart is beating, extremities have developed, and facial features are discernible.
   b. Tylenol is generally not considered to be teratogenic and is safe to use during pregnancy in moderation. Explain that she is right to be concerned about substances that she ingests or is exposed to in the environment. Encourage her to consult with her physician before taking any type of over-the-counter medication.
2. *Suggested answers:*
   a. The fetus is 7 to 8 centimeters in length and weighs approximately 45 grams. It is possible to tell the sex of the fetus by looking at it. The heart beat should be audible with a Doppler. Offer to find the heart beat and let Rebecca listen to it.
   b. Explain to Rebecca that it may be difficult to tell if the twins are identical or fraternal until they are born. The physician may be able to give her an idea after looking at the sonogram. If there is only one amniotic sac and one placenta, then the

twins probably are identical. If the sonogram shows that one is a boy and one is a girl, then it is clear the twins are fraternal. If an amniocentesis is done, it is possible to tell whether or not the twins are identical because identical twins share the same genetic material.

CHAPTER 6

NCLEX-Style Review Questions

1. b
   Rationale. Amenorrhea, nausea, and fatigue are all presumptive signs of pregnancy because they can be caused by many conditions other than pregnancy. Positive signs of pregnancy, such as sonographic evidence of a fetal outline, audible fetal heart sounds, and fetal movement felt by the examiner, confirm pregnancy because they cannot be attributed to other conditions. Probable signs of pregnancy, such as positive laboratory tests, ballottement, and Braxton Hicks contractions strongly suggest pregnancy.
2. d
   Rationale. Softening of the uterine isthmus is called Hegar's sign and is a probable sign of pregnancy. It is more objective than the presumptive signs; however, there are conditions, other than pregnancy, that can cause this sign, so it is considered probable, rather than positive. Chadwick's sign is a bluish/purple color to the vagina and cervix due to pelvic congestion. Goodell's sign is a softening of the cervix. All of these are probable signs.
3. b
   Rationale. At 16 weeks the uterine fundus should measure halfway between the pubic bone and umbilicus. At approximately 12 weeks the fundus is just above the pubic bone. At 20 weeks, it should be at the umbilicus.
4. a
   Rationale. During pregnancy a woman's caloric needs increase by approximately 300 calories per day. Five hundred extra calories are needed during lactation. Eating for two does not mean that the caloric intake should be doubled. This practice would result in too much weight gain and possibly lead to fetal macrosomia. The pregnant woman should not restrict calories during pregnancy.

Critical Thinking: What Would You Do?

1. *Suggested answers:*
   a. You should find Carla's fundus at the umbilicus.
   b. Yes. You should be able to easily find the heart beat with a Doppler device. In fact the heart beat should be detectable with a Doppler by 10 to 12 weeks.
   c. Carla is adapting well to her pregnancy. The 2nd trimester is generally a time when the woman enjoys being pregnant. The psychological task of this trimester is to accept the baby. She is progressing well toward that goal as evidenced by her preparations of the nursery.
2. *Suggested answers:*
   a. Carla is experiencing supine hypotensive syndrome.
   b. Immediately assist Carla to turn to her left side. Advise her not to lie flat on her back because this compresses the major blood vessels.
   c. Carla's weight gain is on track for a healthy pregnancy. Advise her to continue eating healthy, well-balanced meals.
3. *Suggested answers:*
   a. Vegans can get sufficient protein by paying careful attention to combining foods. Advise Monica to combine legumes with grains each day to meet her needs for complete protein. She can add fortified soy or rice milk to her diet, as well. Seeds and nuts are additional important sources of protein for Monica.
   b. Iron is necessary to build red blood cells. It is difficult for pregnant women to get enough iron from diet alone to meet the requirements. In addition, because Monica is a vegan, all her food sources of iron are from plant sources, which are less well absorbed than are animal sources of iron. Monica should continue to take her iron pills, or she is at risk for developing anemia.
   c. Carrot juice will not likely be harmful for her baby, even in fairly large amounts. Vitamin A from plant sources is in the form of beta carotene. The body converts this substance to vitamin A. Beta carotene is not as likely to be toxic as are megadoses of pre-formed vitamin A.

CHAPTER 7

NCLEX-Style Review Questions

1. a
   Rationale. Nagele's rule states to first add 7 days to the date of the LMP, then subtract 3 months, which would give a due date of October 17 of the current year.
2. d
   Rationale. The woman has been pregnant five times (current pregnancy, three living children, and one abortion). She had two children at term (T2), one preterm child (P1), one abortion (A1), and three living children (L3).

3. b
Rationale. The woman is larger than expected for her dates. Normally the fundal height should measure 28 centimeters at 28 weeks. A sonogram is the best method to determine the likely cause of the discrepancy. A multiple marker screening test is a variation of the MSAFP test that is routinely offered to all women between 16 and 18 weeks' gestation. It is possible that the woman will need more frequent prenatal visits; however, before this plan is carried out, the cause of the discrepancy must be identified.
4. b
Rationale. Group B streptococcus is a bacterium that often colonizes the vagina and rectum. It can cause serious neonatal infection if contracted during labor. All women are routinely screened for group B streptococcus after 35 weeks' gestation and before delivery, so that women who are positive can be treated with antibiotics during labor. It is no longer recommended that only women with risk factors be checked for group B streptococcus. If this question was difficult for you, review the section Subsequent Prenatal Visits.
5. d
Rationale. Telling the woman to think it over and discuss it with her family and then providing support regardless of her decision is the most supportive answer. It also allows the woman time to discuss her options with her family before she makes a decision. It is not dangerous to the mother to carry a child with a chromosomal abnormality to term. Giving the mother advice one way or the other is not therapeutic. It is better to explain options and give information regarding the likely outcome for each available option.

Critical Thinking: What Would You Do?

1. *Suggested answers:*
   a. It is important to get a thorough history from Theresa. First explore with her the chief complaint. What symptoms is she having that lead her to believe that she is pregnant? In addition to the chief complaint, a history includes reproductive, medical–surgical, family, and social histories.
   b. Explain to Theresa that this is important information because the primary care provider will want to follow up more closely because she is at higher risk for gestational diabetes. Be certain to make the RN and the primary care provider aware of this information. Any part of the history that varies from expected should be reported.
   c. You will need to place the patient in a room with an examination table. You will need drapes, sterile gloves, speculum, a swab for the Pap test, a glass slide, fixative, and sterile lubricant.
2. *Suggested answers:*
   a. First you should instruct Amanda to do a fetal kick count. This is an objective way to measure if the baby is moving less than normal. If the baby moves less than 10 times in 2 hours, instruct Amanda to come to the clinic to be checked.
   b. The priority nursing assessment is to take the fetal heart rate (FHR). This assessment will give immediate feedback as to the status of the fetus. A normal FHR is between 110 and 160 bpm.
   c. The BPP combines the NST and ultrasound measurements to predict fetal well-being. Instruct her that it is best for her to have a full bladder for the ultrasound examination. Tell her that the examiner will estimate the amount of amniotic fluid, count fetal movements, and observe fetal tone and respiratory movements. An NST will be done to determine if the fetal heart is reactive. A total score will be assigned, which will give the primary care provider information upon which to make treatment decisions. The NST is normally done by the nurse. The ultrasound portion of the examination is done by a trained radiology technician, the physician, or a specially trained nurse.
3. *Suggested answers:*
   a. Both tests are invasive and carry risks. The advantage to CVS is that it can be performed earlier in the pregnancy (10 to 12 weeks versus 15 to 20 weeks for amniocentesis). Early diagnosis allows for treatment decisions to be made earlier in the pregnancy. Results are back within 7 to 10 days for CVS; whereas, amniocentesis results may not be available for 2 to 3 weeks. One disadvantage of CVS is that some authorities report a higher rate of spontaneous abortion after CVS than after amniocentesis. Another disadvantage is that because no amniotic fluid is withdrawn, neural tube defects might be missed; whereas, amniocentesis shows increased alpha-fetoprotein levels if a neural tube defect were present. Another disadvantage of CVS is that there is a small risk of placental mosaicism, which could indicate an abnormal fetus, even if the fetus were normal.
   b. Explain to Rebecca that some women decide to proceed with genetic testing even if they will not consider abortion. The information gained can be used to research the disorder so that the parents can be better prepared to deal with it after birth. It also allows the primary care provider to determine treatment options other than abortion.
   c. The fetus with thrombocytopenia can receive platelet transfusions via cordocentesis if the disorder is severe enough to warrant this

therapy. Rebecca will be prepared as for an amniocentesis. Ultrasound will be used to locate the umbilical cord vessels. A needle is used to pierce the blood vessel and infuse platelets. This therapy will likely be done every week until delivery.

CHAPTER 8

NCLEX-Style Review Questions

1. c
   Rationale. The powers are the only component that is unexpected at this time. Because she is dilated 4 centimeters, she is considered to be in active labor. In active labor the contractions are generally closer together and are of at least moderate intensity. The contraction pattern described in this scenario is likely to be inefficient, causing the labor process to slow. All of the other components are favorable to the progress of labor. The passageway is roomy. The passenger is in a good position, and the maternal psyche is relaxed, a state that makes coping with contractions less difficult.
2. b
   Rationale. The most accurate answer is the one that explains that several factors work together to cause labor to begin. Telling the woman that it is a mystery is not entirely accurate because, although we don't have all the answers, scientists do have a partial understanding of the forces that affect labor. If there is a special hormone that signals labor to begin, it has not been discovered. Telling the woman not to worry about it is not therapeutic and dismisses her concern unnecessarily.
3. c
   Rationale. The description fits that of a fetus in the right occiput anterior (ROA) position.
4. c
   Rationale. This scenario describes the third stage of labor. The third stage begins just after the baby is born and lasts through delivery of the placenta. The first stage is from the beginning of cervical dilation to full dilation at 10 centimeters. The second stage begins with full dilation and ends with birth of the baby.

Critical Thinking: What Would You Do?

1. *Suggested answers:*
   a. Although the bony passageway (the pelvis) is adequate to accommodate a vaginal delivery, if the soft tissue of the passageway (the cervix, in this instance) does not dilate, the fetus cannot travel through. If the cervix does not eventually begin to dilate, the baby will have to be delivered by cesarean section.
   b. Because uterine contractions are the power that causes cervical dilation, an ineffective contraction pattern can be one cause of failure to dilate. Perhaps the contractions are too far apart, or they are not strong enough. Another possible explanation for failure to dilate is that the fetus is unusually large, so even if the pelvis is adequate for a normal size fetus, an abnormally large fetus may be too big to fit or may be in an unusual position. This situation could result in failure of the cervix to dilate. Another possible factor is that Anna might be tense, and she might be "fighting" the contractions. The fear-tension-pain cycle also can interfere with labor progress.
2. *Suggested answers:*
   a. Normally, the fetus starts out with the back of his head (his occiput) facing to one side of the maternal pelvis (either right or left occiput transverse). If he starts in an occiput transverse position, he must rotate so that the back of his head (the occiput) faces toward the front of the maternal pelvis, an anterior position. Because Anna's fetus is occiput posterior, the back of his head is positioned toward the back of Anna's pelvis. This means the fetus will have to rotate 180° or deliver face up.
   b. The labor likely will be longer and involve more back pain than would be the case if the fetus were occiput transverse or occiput anterior.
3. *Suggested answers:*
   a. From the description, it sounds as if Anna is entering the transition phase of labor, so the nurse will probably find that she is dilated between 8 and 9 centimeters.
   b. It would be helpful to explain to Anna's partner that her outburst is normal at this time because she is entering the most intense, but fortunately, the shortest phase of labor. The partner can continue to be supportive if he or she knows that Anna's behavior is expected and not to be taken personally.
4. *Suggested answers:*
   a. When a baby is delivered face up, the condition is recorded as "persistent occiput posterior."
   b. He will likely have molding and overriding sutures. Many lay people describe this condition as the baby having a "cone head." He may also have some soft tissue swelling known as caput succedaneum.
   c. Anna will probably be excited and want to hold the baby. She will likely explore his body with her fingertips and count his fingers and toes. The pain of contractions will be forgotten quickly.

CHAPTER 9

NCLEX-Style Review Questions

1. b
Rationale. Rarely is there a pain-free labor. This woman needs to know that she will likely have some pain before she is far enough dilated to receive an epidural. Discussing pain relief options with the physician and childbirth educator indicates that the woman is taking responsibility for pain relief during labor. It would be appropriate to ask this woman if she has any additional questions about any of the options discussed. Practicing relaxation techniques and asking for IV pain medications are both appropriate actions.
2. a
Rationale. Caregivers often underrate the woman's pain. Although observing for nonverbal indicators, taking the vital signs, and observing interactions with visitors may give clues as to whether or not the woman is experiencing pain, the only way to know for sure is for the nurse to directly ask the woman to describe her pain and to rate it. The nurse should not wait until the woman complains of pain before doing a thorough pain assessment because some women will attempt to endure the pain without complaining.
3. c
Rationale. Each woman experiences labor pain in a unique way. The "best" method is the method that coincides with the woman's belief system and works for the woman. It is best to learn several methods because it is difficult to predict which method will be most beneficial for the woman until she actually experiences labor. Stating that an epidural is the best or that natural childbirth is best attempts to impose the nurse's beliefs about labor pain management on the woman. Stating that most women require some type of IV pain medication during labor is incorrect. Many women go through labor without IV pain medications.
4. b
Rationale. Counter-pressure on the lower back and intradermal water injections are interventions that are specifically indicated for intense back labor. Intermittent labor support and reassurance that the pain is temporary are not particularly helpful for any type of labor pain. Effleurage and ambulation generally are more helpful in early labor and are not specific to back labor. Hypnosis and imagery require special training and are not specific to back labor.
5. d
Rationale. An IV fluid bolus is given before epidural anesthesia to help prevent hypotension. Telling the woman that it is a routine procedure in preparation for an epidural does not adequately answer the question. It would be inappropriate for the nurse to slow the IV fluids simply because the woman complained that the fluids felt cold. IV hydration is not given to prevent spinal headaches. If you had trouble with this question, review the section Epidural Anesthesia.

Critical Thinking: What Would You Do?

1. *Suggested answers:*
   a. You should advise Betty to take childbirth classes. It will be best if she chooses an instructor who teaches and has the woman practice relaxation techniques. She may want to attend a Lamaze or Bradley method class. Suggest that she ask about the use of a birthing ball. Recommend a doula. Research has shown that women are more successful with natural childbirth if they have continuous labor support, which a doula provides. Encourage her to pack lip balm and hard candy to treat and prevent dry lips and mouth. Suggest that she explore water therapy options.
   b. Explain to Betty that she may change her mind once she is in labor. Tell her that changing her mind is OK and does not represent a failure on her part. Many women attempt natural childbirth and then elect to use some type of analgesia or anesthesia. If her labor is prolonged or she requires oxytocin augmentation, she may need additional methods of pain relief.
2. *Suggested answers:*
   a. It may be helpful for Betty to ambulate or at least change positions frequently at this point in labor. Engaging in activities that distract her from the contractions may also be helpful. Slow chest breathing and effleurage probably will be helpful in coping with contractions. Using a focal point that she practiced in childbirth classes is often helpful at this stage of labor. Water therapy may be used, although many experts recommend waiting until a more advanced stage of labor to use this method.
   b. Your reply should be supportive of Betty's request. Give her encouragement about the progress she has made thus far. Remind her that IV analgesia won't completely relieve the pain, but it should take the edge off the pain and help her to relax between contractions, which may help her progress. Encourage her to use the call bell before attempting to ambulate

after you administer the medication. Explain to her coach/partner that it is normal for her to sleep between contractions after IV analgesia.

c. Again, your reply should be supportive of Betty's request. Explain that it is OK to change her mind and that you will contact the physician about her request. When you give report to the anesthesiologist, inform him or her that Betty initially desired natural childbirth and that this is a change of plans for her. This information will be useful when the anesthesiologist interviews Betty for the epidural.

CHAPTER 10

NCLEX-Style Review Questions

1. b
   Rationale. The water running down the woman's legs is an indication that the membranes have ruptured. The fern test would confirm that the fluid is amniotic fluid versus urine.
2. c
   Rationale. The woman should not push until the cervix is dilated completely. Otherwise her cervix may swell, a condition that will slow the progress of labor. Blowing at the peak of contractions (when the urge to push is most intense) helps the woman not to push.
3. c
   Rationale. The woman is low risk, in active labor, and the monitor tracing is reassuring; therefore, her monitor strip should be evaluated every 30 minutes.
4. a
   Rationale. Intermittent auscultation is within the standard of care for low-risk laboring women, so it is appropriate to comply with the woman's request. She will need to be on the monitor for an initial 20-minute period to obtain a baseline recording of the FHR. Although many labor units prefer continuous EFM because intermittent auscultation takes more of the staff member's time, it would not be appropriate to deny the woman her request solely for this reason.
5. d
   Rationale. Amnioinfusion is done in an attempt to relieve cord compression when persistent variables are present, particularly if they are worrisome. The pattern described in answer d is worrisome because the fetal heart tones fall significantly (the variables are "deep") and they are occurring with each contraction.

Critical Thinking: What Would You Do?

1. *Suggested answers:*
   a. All admission assessments should be completed. This includes an evaluation of current labor status, an obstetric, medical–surgical, and social history, and determining desires/plans for labor and birth and for care of the newborn. Current weight and vital signs should be obtained, and a vaginal examination should be done. A urine specimen is collected, and the EFM applied.
   b. Because she is excited and talkative, it appears that Priscilla is in the latent phase of labor (early labor).
   c. The cervix will most likely be dilated 1 to 3 cm and be partially effaced with a vertex at −1 to +1 station.
   d. Breathing and relaxation techniques and the stages of labor can be reviewed with Priscilla and her husband. Once it is determined that the fetus is doing well per the monitor tracing, the nurse encourages Priscilla to ambulate. Distraction techniques work best during early labor. The nurse could suggest that Priscilla watch a favorite TV show, do crossword puzzles, or talk with friends on the telephone.
   e. If the couple had not attended childbirth preparation classes, education about the birth process and what to expect would be appropriate. The nurse could teach a few breathing and relaxation techniques to the woman and her partner. Throughout labor, education and support are a priority. If the woman is extremely anxious, interventions would focus on helping her to cope with the particular phase/stage of labor that she is in. Explanations should be simple and to the point. Overly detailed explanations and instructions might increase her anxiety.
2. *Suggested answers:*
   a. Because Priscilla is dilated 5 cm, she is in the active phase of the first stage of labor. A woman is in active labor when the cervix is dilated from 4 to 8 cm.
   b. The nurse takes vital signs every 30 to 60 minutes. It is important for the nurse to evaluate hydration status by assessing the mucous membranes and intake and output. The nurse evaluates FHR and contraction pattern every 15 to 30 minutes.
   c. Priscilla and her husband are using a ritual to cope with contractions. It appears that the ritual is helping.
   d. The nurse offers comfort measures, such as ice chips and lip balm; a cool, damp washcloth for the forehead; back rubs; effleurage; and frequent perineal care and change of absorbent pads. It is

important for the nurse to encourage Priscilla to void at least every 2 hours. Because the ritual is working, the nurse encourages the couple to continue using it. The nurse ensures privacy for the couple and keeps the environment quiet and nonstimulating. The nurse also periodically offers to take over the role of the coach for a few minutes so that Priscilla's husband can take a break.

3. *Suggested answers:*
   a. The practical nurse assists the RN to perform a vaginal examination. Priscilla's behavior indicates that she has probably reached the transition phase of labor.
   b. The nurse informs the couple of the results of the vaginal examination. The focus of interventions should be to help Priscilla relax between contractions. The nurse encourages the husband in his role as coach and reminds him that Priscilla's behavior is normal during the transition phase. It is important for the nurse and the husband to work together to help find the breathing and relaxation techniques that will help Priscilla cope with her labor. The nurse assists Priscilla to change positions and changes the under-buttocks pad frequently to keep her as dry and comfortable as possible.
   c. If Priscilla is able to relax between contractions, and her husband continues to be supportive, the nursing interventions have been effective.
4. *Suggested answers:*
   a. Take in a general overview of the situation, noting in particular the coping status of the woman and her partner. Assess the EFM tracing for FHR pattern and uterine contraction pattern. Palpate the uterine contractions. Check the IV infusion and site. Take the vital signs. Listen to lung and bowel sounds (remember this is your initial assessment). Determine time and amount of last voiding. Palpate the bladder for distention. Observe the perineum for bloody show, bleeding, and/or leaking of fluid.
   b. First note the frequency and duration of the pattern on the fetal monitor tracing. Then stand at Martha's side and place your hand on the fundus. Leave your hand on the fundus through at least two contractions. Note the intensity at the acme (peak) of the contraction (mild feels like tip of your nose, moderate feels like your chin, strong feels like your forehead). Determine if the uterus is completely relaxing between uterine contractions. Chart your findings in the labor record.
5. *Suggested answers:*
   a. The baseline is within the normal range and is reassuring. Early decelerations are occurring with each contraction. This pattern is benign. Therefore, the overall pattern is reassuring because there are no nonreassuring patterns.
   b. Report your findings to the charge nurse and ask if he wants to do a vaginal examination. Martha is showing signs that her labor is progressing (increased restlessness and bloody show); therefore, it is important to determine if she is close to delivery so that preparations can be made.

CHAPTER 11

NCLEX-Style Review Questions

1. d
   Rationale. Sutures used to repair an episiotomy are absorbable and do not need to be removed.
2. a
   Rationale. Providing a general explanation of the procedure is the only response that accurately represents the truth to the woman. Asking the doctor is not appropriate. It is not *always* better to have a vaginal delivery. There are times when a cesarean is preferred, but feeling tired of being pregnant is not one of those instances. Using "why" questions and saying "don't you know" are not usually therapeutic.
3. b
   Rationale. Although the procedure can be uncomfortable, it should not be outright painful. If the woman is experiencing too much pain, the physician will stop the procedure. Stating that the woman wants what is best for the baby and telling her that she will be fine with holding the nurse's hand are nontherapeutic responses.
4. b
   Rationale. The cervix must be dilated fully before forceps can be applied. Forceps are not necessarily dangerous. The physician will determine which instrument (forceps versus vacuum extractor) is best indicated for the situation, if any. In this case it is better to give some information rather than to make a blanket statement of "I don't know." The water bag must be ruptured before forceps can be applied.

Critical Thinking: What Would You Do?

1. *Suggested answers:*
   Amy needs to know that although a vaginal delivery is planned and expected, it cannot be guaranteed. There are many conditions that endanger the life of the woman, her fetus, or both that cannot always be anticipated and for which a cesarean delivery might become necessary. Amy needs encouragement to attend the class because

she will be much better prepared to cope if she is prepared versus going into the situation completely uninformed.

2. *Suggested answers:*
   a. A Bishop score of 4 means that her cervix is unripe. It is unlikely that she will go into labor spontaneously within the next few days. It is also unlikely that her body would respond to an induction of labor unless cervical ripening procedures were used first.
   b. The physician would likely recommend that a cervical ripening procedure be used before induction of labor. Mechanical means include membrane stripping, and artificial dilation of the cervix using a balloon catheter or laminaria. Pharmacologic means include prostaglandins such as dinoprostone and misoprostol. Labor induction is more likely to be successful when cervical ripening is done first.
3. *Suggested answers:*
   You will need sterile gloves for the physician, a sterile swab, and a speculum. The test involves collecting a cervical secretion sample during a speculum exam and sending the sample to the lab for testing.
4. *Suggested answers:*
   You should notify the RN and/or the physician immediately and prepare for a cesarean delivery because it is likely Ellen has experienced a uterine rupture. It is imperative that the cesarean be done as quickly as possible to save the baby, as well as Ellen's life.

CHAPTER 12

NCLEX-Style Review Questions

1. c
   Rationale. Suture used to repair episiotomy is absorbable. It is helpful to let the woman know that she is not alone in her fear. This response helps build trust. Because sutures are not removed, telling the woman that she will feel pulling is incorrect information. Although emphasizing the importance of a follow-up checkup, this response is not the best answer because it could be construed as condescending and it does not take into account the woman's feelings. Telling the woman not to worry dismisses the woman's concerns and doesn't give her complete information.
2. c
   Rationale. A shaking chill shortly after delivery is a common occurrence. Placing pre-warmed blankets usually remedies the problem. Finishing vital sign measurement and then making a decision indicates that the nurse doesn't really know what to do. Notifying the RN immediately or summoning assistance is unnecessary because the woman is most likely experiencing a normal postpartum sensation. This is not an emergency situation.
3. a
   Rationale. The woman is experiencing respiratory depression from the narcotic that was given in the spinal anesthesia. It is appropriate to administer naloxone (Narcan), which should be readily available. This medication is usually part of the preprinted or routine orders after this type of anesthesia. It is not appropriate to instruct her to breathe more rapidly because her respiratory drive is being suppressed artificially by the narcotic. Calling the anesthesiologist would be appropriate only if there were no orders, which is unlikely. Performing rescue breathing is too aggressive. The woman likely will have a good response to the Narcan.
4. c
   Rationale. Itching is common after spinal anesthesia in which a narcotic was administered. This is the likely cause of the itching. It is most appropriate for the nurse to inquire first to make sure the woman wants treatment. Benadryl would be the most appropriate first choice. Narcan is reserved for cases of severe itching that do not respond to Benadryl. The nurse shouldn't have to call the anesthesiologist because there is almost always an order available for treating this common occurrence. Observing and waiting is not the best choice. It is better to directly inquire regarding the woman's wishes and to let her know that treatment is available.
5. b
   Rationale. Cold is the treatment for breast engorgement when the woman is bottle-feeding. If she were breast-feeding, warmth would be appropriate. It is not appropriate to encourage a woman to breast-feed simply to treat breast engorgement, particularly after she has already made a decision to bottle-feed. It is also not helpful to empty the breasts of milk because this will simply stimulate more milk production.

Critical Thinking: What Would You Do?

1. *Suggested answers:*
   a. Heather probably fainted secondary to postural hypotension after getting up too quickly out of bed. Careful instructions by the nurse that Heather should be accompanied by the nurse the first time up and instructions to dangle her feet at the side of the bed for several minutes before getting up likely could have prevented this fall.

b. Check her fundus, the lochia, and check for suprapubic distention. The fundus probably will be slightly boggy and deviated to one side. The lochia probably will be moderate to large, and you likely will find suprapubic distention.
c. Assist Heather to the restroom to void. Run water. If possible have her place her hand in warm water. Give her privacy and time to empty her bladder. If noninvasive measures don't work, you might have to catheterize her; however, it is best to avoid this if possible because of the increased risk for infection.
d. You want to do a complete assessment to see if you can find a likely source of infection. Check the breasts for hard, reddened areas. Check the nipples for cracks. Check the lungs for congestion. Check the uterus to see if involution is progressing as expected. Endometritis can interfere with normal involution; it can also make the uterus tender to the touch. Check the lochia. Especially note the odor. A smell like rotting meat is associated with endometrial infection. Check the perineum for signs of infection at the episiotomy site.

2. *Suggested answers:*
   a. Grand multiparity and the difficult, prolonged labor put Marla at risk for uterine atony and subsequent hemorrhage.
   b. She is probably experiencing uterine atony. The first thing you should do is massage the uterus to try to get it to contract. Next you should increase the IV with added Pitocin, if available. Then call for assistance. Someone should take the vital signs. If the bleeding does not come quickly under control, someone needs to call the physician for further orders.
3. *Suggested answers:*
   a. You need to first inquire to find out where Mindy is hurting. There are several potential sources of pain, so you want to find out exactly where she is hurting so that you can better treat her pain.
   b. Incisional pain usually responds well to acetaminophen/narcotic combination products. Gas pain is best relieved by walking, then lying on the left side. Encourage Mindy to release the gas and not hold back because of embarrassment. Mylicon tablets are also helpful. Once you have tried all of these measures without relief, call the physician for an order for a suppository.
   c. First assess to see if there is swelling, redness, and warmth in the leg with the positive Homans' sign. Then report this finding to the RN in charge. This may indicate that there is thrombus formation.

CHAPTER 13

NCLEX-Style Review Questions

1. a
   Rationale. An infant born by cesarean delivery does not have the benefit of passing through the birth canal. Much of the fluid normally present in a fetus' respiratory tract is squeezed out while passing through the birth canal during a vaginal delivery. Surfactant develops in the lungs as the fetus matures. Its presence or absence is not associated with the method of delivery. An infant born by cesarean experiences sensory stimulation during birth, as does the infant born vaginally.
2. c
   Rationale. Telling the mother that this is normal and showing how to clean the area reassures the mother and also teaches her how to deal with the leaking fluid. Although it is a normal finding, telling her "not to worry" is too dismissive of her concerns. Deferring to the charge nurse when you don't know is an acceptable strategy, but the nurse should be familiar with "witch's milk." Leaking fluid from the nipples is not a symptom of infection.
3. c
   Rationale. The base of the cord should be dry without any redness. This finding could indicate that infection is present. Notify the charge nurse of the finding and carry out any orders that are given. Calling the doctor and asking for IV antibiotics is an over-reaction at this point. Additional assessment is needed. A dressing should not be applied unless the physician orders it. Showing the mother how to wash the area may falsely reassure her that this is a normal finding.
4. d
   Rationale. The children running around the bassinet are creating air currents. The baby's blanket is loose, so he has probably lost some heat to convection. The damp T-shirt promotes heat loss by evaporation. Conduction occurs when heat is lost to a cold surface. This scenario does not indicate that the bassinet is cold and the room itself is warm. Radiation occurs when heat is lost to a nearby cold surface. The bassinet is located away from windows and doors, so radiation is not the most likely source of heat loss.

Critical Thinking: What Would You Do?

1. *Suggested answers:*
   a. The mottling and cool extremities indicate that the baby is likely cold. You should immediately wrap the baby in several blankets and make sure he wears a hat.

b. Instruct the parents on the importance of keeping the baby warm. The baby should be snugly wrapped in blankets, or he should be skin to skin with his parents to avoid cold stress. In addition, the bassinet should be positioned away from windows and doors.

2. *Suggested answers:*
   a. The baby's skin is jaundiced. Jaundice in the newborn is usually caused by breakdown of red blood cells. The immature liver cannot handle the bilirubin released from the red blood cells.
   b. Because the baby's jaundice appeared on day 3 and not in the first 24 hours, it is most likely physiologic jaundice and usually does not indicate illness. However, all jaundice should be evaluated, so explain to Mary that you will report the condition to the pediatrician for follow-up.
3. *Suggested answers:*
   a. Explain to Mary that the baby is giving cues that he is sleepy. He has had enough interaction and needs rest. Reassure her that this does not indicate the baby is rejecting her. Rather, he is communicating a need in the only way he knows how. After he has rested, he will be ready to interact again.
   b. The blue-black spot is most likely a Mongolian spot. It should have been noted and described in the nursery. Reassure Mary that this is a birthmark and does not indicate maltreatment. Tell her that the mark will fade with time.

CHAPTER 14

NCLEX-Style Review Questions

1. b
   Rationale. Ovulation can occur in the absence of menstruation and the woman who is exclusively breast-feeding can conceive, therefore she should use some form of contraception. The woman should be offered a nonhormonal type of contraception as a first choice while she is breast-feeding.
2. c
   Rationale. Formula does not have the immunologic properties of breast milk. Although it is the woman's choice whether or not she wants to breast-feed, she should be informed before making her decision. The benefits of formula feeding are not equal to those of breast-feeding. The woman's economic status should not determine how the nurse responds to the woman's question.
3. a
   Rationale. The position, latch, and sucking of the newborn are the priority assessments to be made during a feeding session. The nurse should assess the woman's support systems, but during a feeding session is not the most appropriate time to do so. An increase in lochia flow is a good indicator for effective newborn sucking. However, checking the woman's perineal pad during a breast-feeding session is inappropriate. The woman can verbalize if her flow has increased or if she has cramping. Before determining the need for a lactation consult, the nurse should first assess the newborn's feeding ability.

Critical Thinking: What Would You Do?

1. *Suggested answers:*
   a. First ask Sally some questions to see if she has had any prior exposure to breast-feeding. Then ask questions about Sally's feelings regarding breast-feeding. Explain to Sally the benefits of breast-feeding for both the woman and the newborn.
   b. Tell Betsy that the woman does not have to stop breast-feeding to return to work or school. She can pump at work, and the newborn's caregiver can feed her newborn the expressed breast milk. If she feels that she would be unable to pump at work, advise Betsy that the newborn gets multiple benefits from breast-feeding, even if it only lasts for several weeks. The baby still gets the antibodies from colostrum. Also, bonding is enhanced.
   c. Teach Elizabeth that the breasts do make milk after delivery in response to hormonal changes. To dry up the milk supply after delivery, she should wear a tight bra and avoid expressing any milk. Teach her to avoid warm water from a shower spraying on her breasts. She may experience some engorgement when the milk comes in, and it may be uncomfortable. Cold packs, a tight bra, and analgesics help to lessen the discomfort, and her body will stop making milk because none is being expressed.
2. *Suggested answers:*
   a. The colostrum that the newborn receives each time he or she breast-feeds provides enough calories. The newborn will not starve, and his frequent feedings will help to establish a good milk supply and help the woman's milk to come in.
   b. Ask Alicia how much the newborn is taking at a feeding and how often the newborn is feeding. She may be overfeeding or spacing the feedings too close together. Ask how much the newborn is spitting up and if it occurs with a burp or not. Also ask if there is a history of cow's milk allergies in Alicia's or the father of the baby's family.

The newborn may need a specialty formula, if the pediatrician determines the newborn cannot tolerate a milk-based formula.

c. Lanya should hold her newborn in the football hold or in the side-lying position. Both of these positions keep the newborn off of her abdomen. She can rest easier in the side-lying position while the newborn breast-feeds.

d. Teach Tricia the three ways formula is available: ready-to-feed, powder, and concentrate. Ready-to-feed does not need to be mixed, but powder and concentrate need to be mixed according to package directions. She needs to wash all bottles and nipples before the first use and then after each use. Either hand washing or machine washing is acceptable. She does not need to sterilize the bottles.

e. Breast milk is good at room temperature for as long as 10 hours, in the refrigerator for as long as 8 days, and if frozen in a deep freezer, as long as 6 months. After the milk has been thawed, it should be used within 24 hours.

CHAPTER 15

NCLEX-Style Review Questions

1. c

   Rationale. Baby Boy Alvarez gets a score of 2 for a heart rate greater than 100. All other parameters receive a score of 1 each, for a total score of 6. Apgar scores of 4 to 6 indicate moderate difficulty transitioning. Apgar scores of 1 to 3 indicate severe difficulty making the transition to life outside the womb. Scores of 7 or greater are associated with vigorous newborns.

2. b

   Rationale. The baby is large for gestational age. Although he could have problems in any of the areas listed, hypoglycemia is the likeliest cause of trouble for this baby initially.

3. c

   Rationale. He is most likely to lose heat by evaporation from his head. This situation could be prevented by thoroughly drying the head and putting a cap on the baby. Conductive heat loss occurs with direct contact with a cold surface. Putting him in skin-to-skin contact with his mother prevents this type of heat loss. Convective heat loss occurs through air currents. Covering the baby with a blanket helps prevent this type of heat loss. Radiation of warmth away from the baby to a nearby cold surface is not a likely source of heat loss at this time because the baby is skin to skin with his mother and covered with a blanket.

4. c

   Rationale. It is appropriate to ask to see identification from someone who is not wearing a name badge. You do not want to provoke a possible kidnapper by threatening her in any way. Stating that the person must be the woman's sister makes an assumption that could very well be erroneous. When nurses make incorrect assumptions, it is easier for kidnappers to carry out their plans.

Critical Thinking: What Would You Do?

1. *Suggested answers:*
   a. Quickly dry the newborn to prevent chilling from evaporation while assessing his respiratory effort. Place him on his mother's bare chest and cover them both with blankets. Be sure to cover his head, as well as his body. In addition to respiratory effort, count the heart rate (taken from feeling the base of the umbilical cord), note muscle tone, reflex irritability, and color. Assign the Apgar score.
   b. The newborn may be suffering from hypoglycemia. He should be put to the breast immediately.
   c. The newborn will need erythromycin ointment placed in both eyes, and he will need a vitamin K injection.
2. *Suggested answers:*
   a. Use the bulb syringe to suction the mouth, then the nose.
   b. Use a suction catheter to suction secretions. Place the catheter down the back of the throat. Apply intermittent suction as you pull the catheter out with a steady motion.
3. *Suggested answers:*
   a. It is likely that the newborn is in pain.
   b. The nurse should try several comfort measures. Swaddling, holding, and rocking may be helpful. Allowing the newborn to suck on a pacifier, especially if a little sweetener is added, is comforting. Check the physician's orders for pain medication. It is appropriate to medicate newborns for pain.
4. *Suggested answers:*
   a. Reassure the mother that the yellow crust is a normal finding after a circumcision and indicates healing. Instruct her not to remove the crust. If redness, swelling, or foul-smelling discharge are noted, the baby should be seen by a physician because these are signs of infection.
   b. Reassure the mother that it is normal for babies to cry. Suggest some ways she might use to try to calm the baby. Walking, rocking, singing, and riding in a car are all good things to try. A pacifier might be helpful. Be sure that she knows it's OK to ask someone to help or for her to take a time out if she begins to feel frustrated.

CHAPTER 16

NCLEX-Style Review Questions

1. b
   Rationale. Most adults do not develop type 2 DM until middle adulthood. Most women who enter pregnancy with DM have type 1 DM.
2. b
   Rationale. Persistent rales in the bases of the lungs are most frequently the first indication of impending heart failure. Blood pressure changes and wheezing are usually not associated with heart failure.
3. a
   Rationale. Infection can trigger a crisis. Staying well hydrated, getting plenty of rest, and avoiding infection can help the pregnant women with sickle cell anemia avoid a crisis.
4. d
   Rationale. Multiple bruises in various stages of healing should raise a strong suspicion of IPV. Typically the woman would display possible suspiciousness or anxiety. Bilateral pedal edema may be a typical discomfort associated with this stage of the woman's pregnancy. A small bruise on the thigh is not highly suggestive of abuse.

Critical Thinking: What Would You Do?

1. *Suggested answers:*
   a. The oral glucose tolerance test. At least two of the following parameters were found: fasting blood sugar greater than 95 mg/dL, 1 hour postprandial blood sugar greater than 180 mg/dL, 2 hour postprandial greater than 155 mg/dL, or 3 hour postprandial greater than 140 mg/dL.
   b. History of a large-for-gestational-age infant, history of GDM, previous unexplained fetal demise, advanced maternal age (greater than 35 years), family history of type 2 DM or GDM, obesity (greater than 200 pounds), non-Caucasian ethnicity, fasting blood glucose of greater than 140 mg/dL, and random blood glucose of greater than 200 mg/dL
   c. Monitoring and maintaining strict blood sugar control, diet and exercise, fetal surveillance, and preventing infection
2. *Suggested answers:*
   a. Pregnancy has variable effects on asthma. Sometimes it gets worse. Sometimes it gets better. And sometimes there is no change.
   b. A teaching plan should include the following points: continuing the use of asthma medications; avoiding over-the-counter medications unless the woman has talked with the physician about using them; identifying and protecting herself from asthma triggers; avoiding cigarette smoke, exposure to animals, and dusty, damp environments; staying inside in air-conditioned surroundings during pollen seasons and when the pollution or mold index is high; wearing mask or scarf over mouth on excessively cold days to help warm the air; protecting self from colds and flu because respiratory infections can trigger acute asthma attacks (avoiding crowds where viruses may be prevalent; washing hands frequently; and obtaining the flu shot if you have moderate or severe asthma); avoiding foods or chemicals that might have caused a reaction in the past, such as sulfites or MSG; continuing to take allergy shots; monitoring peak expiratory flow rate (PEFR) regularly; developing a crisis management plan in consultation with the physician; and being able to recognize warning signs, such as lack of rapid improvement when taking rescue medications, improvement not sustained, condition worsens, episode is severe, fetal movement decreases, and other warning signs of an impending attack, possibly including headache, itchy throat, sneezing, coughing, or feeling tired.
3. *Suggested answers:*
   a. The most common method of transmission is unprotected sexual intercourse with an infected partner. Risk factors include blood transfusions, sharing needles, and multiple sex partners.
   b. The two priority goals for Rachel's care are to prevent progression of her disease and prevent perinatal transmission to her fetus.
   c. The physician most likely will prescribe oral zidovudine (ZDV) therapy.
   d. The best way to protect an unborn child from HIV (when the mother is HIV-positive) is for the mother to take zidovudine throughout pregnancy, deliver by cesarean section at 38 weeks' gestation, and avoid breast-feeding and administer zidovudine to the newborn infant.
   e. It would be wise for her to have her other children tested. Although she may have tested negative during her last pregnancy, it can take time after exposure for a person to test positive. Having the children tested would relieve her of unnecessary worry.

CHAPTER 17

NCLEX-Style Review Questions

1. d
   Rationale. Although the woman has a history of habitual or recurrent abortion (she has been pregnant four times and has never carried a pregnancy

to term), the cramps and spotting in the presence of a closed cervix are consistent with a diagnosis of threatened abortion. Symptoms of an ectopic pregnancy often begin before the patient knows for certain that she is pregnant. It is unlikely that she would carry the pregnancy for 12 weeks, if it were not implanted within the uterus (e.g., if it were a tubal pregnancy, the tube already would have ruptured). The pain and closed cervix are inconsistent with a diagnosis of incompetent cervix.

2. c
   Rationale. The woman has an elevated blood pressure. The abdominal pain could be epigastric pain associated with preeclampsia, or it could be pain from a placental abruption. Because her pulse is elevated and she is restless and diaphoretic with dark, red vaginal bleeding, she should first be assessed for signs of placental abruption. This condition presents the greatest immediate danger to mother and baby. The fetal heart tones will give information on the status of the fetus, and palpating the fundus will allow for assessment of uterine irritability, rigidity, tenderness, and/or contractions. Any other assessments would take lower priority.
3. c
   Rationale. The "clumps" in the vaginal discharge probably are pieces of swollen villi being expelled. This finding would be consistent with a molar pregnancy (gestational trophoblastic disease). Bright red painless vaginal bleeding is associated with placenta previa. Brisk deep tendon reflexes occur with preeclampsia, and shoulder pain is most often associated with ectopic pregnancy. Painful uterine contractions occur with labor or placental abruption, and nausea is a nonspecific symptom.
4. b
   Rationale. Limiting fluids with meals will aid in retention of food. The woman with hyperemesis gravidarum should nibble on carbohydrates. Food with high fat content might actually increase feelings of nausea. It is best for a person with nausea to stay away from strong food odors. If possible, someone else should do the cooking, and the food should be served in a pleasant, well-ventilated area. Antiemetics should be given 30 minutes before meals, not after meals.

Critical Thinking: What Would You Do?

1. *Suggested answers:*
   a. The nurse should inquire to see if Maria is experiencing headache, blurred vision, and spots before her eyes, or epigastric pain. Her history of sudden weight gain and elevated blood pressure raise the suspicion that she is developing preeclampsia. Any woman suspected of having preeclampsia should be asked regarding headache, visual disturbances, and abdominal or epigastric pain. A "yes" answer to any of these parameters is a warning sign that she may soon have a convulsion.
   b. Maria's blood pressure should be checked again after lying on her left side for several minutes. Both pressures are recorded. In addition to a complete head-to-toe assessment, Maria's lungs should be auscultated carefully, deep tendon reflexes should be checked for briskness, and the presence of clonus should be determined. The amount of edema is noted and the urine is screened for protein.
   c. She is likely to be placed on bed rest in the hospital with orders for a preeclampsia lab workup and a 24-hour urine for protein.
2. *Suggested answers:*
   a. Maria should be placed in a quiet room with the lights dimmed to decrease sensory stimulation. Seizure precautions should be implemented. The side rails should be up and padded with pillows or blankets. Suction and oxygen equipment are set up and checked to see that each is working. These precautions are taken to help prevent seizures or to intervene quickly to prevent injury if a seizure were to occur.
   b. If Maria has preeclampsia, it is likely that the 24-hour urine specimen will have at least 300 grams of protein. She may have a decreased creatinine clearance and an elevated BUN and creatinine, although these findings are usually associated with severe disease. The hematocrit will likely be elevated because of hemoconcentration, and the platelets will be low or on the low side of normal. In mild preeclampsia, liver enzymes should not be elevated and the coagulation profile should be normal. However, if severe disease is present, liver enzymes will be elevated and the bleeding time prolonged.
   c. The private room is ordered and visitors are limited to decrease sensory stimulation. Bright lights, loud noise, and frequent movements associated with frequent visitors may precipitate a seizure.
3. *Suggested answers:*
   a. Fetal kick counts should be done after every meal; NSTs are done at least twice weekly; and biophysical profiles, sonograms, and amniocentesis are done as ordered.
   b. Record FHR and vital signs at least every 4 hours. Auscultate lungs every 2 to 4 hours to detect evidence of developing pulmonary edema. Ask regarding the presence of headache, visual disturbances, or epigastric pain with each

assessment. Check deep tendon reflexes and clonus every 4 hours. Institute seizure precautions. Maintain strict input and output and report output of less than 120 cc every 4 hours.

c. "Mild" is a term used to differentiate two levels of preeclampsia. However, this is a serious condition that requires continuous monitoring. The condition will not go away until the baby is delivered; therefore, hospitalization should continue for the safety of mother and baby. In addition, the disease can progress rapidly. If progression is noted promptly, seizure activity may be averted. The risk is that she could not make it to the hospital in time to prevent seizures if she were to self-monitor at home.

4. *Suggested answers:*
   a. Maria now has signs of severe preeclampsia.
   b. Maria's lungs should be auscultated. She should be asked regarding the presence of epigastric pain. Deep tendon reflexes and clonus are determined. After the assessment, the charge nurse and physician should be immediately notified of the findings.
   c. Maria will now be on strict bed rest. An IV will be inserted, if she does not already have access. A Foley catheter may be ordered to monitor hourly outputs. The nurse should anticipate an order for magnesium sulfate. Labor will probably be induced soon.

CHAPTER 18

NCLEX-Style Review Questions

1. d
   Rationale. Prolonged rupture of membranes, prolonged labor, and maternal fever place the newborn at risk for neonatal pneumonia. ABO incompatibility relates to the woman's and newborn's blood types. You were not given this information in the scenario. Fistula formation and pelvic floor injury are maternal injuries that can result from prolonged or difficult labor.
2. c
   Rationale. Prolonged labor characterized by back pain is most frequently caused by an occiput posterior position of the fetus. Although breech position, fetal macrosomia, and nongynecoid pelvis can cause labor dystocia, the only one characterized by back labor is occiput posterior position.
3. a
   Rationale. Because this woman has a history of preterm birth, she is at very high risk of delivering prematurely again. Although it may be appropriate for her to have hydration and to lie on her left side, she should come into the hospital to be monitored. The sooner she comes in, the sooner treatment can begin. The goal is to delay birth for as long as possible to allow the fetal lungs time to mature.
4. c
   Rationale. Flexing the woman's thighs is called McRoberts maneuver. This is an appropriate nursing intervention for shoulder dystocia. Rescue breathing is not appropriate. Fundal pressure is contraindicated. Watching the monitor for signs of fetal distress is not indicated because the fetal head has already been delivered. The priority is assisting the woman to deliver the body. If you had difficulty with this question, review the section Shoulder Dystocia.

Critical Thinking: What Would You Do?

1. *Suggested answers:*
   Basically Julia has three options. The physician can attempt to turn the baby using a version procedure; a cesarean delivery can be planned; or, if the physician agrees, Julia can be allowed a trial of labor with a vaginal breech delivery. It is important to remember that not all physicians will perform a vaginal breech delivery. It would be important to know this information before discussing Julia's options with her.
2. *Suggested answers:*
   a. Even though labor is not going to be induced at this time, it is important that Julia and her husband stay in the hospital. Research has shown that women with PROM do better when they are monitored in the hospital versus going home and coming back into the hospital when contractions begin.
   b. Monitor the fetal heart rate as ordered by the primary care practitioner. Be alert for sudden deep variable decelerations of the fetal heart rate that might indicate a prolapsed umbilical cord. Take the woman's temperature at least every 2 hours. Monitor for signs of infection, such as temperature elevation, fetal or maternal tachycardia, and cloudy or foul-smelling amniotic fluid.
   c. Preterm PROM requires expectant management, usually on bed rest, unless there are signs of infection, in which case the fetus will be delivered. Otherwise, administer antibiotics as ordered. Explain pelvic rest to the woman and help her stay on bed rest, as ordered. Do not perform vaginal examinations unless specifically ordered to do so by the primary care practitioner. Instruct the woman to perform fetal kick counts after every meal. Assist the RN to perform daily NSTs, as ordered. Give intramuscular injections of corticosteroids to hasten fetal lung

maturity, as ordered. Other interventions are carried out in the same manner as that used for the woman with term PROM.

3. *Suggested answers:*
Report these findings to the RN right away. The RN will perform a thorough assessment and call report to the physician. An ECG may be ordered. You may have to withhold the next dose of terbutaline, or the physician may decide to try a different tocolytic.

CHAPTER 19

NCLEX-Style Review Questions

1. b
Rationale. The signs and symptoms are those most closely associated with endometritis. Mastitis would involve a localized area of redness on the breast. Subinvolution may occur with endometritis, but the symptoms listed indicate infection. An episiotomy infection probably would not involve such a high fever, and abdominal pain usually is not associated with this diagnosis.
2. c
Rationale. The first action would be to raise the head of the bed. This action may help the woman be able to breathe better. Oxygen should be administered by face mask, not by nasal cannula. Blood gas analysis may be appropriate, but this is not the priority. Telling the woman that she doesn't need to worry is not therapeutic. The woman is in distress.
3. d
Rationale. The only observation of concern is the one in which the woman refers to her baby as "it" and speaks negatively of her crying all the time. These observations may indicate that malattachment is occurring. Actively participating in the newborn's care, comparing the newborn's characteristics with those of a family member, and anticipating discharge indicate positive responses.
4. b
Rationale. A woman who experiences a large amount of bleeding may be experiencing postpartum hemorrhage and is at risk for injury. Changes in vital signs, particularly her blood pressure and pulse, may indicate shock. In this case it would not be appropriate to allow her to ambulate. In addition, complaints of dizziness increase the risk that she might fall. Although it is important to assess attachment, lochia color, degree of responsiveness or level of orientation, fundal location, and support systems, these are not the priority assessments in a woman experiencing a large amount of vaginal bleeding. Obtaining height would be inappropriate. A complete blood count may be ordered later to evaluate the woman's extent of bleeding.

Critical Thinking: What Would You Do?

1. *Suggested answers:*
   a. Josie is not responding to the baby's cues and is ignoring the crying. These signs along with her age put Josie at risk for malattachment with her baby. You need to evaluate for other signs of malattachment, such as turning away from the baby, not interacting or talking to the baby, or making negative comments.
   b. You should pick up the baby and comfort her. Role model healthy behaviors to Josie and encourage her to interact with the baby. Give her positive feedback when she interacts positively with the baby. Teach Josie how to read the baby's cues. You should involve social services or a clinical psychologist in the discharge planning process.
2. *Suggested answers:*
   a. Tiffany's bladder is probably full. First massage the fundus, and then assist Tiffany to empty her bladder.
   b. If the fundus remains firm and in the midline, but a steady flow of lochia is noted despite fundal massage, Tiffany may have a laceration. Notify the primary care provider of your suspicions because the laceration may require repair. Continue to monitor vital signs and bleeding.
3. *Suggested answers:*
   a. The woman may have an incisional infection. Take the woman's temperature, and then call the primary care provider for additional orders.
   b. Assess any hardened areas for redness, warmth, and tenderness. Instruct the woman to breast-feed frequently and completely empty the affected breast with each feeding. Warm compresses immediately before breast-feeding will help the milk to let down. In addition, it may help to massage the hardened area while the baby is suckling to help unclog the duct. She should use careful handwashing and get plenty of rest.

CHAPTER 20

NCLEX-Style Review Questions

1. d
Rationale. Based on the Ballard scoring tool, bald areas, plantar creases covering the sole, and 3- to 4-mm breast buds are characteristics found in an older gestational age newborn. Abundant or absent lanugo, flat areola, flat pinna, anterior transverse

plantar crease, ear recoil, few scrotal rugae, transparent skin, and prominent clitoris are findings associated with a younger gestational age newborn.

2. c
   Rationale. Maternal diabetes is the most widely known contributing factor for newborns who are LGA. Having no other children and gaining little weight during pregnancy are not associated factors contributing to the size of the newborn. A history of smoking during pregnancy is a contributing factor for newborns who are SGA (small for gestational age).
3. b
   Rationale. The preterm newborn may experience thermoregulation problems (difficulty maintaining body temperature), and as a result, the newborn may develop hypothermia. Therefore, monitoring body temperature would be a priority. Although repositioning every 2 hours, promoting rest between procedures, and recording urinary output would be important, these interventions would not be as high a priority as monitoring the newborn's temperature.
4. c
   Rationale. The newborn of a mother who abused cocaine during pregnancy would most likely experience withdrawal symptoms, including tremors, restlessness, hyperactivity, disorganized or hyperactive reflexes, increased muscle tone, sneezing, tachypnea, vomiting, diarrhea, disturbed sleep patterns, a shrill high-pitched cry, and commonly, feeding problems. Above average weight is not associated with newborns born to cocaine-using mothers. Normally, a newborn sleeps for the majority of hours in a day. However, the newborn of a cocaine-using mother most likely would experience disturbed sleeping patterns. Facial deformities are associated with fetal alcohol syndrome.
5. a, c, d, f
   Rationale. Preterm newborns typically exhibit thin extremities with little muscle or subcutaneous fat, a disproportionately large head and abdomen, visible veins in the abdomen and scalp, and soft, pliable ears with minimal cartilage. In addition, the skin is thin, relatively translucent, and usually wrinkled, and the newborn has plentiful lanugo over the extremities, back, and shoulders.

Critical Thinking: What Would You Do?

1. *Suggested answers:*
   a. The nurse needs to support this mother by listening to her, spending time with her, and answering any questions she has. The nurse needs to reassure this mother that she did not cause the infant's bilirubin to be elevated and that the condition can be treated.
   b. The purpose of the phototherapy is to use special lights to help reduce bilirubin levels.
   c. While the infant is under the lights, the infant's eyes will be covered and he will be nude. The infant may have skin rashes; loose, greenish stools; increased temperature; loss of water; and priapism (a perpetual abnormal erection of the penis).
2. *Suggested answers:*
   a. No amount of alcohol is believed to be safe, and women should stop drinking at least 3 months before they plan to become pregnant.
   b. Fetal alcohol syndrome is often apparent in newborns of mothers with chronic alcoholism and sometimes appears in newborns whose mothers are low to moderate consumers of alcohol.
   c. The infant with fetal alcohol syndrome may have low birth weight, smaller length and head circumference, short palpebral fissures (eyelid folds), reduced ocular growth, and a flattened nasal bridge.
   d. The child's growth may be slow and his or her mental development may be retarded.

CHAPTER 21

NCLEX-Style Review Questions

1. d
   Rationale. The balance of formation and absorption of cerebrospinal fluid found within the ventricles and subarachnoid spaces of the cranial cavity is disturbed in hydrocephalus, thus causing an increase in the head circumference of the child. A sac protruding on the lower back suggests a neural tube defect. Normal respiratory rates for newborns range from 30 to 50 breaths per minute. Gluteal folds higher on one side might suggest developmental hip dysplasia.
2. b
   Rationale. The newborn with tetralogy of Fallot has a decreased oxygen saturation and thus has cyanosis, dyspnea, and tachycardia. The child is easily fatigued and often cannot expend enough energy to eat enough to have normal growth and development. Spina bifida, congenital rubella, and hip dysplasia are not associated with these findings.
3. b
   Rationale. After repair of a cleft lip and cleft palate, the risk for infection is high. Therefore the nurse's priority would be to monitor the incision and repair site closely for signs of infection, such as redness or drainage at the incision site, and keep the suture line clean and free of infection, thereby promoting optimal healing without scarring. Although documenting the time period the

restraints are on and off, teaching the caregivers about dental care and hygiene, and providing sensory stimulation and age-appropriate toys are important, these are interventions appropriate for any newborn who has had a cleft lip/cleft palate repair but would not be the priority at this time.

4. a

   Rationale. Promoting skin integrity and monitoring closely for any signs of skin irritation or breakdown are important in a child with any type of cast, but especially for the child with a spica cast because of the size of the cast and possible soiling from urine or bowel elimination. Changing bedding and clothing every 4 hours, weighing every morning and evening using the same scale, and monitoring temperature and pulse every 2 hours would not necessarily be included in the plan of care for the newborn who has a hip spica cast.

5. a, b, d

   Rationale. Antibiotics may be given to prevent possible infection, and the child is monitored closely for any signs of infection. Before surgery, the sac is kept moist and covered to prevent the sac from becoming dry. A prone, not supine, position is maintained to prevent injury to the sac. The dressing is changed every 2 hours to keep it moist.

Critical Thinking: What Would You Do?

1. *Suggested answers:*
   a. The nurse offers support and acceptance of this mother by staying with her, putting a hand on her shoulder or gently touching her, and either staying silent or using therapeutic statements to show acceptance of this mother's feelings.
   b. The mother might be feeling sadness, guilt, a feeling of loss of having the "perfect" child, and fear of the child's future.
   c. The nurse might respond with a comment such as, "this must be difficult for you." After the mother has had time to adjust to the appearance of her child, the nurse can further support her with more information about the correction that can be done.
2. *Suggested answers:*
   a. Hydrocephalus occurs when there is an imbalance of the amount of cerebrospinal fluid being formed and the amount being reabsorbed. The child has an excess of cerebrospinal fluid in his cranial cavity. This can happen because of a blockage, an obstruction, or an injury or infection.
   b. Cody will have a tube placed just under the skin in his head to drain the excess fluid from his brain into his peritoneal cavity, where it will be absorbed. If untreated, the outcome is poor and can result in death.
   c. Cody will need continued follow-up care and shunt revisions, but depending on the cause, treatment, brain damage sustained, and complications, children can lead relatively normal lives.
3. *Suggested answers:*
   a. The infant weighs 4.5 kg.
   b. The low dose would be 4.5 mg.
   c. The high dose would be 9.9 mg.

Appendix A

Standard and Transmission-Based Precautions

Use Standard Precautions, or the equivalent, for the care of all patients. *Category IB**

A. Handwashing

(1) Wash hands after touching blood, body fluids, secretions, excretions, and contaminated items, whether or not gloves are worn. Wash hands immediately after gloves are removed, between patient contacts, and when otherwise indicated to avoid transfer of microorganisms to other patients or environments. It may be necessary to wash hands between tasks and procedures on the same patient to prevent cross-contamination of different body sites. *Category IB*

(2) Use a plain (nonantimicrobial) soap for routine handwashing. *Category IB*

(3) Use an antimicrobial agent or a waterless antiseptic agent for specific circumstances (e.g., control of outbreaks or hyperendemic infections), as defined by the infection control program. *Category IB* (See Contact Precautions for additional recommendations on using antimicrobial and antiseptic agents.)

B. Gloves

Wear gloves (clean, nonsterile gloves are adequate) when touching blood, body fluids, secretions, excretions, and contaminated items. Put on clean gloves just before touching mucous membranes and nonintact skin. Change gloves between tasks and procedures on the same patient after contact with material that may contain a high concentration of microorganisms. Remove gloves promptly after use, before touching noncontaminated items and environmental surfaces, and before going to another patient, and wash hands immediately to avoid transfer of microorganisms to other patients or environments. *Category IB*

(From Recommendations for Isolation Precautions in Hospitals developed by the Centers for Disease Control and Prevention and the Hospital Control Practices Advisory Committee [HICPAC], February 18, 1997.)

**Category IB*. Strongly recommended for all hospitals and reviewed as effective by experts in the field and a consensus of HICPAC members on the basis of strong rationale and suggestive evidence, even though definitive studies have not been done.

C. Mask, Eye Protection, Face Shield

Wear a mask and eye protection or a face shield to protect mucous membranes of the eyes, nose, and mouth during procedures and patient-care activities that are likely to generate splashes or sprays of blood, body fluids, secretions, and excretions. *Category IB*

D. Gown

Wear a gown (a clean, nonsterile gown is adequate) to protect skin and to prevent soiling of clothing during procedures and patient-care activities that are likely to generate splashes or sprays of blood, body fluids, secretions, or excretions. Select a gown that is appropriate for the activity and amount of fluid likely to be encountered. Remove a soiled gown as promptly as possible, and wash hands to avoid transfer of microorganisms to other patients or environments. *Category IB*

E. Patient-Care Equipment

Handle used patient-care equipment soiled with blood, body fluids, secretions, and excretions in a manner that prevents skin and mucous membrane exposures, contamination of clothing, and transfer of microorganisms to other patients and environments. Ensure that reusable equipment is not used for the care of another patient until it has been cleaned and reprocessed appropriately. Ensure that single-use items are discarded properly. *Category IB*

F. Environmental Control

Ensure that the hospital has adequate procedures for the routine care, cleaning, and disinfection of environmental surfaces, beds, bedrails, bedside equipment, and other frequently touched surfaces, and ensure that these procedures are being followed. *Category IB*

G. Linen

Handle, transport, and process used linen soiled with blood, body fluids, secretions, and excretions in a manner that prevents skin and mucous membrane exposures and contamination of clothing, and that avoids transfer of microorganisms to other patients and environments. *Category IB*

H. Occupational Health and Bloodborne Pathogens

(1) Take care to prevent injuries when using needles, scalpels, and other sharp instruments or devices; when handling sharp instruments after procedures;

when cleaning used instruments; and when disposing of used needles. Never recap used needles, or otherwise manipulate them using both hands, or use any other technique that involves directing the point of a needle toward any part of the body; rather, use either a one-handed "scoop" technique or a mechanical device designed for holding the needle sheath. Do not remove used needles from disposable syringes by hand, and do not bend, break, or otherwise manipulate used needles by hand. Place used disposable syringes and needles, scalpel blades, and other sharp items in appropriate puncture-resistant containers, which are located as close as practical to the area in which the items were used, and place reusable syringes and needles in a puncture-resistant container for transport to the reprocessing area. *Category IB*

(2) Use mouthpieces, resuscitation bags, or other ventilation devices as an alternative to mouth-to-mouth resuscitation methods in areas where the need for resuscitation is predictable. *Category IB*

I. Patient Placement

Place a patient who contaminates the environment or who does not (or cannot be expected to) assist in maintaining appropriate hygiene or environmental control in a private room. If a private room is not available, consult with infection control professionals regarding patient placement or other alternatives. *Category IB*

J. Respiratory Hygiene/Cough Etiquette

Instruct symptomatic persons to cover mouth/nose when sneezing/coughing; use tissues and dispose in no-touch receptacle; observe hand hygiene after soiling of hands with respiratory secretions; wear surgical masks if tolerated or maintain spatial separation, >3 feet if possible. *Category IB*.[†]

[†]Guidelines for respiratory hygiene/cough etiquette have been added to the 2004 **DRAFT** *CDC guidelines for isolation precautions: Preventing transmission of infectious agents in healthcare settings. 2004.* https://www.cdc.gov/nicdod/hip/isoguide.htm

Appendix B

NANDA-Approved Nursing Diagnoses

This list represents the NANDA-approved nursing diagnoses for clinical use and testing.

Domain 1: Health Promotion

Description

The awareness of well-being or normality of function and the strategies used to maintain control of and enhance that well-being or normality of function

Approved Diagnoses

Effective Therapeutic Regimen Management
Ineffective Therapeutic Regimen Management
Ineffective Family Therapeutic Regimen Management
Ineffective Community Therapeutic Regimen Management
Health-Seeking Behaviors (specify)
Ineffective Health Maintenance
Impaired Home Maintenance
Readiness for Enhanced Management of Therapeutic Regimen
Readiness for Enhanced Nutrition

Domain 2: Nutrition

Description

The activities of taking in, assimilating, and using nutrients for the purpose of tissue maintenance, tissue repair, and the production of energy

Approved Diagnoses

Ineffective Infant Feeding Pattern
Impaired Swallowing
Imbalanced Nutrition: Less Than Body Requirements
Imbalanced Nutrition: More Than Body Requirements
Risk for Imbalanced Nutrition: More Than Body Requirements
Deficient Fluid Volume
Risk for Deficient Fluid Volume
Excess Fluid Volume
Risk for Imbalanced Fluid Volume
Readiness for Enhanced Fluid Balance

Domain 3: Elimination

Description

Secretion and excretion of waste products from the body

Approved Diagnoses

Impaired Urinary Elimination
Urinary Retention
Total Urinary Incontinence
Functional Urinary Incontinence
Stress Urinary Incontinence
Urge Urinary Incontinence
Reflex Urinary Incontinence
Risk for Urge Urinary Incontinence
Readiness for Enhanced Urinary Elimination
Bowel Incontinence
Diarrhea
Constipation
Risk for Constipation
Perceived Constipation
Impaired Gas Exchange

Domain 4: Activity/Rest

Description

The production, conservation, expenditure, or balance of energy resources

Approved Diagnoses

Disturbed Sleep Pattern
Sleep Deprivation
Readiness for Enhanced Sleep
Risk for Disuse Syndrome
Impaired Physical Mobility
Impaired Bed Mobility
Impaired Wheelchair Mobility
Impaired Transfer Ability
Impaired Walking
Deficient Diversional Activity
Dressing/Grooming Self-Care Deficit
Bathing/Hygiene Self-Care Deficit
Feeding Self-Care Deficit
Toileting Self-Care Deficit
Delayed Surgical Recovery
Disturbed Energy Field
Fatigue
Decreased Cardiac Output
Impaired Spontaneous Ventilation
Ineffective Breathing Pattern
Activity Intolerance
Risk for Activity Intolerance
Dysfunctional Ventilatory Weaning Response
Ineffective Tissue Perfusion (specify type: Renal, Cerebral, Cardiopulmonary, Gastrointestinal, Peripheral)

Domain 5: Perception/Cognition

Description

The human information-processing system, including attention, orientation, sensation, perception, cognition, and communication

(box continues on page 580)

Approved Diagnoses
Unilateral Neglect
Impaired Environmental Interpretation Syndrome
Wandering
Disturbed Sensory Perception (specify: Visual, Auditory, Kinesthetic, Gustatory, Tactile, Olfactory)
Deficient Knowledge (specify)
Readiness for Enhanced Knowledge
Acute Confusion
Chronic Confusion
Impaired Memory
Disturbed Thought Processes
Impaired Verbal Communication
Readiness for Enhanced Communication

Domain 6: Self-Perception

Description
Awareness about the self

Approved Diagnoses
Disturbed Personal Identity
Powerlessness
Risk for Powerlessness
Hopelessness
Risk for Loneliness
Readiness for Enhanced Self-Concept
Chronic Low Self-Esteem
Situational Low Self-Esteem
Risk for Situational Low Self-Esteem
Disturbed Body Image

Domain 7: Role Relationships

Description
The positive and negative connections or associations between persons or groups of persons and the means by which those connections are demonstrated

Approved Diagnoses
Caregiver Role Strain
Risk for Caregiver Role Strain
Impaired Parenting
Risk for Impaired Parenting
Readiness for Enhanced Parenting
Interrupted Family Processes
Readiness for Enhanced Family Processes
Dysfunctional Family Processes: Alcoholism
Risk for Impaired Parent/Infant/Child Attachment
Effective Breastfeeding
Ineffective Breastfeeding
Interrupted Breastfeeding
Ineffective Role Performance
Parental Role Conflict
Impaired Social Interaction

Domain 8: Sexuality

Description
Sexual identity, sexual function, and reproduction

Approved Diagnoses
Sexual Dysfunction
Ineffective Sexuality Patterns

Domain 9: Coping/Stress Tolerance

Description
Contending with life events/life processes

Approved Diagnoses
Relocation Stress Syndrome
Risk for Relocation Stress Syndrome
Rape-Trauma Syndrome
Rape-Trauma Syndrome: Silent Reaction
Rape-Trauma Syndrome: Compound Reaction
Post-Trauma Syndrome
Risk for Post-Trauma Syndrome
Fear
Anxiety
Death Anxiety
Chronic Sorrow
Ineffective Denial
Anticipatory Grieving
Dysfunctional Grieving
Impaired Adjustment
Ineffective Coping
Disabled Family Coping
Compromised Family Coping
Defensive Coping
Ineffective Community Coping
Readiness for Enhanced Coping
Readiness for Enhanced Family Coping
Readiness for Enhanced Community Coping
Autonomic Dysreflexia
Risk for Autonomic Dysreflexia
Disorganized Infant Behavior
Risk for Disorganized Infant Behavior
Readiness for Enhanced Organized Infant Behavior
Decreased Intracranial Adaptive Capacity

Domain 10: Life Principles

Description
Principles underlying conduct, thought, and behavior about acts, customs, or institutions as being true or having intrinsic worth

Approved Diagnoses
Readiness for Enhanced Spiritual Well-Being
Spiritual Distress
Risk for Spiritual Distress
Decisional Conflict (specify)
Noncompliance (specify)

Domain 11: Safety/Protection

Description
Freedom from danger, physical injury, or immune-system damage; preservation from loss; and protection of safety and security

Approved Diagnoses
Risk for Infection
Impaired Oral Mucous Membrane
Risk for Injury
Risk for Perioperative Positioning Injury
Risk for Falls
Risk for Trauma
Impaired Skin Integrity
Risk for Impaired Skin Integrity
Impaired Tissue Integrity
Impaired Dentition
Risk for Suffocation
Risk for Aspiration
Ineffective Airway Clearance
Risk for Peripheral Neurovascular Dysfunction
Ineffective Protection

Risk for Sudden Infant Death Syndrome
Risk for Self-Mutilation
Self-Mutilation
Risk for Other-Directed Violence
Risk for Self-Directed Violence
Risk for Suicide
Risk for Poisoning
Latex Allergy Response
Risk for Latex Allergy Response
Risk for Imbalanced Body Temperature
Ineffective Thermoregulation
Hypothermia
Hyperthermia

Domain 12: Comfort

Description
Sense of mental, physical, or social well-being or ease

Approved Diagnoses
Acute Pain
Chronic Pain
Nausea
Social Isolation

Domain 13: Growth/Development

Description
Age-appropriate increase in physical dimension, organ systems, and/or attainment of developmental milestones

Approved Diagnoses
Risk for Disproportionate Growth
Adult Failure to Thrive
Delayed Growth and Development
Risk for Delayed Development

Appendix C

JCAHO List of "Do Not Use" Abbreviations

The Joint Commission on Accreditation of Healthcare Organizations and the Institute for Safe Medication Practices have listed the following abbreviations as dangerous, due to the potential of medication and other errors being made if these are used.

Abbreviation	Potential Problem	Preferred Term
U (for unit)	Mistaken as zero, four or cc.	Write "unit."
IU (for International Unit)	Mistaken as IV (intravenous) or 10 (ten).	Write "International Unit."
Q.D., Q.O.D (Latin abbreviation for once, and the "O" can be mistaken for "I," daily and every other day)	Mistaken for each other. The period after the Q can be mistaken for an "I."	Write "daily" and "every other day."
Trailing zero (X.0 mg), Lack of leading zero (.X mg)	Decimal point is missed.	Never write a zero by itself after a decimal point (X mg), and always use a zero before a decimal point (0.X mg).
MS MSO_4 $MgSO_4$	Confused for one another. Can mean morphine sulfate or magnesium sulfate.	Write "morphine sulfate" or "magnesium sulfate."
μg (for microgram)	Mistaken for mg (milligrams) resulting in 1,000-fold dosing overdose.	Write "mcg."
H.S. (for half-strength or Latin abbreviation for bedtime)	Mistaken for either half-strength or hour of sleep (at bedtime). q.H.S. mistaken every hour. All can result in dosing error.	Write out "half-strength" or "at bedtime."
T.I.W. (for three times a week)	Mistaken for three times a day or twice weekly, resulting in an overdose.	Write "3 times weekly" or "three times weekly."
S.C. or S.Q. (for subcutaneous)	Mistaken as SL for sublingual, or "5 every."	Write "Sub-Q", "subQ", or "subcutaneously."
D/C (for discharge)	Interpreted as discontinue or whatever medications follow (typically discharge meds).	Write "discharge."
c.c. (for cubic centimeter)	Mistaken for U (units) when poorly written.	Write "ml" for milliliters.
A.S., A.D., A.U. (Latin abbreviation for left, right, or both ears)	Mistaken for OS, OD, OU, etc.	Write: "left ear," "right ear," or "both ears."

An abbreviation on the "Do Not Use" list should not be used in any of its forms—upper or lower case, with or without periods. For example, if Q.D. is on your list, you can't use "QD" or "qd." Any of those variations are confusing and can be misinterpreted. Retrieved June 18, 2004, from www.jcaho.org.

Appendix D

Good Sources of Essential Nutrients

Protein	Vitamin A	Vitamin B			Vitamin C	Vitamin D	Minerals		
		Thiamine	Riboflavin	Niacin			Calcium	Iron	Iodine
Meat, poultry, fish, milk products and eggs. Whole wheat grains, nuts, peanut butter, legumes are also good sources of protein, but need to be supplemented by some animal protein, such as meat, eggs, milk, cheese, cottage cheese or yogurt.	Green leafy vegetables, deep yellow vegetables and fruits, whole milk or whole milk products, egg yolk.	Meat, fish, poultry, eggs, whole grain, legumes, potatoes, green leafy vegetables.	Milk (best source), meat, egg yolk, green vegetables.	Meat, fish, poultry, peanut butter, wheat germ, brewer's yeast. Although the amount in milk is small, children whose intake of milk is adequate do not develop pellagra.	Citrus fruits and tomatoes, fresh or frozen citrus fruit juices, strawberries, cantaloupe. Breast milk is an adequate source of vitamin C for young infants only if the mother's diet contains sufficient vitamin C.	Sunlight, fish liver oils, fortified milk and synthetic vitamin D.	Milk and milk products, squash, sweet potatoes, raisins, rhubarb, well-cooked dried beans, turnip greens, Swiss chard, mustard greens.	Green leafy vegetables, liver, meats and eggs, dried fruits, whole grain or enriched bread and cereals.	Seafoods, plants grown on soil near the sea, iodized salt.

Appendix E

Breast-feeding and Medication Use

GENERAL CONSIDERATIONS

- Most medications are safe to use while breast-feeding; however, the woman should always check with the pediatrician, physician, or lactation specialist before taking any medications, including over-the-counter and herbal products.
- Inform the woman that she has the right to seek a second opinion if the physician does not perform a thoughtful risk-versus-benefit assessment before prescribing medications or advising against breast-feeding.
- Most medications pass from the woman's bloodstream into the breast milk. However, the amount is usually very small and unlikely to harm the baby.
- A preterm or other special needs neonate is more susceptible to the adverse effects of medications in breast milk. A woman who is taking medications and whose baby is in the neonatal intensive care unit or special care nursery should consult with the pediatrician or neonatologist before feeding her breast milk to the baby.
- If the woman is taking a prescribed medication, she should take the medication just after breast-feeding. This practice helps ensure that the lowest possible dose of medication reaches the baby through the breast milk.
- Some medications can cause changes in the amount of milk the woman produces. Teach the woman to report any changes in milk production.

LACTATION RISK CATEGORIES (LRC)

Lactation Category	Risk	Rationale
L1	Safest	Clinical research or long-term observation of use in many breast-feeding women has not demonstrated risk to the infant.
L2	Safer	Limited clinical research has not demonstrated an increase in adverse effects in the infant.
L3	Moderately safe	There is possible risk to the infant; however, the risks are minimal or nonthreatening in nature.These medications should be given only when the potential benefit outweighs the risk to the infant.
L4	Possibly hazardous	There is positive evidence of risk to the infant; however, in life-threatening situations or for serious diseases, the benefit might outweigh the risk.
L5	Contraindicated	The risk of using the medication clearly outweighs any possible benefit from breast-feeding.

POTENTIAL EFFECTS OF SELECTED MEDICATION CATEGORIES ON THE BREAST-FED INFANT

Narcotic Analgesics

- Codeine and hydrocodone appear to be safe in moderate doses. Rarely the neonate may experience sedation and/or apnea. (LRC: L3)
- Meperidine (Demerol) can lead to sedation of the neonate. (LRC: L3)
- Low to moderate doses of morphine appear to be safe. (LRC: L2)

- Trace-to-negligible amounts of fentanyl are found in human milk. (LRC: L2)

Non-narcotic Analgesics and NSAIDs

- Acetaminophen and ibuprofen are approved for use. (LRC: L1)
- Naproxen may cause neonatal hemorrhage and anemia if used for prolonged periods. (LRC: L3 for short-term use and L4 for long-term use)
- The newer COX2 inhibitors, such as celecoxib (Celebrex), appear to be safe for use. (LRC: L2)

Antibiotics

- Levels in breast milk are usually very low.
- The penicillins and cephalosporins are generally considered safe to use. (LRC: L1 and L2)
- Tetracyclines can be safely used for short periods but are not suitable for long-term therapy (e.g., for treatment of acne). (LRC: L2)
- Sulfonamides should not be used during the neonatal stage (the first month of life). (LRC: L3)

Antihypertensives

- A high degree of caution is advised when antihypertensives are used during breast-feeding.
- Some beta blockers can be used.
- Hydralazine and methyldopa are considered to be safe. (LRC: L2)
- ACE inhibitors are not recommended in the early postpartum period.

Sedatives and Hypnotics

- Neonatal withdrawal can occur when antianxiety medications, such as lorazepam, are taken. Fortunately withdrawal is generally mild.
- Phenothiazines, such as Phenergan and Thorazine, may lead to sleep apnea and increase the risk for sudden infant death syndrome.

Antidepressants

- The risk to the baby often is higher if the woman is depressed and remains untreated, rather than taking the medication.
- The older tricyclics are considered to be safe; however they cause many bothersome side effects, such as weight gain and dry mouth, which may lead to noncompliance on the part of the woman.
- The selective serotonin uptake inhibitors (SSRIs) also are considered to be safe and have a lower side effect profile, which makes them more palatable to the woman. (LRC: L2 and L3)

Mood Stabilizers (Antimanic Medication)

- Lithium is found in breast milk and is best not used in the breast-feeding woman. (LRC: L4)
- Valproic acid (Depakote) seems to be a more appropriate choice for the woman with bipolar disorder. The infant will need periodic lab studies to check platelets and liver function.

Corticosteroids

- Corticosteroids do not pass into the milk in large quantities.
- Inhaled steroids are safe to use because they don't accumulate in the bloodstream.

Thyroid Medication

- Thyroid medications, such as levothyroxine (Synthroid), can be taken while breast-feeding.
- Most are in LRC category L1.

MEDICATIONS THAT USUALLY ARE CONTRAINDICATED FOR THE BREAST-FEEDING WOMAN

- Amiodarone
- Antineoplastic agents
- Chloramphenicol
- Doxepin
- Ergotamine and other ergot derivatives
- Iodides
- Methotrexate and immunosuppressants
- Lithium
- Radiopharmaceuticals
- Ribavirin
- Tetracycline (prolonged use—more than 3 weeks)
- Pseudoephedrine (found in many over-the-counter medications)

Material in this Appendix was adapted from information found on the American Academy of Pediatrics website (www.aap.org) and from Riordan, J. (2005). *Breastfeeding and human lactation*, 3rd ed. Jones and Bartlett Publishers: Boston; Hale, T. W. (2004). *Medications and mother's milk*, 11th ed. Amarillo, TX: Pharmasoft Publishing.

Appendix F

Cervical Dilation Chart

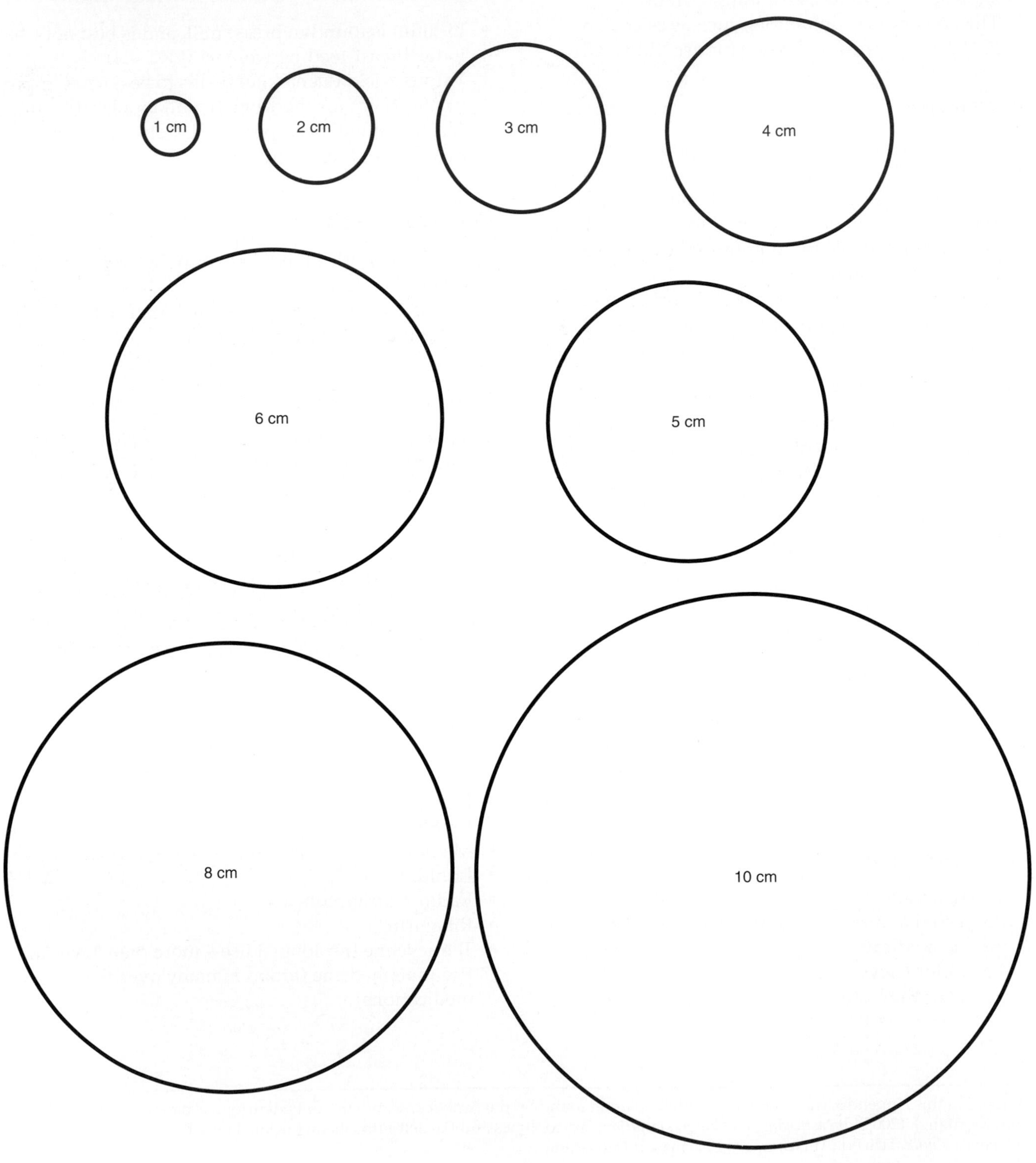

Appendix G

Temperature and Weight Conversion Charts

Conversion of Pounds to Kilograms

Pounds	0	1	2	3	4	5	6	7	8	9
0	—	0.45	0.90	1.36	1.81	2.26	2.72	3.17	3.62	4.08
10	4.53	4.98	5.44	5.89	6.35	6.80	7.25	7.71	8.16	8.61
20	9.07	9.52	9.97	10.43	10.88	11.34	11.79	12.24	12.70	13.15
30	13.60	14.06	14.51	14.96	15.42	15.87	16.32	16.78	17.23	17.69
40	18.14	18.59	19.05	19.50	19.95	20.41	20.86	21.31	21.77	22.22
50	22.68	23.13	23.58	24.04	24.49	24.94	25.40	25.85	26.30	26.76
60	27.21	27.66	28.12	28.57	29.03	29.48	29.93	30.39	30.84	31.29
70	31.75	32.20	32.65	33.11	33.56	34.02	34.47	34.92	35.38	35.83
80	36.28	36.74	37.19	37.64	38.10	38.55	39.00	39.46	39.91	40.37
90	40.82	41.27	41.73	42.18	42.63	43.09	43.54	43.99	44.45	44.90
100	45.36	45.81	46.26	46.72	47.17	47.62	48.08	48.53	48.98	49.44
110	49.89	50.34	50.80	51.25	51.71	52.16	52.61	53.07	53.52	53.97
120	54.43	54.88	55.33	55.79	56.24	56.70	57.15	57.60	58.06	58.51
130	58.96	59.42	59.87	60.32	60.78	61.23	61.68	62.14	62.59	63.05
140	63.50	63.95	64.41	64.86	65.31	65.77	66.22	66.67	67.13	67.58
150	68.04	68.49	68.94	69.40	69.85	70.30	70.76	71.21	71.66	72.12
160	72.57	73.02	73.48	73.93	74.39	74.84	75.29	75.75	76.20	76.65
170	77.11	77.56	78.01	78.47	78.92	79.38	79.83	80.28	80.74	81.19
180	81.64	82.10	82.55	83.00	83.46	83.91	84.36	84.82	85.27	85.73
190	86.18	86.68	87.09	87.54	87.99	88.45	88.90	89.35	89.81	90.26
200	90.72	91.17	91.62	92.08	92.53	92.98	93.44	93.89	94.34	94.80

Conversion of Pounds and Ounces to Grams for Newborn Weights

Pounds	Ounces 0	1	2	3	4	5	6	7	8	9	10	11	12	13	14	15
0	—	28	57	85	113	142	170	198	227	255	283	312	430	369	397	425
1	454	482	510	539	567	595	624	652	680	709	737	765	794	822	850	879
2	907	936	964	992	1021	1049	1077	1106	1134	1162	1191	1219	1247	1276	1304	1332
3	1361	1389	1417	1446	1474	1503	1531	1559	1588	1616	1644	1673	1701	1729	1758	1786
4	1814	1843	1871	1899	1928	1956	1984	2013	2041	2070	2098	2126	2155	2183	2211	2240
5	2268	2296	2325	2353	2381	2410	2438	2466	2495	2523	2551	2580	2608	2637	2665	2693
6	2722	2750	2778	2807	2835	2863	2892	2920	2948	2977	3005	3033	3062	3090	3118	3147
7	3175	3203	3232	3260	3289	3317	3345	3374	3402	3430	3459	3487	3515	3544	3572	3600
8	3629	3657	3685	3714	3742	3770	3799	3827	3856	3884	3912	3941	3969	3997	4026	4054
9	4082	4111	4139	4167	4196	4224	4252	4281	4309	4337	4366	4394	4423	4451	4479	4508
10	4536	4564	4593	4621	4649	4678	4706	4734	4763	4791	4819	4848	4876	4904	4933	4961
11	4990	5018	5046	5075	5103	5131	5160	5188	5216	5245	5273	5301	5330	5358	5386	5415
12	5443	5471	5500	5528	5557	5585	5613	5642	5670	5698	5727	5755	5783	5812	5840	5868
13	5897	5925	5953	5982	6010	6038	6067	6095	6123	6152	6180	6209	6237	6265	6294	6322
14	6350	6379	6407	6435	6464	6492	6520	6549	6577	6605	6634	6662	6690	6719	6747	6776
15	6804	6832	6860	6889	6917	6945	6973	7002	7030	7059	7087	7115	7144	7172	7201	7228

Conversion of Fahrenheit to Celsius

Celsius	Fahrenheit	Celsius	Fahrenheit	Celsius	Fahrenheit
34.0	93.2	37.0	98.6	40.0	104.0
34.2	93.6	37.2	99.0	40.2	101.4
34.4	93.9	37.4	99.3	40.4	104.7
34.6	94.3	37.6	99.7	40.6	105.2
34.8	94.6	37.8	100.0	40.8	105.4
35.0	95.0	38.0	100.4	41.0	105.9
35.2	95.4	38.2	100.8	41.2	106.1
35.4	95.7	38.4	101.1	41.4	106.5
35.6	96.1	38.6	101.5	41.6	106.8
35.8	96.4	38.8	101.8	41.8	107.2
36.0	96.8	39.0	102.2	42.0	107.6
36.2	97.2	39.2	102.6	42.2	108.0
36.4	97.5	39.4	102.9	42.4	108.3
36.6	97.9	39.6	103.3	42.6	108.7
36.8	98.2	39.8	103.6	42.8	109.0

$(°C) \times (9/5) + 32 = °F$

$(°F - 32) \times (5/9) = °C$

INDEX

Page numbers followed by *f* indicate figures; those followed by *t* indicate tables.

A

C

D

E

F

G

H

J

K

L

M

N

U